Bennett & Brachman's Hospital Infections

FIFTH EDITION

EDITOR

━━ **WILLIAM R. JARVIS, MD**

President, Jason and Jarvis Associates
Hilton Head Island, South Carolina;
Port Orford, Oregon;
San Francisco, California

◼ Wolters Kluwer | Lippincott Williams & Wilkins
Health
Philadelphia · Baltimore · New York · London
Buenos Aires · Hong Kong · Sydney · Tokyo

Acquisitions Editor: Frances R. DeStefano
Managing Editor: Michelle LaPlante
Production Manager: Jennifer Harper
Manufacturing Coordinator: Kathleen Brown
Marketing Manager: Kimberly Schonberger
Creative Director: Doug Smock
Production Services: Pine Tree Composition, Inc.

Library of Congress Cataloging-in-Publication Data
Bennett & Brachman's hospital infections.—5th ed. / edited by William R. Jarvis.
   p. ; cm.
  Rev. ed. of: Hospital infections / edited by John V. Bennett, Philip S. Brachman. 4th ed. c1998.
  Includes bibliographical references and index.
  ISBN-13: 978-0-7817-6383-7
  ISBN-10: 0-7817-6383-5
  1. Nosocomial infections. 2. Nosocomial infections—Prevention. I. Bennett, John V. II. Jarvis, William R. (William Robert), 1948- III. Hospital infections. IV. Title: Hospital infections. V. Title: Bennett and Brachman's hospital infections.
  [DNLM: 1. Cross Infection—prevention & control. 2. Cross Infection—etiology. WX 167 B4705 2007]
  RA969.H64 2007
  614.4'4—dc22
                  2007017615

Care has been taken to confirm the accuracy of the information presented and to describe generally accepted practices. However, the authors, editors, and publisher are not responsible for errors or omissions or for any consequences from application of the information in this book and make no warranty, expressed or implied, with respect to the currency, completeness, or accuracy of the contents of the publication. Application of this information in a particular situation remains the professional responsibility of the practitioner.

The authors, editors, and publisher have exerted every effort to ensure that drug selection and dosage set forth in this text are in accordance with current recommendations and practice at the time of publication. However, in view of ongoing research, changes in government regulations, and the constant flow of information relating to drug therapy and drug reactions, the reader is urged to check the package insert for each drug for any change in indications and dosage and for added warnings and precautions. This is particularly important when the recommended agent is a new or infrequently employed drug.

Some drugs and medical devices presented in this publication have Food and Drug Administration (FDA) clearance for limited use in restricted research settings. It is the responsibility of the health care provider to ascertain the FDA status of each drug or device planned for use in their clinical practice.

To purchase additional copies of this book, call our customer service department at (800) 638-3030 or fax orders to (301) 223-2320. International customers should call (301) 223-2300.

Visit Lippincott Williams & Wilkins on the Internet: at LWW.com. Lippincott Williams & Wilkins customer service representatives are available from 8:30 am to 6 pm, EST.

10 9 8 7 6 5 4 3 2 1

To my wife, Janine, and our children, Danielle and Ashley, for their love, friendship, and never-ending support and encouragement, as well as their unique ability to keep me balanced, grounded, and to put everything into perspective.

Contents

SECTION III: ENDEMIC AND EPIDEMIC HOSPITAL INFECTIONS 481

Contributors

BENEDETTA ALLEGRANZI, MD Consultant, Infection Control Program, University of Geneva Hospitals

MARY ANDRUS, BA, RN, CIC Nurse Epidemiologist, Northrop Grumman Contractor, Division of Healthcare Quality Promotion, Centers for Disease Control and Prevention

LENNOX K. ARCHIBALD, MBBS, FRCP, DTM&H Hospital Epidemiologist, Division of Infectious Diseases, University of Florida, College of Medicine, Department of Medicine, Shands Hospital at the University of Florida

MATTHEW J. ARDUINO, MS, Dr PH Lead Microbiologist, Division of Healthcare Quality Promotion, Centers for Disease Control and Prevention

ELISE BELTRAMI, MD, MPH Technical Information Specialist, Division of Healthcare Quality Promotion, Centers for Disease Control and Prevention

JOAN BLANCHARD, RN, BSN, MSS, CNOR, CIC Perioperative Nursing Specialist, Center for Nursing Practice, Association of periOperative Nurses

DAVID B. BLOSSOM, MD, MS Epidemic Intelligence Service Officer, Division of Healthcare Quality Promotion, Centers for Disease Control and Prevention

ELIZABETH A. BOLYARD, RN, MPH Technical Information Specialist, Division of Healthcare Quality Promotion, Centers for Disease Control and Prevention

MICHAEL A. BORG, MD, DipHIC, FMC (Path) Lecturer, Faculty of Medicine and Surgery, University of Malta, Msida, Malta, Consultant, Infection Control, Infection Control Unit, St. Luke's Hospital

DOUGLAS C. CHANG, MD Mycotic Diseases Branch, Division of Foodborne, Bacterial, and Mycotic Diseases, National Center for Zoonotic, Vector-Borne, and Enteric Diseases, Centers for Disease Control and Prevention

CAROL E. CHENOWETH, MD Associate Professor, Clinical Track, Division of Infectious Diseases, Department of Internal Medicine, University of Michigan Health System, Medical Director, Departments of Infection Control and Epidemiology, University of Michigan Hospitals and Health Centers

RAYMOND CHINN, MD, FACP Hospital Epidemiologist, Department of Infectious Diseases and Epidemiology, Sharp Memorial Hospital

NANCY CHOBIN, R.N., AAS, ACSP, CSPDM Educator, Corporate Consultant/Sterile Processing, Saint Barnabas Health Care System

SARA E. COSGROVE, MD, HS Assistant Professor, Department of Medicine, Johns Hopkins University, School of Medicine, Baltimore, Maryland, Director, Antibiotic Management Program, Associate Hospital Epidemiologist, Johns Hopkins Medical Institution

DONALD E. CRAVEN, MD Professor, Department of Medicine, Tufts University School of Medicine, Chief, Division of Infectious Diseases, Lahey Medical Clinic

E. PATCHEN DELLINGER, MD Professor and Vice Chairman, Department of Surgery, Chief, Division of General Surgery, University of Washington

ROBERT A. DUNCAN, MD, MPH Instructor, Department of Medicine, Harvard Medical School, Hospital Epidemiologist & Senior Staff, Center for Infectious Diseases and Prevention, Lahey Medical Clinic

MICHAEL EDMOND, MD, MPH, MPA Professor, Internal Medicine, Epidemiology and Community Health, Virginia Commonwealth University School of Medicine, Hospital Epidemiologist/Medical Director, Performance Improvement, Virginia Commonwealth University Medical Center

N. JOEL EHRENKRANZ, MD Emeritus Fellow, Florida Consortium for Infectious Diseases

SERGEY R. EREMIN, MD, PhD Associate Professor, Department of Epidemiology, Mechnikov State Medical Academy

BARRY M. FARR, MD, MSc Professor Emeritus, Department of Medicine, University of Virginia

SCOTT K. FRIDKIN, MD Deputy Chief, Surveillance Branch, Division of Healthcare Quality Promotion, Centers for Disease Control and Prevention

CANDACE FRIEDMAN, MPH, CIC Director, Infection Control and Epidemiology, University of Michigan Health System

ROBERT PAUL GAYNES, MD Associate Professor of Medicine, Emory University School of Medicine, Division of Healthcare Quality Promotion, Centers for Disease Control and Prevention

JOY S. GOULDING, BA Coordinating Center for Infectious Diseases, Strategic Science and Program Unit, Office Informatics, Customer Service and IT Assets Team, Centers for Disease Control and Prevention

STEPHAN A. HARBARTH, MD, M.S. Senior Research Associate (Privat-Docent), Department of Internal Medicine, Geneva University Medical School, Associate Hospital Epidemiologist, Infection Control Program, Geneva University Hospitals

MARY K. HAYDEN, MD Attending Physician, Rush Medical Laboratories, Director, Division of Clinical Microbiology, Associate Professor of Medicine and Pathology, Internal Medicine, Infectious Diseases, and Pathology, Rush University Medical Center

DAVID K. HENDERSON, MD Deputy Director for Clinical Care, Clinical Center, National Institutes of Health

TERESA HORAN, MPH Division of Healthcare Quality Promotion, Centers for Disease Control and Prevention

WILLIAM R. JARVIS, MD President, Jason and Jarvis Associates, Hilton Head Island, South Carolina 29938

MARILYN JONES, RN, BSN, MPH, CIC Director, Interventional Epidemiology for Patient Safety and Infection Control Program, Center for Healthcare Quality and Effectiveness, BJC HealthCare

EBBING LAUTENBACH, MD, MPH, MSCE Assistant Professor of Medicine and Epidemiology, Associate Hospital Epidemiologist, Hospital for the University of Pennsylvania, Senior Scholar, Center for Clinical Epidemiology and Biostatistics, University of Pennsylvania

DANIEL P. LEW, MD Professor, Internal Medicine, University of Geneva Faculty of Medicine, Chief, Division of Infectious Diseases, University of Geneva Hospitals

DONNA R. LEWIS, NP, MSN Adjunct Faculty, Nell Hodgson Woodruff School of Nursing, Emory University, Clinical Nurse Research Coordinator, Birmingham/Atlanta VA Geriatric Research, Education, and Clinical Care Center (GRECC), Atlanta Veterans Affairs Medical Center

WILINA LIM, MB, BS, MRC (Path) Chief, Virology Division, Public Health Laboratory Services Branch, Centre for Health Protections, Hong Kong Department of Health, Department of Microbiology, Queen Mary Hospital

MICHAEL Y. LIN, MD Department of Infectious Diseases, Rush Medical College and John H. Stroger Jr. Hospital

MOI LIN LING, MBBS, FRCPA, CPHQ Director, Infection Control, Singapore General Hospital

TAMMY LUNDSTROM, MD, JD Sr. VP, Chief Quality and Safety Officer, Detroit Medical Center, Associate Professor of Medicine, Division of Infectious Diseases, Wayne State University

PATRICIA LYNCH, RN, MBA Principal, Epidemiology Associates

DENNIS G. MAKI, MD Ovid O. Meyer Professor, Department of Medicine, University of Wisconsin School of Medicine and Public Health, Head, Section of Infectious Diseases, Hospital Epidemiologist, Attending Physician, Center for Trauma and Life Support, University of Wisconsin Hospital & Clinics

L. CLIFFORD MCDONALD, MD Medical Epidemiologist, Division of Healthcare Quality Promotion, Centers for Disease Control and Prevention

ALBERT T. MCMANUS, PhD Assistant Professor, US Army Institute of Surgical Research, Brooke Army Medical Center

LEONARD A. MERMEL, DO, ScM, AM (Hon), FACP, FIDSA, FSHEA Professor, Department of Medicine, Brown Medical School, Providence, RI 02912, Medical Director, Department of Infection Control, Rhode Island Hospital

CHRISTOPHER C. MOORE, MD Assistant Professor, Department of Internal Medicine, Division of Infectious Diseases and International Health, University of Virginia

DAVID W. MOZINGO, MD Professor of Surgery and Anesthesiology, University of Florida, Director, Shands Burn Center, Department of Surgery, Shands Hospital

BELINDA OSTROWSKY, MD Freelance Consultant

ROBERT C. OWENS, Jr., PharmD Department of Medicine, University of Vermont, College of Medicine, Co-Director, Antimicrobial Stewardship Program, Department of Clinical Pharmacy and the Division of Infectious Diseases, Maine Medical Center

ELI N. PERENCEVICH, MD, MS Associate Professor, Department of Epidemiology and Preventive Medicine, University of Maryland, Baltimore, VA Maryland Healthcare System

KATHLEEN H. PETERSEN, MS, CIC Infection Control Practitioner, Departments of Infection Control and Epidemiology, University of Michigan Health System

DIDIER PITTET, MD, MS Professor, Internal Medicine, University of Geneva Faculty of Medicine, Director, Infection Control Program, Department of Internal Medicine, University of Geneva Hospitals

BASIL A. PRUITT, JR., MD Clinical Professor, Department of Surgery, University of Texas Health Sciences Center at San Antonio, Surgical Consultant, Burn Center, U.S. Army Institute of Surgical Research

BARTH L. RELLER, MD, DTM&H Professor, Medicine and Pathology, Duke University School of Medicine, Consultant in Infectious Diseases, Director, Clinical Microbiology, Departments of Medicine and Pathology, Duke University Hospital, Duke University Health System

FRANK SCORGIE RHAME, MD Adjunct Professor, Division of Infectious Diseases, University of Minnesota, School of Medicine, Research Director, Abbott Northwestern Hospital

CHELSEY L. RICHARDS, MD, MPH   Deputy Director, Division of Healthcare Quality Promotion, Centers for Disease Control and Prevention

VICTOR D. ROSENTHAL, MD, MSc, CIC   Professor, Infection Control and Hospital Epidemiology, Medical College of Buenos Aires, Chief, Infectious Diseases and Infection Control, Bernal Medical Center

VIRGINIA R. ROTH, MD, FRCPC   Director, Infection Prevention and Control Program, The Ottawa Hospital, General Campus

ROBERT H. RUBIN, MD, FACP, FCCP   Associate Director, Division of Infectious Diseases, Brigham and Women's Hospital, Chief, Surgical and Transplant Infectious Diseases, Massachusetts General Hospital

WILLIAM A. RUTALA, MD   Professor, Department of Medicine, University of North Carolina School of Medicine, Chapel Hill, North Carolina, Director, Hospital Epidemiology, Occupational Health, and Safety Program, University of North Carolina Healthcare System, Manning Drive, Chapel Hill, North Carolina

CASSANDRA D. SALGADO, MD, MS   Assistant Professor, Department of Medicine, Division of Infectious Diseases, Medical University of South Carolina, Hospital Epidemiologist, Department of Infection Control, Medical University of South Carolina

SANJAY SAINT, MD, MPH   Professor, Internal Medicine, University of Michigan Medical School

HUGO SAX, MD   Tutor, Department of Medicine, University of Geneva Faculty of Medicine, Deputy Director, Infection Control Program, Department of Internal Medicine, University of Geneva Hospitals

WILLIAM E. SCHECKLER, MD   Professor Emeritus, Family Medicine and Medicine, University of Wisconsin School of Medicine and Public Health, Hospital Epidemiologist, Department of Infection Control, St. Mary's Hospital

MICHAEL SCHELD, MD   Professor of Medicine, Bayer-Gerald N. Mandell Professor of Infections Diseases, Division of Infectious Diseases and International Health, University of Virginia

WING-HONG SETO, MBBS, MRCP   Honorary Professor, Department of Microbiology, University of Hong Kong, Pokfulam, Hong Kong, China, Chief of Service, Department of Microbiology, Queen Mary Hospital

JANE D. SIEGEL, MD   Professor of Pediatrics, University of Texas Southwestern Medical Center, Medical Director, Department of Infection Control, Children's Medical Center Dallas

BRYAN P. SIMMONS, MD, FACP   Clinical Professor, Internal Medicine, University of Tennessee Health Sciences Center, Medical Director, Infection Control, Methodist Le Bonheur Healthcare

LAURENCE SLUTSKER, MD, MPH   Chief, Malaria Branch, Division of Parasitic Diseases, National Center for Zoonotic, Vectorborne and Enteric Diseases, Coordinating Center for Infectious Diseases, Centers for Disease Control and Prevention

BARBARA SOULE, RN, MPA, CIC   Practice Leader, Infection Prevention and Control, Joint Commission Resources & Joint Commission International

KATHLEEN STEGER CRAVEN, RN, MPH   Section Head, Director, Research Practice Institute, Inc., Senior Management, Styllus, LLC

REBECCA H. SUNENSHINE, MD   Division of Healthcare Quality Promotion, Centers for Disease Control and Prevention

FRED C. TENOVER, PhD, D (ABMM)   Associate Director for Laboratory Science, Division of Healthcare Quality Promotion, Centers for Disease Control and Prevention

ILKER UÇKAY, MD   Resident, Service of Infectious Diseases, Geneva University Hospitals

AUGUST JOHN VALENTI, MD, FACP, FSHEA, FIDSA   Clinical Professor of Medicine, Departments of Medicine and Infectious Diseases, University of Vermont College of Medicine, Director, Epidemiology and Infection Prevention, Maine Medical Center

MARGARITA A. VILLARINO, MD, MPH   Medical Epidemiologist, Division of Tuberculosis Elimination, Centers for Disease Control and Prevention

DAVID A. WEBER, MD   Professor, Departments of Medicine, Pediatrics, Epidemiology, University of North Carolina, Medical Director, Hospital Epidemiology and Occupational Health, UNC Health Care System

SHARON WELBEL, MD   Assistant Professor, Departments of Internal Medicine and Infectious Diseases, Rush University Medical Center, Hospital Epidemiologist, Departments of Internal Medicine and Infectious Diseases, John H. Stroger, Jr. Hospital

MICHAEL L. WILSON, MD   Professor and Associate Professor, Departments of Internal Medicine and Infectious Diseases, Washington University School of Medicine, Professor and Vice-Chair, Department of Pathology, University of Colorado School of Medicine, Director, Department of Pathology and Laboratory Services, Denver Health

KEITH F. WOELTJE, MD, PhD   Associate Professor, Departments of Internal Medicine and Infectious Diseases, Washington University School of Medicine, Medical Director, Infection Control and HealthCare, BJC HealthCare

EILEEN L. YEE, MD   Division of Viral Diseases/Epidemiology Branch, National Center for Immunization and Respiratory Diseases, Centers for Disease Control and Prevention

Preface

Prevention and control of healthcare-associated infections or HAIs has become the focus of many efforts at the local, national, and international level. Although for decades, infection control professionals and others interested in healthcare epidemiology in healthcare facilities have focused their attention on surveillance and control of HAIs, it is only most recently that the public is demanding accountability for the prevention and control of preventable HAIs. This has led to a movement for public reporting of HAI rates, the passing of legislation in many states requiring public reporting of HAIs, and an intensification of efforts to prevent and control these infections.

In the past, most in infection control used "benchmarking" to self-assess. That is, if their healthcare facilities HAI rate was at or below the median reported rate for other similar facilities (often compared with the Centers for Disease Control and Prevention's [CDC's] National Nosocomial Infections Surveillance [NNIS] system data), then no further action was necessary. However, recent interventions suggest that an even greater proportion of HAIs are preventable than previously estimated. The goal of this fifth edition of *Hospital Infections* is to provide the reader with the latest in the field of healthcare epidemiology and HAI prevention and control and to provide the tools to move the field of healthcare epidemiology and infection control to zero tolerance, i.e., the goal of preventing all the preventable HAIs that we possibly can.

Over the past several decades, there have been tremendous advances in the field of healthcare epidemiology and infection control. Like the delivery of healthcare, the field of healthcare epidemiology and infection control has moved from surveillance and control of HAIs in hospitals to include all inpatient and outpatient healthcare settings, including long-term care, rehabilitative care, acute, acute step-down, transitional care, etc. Each of these settings has unique issues to address in healthcare epidemiology and infection control. In addition, the field of healthcare epidemiology has advanced to include infectious and non-infectious processes. In this new edition of *Hospital Infections*, we address many of these issues.

Over half of the authors of chapters in this edition of *Hospital Infections* are new. Thus, the material is new and updated to include the latest in the field. We have tried to address healthcare epidemiology and infection control issues in surveillance, prevention, patient safety, and more in all settings from the small community hospital

to large referral centers, inpatient and outpatient settings. We provide the approaches to surveillance as outlined from the CDC's National Healthcare Safety Network or NHSN; approaches to cost and cost benefit analyses of HAI prevention programs; the risk factors for HAIs and the measures proven to prevent or reduce these infections—focusing on the evidence upon which these recommendations are based.

Antimicrobial-resistant pathogens or ARPs have become a major public health crisis. Since the late 1970s, methicillin-resistant *Staphylococcus aureus* (MRSA) has become endemic in most healthcare facilities throughout the world (with a few exceptions—such as facilities in Northern Europe and West Australia). During the 1990s, we saw the emergence of vancomycin-resistant enterococcus (VRE) in the United States and, within a decade, it also has become endemic in many healthcare facilities. Increasingly HAIs are being caused by pathogens with greater and greater resistance to antimicrobials. We no longer can rely on the pharmaceutical industry to develop the next great antimicrobial to treat patients with ARP infections. We are returning to the pre-antibiotic era for some of our HAI pathogens—such as the emergence of vancomycin-intermediate or vancomycin-resistant *S. aureus* or pan-resistant *Acinetobacter* spp.! The prevention of transmission of these and other ARPs will be dependent upon the implementation of proven infection control measures. Improving the stewardship of antimicrobials may reduce the emergence of such strains, but only the complete adherence to proven infection control measures will prevent the transmission of such strains in our healthcare facilities. Because of the importance of this issue, we have included several chapters addressing the topic from the microbiologic (mechanisms of resistance and how to detect them), epidemiologic (risk factors and modes of transmission) and interventional (evidence-based methods to prevent the emergence or transmission of these pathogens) perspective.

Healthcare epidemiology and infection control activities no longer are just important in developed countries. Rather, the prevention and control of HAIs is a critical component of effective patient safety programs in all healthcare settings in the world. For that reason, we have invited renowned authors from around the world to address critical elements of successful infection prevention and control programs, such as hand hygiene, pandemic influenza, and patient safety. We hope that by including the perspective of those throughout the world that we can bring the healthcare epidemiology and infection control communities together and enhance the speed of improvement of infection control and healthcare epidemiology activities in all healthcare facilities throughout the world.

Finally, over the last several years, two areas of infection control have surfaced with great fanfare and media attention. The first is medical errors and patient safety and the second is public reporting of HAI rates. Since the Institute of Medicine (IOM) Report on Medical Errors, greater emphasis has been focused in healthcare facilities on surveillance of and prevention of non-infectious disease adverse events. We have included a chapter on patient safety to increase knowledge in this area and to illustrate how healthcare epidemiology and infection control processes can easily be applied to non-infectious disease adverse events. Many healthcare epidemiology and infection control programs have assumed responsibility for the patient safety program. It is important to remember that HAIs are the major cause of adverse patient events causing morbidity and mortality and the advances made in infection control are testimony to the cost-efficacy of investing over the years in infection prevention and control programs. Despite these advances, the public demands more access to HAI rate data to make informed decisions about their healthcare. Thus, the movement for public reporting of HAI rates was born. We have included a chapter on public reporting of HAI rates. This chapter emphasizes the importance of providing the consumer with validated and risk adjusted rates. We should take the lead in educating legislators, consumers, and others on the advances we have made in the past two decades on calculating risk-adjusted HAI rates for valid inter- or intra-healthcare facility rate comparisons. We are entering an era of zero tolerance for HAIs. The healthcare epidemiology and infection control community should take the enormous advances in knowledge contained in this edition of *Hospital Infections* and insure that the prevention interventions are fully implemented, so that as many preventable HAIs as possible are prevented, with the ultimate goal being that all preventable HAIs are being prevented. If prevention is primary, action is essential!

—William R. Jarvis, MD

General Considerations of Hospital Infections

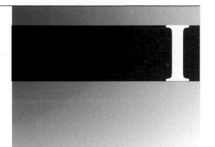

I

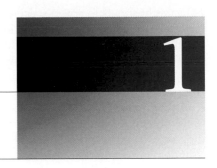

Epidemiology of Healthcare-Associated Infections

Belinda Ostrowsky

INTRODUCTION AND IMPORTANCE/EXPANDING ROLE OF EPIDEMIOLOGY IN THE HEALTHCARE FACILITIES

The term epidemiology is derived from the Greek epi (on or upon), demos (people or population), and logos (word or reason). Literally, it means "the study of things that happen to people"; historically, it has involved the study of epidemics [1,2]. The Harvard School of Public Health defines epidemiology as "the study of the frequency, distribution and determinants of disease in humans.... Epidemiologists use many approaches, but the ultimate aim of epidemiologic research is the prevention or effective control of human disease." [3] For many years, the population for discussion in this text would have been solely/predominately hospitalized patients and the terms hospital-acquired or nosocomial infection would have been used. Since the spectrum of healthcare and the interaction of different types of healthcare facilities (including hospital, long-term care, rehabilitation, or ambulatory care facilities) have expanded in recent years, a more appropriate term healthcare-associated infections (HAI) will be used in this chapter (still used interchangeably with nosocomial as appropriate)[4].

In hospitals alone, HAIs account for an estimated 2 million infections, 90,000 deaths, and $4.5 billion in excess health care costs annually [4,5]. There has been a shift in the patient population that healthcare facilities care for, especially in hospitals, to more complicated patients, including those who are more severely ill (multiple comorbidities and the need for intensive care unit [ICU] level of care) and an increasing number of patients who are severely immunocompromised. More devices and procedures are used in patients and for longer durations of time. In recent cost-conscious times, there are been staffing shortages (decreasing staff to patient ratios). In addition, over several decades, antimicrobial resistant pathogens (ARPs) and emerging infectious diseases have emerged. All of these have added to the challenge of preventing and controlling HAIs [6].

In addition, in the last several years, broadened concerns for medically adverse events by reports such as the Institutes of Medicine's (IOM) To Err is Human: Building a Safer Health System [7], including medical errors, have illustrated the use of basic epidemiological methods and the expansion of the role of those in infection control and healthcare epidemiology. Recently, there also has been a campaign by the Consumer's Union for the public disclosure of HAI rates [8]. This organization states that the goal of its campaign is to help consumers find the best quality of care by promoting the public disclosure of HAI rates. If hospitals disclose this key information, it says, consumers and employers can select the safest hospitals, and competition among hospitals will quickly force the worst to improve. In several states, legislation that obligates hospitals to report specific infection information has been passed. Professional infection control and healthcare epidemiology organizations and healthcare epidemiologists throughout the United States are assisting in framing model legislation and helping hospitals how to comply with these legislations [8,9]. Concerns are that state reporting systems should be based on reliable data, adhere to recommended practices that have been shown to reduce the risk of HAIs and improve patient care, protect patient confidentiality, and reflect the fact that some institutions treat more seriously ill patients.

All of these challenges illustrate the important and evolving role that those in infection control and healthcare epidemiology have in healthcare facilities. Although the circumstances may change, it is the working knowledge of the principals of epidemiology and especially of the subtleties that apply to HAI/adverse events that is essential and sets us apart from other healthcare workers (HCWs). The healthcare epidemiologist will be the one person who has the skills to analytically review occurrences and design studies to evaluate risk factors and interventions (i.e., wielding the power of epidemiology to impact prevention and control of HAIs).

It is with this in mind that the focus of this chapter is to review the basic principles of epidemiology with special emphasis on the relationship of these to HAIs. This first chapter in previous editions of this text, *Hospital Infections* [1] had been relatively stable and written by one of the fathers of infectious diseases epidemiology and nosocomial infections. Although much of the basic format of this chapter is unchanged, the authors hope to update this classic chapter including new nomenclature, advanced epidemiological methods and updated examples, and references for the basic epidemiological principals related to HAI.

DEFINITIONS

Infection and Colonization

Although terms such as infection, infectious disease, subclinical infection, and colonization are used frequently, the subtleties of these terms often are confusing. The term infection implies the successful multiplication of a microbe on or within a host. The term infectious disease applies when signs and symptoms result from infection and its associated damage or altered physiology [1,10].

If the infection provokes an immune response only, without overt clinical disease, it is a subclinical or inapparent infection. Colonization implies the presence of a microorganism in or on a host with growth and multiplication of the microorganism but without any overt clinical expression or detected immune reaction at the time it is isolated [1]. Subclinical or inapparent infection refers to a relation between the host and microorganism in

which the microorganism is present; there is no overt expression of the presence of the microorganism, but there is interaction between the host and microorganism that results in a detectable immune response, such as a serologic reaction, a skin test conversion, or a proliferative response of white blood cells to antigens from infecting organisms [1]. Therefore, special tests to detect immune responses may be needed to differentiate colonization from subclinical infection. In many instances, there is an absence of such data and the situation is considered colonization.

A carrier (or colonized person) is an individual colonized with a specific microorganism and from whom the organism can be recovered (i.e., cultured) but who shows no overt expression of the presence of the microorganism at the time it is isolated [1,11]; a carrier may have a history of previous disease due to that organism, such as typhoid.

Colonization is a natural process in the development of natural flora. In the neonate, this process occurs within days to weeks of delivery after which the neonate's normal flora is similar to that seen in adults [11]. Whether colonization occurs long or immediately before infection, it can play a major role in the development of HAIs. In many instances, colonization is a necessary precedent to infection. It is worth discussing colonization in more detail since there is heated discussion in the infection control/healthcare epidemiology community about screening for colonization with ARPs and the role and extent of isolation policies/practices. Those who advocate screening and aggressive infection control practices/isolation contend that colonized patients represent a large predominately unrecognized population who can serve as an unchecked reservoir for infection and that once the proportion of colonization patients reaches a threshold, this may lead to high burden of infection with these ARPs for which antimicrobial treatments are limited [12,13]. Those who oppose these screening programs point to limited resources/cost, competing emerging issues and the concerns about the strength of studies/data to support these efforts and practices [14].

Dissemination and Related Concepts

Dissemination, or shedding of microorganisms, refers to the movement of organisms from a person carrying them into the immediate environment [1]. This could be illustrated by culture samples of air or surfaces or other inanimate objects onto which microorganisms from the carrier may have been deposited. Shedding studies may be conducted in specially constructed chambers designed to quantitate dissemination. While shedding studies occasionally have been useful to document unusual dissemination [15], they have generally not been useful in identifying carriers whose dissemination has resulted in infection in other persons. In the hospital setting, dissemination is most effectively identified by means of surveillance in which the occurrence of infection among contacts is noted.

In some hospitals, culture surveys of all or selected asymptomatic staff may be conducted in an attempt to identify carriers of certain organisms. Even in outbreak settings, such surveys lack practical relevance, can be costly, and can actually be misleading. This practice identifies only those who are culture positive and does not in itself reliably separate colonized persons into disseminators versus nondisseminators. The practice could erroneously identify a HCW as the source and have serious ramifications for his or her future. Instead, culture surveys should be directed by sound surveillance and epidemiological investigation to identify the potential source [16]. Additional laboratory studies to confirm the presence of a suspected HCW or patient disseminator may then be undertaken.

In some instances, dissemination from a carrier has been reported to be influenced by the occurrence of an unrelated disease such as a second infection [17]. One report, for example, suggested that infants carrying staphylococci in their nares disseminate staphylococci only after the onset of a viral respiratory infection. Such infants are called cloud babies. In another instance, a physician disseminated staphylococci from his skin because of a reactivation of chronic dermatitis. Desquamation of his skin led to the transmission of staphylococci (probably by skin squames) to patients with whom he had contact. Dissemination of tetracycline-resistant *Staphylococcus aureus* from individuals carrying this organism who were treated with tetracycline has been reported. The risk of dissemination is generally greater from individuals with disease caused by that organism than from individuals with subclinical infection or colonization with the organism [17].

Contamination refers to microorganisms that are transiently present on body surface (e.g., hands) without tissue invasion or physiologic reaction. Contamination also refers to the presence of microorganisms on or in an inanimate object.

Healthcare-Associated/Nosocomial Infections

In previous editions of this text, the terms hospital-acquired or nosocomial infections would have been used. With the definition for hospital-acquired/nosocomial infections as infections that develop within a hospital or are produced by microorganisms acquired during hospitalization. As discussed previously, the delivery and scope of healthcare and healthcare epidemiology is expanding. The Centers for Disease Control and Prevention (CDC) defines HAIs as infections that patients acquire during the course of receiving treatment for other conditions or that HCWs acquire while performing their duties within a healthcare setting [4]. Even the branch of CDC that was formally the Hospital Infections Program broadened its name to the Division of Healthcare Quality Promotion to reflect this sentiment [4].

The CDC's National Nosocomial Infections Surveillance (NNIS) system was developed in the early 1970s to monitor the incidence of HAIs and their associated risk factors

and pathogens. NNIS is the only national system for tracking HAIs [18]. The NNIS system currently is undergoing a major redesign as a Web-based knowledge management and adverse events reporting system. Once implemented, the redesigned system (to be called the National Healthcare Safety Network [NHSN]) will cover new areas of patient safety monitoring and evaluation. Although the NNIS system is for surveillance purposes and NNIS definitions are not necessarily to be held as a gold standard for clinical/therapeutic decisions, some important points about HAIs can be illustrated by NNIS experience and definitions [19]. The first is that a major factor that specifically separates epidemiology and HAIs from other infectious diseases is that there is a quest to step away from a single patient and to standardize definitions to consistently identify trends in HAIs. In beginning to identify a cluster or outbreak, one of the early and consistent steps is to try to find a definition as to what constitutes a case of the HAI in question. Use of uniform definitions is critical if data collected are to be used for inter- or intrafacility comparisons, or to data from aggregated systems (e.g., NNIS) [16,19].

The NNIS/NHSN system defines an HAI as a localized or systemic condition that results from adverse reaction to the presence of an infectious agent (s) or its toxin(s), which was not present or incubating at the time of admission to the hospital/facility. For bacterial HAIs, this means that the infection usually becomes evident ≥48 hours (i.e., the typical incubation period) after admission. Since incubation periods vary with type of pathogen and patient's underlying disease, each infection must be assessed individually.

Two special situations that are usually HAIs are infection in a neonate that results from passage through the birth canal and infection that is acquired in the hospital but does not become evident until after hospital discharge. The majority of HAIs becomes clinically apparent while the patients are still in the facility; however, different studies have given widely varying estimates that between 12%–84% of surgical site infections (SSIs) are detected after discharge from the hospital [20]. Since the length of postoperative stay continues to decrease, many SSIs may not be detected for several weeks after discharge and may not require readmission to the hospital where the operation occurred. In these instances, the patient became colonized/infected while in the hospital, but the incubation period was longer than the patient's hospital stay. This sequence also is seen in some infections of newborns and in most breast abscesses of new mothers (since the length of postpartum stay also is brief).

Two special situations that usually are not considered HAIs are the complication or extension of infection(s) already present on admission unless a change in pathogen or symptoms strongly suggests the acquisition of new infection and the infection in an infant that is known or proven to have been acquired transplacentally (e.g., toxoplasmosis, syphilis) and becomes evident ≤48 hours after birth. Infections incubating at the time of the patient's admission to the facility are not HAIs; they are community acquired unless they result from a previous healthcare exposure. However, community-acquired infections can serve as a ready source of infection for other patients or HCWs and thus must be considered in the total scope of hospital-related infections.

Two important principles of HAIs relate to infections that are preventable versus those that are nonpreventable. The term preventable HAI implies that some event related to the infection could have been altered and that such alteration would have prevented the infection from occurring. A HCW who does not perform hygiene on his or her hands between contacts with the urinary collection equipment of two patients, for example, may transmit pathogens from the first patient to the second, which may result in a urinary tract infection. Hand hygiene might have prevented this infection from occurring. The identification of such an event in retrospect, however, is difficult; it is necessary to distinguish this situation from circumstances in which both patients developed infections from their own endogenous flora (e.g., from *Escherichia coli*). It often is impossible to identify the precise mode of acquisition of individual HAIs. More than one mode of transmission may contribute to the development of the same infection, and not all modes may be preventable.

A nonpreventable infection is one that will occur despite all possible precautions, for example, infection in an immunosuppressed patient due to endogenous flora. It has been estimated that approximately 30% of all reported HAIs are preventable [1]; however, more recent studies documenting the near elimination of catheter-related bloodstream infections (BSIs) in ICU patients suggest that an even higher percentage of HAIs may be preventable. Outbreaks, especially those caused by a common vehicle, potentially are preventable; however, outbreaks/clusters account for only a small number of HAIs (5–10% of all HAIs) [21,22]. Prompt investigation and the institution of rational control measures should reduce the extent of the epidemic. Endemic infections account for the majority of HAIs, and the consistent application of recognized, effective control and prevention measures for endemic infections probably is the single most important factor in reducing the overall level of HAIs.

Source: Endogenous (Autogenous) or Exogenous

Two terms endogenous (autogenous) and exogenous, are helpful in understanding HAIs. Endogenous infections are caused by the patient's own flora; exogenous infections result from transmission of organisms from a source other than the patient. For endogenous infections, that patient either was admitted to the facility colonized with these microorganisms or became colonized at some point during his or her stay at the hospital/facility after admission. It may

not always be possible to determine whether a particular organism isolated from a patient with an HAI caused by that organism is exogenous or endogenous, and the term autogenous should be used in this situation. Autogenous infection indicates that the infection was derived from the flora of the patient, whether or not the infecting organism became part of the patient's flora subsequent to admission [1]. Information about current infectious diseases/microorganism problems in the community or in hospital contacts may be useful in differentiating the two sources. For example, in the past, if a patient had an infection with methicillin-resistant *S. aureus* (MRSA), it probably would have been assumed that this infection was related to acquisition in the healthcare facility. In the last several years, however, episodes of community-acquired MRSA [23,24], have increased and it may be helpful to know the local occurrence of these community-acquired isolates in addition to the patient's recent healthcare-related and antimicrobial exposures. Microbiologic characteristics of the organism such as antibiograms, biochemical testing, and molecular typing (staphylococcal cassette or genotype) may provide additional evidence to support nosocomial versus community origin of these strains/infections.

Spectrum of Occurrence of Cases

Often possible clusters of HAIs are detected through clinical microbiology or infection control surveillance data or by an astute laboratorian or clinician [16,25]. Once a cluster is detected, one must evaluate whether this represents a problem, such as an outbreak. As discussed previously, exploring cases and arriving at a case definition is essential to identify as many cases as possible. Comparing the rate of the event during the cluster to a period before the cluster can establish whether an outbreak is occurring. A few definitions are helpful to characterize disease frequency, including sporadic, endemic (hyperendemic), outbreak, and epidemic.

Sporadic means that episodes occur occasionally and irregularly without any specific pattern. Endemic means that the disease occurs with ongoing frequency in a specific geographic area in a finite population and over a defined time period. Hyperendemic refers to what appears to be a gradual increase in the occurrence of a disease in a defined area beyond the expected number; however, it may not be certain whether the disease will occur at epidemic proportions. An epidemic is a definite increase in the incidence of a disease above its expected endemic occurrence. Outbreak often is used interchangeably with epidemic; however, many use outbreak to mean an increased rate of occurrence but not at levels as serious as an epidemic [1].

An occasional gas gangrene infection among postoperative patients is an example of a sporadic infection. An endemic HAI is represented by the regular occurrence of infections either in a particular site or at different sites that are due to the same organism, occur at a nearly constant rate, and are generally considered by the hospital staff to be within expected and acceptable limits. SSIs due to a single organism that follow operations classified as "contaminated surgery," for example, could represent the endemic level of SSIs.

Plotting a histogram of the distribution of "cases" by time in an "epidemic curve" may aid in confirming the existence of an outbreak (versus sporadic or endemic infections) and developing hypotheses about the mode of transmission [16,26,27]. This can be simply executed on graph paper or by using a variety of software packages, such as Microsoft Excel or PowerPoint. Details on the construction of an epidemic curve are described in the descriptive epidemiology section (also Table 1-2 and Figure 1-1).

Measures of Disease Frequency-Incidence and Prevalence and Related Measures

To identify that a problem with HAIs exists, it is important to be able to quantify the frequency of disease/event

occurrence. The two most commonly used measures of disease frequency are prevalence and incidence. Some unique issues that may occur with HAIs related to these measures of frequency will be reviewed, and some additional measures of incidence (incidence density and cumulative incidence) and prevalence are discussed. Each of these measures has uses in healthcare epidemiology and advantages and disadvantages (Table 1-1).

Incidence is the number of new cases in a specific population in a defined time period [28]. Prevalence is a measure of status rather than newly occurring disease and of people who have the disease at a specific time [28].

Incidence can be described in several ways. Incidence density (also known as the incidence rate) is the number of new events (disease onset) in a specified amount of person-time (hospital or healthcare facility days) in a population at risk [28,29]. Incidence density usually is restricted to the first event (first HAI, i.e., BSI), since second events are not statistically independent events in the same individual

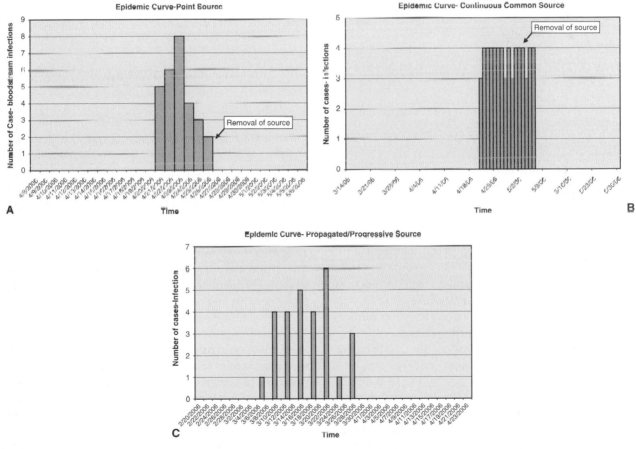

Figure 1-1 Examples of epidemic curves. (A) Point-source: This epidemic curve represents a point-source exposure. The patients are all exposed to the same source and the curve rapidly rises to a peak and then resolves when the source is removed. (B) Continuous Common source: This epidemic curve represents a continuous common source outbreak. Exposure to the source is prolonged and thus the curve is less peaked than the point-source curve. Here the downward slope of the curve quickly decreases with removal of the exposure. (C) Propagated/Progressive source: This epidemic curve represents a propagated/progressive source. Each case is a source of infection for the subsequent case. There are usually several peaks caused by person-to-person transmission.

TABLE 1-1

MEASUREMENTS OF OCCURRENCE (TERMS FOR INCIDENCE AND PREVALENCE)

Measure of Association	Additional Names	Definition/ Formula	Units	Uses in Health Care Epidemiology/ Advantages	Disadvantages
Incidence		Number of new events or disease during a time	Cases/time, rate		
Incidence Density	Incidence rate	Number of *first events* Observed time at risk for a first event	1/time	First events/1,000 facility-days Allows for correction for time and separates out duration of exposure	Not clear what to do with second and subsequent events
Cumulative Inci- dence	Attack rate	Sum of all *first events* Sum of all person-time at risk for first events	No units, expressed as %	Helpful when point source considered	Does not distinguish first from other events, does not take into account different risk with time
Prevalence	Point prevalence Prevalence proportion, prevalence rate	Proportion of individuals with disease or condition at one point in time	Proportion, %	For point-prevalence surveys such as cross-sectional studies	Influenced by incidence and duration

(i.e., once the patient has had one HAI, he or she is more likely to have a second one). The population at risk includes all patients who have not yet had the first event. Once a patient acquires the first HAI, he or she would not still be a part of the population at risk and would be withdrawn. Patients who never have an HAI would contribute all their hospital-/facility-days to the pool of days at risk for a first event, but patients who became infected would contribute only those hospital-days before the onset of the infection.

Since the first event is just a number, incidence density has the units of (1/time). In practical use in healthcare epidemiology, HAI rates usually are expressed as number of first events in 1,000 hospital-/facility-days (usually gives a single or double-digit number of events per 1,000 hospital days) [29,30]. The advantage of using incidence density is that it allows a way to correct for time and separat out the duration of exposure from the effect of daily risk. Examples where this is particularly useful in healthcare epidemiology are in comparisons of those with short versus long hospital stays and for peripheral intravenous lines versus central venous catheters [29,30]. In each of these instances, the time at risk is substantially longer for the second group versus the first.

A question that arises with the incidence density is what to do with a second or additional event (e.g., second HAI; i.e., second healthcare-associated BSI) since multiple studies have shown that the subsequent events are not independent. The first guidance is that for quantitative analysis of HAIs, it would be overly simplistic and misleading to sum these nonindependent events and put them over the denominator [29]. The first and each subsequent event actually would be a risk factor for the next infection, which is why it is best to restrict analysis to the first event.

There are more complex methods to include first and multiple/subsequent events in a study using different stratum [31]. For example, one approach is to define the population at risk differently for each occurrence [28]: The population at risk for the first event would consist of individuals who have not experienced the disease before; the population at risk for the second event or first recurrence would be limited to those who have experienced the event (infection) once and once only, and so on. An individual should contribute time to the denominator of the incidence rate for first events only until the time that the disease first occurs. At that point, the individual should cease contributing time to the denominator of that rate and should begin contributing time to the denominator of the rate measuring the second occurrence. If and when there is a second event, the individual should stop contributing time to the rate measuring the second occurrence and begin contributing to the denominator of the rate measuring the third occurrence, and so forth.

Cumulative incidence is the proportion of all those at risk who ultimately suffer a first event [28–30]. In traditional infectious disease epidemiology, this has been termed the attack rate [29]. This is actually not a rate but a proportion. Cumulative incidence is derived from the incidence density and in simple terms could be thought of as the sum of all incidence densities for first events over all of the person-time at risk for the first event. This is a simple proportion and thus has no units. For overall HAIs, the time implied is the course of hospitalization (duration in the facility) until the first event or discharge without first event. There are a few limitations to the cumulative incidence. First, there should be follow-up for all at risk to determine whether they have the first event. However, patients do not all have the same length of hospital stay or remain at risk for the same amount of time. Also, HAIs are time related, and comparing HAI rates among patients with differing lengths of stay can be misleading. The cumulative incidence could be of particular use with an HAI considered to be from a point-source, such as a contaminated fluid or SSI (operation as the point-source) [29,30].

In the past, HAIs were reported as a cumulative incidence of number of infections per 100 discharges. One disadvantage of this aggregation and presentation is that there was no distinction between separate first infection from multiple infections in the same patients (thus, 10 infections per 100 discharges could be 10 infections from one very complicated patient, 10 from 10 different healthy patients, or some description between these extremes; the extremes illustrate how this summary term could be quite different in its clinical and epidemiological relevance and in what intervention methods might be necessary). Another disadvantage is that since one patient could be counted multiple times, this would not take into account lack of statistical independence, thus making comparisons difficult [29].

Unlike incidence measures, which focus on events, prevalence focuses on disease status. Prevalence is defined as the proportion of a population that has disease at a specific point in time [30]. Several terms, such as point prevalence, prevalence proportion, and prevalence rate, often are used interchangeably. Prevalence depends on the incidence and the duration of the disease. As either of these increases, the prevalence increases. The main useful measure for healthcare epidemiology would be point prevalence for studies such as a cross-sectional study [30] (i.e., a point prevalence survey on a day using cultures to detect colonization/infections with an ARP, such as vancomycin-resistant enterococcus (VRE) or MRSA). This could give an idea of the burden of a problem at a particular point in time to assist in defining that a problem exists, guide decisions to pursue additional studies, and allow for allocation of resources. Of note, populations are dynamic and since individuals are entering and leaving the population, the prevalence can vary based on when it is measured.

EPIDEMIOLOGICAL METHODS

Generally, three techniques are used in epidemiologic studies: descriptive, analytic, and experimental; all may be used in investigating HAIs. Descriptive epidemiology is the foundation for evaluation of HAIs and is used in both surveillance and most investigations of potential problems/outbreaks. Once the initial problem has been defined by descriptive epidemiology, additional studies using analytic and/or experimental methods can be conducted to develop more information about the problem, confirm initial impressions, prove/disprove hypotheses (including identifying risk factors/potential associations/sources or causes), and evaluate the effectiveness of control measures and/or prevention measures.

The presentation of descriptive epidemiology can include case report/case series. A case report is the clinical description of a single patient. A case series is a report of >1 patient. These types of studies/publications are easy to prepare and can serve as examples to other healthcare epidemiologists. These studies also can serve as a resource to generate hypotheses and ideas for additional studies. The disadvantage of this type of study is that patient numbers are small, and the findings may not be generalizable to other populations. In addition, no comparison to other groups has been made.

The analytic study section will discuss case-control and cohort studies, which are the comparative studies frequently used in healthcare epidemiology, especially to explore outbreaks and healthcare epidemiology problems to identify risk factors and potential associations. Additional analytic-type studies that can be used for healthcare epidemiological studies are ecological or cross-sectional studies. Experimental methods of studies include randomized control trials (rarely used in healthcare epidemiology) and quasi-experimental studies (to evaluate an intervention without randomization).

DESCRIPTIVE EPIDEMIOLOGY

Descriptive epidemiologic studies evaluate the occurrence of disease in terms of time, place, and person [1,26]; each "case" of a disease is first characterized by describing these three attributes. When data from the individual cases are combined and analyzed, the parameters of the outbreak or disease problem should be characterized. Issues that arise regarding time, place, and person in general descriptive epidemiology and specifics to healthcare epidemiology are discussed next.

Time

There are four time trends to consider: secular, periodic, seasonal, and acute [1]. Secular trends are long-term trends in the occurrence of a disease—that is, variations that occur over a period of years. An example in HAIs would be the gradual increase in fungal BSIs, including those that are nonalbicans Candida and azol resistant [32]. Periodic trends are temporal interruptions of the secular trend and usually reflect changes in the overall susceptibility to the disease in the population. The upsurge in Influenza A activity every 2 to 3 years, for instance, reflects the periodic trend of this disease and generally is the result of antigenic drift of the Influenza A virus. Seasonal trends are the annual variations in disease incidence related in part to seasons. In general, the occurrence of a particular communicable disease increases when the circumstances that influence its transmission are favorable. The seasonal pattern of both community-acquired and healthcare-associated respiratory disease, for example, is high incidence in the fall and winter months when transmission is enhanced because people are together in rooms with closed windows and are breathing unfiltered, recirculating air. Thus, they have more contact with one another and with droplets/droplet nuclei. There also may be agent and host factors that influence the seasonal trends. Another example is that healthcare-associated *Acinetobacter spp.* infections have a seasonal trend, increasing in the summer and fall [33]. The fourth type of time variation is the acute or epidemic/outbreak occurrence of a disease with its characteristic upsurge in incidence.

As described previously, a graphic representation of the "cases" can assist in confirming the existence of an outbreak, its source, its transmission, the point of an outbreak you are in, and evaluating interventions. The overall shape of the epidemic curve depends on the interaction of many factors: characteristics of the agent (i.e., pathogenicity, concentration, and incubation period), the method of transmission, host factors (i.e., susceptibility and concentration of susceptible individuals), and environmental factors (i.e., temperature, humidity, movement of air, and general housekeeping). A step-by-step guide to creating an epidemic curve is included in Table 1-2 [16,26,27].

The following are a few points to keep in mind while attempting to create/interpret an epidemic curve. The time scale will vary according to the incubation or latency period, ranging from minutes, as in an outbreak of disease following exposure to a toxin or a chemical, to months, as in an epidemic of hepatitis B. The time scale (abcissa, hortizontal scale, *x* axis) should be selected with three facts in mind: (1) The unit time interval should be less than the average incubation period (commonly one-fourth to one-third of the probable incubation period) so that the true nature of the epidemic curve will be apparent (i.e., all the cases will not be bunched together); (2) the scale should be extended far enough in time to allow all cases to be plotted; and (3) any cases that occurred before the epidemic should be plotted to give a basis for comparison with the epidemic/outbreak experience [1,26,27]

If the epidemic curve starts with the index case (i.e., the first case in the outbreak), the time between the index case and onset of the next case reflects the incubation period if transmission was from the index case directly to the next case—that is, from person to person. The upslope in the curve is determined by the incubation period, the number and concentration of exposed susceptible persons, the number of infected sources, and the ease of transmission. The height of the peak of the curve is influenced by the total number of exposed susceptible individuals and the time interval over which they occur. The downslope of the curve is usually more gradual than the upslope; its gradual change reflects cases with longer incubation periods and the decreasing number of susceptible individuals. The initiation of control measures may contribute to the gradual decline or to a sudden decrease in the appearance of new cases [1].

When interpreting an epidemic curve, it is useful to look at the overall shape of the curve to assist in determining how the outbreak spread throughout the population and, potentially, if the disease is unknown, the initial diagnosis of the disease. For simplicity, there are three main patterns the epidemic curve can take (Figure 1-1) [27]. In a point-source epidemic, persons are exposed to the same exposure over a limited, defined period of time, usually within one incubation period. The shape of this curve commonly rises rapidly and contains a definite peak at the top followed by a gradual decline. Sometimes cases also may appear as a wave that follows a point-source by one incubation period or time interval. This is called a point-source with secondary transmission.

In a continuous common-source epidemic, exposure to the source is prolonged over an extended period of time and may occur over >1 incubation period. The downward slope of the curve may be very sharp if the common source is removed or gradual if the outbreak is allowed to exhaust itself (i.e., affect all susceptible persons).

A propagated (progressive source) epidemic occurs when a case of disease serves as a source of infection for subsequent cases, and those subsequent cases, in turn, serve as sources for later cases. The shape of the curve usually contains a series of successively larger peaks, reflective of the increasing number of cases caused by person-to-person contact until the pool of susceptibles is exhausted or control measures are implemented.

In reality, mixed modes of transmission may occur, and the epidemic curve could include both point-source and propagated cases.

Place

Although outbreaks of HAI occur infrequently in some settings, such as ICUs, they can account for a substantial percentage of the HAIs. In an investigation of HAIs, three different places may be involved. The first is where the patient is when the disease is diagnosed, and the second is where contact occurred between the patient and the agent. If a vehicle of infection is involved, the third place is where

TABLE 1-2
STEPS IN CONSTRUCTING AN EPIDEMIC CURVE

Steps	Details	Examples/Comments Specific for Healthcare-Associated Infections
Step 1: Identify the Date of Onset	Identify the date of onset of illness for each case. For a disease with a very short incubation period, identify the time of onset to produce an epidemic curve with enough detail to discern patterns in the outbreak. If the date of onset is unknown, use one of the following dates: date of report, date of death, or date of diagnosis.	Likely date of diagnosis used such as in an outbreak of healthcare-associated bloodstream infections, the date of the culture collection would be used.
Step 2ª: Set the Time Interval	Set the time interval for the x axis. The time intervals are preferably based on the incubation period of the disease, if known. The time interval is critical because intervals that are too short (e.g., hours, for diseases with long incubation periods) or too long may obscure the underlying pattern of the outbreak. As a rule of thumb, select a unit of about 1/3–1/4 of the incubation period for the time interval on the x axis.	
Step 3ª: Create x-Axis Lead and End Periods	Illustrate the time period before and after the concentration of cases to possibly reveal source cases, secondary transmission, and other outliers of interest. The following steps can be used when establishing lead and end periods. 1. From the line listing, find the first and last dates of onset. 2. To create the *lead* period, extend the scale back two incubation periods from the first date of onset. 3. To create the *end* period, extend the scale forward two incubation periods after the last case.	
Step 4: Draw Tick Marks and Label Time Intervals	Draw the tick marks on the x axis according to the interval chosen. Begin putting labels, such as the interval or date markers (i.e., dates of onset) on the x axis,	
Step 5: Assign Area Equal to One Case	If drawn on paper, assign the area that will be equal to one case on the x axis, which is usually square or rectangular.	
Step 6: Plot the Cases on the Graph	Now plot the cases on the graph. There should be no gaps between adjacent time intervals because this is a histogram, not a bar graph.	
Step 7: Mark the Critical Events on the Graph and Add Graph Labels	Labels are useful tools to identify or highlight events and cases of importance. In addition, title, legend, and axis labels provide the reader visual aids to assist in interpreting the curve.	Important events may include when a control of intervention was put into place.
Step 8: Interpreting an Epidemic Curve	Through review of the different patterns illustrated in an epidemic curve, it is possible to hypothesize: ■ How an epidemic spread throughout a population. ■ At what point an epidemic currently is. ■ The diagnosis of the disease by establishing the potential incubation period. When analyzing an epidemic curve, consider the following factors to assist in interpreting an outbreak. ■ The overall pattern of the epidemic. ■ The time period when the persons were exposed. ■ Whether there any outliers. Typically, epidemic curves fall into three different classifications: ■ Point-source. ■ Continuous common source. ■ Propagated (progressive source).	

(continued)

		TABLE 1-2

		(CONTINUED)

Steps	Details	Examples/Comments Specific for Healthcare-Associated Infections
Step 9: Viewing an Epidemic Curve by Characteristics	Stratification is a mainstay of epidemiologic analysis because it provides an investigator a different perspective on key variables. In the process of viewing an epidemic curve, it can be helpful to divide a population into several subgroups to ■ Illustrate a pattern contained in potentially unmeasured characteristics such as geography or job classification. ■ Provide a uniform baseline for comparison.	This may include cases that fit a possible/probable vs. confirmed case definition

Adapted from CDC, Division of Epidemiology and Surveillance Capacity Development DESCP, *Training resources modular learning components (mini-modules) constructing an epidemic curve, also available online at* **http://www.cdc.gov/descd/MiniModules/Epidemic_Curve/page01.htm** *[27]*

[a]When the disease and incubation periods are unknown, it is often necessary to draw an epidemic curve. Step 2 (setting the time interval) and step 3 (creating the lead and end periods on the x axis) will be slightly different in that case. Lead and end periods. When the incubation period is unknown, use 1 to 2 weeks for the lead and end periods. Time intervals. If the disease is unknown, a good way to set the time interval is to create at least three epidemic curves, each with a different time interval.

the vehicle became contaminated. To implement the most appropriate control and preventive measures, it is necessary to distinguish between these three geographic areas; certain actions may control additional spread from a specific focus but may not prevent new cases from occurring if the source continues to contaminate/infect new vehicles.

An example will help to emphasize the importance of carefully describing the place or places involved in disease outbreaks. In an outbreak of nosocomial salmonellosis, the patients were located on various wards throughout the hospital at the time they developed disease. Individual control measures were directed at each patient on the various wards; however, the place of infection was the radiology department, where barium used for gastrointestinal tract roentgenographic examinations was contaminated with salmonella. The barium had been contaminated in the radiology department, and thus preventive measures directed there terminated the outbreak.

Because transfer of patients between hospital wards or units is common, it may be difficult to attribute an outbreak to a particular geographic area. Infection rates can be calculated for other areas of the hospital and compared to the area(s) with the cluster to aid in identifying the location of the outbreak [16]. In addition, a review of the geographic location of cases using a spot map of the hospital or ICU may suggest the location or pattern of transmission [16,26].

Person

The third major component of descriptive epidemiology is person. Careful evaluation of host factors related to the individual person includes consideration of age,

gender, race, immunization status, immunocompetence, and presence of underlying disease that may influence susceptibility (acute or chronic), therapeutic or diagnostic procedures, medications, and nutritional status. In essence, any host factor that can influence the development of disease must be considered and described. Those factors that increase the patient's chance of developing disease are known as risk factors.

Age also can be an important clue to the source of an outbreak of disease. If, in an apparent common-source outbreak, for example, all ages are involved, the source of the outbreak must have been exposed patients scattered through at least several wards. On the other hand, if all the patients involved in an epidemic are women of child-bearing age, in attempting to identify the place of the exposure, the investigation can be narrowed to the obstetric or, possibly, the gynecology ward.

Consideration of therapeutic procedures may be of similar importance. If all patients who developed BSIs due to the same organism have received intravenous fluid therapy, a common source of intravenous fluids could be suspected as the cause of the outbreak.

In addition, knowledge of intrinsic host risk factors is useful because separate risk-specific rates can be calculated, which allows for the comparison of HAIs among patients with similar risk. Severity of illness is a strong confounding variable in outbreaks in healthcare settings. The Acute Physiology and Chronic Health Evaluation (APACHE II) and Diagnostic Related Groups (DRGs) are well-known indices used to assess and control the severity of illness [35, 36]. These indices are used to predict the risk of death among ICU patients and for staff resource utilization. In pediatrics, severity of illness scores including the modified abbreviated injury severity score (MISS) and Score for Neonatal Acute Physiology (SNAP) have been used to assess neonatal/pediatric populations [36,37].

ANALYTIC EPIDEMIOLOGY

After descriptive epidemiologic review has been performed and hypotheses have been generated, one may need additional studies to identify the source of a problem/outbreak. Settings in which additional efforts should be considered are when resources are available, when the problem/outbreak is associated with high mortality or severe disease, when new or unusual pathogens or methods of transmission are identified, or when the problem/outbreak continues despite implementing control measures. Additionally, the principles involved in these methods have application to surveillance; surveillance data commonly are analyzed by the descriptive method, and such analysis may suggest the need for analytic studies to identify certain features of a disease. The choice of analytical/comparative study depends on resources, time, and size of the problem/outbreak.

A few basic epidemiological principles should be reviewed with an emphasis on how these concepts vary or apply to HAIs. These are study designs/methods (emphasizing case-control or cohort studies but also including ecologic and cross-sectional studies), measures of association, strength of association, and bias/confounding. Although this chapter is not meant to be a primer on general epidemiology, some key points will be reviewed.

Study Designs/Methods

Two frequently used analytic methods include case-control or cohort studies. In both instances, associations that may identify causes and effects are sought. The case-control method starts with the effect (cases) and searches for causative host and exposure factors, and the cohort method starts with potential causative factors and evaluates the effect. The case-control and cohort methods also have been referred to as retrospective or prospective studies, respectively; both methods, however, can be either retrospective or prospective. These terms indicate the temporal frame of reference for the collection of specific data: in a retrospective study, data are collected after the event has occurred; in a prospective study, the data are collected as the event occurs.

Case-Control Study

In a case-control study, case-patients are compared with (a set ratio usually of 1:2 or 1:3) control-patients who do not have the adverse outcome or infection but have had the opportunity for the exposure. The case-control approach has the advantages of being inexpensive, relatively quick, and easily reproducible. It is used most often in acute

disease investigations, since the epidemiologist usually arrives after a problem is recognized and often after the peak of the epidemic has passed. It also allows evaluation of many potential associated exposures and for outbreaks/problems that may have persisted for lengthy periods of time.

One of the main controversies with this type of study is the appropriate choice of control-patients [38]. In one investigation of transmission of VRE in 32 hospitals and long-term care facilities, we wanted to explore the characteristics and exposures of those patients with VRE-colonization. The facilities varied in size and provided a range of intensity of medical care. VRE-colonized patients were identified from several different facilities. Thus, for each case-patient, we chose a control-patient from the same facility, and the analysis was matched for the facility [39].

In ICU outbreaks, since the patients are very different (e.g., more severely ill, have more devices, experience more procedures, take more medications) from non-ICU patients, other ICU patients may be the most appropriate controls [25,40,41]. In some studies, controls may be matched to cases on certain factor(s), such as age, gender, or other factors known to predispose to the outcome. In general, random selection of controls is preferred [42,43]. Two concerns about matching are that special statistics are needed for matched analyses and that when matching is performed, no comparisons can be made between case- and control-patients on the factors on which matching was done [42].

Review of the case-patients' medical records should identify several potential sources/risk factors. In the case-control study, a comparison of the presence or absence of these factors in the case-patients and controls is performed to see whether any of these exposures is more likely to be present in cases, suggesting that this may be associated with the outbreak. Use of standardized data collection forms facilitates the systematic review of exposures.

A pitfall in some healthcare outbreaks is that many exposures can be collected. Only biologically plausible exposures should be evaluated. A rule of thumb is that if an exposure is not present in at least 30%–40% of the cases, even if it is more common in cases than controls, it will not account for enough cases to be the source of the outbreak (attributable risk—the amount or proportion of disease incidence/risk that can be attributed to a specific exposure) [40,44,45].

Two important statistical principles should be reviewed at this point relating to errors. Type I error (α error) relates to concluding that a statistical relationship exists when it does not. This may occur in a case-control study when many factors/exposures are evaluated. With multiple tests, a relationship may be found to be statistically significant but represents a false positive. Often these false positive relationships have only borderline significance (p values near 0.05) with weaker magnitudes of association and lack of biological plausibility. The take-home message is not to examine factors that are not clinically relevant or biologically plausible since a relationship may be identified purely by performing multiple tests looking at multiple variables [46]. For other studies not related to outbreaks, it best to make an a priori plan in which variables are to be collected and analyzed to prevent this problem.

Type II error (β error) relates to concluding that a factor is not significantly associated with becoming a case when it in fact is related. This error is related to the concept of power. Power is $1 - \beta$ error. These concepts are greatly affected by the sample size in a study. In a planned research protocol, set numbers of cases and controls can be enlisted. In an outbreak situation, the number of cases is obviously limited. The main points are that HAI outbreaks/studies may be of a smaller scale and that certain associations may not reach statistical significance; however, trends may still have clinical significance [46].

Another area of controversy is how long variables of interest should be collected in case-and control-patients. This needs to be clear for those reviewing charts/medical records. In one ICU outbreak we investigated, exposure data were collected for the case-patients from SICU admission until the day of diagnosis of their *S. marcescens* BSI and for controls from the date of SICU admission to the median time that the case-patients developed their *S. marcescens* BSI (7 days) or discharge date from the SICU if the controls' SICU length of stay was < 7 days. The exposure period for case-patients and controls should be similar [40]. For case-patients only, exposure until the onset of illness should be collected. For example, antimicrobial exposures for acquisition of VRE probably should be collected for the proceeding days or weeks rather than months before onset of colonization. Exposure months before onset of a disease may be present but have no relationship to disease acquisition. Similarly, exposure data should be collected for a preceding biologically plausible period of time. Control exposures to case-patients should be collected for a similar period, not for the entire hospitalization. Often, this process will lead to a difference with case-patients that really represents the fact that the exposure period in controls (admission to discharge) is longer than in case-patients (admission until onset of disease).

Case-control studies establish only that case-patients were more likely to have been exposed to potential risk factors than were controls. In case-control studies, one can calculate an odds ratio (abbreviated OR), which estimates the relative risk (RR) and measures the strength of the association between the condition and the exposure/risk factor (Figure 1-2) [42,47].

		OUTCOME	
		Present (cases)	Absent (controls)
FACTOR	Present (exposed)	A	B
	Absent (unexposed)	C	D

Relative Risk

Risk of disease among exposed = A / (A+B)

Risk of disease among unexposed = C/ (C+D)

$$\text{Relative Risk} = \frac{A / (A+B)}{C / (C+D)}$$

Odds Ratio

Odds of exposure given disease = A / C

Odds of exposure given no disease = B / D

$$\text{Disease Odds Ratio} = \frac{A/C}{B/D} = \frac{AD}{BC}$$

Relationship between relative risk and odds ratio

When disease is rare, B>>A, and D>>>C

$$\text{Relative Risk} = \frac{A / (A+B)}{C / (C+D)} \sim \frac{AD}{BC} = \text{Odds ratio}$$

Figure 1-2 Example of a two by two table and definitions for measures of effect or association, relative risk and odds ratio.

Cohort Study

In a cohort study, one assesses the entire population (e.g., all ICU patients from June 2000–December 2001) and evaluates what exposures are more common among those who develop disease/infection than those who do not. As mentioned earlier, a cohort study may be either prospective or retrospective. This distinction depends on when the study is conducted with regard to when the outcome of interest occurs. If patients are identified as exposed and unexposed and then followed forward in time to determine whether they develop the disease, this is a prospective cohort study. If the study is conducted after the time of outcome has already occurred, this is a retrospective cohort study. In either study, subjects are selected based on their exposure to the variable of interest, and these groups are compared based on the outcome.

The main advantage of the cohort study (versus the case-control study) is that if significantly more exposed patients than unexposed patients develop the outcome, this factor may be not only associated but also causally related to the outbreak. In a cohort study, one can quantify the extent to which the exposure increases the risk of developing the condition in a summary term RR (Figure 1-2) [47]. Several cohorts may be followed, each representing a different level of exposure to a factor, thus allowing for the determination of a dose response. Unlike the OR, the RR not only describes that the exposure is associated with the outcome but also denotes causation.

Disadvantages of the cohort study are that they may be costly and time-consuming since patients must be followed in time until a sufficient number develop the outcome of interest (which could be a lengthy period of time if the disease course is slow or the disease is rare). This could lead to loss of follow-up of some in the cohort. Some of these limitations are lessened by performing a cohort study retrospectively because the outcome has already happened.

A variant on the traditional case-control and cohort design can be helpful in the evaluation of HAIs. A case-control study within an identified cohort is sometimes termed a "nested case-control" study.

Other Analytics Epidemiology Methods

Ecologic Studies

The studies described so far share the characteristic that the observations made pertain to individuals. Ecologic or aggregate studies conduct research in which the unit of observation is a group of people rather than an individual. The requirement is that information on the population studies be available to measure the exposure and disease distributions in each group. Because the data in ecologic studies are measurements averaged over individuals, the degree of association between exposure and disease need not reflect individual associations. These data may be more easily obtainable than individual-level patient data but as discussed cannot be extrapolated to an individual patient and, in fact, if done could lead to an ecologic fallacy, an error in the interpretation of statistical data, in which inferences about the nature of individuals are based solely on aggregate statistics collected for the group to which those individuals belong. This fallacy assumes that all members of a group exhibit characteristics of the group at large.

In healthcare epidemiology, some examples of ecologic studies are the use of data aggregated for other purposes, such as drug dispending data from hospital pharmacies, and the antimicrobial susceptibility data from the hospital clinical microbiology laboratory. A good example would be hospital data that could show an increase in use of the antimicrobial vancomycin and VRE in enterococcal isolates, but it will not be possible to know whether the patients who received vancomycin were the patients who acquired VRE. This type of data, however, may serve as exploratory data on which to base additional studies.

An interesting use of ecologic data is the CDC's NNIS Intensive Care Antimicrobial Resistance Epidemiology (ICARE) project [48]. During this 4-year study, a subset of NNIS hospitals (50 ICUs at 20 U.S. hospitals) monitored antimicrobial use and ARPs. Participating hospitals reported the grams of select antimicrobial agents administered to patients and the antimicrobial susceptibility results of isolates recovered from clinical specimens from hospitalized patients each month. Microbiologic data were aggregated for each ICU separately, all non-ICU inpatient wards combined, and all outpatient areas combined. Pharmacy data were reported for the same hospital strata except for outpatient areas for which pharmacy data were not available. Amounts of antimicrobial agents reported were standardized by conversion to defined daily doses; for parenteral vancomycin, one daily dose was defined as 2 grams.

The study found that after data were adjusted for changes in MRSA prevalence, changes in specific prescriber practice at ICUs were associated with significant decreases in vancomycin use (mean decrease −48 defined daily doses per 1,000 patient days, $p < 0.001$). These ICUs also reported significant decreases in VRE prevalence compared with those not using unit-specific changes in practice (mean decrease of 7.5% compared with mean increase of 5.7%, $p < 0.001$). In this study, practice changes that focused on specific ICUs were associated with decreases in ICU vancomycin use and VRE prevalence. This example illustrates how HAI data may be aggregated for ecologic study, such as the development of defined daily doses and which hospital units' data were compared.

Cross-Sectional Studies

A cross-sectional study is a survey or sampling of a population in which the status of the exposure and the outcome are ascertained at the same time. In healthcare epidemiology, this study type is frequently used to assess the prevalence of a specific disease, such as amount of antimicrobial resistance. A disadvantage to this type of study is that it does not give an idea about transition of status over time. Depending on the populations, a cross-sectional study may be analyzed as a cohort or case-control study.

Measures of Association and Related Concepts

A measure of association provides an index of how strongly two factors under study vary in concert [49]. The more tightly they are linked, the more evidence exists that they are causally related to each other (though not necessarily that one causes the other, since they might both be caused by a third factor). Although this term and "measure of effect" have frequently been used interchangeably, Rothman and Greenland draw the following distinction: associations involve comparisons between groups or populations; effects involve comparisons of the same population (hypothetically) observed in two different conditions; measures of association are typically used to estimate measures of effect [49].

In Figure 1-2, a two-by-two table is constructed and the calculation for relative risk and odds ratio [43,47], the two main measures of association that healthcare epidemiologists deal with on a regular basis, are illustrated. The calculations are not the difficult part; it is understanding what these measures elude about the study and the two populations being compared (and what they do not mean).

Depending on the study performed, either an RR or OR usually will be calculated. First, it is worth distinguishing between risk versus odds. Risk refers to probability and has a numerator with the event/occurrence of interest and a denominator with all possible outcomes including the event of interest. The odds has the same numerator, but the denominator includes all possibilities minus the event/outcome of interest.

The RR is the ratio of two probabilities of the outcome in the exposed over the probability of the outcome in the unexposed [49]. The RR can be calculated in cohort studies (and randomized control trials). If there is not a difference in the risk of the exposed versus the unexposed, then the RR = 1. RR >1.0 implies that the exposed group is more likely to have the outcome than those without the exposure (no effect). An RR <1 implies that the exposed group was less likely to have the outcome than the nonexposed group (protective) [49].

A study of pyrogenic reactions associated with single daily dosing of intravenous gentamicin illustrates the use of RR in a cohort study [50]. The authors conducted cohort studies in an inpatient service of a large community hospital in Los Angeles, California, following patients for the occurrence of pyrogenic reactions (chills, rigors, or shaking chills) within 3 hours after the initiation of gentamicin. During the epidemic period, 22/152 (15%) patients developed documented pyrogenic reactions following receipt of gentamicin. Pyrogenic reactions were more likely among patients receiving single daily dosing than multiple daily dosing of gentamicin (20/73 [27%] versus 2/79 [3%]; relative risk was 10.8%). Thus, in simple terms, those receiving single daily dosing of gentamicin had a risk of developing a pyrogenic reaction that was 10.8 times higher than the risk of those who received multiple daily dosing.

The OR is less intuitive in its interpretation but is the measure that will be available from a case-control study [49]. In this type of study, the subjects are enrolled based on the outcome of interest (comparing a group with the outcome to a group without the outcome) to determine what proportion in each group has an exposure/risk of interest. An RR cannot be directly calculated, because how common the outcomes/exposures are in the entire population cannot be measured. Only an OR can be calculated. An OR reflects the odds of exposure with the outcome divided by the odds of exposure in study subjects without the outcome. An OR = 1.0 implies no effect.

An RR cannot be calculated from a case-control study in usual situations; however, if a disease is rare, the OR can closely approximate the RR that would have been derived from a cohort study [30,49]. The calculations to support this are in Figure 1-2.

An outbreak of *Serratia marcescens* BSI traced to an infused narcotic by using a case-control study illustrates the interpretation of OR [51]. To identify risk factors for the BSIs, patients with *S. marcescens* BSIs were compared to randomly selected controls. Patients with *S. marcescens* BSIs were more likely to have received fentanyl in the surgical ICU (odds ratio, 31; $p < 0.001$) and were more likely to have been exposed to two particular respiratory therapists (odds ratios, 13.1 and 5.1; $p < 0.001$ for both comparisons). One respiratory therapist had been reported for tampering with fentanyl, and his hair sample tested

positive for it. Cultures of fentanyl infusions from two case-patients yielded *S. marcescens* and *E. cloacae*. The isolates from the case-patients and from the fentanyl infusions had similar patterns on pulsed-field gel electrophoresis. After removal of the implicated respiratory therapist, no further cases occurred. To translate some of the ORs into understandable statements, for the odds ratio of 31, 13.1, and 5.1 above, cases (patients with Serratia BSI) were 31 times more likely than controls to have received fentanyl in the surgical ICU, cases were 13.1 times more likely than controls to have been exposed to/received care from respiratory therapist X, and 5.1 times more likely to have been exposed to/received care from respiratory therapist Y.

Strength of Association and Confidence Intervals

Analysis should begin with simple univariate frequencies followed by two-by-two tables for binary outcomes with bivariate analysis (Fisher's exact or chi-square tests) or appropriate tests for continuous variables (parametric *t* tests or nonparametric tests); (Figure 1-2) [43]. A software package, Epi-Info, is available from the CDC at no cost. This software package is very useful for acquiring, organizing, and interpreting epidemiologic data from questionnaire to final analysis (**http://www.cdc.gov/epiinfo/**).

It is not the intent of this chapter to discuss the background or derivation of these tests for significance. However, interpreting the results for everyday use in healthcare epidemiology is helpful. The idea of these tests is to assess whether a difference seen between groups compared in the studies is real or could be based on chance alone and to assign a probability that the difference is real. By convention, a *p* value of <0.05 is usually considered statistically significant [29,30]. This suggests that there is a ≤5% chance that the difference between the groups is due to chance alone. The 0.05 is the convention but somewhat arbitrary, and there may be cases where a less stringent cut off of 0.1 is used. The *p* value can be affected by sample size; with a large enough sample, even small differences may be statistically significant but may not have clinical relevance (a problem in large database analysis, that is, pooled data such as a nationwide database). On the other hand, a larger difference may not reach statistical significance if the sample size is small (a problem in some HAI outbreaks if small numbers of cases are seen).

In the Serratia outbreak linked to fentanyl contamination described earlier [51], patients with *S. marcescens* BSI were more likely to have received fentanyl in the surgical ICU (odds ratio, 31; $p < 0.001$). The *p* value was actually much smaller <0.000001, thus, there was a less than 1 in 1,000,000 chance that the results seen (that cases were more likely to have received fentanyl in the surgical ICU than controls) is by chance alone.

Due to the limitations of the *p* value, a 95% confidence interval for the measures of association (ORS and RRs, depending on the study performed) provides a range within which the true magnitude of the association lies with a certain degree of assurance. If the range includes 1.0, the p value often is nonsignificant or close to 0.05. Sample size also affected these confidence intervals. Especially since HAI outbreaks may be small, studies often suffer from wide confidence intervals [30]. For example, in the study described earlier, pyrogenic reactions were more likely among patients receiving single daily dosing than there receiving multiple daily dosing gentamicin (20/73 [27%] versus 2/79 [3%]; $RR = 10.8, p < 0.01$ with a 95% confidence interval of 2.6 to 44.7) [50]. Thus, those receiving single daily dosing had a risk to develop a pyrogenic reaction that was higher than the risk of those who received multiple daily dosing of gentamicin, but it is not clear whether it was 2.6 times higher, 44.7 times higher, or somewhere in between.

Bias and Confounding

Bias is defined as any systematic error in an epidemiologic study that results in an incorrect estimate of the association between exposure and risk of disease [52]. Evaluating the role of bias as an alternative explanation for an observed association is necessary in interpreting any study result. Unlike chance and confounding, which can be evaluated quantitatively, the effects of bias are far more difficult to evaluate and may even be impossible to consider in the analysis. There are two general classes of bias. Selection bias refers to any error that arises in the process of identifying the study populations (discussed in the case-control section regarding appropriate controls). The second general category, observation or information bias, includes any systemic error in the measurement of information on exposure or outcome (discussed in the case-control section regarding how long to collect exposure information for cases and controls). The prevention and control of potential biases must be accomplished through careful study design and meticulous conduct of the study. Once a potential source of bias is introduced, it usually is extremely difficult to correct for its effects analytically. However, it is necessary to estimate both the direction and magnitude that the bias would have on the effect, and investigators should discuss all of these issues fully in published reports to provide readers the maximum opportunity to judge for themselves whether the bias accounts for the observed findings.

Confounding can be thought of as a mix of the effect of the exposure under study on the disease with that of a third factor [53]. This third factor must be associated with the exposure and be independent of that exposure, that is, be a risk factor for the disease. Confounding can lead to an overestimate or underestimate of the true association between exposure and disease and can even change the direction of the observed effect. A number of methods are available to control confounding in the design or analysis of any study. These include restriction, matching, or randomization (in clinical trials) in the design and stratification and multivariate techniques in the analysis. No single method can be considered optimal in every situation. Each has strengths and limitations, which must be carefully considered at the beginning of the study. In most situations, a combination of strategies will provide better insight into the nature of the data and more efficiently control for confounding than a single approach [53]. Common examples of confounders in HAIs are length of stay and severity of illness.

EXPERIMENTAL EPIDEMIOLOGY

Randomized Control Trials

The third method of epidemiologic investigation is the experimental method, which is a definitive method of proving or disproving a hypothesis. The experimental method assumes that risk or protective factors are followed by effects on outcomes and that a deliberate manipulation of these factors is predictably followed by an alteration in the outcomes that could rarely be explained by chance. The two groups selected for study are ideally similar in all respects except for the presence of the study factor in one group. Either the case-control or the cohort method is used to evaluate the interaction between the cause and the effect.

An example of the experimental method is the evaluation of a new drug as treatment for a disease: A group of patients with the disease is randomly divided into two subgroups that are equal in all respects except that one of the subgroups is treated with the experimental drug and the other subgroup (the control group) is given a placebo or another agent known to be effective in treating or preventing the disease. If there is no other variation between the two groups, any differences in the course of the disease may be ascribed to the use of the drug.

The experimental method has less direct use in the investigation of HAI outbreaks today than the other analytic methods such as case-control or cohort studies. The experimental method, however, is useful in assessing general patient care practices and in evaluating new methods to control and prevent disease. Placebo-controlled trials have less use in therapeutic studies because of the needs for informed consent and for preventing the placement of the patient at an unjustified or greater risk in attempting to conduct a specific study.

Thus, while the healthcare epidemiologist may not perform these studies, it is important to have a working knowledge of these types of studies as a comparison to the descriptive and analytic methods described previously so that the strengths and weaknesses of these other designs can be acknowledged (since experimental trials such as random control trials provide the best support for causality). In addition, healthcare epidemiologists play multiple roles at facilities and may be asked to aid in the assessment of new products for which experimental trials may have been performed and should be able to read the literature and interpret studies for others at the facility.

Quasi-Experimental Studies (Pre- and Postinterventions)

Quasi experimental studies, however, are used in infection control, particularly when a nonrandomized intervention is put into place, assessments of a baseline are taken before the intervention, and similar data are collected before and after the intervention [30,54]. The advantages of these methods include allowance for study of an intervention when a randomized control trial is not feasible for a number of reasons including ethics (in an outbreak setting, the first priority is to protect patients and control the outbreak, withholding treatment/control measures) may be unethical, logistics (it may be impossible to randomize changes to different patients/units), cost, and acceptability.

One disadvantage of quasi experimental studies is that it may be difficult to control for potential confounding variables that may have changed over the same/similar time as the intervention that could account for the change in outcome in part or in full rather than the intervention. Another disadvantage may be a natural change/range in outcomes that may have happened even without the intervention; thus, it may be difficult to attribute the change to the intervention.

An example of this type of study is described in relationship to preventing transmission of the multidrug-resistant *Mycobacteria tuberculosis* to patients and HCWs [55]. It was a retrospective cohort study measuring the proportion of case-patients with nosocomial acquired *M. tuberculosis* and the rate of tuberculin skin test conversion among HCWs before and after implantation of control measures (from the 1990 CDC guidelines: prompt isolation and treatment of patients, rapid diagnostic techniques, negative pressure isolation, and molded surgical masks for HCWs). The study found that the proportion of patients with multidrug resistant strains of *M. tuberculosis* decreased after the intervention (10/70 [14%] compared to 30/95 [32%] patients before the intervention; RR = 0.5, 95% CI, 0.2 to 0.9).

CHAIN OF INFECTION

General Aspects

Infection results from the interaction between an infectious agent and a susceptible host. This interaction—called transmission—occurs by means of contact between the agent and the host. Three interrelated factors—the agent, transmission, and host—represent the chain of infection.

The links interrelate with and are affected by the environment; this relation is referred to as the ecology of infection, that is, the relation of microorganisms to disease as affected by the factors of their environment. In attempting to control and/or prevent HAIs, an attack on the chain of infection at its weakest link is generally the most effective procedure. With definition of the links in the chain for each HAI, future trends of the disease should be predictable, and it should be possible to develop effective control and prevention techniques. Defining the chain of infection leads to specific action in contrast to the incorporation of nonspecific actions in an attempt to control a HAI problem.

Disease causation is multifactorial; that is, disease results from the interaction of many factors related to the agent, transmission, and host. The development of disease reflects the interaction of these factors as they affect a person. Thus, some people exposed to an infectious agent develop disease and others do not.

Agent

Agent characteristics

The first link in the chain of infection is the microbial agent, which may be a bacterium, virus, fungus, or parasite. The majority of HAIs is caused by bacteria and viruses; fungi are assuming a greater role and parasites a rare cause. A number of factors help to characterize the agent, including infectiousness, pathogenicity (including virulence and invasiveness), dose, specificity, infectivity, and other agent factors (including antimicrobial resistance) [1,10].

The determination of the number of the susceptible individuals who become infected with an organism to which they are exposed is a measure of the infectiousness of that organism. Host factors can influence the infectiousness of an organism.

The measure of the ability of microorganisms to induce disease is referred to as pathogenicity, and it may be assessed by disease-colonization ratios. An organism with low pathogenicity is alpha-hemolytic streptococcus; it commonly colonizes humans but only rarely causes clinical disease. The pathogenicity of an organism is additionally described by characterizing the organism's virulence and invasiveness.

Virulence is the measure of the severity of the disease. In epidemiologic studies, virulence is defined more specifically by assessing morbidity and mortality rates and the degree of communicability. The virulence of organisms ranges from slightly to highly virulent. Although some organisms are described as avirulent, it appears that any organism can cause disease under certain circumstances. Some naturally occurring organisms have been considered avirulent or of low virulence; however, under certain conditions, such as high doses, host immunodeficiency, or both, disease has resulted from contact with these organisms. For years, *Serratia marcescens*, for example, was considered to be an avirulent organism; because of this and the easily recognizable red pigment produced by certain strains, these organisms were used for environmental studies in hospitals. However, as hospitalized patients became more susceptible to developing infections due to advancing age, comorbid conditions, immunosuppression, and the effects of new diagnostic and therapeutic measures, HAIs due to *S. marcescens* organisms subsequently became recognized and reported. Invasiveness describes the ability of microorganisms to invade tissues. Some organisms can penetrate the intact integument whereas other microorganisms can enter only through a break in the skin or mucous membranes.

Another important agent factor is dose, that is, the number of organisms available to cause infection. The infective dose of an agent is that quantity of it necessary to cause infection. The number of organisms necessary to cause infection varies from organism to organism and from host to host and is influenced by the mode of transmission.

Microorganisms may be specific with respect to their range of hosts. *Brucella abortus* is highly communicable in cattle but not in humans. Some Salmonella spp. are common to both animals and humans, but others have a narrow range of specificity; for example, *S. typhosa* is known to infect only humans.

Infectivity refers to the ability of an organism to spread from a source to a host [1,10]. An infected human may be infective during the incubation period (e.g., hepatitis A), the clinical disease state (e.g., Influenza A), convalescence (e.g., salmonellosis, shigellosis), or some combination of the three. Additionally, an asymptomatic carrier (or colonized person) who does not show evidence of clinical disease may be infective. In some diseases, such as typhoid fever or hepatitis B, a chronic carrier state may develop in which the individual may be infective for a long time, possibly years, while showing no symptoms of illness. However, the microorganisms that most commonly cause HAIs, such as *E. coli*, Klebsiella, Enterobacter, and Pseudomonas spp., do not demonstrate the same patterns of infectivity or evoke the protective immune responses that typhoid fever or hepatitis B does.

Asymptomatic or subclinical carriers may be the more important source of infection than the clinically infected individual. The staphylococcus carrier provides a classic example of the asymptomatic dissemination of infectious organisms; in this instance, the site of dissemination may be the anterior nares or, at times, the skin. Similarly, the site of asymptomatic streptococcal carriage may be in the pharynx, perianal area, or vagina.

The source of an infection may be an atypical case of a specific disease whose clinical course has been modified by therapy, vaccine (as in measles), or prophylaxis (such as the use of immune serum globulin in hepatitis A). Animals also may provide a source of infection, although this is of less concern in the healthcare settings.

Additional characteristics of the agent that may affect their ability to produce disease are the production of virulence factors/enzymes, antigenic shift and drift (such

as seen by Influenza A), and development/acquisition of antimicrobial resistance (via plasmid or gene mutation).

The increase in antimicrobial resistance has had a dramatic affect on HAIs. Changes in antimicrobial sensitivity may make therapy difficult; it can result in an increasing prevalence of the resistant strain, reduce the necessary infecting or colonizing doses of the organism in those receiving drugs to which these strains are resistant, increase the numbers of organisms disseminated from persons colonized with these strains, and potentially increase the frequency of HAIs due to this more resistant strain [1].

Reservoir, Source, and Portal of Exit

All organisms have a reservoir and a source; these may be the same or different, and it is important to distinguish between these potentially different sites if control and/or prevention measures are to be directed at this aspect of the chain of infection. The reservoir is the place where the organism maintains its presence, metabolizes, and replicates. Viruses generally survive better in human reservoirs; the reservoir of gram-positive bacteria is usually a human, whereas gram-negative bacteria may have either a human or an animal reservoir (e.g., Salmonella) or an inanimate reservoir (e.g., Pseudomonas in water).

The source is the place from which the infectious agent passes to the host, either by direct or indirect contact, droplet, airborne, common vehicle, or a vector as the means of transmission. Sources also may be animate or inanimate. The source may become contaminated from the reservoir. For example, a reservoir for Pseudomonas spp. may be the tap water in a hospital; however, the source from which it is transmitted to the patient may be a humidifier that has been filled with contaminated tap water.

The portal of exit for organisms from humans usually is single, although it may be multiple. In general, the major portals of exit are the respiratory and gastrointestinal tracts and the skin and wounds. Blood also may be the portal of exit, as in hepatitis B or human immunodeficiency virus (HIV) infections. However, depending on the organism, any bodily secretion or excretion can be infectious.

Transmission

Transmission, the second link in the chain of infection, describes the movement of organisms from the source to the host. Spread may occur through one or more of five different routes: contact (either direct or indirect), droplet, airborne, common vehicle, and vectorborne (described later based on CDC Guidelines for isolation precautions in hospitals) [56]. An organism may have a single route of transmission, or it may be transmissible by two or more routes. *M. tuberculosis*, for example, is almost always transmitted by the airborne route; measles is primarily a contact-spread disease but may also be transmitted through the air; salmonellae may be transmitted by contact or by the common-vehicle, airborne, or vector-borne routes. Thus, in defining the route of transmission, although one route may be the obvious one involved in an HAI problem, another route also may be operative. Knowledge regarding the route of transmission for a specific pathogen can be very helpful in the investigation of an HAI problem. Such information can point to the source and may allow control measures to be introduced more rapidly.

Contact Transmission

Contact transmission is the most important and frequent mode of transmission of HAI pathogens. Contact transmission can be divided into two subgroups, direct-contact transmission and indirect-contact transmission [56]. Direct-contact transmission involves a direct body surface-to-body surface contact and physical transfer of microorganisms between a susceptible host and an infected or colonized person as occurs when a person turns a patient, bathes a patient, or performs other patient-care activities that require direct personal contact. Direct-contact transmission also can occur between two patients with one serving as the source of the infectious microorganisms and the other as a susceptible host.

Indirect-contact transmission involves contact of a susceptible host with a contaminated intermediate object, usually inanimate, such as contaminated instruments, needles, or dressings, or contaminated hands that are not washed and gloves that are not changed between patients. The intermediate object may become contaminated from an animate or inanimate source. An example is the transfer to susceptible hosts of enteric organisms on an endoscope that initially became contaminated when brought in contact with an infected patient (the index patient). Examples of organisms that can be transmitted via contact are VRE and MRSA.

Droplet Transmission

Droplet transmission, theoretically, is a form of contact transmission. However, the mechanism of transfer of the pathogen to the host is quite distinct from either direct- or indirect-contact transmission. Thus, in the 1996 Guidelines for Isolation Precautions in Hospitals, droplet transmission was considered a separate route of transmission [56]. Droplets are generated from the source person primarily during coughing, sneezing, talking, and performing certain procedures such as suctioning and bronchoscopy. Transmission occurs when droplets (large-particle droplets, >5 µm in size) containing microorganisms generated from the infected person are propelled a short distance through the air and deposited on the host's conjunctivae, nasal mucosa, or mouth. Transmission via large-particle droplets requires close contact between source and recipient persons, because droplets do not remain suspended in the air and generally travel only short distances, usually 3 feet or less, through the air. Because droplets do not remain suspended in the air, special air handling and ventilation are not required to prevent droplet transmission (as opposed to airborne transmission). Examples of pathogens transmitted by the droplet route are *Bordetella pertussis* and *Neisseria meningitides*.

Airborne Transmission

Airborne transmission occurs by dissemination of either airborne droplet nuclei (small-particle residue [≤5 µm in size] of evaporated droplets containing microorganisms that remain suspended in the air for long periods of time—hours or possibly days) or dust particles containing the infectious agent. Microorganisms carried in this manner can be dispersed widely by air currents and may be inhaled by a susceptible host within the same room or over a longer distance from the source-patient, depending on environmental factors; therefore, special air handling and ventilation are required to prevent airborne transmission. Microorganisms transmitted by airborne transmission include *M. tuberculosis*, rubeola, and varicella viruses (including disseminated zoster) [56]. In the last several years, there has been controversy as to whether other emerging pathogens/diseases (SARS, smallpox) might be transmitted via airborne route (which would have implications for isolation and personal protective equipment) [57–59]. The airborne route of transmission is more frequently assumed to be the route of an infection than is the case [1]. Creation of an infectious aerosol is more difficult than is usually recognized.

Common-Vehicle Transmission

In common-vehicle-spread infection, a contaminated inanimate vehicle, such as food, water, medications, devices, and equipment, serves as a vector for transmission of the agent to multiple persons [56]. The susceptible host becomes infected after contact with the common vehicle. This transmission may be active if the organisms replicate while in the vehicle, such as salmonellae in food, or passive if the organisms are passively carried by the vehicle, such as hepatitis A in food. Other types of common vehicles include blood and blood products (hepatitis B and HIV), intravenous fluids (gram-negative septicemia), and medications (gram-negative septicemia, fungal infections) in which units or batches of a product become contaminated from a common source and serve as a common vehicle for multiple infections.

Vector-Borne Spread

vector-borne transmission occurs when vectors such as mosquitoes, flies, rats, and other vermin transmit microorganisms [56]; this route of transmission is of less significance in U.S. hospitals than in other regions of the world.

Host

The third link in the chain of infection is the host. Disease does not always follow the transmission of infectious agents to a host. As previously discussed, various agent factors play a part; similarly, a variety of host factors must also be surmounted before infection occurs and disease develops. Host factors that influence the development of infections are the site of deposition of the agent and the host's defense mechanisms, referred to as immunity, either specific or nonspecific.

Portal of Entrance

Sites of deposition include the skin, mucous membranes, and respiratory, gastrointestinal, and urinary tracts. *Staphylococci spp.* need a minute breach in the integrity of the skin to gain entrance to the body. Mechanical transmission may occur through the normal skin, as with hepatitis B or HIV viruses on a contaminated needle or in contaminated blood. Abnormal skin, such as a preexisting wound, may be the site of deposition of organisms such as *Pseudomonas aeruginosa.* Mucous membranes may be the site of entrance, as the conjunctiva is for adenovirus.

Another site of deposition is the respiratory tract. The exact area of deposition depends on the size of the airborne particle and the aerodynamics at the time of transmission. Generally, particles $\geq 5/lm$ in diameter will be deposited in the upper respiratory tract, whereas those $<5/lm$ in diameter will be deposited in the lower respiratory tract.

Infectious agents may gain entrance to the body through the intestinal tract by means of ingestion of contaminated foods or liquids, contaminated supplemental feedings, and contaminated medications or through contaminated equipment, such as endoscopes inserted into the intestinal tract. The urinary tract may become infected from contaminated foreign objects such as catheters or cystoscopes inserted into the urethra or by the retrograde movement of organisms on the external surface of a catheter inserted into the bladder.

Organisms may gain entrance into the host via the placenta, as occurs in rubella and toxoplasmosis. Transplantation is another method by which microorganisms enter the host; infection may follow renal transplantation if the donated kidney is infected with cytomegalovirus.

An organism may colonize one site and cause no disease, but the same organism at another site may result in clinical disease. *E. coli,* for example, routinely colonizes the gastrointestinal tract and under normal circumstances does not cause disease; however, the same organism in the urinary tract may cause infection. *S. aureus* may colonize the external nares without any evidence of disease, but when the same organism colonizes a fresh surgical wound, an SSI may develop.

Nonspecific and Specific Defense Mechanisms

Humans have extensive nonspecific and specific defense mechanisms to protect against infection [1]. Nonspecific defense mechanisms include the skin, mucous membranes, and certain bodily secretions (tears, mucus, enzymes). The local inflammatory response provides another nonspecific host defense mechanism. Other nonspecific protective mechanisms include genetic, hormonal, nutritional, behavioral, and personal hygiene factors. Age, as influenced by these nonspecific factors, is associated with decreased resistance at either end of the spectrum; the very young and the very old frequently are more susceptible to infection. Surgery and the presence of chronic diseases, such as diabetes, blood disorders, certain lymphomas, and collagen diseases, alter host resistance.

Specific immunity results from either natural or artificially induced (i.e., vaccines, immunoglobulin) events. Over the last several decades, medical therapies for conditions such as cancers, solid organ/bone marrow transplantation, and HIV have increased the population of hosts with significant immunosuppression. These hosts have added to the challenges of HAIs.

Host Response

The spectrum of the host's response to a microorganism may range from a subclinical (or inapparent) infection to a clinically apparent illness, the extreme being death. The host may become a carrier of the organism. The clinical spectrum of disease varies from mild to a typical course (although a disease may typically be mild) to severe disease and possible death. The degree of host response is determined by both agent and host factors and includes the dose of the infecting organism, its organ specificity, the pathogenicity of the infecting organism, its virulence and invasiveness, and its portal of entry. Host factors include the quantitative and qualitative level of the specific and nonspecific immunologic factors previously discussed.

The same organism infecting different hosts can result in a clinical spectrum of disease that is the same, similar, or different in various individuals. For example, many cases of what appears to be the outbreak disease may meet the clinical case definition, whereas other cases that epidemiologically are related to the same epidemic may not meet the same case definition. They may, in fact, be cases of the outbreak disease but with a different clinical spectrum (as can occasionally be demonstrated by serologic tests). They also may be cases of other diseases occurring concurrently with the outbreak.

Environment

Patients at healthcare facilities often are confined to a hospital bed and surrounded by multiple medical devices, equipment, and environmental surfaces. Thus, there is concern that the facility environment may play a role in the chain of infection. At times, too much emphasis is placed on the role of the environment; for example, it is inappropriate to take environmental cultures routinely throughout a hospital. However, in investigating HAIs, it may be appropriate to obtain environmental cultures as suggested by the circumstances of the specific problem under investigation [1,16,60]. A compromise and a healthy respect for the environment are needed with maintenance that does not deliberately promote the transmission of disease-causing agents to hosts but without excessive control measures that impose unnecessary and ineffective actions on the hospital staff and a consequent loss of efficiency and effectiveness, and a wasting of resources such as personnel time and money [1,16].

Some environmental factors can influence all of the links in the chain of infection, whereas others are more limited in their range of action. Humidity, for example, can influence a multiplicity of factors; it can affect the persistence of an agent at its source, its transmission through the air, and the effectiveness of a host's mucous membranes in resisting infection.

Replication of the agent at its reservoir may depend on certain substances in the environment. The agent's survival is influenced by the temperature, humidity, pH, and radiation at its reservoir or source.

The transmission of agents will be affected by environmental factors such as temperature and humidity as mentioned earlier. Airborne transmission is influenced by air velocity and the direction of its movement. The stability and concentration of an aerosol are directly related to environmental factors. In winter, people tend to be indoors with closed windows and reduced air circulation, and this increases the risk of airborne disease; in summer, room air is air conditioned or diluted with outside air. In outbreaks associated with common vehicle transmission, the temperature of the environment will influence the level of contamination in the vehicle.

The host's resistance mechanisms are affected by environmental factors; for example, in an excessively dry atmosphere, mucous membranes become dry and are less able to protect against microbial invasion. Also, the host's behavioral patterns are influenced by temperature.

Ultimately, the reason to discuss the links in the chain of infection and their modulators, for example, the environment, in such detail is that once these factors have been examined, the most appropriate methods of control and prevention can be determined.

CONCLUSIONS

The intent of this chapter was to review some of the basic epidemiological concepts and methods with an emphasis on HAIs. Many of the concepts are expanded upon in later chapters. However, the reader may wish to seek additional resources and references on specific general epidemiology concepts.

REFERENCES

1. Brachman PS. Epidemiology of Nosocomial Infections. In: Bennett JV, Brachman PS, eds. *Hospital infections*. Philadelphia: Lippincott-Raven, 1998:3–16.
2. Schoenbach VJ, Rosamond WD. *Understanding the fundamentals of epidemiology: an evolving text*. Chapel Hill, NC: Department of Epidemiology, School of Public Health, University of North Carolina at Chapel Hill, 2000.
3. Harvard School of Public Health, Department of Epidemiology. http://www.hsph.harvard.edu/epidemiology/index.html. 2006.
4. Centers for Disease Control; healthcare-associated infections. http://www.cdc.gov/ncidod/dhqp/healthDis.html. 2006.
5. Weinstein RA. Nosocomial infection update. *Emerg Infect Dis* 1998; 4:416–420.
6. Burke JP. Infection control—a problem for patient safety. *N Engl J Med* 2003; 348:651–656.
7. Kohn LT, Corrigan JM, Donaldson MS. To err is human: building a safer health system. A report to Institute of Medicine, Committee on Quality of Health Care in America 2000. 2006.
8. McKibben L, Horan T, Tokars JI, et al. Guidance on public reporting of healthcare-associated infections: recommendations of the Healthcare Infection Control Practices Advisory Committee. *Am J Infect Control* 2005; 33:217–226.
9. Wong ES, Rupp ME, Mermel L, et al. Public disclosure of healthcare-associated infections: the role of the Society for Healthcare Epidemiology of America. *Infect Control Hosp Epidemiol* 2005; 26:210–212.
10. Relman DA, Falkow S. Microbial virulence factors. In: Mandell GL, Douglas RG, Bennett JE, Dolin R, eds. *Mandell, Douglas, and Bennett's principles and practice of infectious diseases*. Philadelphia: Churchill Livingstone, 2000:2.
11. Jarvis WR. The epidemiology of colonization. *Infect Control Hosp Epidemiol* 1996; 17:47–52.
12. Jarvis WR, Ostrowsky B. Dinosaurs, methicillin-resistant Staphylococcus aureus, and infection control personnel: survival through translating science into prevention. *Infect Control Hosp Epidemiol* 2003; 24:392–396.
13. Muto CA, Jernigan JA, Ostrowsky BE, et al. SHEA guideline for preventing nosocomial transmission of multidrug-resistant strains of *Staphylococcus aureus* and enterococcus. *Infect Control Hosp Epidemiol* 2003; 24:362–386.
14. Ostrowsky B, Steinberg JT, Farr B, et al. Reality check: should we try to detect and isolate vancomycin-resistant enterococci patients? *Infect Control Hosp Epidemiol* 2001; 22:116–119.
15. Sherertz RJ, Bassetti S, Bassetti-Wyss B. "Cloud" health-care workers. *Emerg Infect Dis* 2001; 7:241–244.
16. Beck-Sague C, Jarvis WR, Martone WJ. Outbreak investigations. *Infect Control Hosp Epidemiol* 1997; 18(2):138–145.
17. Kluytmans J, van Belkum A, Verbrugh H. Nasal carriage of *Staphylococcus aureus*: epidemiology, underlying mechanisms, and associated risks. *Clin Microbiol Rev* 1997; 10:505–520.
18. Emori TG, Culver DH, Horan TC, et al. National nosocomial infections surveillance system (NNIS): description of surveillance methods. *Am J Infect Control* 1991; 19:19–35.
19. Horan TC, Gaynes RP. Surveillance of nosocomial infections. In: Mayhall CG, ed. *Hospital epidemiology and infection control*. Philadelphia: Lippincott Williams & Wilkins, 2004: 1659–1702.
20. Mangram AJ, Horan TC, Pearson ML, et al. Guideline for prevention of surgical site infection, 1999. Hospital Infection Control Practices Advisory Committee. *Infect Control Hosp Epidemiol* 1999; 20:250–278.
21. Jarvis WR. Nosocomial outbreaks: the Centers for Disease Control's Hospital Infections Program experience, 1980–1990. Epidemiology Branch, Hospital Infections Program. *Am J Med* 1991; 91(3B):101S–106S.
22. Jarvis WR. Hospital Infections Program, Centers for Disease Control and Prevention On-site Outbreak Investigations, 1990 to 1999. *Seminars in infection control*. 2001:73–84.
23. Naimi TS, LeDell KH, Boxrud DJ, et al. Epidemiology and clonality of community-acquired methicillin-resistant *Staphylococcus aureus* in Minnesota, 1996–1998. *Clin Infect Dis* 2001; 33:990–996.
24. Naimi TS, LeDell KH, Como-Sabetti K, et al. Comparison of community- and health care-associated methicillin-resistant *Staphylococcus aureus* infection. *JAMA* 2003; 290:2976–2984.
25. Tafuro P, Ristuccia P. Recognition and control of outbreaks of nosocomial infections in the intensive care setting. *Heart Lung* 1984; 13:486–495.

26. Gregg MB, Dicker RC, Goodman RA. *Field epidemiology*. New York: Oxford University Press, 1996.
27. Centers for Disease Control. Training resources modular learning components (mini-modules) constructing an epidemic curve. http://www.cdc.gov/descd/MiniModules/Epidemic_Curve/page09.htm. 2006.
28. Rothman KS, Greenland S. Measures of disease frequency. In: Rothman KJ, Greenland S, eds. *Modern epidemiology*. Philadelphia: Lippincott-Raven, 1998:29–46.
29. Freeman J. Quantitative epidemiology. In: Herwaldt LA, Decker MD, eds. *The Society for Healthcare Epidemiology of America—A practical handbook for hospital epidemiologists*. Thorofare, NJ: Slack, 1998:205–213.
30. Ebbing L. Epidemiologic methods in infection control. In: Lautenbach E, Woeltje KF, Society for Healthcare Epidemiology of America, ed. *Practical handbook for healthcare epidemiologists*. Thorofare, NJ: Slack, 2004.
31. Brawley RL, Weber DJ, Samsa GP, Rutala WA. Multiple nosocomial infections: an incidence study. *Am J Epidemiol* 1989; 130: 769–780.
32. Edwards JE. Candida species. In: Mandell GL, Douglas RG, Bennett JE, Dolin R, eds. *Mandell, Douglas, and Bennett's principles and practice of infectious diseases*. Philadelphia: Churchill Livingstone, 2000:2656–2674.
33. McDonald LC, Banerjee SN, Jarvis WR. Seasonal variation of Acinetobacter infections: 1987–1996: nosocomial infections surveillance system. *Clin Infect Dis* 1999; 29:1133–1137.
34. Gross PA. Basics of stratifying for severity of illness. *Infect Control Hosp Epidemiol* 1996; 17:675–686.
35. Knaus WA, Wagner DP, Draper EA, et al. The APACHE III prognostic system: risk prediction of hospital mortality for critically ill hospitalized adults. *Chest* 1991; 100:1619–1636.
36. Furnival RA, Schunk JE. ABCs of scoring systems for pediatric trauma *Pediatr Emerg Care* 1999; 15:215–223.
37. Richardson DK, Corcoran JD, Escobar GJ, Lee SK. SNAP-II and SNAPPE-II: simplified newborn illness severity and mortality risk scores. *J Pediatr* 2001; 138:92–100.
38. Harris AD, Samore MH, Lipsitch M, et al. Control-group selection importance in studies of antimicrobial resistance: examples applied to Pseudomonas aeruginosa, Enterococci, and *Escherichia coli*. *Clin Infect Dis* 2002; 34:1558–1563.
39. Ostrowsky BE, Trick WE, Sohn AH, et al. Control of vancomycin-resistant enterococcus in health care facilities in a region. *N Engl J Med* 2001; 344:1427–1433.
40. Ostrowsky B, Jarvis WR. Efficient management of outbreak investigations. In: Wenzel RP, ed. *Prevention and control of nosocomial infections*. Philadelphia: Lippincott Williams & Wilkins, 2003:500–523.
41. Wenzel RP, Thompson RL, Landry SM, et al. Hospital-acquired infections in intensive care unit patients: an overview with emphasis on epidemics. *Infect Control* 1983; 4:371–4375.
42. Gordis L. Case-control and cross-sectional studies. In: Gordis L, ed. *Epidemiology*. Philadelphia. W.B. Saunders, 2000:140–157.
43. Freeman J. Modern quantitative epidemiology in the hospital. In: Mayhall CG, ed. *Hospital epidemiology and infection control*. Baltimore: Williams & Wilkins, 1996:11–40.
44. Gordis L. More on risk: estimating the potential for prevention. In: Gordis L, ed. *Epidemiology*. Philadelphia: W.B. Saunders, 2000:172–179.
45. Leviton A. Letter: definitions of attributable risk. *Am J Epidemiol* 1973; 98:231.
46. Gordis L. Randomized trials: some further issues. In: Gordis L, ed. *Epidemiology*. Philadelphia: W.B. Saunders, 2000:110–128.
47. Gordis L. A pause for review: comparing cohort and case-control studies. In: Gordis L, ed. *Epidemiology*. Philadelphia: W.B. Saunders, 2000:180–183.
48. Fridkin SK, Lawton R, Edwards JR, et al. Monitoring antimicrobial use and resistance: comparison with a national benchmark on reducing vancomycin use and vancomycin-resistant enterococci. *Emerg Infect Dis* 2002; 8:702–707.
49. Greenland S, Rothman KS. Measures of effect and measures of association. In: Rothman KJ, Greenland S, eds. *Modern epidemiology*. Philadelphia: Lippincott-Raven, 1998:47–64.
50. Buchholz U, Richards C, Murthy R, et al. Pyrogenic reactions associated with single daily dosing of intravenous gentamicin. *Infect Control Hosp Epidemiol* 2000; 21:771–774.
51. Ostrowsky BE, Whitener C, Bredenberg HK, et al. *Serratia marcescens* bacteremia traced to an infused narcotic. *N Engl J Med* 2002; 346:1529–1537.
52. Hennekens CH, Buring JE. Analysis of epidemiological studies: evaluating the role of bias. In: Hennekens CH, Buring JE, Mayrent SL, eds. *Epidemiology in medicine*. Boston: Little, Brown, 1987:272–286.
53. Hennekens CH, Buring JE. Analysis of epidemiological studies: evaluating the role of confounding. In: Hennekens CH, Buring JE, Mayrent SL, eds. *Epidemiology in medicine*. Boston: Little, Brown, 1987:287–323.
54. Rothman KS, Greenland S. Types of epidemiological studies. In: Rothman KJ, Greenland S, eds. *Modern epidemiology*. Philadelphia: Lippincott Raven, 1998:67–68.
55. Maloney SA, Pearson ML, Gordon MT, et al. Efficacy of control measures in preventing nosocomial transmission of multidrug-resistant tuberculosis to patients and health care workers. *Ann Intern Med* 1995; 122:90–95.
56. Garner JS. Guideline for isolation precautions in hospitals. The Hospital Infection Control Practices Advisory Committee. *Infect Control Hosp Epidemiol* 1996; 17:53–80.
57. Varia M, Wilson S, Sarwal S, et al. Investigation of a nosocomial outbreak of severe acute respiratory syndrome (SARS) in Toronto, Canada. *CMAJ* 2003; 169:285–292.
58. Shaw K. The 2003 SARS outbreak and its impact on infection control practices. *Public Health* 2006; 120:8–14.
59. Henderson DA, Inglesby TV, Bartlett JG, et al. Smallpox as a biological weapon: medical and public health management. Working Group on Civilian Biodefense. *JAMA* 1999; 281:2127–2137.
60. Jarvis WR. Usefulness of molecular epidemiology for outbreak investigations. *Infect Control Hosp Epidemiol* 1994; 15:500–503.

The Healthcare Epidemiologist

Virginia R. Roth and Bryan P. Simmons

DEFINITION

A healthcare epidemiologist investigates the rates and determinants of adverse outcomes in the healthcare environment with a primary focus on healthcare-acquired infections (HAIs). A healthcare epidemiologist is not solely an investigator but also implements preventative measures to improve outcomes.

HISTORY

Healthcare epidemiology has been practiced since the mid-1800s; Nightingale, Semmelweis, Lister, and Holmes all made significant contributions to the field. Modern healthcare epidemiology began in the 1950s in Great Britain when infection control systems were used to address hospital outbreaks of staphylococcal infections. In the 1960s, the American Hospital Association (AHA) formed the Committee on Infections within Hospitals, and the Communicable Disease Center (CDC, now the Centers for Disease Control and Prevention) formed the Hospital Infections Unit. These two organizations supported an organized approach to addressing HAIs in the United States, and the AHA published a manual on prevention of HAIs that was used extensively for almost two decades [1].

Because of the need to organize and promote the scientific basis of hospital infection control programs and to encourage expansion of such programs, the CDC convened the first International Conference on Nosocomial Infections in 1970 [2–4]. In 1980, a group of physicians practicing healthcare epidemiology formed the Society for Hospital Epidemiology of America (SHEA), now called the Society for Healthcare Epidemiology of America (see Chapter 11). Similar organizations were formed in other countries. The first hospital epidemiologists concentrated their efforts on preventing HAIs, and the landmark Study on the Efficacy of Nosocomial Infection Control (SENIC) project reinforced their efforts by demonstrating that a physician specially trained in infection control could reduce the HAI rate [5]. The boundaries of hospital epidemiology have now expanded beyond infection control into clinical performance, quality management, and disaster planning. Furthermore, the settings in which healthcare epidemiology is practiced have now expanded beyond hospitals into long-term care, continuing care, outpatient and ambulatory care, and community based settings.

ROLES AND RESPONSIBILITIES

Healthcare epidemiologists play a key role in the prevention and control of adverse healthcare outcomes with a particular focus on HAIs. This is accomplished through surveillance, outbreak investigation, quality management and patient safety initiatives, educational programs, research, and committee representation (Table 2-1). The healthcare epidemiologist usually works alongside one or more infection control professionals (ICPs) and may be responsible for administering the infection control program. The healthcare epidemiologist also is responsible for maintaining close communication with other programs within the healthcare environment as well as public health and governmental agencies. More recently,

| **TABLE 2-1** |
| **THE HEALTHCARE EPIDEMIOLOGIST'S ROLES** |

- Surveillance
- Outbreak investigation
- Quality management and patient safety initiatives
- Education
- Research
- Committee representation
- Administration of infection control program
- Consultation and communication
- Disaster planning

healthcare epidemiologists have been involved in contingency planning for pandemics and other disasters.

Surveillance

Surveillance is one of the single most important functions of the healthcare epidemiologist [5]. As more jurisdictions mandate public disclosure of HAI rates, healthcare epidemiologists are increasingly being called on to design and implement mandatory reporting systems and monitor their results [6] (see Chapter 15). The primary objectives of surveillance are to identify problems for correction, order priorities, and take measures to reduce adverse outcomes (see Chapter 4). The healthcare epidemiologist is responsible for setting surveillance priorities and overseeing data collection, analysis, interpretation, and reporting. When possible, surveillance methodology should be consistent with national or international surveillance systems to allow for benchmarking. Surveillance data are most useful when compared against historical rates within the same facility or against national benchmarks. It has been suggested that many HAIs are preventable [7], and several centers have shown that multifaceted system interventions can reduce central line–associated bloodstream infections and ventilator-associated pneumonia rates to almost zero [8,9]. The healthcare epidemiologist should lead multidisciplinary intervention teams to implement the system changes necessary to reduce infection rates.

Outbreak Investigation

The healthcare epidemiologist plays a key role in confirming the existence of an outbreak and overseeing data collection, data analysis, and implementation of control measures by the outbreak management team. As part of the outbreak investigation, the healthcare epidemiologist should determine what patient and environmental testing is required and assist in interpreting the results. Additional responsibilities during an outbreak include communication with administrators, physicians, the local public health department, and the media.

Quality Management and Patient Safety

Many healthcare epidemiologists have become involved in quality management and patient safety initiatives because epidemiology is as useful to these areas as it is to infection control (see Chapter 14) [10–12]. Continuous quality improvement (CQI) programs depend on data management and statistical analysis that can be provided by healthcare epidemiologists [10,13]. The healthcare epidemiologist also can expand into other areas of quality management, such as clinical practice guideline development [14]. The use of such guidelines can minimize unwanted practice variation and healthcare costs. The tools of CQI also can be applied to infection control programs to reduce the rate of endemic infections, which constitute the majority of HAIs [15,16] (see Chapter 30). Finally, the U.S. National Healthcare Safety Network (formally the National Nosocomial Infections Surveillance System, or NNIS) demonstrates the value of a national surveillance system in promoting patient safety [17].

Education Programs

Good infection control practices can reduce both patient and provider risk of HAIs [18,19]. Unfortunately, healthcare providers often fail to follow these basic practices, and compliance among physicians is generally much lower than among other providers [20–26]. Several recent studies have shown an alarming lack of infection control training and knowledge in this provider group [27–30]. The healthcare epidemiologist is in a unique position to promote and reinforce proper infection control measures among physicians and medical trainees. In academic settings, healthcare epidemiologists are often responsible for providing formal infection control training to infectious diseases residents and other physicians. Finally, the healthcare epidemiologist should support and promote the development of an infection control orientation and training program for all healthcare personnel.

Research

Healthcare epidemiologists have a well-established history of identifying and quantifying infection control measures that reduce adverse patient outcomes. The infection control literature accounts for many of the patient safety practices for which there is strong supporting evidence [31,32]. However, many research gaps have been identified [31,33,34], and healthcare epidemiologists must play a pivotal role in addressing these gaps.

Committee Representation

The healthcare epidemiologist should be an active standing member, and may serve as chair, of the infection control committee. This committee is responsible for approving infection control policies, highlighting infection control issues to the medical and senior administration of the facility, and reviewing infection control surveillance and outbreak data to develop an appropriate action plan. In addition to infection control committee membership, the healthcare epidemiologist provides valuable input to other committees including occupational health and safety, product evaluation and standardization, pharmacy and therapeutics (particularly with respect to antimicrobial selection and use), and sterilization/disinfection. Membership on these committees may be on an ad hoc basis. Finally, healthcare epidemiologists provide valuable technical and clinical expertise to national and international committees responsible for developing infection control and patient safety-related guidelines.

Administration of an Infection Control Program

In some settings, the healthcare epidemiologist is responsible for the human and financial resources of the infection control program. These responsibilities include developing and implementing the program's goals and objectives, recruiting and selecting staff, delegating responsibilities, developing and controlling the budget, and reporting to administration. Administrative responsibilities also include advocating for additional infection control resources depending on local need and ensuring an appropriate reporting mechanism to allow for timely administrative action when infection control issues are identified.

Communication

The healthcare epidemiologist must maintain close communication with all other members of the infection control team. Furthermore, healthcare epidemiology impacts nearly every area of healthcare delivery including medical, nursing, occupational health, microbiology, pharmacy, housekeeping, logistical services, risk management, and patient relations. Thus, the healthcare epidemiologist must maintain good communication with these areas. Informal communication during clinical rounds or hallway conversations is often as effective as formal consultations or meetings. Thus, the healthcare epidemiologist should be a visible and approachable member of the infection control team. Finally, the healthcare epidemiologist should ensure good external communication on infection control related issues. This includes informing the local public health department and the surrounding community of outbreaks, disaster planning efforts, and other infection control issues of general concern. Communication with the general public should be in conjunction with the public relations department.

Disaster Planning

The healthcare epidemiologist should play a lead role in emergency preparedness and response to pandemics, incidents of bioterrorism, natural disasters, and other emergencies [35–37]. The healthcare epidemiologist should be involved in developing the healthcare facility's response plan, providing information and education on protective measures for staff, stockpiling of medications and supplies, and ensuring that robust surveillance systems are in place for prompt detection of an emerging infectious disease or potential emergency events or bioterrorism attacks.

SKILLS AND SUPPORT NEEDED

The healthcare epidemiologist needs many skills to succeed (Table 2-2). The discipline of infection control has increasingly incorporated epidemiologic principles and statistical analyses that are generally not learned in clinical training. Thus, formal training in healthcare epidemiology has become important. Few countries have established standards or certified training programs for healthcare epidemiology although early efforts are underway in Europe [34,38]. In the absence of training standards, healthcare epidemiologists must have sufficient knowledge and training to be viewed locally as credible authorities on infection control and epidemiology, particularly by physicians and health administrators.

Epidemiology Skills

The healthcare epidemiologist's most valuable tool is a thorough knowledge of the science of epidemiology and its associated statistical tools. Those who treat hospital epidemiology as a hobby are unlikely to make the impact

TABLE 2-2
WHAT YOU NEED TO SUCCEED AS A HOSPITAL EPIDEMIOLOGIST

Skills
- Infection control knowledge
- Epidemiology and statistical skills
- Leadership skills
- Interpersonal skills
- Clinical skills

Support
- Partnership with infection control professionals
- Effective reporting structure
- Network of colleagues
- Computer/software support
- Administrative support
- A contract

necessary for their healthcare systems to compete in the future. Scientific skills will allow the epidemiologist to prevent infections and other complications and to seek out and eliminate costly but ineffective infection control traditions (ritual) and quality management busywork. These skills also should help in product evaluation and selection. Most new products cost more than the products that they are designed to replace, but few are worth the extra cost. Good epidemiology skills also are needed to present accurate data to the administration and the medical committees in a concise and forceful format. Such data are difficult to ignore and can drive necessary change and improvement.

Leadership Skills

The healthcare epidemiologist requires leadership skills to be effective in the complex healthcare environment. Effecting change and implementing policy, sometimes over the objections of many other physicians and hospital employees, requires an effective leader. Leadership skills are necessary to develop a vision and goals for the infection control program and to foster team building to achieve these goals. Healthcare epidemiologists who are responsible for program administration also require time management, budgeting, planning, and human resource management skills. The healthcare epidemiologist should consider leadership and management training.

Interpersonal Skills

It is essential to know how to interact with people to get things done. The healthcare epidemiologist should be friendly, visible, approachable, and known. The healthcare epidemiologist must have the confidence of the medical staff to persuade physicians to change their ways when necessary. Negotiation skills are a valuable asset because change must often be negotiated rather than mandated. The healthcare epidemiologist must also have the confidence of administration and be able to negotiate the monetary and other support necessary to implement change. It is important that administration be kept informed of the activities, successes, and needs of the infection control department.

Clinical Skills

A clinical background, while not essential, proves very useful to the healthcare epidemiologist. It allows for more seamless integration into the healthcare delivery environment and enhances credibility with physicians and other clinical leaders. It also creates opportunities to interact with, and provide immediate feedback to, other healthcare workers in the clinical setting (e.g., during "ward rounds") rather than adopting a purely administrative approach.

Infrastructure Requirements

One of the first management decisions a healthcare epidemiologist should make is to determine what support is needed to do a good job. The healthcare epidemiologist is likely to be most effective when surrounded by a team of ICPs and provided administrative support. He/She should report to both a senior administrator (e.g., vice president of medical affairs) and an influential infection control committee [39]. Developing a network of other healthcare epidemiologists through professional societies and scientific conferences is another valuable resource.

Computers and software are very important to the modern infection control program [40] (see Chapter 8). Computers allow management of surveillance data to assess trends and find solutions to problems. Computers can eliminate the need for a retrospective chart review for all but the most complex problem. In addition, computers can be programmed to prevent problems rather than just count them. The healthcare epidemiologist in partnership with the ICP needs to select the best software for the hospital's needs. Thus, the healthcare epidemiologist must be familiar with the advantages and disadvantages of various software programs.

Networks

Infection control networks are becoming an invaluable resource for healthcare facilities without access to a well-trained hospital epidemiologist, particularly at many community hospitals (see Chapter 10). Infection control networks can favorably impact HAI rates [41]. Policies, surveillance techniques, data analysis, education, outbreak investigation, and product evaluations are additional aspects of the infection control program that can be provided effectively by a network [42].

GETTING PAID

Some administrators are unwilling to pay for healthcare epidemiology services and consider them part of the duties that the medical staff provides to the hospital through committee activities [43]. However, there is a premium on preventing HAIs and other complications, because they represent a source of monetary loss for the organization (see Chapter 17) [44–46]. Haley et al. used SENIC data to devise a formula for calculating cost savings by instituting various components of a well-run infection control program [47]. In addition to the costs saved by preventing HAIs, the knowledgeable hospital epidemiologist can save the hospital money by eliminating unnecessary ritual, controlling unnecessary antibiotic use, and rejecting expensive new products that are not cost effective. In both resourced and underresourced

TABLE 2-3
FUTURE OPPORTUNITIES FOR THE HEALTHCARE EPIDEMIOLOGIST

- Control of multidrug-resistant organisms
- Disaster planning
- Public reporting
- Increased outpatient focus
- Clinical performance management and assessment
- New product/new technology assessment
- Quality service despite reduced resources

countries, these savings can be presented to administration when seeking reimbursement [48]. In many instances, improving the quality of care and reducing adverse patient outcomes is more easily demonstrated than cost savings associated with healthcare epidemiology initiatives. These initiatives also may help negate the legal liability of a healthcare facility in the face of an adverse patient outcome. Thus, quality, not cost, may be the primary incentive for administrators to retain healthcare epidemiology expertise.

THE FUTURE

There will be many opportunities for hospital epidemiologists to apply their skills in the future (Table 2-3) provided that they are willing to adapt to meet the needs created by changing healthcare delivery systems [49–51]. This may be especially true for infectious diseases physicians [52,53]. Perhaps the most pressing of these needs will be controlling the spread of multidrug-resistant organisms, but improving quality in the face of declining resources represents a major challenge. Mandated public reporting, emerging infectious diseases (e.g., severe acute respiratory syndrome, or SARS), and pandemic planning have increased demands for healthcare epidemiology expertise. Clearly, the well-trained and experienced epidemiologist will have many challenges and opportunities ahead.

REFERENCES

1. Weinstein RA, Pugliese G. The American Hospital Association. *Infect Control Hosp Epidemiol* 1994;15:269–273.
2. Brachman P, Eickhoff T. *Proceedings of the International Conference on Nosocomial Infections.* Chicago: American Hospital Association, 1971.
3. Eickhoff TC. The Third Decennial International Conference on Nosocomial Infections: historical perspective: the landmark conference in 1970. *Am J Med* 1991;91:3S–5S.
4. Williams REO. Summary of conference. In: Brachman PS, Eickhoff TC, eds. *Proceedings of the International Conference on Nosocomial Infections.* Chicago: American Hospital Association, 1971.
5. Haley RW, Culver DH, White JW, et al. The efficacy of infection surveillance and control programs in preventing nosocomial infections in US hospitals. *Am J Epidemiol* 1985;121:182–205.
6. McKibben L, Horan T, Tokars JI, et al. Guidance on public reporting of healthcare-associated infections: recommendations of the Healthcare Infection Control Practices Advisory Committee. *Am J Infect Control* 2005;33:217–226.
7. Kohn LT, Corrigan JM, Donaldson MS. *To err is human: building a safer health system.* The National Academies Press, 2000.
8. Centers for Disease Control and Prevention. Reduction in central line-associated bloodstream infections among patients in intensive care units—Pennsylvania, April 2001–March 2005. *MMWR Morb Mortal Wkly Rep* 2005;54:1013–1016.
9. Berenholtz SM, Pronovost PJ, Lipsett PA, et al. Eliminating catheter-related bloodstream infections in the intensive care unit. *Crit Care Med* 2004;32:2014–2020.
10. Kritchevsky SB, Simmons BP. The tools of quality improvement: CQI versus epidemiology. *Infect Control Hosp Epidemiol* 1995;16:499–502.
11. Simmons BP, Kritchevsky SB. Epidemiologic approaches to quality assessment. *Infect Control Hosp Epidemiol* 1995;16:101–104.
12. Wenzel RP, Pfaller MA. Infection control: the premier quality assessment program in United States hospitals. *Am J Med* 1991;91:27S–31S.
13. Kritchevsky SB, Simmons BP. Continuous quality improvement: concepts and applications for physician care. *JAMA* 1991;266:1817–1823.
14. Epstein PE. Cassandra and the clinician: are clinical prediction rules changing the practice of medicine? *Ann Intern Med* 1990;113:646–647.
15. Haley RW, Tenney JH, Lindsey JO, II et al. How frequent are outbreaks of nosocomial infection in community hospitals? *Infect Control* 1985;6:233–236.
16. An approach to the evaluation of quality indicators of the outcome of care in hospitalized patients, with a focus on nosocomial infection indicators. The Quality Indicator Study Group. *Infect Control Hosp Epidemiol* 1995;16:308–316.
17. Centers for Disease Control and Prevention. Monitoring hospital-acquired infections to promote patient safety. United States, 1990–1999. *MMWR Morb Mortal Wkly Rep* 2000;49:149–153.
18. Boyce JM, Pittet D. Guideline for hand hygiene in health-care settings. Recommendations of the Healthcare Infection Control Practices Advisory Committee and the HICPAC/SHEA/APIC/IDSA Hand Hygiene Task Force. *MMWR Recomm Rep* 2002;51:1–45
19. Pittet D, Hugonnet S, Harbarth S, et al. Effectiveness of a hospital-wide programme to improve compliance with hand hygiene. *Lancet* 2000;356:1307–1312.
20. Afif W, Huor P, Brassard P, Loo VG. Compliance with methicillin-resistant Staphylococcus aureus precautions in a teaching hospital. *Am J Infect Control* 2002;30:430–433.
21. Kaplan LM, McGuckin M. Increasing handwashing compliance with more accessible sinks. *Infect Control* 1986;7:408–410.
22. Larson E, Killien M. Factors influencing handwashing behavior of patient care personnel. *Am J Infect Control* 1982;10:93–99.
23. Larson EL, McGinley KJ, Foglia A, et al. Handwashing practices and resistance and density of bacterial hand flora on two pediatric units in Lima, Peru. *Am J Infect Control* 1992;20:65–72.
24. Michalsen A, Delclos GL, Felknor SA, et al. Compliance with universal precautions among physicians. *J Occup Environ Med* 1997;39:130–137.
25. Pittet D, Mourouga P, Perneger TV. Compliance with handwashing in a teaching hospital. *Ann Intern Med* 1999;130:126–130.
26. Weinstein RA. Nosocomial infection update. *Emerg Infect Dis* 1998;4:416–420.
27. Askarian M, Honarvar B, Tabatabaee HR, Assadian O. Knowledge, practice and attitude towards standard isolation precautions in Iranian medical students. *J Hosp Infect* 2004;58:292–296.
28. Askarian M, Mirzaei K, Mundy LM, McLaws ML. Assessment of knowledge, attitudes, and practices regarding isolation precautions among Iranian healthcare workers. *Infect Control Hosp Epidemiol* 2005;26:105–108.
29. Feather A, Stone SP, Wessier A, et al. 'Now please wash your hands': the handwashing behaviour of final MBBS candidates. *J Hosp Infect* 2000;45:62–64.

30. Stein AD, Makarawo TP, Ahmad MF. A survey of doctors' and nurses' knowledge, attitudes and compliance with infection control guidelines in Birmingham teaching hospitals. *J Hosp Infect* 2003;54:68–73.

31. Shojania KG, Duncan BW, McDonald KM, et al. Making health care safer: a critical analysis of patient safety practices. *Evid Rep Technol Assess* 2001 (Summ):i–x,1–668.

32. Berwick DM, Calkins DR, McCannon CJ, Hackbarth AD. The 100,000 lives campaign: setting a goal and a deadline for improving health care quality. *JAMA* 2006;295:324–327.

33. Lynch P, Jackson M, Saint S. Research Priorities Project, Year 2000: establishing a direction for infection control and hospital epidemiology. *Am J Infect Control* 2001;29:73–78.

34. Daschner FD, Cauda R, Grundmann H, et al. Hospital infection control in Europe: evaluation of present practice and future goals. *Clin Microbiol Infect* 2004;10:263–266.

35. Association for Professionals in Infection Control and Epidemiology Inc. and Centers for Disease Control and Prevention. Bioterrorism readiness plan—a template for healthcare facilities. *ED Manag* 1999;11 (suppl):1–16.

36. Petrosillo N, Puro V, Di Caro A, Ippolito G. The initial hospital response to an epidemic. *Arch Med Res* 2005;36:706–712.

37. Smith AF, Wild C, Law J. The Barrow-in-Furness legionnaires' outbreak: qualitative study of the hospital response and the role of the major incident plan. *Emerg Med J* 2005;22:251–255.

38. Voss A, Allerberger F, Bouza E, et al. The training curriculum in hospital infection control. *Clin Microbiol Infect* 2005;111 (Suppl):33–35.

39. Scheckler WE, Brimhall D, Buck AS, et al. Requirements for infrastructure and essential activities of infection control and epidemiology in hospitals: a consensus panel report. *Infect Control Hosp Epidemiol* 1998;19:114–124.

40. Classen DC. Information management in infectious diseases: survival of the fittest. *Clin Infect Dis* 1994;19:902–909.

41. Kaye KS, Engemann JJ, Fulmer EM, et al. Favorable impact of an infection control network on nosocomial infection rates in community hospitals. *Infect Control Hosp Epidemiol* 2006;27:228–232.

42. Ehrenkranz NJ. Starting an infection control network. *Infect Dis Clin Pract* 1995;4:194–198.

43. Deery HG, II. Negotiating with administration—or how to get paid for doing hospital epidemiology. *Infect Control Hosp Epidemiol* 1997;18:209–214.

44. Haley RW, White JW, Culver DH, Hughes JM. The financial incentive for hospitals to prevent nosocomial infections under the prospective payment system: an empirical determination from a nationally representative sample. *JAMA* 1987;257:1611–1614.

45. Miller PJ, Farr BM, Gwaltney JM, Jr. Economic benefits of an effective infection control program: case study and proposal. *Rev Infect Dis* 1989;11:284–288.

46. Dunagan WC, Murphy DM, Hollenbeak CS, Miller SB. Making the business case for infection control: pitfalls and opportunities. *Am J Infect Control* 2002;30:86–92.

47. Haley RW. *Managing hospital infection control for cost-effectiveness: a strategy for reducing infectious complications.* Chicago: American Hospital Association Publications, 1986.

48. Starling C. Infection control in developing countries. *Curr Opin Infect Dis* 2001;14:461–466.

49. Ruef C. Prospective evaluation of a hospital epidemiologist's activities at a European tertiary-care medical center. *Infect Control Hosp Epidemiol* 1999;20:604–606.

50. Wenzel RP. Instituting health care reform and preserving quality: role of the hospital epidemiologist. *Clin Infect Dis* 1993;17:831–834.

51. Simmons BP, Parry MF, Williams M, Weinstein RA. The new era of hospital epidemiology: what you need to succeed. *Clin Infect Dis* 1996;22:550–553.

52. Sande MA. Health care reform: implications for professions related to infectious diseases. *J Infect Dis* 1994;169:1197–1200.

53. Tice AD, Slama TG, Berman S, et al. Managed care and the infectious diseases specialist. *Clin Infect Dis* 1996;23:341–368.

Hand Hygiene

3

Didier Pittet, Benedetta Allegranzi, and Hugo Sax

HISTORY OF HAND HYGIENE

Handwashing with soap and water has been considered a measure of personal hygiene for centuries [1,2], but the link between handwashing and the spread of disease was established only in the last 200 years. In the mid-1800s, decades before the discoveries of Pasteur and Lister, studies by Ignaz Semmelweis in Vienna and Oliver Wendell Holmes in Boston established that hospital-acquired diseases were transmitted via the hands of healthcare workers (HCWs). In 1847, Semmelweiss was appointed as a house officer in one of the two obstetric clinics located at the University of Vienna Allgemeine Krankenhaus (General Hospital). He observed that maternal mortality rates, mostly due to puerperal fever, were substantially higher in one clinic compared to the other (16% vs 7%) [3]. He also noted that physicians and medical students often went directly to the delivery suite after performing autopsies and had a disagreeable odor on their hands despite handwashing with soap and water before entering the clinic. He hypothesized that "cadaverous particles" were transmitted via the hands of students and physicians and caused puerperal fever. As a consequence, Semmelweis recommended that hands be scrubbed in a chlorinated lime solution before every patient contact and particularly after leaving the autopsy room. Following the implementation of this measure, the mortality rate dropped dramatically to 3% in the clinic most affected.

This intervention represents the first evidence that cleansing heavily contaminated hands with an antiseptic agent can reduce nosocomial transmission of germs more effectively than handwashing with plain soap and water. Unfortunately, both Holmes and Semmelweis failed to observe a sustained change in their colleagues' behavior.

A prospective controlled trial conducted in a hospital nursery [4] and investigations conducted during the past 40 years have confirmed the important role that contaminated HCWs' hands play in the transmission of healthcare-associated infection (HAI) pathogens [5].

The 1980s represented a landmark in the evolution of concepts of hand hygiene in health care. The first national hand hygiene guidelines were published in the 1980s [6–8], followed by several others in more recent years in different countries.

In 1995 and 1996, the U.S. Centers for Disease Control and Prevention (CDC)/Healthcare Infection Control Practices Advisory Committee (HICPAC) recommended that either antimicrobial soap or a waterless antiseptic agent be used for cleansing hands upon leaving the rooms of patients with multidrug-resistant pathogens [9,10]. More recently, the CDC/HICPAC guidelines issued in 2002 [11] and the current advanced draft of the World Health Organization (WHO) Guidelines on Hand Hygiene in Healthcare [5] have defined alcohol-based handrubbing, where available, as the standard of care for hand hygiene practices in healthcare settings, whereas handwashing is reserved for particular situations only [5].

DEFINITIONS

Hand hygiene during healthcare delivery can be performed either by handwashing or by handrubbing. The purpose of performing hand hygiene for routine patient care is to remove microbial contamination acquired by recent contact with infected or colonized patients or with environmental sources and, in some instances, to remove organic matter from the hands.

Standard handwashing with plain soap and water removes lipid and adhering dirt, soil, and various organic substances from the hands. Plain soap has minimal antimicrobial activity but after 30 seconds can reduce counts by 1.8–2.8 $\log_{10}$ [1]. In several studies, however, handwashing

TABLE 3-1

INDICATIONS FOR HANDWASHING AND HAND ANTISEPSIS

Washing hands with soap and water when visibly dirty or contaminated with proteinaceous material, visibly soiled with blood or other body fluids, or if exposure to potential spore-forming organisms is strongly suspected or proven (IB) or after using the restroom (II).

Preferably use an alcohol-based handrub for routine hand antisepsis in all other clinical situations described in items (a) to (f) listed if hands are not visibly soiled (IA). Alternatively, wash hands with soap and water (IB).

Perform hand hygiene:

a. Before and after having direct contact with patients (IB).
b. After removing gloves (IB).
c. Before handling an invasive device for patient care regardless of whether or not gloves are used (IB).
d. After contact with body fluids or excretions, mucous membranes, nonintact skin, or wound dressings (IA).
e. If moving from a contaminated body site to a clean body site during patient care (IB);
f. After contact with inanimate objects (including medical equipment) in the immediate vicinity of the patient (IB).

Wash hands with either plain or antimicrobial soap and water or rub hands with an alcohol-based formulation before handling medication or preparing food (IB).

When alcohol-based handrub is already used, do not use antimicrobial soap concomitantly (II).

Adapted from World Health Organization. WHO Guidelines for Hand Hygiene in Health Care (Advanced Draft). Geneva: World Health Organization, 2006 (**http://www.who.int/patientsafety/information_ centre/Last_April_versionHH_Guidelines%5b3%5d.pdf**) accessed 19 July 2006.

with plain soap failed to remove pathogens from HCW's hands [12–14].

Hygienic hand antisepsis is significantly more efficient than standard handwashing and can be performed either by washing with an antimicrobial soap or a detergent and water (antiseptic handwashing) or by handrubbing with antiseptic preparations (antiseptic handrubbing). Antiseptic handrubs are available as different formulations (liquid, gels, foams) and bypass the need for an exogenous source of water and towels or other hand-drying devices.

Indications for performing hand hygiene and for opting for handwashing rather than handrubbing are discussed in the following sections and listed in Table 3-1.

MODEL OF HAND TRANSMISSION OF MICROORGANISMS IN HEALTH CARE

A clear understanding of the process of hand transmission is critical to successful education strategies, assessment of HCWs' hand hygiene performance, and research. According to existing scientific evidence [5], a model of hand

transmission has been proposed and serves as a basis for the recently reviewed recommendations on indications for hand hygiene action [5].

Transmission of HAI pathogens from one patient to another or within the same patient from one body site to another via HCWs' hands requires five sequential steps described in more detail below and illustrated in Figure 3-1.

Step 1: Organisms Present on Patient Skin or the Inanimate Environment

Both the patient's skin [12,15–21] and the inanimate environment [13,21–24] harbor large amounts of germs including multiresistant bacteria, fungi, and viruses. Of importance, HAI pathogens can be recovered not only from infected or draining wounds but also from frequently colonized areas of normal, intact patient skin. Exogenous and endogenous factors, such as exposure to antibiotics and medical devices, host immunity deficiency and patient comorbidities as well as the frequency and efficacy of hand cleansing by HCWs determine the type of skin flora and its burden. The microbial load on surfaces in the hospital environment will equally vary in an unpredictable way due to type of surface and environmental cleaning, patient characteristics, hand hygiene, and humidity.

Step 2: Organism Transfer on Healthcare Workers' Hands

In addition to resident flora, hand skin acquires transient flora by exposure to colonized objects, inanimate surfaces, and patients. Contamination of HCWs' hands before and after direct patient contact, wound care, intravascular catheter care, respiratory tract care, and handling patient secretions [25] revealed that the number of bacteria recovered ranged from 0 to 300 colony-forming units. Hand colonization occurs also following "clean procedures" or touching intact areas of skin of hospitalized patients [13,18,24,26]. Furthermore, gloves do not provide complete protection against hand contamination [27–30].

Step 3: Organism Survival on Hands

Hand colonization with commensal flora and with potential pathogens progressively increases during patient care due to germ capacity to survive on skin [25,31]. Several studies have shown the ability of microorganisms to survive on hands for differing times [32–35]. For example, according to Noskin et al., both *Enterococcus faecalis* and vancomycin-resistant *E. faecium* survived for at least 60 minutes on gloved and ungloved fingertips [36]. Studies by Ansari et al. using rotavirus, rhinovirus, and human parainfluenza virus 3 showed survival up to 60 minutes [37,38].

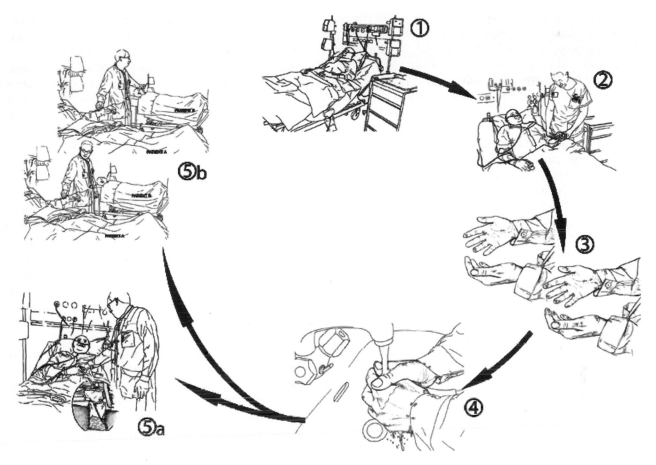

Figure 3-1 Model for hand transmission of microbial pathogens. (Reproduced with permission from Pittet D, Allegranzi B, Sax H, Dharan S., Pessoa-Silva CL, Donaldson L, Boyce JM, WHO Global Patient Safety Challenge, World Alliance for Patient Safety. Evidence-based model for hand transmission during patient care and the role of improved practices. *Lancet Infect Dis* 2006; 6:641–652.)

Step 4: Defective Hand Hygiene Results in Hands Remaining Contaminated

When HCWs fail to clean their hands between touching different patients or during the sequence of patient care, particularly when hands move from a microbiologically contaminated to a clean body site in the same patient, microbial transfer is likely to occur. Adequate and timely hand hygiene technique is essential for effective removal of contamination and to prevent persistent colonization.

Wearing rings and artificial fingernails increases the frequency of hand contamination with potential HAI pathogens, even after use of either soap or alcohol-based hand gel [39,40] and has been associated with HAI outbreaks [41].

Step 5: Contaminated Hands Cross-Transmit Organisms

Failure to practice hand hygiene between sequential hand-surface exposures results in HCWs' hands acting as organism carriers ready to spread potentially harmful pathogens onto another surface. Once deposited on patients, the cross-transmitted organisms will establish either a carrier state or lead directly to infection (Figure 3.1).

Of importance, pathogen transfer also can occur within the same patient from a colonized area to a clean body site or onto an invasive medical device. Given that most HAIs are of endogenous nature, this latter pathway of transmission by HCWs' hands is of the utmost etiologic importance.

INDICATIONS FOR HAND HYGIENE DURING HEALTHCARE

Effective hand hygiene should remove transient flora on HCWs' hands at critical moments during care activity with the clear objective to prevent cross-transmission of potentially harmful organisms and infection. A set of indications for hand hygiene has been established according to scientific evidence and is congruent with the model of transmission (as noted previously). These indications are listed in the most recent international guidelines and weighed according to supporting evidence (Table 3-1) [5]. The first indications on the list (i.e., before and after having direct contact with a patient) are easy to remember for HCWs because they are linked to approaching or leaving the patient. Other indications, more difficult to identify, are linked to specific tasks and occur mostly during a care sequence in the same patient (i.e., before handling an invasive device or after a task associated with the risk of exposure to body fluids). According to the model of transmission, hand hygiene before a patient contact or an invasive procedure is aimed at protecting the patient. In contrast, hand hygiene after tasks or contact with patients and their immediate surroundings serves to protect the HCW against colonization and infection and to prevent germ spread to the environment. Intriguingly, HCWs more often comply with the indication after a patient contact or after a care task.

For practical purposes, it is important to recognize that ≥2 of the listed indications might occur simultaneously during a sequence of care requiring only a single hand hygiene action. The guidelines also describe optimal techniques for handrubbing and handwashing and specify that the latter be reserved only for situations when hands are visibly soiled and transmission of spores is strongly suspected or proven and after using the restroom [5] (Table 3-1).

Hand hygiene should be performed after glove removal because wearing gloves does not completely prevent hand colonization [31] and/or contamination. Moreover, hand hygiene should be performed when an indication occurs, regardless of whether gloves are worn or not [5,11].

PROPERTIES OF HAND ANTISEPSIS AGENTS

Antiseptic agents (both soap and handrubs) contain an antimicrobial substance, which reduces or inhibits the growth of microorganisms on living tissues. The most popular agents are briefly described next (Table 3-2).

Considering antimicrobial activity, alcohols have the broadest antimicrobial spectrum compared to other agents, with excellent *in vitro* and *in vivo* activity against Gram-positive and Gram-negative vegetative bacteria (including multidrug-resistant pathogens such as methicillin-resistant *Staphylococcus aureus* and vancomycin-resistant enterococci), *Mycobacterium tuberculosis*, and a variety of fungi [42–50]. Mycobacteria and fungi also are killed by iodophors and less effectively by chlorhexidine, chloroxylenol, or hexachlorophene. Most enveloped (lipophilic) viruses (e.g., herpes simplex virus, human immunodeficiency virus, influenza virus, respiratory syncytial virus, and vaccinia virus) are susceptible to alcohols, chlorhexidine, and iodophors [42,51–59]. Other enveloped viruses (hepatitis B virus and probably hepatitis C virus) are somewhat less susceptible to alcohols but are killed by concentrations as high as 60–70% (*v/v*) [60]. In some *in vivo* studies, alcohols showed some activity also against a number of non-enveloped viruses (rotavirus, adenovirus,

rhinovirus, hepatitis A virus, and enteroviruses) [61–65]. In general, ethanol has stronger activity against viruses than isopropanol [66]. Iodophors and, to a minor extent, chlorhexidine also are active against some non-enveloped viruses. None of the listed antiseptic agents has an activity against bacterial spores or protozoan oocysts. Iodophors are only slightly sporicidal but at higher concentrations than the ones used in antiseptics [67].

Alcohols are the most frequently used antimicrobial component of handrubs. Alcohol-based handrubs are considered the most effective antiseptic agents for hand hygiene, and they generally contain either ethanol, isopropanol or n-propanol or a combination of two of these products. Alcohol solutions containing 60–80% (*v/v*) alcohol are most effective with higher concentrations being less potent [43,44]. In all published studies, alcohols were more effective than plain soap; furthermore, in the vast majority of trials, they reduced bacterial counts on hands to a greater extent than washing hands with soaps or detergents containing hexachlorophene, povidone-iodine, 4% chlorhexidine, or triclosan [68].

Chlorhexidine gluconate has been incorporated into a number of hand hygiene preparations. Aqueous or detergent formulations containing 0.5%, 0.75%, or 1% chlorhexidine are more effective than plain soap but less effective than antiseptic detergent preparations containing 2% and 4% chlorhexidine gluconate [69,70]. Chlorhexidine's immediate antimicrobial activity is slower than that of alcohols, but it has significant residual activity [69–76].

Iodophors are composed of elemental iodine, iodide, or triiodide, and a polymer carrier of high molecular weight, such as polyvinyl pyrrolidone (povidone) and ethoxylated nonionic detergents (poloxamers) [55,77]. Their persistent antimicrobial activity is controversial. Most iodophor preparations used for hand hygiene contain 7.5–10.0% povidone-iodine.

Chloroxylenol has been widely used in antimicrobial soaps and as a preservative in cosmetics and other products. It has good *in vitro* activity against Gram-positive organisms and fair activity against Gram-negative bacteria, mycobacteria, and some viruses [1,78,79]; in particular, the activity against *Pseudomonas aeruginosa* is limited. Chloroxylenol is considered to be less rapidly active than chlorhexidine gluconate or iodophors, and its residual activity is less pronounced than that of chlorhexidine [78,79].

Hexachlorophene is a bisphenol contained in emulsions used for hygienic handwashing and patient bathing. It has residual activity for several hours after use and a cumulative effect [1,80–82]. Because of its high rates of dermal absorption and subsequent toxic effects, including neurotoxicity [83], the agent is classified by the U.S. Food and Drug Administration (FDA) as not safe and effective for use as an antiseptic agent for handwashing and has been banned worldwide [66,84,85].

Quaternary ammonium compounds belong to a large group; alkyl benzalkonium chlorides have been the most

TABLE 3-2
PREPARATIONS FOR HAND HYGIENE

Agent	Gram+ Bacteria	Gram− Bacteria	Mycobacteria	Fungi	Enveloped Virus	Non-enveloped Virus	Spores	Speed of Action	Residual Activity	Use
Alcohols	++	+++	+++	++	++	+	−	Fast	No	HR
Chlorhexidine	+++	++	+	+	++	+	−	Intermediate	Yes	HR, HW
Chloroxylenol	+++	+	+	+	+	±	−	Slow	Contradictory	HW
Hexachlorophene[a]	+++	+	+	+	?	?	−	Slow	Yes	HW, but not recommended
Iodophors	+++	+++	++	−+	++	++	±[b]	Intermediate	Contradictory	HW
Quaternary ammonium compounds[c]	++	+	±	±	+	?	−	Slow	No	HR, HW; seldom;+alcohols
Triclosan[d]	+++	++	±	±[e]	?	?	−	Intermediate	Yes	HW; seldom

HR, handrubbing; HW, handwashing

Activity: +++ excellent; ++ good, but does not include the entire bacterial spectrum; + fair; ± controversial; − no activity

[a]Bacteriostatic.

[b]In concentrations used in antiseptics, iodophors are not sporicidal.

[c]Bacteriostatic, fungistatic, microbicidal at high concentrations.

[d]Mostly bacteriostatic.

[e]Activity against Candida spp., but little activity against filamentous fungi.

widely used as antiseptics. They are primarily bacteriostatic and fungistatic, though microbicidal at high concentrations against some organisms [1]. They are more active against Gram-positive bacteria than against Gram-negative bacilli and have relatively weak activity against mycobacteria and fungi and stronger activity against lipophilic viruses.

Triclosan is a nonionic, colorless substance that has antimicrobial activity at concentrations ranging from 0.2% to 2% but tends to be bacteriostatic [1]. Like chlorhexidine, triclosan has persistent activity on the skin. According to the FDA, available data are insufficient to classify it as safe and effective for hand antisepsis [84].

METHODS TO EVALUATE THE ANTIMICROBIAL EFFICACY OF ANTISEPTIC AGENTS

Every new formulation for hand antisepsis should be tested for its antimicrobial efficacy to demonstrate that it has superior efficacy over normal soap or meets an agreed performance standard. The most appropriate method is to artificially contaminate volunteers' hands with the test organism before applying the test formulation. In Europe, the most commonly used test methods (EN 1499 [86] for antiseptic soaps and EN 1500 [87] for handrubs) are those of the European Committee for Standardization (CEN). These use a randomized, crossover design and compare the product with a standardized reference agent. The EN 1499 [86] norm requires that the mean $\log_{10}$ reduction of microbial hand contamination by the antiseptic soap be significantly higher than that obtained with the control (soft soap). For the EN 1500, the efficacy of the tested handrub should not be significantly lower than that of the reference alcohol-based rub (isopropyl alcohol or isopropanol 60% volume).

In the United States, antiseptics are regulated by the FDA [84] which refers to the standards of the American Society for Testing and Materials (ASTM). The most frequently used method for testing handwashing and handrubbing agents is the ASTM E-1174 [88]. Criteria for efficacy are a 2-$\log_{10}$ reduction of the indicator organism on each hand within 5 minutes after the first use and a 3-$\log_{10}$ reduction within 5 minutes after the tenth use.

Shortcomings of current test methods are discussed in detail elsewhere [5].

SKIN REACTIONS

The tolerability of hand hygiene products is a major factor that influences acceptance and ultimate usage by HCWs and is a key determinant to the success of hand hygiene promotion [89].

Two major types of skin reactions are associated with hand hygiene: irritant contact dermatitis and allergic contact dermatitis.

Irritant Contact Dermatitis

The first reaction type is the most common and includes symptoms such as dryness, burning sensation, itching, skin that feels "rough," erythema, scaling, cracking, and bleeding. Frequent and repeated use of hand hygiene products, particularly soaps and other detergents, is an important cause of chronic irritant contact dermatitis among HCWs [90]. In one study, approximately 25% of nurses reported symptoms or signs of dermatitis on their hands, but 85% gave a history of skin problems [91]. Skin that is damaged by repeated exposure to detergents may be more susceptible to irritation by all types of hand antiseptic formulations [92]. Hot water, incomplete drying of hands, and the quality of paper towels can contribute to dermatitis. Low relative humidity associated with failure to use supplementary hand lotion or cream contributes to dermatitis with both hand rubbing and washing [93,94].

Shearing forces when wearing or removing gloves and allergy to latex proteins also are risk factors for hand dermatitis among HCWs [95]. Routinely washing hands with soap and water immediately before or after using an alcohol-based formulation not only is unnecessary but also may lead to dermatitis. Additionally, frequent glove use and donning gloves while hands are still wet can increase the risk of skin irritation.

Antimicrobial soaps may cause irritation due to the antimicrobial agent or to other ingredients of the formulation. Several studies have demonstrated that alcohol-based preparations are better tolerated and associated with better skin condition when compared with either plain or antiseptic hand products [89]. Irritant contact dermatitis is more commonly reported with iodophors [96] and less frequently with chlorhexidine, chloroxylenol, triclosan, or alcohol-based products. The variable potential of detergents to cause skin irritation can be reduced by adding emollients and humectants.

Allergic Contact Dermatitis

Allergic contact dermatitis is rare and results from an allergy to an ingredient in the hand hygiene product; clinical symptoms can be mild and localized or severe, such as anaphylaxis. Allergic reactions to products applied to the skin (contact allergy) can present as a delayed type of reaction (allergic contact dermatitis) or less commonly as an immediate reaction (contact urticaria). The most common causes of contact allergies are fragrances and preservatives with emulsifiers being less common triggers [97–100]. Liquid soaps, hand lotion, ointments, or creams used by HCWs can contain ingredients causing contact allergies [98,99].

Allergic reactions to antiseptic agents including quaternary ammonium compounds, iodine or iodophors, chlorhexidine, triclosan, chloroxylenol, and alcohols and possible toxicity in relation to dermal absorption of products have been reported [89]. Allergic contact dermatitis due to alcohol-based handrubs is very uncommon, however, and could represent true allergy to the alcohol, to an impurity or aldehyde metabolite, or to another product constituent [89,97,101]. There are few reports of allergic dermatitis resulting from contact with ethanol [102–104] and only one report of ethanol-related contact urticaria syndrome [105]. More recently, Cimiotti et al. reported adverse reactions, mostly reversible, associated with an alcohol-based handrub preparation [106].

There are three primary strategies to minimize hand hygiene-related irritant contact dermatitis among HCWs: selection of less irritating hand hygiene products, education regarding proper skin care management, and routine use of moisturizing skin care products.

MONITORING HAND HYGIENE PRACTICES AND DETERMINANTS OF COMPLIANCE

Monitoring hand hygiene performance is an activity of crucial importance to assess baseline compliance by HCWs, provide feedback to HCWs, evaluate the impact of promotion interventions, investigate outbreaks, and answer research questions [107–117].

Hand hygiene practices during routine healthcare delivery can be evaluated directly or indirectly. Direct methods include observation, patient assessment, and self-reports. Direct observation by trained and validated observers is regarded as the gold standard because it quantifies the need for hand hygiene and the actual performance. To calculate the compliance rate, the number of hand hygiene actions performed by HCWs is divided by the number of opportunities for hand hygiene. The method should respect basic epidemiological principles (e.g., sample size calculation, exclusion of selection, observer, and observation bias). Eventually, adjustment for confounders (e.g., professional category or healthcare setting) could be needed.

Indirect methods include monitoring consumption of products (e.g., soap, handrub, and paper towels) and electronic monitoring of the use of wash basins or handrub dispensers. These methods can be attractive as less time consuming and resource demanding than direct observation. Lack of a quantification of the need for hand hygiene can partially be surrogated by relating consumption to patient-days or workload measures [118] or estimating the required amount using a computerized database of nursing activities [119]. Some studies [107,120,121] have shown that the consumption of products used for hand hygiene correlated with observed hand hygiene compliance; others established no correlation [122]. Thus, the use of this measure as a surrogate for monitoring hand hygiene practices deserves further validation.

Recent epidemiologic investigations on HCWs' compliance with hand hygiene have revealed key findings.

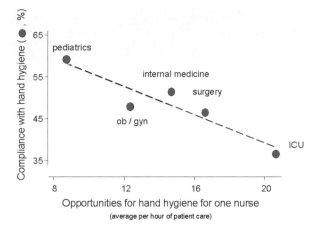

Figure 3-2 Relation between opportunities for hand hygiene and compliance across hospital wards. (Modified with permission from Pittet D, Mourouga P, Perneger TV. Compliance with handwashing in a teaching hospital. Ann Intern Med 1999; 130: 126–130.)

Adherence has been unacceptably poor with mean baseline rates ranging from 5% to 81% and an overall average of about 40% (reviewed in detail in [5]). In the largest survey conducted so far [123], the investigators identified hospital-wide predictors of poor adherence to recommended hand hygiene measures during routine patient care. Predicting variables included professional category, hospital ward (Figure 3-2), time of day/week, and type and intensity of patient care defined as the number of opportunities for hand hygiene per hour of patient care (Table 3-3). Moreover, perceived barriers to adherence with hand hygiene guidelines have been assessed or quantified in observational studies. Among others, they include skin irritation caused by hand hygiene agents, inaccessible hand hygiene supplies, interference with HCW–patient relationships, patient needs perceived as a priority over hand hygiene, wearing of gloves, forgetfulness, lack of knowledge of guidelines, insufficient time for hand hygiene, and high workload and understaffing (Table 3-3).

Recent studies have confirmed an inverse relation between intensity of patient care and adherence to hand hygiene (Figure 3-3) [124–126]. Thus, time required for traditional handwashing could make optimal compliance with earlier guidelines unrealistic. The system change from time-consuming handwashing to handrub with an alcohol-based preparation has revolutionized hand hygiene practices and now is considered the standard of care [5,127].

STRATEGIES TO PROMOTE HAND HYGIENE

HCW education is an inherent component of the work of the infection control team. However, it is now recognized that education alone may not be sufficient to achieve hand

TABLE 3-3

MAIN FACTORS INFLUENCING ADHERENCE TO HAND HYGIENE PRACTICES

Individual level
- Lack of education or experience
- Being a physician, compared to other health-care professionals
- Lack of knowledge of guidelines
- Being a refractory noncomplier
- Skin irritation by hand hygiene agents

Group level
- Lack of education or lack of performance feedback
- Working in critical care or in high workload conditions
- Downsizing or understaffing
- Lack of encouragement or role model from key staff

Institutional level
- Lack of written guidelines
- Lack of suitable hand hygiene agents
- Lack of skin-care promotion or agents
- Lack of culture or tradition of compliance
- Lack of administrative leadership, sanctions, rewards, or support

Governmental level
- Lack of awareness and commitment regarding the importance of health care-associated infection
- Lack of specific regulations and policies on prevention of healthcare-associated infection
- Lack of national guidelines on hand hygiene in health care
- Lack of promotion of national or regional campaigns to improve hand hygiene in health care
- Insufficient allocation of financial resources for this purpose

hygiene improvement. HCWs' behavioral attitudes toward compliance with recommended practices are extremely complex and multifactorial [128–132], and experts agree that a successful program must be multidisciplinary and multifaceted to counteract most reasons for poor compliance [115,131].

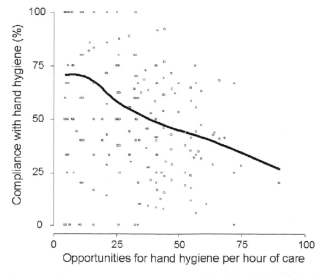

Figure 3-3 Relation between the number of opportunities for hand hygiene and compliance. (Modified with permission from Pittet D, Mourouga P, Perneger TV. Compliance with handwashing in a teaching hospital. *Ann Intern Med* 1999; 130:126–130.)

Several studies showed a significant increase in hand hygiene compliance after the introduction of handrubs [107,113,120,121,123,133–140]. Moreover, availability of handrub dispensers at the point of care or individual pocket dispensers is now considered the standard of care [5,127].

Table 3-4 presents published strategies for the promotion of hand hygiene in hospitals. Some of the strategies could be unnecessary in certain settings but could be helpful in others. To establish whether single factors (e.g., increased education, individual reinforcement technique, appropriate rewarding, administrative sanction, enhanced self-participation, active involvement of a larger number of organizational leaders, enhanced perception of health threat, self-efficacy, and perceived social pressure) [129,141–144] or combinations of these factors actually determine improvement of HCWs' adherence to hand hygiene requires further research. Ultimately, adherence to recommended hand hygiene practices should become part of a culture of patient safety in which a set of interdependent elements of quality interact to achieve the shared objective [145].

IMPACT OF HAND HYGIENE PROMOTION

The impact of strategies and/or campaigns to promote hand hygiene in healthcare settings can be measured primarily by

TABLE 3-4
STRATEGIES FOR SUCCESSFUL PROMOTION OF HAND HYGIENE IN HOSPITALS

Strategy	Selected References*
1. Education	[107,110,112–117,119,121,136,137,156]
2. Routine observation and feedback	[107,112,113,115,116,121,137,156,157]
3. Engineering control	
Make hand hygiene possible, easy, convenient	[107,114–116,119,136,156,158,159]
Make alcohol-based handrub available	[107,113,117,120,134,136,137]
4. Patient education	[120,160,161]
5. Reminders in the workplace	[107,109,113,114,116,117,134,136,162–165]
6. Administrative sanction/rewarding	[117,141,142]
7. Change in hand hygiene agent	[113,117,120,123,134,136,137,166,167]
8. Promote/facilitate skin care for HCWs' hands	[107,166,168,169]
9. Active participation at individual & institutional level	[107,108,116,136,142,170]
10. Improve institutional safety climate	[107,108,116,136,142]
11. Enhance individual & institutional self-efficacy	[107,108,116,136,142]
12. Avoid overcrowding, understaffing, excessive workload	[107,123,139,171,172]
13. Combine several of above strategies	[107,108,110,112,113,115,116,136,137,142]

*Only selected references have been listed; readers should refer to more extensive reviews for exhaustive reference lists [1,54,128,142,173].
Adapted with permission from World Health Organization. WHO Guidelines for Hand Hygiene in Health Care (Advanced Draft). Geneva: World Health Organization, 2006.
(**http://www.who.int/patientsafety/information_centre/Last_April_versionHH_Guidelines%5b3%5d.pdf**)
accessed 19 July 2006.

monitoring hand hygiene compliance in daily care practice before and after the intervention. Over the past 12 years, several studies have demonstrated the effectiveness of such strategies on improving this process indicator, mostly based on a multimodal approach [107,113,114,116,120, 135,146–151]. In most of these interventional studies, the introduction of alcohol-based handrubs at the point of care as a system change was the crucial component of the promotional strategy [107,113,114,116,120,135, 146–151].

It is evident that the most valuable method to demonstrate the impact of hand hygiene improvement is to detect a significant reduction of HAI rates in the study intervention setting. Unfortunately, a limited number of studies monitored the effect on this crucial outcome indicator because active surveillance of infection is highly resource demanding and complex to perform in a reliable manner (Table 3-5). Despite study limitations, most reports based on multimodal strategies, including the introduction of an alcohol-based handrub, showed a temporal relation between improved hand hygiene practices and reduced HAI rates. However, only a few reported a sustained effect over a prolonged period of time [107,117,152–155]. Although it remains important to generate additional scientific and causal evidence for the impact of enhanced adherence with hand hygiene on HAI rates, these results strongly suggest that improved hand hygiene practices reduce the risk of transmission of pathogenic microorganisms.

GLOBAL PERSPECTIVE AND RESEARCH AGENDA

Poor compliance with hand hygiene affects facilities at any level of country development. Improvement relies not only on individual HCW awareness and knowledge but also on involvement at institutional and governmental levels, thus implying the need for system and policy changes. Recent or potential pandemics (e.g., severe acute respiratory syndrome [SARS] and Avian Influenza) have amply demonstrated that standard precautions, including hand hygiene, are not implemented in an optimal manner in many healthcare facilities worldwide. In a global perspective, hand hygiene promotion may imply different approaches depending on where the intervention is conducted. In developed countries, the issue could be for hospitals to find innovative strategies for previous campaign reinforcement or the introduction of new sophisticated solutions, whereas in resource-poor facilities in developing countries, a stronger effort should be made to convey messages in the simplest way and to seek low-cost practical solutions. The recently issued WHO Guidelines on Hand Hygiene in Health Care (Advanced Draft) and their implementation strategy represent an unprecedented effort to promote hand hygiene with an evidence-based approach adapted to local needs and resources in a global perspective [5].

Although the published scientific evidence on hand hygiene has increased considerably in recent years, many

TABLE 3-5

ASSOCIATION BETWEEN HAND HYGIENE IMPROVEMENT AND HEALTH CARE–ASSOCIATED INFECTION RATES: HOSPITAL-BASED STUDIES, 1995–2005

Year	Authors	Hospital Setting	Significant Results	Duration of Follow-up
1995	Zafar et al. [138]	Newborn nursery	Control of a MRSA outbreak using a triclosan preparation for hand antisepsis in addition to other infection control measures	3.5 years
2000	Larson et al. [108]	MICU/NICU	Significant (85%) relative reduction of VRE rate in the intervention hospital; statistically insignificant (44%) relative reduction in control hospital; no significant change in MRSA	8 months
2000	Pittet et al. [107]	Hospitalwide	Significant reduction in the annual overall prevalence of healthcare-associated infections (41.5%) and MRSA cross-transmission rates (87%). Active surveillance cultures and contact precautions were implemented during same time period.	5 years
2003	Hilburn et al. [174]	Orthopedic surgical unit	36.1% decrease in infection rates (from 8.2% to 5.3%)	10 months
2004	MacDonald et al. [165]	Hospitalwide	Significant reduction in hospital-acquired MRSA cases (from 1.9% to 0.9%)	1 year
2004	Swoboda et al. [159]	Adult intermediate care unit	Reduction in health care–associated infection rates (not statistically significant)	2.5 months
2004	Lam et al. [114]	NICU	Reduction (not statistically significant) in health care–associated infection rates (from 11.3/1000 patient-days to 6.2/1000 patient-days)	6 months
2004	Won et al. [117]	NICU	Significant reduction in health care–associated infection rates (from 15.1/1000 patient-days to 10.7/1000 patient-days), in particular of respiratory infections	2 years
2005	Gordin et al. [152]	Hospitalwide	Significant reduction in nosocomially acquired MRSA (21%) and VRE (41%)	3 years
2005	Zerr et al. [153]	Hospitalwide	Significant reduction in hospital-associated rotavirus infections	4 years
2005	Rosenthal et al. [154]	Adult ICUs	Significant reduction in health care–associated infection rates (from 47.5/1000 patient-days to 27.9/1000 patient-days)	21 months
2005	Johnson et al. [155]	Hospitalwide	Significant reduction (57%) in MRSA bacteremia	36 months

ICU, intensive care unit; NICU, neonatal ICU; MRSA, methicillin-resistant *Staphylococcus aureus*; MICU, medical ICU.

controversial issues remain unsolved. The main areas for research are optimal products and practical technique, clinical efficacy and cost effectiveness, and laboratory-based and epidemiologic models to link hand hygiene practices with microbial transmission, standardization of monitoring, and system evolution. From a global perspective of hand hygiene implementation, international experts acknowledge the need for field testing to identify practical solutions concerning water quality for hand hygiene, soap contamination during use, hand drying, microbicidal activity against Norwalk virus and multiresistant bacteria, hand hygiene and use/re-use of gloves, surgical hand antisepsis, and hand hygiene behavior and promotion in different cultural settings [5].

Among the most important issues for research are the impact of specific hand hygiene indications on specific infectious outcomes and risk level in case of negligence, relation between compliance and infectious outcomes, impact of glove use on transmission between patients and within the same patient, and the most effective promotion strategies to guarantee sustained improvement.

ACKNOWLEDGMENTS

The authors thank Rosemary Sudan for outstanding editorial support.

REFERENCES

1. Rotter M. Hand washing and hand disinfection. In: Mayhall CG, ed. *Hospital epidemiology and infection control.* 2ed. Philadelphia: Lippincott Williams & Wilkins, 1999; 1339–1355.

2. Jumaa PA. Hand hygiene: simple and complex. *Int J Infect Dis* 2005; 9(3)14.

3. Semmelweis I. Die Aetiologie, der Begriff und die Prophylaxis des Kindbettfiebers [*The etiology, concept and prophylaxis of childbed fever*]. Pest, Wien, und Leipzig: C.A.Hartleben's Verlag-Expedition, 1861.

4. Mortimer EA, Lipsitz PJ, Wolinsky E, et al. Transmission of *Staphylococci* between newborns. *Am J Dis of Child* 1962; 104:289–295.

5. World Health Organization. WHO guidelines for hand hygiene in health care (advanced draft). Geneva: World Health Organization, 2006 (www.who.int/patientsafety/information_centre/Last_April_versionHH_Guidelines%5b3%5d.pdf) accessed 19 July 2006.

6. Bryan P, Simmons B. Guidelines for hospital environmental control, section 1. Antiseptics, handwashing, and handwashing facilities. In: Centers for Diseases Control and Prevention (CDC), ed. *CDC Hospital Infections Program (HIP) Guidelines for Prevention and Control of Nosocomial Infections*, Atlanta: Springfield, 1981:6–10.

7. Garner JS, Favero MS. CDC guideline for handwashing and hospital environmental control, 1985. *Infect Control* 1986; 7:231–243.

8. Bjerke NB. The evolution: handwashing to hand hygiene guidance. *Crit Care Nurs Q* 2004; 27:295–307.

9. Hospital Infection Control Practices Advisory Committee (HICPAC). Recommendations for preventing the spread of vancomycin resistance. *Infect Control Hosp Epidemiol* 1995; 16:105–113.

10. Garner JS. Guideline for isolation precautions in hospitals. *Infect Control Hosp Epidemiol* 1996; 17:53–80.

11. Boyce JM, Pittet D. Guideline for hand hygiene in health-care settings. Recommendations of the Healthcare Infection Control Practices Advisory Committee and the HICPAC/SHEA/APIC/IDSA Hand Hygiene Task Force. *MMWR* 2002; 51 (RR-16):1–45.

12. Ehrenkranz NJ, Alfonso BC. Failure of bland soap handwash to prevent hand transfer of patient bacteria to urethral catheters. *Infect Control Hosp Epidemiol* 1991;12:654–662.

13. McFarland LV, Mulligan ME, Kwok RY, Stamm WE. Nosocomial acquisition of *Clostridium difficile* infection. *New Engl J Med* 1989, 320:204–210.

14. Bottone EJ, Cheng M, Hymes S. Ineffectiveness of handwashing with lotion soap to remove nosocomial bacterial pathogens persisting on fingertips. a major link in their intrahospital spread. *Infect Control Hosp Epidemiol* 2004; 25:262–264

15. Casewell MW. The role of hands in nosocomial gram negative infection. In: Maibach HI, Aly R, eds. *Skin Microbiology Relevance to Clinical Infection*. New York: Springer-Verlag, 1981; 192–202.

16. Larson EL, Cronquist AB, Whittier S, Lai L, et al. Differences in skin flora between inpatients and chronically ill patients. *Heart Lung* 2000; 29:298–305.

17. Larson EL, McGinley KJ, Foglia AR, et al. Composition and antimicrobic resistance of skin flora in hospitalized and healthy adults. *J Clin Microbiol* 1986; 23:604–608.

18. Sanderson PJ, Weissler S. Recovery of coliforms from the hands of nurses and patients: activities leading to contamination. *J Hosp Infect* 1992; 21:85–93.

19. Coello R, Jiminez J, Garcia M, et al. Prospective study of infection, colonization and carriage of methicillin-resistant *Staphylococcus aureus* in an outbreak affecting 990 patients. *Eur J Clin Microbiol* 1994; 13:74–81.

20. Bertone SA, Fisher MC, Mortensen JE. Quantitative skin cultures at potential catheter sites in neonates. *Infect Control Hosp Epidemiol* 1994;15:315–318.

21. Bonten MJM, Hayden MK, Nathan C, et al. Epidemiology of colonisation of patients and environment with vancomycin-resistant *Enterococci*. *Lancet* 1996; 348:1615–1619.

22. Walter CW, Kundsin RB, Shilkret MA, Day MM. The spread of *Staphylococci* to the environment. *Antibiot Annu* 1958–1959; 6:952–957.

23. Boyce JM, Opal SM, Chow JW, et al. Outbreak of multidrug-resistant *Enterococcus faecium* with transferable *vanB* class vancomycin resistance. *J Clin Microbiol* 1994; 32:1148–1153.

24. Samore MH, Venkataraman L, DeGirolami PC, et al. Clinical and molecular epidemiology of sporadic and clustered cases of nosocomial *Clostridium difficile* diarrhea. *Am J Med* 1996; 100:32–40.

25. Pittet D, Dharan S, Touveneau S, et al. Bacterial contamination of the hands of hospital staff during routine patient care. *Arch Int Med* 1999; 159:821–826.

26. Ojajarvi J. Effectiveness of hand washing and disinfection methods in removing transient bacteria after patient nursing. *J Hyg* (London) 1980; 85:193–203.

27. Olsen RJ, Lynch P, Coyle MB, et al. Examination gloves as barriers to hand contamination in clinical practice. *JAMA* 1993; 270:350–353.

28. Tenorio AR, Badri SM, Sahgal NB, et al. Effectiveness of gloves in the prevention of hand carriage of vancomycin-resistant *Enterococcus* species by health care workers after patient care. *Clin Infect Dis* 2001; 32:826–829.

29. Lucet JC, Rigaud MP, Mentre F, et al. Hand contamination before and after different hand hygiene techniques: a randomized clinical trial. *J Hosp Infect* 2002; 50:276–280.

30. Doebbeling BN, Pfaller MA, Houston AK, Wenzel RP. Removal of nosocomial pathogens from the contaminated glove: implications for glove reuse and handwashing. *Ann Intern Med* 1988;109:394–398.

31. Pessoa-Silva CL, Dharan S, Hugonnet S, et al. Dynamics of bacterial hand contamination during routine neonatal care. *Infect Control Hosp Epidemiol* 2004; 25:192–197.

32. Musa EK, Desai N, Casewell MW. The survival of *Acinetobacter calcoaceticus* inoculated on fingertips and on formica. *J Hosp Infect* 1990; 15:219–227.

33. Fryklund B, Tullus K, Burman LG. Survival on skin and surfaces of epidemic and non epidemic strains of *Enterobacteria* from neonatal special care units. *J Hosp Infect* 1995; 29:201–208.

34. Doring G, Jansen S, Noll H, et al. Distribution and transmission of *Pseudomonas aeruginosa* and *Burkholderia cepacia* in a hospital ward. *Pediatr Pulmonol* 1996; 21:90–100.

35. Islam MS, Hossain MZ, Khan SI, et al. Detection of nonculturable *Shigella dysenteriae* 1 from artificially contaminated volunteers' fingers using fluorescent antibody and PCR techniques. *J Diarrhoeal Dis Rese* 1997; 15:65–70.

36. Noskin GA, Stosor V, Cooper I, Peterson LR. Recovery of vancomycin-resistant *Enterococci* on fingertips and environmental surfaces. *Infect Control Hosp Epidemiol* 1995; 16:577–581.

37. Ansari SA, Springthorpe VS, Sattar SA, et al. Potential role of hands in the spread of respiratory viral infections. studies with human *Parainfluenza virus 3* and *Rhinovirus 14*. *J Clin Microbiol* 1991; 29:2115–2119.

38. Ansari SA, Sattar SA, Springthorpe VS, et al. *Rotavirus* survival on human hands and transfer of infectious virus to animate and nonporous inanimate surfaces. *J Clin Microbiol* 1988; 26:1513–1518.

39. Trick WE, Vernon MO, Hayes RA, et al. Impact of ring wearing on hand contamination and comparison of hand hygiene agents in a hospital. *Clin Infect Dis* 2003; 36:1383–1390.

40. McNeil SA, Foster CL, Hedderwick SA, Kauffman CA. Effect of hand cleansing with antimicrobial soap or alcohol-based gel on microbial colonization of artificial fingernails worn by health care workers. *Clin Infect Dis* 2001; 32:367–72.

41. Gupta A, Della-Latta P, Todd B, et al. Outbreak of extended-spectrum beta-lactamase-producing *Klebsiella pneumoniae* in a neonatal intensive care unit linked to artificial nails. *Infect Control Hosp Epidemiol* 2004; 25:210–215.

42. Larson EL, Morton HE. Alcohols. In: Block SS, ed. *Disinfection, sterilization and preservation*. 4th ed. Philadelphia: Lea & Febiger, 1991; 191–203.

43. Price PB. Ethyl alcohol as a germicide. *Arch Surg* 1939; 38:528–542.

44. Harrington C, Walker H. The germicidal action of alcohol. *Boston Med Surg J* 1903; 148:548–552.

45. Coulthard CE, Sykes G. The germicidal effect of alcohol with special reference to its action on bacterial spores. *Pharm J* 1936; 137:79–81.

46. Pohle WD, Stuart LS. The germicidal action of cleaning agents—a study of a modification of Price's procedure. *J Infect Dis* 1940; 67:275–281.

47. Gardner AD. Rapid disinfection of clean unwashed skin. *Lancet* 1948:760–763.

48. Sakuragi T, Yanagisawa K, Dan K. Bactericidal activity of skin disinfectants on methicillin-resistant *Staphylococcus aureus*. *Anesthes Analg* 1995; 81:555–558.

49. Kampf G, Jarosch R, Ruden H. Limited effectiveness of chlorhexidine-based hand disinfectants against methicillin-resistant *Staphylococcus aureus* (MRSA). *J Hosp Infect* 1998; 38:297–303.

50. Kampf G, Hofer M, Wendt C. Efficacy of hand disinfectants against vancomycin-resistant *Enterococci in vitro*. *J Hosp Infect* 1999; 42:143–150.

51. Platt J, Bucknall RA. The disinfection of respiratory syncytial virus by isopropanol and a chlorhexidine-detergent handwash. *J Hosp Infect* 1985; 6:89–94.

52. Krilov LR, Hella Harkness S. Inactivation of respiratory syncytial virus by detergents and disinfectants. *Pediatr Infect Dis* 1993; 12:582–584.

53. Narang HK, Codd AA. Action of commonly used disinfectants against enteroviruses. *J Hosp Infect* 1983; 4:209–212.

54. Larson EL. APIC guideline for handwashing and hand antisepsis in health care settings. *Am J Infect Control* 1995; 23:251–269.

55. Gottardi W. Iodine and iodine compounds. In: Block SS, ed. *Disinfection, sterilization and preservation*. 4th ed. Philadelphia: Lea & Febiger, 1991; 152–166.

56. Goldenheim PD. *In vitro* efficacy of povidone-iodine solution and cream against methicillin-resistant *Staphylococcus aureus*. *Postgrad Med J* 1993; 69 (Suppl 3):S62–S65.

57. Traore O, Fournet F, Laveran H. An *in-vitro* evaluation of the activity of povidone-iodine against nosocomial bacterial strains. *J Hosp Infect* 1996; 34:217–222.

58. McLure AR, Gordon J. In-vitro evaluation of povidone-iodine and chlorhexidine against methicillin-resistant *Staphylococcus aureus*. *J Hosp Infect* 1992; 21:291–299.

59. Davies JG, Babb JR, Bradley CR. Preliminary study of test methods to assess the virucidal activity of skin disinfectants using *Poliovirus* and *bacteriophages*. *J Hosp Infect* 1993; 25:125–131.

60. Sattar SA, Tetro J, Springthorpe VS, Giulivi A. Preventing the spread of *Hepatitis B* and *C viruses*: where are germicides relevant? *Am J Infect Control* 2001; 29:187–197.

61. Ansari SA, Springthorpe VS, Sattar SA, et al. Comparison of cloth, paper, and warm air drying in eliminating viruses and bacteria from washed hands. *Am J Infect Control* 1991; 19:243–249.

62. Ansari SA, Sattar SA, Springthorpe VS, et al. *In vivo* protocol for testing efficacy of hand-washing agents against viruses and bacteria: experiments with *Rotavirus* and *Escherichia coli*. *App Environ Microbiol* 1989; 55:3113–3118.

63. Sattar SA, Abebe M, Bueti AJ, et al. Activity of an alcohol-based hand gel against human *Adeno-, Rhino-*, and *Rotaviruses* using the fingerpad method. *Infect Control Hosp Epidemiol* 2000; 21:516–519.

64. Wolff MH. *Hepatitis A virus*: a test method for virucidal activity. *J Hosp Infect* 2001; 48(Suppl A):S18–S22.

65. Steinmann J, Nehrkorn R, Meyer A, Becker K. Two in-vivo protocols for testing virucidal efficacy of handwashing and hand disinfection. *Zentralbl Hyg Umweltmed* 1995; 196:425–436.

66. Kampf G, Kramer A. Epidemiologic background of hand hygiene and evaluation of the most important agents for scrubs and rubs. *Clin Microbiol Rev* 2004;17:863–893.

67. Rotter ML. Hand washing and hand disinfection. In: Mayhall G, ed. *Hospital epidemiology and infection control*. Baltimore: Williams & Wilkins, 1996; 1052–1068.

68. Picheansathian W. A systematic review on the effectiveness of alcohol-based solutions for hand hygiene. *Int J Nurs Pract* 2004; 10:3–9.

69. Lowbury EJL, Lilly HA, Ayliffe GAJ. Preoperative disinfection of surgeon's hands: use of alcoholic solutions and effects of gloves on skin flora. *BMJ* 1974; 4:369–372.

70. Lowbury EJL, Lilly HA. Use of 4% chlorhexidine detergent solution (hibiscrub) and other methods of skin disinfection. *BMJ* 1973; 1:510–515.

71. Ayliffe GAJ, Babb JR, Quoraishi AH. A test for "hygienic" hand disinfection. *J Clin Pathol* 1978; 31:923–928.

72. Pereira LJ, Lee GM, Wade KJ. An evaluation of five protocols for surgical handwashing in relation to skin condition and microbial counts. *J Hosp Infect* 1997; 36:49–65.

73. Larson EL, Butz AM, Gullette DL, Laughon BA. Alcohol for surgical scrubbing? *Infect Control Hosp Epidemiol* 1990;11:139–143.

74. Aly R, Maibach HI. Comparative study on the antimicrobial effect of 0.5% chlorhexidine gluconate and 70% isopropyl alcohol on the normal flora of hands. *Appl Environmen Microbiol* 1979; 37:610–613.

75. Rosenberg A, Alatary SD, Peterson AF. Safety and efficacy of the antiseptic chlorhexidine gluconate. *Surg Gynecol Obstet* 1976; 143:789–792.

76. Rotter ML. Hygienic hand disinfection. *Inf Control* 1984; 1:18–22.

77. Anderson RL. Iodophor antiseptics: intrinsic microbial contamination with resistant bacteria. *Infect Control Hosp Epidemiol* 1989; 10:443–446.

78. Larson E. Guideline for use of topical antimicrobial agents. *Am J Infect Control* 1988; 16:253–266.

79. Larson E, Talbot GH. An approach for selection of health care personnel handwashing agents. *Inf Control* 1986; 7:419–424.

80. Gravens DL, Butcher HR, Jr., Ballinger WF, Dewar NE. Septisol antiseptic foam for hands of operating room personnel: an effective antibacterial agent. *Surgery* 1973; 73:360–367.

81. Lowbury EJL, Lilly HA, Bull JP. Disinfection of hands: removal of resident bacteria. *BMJ* 1963; 1:1251–1256.

82. Kundsin RB, Walter CW. The surgical scrub-practical consideration. *Arch Surg* 1973; 107:75–77.

83. Shuman RM, Leech RW, Alvord ECJ. Neurotoxicity of hexachlorophene in humans. II. A clinicopathological study of 46 premature infants. *Arch Neurol* 1975; 32:320–325.

84. Food and Drug Administration. Tentative final monograph for healthcare antiseptic drug products; proposed rule. *Fed Reg* 1994;59:31441–31452.

85. Kimbrough RD. Review of recent evidence of toxic effects of hexachlorophene. *Pediatr* 1973; 51:391–394.

86. EN 1499. Chemical disinfectants and antiseptics—hygienic hand wash—test method and requirements. In: European Committee for Standardization. 1997.

87. EN 1500. Chemical disinfectants and antiseptics—hygienic handrub—test method and requirements. In: European Committee for Standardization. 1997.

88. E 1174. Standard test method for evaluation of the effectiveness of health care personnel or consumer hand wash formulations. In: ASTM International. 1999.

89. Larson EGR, Pessoa-Silva CL, Boyce J, et al. Skin reactions related to hand hygiene and selection of hand hygiene products. *Am J Infect Control* 2006;34:627–635.

90. Tupker RA. Detergent and cleansers. In: van der Valk PGM, Maibach H., eds. *The irritant contact dermatitis syndrome*. New York: CRC Press, 1996; 71–76.

91. Larson E, Friedman C, Cohran J, et al. Prevalence and correlates of skin damage on the hands of nurses. *Heart Lung* 1997; 26:404–412.

92. Lubbe J, Ruffieux C, Van Melle G, Perrenoud D. Irritancy of the skin disinfectant n-propanol. *Contact Dermatitis* 2001; 45:226–231.

93. Ohlenschlaeger J, Friberg J, Ramsing D, Agner T. Temperature dependency of skin susceptibility to water and detergents. *Acta Derm Venereol* 1996; 76:274–276.

94. Emilson A, Lindbert M, Forslind B. The temperature effect of *in vitro* penetration of sodium lauryl sulfate and nickel chloride through human skin. *Acta Derm Venereol* 1993; 73:203–207.

95. Kownatzki E. Hand hygiene and skin health. *J Hosp Infect* 2003; 55:239–245.

96. Larson E, Leyden JJ, McGinley KJ, et al. Physiologic and microbiologic changes in skin related to frequent handwashing. *Infect Control* 1986; 7:59–63.

97. De Groot AC. Contact allergy to cosmetics: causative ingredients. *Contact Dermatitis* 1987;17:26–34.

98. Schnuch A, Uter W, Geier J, et al. Contact allergies in healthcare workers—results from the IVDK. *Acta Derm Venereol* 1998; 78:358–363.

99. Rastogi SC, Heydorn S, Johansen JD, Basketter DA. Fragrance chemicals in domestic and occupational products. *Contact Dermatitis* 2001; 45:221–225.

100. Uter W, Schnuch A, Geier J, et al. Association between occupation and contact allergy to the fragrance mix: a multifactorial analysis of national surveillance data. *Occup Environ Med* 2001; 58:392–398.

101. Ophaswongse S, Maibach HI. Alcohol dermatitis: allergic contact dermatitis and contact urticaria syndrome: a review. *Contact Dermatitis* 1994; 30:1–6.

102. Kanzaki T, Sakakibara N. Occupational allergic contact dermatitis from ethyl-2-bromo-p-methoxyphenylacetate. *Contact Dermatitis* 1992; 26:204–205.

103. Patruno C, Suppa F, Sarracco G, Balato N. Allergic contact dermatitis due to ethyl alcohol. *Contact Dermatitis* 1994; 31:124.

104. Okazawa H, Aihara M, Nagatani T, Nakajima H. Allergic contact dermatitis due to ethyl alcohol. *Contact Dermatitis* 1998; 38:233.

105. Rilliet A, Hunziker N, Brun R. Alcohol contact urticaria syndrome (immediate-type hypersensitivity). *Dermatol* 1980; 61:361–364.

106. Cimiotti J, Marmur ES, Nesin M, et al. Adverse reactions associated with an alcohol-based hand antiseptic among nurses in a neonatal intensive care unit. *Am J Infect Control* 2003; 31:43–48.

107. Pittet D, Hugonnet S, Harbarth S, et al. Effectiveness of a hospital-wide programme to improve compliance with hand hygiene. *Lancet* 2000; 356:1307–1312.

108. Larson EL, Early E, Cloonan P, et al. An organizational climate intervention associated with increased handwashing and decreased nosocomial infections. *Behavior Med* 2000; 26:14–22.

109. Conly JM, Hill S, Ross J, et al. Handwashing practices in an intensive care unit: the effects of an educational program and its relationship to infection rates. *Am J Infect Control* 1989; 17:330–339.

110. Dubbert PM, Dolce J, Richter W, et al. Increasing ICU staff handwashing: effects of education and group feedback. *Infect Control Hosp Epidemiol* 1990; 11:191–193.

111. Raju TN, Kobler C. Improving handwashing habits in the newborn nurseries. *Am J Med Sci* 1991; 302:355–358.

112. Tibballs J. Teaching hospital medical staff to handwash. *Med J Aust* 1996; 164:395–398.

113. Harbarth S, Pittet D, Grady L, et al. Interventional study to evaluate the impact of an alcohol-based hand gel in improving hand hygiene compliance. *Pediatr Inf Dis J* 2002; 21:489–495.

114. Lam BC, Lee J, Lau YL. Hand hygiene practices in a neonatal intensive care unit: a multimodal intervention and impact on nosocomial infection. *Pediatrics* 2004; 114:e565–571.

115. Larson EL, Bryan JL, Adler LM, Blane C. A multifaceted approach to changing handwashing behavior. *Am J Infect Control* 1997; 25:3–10.

116. Rosenthal VD, McCormick RD, Guzman S, et al. Effect of education and performance feedback on handwashing: the benefit of administrative support in Argentinean hospitals. *Am J Infect Control* 2003; 31:85–92.

117. Won SP, Chou HC, Hsieh WS, et al. Handwashing program for the prevention of nosocomial infections in a neonatal intensive care unit. *Infect Control Hosp Epidemiol* 2004; 25:742–746.

118. Pittet D, Boyce JM. Revolutionising hand hygiene in health-care settings: guidelines revisited. *Lancet Infect Dis* 2003; 3:269–270.

119. Colombo C, Giger H, Grote J, et al. Impact of teaching interventions on nurse compliance with hand disinfection. *J Hosp Infect* 2002; 51:69–72.

120. Bischoff WE, Reynolds TM, Sessler CN, et al. Handwashing compliance by health care workers: The impact of introducing an accessible, alcohol based hand antiseptic. *Arch Intern Med* 2000; 160:1017–1021.

121. Hugonnet S, Perneger TV, Pittet D. Alcohol-based handrub improves compliance with hand hygiene in intensive care units. *Arch Intern Med* 2002; 162:1037–1043.

122. van de Mortel T, Murgo M. An examination of covert observation and solution audit as tools to measure the success of hand hygiene interventions. *Am J Infect Control* 2006; 34:95–99.

123. Pittet D, Mourouga P, Perneger TV. Compliance with handwashing in a teaching hospital. *Ann Intern Med* 1999; 130:126–130.

124. Pittet D, Stephan F, Hugonnet S, et al. Hand-cleansing during postanesthesia care. *Anesthesiol* 2003; 99:530–535.

125. Pittet D, Simon A, Hugonnet S, et al. Hand hygiene among physicians: performance, beliefs, and perceptions. *Ann Intern Med* 2004; 141:1–8.

126. O'Boyle CA, Henly SJ, Larson E. Understanding adherence to hand hygiene recommendations: the theory of planned behavior. *Am J Infect Control* 2001; 29:352–360.

127. NPSA/PASA. Hand hygiene project. In: *NPSA/PASA Reports & Documents*, 2004 (http://www.npsa.nhs.uk/cleanyourhands/ resources/documents) accessed 19 July 2006.

128. Pittet D. Improving compliance with hand hygiene in hospitals. *Infect Control Hosp Epidemiol* 2000; 21:381–386.

129. Pittet D. The Lowbury lecture: behaviour in infection control. *J Hosp Infect* 2004; 58:1–13.

130. Pittet D. Promotion of hand hygiene: magic, hype, or scientific challenge? *Infect Control Hosp Epidemiol* 2002; 23:118–119.

131. Pittet D. Improving adherence to hand hygiene practice: a multidisciplinary approach. *Emerg Infect Dis* 2001; 7:234–240.

132. Naikoba S, Hayward A. The effectiveness of interventions aimed at increasing handwashing in healthcare workers—a systematic review. *J Hosp Infect* 2001; 47:173–180.

133. Muto CA, Sistrom MG, Farr BM. Hand hygiene rates unaffected by installation of dispensers of a rapidly acting hand antiseptic. *Am J Infect Control* 2000; 28:273–276.

134. Maury E, Alzieu M, Baudel JL, et al. Availability of an alcohol solution can improve hand disinfection compliance in an intensive care unit. *Am J Resp Crit Care Med* 2000; 162:324–327.

135. Girard R, Amazian K, Fabry J. Better compliance and better tolerance in relation to a well-conducted introduction to rub-in hand disinfection. *J Hosp Infect* 2001; 47:131–137.

136. Gopal Rao G, Jeanes A, Osman M, et al. Marketing hand hygiene in hospitals—a case study. *J Hosp Infect* 2002; 50:42–47.

137. Brown SM, Lubimova AV, Khrustalyeva NM, et al. Use of an alcohol-based hand rub and quality improvement interventions to improve hand hygiene in a Russian neonatal intensive care unit. *Infect Control Hosp Epidemiol* 2003; 24:172–179.

138. Zafar AB, Butler RC, Reese DJ, et al. Use of 0.3% triclosan (Bacti-Stat) to eradicate an outbreak of methicillin-resistant *Staphylococcus aureus* in a neonatal nursery. *Am J Infect Control* 1995; 23:200–208.

139. Harbarth S, Sudre P, Dharan S, et al. Outbreak of *Enterobacter cloacae* related to understaffing, overcrowding, and poor hygiene practices. *Infect Control Hosp Epidemiol* 1999; 20:598–603.

140. Webster J. Handwashing in a neonatal intensive care nursery: product acceptability and effectiveness of chlorhexidine gluconate 4% and triclosan 1%. *J Hosp Infect* 1992; 21:137–141.

141. Boyce JM. It is time for action: improving hand hygiene in hospitals. *Ann Intern Med* 1999; 130:153–155.

142. Kretzer EK, Larson EL. Behavioral interventions to improve infection control practices. *Am J Infect Control* 1998; 26:245–253.

143. Kelen GD, Green GB, Hexter DA, Fortenberry DC. Substantial improvement in compliance with universal precautions in an emergency department following institution of policy. *Arch Intern Med* 1991; 151:2051–2056.

144. Lundberg GD. Changing physician behavior in ordering diagnostic tests. *JAMA* 1998; 280:2036.

145. Phillips DF. "New look" reflects changing style of patient safety environment. *JAMA* 1999; 281:217–219.

146. Berg DE, Hershow RC, Ramirez CA. Control of nosocomial infections in an intensive care unit in Guatemala City. *Clin Infect Dis* 1995; 21:588–593.

147. Avila-Aguero ML, Umana MA, Jimenez AL, et al. Handwashing practices in a tertiary-care, pediatric hospital and the effect on an educational program. *Clin Perform Qual Health Care* 1998; 6:70–2.

148. Maury E, Alzieu M, Baudel JL, et al. Availability of an alcohol solution can improve hand disinfection compliance in an intensive care unit. *Am J Respir Crit Care Med* 2000; 162:324–7.

149. Girou E, Oppein F. Handwashing compliance in a French university hospital: new perspective with the introduction of hand-rubbing with a waterless alcohol-based solution. *J Hosp Infect* 2001; 48 (Suppl A):S55–S57.

150. Creedon SA. Health care workers' hand decontamination practices: an Irish study. *Clin Nurs Res* 2006; 15:6–26.

151. Eldridge NE, Woods SS, Bonello RS, et al. Using the six sigma process to implement the Centers for Disease Control and

Prevention Guideline for Hand Hygiene in 4 intensive care units. *J Gen Intern Med* 2006; 21 (Suppl 2):S35–S42.

152. Gordin FM, Schultz ME, Huber RA, Gill JA. Reduction in nosocomial transmission of drug-resistant bacteria after introduction of an alcohol-based handrub. *Infect Control Hosp Epidemiol* 2005; 26:650–3.

153. Zerr DM, Allpress AL, Heath J, et al. Decreasing hospital-associated rotavirus infection: a multidisciplinary hand hygiene campaign in a children's hospital. *Pediatr Infect Dis J* 2005; 24:397–403.

154. Rosenthal VD, Guzman S, Safdar N. Reduction in nosocomial infection with improved hand hygiene in intensive care units of a tertiary care hospital in Argentina. *Am J Infect Control* 2005; 33:392–7.

155. Johnson PD, Martin R, Burrell LJ, et al. Efficacy of an alcohol/chlorhexidine hand hygiene program in a hospital with high rates of nosocomial methicillin-resistant *Staphylococcus aureus* (MRSA) infection. *Med J Aust* 2005; 183:505–514.

156. Aspock C, Koller W. A simple hand hygiene exercise. *Am J Infect Control* 1999; 27:370–372.

157. Graham M. Frequency and duration of handwashing in an intensive care unit. *Am J Infect Control* 1990; 18:77–81.

158. Resnick L, Veren K, Salahuddin SZ, et al. Stability and inactivation of HTLV-III/LAV under clinical and laboratory environments. *JAMA* 1986; 255:1887–1891.

159. Swoboda SM, Earsing K, Strauss K, et al. Electronic monitoring and voice prompts improve hand hygiene and decrease nosocomial infections in an intermediate care unit. *Crit Care Med* 2004; 32:358–363.

160. McGuckin M, Waterman R, Porten L, et al. Patient education model for increasing handwashing compliance. *Am J Infect Control* 1999; 27:309–314.

161. McGuckin M, Waterman R, Storr IJ, et al. Evaluation of a patient-empowering hand hygiene programme in the UK. *J Hosp Infect* 2001; 48:222–227.

162. Simmons B, Bryant J, Neiman K, et al. The role of handwashing in prevention of endemic intensive care unit infections. *Infect Control Hosp Epidemiol* 1990; 11:589–594.

163. Avila-Aguero ML, Umana MA, Jimenez AL, et al. Handwashing practices in a tertiary-care, pediatric hospital and the effect on an educational program. *Clin Perform Qual Health Care* 1998; 6:70–72.

164. Khatib M, Jamaleddine G, Abdallah A, Ibrahim Y. Hand washing and use of gloves while managing patients receiving mechanical ventilation in the ICU. *Chest* 1999; 116:172–175.

165. MacDonald A, Dinah F, MacKenzie D, Wilson A. Performance feedback of hand hygiene, using alcohol gel as the skin decontaminant, reduces the number of inpatients newly affected by MRSA and antibiotic costs. *J Hosp Infect* 2004; 56:56–63.

166. Larson E. Skin hygiene and infection prevention: more of the same or different approaches? *Clin Infect Dis* 1999; 29:1287–1294.

167. Doebbeling BN, Stanley GL, Sheetz CT, et al. Comparative efficacy of alternative hand-washing agents in reducing nosocomial infections in intensive care units. *New Engl J Med* 1992; 327:88–93.

168. Larson E, Killien M. Factors influencing handwashing behavior of patient care personnel. *Am J Infect Control* 1982; 10: 93–99.

169. Zimakoff J, Kjelsberg AB, Larsen SO, Holstein B. A multicenter questionnaire investigation of attitudes toward hand hygiene, assessed by the staff in fifteen hospitals in Denmark and Norway. *Am J Infect Control* 1992; 20:58–64.

170. Thomas M, Gillespie W, Krauss J, Harrison S, et al. Focus group data as a tool in assessing effectiveness of a hand hygiene campaign. *Am J Infect Control* 2005; 33:368–373.

171. Pettinger A, Nettleman MD. Epidemiology of isolation precautions. *Infect Control Hosp Epidemiol* 1991; 12:303–307.

172. Haley RW, Bregman D. The role of understaffing and overcrowding in recurrent outbreaks of staphylococcal infection in a neonatal special-care unit. *J Infect Dis* 1982; 145:875–885.

173. Pittet D, Boyce JM. Hand hygiene and patient care: pursuing the Semmelweis legacy. *Lancet Inf Dis* 2001:9–20.

174. Hilburn J, Hammond BS, Fendler EJ, Groziak PA. Use of alcohol hand sanitizer as an infection control strategy in an acute care facility. *Am J Infect Control* 2003; 31:109–116.

Personnel Health Services

4

Elise M. Beltrami and Elizabeth A. Bolyard

Healthcare personnel (HCP) are at risk of exposure to infectious diseases in both the workplace and the community. If they develop an infection, they may pose a risk for transmission of that infectious pathogen to patients, other HCP, members of their households, or other community contacts. In this chapter, the term health care personnel refers to all paid and unpaid persons working in healthcare settings who have the potential for exposure to infectious materials, including body substances and contaminated medical supplies, equipment, environmental surfaces, or air. In general, HCP inside or outside hospitals who have contact with patients, body fluids, or specimens have a higher risk of acquiring or transmitting pathogens than do other HCP who have only brief casual contact with patients and their environment (e.g., beds, furniture, bathrooms, food trays, or medical equipment).

This chapter outlines the infection control elements of a personnel health service and discusses important aspects of selected transmissible diseases excluding hepatitis B virus (HBV) infection, hepatitis C virus infection, and human immunodeficiency virus (HIV) infection, which are discussed in Chapter 42, Bloodborne Pathogen Prevention.

INFECTION CONTROL ELEMENTS OF A PERSONNEL HEALTH SERVICE

Whether performed "in house" or contracted out, certain elements are necessary for the appropriate functioning of a personnel health service: (a) coordination with other departments, (b) pre-employment or placement medical evaluations, (c) health and safety education, (d) immunization programs, (e) management of job-related illnesses and exposures to infectious pathogens, including policies for work restrictions for infected or exposed personnel, (f) counseling services for personnel on infection risks related to employment or special conditions, and (g) maintenance and confidentiality of personnel health records.

The organization of a personnel health service can be influenced by the size of the institution, the number of personnel, and the services offered. To ensure that contractual personnel who are not paid by the healthcare facility receive appropriate personnel health services, contractual agreements with their employers should contain provisions consistent with the policies of the facility that uses those employees. Personnel with specialized training and qualifications in occupational health can facilitate the provision of effective services.

Coordination with Other Departments

For infection control objectives to be achieved, the activities of the personnel health service must be coordinated with infection control and other appropriate departmental personnel. This coordination will help ensure adequate surveillance of infections in personnel and provision of preventive services. Coordination of activities also will help to ensure that investigations of exposures and outbreaks are conducted efficiently and preventive measures implemented promptly.

Placement Medical Evaluations

Medical evaluations before employee placement can ensure that personnel are not placed in jobs that would pose undue risk of infection to them, other personnel, patients, or visitors. An important component of the placement evaluation is a health inventory. This includes determining immunization status and obtaining histories of any conditions that could predispose personnel to acquiring or transmitting infectious diseases.

A physical examination can be used to screen personnel for conditions that could increase the risk of transmitting pathogens or acquiring work-related diseases and can serve as a baseline for determining whether future diseases are work related. However, the cost effectiveness of routine physical examinations, including laboratory testing (e.g., complete blood cell counts, urinalysis, and chest radiographs) and screening for enteric or other pathogens for infection control purposes, has not been demonstrated. Conversely, screening for some vaccine-preventable diseases, such as HBV, measles, mumps, rubella, or varicella, could be cost effective. In general, the health inventory can be used to guide decisions regarding physical examinations or laboratory tests. However, some local public health ordinances could mandate that certain screening procedures be used. Periodic evaluations may be done as indicated for job reassignment, for ongoing programs (e.g., tuberculosis [TB] screening), or for evaluation of work-related problems.

Personnel Health and Safety Education

Personnel are more likely to comply with an infection control program if they understand its rationale. Thus, personnel education is an important element of an effective infection control program. Clearly written policies, guidelines, and procedures ensure uniformity, efficiency, and effective coordination of activities. However, because the risk of infection varies by job category, infection control education should be tailored accordingly. In addition, some HCP may need specialized education on infection risks related to their employment and on preventive measures that will reduce those risks. Furthermore, educational materials need to be appropriate in content and vocabulary to the educational level, literacy, and language of the employee. The training should comply with existing federal, state, and local regulations regarding requirements for employee education and training. All HCP need to be educated about the organization's infection control policies and procedures.

Immunization Programs

Ensuring that personnel are immune to vaccine-preventable diseases is an essential part of successful personnel health programs. Optimal use of vaccines can prevent transmission of vaccine-preventable diseases and eliminate unnecessary work restriction. Prevention of illness through comprehensive personnel immunization programs is far more cost-effective than case management and outbreak control. In particular, interventions to increase influenza vaccination of HCP have been shown to be effective [1]. Mandatory immunization programs, which include both newly hired and currently employed persons, are more effective than voluntary programs in ensuring that susceptible persons are vaccinated [2].

National guidelines for immunization of and postexposure prophylaxis (PEP) for HCP are provided by the U.S. Public Health Service's Advisory Committee on Immunization Practices (ACIP) [3–18].

Screening tests are available to determine susceptibility to certain vaccine-preventable diseases (e.g., HBV, measles, mumps, rubella, and varicella). Such screening programs should be combined with tracking systems to ensure accurate maintenance of personnel immunization records. Accurate immunization records ensure that susceptible personnel are promptly identified and appropriately vaccinated. For more details about vaccinations for HCP, see Vaccinations in Patients and Healthcare Workers.

Management of Job-Related Illnesses and Exposures

Primary functions of the personnel health service are to arrange for prompt diagnosis and management of job-related illnesses and to provide appropriate PEP after job-related exposures. It is the responsibility of the healthcare organization to implement measures to prevent further transmission of pathogens, which sometimes warrants exclusion of personnel from work or patient contact [19]. Decisions about work restrictions are based on the mode of transmission and the epidemiology of the disease (Table 4-1). The term exclude from duty in this chapter should be interpreted as exclusion from the healthcare facility and from healthcare activities outside the facility. Personnel who are excluded should avoid contact with susceptible persons both in the facility and in the community. Exclusion policies should include a statement of authority defining who may exclude personnel. The policies also need to be designed to encourage personnel to report their illnesses or exposures, not to penalize them with loss of wages, benefits, or job status. Workers' compensation laws do not cover exclusion from duty for exposures to infectious diseases; therefore, policies should include a method for providing wages during the period that HCP are not able to work. In addition, exclusion policies must be enforceable, and all HCP, especially department heads, supervisors, and nurse managers, should know which infections warrant exclusion and where to report the illnesses 24 hours a day, 7 days a week. HCP who have contact with infectious patients outside the healthcare setting also need to be included in the postexposure program and encouraged to report any suspected or known exposures promptly.

TABLE 4-1

SUMMARY OF SUGGESTED WORK RESTRICTIONS FOR HEALTHCARE PERSONNEL EXPOSED TO OR INFECTED WITH INFECTIOUS DISEASES OF IMPORTANCE IN HEALTHCARE SETTINGS, IN THE ABSENCE OF STATE AND LOCAL REGULATIONS. (MODIFIED FROM BOLYARD EA, TABLAN OC, WILLIAMS WW, ET AL. GUIDELINE FOR INFECTION CONTROL IN HEALTH CARE PERSONNEL, 1998. *INFECT CONTROL HOSP EPIDEMIOL* 1998;19:407–63)

Disease/Problem	Work Restriction	Duration
Conjunctivitis	Restrict from patient contact and contact with the patient's environment	Until discharge ceases
Cytomegalovirus infections	No restriction	
Diarrheal diseases		
Acute stage (diarrhea with other symptoms)	Restrict from patient contact, contact with the patient's environment, or food handling	Until symptoms resolve
Convalescent stage, *Salmonella* spp.	Restrict from care of high-risk patients	Until symptoms resolve; consult with local and state health authorities regarding need for negative stool cultures
Hepatitis A	Restrict from patient contact, contact with patient's environment, and food handling	Until 7 days after onset of jaundice
Herpes simplex Hands (herpetic whitlow)	Restrict from patient contact and contact with the patient's environment	Until lesions heal
Measles Active	Exclude from duty	Until 7 days after the rash appears
Postexposure (susceptible personnel)	Exclude from duty	From the 5th day after the 1st exposure through the 21st day after last exposure
Meningococcal infections	Exclude from duty	Until 24 hours after start of effective therapy
Mumps Active	Exclude from duty	Until 9 days after onset of parotitis
Postexposure (susceptible personnel)	Exclude from duty	From 12th day after 1st exposure through until 25 days after last exposure or until 9 days after onset of parotitis
Pertussis Active	Exclude from duty	From beginning of catarrhal stage through 3rd week after onset of paroxysms or until 5 days after start of effective antimicrobial therapy
Postexposure (asymptomatic personnel)	No restriction, prophylaxis recommended	
Postexposure (symptomatic personnel)	Exclude from duty	Until 5 days after start of effective antimicrobial therapy
Rubella Active	Exclude from duty	Until 5 days after rash appears
Postexposure (susceptible personnel)	Exclude from duty	From 7th day after 1st exposure through 21st day after last exposure
Staphylococcus aureus infection	Restrict from contact with patients and patient's environment or food handling	Until lesions have resolved
Active, draining skin lesions		
Tuberculosis		
Active disease	Exclude from duty	Until proved noninfectious
TST converter	No restriction	
Varicella Active	Exclude from duty	Until all lesions dry and crust
Postexposure (susceptible personnel)	Exclude from duty	From 10th day after 1st exposure through 21st day (28th day if VZIG given) after last exposure
Viral respiratory infections, acute febrile	Consider excluding from the care of high risk patients or contact with their environment during community outbreak of RSV and influenza	Until acute symptoms resolve
Zoster		
Localized, in healthy person	Cover lesions; restrict from care of high-risk patients	Until all lesions dry and crust
Generalized or localized in immunosuppressed person	Restrict from patient contact	Until all lesions dry and crust
Postexposure (susceptible personnel)	Restrict from patient contact	From 10th day after 1st exposure through 21st day (28th day if VariZIG given) after last exposure or, if varicella occurs, until all lesions dry and crust

Health Counseling

Access to adequate health counseling for HCP is another crucial element of an effective personnel health service. Health counseling allows personnel to receive individually targeted information regarding (a) the risk and prevention of occupationally acquired infections, (b) the risk of illness or other adverse outcome after exposure, (c) management of exposure, including the risks and benefits of PEP regimens, and (d) the potential consequences of exposure or communicable disease for family members, patients, or other personnel, both inside and outside the healthcare facility.

Maintenance of Records, Data Management, and Confidentiality

Maintenance of records related to medical evaluations, immunizations, exposures, PEP, and screening tests in a retrievable, preferably computerized, database allows efficient monitoring of the health status of HCP. Such record keeping also helps to ensure that the organization will provide consistent and appropriate services to HCP.

Individual records for all HCP should be maintained in accordance with the Occupational Safety and Health Administration (OSHA) medical records standard, which requires the employer to retain records, maintain employee confidentiality, and provide records to employees when they ask to review them [20]. In addition, the OSHA "Occupational Exposure to Bloodborne Pathogens; Final Rule" [21] requires employers, including healthcare facilities, to establish and maintain an accurate, confidential record for each employee with occupational exposure to bloodborne pathogens. The standard also requires that each employer ensure that it maintain employee medical records for at least the duration of the worker's employment plus 30 years.

Occupational health departments need to protect and safeguard protected health information as defined by the Health Insurance Portability and Accountability Act of 1996 (HIPAA) and the American Disabilities Act (ADA) [22]. Information about injuries and communicable diseases may be disclosed to public health authorities for the purpose of preventing or controlling disease, injury, or disability.

EPIDEMIOLOGY AND CONTROL OF SELECTED INFECTIONS TRANSMITTED AMONG HOSPITAL PERSONNEL AND PATIENTS

The following section provides more detail about selected infectious pathogens and conditions that can be transmitted in the healthcare setting. These pathogens and conditions could require consideration for employee placement or work restrictions. Bloodborne pathogens, including HBV, hepatitis C virus, and HIV, are not included here but are discussed in Chapter 42, Bloodborne Pathogen Prevention.

Conjunctivitis

Although conjunctivitis can be caused by a variety of bacteria and viruses, adenovirus has been the primary cause of healthcare-associated outbreaks of conjunctivitis. Healthcare-associated outbreaks have primarily occurred in eye clinics or offices but also have been reported in neonatal intensive care units and long-term care facilities [23–27]. The incubation period ranges from 5 to 12 days, and shedding of virus occurs from late in the incubation period to as long as 14 days after onset of disease [24]. Adenovirus survives for long periods on environmental surfaces; ophthalmologic instruments and equipment can become contaminated and be a source of transmission. Contaminated hands also are a major source of person-to-person transmission of adenovirus, both from patients to HCP and from HCP to patients. Hand hygiene, glove use, and disinfection of instruments can prevent the transmission of adenovirus [23,24]. Infected personnel should not provide patient care for the duration of symptoms after onset of purulent conjunctivitis caused by adenovirus or other pathogens [24,25].

Cytomegalovirus

There are two principal reservoirs of cytomegalovirus (CMV) in healthcare institutions: (a) infants and young children infected with CMV and (b) immunocompromised patients for example, those undergoing solid-organ or bone-marrow transplantation or those with acquired immunodeficiency syndrome (AIDS) [28,29]. However, HCP who provide care to such high-risk patients have a rate of primary CMV infection that is no higher than that among personnel without such patient contact (3% vs. 2%) [30–34].

CMV transmission appears to occur directly either through close, intimate contact with a person excreting CMV or through contact with contaminated secretions or excretions, especially saliva or urine [33,35,36]. Transmission by the hands of HCP or infected persons also has been suggested [29,37]. The incubation period for person-to-person transmission is not known. Although CMV can survive on environmental surfaces and other objects for short periods [38], there is no evidence that the environment plays a role in the transmission of this pathogen [29].

Because infection with CMV during pregnancy may have adverse effects on the fetus, women of childbearing age need to be counseled regarding the risks and prevention of transmission of CMV in both nonoccupational and occupational settings [39]. No studies clearly indicate that sero-negative HCP can be protected from infection by transfer to areas with less contact with patients likely to be reservoirs for CMV [28–30,34].

Serologic or virologic screening programs to identify CMV-infected patients or sero-negative female personnel of childbearing age are impractical and costly for the following reasons: (a) the virus can be intermittently shed [40], and repeated screening tests could be needed to identify shedders, (b) sero-positivity for CMV does not offer complete protection against maternal re-infection or reactivation and subsequent fetal infection [28], and (c) no currently available vaccines or prophylactic therapy for HCP can provide protection against primary infection.

Work restrictions for personnel who contract CMV illnesses are not necessary. The risk of transmission of CMV can be reduced by careful adherence to hand hygiene and Standard Precautions [28,41].

Diphtheria

Healthcare-associated transmission of diphtheria among patients and personnel has been reported [42–44]. HCP are not at substantially higher risk than the general adult population for acquiring diphtheria.

Prevention of diphtheria is best accomplished by maintaining high levels of diphtheria immunity among children and adults [13,45,46]. Immunization with tetanus and diphtheria toxoid (Td) is recommended every 10 years for all adults who have completed the primary immunization series [4,13]. HCP directly exposed to oral secretions of patients infected with *Corynebacterium diphtheriae* should be evaluated in consultation with local public health authorities.

Gastroenteritis

Gastrointestinal infections may be caused by a variety of agents, including bacteria, viruses, and protozoa. However, only a few agents have been documented in healthcare-associated transmission, such as *Salmonella typhimurium*, *Yersinia enterocolitica*, *Escherichia coli*, and norovirus [47–58]. Healthcare-associated transmission of agents that cause gastrointestinal infections usually results from contact with infected individuals [47,53,59], from consumption of contaminated food, water, or other beverages [47,59,60], or from exposure to contaminated objects or environmental surfaces [48,61]. Inadequate HCP hand hygiene [62] and inadequate sterilization or disinfection of patient-care equipment and environmental surfaces increase the likelihood of transmission of agents that cause gastrointestinal infections. Generally, adherence to good hand hygiene by HCP before and after all contacts with patients and food and to either Standard or Contact Precautions [4] will minimize the risk of transmitting enteric pathogens [55,63].

Laboratory personnel who handle infectious materials also may be at risk for occupational acquisition of gastrointestinal infections, most commonly with *Salmonella typhi*.

Personnel who acquire an acute gastrointestinal illness (defined as vomiting, diarrhea, or both, with or without associated symptoms such as fever, nausea, and abdominal pain) are likely to have high concentrations of the infecting agent in their feces (bacteria, viruses, and parasites) or vomitus (viruses and parasites). It is important to determine the etiology of gastrointestinal illness in HCP who care for patients at high risk for severe disease (e.g., neonates, elderly persons, and immunocompromised patients). The initial evaluation of personnel with gastroenteritis needs to include a thorough history and determination of the need for specific laboratory tests, such as stool or blood cultures, stool staining procedures, or serologic or antigen-antibody tests [54,61,64].

Restriction from patient care and the patient's environment or from food handling is indicated for HCP with diarrhea or acute gastrointestinal symptoms regardless of the causative agent [41,61]. Some local and state agencies have regulations that require work exclusion for HCP, food handlers, or both who have gastrointestinal infections caused by *Salmonella* or *Shigella* spp. These regulations may require such personnel to be restricted from duty until results of at least two consecutive stool cultures obtained at least 24 hours apart are negative.

Hepatitis A

Healthcare-associated hepatitis A occurs infrequently, and transmission to HCP usually occurs when the source-patient has unrecognized hepatitis and is fecally incontinent or has diarrhea [65–72]. Other risk factors for hepatitis A virus (HAV) transmission to personnel include activities that increase the risk of fecal-oral contamination such as (a) eating or drinking in patient-care areas [65,67,69,73], (b) not washing hands after handling an infected infant [67,73,74], and (c) sharing food, beverages, or cigarettes with patients, their families, or other staff members [65,67].

HAV is transmitted primarily by the fecal-oral route. The incubation period for HAV is 15 to 50 days. Fecal excretion of HAV is greatest during the incubation period of disease before the onset of jaundice. Once disease is clinically obvious, the risk of pathogen transmission is decreased. However, some patients admitted to the hospital with HAV, particularly immunocompromised patients, can still be shedding virus because of prolonged or relapsing disease, and such patients are potentially infectious [66]. Fecal shedding of HAV, formerly believed to continue only as long as 2 weeks after onset of dark urine, has been shown to occur as late as 6 months after diagnosis of infection in premature infants [65]. Anicteric infection is typical in young children and infants [75].

HCP can protect themselves and others from infection with HAV by adhering to Standard Precautions [41].

Three inactivated HAV vaccines are now available and provide long-term pre-exposure protection against clinical infection with >94% efficacy [75]. Routine administration of HAV vaccine in HCP is not recommended. However, vaccine may be useful for personnel working or living in areas where HAV is highly endemic and is indicated for personnel who handle HAV-infected primates or are exposed to HAV in a research laboratory. The role of HAV vaccine in controlling outbreaks has not been adequately investigated [4]. Immune globulin given within 2 weeks after an HAV exposure is 80% to 90% effective in preventing HAV infection [75] and may be advisable in some outbreak situations [4,75].

Restriction from patient-care areas or food handling is indicated for personnel with HAV infection. They may return to regular duties one week after onset of the illness [4].

Herpes Simplex

Healthcare-associated transmission of herpes simplex virus (HSV) is rare. It has been reported in nurseries [76–78] and intensive care units [79,80] where high-risk patients (e.g., neonates, patients with severe malnutrition, patients with severe burns or eczema, and immunocompromised patients) are located. Healthcare-associated transmission of HSV occurs primarily through contact either with primary or recurrent lesions or with virus-containing secretions, such as saliva, vaginal secretions, or amniotic fluid [77,79,81]. Exposed areas of skin are the most likely sites of infection, particularly when minor cuts, abrasions, or other skin lesions are present [80]. The incubation period of HSV is 2–14 days [82]. The duration of viral shedding has not been well defined [83].

HCP can acquire a herpetic infection of the fingers (herpetic whitlow or paronychia) from exposure to contaminated oral secretions [80,81]. Such exposures are a distinct hazard for nurses, anesthesiologists, dentists, respiratory care personnel, and other personnel who have direct (usually hand) contact with either oral lesions or respiratory secretions from patients [80]. Less frequently, HCP may acquire mucocutaneous infection on other body sites from contact with infectious body secretions [84].

HCP with active HSV infection of the hands (herpetic whitlow) can potentially transmit the pathogen to patients with whom they have contact [81]. Transmission of HSV from HCP with orofacial HSV infection to patients also has been infrequently documented [76]; however, the magnitude of this risk is unknown [78,85]. Although asymptomatic HSV-infected persons can shed the virus, they are less infectious than persons with active lesions [83,86].

HCP can protect themselves from acquiring HSV by adhering to Standard Precautions [41]. The risk of transmission of HSV from personnel with orofacial infections to patients can be reduced by performing hand hygiene before all patient care and by the use of appropriate barriers (e.g., a mask or gauze dressing) to prevent hand contact with the lesion.

Because HCP with orofacial lesions could touch their lesions and potentially transmit HSV, they should be evaluated to determine their potential for transmitting HSV to patients at high risk for serious disease (e.g., neonates, patients with severe malnutrition, patients with severe burns or eczema, and immunocompromised patients) and excluded from the care of such patients as indicated. The evaluation also should consider the extent of the lesion and the severity of illness in the patient population that personnel will contact. Personnel with HSV infections of the fingers or hands can more easily transmit HSV and therefore need to be excluded from patient care until their lesions have crusted. In addition, herpetic lesions can be secondarily infected by *Staphylococcus* or *Streptococcus spp.*, and HCP with such infections should be evaluated to determine whether they need to be excluded from patient contact until the secondary infection has resolved. There have been no reports that personnel with genital HSV infections have transmitted HSV to patients; therefore, work restrictions for personnel with genital herpes are not indicated.

Measles

Healthcare-associated transmission of measles virus has been well described [87–92]. Measles is transmitted both by large droplets during close contact between infected and susceptible persons and by the airborne route [93]. Measles is highly transmissible and frequently misdiagnosed during the prodromal stage. The incubation period for measles is 5–21 days. Immunocompetent persons with measles shed the virus from the nasopharynx, beginning with the prodrome until 3 to 4 days after rash onset; immunocompromised persons with measles could shed virus for extended periods [94].

Strategies to prevent healthcare-associated transmission of measles include (a) documentation of measles immunity in HCP, (b) prompt identification and isolation of persons with fever and rash, and (c) adherence to airborne precautions for suspected and proven patients with measles [41].

It is essential that all HCP have documentation of measles immunity regardless of their length of employment or whether they are involved in patient care. Although persons born before 1957 are generally considered to be immune to measles, serologic studies indicate that 5% to 9% of HCP born before 1957 may not be immune [4,95]. Consideration should be given to recommending a dose of measles-mumps-rubella trivalent vaccine (MMR) to personnel born before 1957 who are unvaccinated and who lack (a) a history of previous measles disease, (b) documentation of receipt of one dose of live measles vaccine, or (c) serologic evidence of measles immunity [3]. HCP born during or after 1957 should be considered immune to measles when they have (a) documentation of physician-diagnosed measles, (b) documentation of two doses of live measles vaccine on or after their first birthday, or (c) serologic evidence of measles immunity (persons with an "indeterminate" level of immunity on testing should be considered susceptible). Persons born between 1957 and 1984 who received childhood measles immunization and were given only one dose of vaccine during infancy could require a second dose of vaccine [2].

Work restrictions are necessary for HCP who acquire measles; they need to be excluded from duty for 7 days after the rash appears. Likewise, HCP not immune to measles need to be excluded from duty from 5 days after the first exposure to 21 days after the last exposure to measles.

Meningococcal Disease

Healthcare-associated transmission of *Neisseria meningitidis* is rare. When proper precautions were not used, *N. meningitidis* has been transmitted from patient to personnel through contact with the respiratory secretions of patients with meningococcemia or meningococcal meningitis or through handling laboratory specimens [96].

N. meningitidis infection usually is transmitted by close contact with aerosols or secretions from the human nasopharynx; the incubation period is from 2–10 days, and patients infected with *N. meningitidis* are rendered noninfectious by 24 hours of effective therapy. HCP who care for patients with suspected *N. meningitidis* infection can decrease their risk of infection by adhering to Droplet Precautions [41].

PEP is advised for persons who have had intensive, unprotected contact (i.e., without wearing a mask) with infected patients (e.g., mouth-to-mouth resuscitation, endotracheal intubation, endotracheal tube management, or close examination of the oropharynx of patients) [8]. Antimicrobial prophylaxis can eradicate carriage of *N. meningitidis* and prevent infections in HCP who have unprotected exposure to patients with meningococcal infections [97].

Because secondary episodes of *N. meningitidis* occur rapidly (within the first week) after exposure to persons with meningococcal disease [98], it is important to begin prophylactic therapy immediately after an intensive, unprotected exposure, often before results of antimicrobial testing are available. Rifampin (600 mg orally every 12 hours for 2 days) is effective in eradicating nasopharyngeal carriage of *N. meningitidis* [97]. Ciprofloxacin (500 mg orally) and ceftriaxone (250 mg intramuscularly) in single-dose regimens also are effective in reducing nasopharyngeal carriage of *N. meningitidis* and are reasonable alternatives to the multidose rifampin regimen [8]. These antimicrobials may be useful when infections are caused by rifampin-resistant meningococci or rifampin is contraindicated. Rifampin and ciprofloxacin are not recommended for pregnant women [8,99,100].

The quadrivalent A,C,Y,W-135 polysaccharide vaccine has been used successfully to control community outbreaks caused by serogroup C [8,99], but its use is not recommended for PEP in healthcare settings [8]. Pre-exposure vaccination can be considered for laboratory personnel who routinely handle soluble preparations of *N. meningitidis* [8,96].

In the absence of exposures to patients with *N. meningitidis* infection, personnel who are asymptomatic carriers of *N. meningitidis* need not be identified, treated, or removed from patient-care activities. However, HCP with meningococcal infection need to be excluded from duty until 24 hours after the start of effective therapy.

Mumps

Mumps transmission has occurred in healthcare facilities housing adolescents and young adults [100,101]. Most episodes of mumps in HCP have been community acquired.

Mumps is transmitted by contact with virus-containing respiratory secretions, including saliva; the portals of entry are the nose and mouth. The incubation period varies from 12–25 days and usually is 16–18 days. The virus can be present in saliva for 6–7 days before parotitis and can persist for as long as 9 days after onset of disease. Exposed HCP may be infectious for 12–25 days after their exposure, and many infected persons remain asymptomatic [103]. Droplet Precautions are recommended for patients with mumps; such precautions should be continued for 9 days after the onset of parotitis [41].

An effective vaccination program is the best approach to the prevention of healthcare-associated mumps transmission [6]. Vaccination with mumps virus vaccine is recommended, unless otherwise contraindicated, for all those who are susceptible to mumps [6,104]; combined MMR is the vaccine of choice [105], especially when the recipient also is likely to be susceptible to measles, rubella, or both.

HCP should be considered immune to mumps if they have (a) documentation of physician-diagnosed mumps, (b) documentation of receipt of two doses of live mumps vaccine on or after their first birthday, or (c) serologic evidence of immunity (individuals who have an "indeterminate" antibody level should be considered susceptible) [6,106]. Although most persons born before 1957 are likely to have been infected naturally, they should receive one dose of live mumps vaccine if they do not meet criteria (a) or (c). Persons born after 1957 should have documentation of two doses of live mumps vaccine on or after their first birthday. Outbreaks among highly vaccinated populations have occurred and have been attributed to primary vaccine failure [107].

Work restrictions are necessary for HCP who acquire mumps; such restrictions should be imposed for 9 days after the onset of parotitis. Likewise, susceptible personnel who are exposed to mumps need to be excluded from duty from the 12th day after the first exposure until 25 days after the last exposure [4,102].

Parvovirus

Transmission of human parvovirus B19 (B19), the cause of erythema infectiosum (fifth disease), to HCP from infected patients appears to be rare but has been reported [108–112]. HCP have acquired infection while working in laboratories or during the care of patients with B19-associated sickle-cell aplastic crises [109–115].

B19 can be transmitted through contact with infected persons, fomites, or large droplets [116]. The incubation period varies, depending on the clinical manifestation of disease, and ranges from 6–10 days [117]. The period of infectivity also varies, depending on the clinical presentation or stage of disease. Persons with erythema infectiosum are infectious before the appearance of the rash, those with infection and aplastic crises for as long as 7 days after the onset of illness, and persons with chronic infection for years.

Pregnant HCP are at no greater risk of acquiring B19 infection than are nonpregnant HCP; however, if a woman does acquire B19 infection during the first half of pregnancy, the risk of fetal death is increased. Female HCP of childbearing age should be counseled regarding the risk of transmission of B19 and appropriate infection control precautions [41].

Most patients with erythema infectiosum are past their period of infectiousness at the time of clinical illness [115]. However, patients in aplastic crisis from B19 or patients with chronic B19 infection can transmit the virus to susceptible HCP or other patients; therefore, patients with pre-existing anemia who are admitted to the hospital with febrile illness and transient aplastic crises should remain on Droplet Precautions for 7 days, and patients with known or suspected chronic infection with B19 should be placed on Droplet Precautions on admission and for the duration of hospitalization [41,110]. Work restrictions are not necessary for HCP exposed to B19.

Pertussis

Healthcare-associated transmission of *Bordetella pertussis* has involved both patients and personnel; non-immunized children are at greatest risk [118–122]. *B. pertussis* transmission occurs by contact with respiratory secretions or large aerosol droplets from the respiratory tracts of infected persons. The incubation period usually is 7–10 days. The period of communicability starts at the onset of the catarrhal stage and extends into the paroxysmal stage up to 3 weeks after onset of symptoms. Pertussis is highly communicable in the catarrhal stage, when the symptoms are nonspecific.

Prevention of transmission of *B. pertussis* in healthcare settings involves (a) early diagnosis and treatment of patients with clinical infection, (b) implementation of Droplet Precautions for infectious patients [41], (c) exclusion of infectious HCP from work, and (d) administration of PEP to persons exposed to infectious patients [121]. Patients with suspected or confirmed pertussis who are admitted to the hospital need to be placed on Droplet Precautions until they have clinical improvement and have received antimicrobial therapy for at least 5 days.

Because immunity among vaccine recipients wanes 5–10 years after the last vaccine dose, HCP can play an important role in transmitting *B. pertussis* to susceptible infants. A single dose of Tetanus, diphtheria, and acellular pertussis (Tdap) vaccine is now recommended for persons age 11–64 years [14]. Acellular pertussis vaccine is immunogenic in adults and carries a lower risk of adverse events than does whole-cell vaccine [122,123].

PEP is indicated for exposed HCP who have not received a recent dose of Tdap. A course of azithromycin (one 500 mg single dose on day 1 then 250 mg per day on days 2–5), erythromycin (2 g per day in four divided doses for 14 days), clarithroymcin (1 g per day in two divided doses for 7 days), or trimethoprim-sulfamethoxazole (one tablet twice daily for 14 days) has been used for this purpose [14,124].

Restriction from duty is indicated for HCP with pertussis from the beginning of the catarrhal stage through the third week after onset of paroxysms, or until 5 days after the start of effective antimicrobial therapy. Exposed HCP do not need to be excluded from duty.

Poliomyelitis

Poliovirus is transmitted through contact with feces or urine of infected persons but can be spread by contact with respiratory secretions and, in rare instances, through items contaminated with feces. The incubation period for nonparalytic poliomyelitis is 3–6 days, but usually is 7–21 days for paralytic polio [125]. Communicability is greatest immediately before and after the onset of symptoms when the virus is in the throat and excreted in high concentration in feces. The virus can be recovered from the throat for 1 week and from feces for several weeks to months after onset of symptoms.

Poliomyelitis associated with oral polio vaccine (OPV) can occur in the recipient (7–21 days after vaccine administration) or susceptible contacts of the vaccine recipient (20–29 days after vaccine administration) [126]. Inactivated poliovirus vaccine (IPV) should be used when adult immunization is warranted, including immunization of pregnant or immunocompromised personnel and personnel who may have contact with immunocompromised patients [4,9,16,125].

HCP who have contact with patients who could be excreting wild virus (e.g., imported poliomyelitis patient) and laboratory personnel handling specimens containing poliovirus or performing cultures to amplify virus should receive a complete series of polio vaccine; if previously vaccinated, they could require a booster dose of IPV [16].

Rabies

Human rabies episodes occur primarily from exposure to rabid animals. Laboratory and animal care personnel who are exposed to infected animals, their tissues, or their excretions are at risk for the disease. Also, rabies transmission to laboratory personnel has been reported in vaccine production and research facilities after exposure to high-titered infectious aerosols [127,128]. Theoretically, rabies can be transmitted to HCP from exposures to saliva from infected patients, but no episodes have been documented after bite or nonbite exposures [129,130].

It also is possible for rabies to be transmitted when other potentially infectious material (e.g., brain tissue or transplanted tissue) comes into contact with non-intact skin or mucous membranes [17,129]. Bites that penetrate the skin, especially bites to the face and hands, pose the greatest risk of transmission of rabies virus from animals to human beings [17]. The incubation period for rabies usually is 1–3 months, but longer periods have been reported.

Except for corneal transplants, exposures inflicted by infected humans could theoretically transmit rabies, but no laboratory-diagnosed instances occurring under such situations have been documented [17]. Two nonlaboratory confirmed episodes of human-to-human rabies transmission in Ethiopia have been described [17]. The reported route of exposure in both instances was direct salivary contact from another human (a bite and a kiss). Routine delivery of health care to a patient with rabies is not an indication for PEP unless exposure of mucous membranes or non-intact skin to potentially infectious body fluids has occurred.

Exposures to rabies virus can be minimized by adhering to Standard Precautions when caring for persons with suspected or confirmed rabies [41] and by using proper biosafety precautions in laboratories [5]. Pre-exposure vaccination has been recommended for all personnel who (a) work with rabies virus or infected animals or (b) engage in diagnostic, production, or research activities with rabies virus [17,130,131]. Consideration also can be given to providing pre-exposure vaccination to animal handlers when research animals are obtained from the wild rather than from a known supplier that breeds the animals.

Rubella

Healthcare-associated transmission of rubella has occurred from HCP to other susceptible HCP and patients, and from patients to susceptible HCP and other patients [132,133].

Rubella is transmitted by contact with nasopharyngeal droplets from infected persons. The incubation period is variable but can range from 12–23 days; most persons have the rash 14–16 days after exposure. The disease is most contagious when the rash is erupting, but virus may be shed from 1 week before to 5–7 days after the onset of the rash [134]. Rubella in adults is usually a mild disease, lasting only a few days; 30% to 50% of patients may be subclinical or inapparent.

Droplet Precautions are used to prevent transmission of rubella. Infants with congenital rubella can excrete virus for months to years; when caring for such patients, it is advisable to use contact precautions for the first year of life unless nasopharyngeal and urine culture results are negative for rubella virus after 3 months of age [41].

Ensuring immunity among all HCP (male and female) is the most effective way to eliminate healthcare-associated transmission of rubella [3,4,6]. HCP should be considered susceptible to rubella if they lack (a) documentation of one dose of live rubella vaccine on or after their first birthday and (b) laboratory evidence of immunity (persons with indeterminate levels are considered susceptible). A history of previous rubella infection is unreliable and should not be considered indicative of immunity to rubella. Although birth before 1957 is generally considered acceptable evidence of rubella immunity, a dose of MMR has been recommended for those HCP who do not have laboratory evidence of immunity [4]. In addition, birth before 1957 is not considered acceptable evidence of rubella immunity for women of childbearing age; history of vaccination or laboratory evidence of rubella immunity is particularly important for women who may become pregnant [4]. Voluntary immunization programs usually are inadequate to ensure personnel protection [1,135]. Because many health departments mandate rubella immunity for HCP, personnel health programs should consult with their local or state health departments before establishing policies for their facilities.

Work restrictions are necessary for HCP who acquire rubella; ill HCP need to be excluded from duty for 5 days after the rash appears. Likewise, HCP susceptible to rubella require exclusion from duty from the seventh day after the first exposure through the 21st day after the last exposure [136].

Scabies and Pediculosis

Scabies

Scabies is caused by infestation with the mite *Sarcoptes scabiei*. The conventional (typical) clinical presentation of scabies includes intense pruritus and cutaneous tracks where mites have burrowed into the skin. Crusted or "Norwegian" scabies can develop among immunocompromised and elderly individuals in which their skin may become hyperkeratotic; pruritus may not be present. In conventional scabies, 10–15 mites are present; in crusted scabies, thousands of mites are harbored in the skin, increasing the potential for transmission [137,138].

Healthcare-associated outbreaks of scabies have occurred in a variety of healthcare settings. Healthcare-associated transmission of scabies occurs primarily through prolonged skin-to-skin contact with an infested person who has conventional scabies [137,139]. Shorter periods of skin-to-skin contact with persons who have crusted scabies can result in transmission. HCP have acquired scabies while performing patient care duties such as sponge bathing, lifting, or applying body lotions [137,138,140]. Transmission by casual contact (e.g., by holding hands) or through inanimate objects, such as infested bedding, clothes, or other fomites, has been reported infrequently [141].

The use of Contact Precautions when taking care of infested patients before application of scabicides can decrease the risk of transmission to HCP [41,138]. Routine cleaning of the environment of patients with typical scabies, especially bed linens and upholstered furniture, will aid in eliminating the mites. Additional environmental cleaning procedures could be warranted for crusted scabies [137,138,142,143].

Most infested HCP have typical scabies with low mite loads [144]; a single correct application of a scabicide is adequate and immediately decreases the risk of transmission [19]. Several lotions are available to treat scabies. The treatment of choice is the topical use of permethrin (5%). Crotamiton and ivermectin are alternative drugs; ivermectin is taken orally and is effective for treating crusted scabies in immunocompromised persons [145]. There are no controlled evaluations of the efficacy of prophylactic scabicide therapy among HCP, and some experts recommend two applications of scabicide for all infested HCP [138,146,147]. If HCP continue to have symptoms after initial treatment, another application of scabicide could be needed. Persistent symptoms likely represent newly hatched mites rather than new infestation; however, pruritus after scabies infestation and treatment can persist for as long as 2 weeks, even without infestation [19]. In outbreak situations in which transmission continues to occur, prophylaxis can be warranted for both patients and exposed HCP [138,146].

Restrictions from patient care are indicated for HCP infested with scabies until after they receive initial treatment and have been medically evaluated and determined to be free of infestation. They should be advised to report for further evaluation if symptoms do not subside.

Pediculosis

Pediculosis is caused by infestation with any of three species of lice: *Pediculus humanus capitus* (human head louse), *Pediculus humanus corporis* (human body louse), or *Phthirus pubis* (pubic or crab louse). Head lice are transmitted by head-to-head contact or by contact with infested fomites such as hats, combs, or brushes. Healthcare-associated transmission, although not common, has occurred [137].

The recommended treatment of pediculosis includes permethrin cream 1%, pyrethrins with piperonyl butoxide, malathion 0.5%, or ivermectin [145,148]. Resistance to various drugs has been reported. HCP exposed to patients with pediculosis do not require treatment unless they show evidence of infestation.

Restriction from patient care is indicated for personnel with pediculosis until after they receive initial treatment and are found to be free of adult and immature lice. If symptoms do not subside after initial treatment, personnel should be advised to report for further evaluation.

Staphylococcal Infection or Carriage, Including Methicillin-Resistant *Staphylococcus aureus*

Staphylococcal infection and carriage occur frequently in human beings. In healthcare settings, the most important sources of *S. aureus* are infected or colonized patients. In recent years, healthcare-associated methicillin-resistant *S. aureus (HA-MRSA)* has accounted for approximately 80% of all *S. aureus* isolates reported to the National Nosocomial Infections Surveillance (NNIS) system [149,150]. The epidemiology of MRSA does not appear to differ from that of methicillin-susceptible, penicillin-resistant *S. aureus* except that outbreaks of MRSA tend to occur more frequently among elderly or immunocompromised patients or among patients with severe underlying conditions [151,152].

Although once found almost exclusively in healthcare settings, strains of *S. aureus* resistant to beta-lactam antibiotics (i.e., MRSA) are becoming increasingly common as a cause of skin and soft tissue infections in persons with no previous contact with the healthcare system. These strains are sometimes referred to as "community-associated MRSA (CA-MRSA)." There is no difference in recommended infection control measures for prevention of transmission of infection when caring for patients infected with either -MRSA or CA-MRSA.

Healthcare-associated transmission of *S. aureus* occurs primarily via the hands of HCP, which can become contaminated by contact with the colonized or infected body sites of patients or their surrounding contaminated environment [152,153]. HCP who are infected or colonized with *S. aureus* also can serve as reservoirs and disseminators of *S. aureus* [154–157]. The role of contaminated environmental surfaces in transmission of *S. aureus* has rarely been well documented [158] and remains controversial, although heavy contamination of fomites could facilitate transmission to patients by hands of HCP [152]. The incubation period for *S. aureus* infections varies by type of disease [159].

Carriage of *S. aureus* is most common in the anterior nares, but other sites, such as the hands, axilla, perineum, nasopharynx, or oropharynx, also can be involved [152]. Carriage of *S. aureus* in the nares has been shown to correspond to hand carriage [149], and persons with skin lesions caused by it are more likely than asymptomatic nasal carriers to disseminate the organism.

Culture surveys of HCP can detect carriers of *S. aureus* but do not indicate which carriers are likely to disseminate organisms. Thus, such surveys are not cost effective and can subject HCP with positive culture results to unnecessary treatment and removal from duty. Culture surveys could be indicated if, after a thorough epidemiologic investigation, HCP are linked to infections. Such implicated HCP then can be removed from clinical duties until carriage has been eradicated [152,154,160–162].

Several antimicrobial regimens have been used successfully to eradicate staphylococcal carriage in HCP. These regimens include orally administered antimicrobial agents (e.g., rifampin, clindamycin, or ciprofloxacin) alone or in combination with another oral (e.g., trimethoprim-sulfamethoxazole) or topical (mupirocin) antimicrobial [163,164]. Resistant *S. aureus* strains have emerged after the use of these oral or topical antimicrobial agents for eradication of colonization [163,164]. Thus, antimicrobial treatment to eradicate carriage should be limited to HCP who are carriers epidemiologically linked to disease transmission. Healthcare-associated transmission of *S. aureus* can be prevented by adherence to Standard Precautions and other forms of Transmission-Based Precautions as needed [41].

Restriction from patient-care activities or food handling is indicated for HCP who have draining *S. aureus* skin lesions until they have received appropriate therapy and the infection has resolved. No work restrictions are necessary for HCP colonized with *S. aureus* unless they have been epidemiologically implicated in *S. aureus* transmission within the facility.

Group A *Streptococcus* Infections

Group A *Streptococcus* (GAS) has been transmitted from infected patients to HCP after contact with infected secretions [165–167], and the infected personnel have subsequently acquired a variety of GAS-related illnesses (e.g., toxic shocklike syndrome, cellulitis, lymphangitis, and pharyngitis). HCP who were GAS carriers have infrequently been linked to sporadic outbreaks of surgical site, postpartum, or burn wound infections [168–174]. The incubation period is variable for other GAS infections [175].

Culture surveys to detect GAS carriage among HCP are not warranted unless HCP are epidemiologically linked to episodes of healthcare-associated infection (HAI). When thorough epidemiologic investigation has implicated HCP in HAI transmission, cultures can be obtained from skin lesions, pharynx, rectum, and vagina; GAS isolates obtained from HCP and patients can be serotyped to determine strain relatedness. Treatment of HCP carriers needs to be individually determined because (a) experience is limited regarding the treatment of HCP carriers implicated in GAS outbreaks and (b) carriage of GAS by HCP could recur through long periods [167–169,171]. Contact is the major mode of transmission of GAS in healthcare settings. Healthcare-associated transmission of GAS to HCP can be prevented by adherence to standard precautions or other Transmission-Based Precautions as needed [41].

Restriction from patient care activities and food handling is indicated for HCP with GAS infections until 24 hours after they have received appropriate therapy. However, no work restrictions are necessary for HCP colonized with GAS unless they have been epidemiologically linked to transmission of infection within the facility.

Tuberculosis

Healthcare-associated transmission of *Mycobacterium tuberculosis* (MTB) is well documented, but such transmission in the United States is generally low. However, the risk can be increased in healthcare facilities located in communities with (a) high rates of HIV, (b) high numbers of persons from tuberculosis (TB)-endemic countries, and (c) communities with a high prevalence of TB infection) [176,177]. In some areas in the United States, the incidence and prevalence of multidrug-resistant *M. tuberculosis* (MDR-TB) also have increased, and healthcare-associated MDR-TB outbreaks have occurred [178–186].

Transmission of MTB can be minimized by developing and implementing an effective TB control program that is based on a hierarchy of controls: (a) administrative controls, (b) engineering controls, and (c) respiratory protection [177,179,187–190].

A TB screening program for personnel is an integral part of a healthcare facility's comprehensive TB control program. Baseline tuberculin skin test (TST) testing of all personnel (including personnel with a history of bacille Calmette-Guérin [BCG] vaccination) during their placement evaluation will identify HCP who have been previously infected. For base-line testing, a two-step tuberculin skin test (TST) procedure for personnel without a TST in the past 12 months can be used to minimize the likelihood of confusing reactivity from an old infection (boosting) with reactivity from a recent infection (conversion). Decisions concerning the use of the two-step procedure for baseline testing in a particular facility should be based on the frequency of boosting in that facility. Criteria used for interpretation of a TST reaction can vary depending on (a) the purpose (diagnostic or epidemiologic) of the test, (b) the prevalence of TB in the population being tested, (c) the immune status of the host, and (d) any previous receipt of BCG immunization. At a minimum, annual TST testing is indicated for personnel with the potential for exposure to TB.

It also is important to obtain an initial chest radiograph for HCP with positive TST reactions, documented TST conversions, or pulmonary symptoms suggestive of TB. In addition, HCP who have positive TST reactions but also received adequate preventive treatment do not need repeat chest films unless they have pulmonary symptoms suggestive of TB.

It is important to administer TSTs to personnel as soon as possible after MTB exposures are recognized. Such immediate TST testing establishes a baseline with which subsequent TSTs can be compared. A TST performed 8–10 weeks after the last exposure will indicate whether infection has occurred. Persons already known to have reactive TSTs need not be retested. HCP with evidence of new infection (i.e., TST conversions) need to be evaluated for active TB. If active TB is not diagnosed, preventive therapy should be considered [177].

For HCP with positive TST results who were probably exposed to drug-susceptible MTB, preventive therapy with isoniazid is indicated unless there are contraindications to such therapy [177]. Alternative preventive regimens have been proposed for persons who have positive TST-test results after exposure to drug-resistant MTB [190,191].

HCP with active pulmonary or laryngeal TB can be highly infectious; exclusion from duty is indicated until they are noninfectious. Work restrictions are not necessary for HCP receiving preventive treatment for latent TB (i.e., positive TST result without active disease) or for HCP with latent TB who do not accept preventive therapy. However, these HCP should be instructed to seek evaluation promptly if symptoms suggestive of TB develop.

Vaccinia

Through aggressive surveillance for smallpox combined with the effective use of smallpox vaccine (vaccinia virus vaccine), the World Health Organization was able to declare the world free of smallpox in 1980. The smallpox vaccine licensed for use in the United States is derived from infectious vaccinia virus. After vaccination, the virus can be cultured from the vaccination site until the scab has separated from the skin (2–21 days after vaccination); thus, susceptible persons could acquire vaccinia from a recently vaccinated person [192–195]. Covering the vaccination site and washing hands after contact with the vaccination site (including bandages) will prevent transmission.

Smallpox vaccination (every 10 years) is indicated for personnel who work directly with orthopox viruses (e.g., monkeypox, vaccinia, variola) or in animal care areas where orthopox viruses are studied. In selected instances, vaccination should be considered for HCP who provide care to recipients of recombinant vaccinia vaccine [4,12]. HCP who receive the vaccine may continue to have contact with patients if the vaccination site is covered and hand hygiene is strictly observed [12]. Vaccine is not recommended for HCP with immunosuppression or eczema or for HCP who are pregnant.

Varicella

Healthcare-associated transmission of varicella-zoster virus (VZV) is well recognized [196–200]. Sources for healthcare exposures have included patients, HCP, and visitors (including the children of HCP) with either varicella or herpes zoster.

The incubation period for varicella is usually 14–16 days but can be from 10–21 days after exposure, although the incubation period can be shorter in immunocompromised persons [201]. In persons who receive postexposure VZV immune globulin, the incubation period can be as long as 28 days after exposure. Transmission of infection may occur from 2 days before rash onset and usually as long as 5 days after rash onset [201].

VZV is transmitted by contact with infected lesions and, in hospitals, airborne transmission has occurred from patients with varicella or zoster to susceptible persons who had no direct contact with the infected patient [202–206]. Adherence to Airborne and Contact Precautions when caring for patients with known or suspected VZV infection can reduce the risk of transmission to HCP [41].

It generally is advisable to allow only HCP who are immune to varicella to take care of patients with VZV. Because of the possibility of transmission to and development of severe illness in high-risk patients, HCP with localized zoster should not take care of such patients until all lesions are dry and crusted [7,206]. HCP with localized zoster are not likely to transmit infection to immunocompetent patients if their lesions can be covered. However, some institutions may exclude HCP with zoster from work until their lesions dry and crust.

Serologic tests have been used to assess the accuracy of reported histories of chickenpox [207]. In adults, a history of varicella is highly predictive of serologic immunity (97% to 99% seropositive). Most adults who have negative or uncertain histories of varicella also are seropositive (71% to 93%). In healthcare institutions, serologic screening of HCP who have negative or uncertain histories is likely to be cost effective, depending on the relative costs of the test and vaccine [4,7].

Administration of varicella vaccine is recommended for all susceptible HCP, especially those who will have close contact with persons at high risk for serious complications [4,7,208]. Persistence of immunity to VZV after vaccination of HCP has been demonstrated up to 8.4 years [209].

Transmission of the vaccine virus is rare and has been documented in immunocompetent persons by polymerase chain reaction (PCR) analysis on only three occasions out of 15 million doses of varicella vaccine distributed. All three episodes resulted in mild disease without complications. Secondary transmission has not been documented in the absence of a vesicular rash postvaccination [7].

When unvaccinated susceptible HCP are exposed to varicella, they are potentially infectious 10–21 days after exposure, and exclusion from duty is indicated from the 10th day after the first exposure through the 21st day after the last exposure, or until all lesions are dry and crusted if varicella occurs. If vaccinated HCP are exposed to varicella, they can be serologically tested immediately after exposure to assess the presence of antibody [208]. If they are seronegative, they may be excluded from duty or monitored daily for development of symptoms. Exclusion from duty is indicated if symptoms (fever, upper respiratory tract symptoms, or rash) develop.

Vaccination should be considered for exposed unvaccinated HCP without documented immunity [200,208]. Because the efficacy of postexposure vaccination is unknown, however, persons vaccinated after an exposure should be managed as previously recommended for unvaccinated persons.

The routine postexposure use of VZV immune globulin (VariZIG) is not recommended among immunocompetent HCP [7]. VariZIG can be costly, does not necessarily prevent varicella, and can prolong the incubation period by a week or more, thus extending the time that HCP will be restricted from duty. The use of VariZIG can be considered for immunocompromised (e.g., HIV-infected) or pregnant HCP [7,210]. Postexposure use of acyclovir can be effective and less costly than the use of VariZIG in some susceptible persons [210]. Antiviral medications are not recommended for routine PEP [201].

Viral Respiratory Infections, Including Influenza, Respiratory Syncytial Virus, and SARS

Healthcare-associated respiratory infections can be caused by a number of viruses, including adenoviruses, influenza virus, parainfluenza viruses, respiratory syncytial virus (RSV), rhinoviruses, or coronavirus (i.e., SARS) [211]. This section focuses on prevention of influenza, RSV, and SARS.

Influenza

Healthcare-associated transmission of influenza has been reported in acute and long-term care facilities [212–215]. Transmission has occurred from patients to HCP [213,214], from HCP to patients [216], and among HCP [215,217–219].

Influenza is believed to be transmitted from person to person by direct deposition of virus-laden large droplets onto the mucosal surfaces of the upper respiratory tract of an individual during close contact with an infected person and by droplet nuclei or small-particle aerosols [10,220].

The incubation period of influenza usually is 1–5 days, and the period of greatest communicability is during the first 3 days of illness. However, virus can be shed before the onset of symptoms and as long as 7 days after illness onset and can be prolonged in young children and immunocompromised persons [221,222]. Adherence to Droplet Precautions can prevent healthcare-associated transmission of influenza [41].

Facilities that employ HCP are strongly encouraged to provide vaccine to HCP by using approaches that maximize vaccination [1,10,223].

During institutional influenza outbreaks, prophylactic antiviral agents (e.g., osetamivir or zanamivir) can be used in conjunction with influenza vaccine to reduce the severity and duration of illness among unvaccinated HCP. Osetamivir or zanamivir may be administered for 2 weeks after HCP vaccination or, in unvaccinated HCP, for the duration of influenza activity in the community [10,211]. Prophylactic antiviral medications can be offered to unvaccinated HCP who provide care to persons at high risk or to all HCP regardless of their vaccination status if the outbreak is suspected to be caused by a strain of influenza virus that is not well matched to the vaccine.

Respiratory Syncytial Virus

Healthcare-associated transmission of respiratory syncytial virus (RSV) is greatest during the early winter when community RSV outbreaks occur; patients, visitors, and HCP can transmit the virus in the healthcare setting. RSV infection is most common among infants and children, who are likely to experience more severe disease. Healthcare-associated transmission has been reported most frequently among newborn and pediatric patients [224, 225], but outbreaks associated with substantial morbidity and mortality have been reported among adults in bone-marrow transplant centers [226], intensive care units [227], and long-term care facilities [228,229].

RSV is present in large numbers in the respiratory secretions of persons symptomatically infected with the virus and can be transmitted directly through large droplets during close contact with such persons or indirectly by hands or fomites that are contaminated with RSV. Hands can become contaminated by handling infected persons' respiratory secretions or contaminated fomites and can transmit RSV by touching the eyes or nose [211]. The incubation period ranges from 2–8 days; 4–6 days is most common. In general, infected persons shed the virus for 3–8 days, but young infants can shed it for as long as 3–4 weeks. Adherence to Contact Precautions effectively prevents healthcare-associated transmission.

SARS

SARS is an emerging respiratory tract infection linked to a novel coronavirus that first appeared in late 2002 in China and spread globally until 2005. In several Asian countries, SARS-coronavirus caused outbreaks in healthcare settings with transmission to large numbers of HCP and patients. Although the most important modes of transmission are by (large) droplet and contact, airborne transmission has not been ruled out. High-risk exposures, such as those associated with aerosolization of respiratory secretions and exposures to "supershedders" have been associated with transmission of the disease to HCP outside the United States [211]. Clinicians evaluating suspected episodes of SARS should use Standard Precautions together with Airborne and Contact Precautions [41,211,230].

Work Restrictions

Because large numbers of HCP can have viral respiratory illnesses during the winter, it might not be possible to restrict infected HCP from all patient-care duties. Nevertheless, it could be prudent to restrict HCP with acute viral respiratory infections from the care of high-risk patients during community outbreaks of RSV and influenza [231].

REFERENCES

 1. Centers for Disease Control and Prevention. Interventions to increase influenza vaccination of health-care workers—California and Minnesota. *MMWR Morb Mortal Wkly Rep* 2005;54: 196–199.
 2. Heseltine PNR, Ripper M, Wohlford P. Nosocomial rubella—consequences of an outbreak and efficacy of a mandatory immunization program. *Infect Control* 1985;6:371–374.
 3. Centers for Disease Control and Prevention. General recommendations on immunization: recommendations of the Advisory Committee on Immunization Practices (ACIP) and the American Academy of Family Physicians (AAFP). *MMWR Morb Mortal Wkly Rep* 2002;51(RR-2):1–36.
 4. Centers for Disease Control and Prevention. Immunization of health-care workers: recommendations of the Advisory Committee on Immunization Practices (ACIP) and the Hospital Infection Control Practices Advisory Committee (HICPAC). *MMWR Morb Mortal Wkly Rep* 1997;46(RR-18):1–42.
 5. Centers for Disease Control. Protection against viral hepatitis: recommendations of the Advisory Committee on Immunization Practices (ACIP). *MMWR Morb Mortal Wkly Rep* 1990:39 (RR-2):1–27.
 6. Centers for Disease Control and Prevention. Measles, mumps, and rubella—vaccine use and strategies for elimination of measles, rubella, and congenital rubella syndrome and control of mumps: recommendations of the Advisory Committee on Immunizations Practices (ACIP). *MMWR Morb Mortal Wkly Rep* 1998;47(RR-7):1–57.
 7. Centers for Disease Control and Prevention. Prevention of varicella: recommendations of the Advisory Committee on Immunizations Practices (ACIP). *MMWR Morb Mortal Wkly Rep* 1996;45(RR-11):1–36.
 8. Centers for Disease Control and Prevention. Prevention and control of meningococcal disease: recommendations of the Advisory Committee on Immunization Practices (ACIP). *MMWR Morb Mortal Wkly Rep* 2000;49(RR-7):1–10.
 9. Centers for Disease Control and Prevention. Update: vaccine side effects, adverse reactions, contraindications and precautions: recommendations of the Advisory Committee on Immunization Practices (ACIP). *MMWR Morb Mortal Wkly Rep* 1996;45 (RR-12):1–35.
10. Centers for Disease Control and Prevention. Prevention and control of influenza: recommendations of the Advisory Committee on Immunization Practices (ACIP). *MMWR Morb Mortal Wkly Rep* 2006;55(RR-10):1–41.
11. Centers for Disease Control and Prevention. Vaccinia (smallpox) vaccine: recommendations of the Immunization Practices Advisory Committee (ACIP). *MMWR Morb Mortal Wkly Rep* 2001;50(RR-10):1–25.
12. Centers for Disease Control and Prevention: Recommendations for using smallpox vaccine in a pre-event vaccination program: supplemental recommendations of the Advisory Committee on Immunizations Practices (ACIP) and the Healthcare Infection Control Practices Advisory Committee (HICPAC). *MMWR Morb Mortal Wkly Rep* 2003;52(RR-7):1–16.
13. Centers for Disease Control. Diphtheria, tetanus, pertussis: recommendations for vaccine use and other preventive measures—recommendations of the Immunization Practices Advisory Committee (ACIP). *MMWR Morb Mortal Wkly Rep* 1991; 40(RR-10):1–28.
14. Centers for Disease Control and Prevention. Recommended antimicrobial agents for treatment and postexposure prophylaxis of pertussis: 2005 CDC guideline. *MMWR Morb Mortal Wkly Rep* 2005:54(RR-14):1–16.
15. Centers for Disease Control and Prevention. Prevention of pneumococcal disease: recommendations of the Advisory Committee on Immunization Practices (ACIP). *MMWR Morb Mortal Wkly Rep* 1997;46(RR-8):1–24.
16. Centers for Disease Control and Prevention. Poliomyelitis prevention in the United States: updated recommendations of the Advisory Committee on Immunization Practices (ACIP). *MMWR Morb Mortal Wkly Rep* 2000;49(RR-5):1–22.
17. Centers for Disease Control. Rabies prevention—United States, 1999: recommendations of the Immunization Practices Advisory Committee (ACIP). *MMWR Morb Mortal Wkly Rep* 1999;49 (RR-1):1–21.
18. Centers for Disease Control and Prevention. Recommendations of the Advisory Committee on Immunization Practices (ACIP): use of vaccines and immune globulins in persons with altered immunocompetence. *MMWR Morb Mortal Wkly Rep* 1993;42 (RR-4):1–18.
19. Herwaldt LA, Pottinger JM, Carter CD, et al. Exposure workups. *Infect Control Hosp Epidemiol* 1997;18:850–871.
20. US Department of Labor, Occupational Health and Safety Administration. Reporting fatalities and multiple hospitalization incidents to OSHA (www.osha.gov/pls/oshaweb/owadisp. show_document?p_table = STANDARDS&p_id = 1278)
21. US Department of Labor, Occupational Safety and Health Administration. Bloodborne pathogens. (www.osha.gov/pls/ oshaweb/owadisp.show_document?p_table = STANDARDS&p _id = 1005).
22. Centers for Disease Control and Prevention. HIPAA privacy rule and public health: guidance from the CDC and the U.S. Department of Health and Human Services. *MMWR Morb Mortal Wkly Rep* 2003;52(Suppl.):1–12.
23. Centers for Disease Control. Epidemic keratoconjunctivitis in an ophthalmology clinic—California. *MMWR Morb Mortal Wkly Rep* 1990;39:598–601.
24. Ford E, Nelson KE, Warren D. Epidemiology of epidemic keratoconjunctivitis. *Epidemiol Rev* 1987;9:244–261.
25. Birenbaum E, Linder N, Varsano N, et al. Adenovirus type 8 conjunctivitis outbreak in a neonatal intensive care unit. *Arch Dis Child* 1993;68:610–611.
26. Warren D, Nelson KE, Farrar JA, et al. A large outbreak of epidemic keratoconjunctivitis: problems in controlling nosocomial spread. *J Infect Dis* 1989;160:938–943.
27. Jernigan JA, Lowry BS, Hayden FG, et al. Adenovirus type 8 epidemic keratoconjunctivitis in an eye clinic: risk factors and control. *J Infect Dis* 1993;167:1307–1313.
28. Onorato IM, Morens DM, Martone WJ, Stansfield SK. Epidemiology of cytomegaloviral infections: recommendations for prevention and control. *Rev Infect Dis* 1985;7:479–497.
29. Demmler GJ, Yow MD, Spector SA, et al. Nosocomial cytomegalovirus infections within two hospitals caring for infants and children. *J Infect Dis* 1987;156:9–16.
30. Ahlfors K, Ivarsson SA, Johnson T, Renmarker K. Risk of cytomegalovirus infection in nurses and congenital infection in their offspring. *Acta Paediatr Scand* 1981;70:819–823.
31. Gerberding JL, Bryant-LeBlanc CE, Nelson K, et al. Risk of transmitting the human immunodeficiency virus, cytomegalovirus, and hepatitis B virus to health care workers exposed to patients with AIDS and AIDS-related conditions. *J Infect Dis* 1987; 156:1–8.
32. Blackman JA, Murph JR, Bale JF. Risk of cytomegalovirus infection among educators and health care personnel serving disabled children. *Pediatr Infect Dis J* 1987;6:725–729.
33. Adler SP. Hospital transmission of cytomegalovirus. *Infect Agents Dis* 1992;1:43–49.
34. Balcarek KB, Bagley R, Cloud G, Pass RF. Cytomegalovirus infection among employees of a children's hospital: no evidence for increased risk associated with patient care. *JAMA* 1990; 263:840–844.
35. Spector SA. Transmission of cytomegalovirus among infants in hospital documented by restriction-endonuclease-digestion analyses. *Lancet* 1983;2:378–381.
36. Adler SP. Cytomegalovirus and child day care: evidence for an increased infection rate among day-care workers. *N Engl J Med* 1989;321:1290–1296.
37. Hutto C, Little EA, Ricks R. Isolation of cytomegalovirus from toys and hands in a day care center. *J Infect Dis* 1986;154:527–530.

38. Faix RG. Survival of cytomegalovirus on environmental surfaces. *J Pediatr* 1985;106:649–652.

39. Finney JW, Miller KM, Adler SP. Changing protective and risky behaviors to prevent child-to-parent transmission of cytomegalovirus. *J Appl Behav Anal* 1993;26:471–472.

40. American Academy of Pediatrics. Summaries of infectious diseases: cytomegalovirus infection. In: Pickering LK, Baker CJ, Long SS, McMillan JA, eds. *Red Book: 2006 Report of the Committee on Infectious Diseases.* 27th ed. Elk Grove Village, IL: American Academy of Pediatrics, 2006, 273–277.

41. Garner JS, Hospital Infection Control Practices Advisor Committee. Guideline for isolation precautions in hospitals. *Infect Control Hosp Epidemiol* 1996;17:53–80.

42. Anderson GS, Penfold JB. An outbreak of diphtheria in a hospital for the mentally subnormal. *J Clin Pathol* 1973;26:606–615.

43. Gray RD, James SM. Occult diphtheria infection in a hospital for the mentally subnormal. *Lancet* 1973;1:1105–1106.

44. Palmer SR, Balfour AH, Jephcott AE. Immunisation of adults during an outbreak of diphtheria. *BMJ* 1983;286:624–626.

45. Centers for Disease Control and Prevention. Update: diphtheria epidemic—new independent states of the former Soviet Union, January 1995–March 1996. *MMWR Morb Mortal Wkly Rep* 1996;45:693–697.

46. Centers for Disease Control and Prevention. Diphtheria epidemic—new independent states of the former Soviet Union, 1990–1994. *MMWR Morb Mortal Wkly Rep* 1995;44:177–181.

47. Steere AC, Craven PJ, Hall WJ III, et al. Person-to-person spread of *Salmonella typhimurium* after a hospital common-source outbreak. *Lancet* 1975;1:319–322.

48. Toivanen P, Toivanen A, Olkkonen L, Aantaa S. Hospital outbreak of *Yersinia enterocolitica* infection. *Lancet* 1973;1:801–803.

49. Ratnam S, Mercer E, Picco B, et al. A nosocomial outbreak of diarrheal disease due to *Yersinia enterocolitica* serotype 0:5, biotype 1. *J Infect Dis* 1982;145:242–247.

50. Kurtz JB, Lee TW, Pickering D. Astrovirus associated gastroenteritis in a children's ward. *J Clin Pathol* 1977;30:948–952.

51. Dryjanski J, Gold JWM, Ritchie MT, et al. Cryptosporidiosis: case report in a health team worker. *Am J Med* 1986;80:751–752.

52. Lewis DC, Lightfoot NF, Cubitt WD, Wilson SA. Outbreaks of astrovirus type 1 and rotovirus gastroenteritis in a geriatric in patient population. *J Hosp Infect* 1989;14:9–14.

53. Koch KL, Phillips DJ, Aber RC, Current WL. Cryptosporidiosis in hospital personnel: evidence for person-to-person transmission. *Ann Intern Med* 1985;102:593–596.

54. Pike RM. Laboratory-associated infections: summary and analysis of 3921 cases. *Health Lab Sci* 1976;13:105–114.

55. Tauxe RV, Hassan LF, Findeisen KO, et al. Salmonellosis in nurses: lack of transmission to patients. *J Infect Dis* 1988;157:370–373.

56. Carter AO, Borczyk AA, Carlson JAK, et al. A severe outbreak of *Escherichia coli* O157:H7-associated hemorrhagic colitis in a nursing home. *N Engl J Med* 1987;317:1496–1500.

57. Zingg W, Colombo C, Jucker T, et al. Impact of an outbreak of norovirus infection on hospital resources. *Infect Control Hosp Epidemiol* 2005;26:263–267.

58. Mattner F, Mattner L, Borck HU, Gastmeier P. Evaluation of the impact of the source (patient vs. staff)on nosocomial norovirus outbreak severity. *Infect Control Hosp Epidemiol* 2005;26:268–272.

59. Schroeder SA, Aserkoff B, Brachman PS. Epidemic salmonellosis in hospitals and institutions: public health importance and outbreak management. *N Engl J Med* 1968;279:674–678.

60. Khuri-Bulos NA, Abu Khalaf M, Shehabi A, Shami K. Foodhandler-associated *Salmonella* outbreak in a university hospital despite routine surveillance cultures of kitchen employees. *Infect Control Hosp Epidemiol* 1994;15:311–314.

61. Centers for Disease Control. Viral agents of gastroenteritis. *MMWR Morb Mortal Wkly Rep* 1990;39(RR-5):1–24.

62. Doebbeling BN, Stanley GL, Sheetz CT, et al. Comparative efficacy of alternative hand-washing agents in reducing nosocomial infections in intensive care units. *N Engl J Med* 1992;327:88–93.

63. Centers for Disease Control and Prevention. Guideline for hand hygiene in health-care settings: Recommendations of the Healthcare Infection Control Practices Advisory Committee and the HICPAC/SHEA/APIC/IDSA Hand Hygiene Task Force. *MMWR Morb Mortal Wkly Rep* 2002;51(RR-16):1–45.

64. Centers for Disease Control. Recommendations for collection of laboratory specimens associated with outbreaks of gastroenteritis. *MMWR Morb Mortal Wkly Rep* 1990;39(RR-14):1–13.

65. Rosenblum LS, Villarino ME, Nainan OV, et al. Hepatitis A outbreak in a neonatal intensive care unit: risk factors for transmission and evidence of prolonged viral excretion among preterm infants. *J Infect Dis* 1991;164:476–482.

66. Carl M, Kantor RJ, Webster HM, et al. Excretion of hepatitis A virus in the stools of hospitalized patients. *J Med Virol* 1982;9:125–129.

67. Drusin LM, Sohmer M, Groshen SL, et al. Nosocomial hepatitis A infection in a paediatric intensive care unit. *Arch Dis Child* 1987;62:690–695.

68. Baptiste R, Koziol D, Henderson DK. Nosocomial transmission of hepatitis A in an adult population. *Infect Control* 1987;8:364–370.

69. Azimi PH, Roberto RR, Guralnik J, et al. Transfusion-acquired hepatitis A in a pre-mature infant with secondary nosocomial spread in an intensive care nursery. *Am J Dis Child* 1986;140:23–27.

70. Skidmore SJ, Gully PR, Middleton JD, et al. An outbreak of hepatitis A on a hospital ward. *J Med Virol* 1985;17:175–177.

71. Klein BS, Michaels JA, Rytel MW, et al. Nosocomial hepatitis A: a multinursery outbreak in Wisconsin. *JAMA* 1984;252:2716–2721.

72. Krober MS, Bass JW, Brown JD, et al. Hospital outbreak of hepatitis A: risk factors for spread. *Pediatr Infect Dis J* 1984;3:296–299.

73. Doebbeling BN, Li N, Wenzel RP. An outbreak of hepatitis A among health care workers: risk factors for transmission. *Am J Public Health* 1993;83:1679–1684.

74. Watson JC, Fleming DC, Borella AJ, et al. Vertical transmission of hepatitis A resulting in an outbreak in a neonatal intensive care unit. *J Infect Dis* 1993;167:567–571.

75. Centers for Disease Control and Prevention. Prevention of hepatitis A through active or passive immunization: recommendations of the Advisory Committee on Immunization Practices (ACIP) *MMWR Morb Mortal Wkly Rep* 2006;55(RR-7):1–23.

76. Van Dyke RB, Spector SA. Transmission of herpes simplex virus type 1 to a newborn infant during endotracheal suctioning for meconium aspiration. *Pediatr Infect Dis J* 1984;3:153–156.

77. Linneman CC, Buchman TG, Light IJ, Ballard JL. Transmission of herpes-simplex virus type 1 in a nursery for the newborn: Identification of isolates by D.N.A. "fingerprinting." *Lancet* 1978;1:964–966.

78. Kleiman MB, Schreiner RL, Fitzen H, et al. Oral herpesvirus infection in nursery personnel: infection control policy. *Pediatrics* 1982;70:609–612.

79. Buchman TG, Roizman B, Adams G, Stover BH. Restriction endonuclease fingerprinting of herpes simplex virus DNA: a novel epidemiological tool applied to a nosocomial outbreak. *J Infect Dis* 1978;138:488–498.

80. Greaves WL, Kaiser AB, Alford RH, Schaffner W. The problem of herpetic whitlow among hospital personnel. *Infect Control* 1980;1:381–385.

81. Adams G, Stover BH, Keenlyside RA, et al. Nosocomial herpetic infections in a pediatric intensive care unit. *Am J Epidemiol* 1981;113:126–132.

82. American Academy of Pediatrics. Summaries of infectious diseases: herpes simplex. In: Pickering LK, Baker CJ, Long SS, McMillan JA, eds. *Red Book: 2006 Report of the Committee on Infectious Diseases.* 27th ed. Elk Grove Village, IL: American Academy of Pediatrics, 2006:361–370.

83. Pereira FA. Herpes simplex: evolving concepts. *J Am Acad Dermatol* 1996;35:503–520.

84. Perl TM, Haugen TH, Pfaller MA, et al. Transmission of herpes simplex virus type 1 infection in an intensive care unit. *Ann Intern Med* 1992;117:584–586.

85. Turner R, Shehab Z, Osborne K, Hendley JO. Shedding and survival of herpes simplex virus from "fever blisters." *Pediatrics* 1982;70:547–549.

86. Spruance SL, Overall JC Jr, Kern ER, et al. The natural history of recurrent herpes simplex labialis: implications for antiviral therapy. *N Engl J Med* 1977;297:69–75.

87. Davis RM, Orenstein WA, Frank JA Jr, et al. Transmission of measles in medical settings, 1980 through 1984. *JAMA* 1986;255:1295–1298.

88. Atkinson WL, Markowitz LE, Adams NC, Seastrom GR. Transmission of measles in medical settings—United States, 1985–1989. *Am J Med* 1991;91(suppl 3B):320S–324S.

89. Raad II, Sheretz RJ, Rains CS, et al. The importance of nosocomial transmission of measles in the propagation of a community outbreak. *Infect Control Hosp Epidemiol* 1989;10:161–166.

90. Istre GR, McKee PA, West GR, O'Mara DJ, Rettig PJ, Stuemky J, et al. Measles spread in hospital settings: an important focus of disease transmission? *Pediatrics* 1987;79:356–358.

91. Rivera ME, Mason WH, Ross LA, Wright HT Jr. Nosocomial measles infection in a pediatric hospital during a community-wide epidemic. *J Pediatr* 1991;119:183–186.

92. Rank EL, Brettman L, Katz-Pollack H, et al. Chronology of a hospital-wide measles out-break: lessons learned and shared from an extraordinary week in late March 1989. *AJIC Am J Infect Control* 1992;209:315–318.

93. Bloch AB, Orenstein WA, Ewing WM. Measles outbreak in a pediatric practice: airborne transmission in an office setting. *Pediatrics* 1985;75:676–683.

94. American Academy of Pediatrics. Summaries of infectious diseases: measles. In: Pickering LK, Baker CJ, Long SS, McMillan JA, eds. *Red Book: 2006 Report of the Committee on Infectious Diseases.* 27th ed. Elk Grove Village, IL: American Academy of Pediatrics, 2006:441–452.

95. Braunstein H, Thomas S, Ito R. Immunity to measles in a large population of varying age. *Am J Dis Child* 1990;144:296–298.

96. Centers for Disease Control. Laboratory-acquired meningococcal disease—United States, 2000. *MMWR Morb Mortal Wkly Rep* 2002;51:141–144.

97. Broome CV. The carrier state: *Neisseria meningitidis. J Antimicrob Chemother* 1986;18(suppl. A)25–34.

98. Gehanno JF, Kohen-Couderc L, Lemeland JG, Leroy J. Nosocomial meningococcemia in a physician. *Infect Control Hosp Epidemiol* 1999;20:564–565.

99. American Academy of Pediatrics. Summaries of infectious diseases: meningococcal disease. In: Pickering LK, Baker CJ, Long SS, McMillan JA, eds. *Red Book: 2006 Report of the Committee on Infectious Diseases.* 27th ed. Elk Grove Village, IL: American Academy of Pediatrics, 2006:452–460.

100. Riedo FX, Plikaytis BD, Broome CV. Epidemiology and prevention of meningococcal disease. *Pediatr Infect Dis J* 1995;14:643–657.

101. Wharton M, Cochi SL, Hutcheson RH, Schaffner W. Mumps transmission in hospitals. *Arch Intern Med* 1990;150:47–49.

102. Fischer PR, Brunetti C, Welch V, Christenson JC. Nosocomial mumps: report of an outbreak and its control. *Am J Infect Control* 1996;24:13–18.

103. American Academy of Pediatrics. Summaries of infectious diseases: mumps. In: Pickering LK, Baker CJ, Long SS, McMillan JA, eds. *Red Book: 2006 Report of the Committee on Infectious Diseases.* 27th ed. Elk Grove Village, IL: American Academy of Pediatrics, 2006:464–468.

104. Williams WW, Preblud SR, Reichelderfer PS, Hadler SC. Vaccines of importance in the hospital setting: problems and developments. *Infect Dis Clin North Am* 1989;3:701–22.

105. Koplan JP, Preblud SR. A benefit-cost analysis of mumps vaccine. *Am J Dis Child* 1982;136:362–364.

106. Centers for Disease Control and Prevention. Notice to readers: updated recommendations of the Advisory Committee on Immunization Practices (ACIP)for the control and elimination of mumps. *MMWR Morb Mortal Wkly Rep* 2006;55:629–630.

107. Hersh BS, Fine PEM, Kent WK, et al. Mumps outbreak in a highly vaccinated population. *J Pediatr* 1991;119:187–193.

108. Shishiba T, Matsunaga Y. An outbreak of erythema infectiosum among hospital staff members including a patient with pleural fluid and pericardial effusion. *J Am Acad Dermatol* 1993;29:265–267.

109. Seng C, Watkins P, Morse D, et al. Parvovirus B19 outbreak on an adult ward. *Epidemiol Infect* 1994;113:345–353.

110. Bell LM, Naides J, Stoffman P, et al. Human parvovirus B19 infection among hospital staff members after contact with infected patients. *N Engl J Med* 1989;321:485–491.

111. Harrison J, Jones DE. Human parvovirus B19 in health care workers. *Occup Med* 1995;45:93–96.

112. Pillay D, Patou G, Hurt S, Kibbler CC, Griffiths PD. Parvovirus B19 outbreak in a children's ward. *Lancet* 1992;339:107–109.

113. Evans JP, Rossiter MA, Kumaran TO, et al. Human parvovirus aplasia: case due to cross infection in a ward. *BMJ* 1984;288:681.

114. Cohen BJ, Courouce AM, Schwartz TF, et al. Laboratory infection with parvovirus B19 [letter]. *J Clin Pathol* 1988;41:1027–1028.

115. Anderson LJ, Gillespie SM, Török TJ, et al. Risk of infection following exposures to human parvovirus B19. *Behring Inst Mitt* 1990;85:60–63.

116. Dowell SF, Török TJ, Thorp JA, et al. Parvovirus B19 infection in hospital workers: community or hospital acquisition. *J Infect Dis* 1995;172:1076–1079.

117. Török TJ. Parvovirus B19 and human disease. *Adv Intern Med* 1992;37:431–455.

118. Centers for Disease Control and Prevention. Outbreaks of pertussis associated with hospitals—Kentucky, Pennsylvania, and Oregon, 2003. *MMWR Morb Mortal Wkly Rep* 2005;54:67–71.

119. Weber DJ, Rutala WA. Pertussis: a continuing hazard for healthcare facilities. *Infect Control Hosp Epidemiol* 2001;22:736–740.

120. Linneman CC Jr, Ramundo N, Perlstein PH, et al. Use of pertussis vaccine in an epidemic involving hospital staff. *Lancet* 1975;2:540–543.

121. Christie C, Glover AM, Willke MJ, et al. Containment of pertussis in the regional pediatric hospital during the greater Cincinnati epidemic of 1993. *Infect Control Hosp Epidemiol* 1995;16:556–563.

122. Shefer A, Dales L, Nelson M, et al. Use and safety of acellular pertussis vaccine among adult hospital staff during an outbreak of pertussis. *J Infect Dis* 1995;171:1053–1056.

123. Orenstein WA. Pertussis in adults: epidemiology, signs, symptoms, and implications for vaccination. *Clin Infect Dis* 1999;28(suppl. 2):S147–S150.

124. Weber DJ, Rutala WA. Management of healthcare workers exposed to pertussis. *Infect Control Hosp Epidemiol* 1994;15:411–415.

125. American Academy of Pediatrics. Summaries of infectious diseases: poliovirus infections. In: Pickering LK, Baker CJ, Long SS, McMillan JA, eds. *Red Book: 2006 Report of the Committee on Infectious Diseases.* 27th ed. Elk Grove Village, IL: American Academy of Pediatrics, 2006:542–547.

126. Centers for Disease Control and Prevention. Paralytic poliomyelitis—United States, 1980–1994. *MMWR Morb Mortal Wkly Rep* 1997;46:79–83.

127. Winkler WG, Fashinell TR, Leffingwell L, et al. Airborne rabies transmission in a laboratory worker. *JAMA* 1973;226:1219–1221.

128. Centers for Disease Control. Rabies in a laboratory worker—New York. *MMWR Morb Mortal Wkly Rep* 1977;26:183–184.

129. Helmick CG, Tauxe RV, Vernon AA. Is there a risk to contacts of patients with rabies? *Rev Infect Dis* 1987;9:511–518.

130. Centers for Disease Control and Prevention. Investigation of rabies infection in organ donor and transplant recipients—Alabama, Arkansas, Oklahoma, and Texas, 2004. *MMWR Morb Mortal Wkly Rep* 2004;53:1–3.

131. Centers for Disease Control and Prevention, National Institutes for Health. *Biosafety in microbiological and biomedical laboratories.* 3rd ed. Atlanta: US Department of Health and Human Services, Public Health Service, 1993.

132. Greaves WL, Orenstein WA, Stetler HC, et al. Prevention of rubella transmission in medical facilities. *JAMA* 1982; 248:861–864.

133. Strassburg MA, Stephenson TG, Habel LA, Fannin SL. Rubella in hospital employees. *Infect Control* 1984;5:123–126.

134. American Academy of Pediatrics. Summaries of infectious diseases: rubella. In: Pickering LK, Baker CJ, Long SS, McMillan JA, eds. *Red Book: 2006 Report of the Committee on Infectious Diseases.* 27th ed. Elk Grove Village, IL: American Academy of Pediatrics, 2006:574–579.

135. Fraser V, Spitznagel E, Medoff G, Dunagan WC. Results of a rubella screening program for hospital employees: a five-year review (1986–1990) *Am J Epidemiol* 1993;138:756–764.

136. Centers for Disease Control and Prevention. Control and prevention of rubella: evaluation and management of suspected outbreaks, rubella in pregnant women, and surveillance for congenital rubella syndrome. *MMWR Morb Mortal Wkly Rep* 2001;50(RR-12):1–23.

137. Lettau LA. Nosocomial transmission and infection control aspects of parasitic and ectoparasitic diseases, part III. Ectoparasites/summary and conclusions. *Infect Control Hosp Epidemiol* 1991;12:179–185.

138. Juranek DD, Currier RW, Millikan LE. Scabies control in institutions. In: Orkin M, Maiback HI, eds. *Cutaneous infestations and insect bites*. New York: Dekker, 1985,139–156.

139. Gooch JJ, Strasius SR, Beamer B, et al. Nosocomial outbreak of scabies. *Arch Dermatol* 1978;114:897–898.

140. Centers for Disease Control. Scabies in health-care facilities—Iowa. *MMWR Morb Mortal Wkly Rep* 1988;37:178–179.

141. Thomas MC, Giedinghagen DH, Hoff GL. Brief report: an outbreak of scabies among employees in a hospital-associated commercial laundry. *Infect Control* 1987;8:427–429.

142. Arlian LG, Estes SA, Vyszenski-Moher DL. Prevalence of *Sarcoptes scabei* in the homes and nursing homes of scabietic patients. *J Am Acad Dermatol* 1988;19:806–811.

143. Estes SA, Estes J. Therapy of scabies: nursing homes, hospitals, and the homeless. *Semin Dermatol* 1993;12:26–33.

144. Hopper AH, Salisbury J, Jegadeva AN, et al. Epidemic Norwegian scabies in a geriatric unit. *Age and Ageing* 1990;19:125–127.

145. Drugs for parasitic infections. *Med Lett Drugs Ther* August 2004, p. 9.

146. Degelau J. Scabies in long-term care facilities. *Infect Control Hosp Epidemiol* 1992;13:421–425.

147. Obasanjo OO, Wu P, Conlon M, Perl TM. An outbreak of scabies in a teaching hospital: lessons learned. *Infect Control Hosp Epidemiol* 2001;22:13–18.

148. Juranek DD. Pediculosis capitis in school children: epidemiologic trends, risk factors, and recommendations for control. In: Orkin M, Maiback HI, eds. *Cutaneous infestations and insect bites*. New York: Dekker, 1985,199–211.

149. Wenzel RP. Healthcare workers and the incidence of nosocomial infection: can treatment of one influence the other? a brief review. *J Chemother* 1994;6(suppl 4):33–37,39–40.

150. Panlilio AL, Culver DH, Gaynes RP, et al. Methicillin resistant *Staphylococcus aureus* in U.S. hospitals, 1975–1991. *Infect Control Hosp Epidemiol* 1992;13:582–586.

151. Boyce JM. Methicillin-resistant *Staphylococcus aureus*: detection, epidemiology and control measures. *Infect Dis Clin North Am* 1989;3:901–913.

152. Boyce JM. Methicillin-resistant *Staphylococcus aureus* in hospitals and long-term care facilities: microbiology, epidemiology, and preventive measures. *Infect Control Hosp Epidemiol* 1992;13:725–737.

153. Henderson DK. Managing methicillin-resistant staphylococci: a paradigm for preventing nosocomial transmission of resistant organisms. *Am J Med* 2006;121(6 suppl 1):S45–S53.

154. Boyce JM, Opal SM, Byone-Potter G, Medeiros AA. Spread of methicillin-resistant *Staphylococcus aureus* in a hospital after exposure to a health care worker with chronic sinusitis. *Clin Infect Dis* 1993;17:496–504.

155. Sherertz RJ, Reagan DR, Hampton KD, et al. A cloud adult: the *Staphylococcus aureus*-virus interaction revisited. *Ann Intern Med* 1996;124:539–547.

156. Belani A, Sherertz RJ, Sullivan ML, et al. Outbreak of staphylococcal infection in two hospital nurseries traced to a single nasal carrier. *Infect Control* 1986;7:487–490.

157. Kreiswirth BN, Kravitz GR, Schlievert PM, Novick RP. Nosocomial transmission of a strain of *Staphylococcus aureus* causing toxic shock syndrome. *Ann Intern Med* 1986;105:704–707.

158. Layton MC, Perez M, Heald P, Patterson JE. An outbreak of mupirocin-resistant *Staphylococcus aureus* on a dermatology ward associated with an environmental reservoir. *Infect Control Hosp Epidemiol* 1993;14:369–375.

159. American Academy of Pediatrics. Summaries of infectious diseases: staphylococcal infections. In: Pickering LK, Baker CJ, Long SS, McMillan JA, eds. *Red Book: 2006 Report of the Committee on Infectious Diseases*. 27th ed. Elk Grove Village, IL: American Academy of Pediatrics, 2006,598–610.

160. Boyce JM, Landry M, Deetz TR, DuPont HL. Epidemiologic studies of an outbreak of nosocomial methicillin-resistant *Staphylococcus aureus* infections. *Infect Control* 1981;2:110–116.

161. Mulligan ME, Murray-Leisure KA, Ribner BS, et al. Methicillin-resistant *Staphylococcus aureus*: a consensus review of the microbiology, pathogenesis, and epidemiology with implications for prevention and management. *Am J Med* 1993;94:313–328.

162. Reboli AC, John JF, Platt CG, Cantley JR. Methicillin-resistant *Staphylococcus aureus* outbreak at a Veterans' Affairs medical center: importance of carriage of the organism by hospital personnel. *Infect Control Hosp Epidemiol* 1990;11:291–296.

163. Boyce JM. MRSA patients: proven methods to treat colonization and infection. *J Hosp Infect* 2001;48(suppl A):S9–S14.

164. Kluytmans JA, Wetheim HF. Nasal carriage of *Staphylococcus aureus* and prevention of nosocomial infections. *Infection* 2005;33:3–8.

165. Valenzuela TD, Hooton TM, Kaplan EL, Schlievert PM. Transmission of toxic strep syndrome from an infected child to a firefighter during CPR. *Ann Emerg Med* 1991;20:90–92.

166. Rammelkamp CH, Mortimer EA, Wolinsky E. Transmission of streptococcal and staphylococcal infection. *Ann Intern Med* 1964;60:753–758.

167. Weber DJ, Rutala WA, Denny FW Jr. Management of health-care workers with pharyngitis or suspected streptococcal infections. *Infect Control Hosp Epidemiol* 1996;17:753–761.

168. Mastro TD, Farley TA, Elliott JA, et al. An outbreak of surgical-wound infections due to group A *Streptococcus* carried on the scalp. *N Engl J Med* 1990;323:968–972.

169. Viglionese A, Nottebart VF, Bodman HA, Platt R. Recurrent group A streptococcal carriage in a health care worker associated with widely separated nosocomial outbreaks. *Am J Med* 1991;91(suppl 3B):329S–333S.

170. Paul SM, Genese C, Spitalny K. Postoperative group A β-hemolytic *Streptococcus* outbreak with the pathogen traced to a member of a healthcare worker's household. *Infect Control Hosp Epidemiol* 1990;11:643–646.

171. Berkelman RL, Martin D, Graham DR, et al. Streptococcal wound infections caused by a vaginal carrier. *JAMA* 1982;247.2680–2682.

172. Schaffner W, Lefkowitz LB Jr, Goodman JS, Koenig MG. Hospital outbreak of infections with group A streptococci traced to an asymptomatic anal carrier. *N Engl J Med* 1969;280:1224–1225.

173. Richman DD, Breton SJ, Goldmann DA. Scarlet fever and group A streptococcal surgical wound infection traced to an anal carrier. *J Pediatr* 1977;90:307–390.

174. Centers for Disease Control and Prevention. Nosocomial group A streptococcal infections associated with asymptomatic health-care workers—Maryland and California, 1997. *MMWR Morb Mortal Wkly Rep* 1999;48:163–166.

175. American Academy of Pediatrics. Summaries of infectious diseases: group A streptococcal infections. In: Pickering LK, Baker CJ, Long SS, McMillan JA, eds. *Red Book: 2006 Report of the Committee on Infectious Diseases*. 27th ed. Elk Grove Village, IL: American Academy of Pediatrics; 2006:610–620.

176. Barnes PF, Bloch AB, Davidson PT, Snider DE. Tuberculosis in patients with human immunodeficiency syndrome. *N Engl J Med* 1991;324:1644–1650.

177. Centers for Disease Control and Prevention. Guidelines for preventing transmission of *Mycobacterium tuberculosis* in health-care settings, 2005. *MMWR Morb Mortal Wkly Rep* 2005;54 (RR-17):1–141.

178. Edlin BR, Tokars JI, Grieco MH, et al. An outbreak of multidrug-resistant tuberculosis among hospitalized patients with the acquired immunodeficiency syndrome. *N Engl J Med* 1992;326:1514–1521.

179. Stroud LA, Tokars JI, Grieco MH, et al. Evaluation of infection control measures in preventing the nosocomial transmission of multidrug-resistant *Mycobacterium tuberculosis* in a New York City hospital. *Infect Control Hosp Epidemiol* 1995;16:141–147.

180. Beck-Sagué CM, Dooley SW, Hutton MD, et al. Hospital outbreak of multidrug-resistant *Mycobacterium tuberculosis* infections: factors in transmission to staff and HIV-infected patients. *JAMA* 1992;268:1280–1286.

181. Wenger PN, Otten J, Breeden A, Orfas E, et al. Control of nosocomial transmission of multidrug-resistant *Mycobacterium tuberculosis* among healthcare workers and HIV-infected patients. *Lancet* 1995;345:235–240.

182. Dooley SW, Villarino ME, Lawrence M, et al. Nosocomial transmission of tuberculosis in a hospital unit for HIV-infected patients. *JAMA* 1992;267:2632–2635.

183. Pearson ML, Jereb JA, Frieden TR, et al. Nosocomial transmission of multidrug-resistant *Mycobacterium tuberculosis*: a risk to patients and health care workers. *Ann Intern Med* 1992;117:191–196.

184. Cleveland JL, Kent J, Gooch BF, et al. Multidrug-resistant *Mycobacterium tuberculosis* in an HIV dental clinic. *Infect Control Hosp Epidemiol* 1995;16:7–11.

185. Ridzon R, Kenyon T, Luskin-Hawk R, et al. Nosocomial transmission of human immuno-deficiency virus and subsequent transmission of multidrug-resistant tuberculosis in a healthcare worker. *Infect Control Hosp Epidemiol* 1997;18:422–423.

186. Jereb JA, Klevens M, Privett TD, et al. Tuberculosis in health care workers at a hospital with an outbreak of multidrug-resistant *Mycobacterium tuberculosis*. *Arch Intern Med* 1995;155:854–859.

187. Pugliese G, Tapper ML. Tuberculosis control in health care. *Infect Control Hosp Epidemiol* 1996;17:819–827.

188. Menzies D, Fanning A, Yuan L, Fitzgerald M. Tuberculosis among health care workers. *N Engl J Med* 1995;332:92–98.

189. Jarvis WR. Nosocomial transmission of multidrug-resistant *Mycobacterium tuberculosis*. *Am J Infect Control* 1995;23:146–151.

190. Maloney SA, Pearson ML, Gordon MT, et al. Efficacy of control measures in preventing nosocomial transmission of multidrug-resistant tuberculosis to patients and health care workers. *Ann Intern Med* 1995;122:90–95.

191. Centers for Disease Control and Prevention. Management of persons exposed to multidrug-resistant tuberculosis. *MMWR Morb Mortal Wkly Rep* 1992;41(RR-11):59–71.

192. Lane JM, Ruben FL, Neff JM, Millar JD. Complications of smallpox vaccination, 1968: results of ten statewide surveys. *J Infect Dis* 1970;122:303–309.

193. Centers for Disease Control. Contact spread of vaccinia from a recently vaccinated Marine—Louisiana. *MMWR Morb Mortal Wkly Rep* 1984;33:37–38.

194. Centers for Disease Control. Contact spread of vaccinia from a National Guard vaccinee—Wisconsin. *MMWR Morb Mortal Wkly Rep* 1985;34:182–183.

195. Centers for Disease Control. Vaccinia outbreak—Newfoundland. *MMWR Morb Mortal Wkly Rep* 1981;30:453–455.

196. Gustafson TL, Shebab A, Brunell PA. Outbreak of varicella in a newborn intensive care nursery. *Am J Dis Child* 1984;138:548–550.

197. Alter SJ, Hammond JA, McVey CJ, Myers MG. Susceptibility to varicella-zoster virus among adults at high risk for exposure. *Infect Control* 1986;7:448–451.

198. Krasinski K, Holzman RS, LaCouture R, Florman A. Hospital experience with varicella-zoster virus. *Infect Control* 1986;7:312–316.

199. Haiduven-Griffiths D, Fecko H. Varicella in hospital personnel: a challenge for the infection control practitioner. *Am J Infect Control* 1987;15:207–211.

200. Weber DJ, Rutala WA. Varicella immunization of health care workers. In: Panlilio A, Cardo D, eds. *Bailliere's clinical infectious diseases: prevention strategies for health care workers.* London: Harcourt, 2000:405–419.

201. American Academy of Pediatrics. Summaries of infectious diseases: varicella-zoster infections. In: Pickering LK, Baker CJ, Long SS, McMillan JA, eds. *Red Book: 2006 Report of the Committee on Infectious Diseases.* 27th ed. Elk Grove Village, IL: American Academy of Pediatrics, 2006:711–725.

202. Asano Y, Iwayama S, Miyata T, et al. Spread of varicella in hospitalized children having no direct contact with an indicator zoster case and its prevention by a live vaccine. *Biken J* 1980;23:157–161.

203. Sawyer MH, Chamberlin CJ, Wu YN, et al. Detection of varicella-zoster virus DNA in air samples from hospital rooms. *J Infect Dis* 1994;169:91–94.

204. LeClair JM, Zaia JA, Levin MJ, et al. Airborne transmission of chickenpox in a hospital. *N Engl J Med* 1980;302:450–453.

205. Gustafson TL, Lavely GB, Brawner ER Jr, et al. An outbreak of airborne nosocomial varicella. *Pediatrics* 1982;70:550–556.

206. Josephson A, Gombert M. Airborne transmission of nosocomial varicella from localized zoster. *J Infect Dis* 1988;158:238–241.

207. Struewing JP, Hyams KC, Tueller JE, Gray GC. The risk of measles, mumps, and varicella among young adults: a sero-survey of US Navy and Marine Corps recruits. *Am J Public Health* 1993;83:1717–1720.

208. Centers for Disease Control and Prevention. Prevention of varicella: updated recommendations of the Advisory Committee on Immunization Practices (ACIP) *MMWR Morb Mortal Wkly Rep* 1999;48(RR-6):1–5.

209. Saiman L, LaRussa P, Steinberg SP, et al. Persistence of immunity to varicella-zoster virus after vaccination of healthcare workers. *Infect Control Hosp Epidemiol* 2001;22:279–283.

210. Centers for Disease Control and Prevention. Varicella-related deaths among adults—United States, 1997. *MMWR Morb Mortal Wkly Rep* 1997;46:409–412.

211. Centers for Disease Control and Prevention. Guideline for preventing health-care–associated pneumonia, 2003. *MMWR Morb Mortal Wkly Rep* 2004;53(RR-03):1–36.

212. Evans ME, Hall KL, Berry SE. Influenza control in acute care hospitals. *AJIC Am J Infect Control* 1997;25:357–362.

213. Kapila R, Lintz DI, Tecson FT, et al. A nosocomial outbreak of influenza. A. *Chest* 1977;71:576–579.

214. Van Voris LP, Belshe RB, Shaffer JL. Nosocomial influenza B virus infection in the elderly. *Ann Intern Med* 1982;96:153–158.

215. Pachucki CT, Walsh Pappas SA, Fuller GF, et al. Influenza A among hospital personnel and patients: implications for recognition, prevention, and control. *Arch Intern Med* 1989;149:77–80.

216. Centers for Disease Control. Suspected nosocomial influenza cases in an intensive care unit. *MMWR Morb Mortal Wkly Rep* 1988;37:3–4, 9.

217. Centers for Disease Control and Prevention. Outbreak of influenza A in a nursing home—New York, December 1991–January 1992. *MMWR Morb Mortal Wkly Rep* 1992;41:129–131.

218. Gross PA, Rodstein M, LaMontagne JR, et al. Epidemiology of acute respiratory illness during an influenza outbreak in a nursing home. *Arch Intern Med* 1988;148:559–561.

219. Cartter ML, Renzullo PO, Helgerson SD, et al. Influenza outbreaks in nursing homes: how effective is influenza vaccine in the institutionalized elderly? *Infect Control Hosp Epidemiol* 1990;11:473–478.

220. Bean B, Moore BM, Sterner B, et al. Survival of influenza viruses on environmental surfaces. *J Infect Dis* 1982;146:47–51.

221. Hall CB, Douglas RG. Nosocomial influenza infection as a cause of intercurrent fevers in infants. *Pediatrics* 1975;55:673–677.

222. Noble GR. Epidemiological and clinical aspects of influenza. In: Beare AS, ed. *Applied influenza research.* Boca Raton, FL: CRC Press, 1982:11–49.

223. Adal KA, Flowers RH, Anglim AM, et al. Prevention of nosocomial influenza. *Infect Control Hosp Epidemiol* 1996;17:641–648.

224. Hall CB. Respiratory syncytial virus: its transmission in the hospital environment. *Yale J Biol Med* 1982;55:219–223.

225. Snydman DR, Greer C, Meissner HC, McIntosh K. Prevention of nosocomial transmission of respiratory syncytial virus in a newborn nursery. *Infect Control Hosp Epidemiol* 1988;9:105–108.

226. Harrington RD, Hooton TM, Hackman RC, et al. An outbreak of respiratory syncytial virus in a bone marrow transplant center. *J Infect Dis* 1992;165:987–993.

227. Guidry GG, Black-Payne CA, Payne DK, et al. Respiratory syncytial virus infection among intubated adults in a university medical intensive care unit. *Chest* 1991;100:1377–1384.

228. Falsey AR. Noninfluenza respiratory virus infection in long-term care facilities. *Infect Control Hosp Epidemiol* 1991;12:602–608.

229. Sorvillo FJ, Huie SF, Strassburg MA, et al. An outbreak of respiratory syncytial virus pneumonia in a nursing home for the elderly. *J Infect* 1984;9:252–256.

230. Centers for Disease Control and Prevention. Outbreak of severe acute respiratory syndrome—worldwide, 2003. *MMWR Morb Mortal Wkly Rep* 2003;52:241–246.

231. Valenti WM, Hruska JF, Menegus MA, Freeburn MJ. Nosocomial viral infections: III. Guidelines for prevention and control of exanthematous viruses, gastroenteritis viruses, picornaviruses, and uncommonly seen viruses. *Infect Control* 1980;2:38–49.

The Development of Infection Surveillance and Control Programs

5

Marilyn Jones and Keith F. Woeltje

INTRODUCTION

The goal of an infection surveillance, prevention, and control program is to prevent healthcare-associated infections (HAIs) in patients, employees and visitors and to achieve that prevention in a cost-effective manner [1]. Therefore, every infection control (IC) program should formally evaluate the effectiveness of prevention efforts and the cost-effectiveness of those efforts [2,3]. These efforts have been expanded to the concept of interventional epidemiology that affirms that the activities and decisions made by IC be viewed from a business perspective including global systems thinking [4].

The term epidemiology in the context of an IC control program refers to enumeration, distribution, and control of infectious diseases in its healthcare population (patients, visitors, and employees). Individuals charged with an IC program must have knowledge in the science of epidemiology including surveillance methodology, study design, statistical methods, infectious agents, and many other competencies [5]. It is no surprise that these skills are the same set used by public health professionals because IC was born out of public health in the late 1950s when there was mounting concern regarding infection agent transmission within the hospital.

In 1958, outbreaks of *Staphylococcus aureus* infections in hospitals prompted the American Hospital Association to recommend that hospitals set up IC programs [6].

A few years later, in the early 1960s, the Centers for Disease Control (now the Centers for Disease Control and Prevention [CDC]) organized an investigations unit section that would assist hospitals in investigating outbreaks. As the 1960s progressed, medical care became increasing complex. Antibiotic-resistant organisms and opportunist pathogens developed as increasing challenges to the infection prevention and control efforts within the hospital setting [4,7]. Nationwide adoption of hospital infection control programs did not occur until the early 1970s when the CDC and the Joint Commission on Accreditation of Hospitals (now Joint Commission on Accreditation of HealthCare Organizations [JCAHO]) recommended that hospitals have IC programs [6,8]. The landmark Study of the Efficacy of Nosocomial Infection Control (SENIC) project demonstrated that an active IC program that included surveillance with feedback of infection rates, along with a physician and nurse with infection control knowledge, resulted in a reduction of HAIs [9,10].

Because the historical development of IC programs had epidemiologic roots, personnel charged with running the IC program traditionally were expected to have strong skills not only in medical and nursing care but also in healthcare epidemiology. More recently, the IC field has appreciated the importance of the business and management skills as well. From a financial perspective, IC departments are viewed as nonrevenue-generating departments because there is no charge to the patient or payor. If careful demonstration of the value to the organization is not documented and shared with key leaders, including those who hold the purse strings, IC may find its financial resources limited if not diminished. To garner resources for the program and mission of preventing HAIs, an IC program must adopt the new approach of "interventional epidemiology" and "give sufficient weight to the economic impact of any project or activity undertaking"[4]. IC program personnel must incorporate effectiveness evaluation into routine project and program planning so that they can demonstrate the value of infection prevention and control to the healthcare organization.

COMPONENTS OF AN INFECTION CONTROL PROGRAM

An infection control program has many facets; however, the central components to be addressed when developing a program are governance, personnel, and the IC plan including the surveillance plan. Also critical to an effective program are the internal and external collaborations, compliance activities, and interventions.

GOVERNANCE

A successful IC program must have both medical and administrative support and participation to accomplish its goals. Often this is accomplished through a formalized IC committee that makes decisions and recommends policies for the facilities' IC program [11]. The IC committee reports to a governing body within the hospital, such as a medical executive group or the hospital's administrative board. This body reviews and acts on the committee's recommendations. The governing body may, in turn, request a review of a current topic in the community or a hospital-specific policy, practice, or issue brought forward from another hospital forum such as a surgical committee. Although JCAHO no longer requires an IC committee per se, the IC standards do call for the demonstration of collaboration between medical staff, administrators, multiple hospital specialties, and IC to assess and develop the IC program [12]. It is necessary for a hospital to demonstrate that infection prevention occurs in all aspects of services rendered throughout the institution and that all employees understand their job-specific infection prevention actions. In addition, some states require that hospitals have a formal IC committee as part of the hospital licensing rules.

DEPARTMENTAL REPORTING STRUCTURE

Like the governance of IC, no single method of departmental reporting structure fits every healthcare facility. Across the country are many examples of effective programs that report to different functions, such as nursing, quality, patient safety, or medical services. Regardless of the chain of command, the critical components are the support of the program during routine operations and an appreciation of critical issues that require immediate attention and added resources, such as sentinel events, outbreaks, or community emergencies.

PERSONNEL

Personnel needs are established based on the size, complexity, services, and the needs of the facility and the community. A hospital epidemiologist and at least one infection control professional (ICP) are the minimum personnel needed for an IC program. The hospital epidemiologist may be a physician and in many instances is an infectious diseases (ID) physician. The expert knowledge of an ID physician is especially useful; however, it is also necessary for the hospital epidemiologist to have specialized training in epidemiology and IC. The Society for Healthcare Epidemiology of America (SHEA) in conjunction with the CDC, some medical schools and other professional organizations offer specific training. The hospital epidemiologist often serves as the chair for the IC committee and is involved in the planning and implementation of the program. The position of hospital epidemiologist is typically not a full-time position or a hospital employee; the physician contracts with the hospital for epidemiology services [13].

The ICP usually is a registered nurse or a medical technologist. Specialized training programs for ICPs are offered by Association for Professionals in Infection Control and Epidemiology (APIC), the Community and Hospital Infection Control Association–Canada (CHICA), other international societies, and other organizations including state hospital associations and health departments. Professional and practice standards define the competency standards and professional accountabilities of the ICP [5]. After two years of IC practice and passing the voluntary, standardized examination demonstrates proficiency in basic infection prevention and control knowledge [14] physicians, technologists, and nurses are eligible to become Certified in Infection Control (CIC) by APIC (other international organizations may have other criteria).

Historically, one ICP for every 250 beds was recommended based on the SENIC study [9]. Advances in medicine, changes in healthcare delivery, and increasing regulatory and compliance requirements have outdated this figure [1]. A Delphi project sponsored by APIC noted that staffing decisions should consider the facility's size, needs, complexity, and patient population. In general, it recommended a ratio of 0.8 to 1.0 ICP for every 100 occupied acute care beds [15].

In addition to the hospital epidemiologist and at least one ICP, support personnel are needed to allow the trained IC staff to focus on surveillance, prevention, and control activities. Secretarial support for scheduling meetings; typing minutes, policies, correspondence, and other documents; and maintaining paperwork, in general, can greatly enhance a program's effectiveness. Additional services for forms creation, data entry, and data management should be available to the IC program [1]. The size of the facility and the complexity of the IC program will determine whether these are dedicated or shared personnel resources. Some facilities have found that sharing secretarial, chart abstraction, data entry, or database management personnel between departments such as IC, quality, and regulatory proves cost effective.

THE INFECTION CONTROL PLAN

The annual IC plan is an essential roadmap for the activities that the IC program will undertake. The annual plan is developed based on the IC program's strategic or long-term plan and the institution's mission and strategic objectives. Strategic planning should encompass traditional business strategies, entrepreneurial thinking, and futurist exercises [16]. Institutional initiatives, new laws and regulatory requirements, and newly published methods for preventing infections should be incorporated. Components of the plan include the overall mission and goal of the program, the goals for the year, and the scope of the IC department including the department hours and the mechanism for providing 24-hour coverage.

Another foundational component of the annual IC plan is the surveillance plan. This plan should include the indicators to be followed during the year (e.g., intensive care unit catheter-associated bloodstream infection rates and surgical site infection rates in cardiac surgery), the rationale for choosing those indicators, case-finding methods, definitions, and data management methods including report distribution. Evaluation of the historical data and a review of services and populations served by the institution will guide the development of the IC surveillance plan [17]. The surveillance plan is not equivalent to the IC plan; that would mistakenly simplify the IC program to only a surveillance program. The IC plan should incorporate activities directly aimed at improving endemic rates. Although IC is charged with protecting against and investigating outbreaks, only approximately 5–10% of all HAIs is associated with outbreaks. The other 90–95% of HAIs is due to endemic or common causes; therefore, the majority of prevention efforts should be focused on reducing endemic HAIs and mitigating HAI risks [18–20].

A plan for IC-related educational activities should be a component of the IC plan. In addition to the routine requirements, such as new employee and annual education, a review of the questions and concerns posed by employees in the past will provide a foundation for new programs or

highlights for the year. It may be helpful for the ICP to log calls to decipher common educational themes.

A schedule for review of policies and procedures should be included in the IC plan as well. Although this review often is seen as a tedious administrative task, it can be turned into a productive activity if it is accompanied with a departmental walk-thru that assesses the environment and practices for their impact on patient and employee HAI risk.

The IC plan should outline special studies and intervention projects. These ventures should be directly related to the missions and goals.

Incorporating routine activities, such as consultation to various committees, product evaluation, and community involvement, into the IC plan is critical because these activities account for considerable amounts of time. Painting a clear picture of the time and resources necessary for all IC activities should be an objective of the plan. However, unexpected circumstances arise, and the plan should have enough flexibility to accommodate unplanned events, such as outbreaks in the institution or community and unexpected regulatory mandates.

In summary, the IC plan includes the mission, goals, and program scope; surveillance plan; education plan; policy and procedure review plan; and special studies.

INTERNAL COLLABORATIONS

Collaborations are critical to the success of the IC program. Although largely immeasurable, the relationships that the ICP develop will positively contribute to its mission. No amount of policies or education will substitute for the trusting relationships that healthcare workers (HCWs) develop with the IC staff. Hospital personnel need to feel that they can be candid about concerns without fear of retribution or shame. Bear in mind that relationships and trust are between individuals, not departments or functions. Therefore, when developing an IC program, the IC staff should concentrate on meeting all department heads and key department leaders including frontline staff. IC employees should focus on understanding the department's issues and attempt to solve concerns even if they may not have a significant impact on HAI rates. When nuisance problems are resolved, individuals are much more likely to have the time, energy, and trust to work on the more challenging issues. Although it may seem elementary, the demonstration of trust and cooperation is the first and foremost critical step in the development of an effective IC program.

Internal departmental partnerships are as extensive as the number of departments within a facility because the IC program is an entitywide function. Each and every department should work with the IC program to incorporate IC activities into their own work. They should recognize that IC is everyone's job, not just the IC's. The affiliations that are paramount and closely aligned with the IC program will be discussed in detail.

Occupational Health

JCAHO and some state regulations mandate the occupational health department's relationship with IC. Even if not required, the overlap of preventing HCWs and patients from being exposed to infectious exposures is an obvious link between the two departments. IC and occupational health work together on the development of the requirements for HCW immunizations, prevention of infectious disease exposures, and postexposure prophylaxis and secondary exposure prevention, including HCW work restrictions [21,22].

The more frequent occupational occurrences necessitate specific and on-going efforts of both IC and occupational health. Specifically, the treatment and prevention of sharps injuries and other body substance exposures through policy and engineering controls is necessary and mandated by the Occupational Safety and Health Administration (OSHA). Predetermined protocols for the treatment of exposures serve to provide rapid management, which is critical for the prevention of bloodborne pathogens, especially those involving human immunodeficiency virus [23]. Some exposure episodes are less straightforward than can be managed with a written protocol. In these instances, the hospital epidemiologist often serves as the consultant for the management of unusual occupational exposures. The prevention of sharps injuries necessitates an epidemiological approach to exposure incidence, including subanalysis within specific groups of HCWs (nurses, operating room personnel, physicians, housekeepers, etc.), specific devices, activities, and work areas. Formal evaluative reports presented to the IC committee or other governing body in addition to providing on-going feedback to the departments where injuries are occurring provides the mechanism for leadership input and resource allocation.

Depending on the community prevalence, tuberculosis prevention and control may account for only a fraction of program time or a significant amount of energy for both the occupational health and IC departments. This is an excellent example of why facility-specific personnel staffing evaluation is necessary and why IC and occupational health must be closely linked either formally through the internal chain of command or informally through collaboration and the IC committee (or similar function).

Patient Safety

Another critical internal collaboration is between IC and patient safety. Although IC is viewed as the first formal effort to protect patients, the discipline of patient safety came into its own after the 1999 publication of *To Err Is Human* by the Institute of Medicine [24,25]. Now JCAHO has incorporated IC into its National Patient Safety Goals by requiring evidence of compliance with the CDC's hand-hygiene recommendations and the reporting of infection-related adverse or sentinel events. Hospitals are now called on to investigate every death caused by an HAI using the specific model of root cause analysis (RCA). Although RCA may be an appropriate tool for rare IC occurrences, such as group A streptococcus surgical infections or an episode of aspergillous HAI, its value has yet to be demonstrated for a specific or single causative factor for infectious deaths due common cause or endemic HAI issues. Nevertheless, the RCA process can be used as a tool to uncover the many suboptimal process issues that contribute to high endemic rates. For example, a death caused by *Clostridium difficile* is likely to be rooted in the on-going, common cause dilemma of horizontal transmission related to suboptimal hand hygiene and isolation precaution compliance, antibiotic treatments, and specific host factors rather than a single "root cause." Because JCAHO mandates RCA for many healthcare facilities, IC personnel must collaborate with their partners in patient safety to perform these analyses. Because JCAHO surveys approximately 82% of acute care hospitals that account for 96% of the hospital beds in the United States [27], most IC personnel will likely participate in RCA procedures. IC personnel can partner with patient safety peers to assist in the epidemiological investigations of process and outcome measures such as falls, venous thrombus embolic events, and medication safety events.

Quality

The quality department and IC also are closely aligned because both departments are charged with improving patient outcomes. Many quality departments are authorized by the hospital to measure quality indicators and report those results to organizations such as the Institute for Healthcare Improvement (IHI) (100,000 lives and impact campaigns) and the Centers for Medicare and Medicaid Services (CMS). At 56 hospitals participating in a collaborative, compliance with the CMS infection prevention indicators in the Surgical Care Improvement Project (SCIP) demonstrated a 27% mean reduction of SSI rates [28,29]. Often the quality measures are based on IC and healthcare epidemiology studies that demonstrated the effectiveness of the individual intervention, such as timely and appropriate surgical prophylactic antibiotics [30–36].

In addition to having overlapping indicator interest with IC, quality personnel often are versed in the models of improvement, such as Continuous Quality Improvement (CQI), Plan-Do-Check-Act (PDCA), Six Sigma, and Lean. IC frequently uses the epidemiologic methods for improving endemic and epidemic HAI rates; however, these quality tools can enhance IC's problem-solving armamentarium. ICPs can lean on the quality professionals who often are proficient in leading and facilitating teams for direct assistance or guidance.

Risk Management

Another hospital department with which IC routinely joins forces is risk management. Every HAI-related death or permanent disability should be reported to the patient safety department and to the risk management department. IC also should report outbreaks and other potentially litigious situations to risk management to protect the institution and its HCWs. In addition to reporting duties, risk management relies on IC departments to implement standards of care that prevent HAIs and thereby reduce liability. Risk management may also request that IC departments review the medical records of patients who have filed or threatened lawsuits that may have infection implications. Policies and procedures from years ago may need to be reviewed to validate that the standard of care for the period is being followed.

Microbiology

A high-quality microbiology department is a true asset to the IC department. Skilled microbiologists and technicians understand the importance of specific clinical specimens, and those individuals will alert IC. Microbiology policies for alerting the IC department should be developed to leave no ambiguity regarding notification of common yet significant pathogens, such as methicillin-resistant *Staphylococcus aureus*, *Clostridium difficile*, or more unusual findings such as acid fast bacilli in respiratory specimens or gram-negative diplococci on a stain of cerebral spinal fluid. Due to the stringent requirements for laboratory certification, most U.S. facilities have reliable methods to identify microbiologic pathogens. External laboratories may be used particularly for specialty tests that require specialized equipment, media, or reagents. During outbreaks, the microbiology staff is consulted for advice regarding environmental sampling and for planning additional specimen processing, such as the heightened screening of a population.

Clinical Care Areas

IC must collaborate with personnel from all clinical areas to ensure that patient care is provided with the utmost attention to infection prevention. Established procedures for IC must be implemented in routine practice. The clinical care areas must be alert for problems that would not be detected by routine surveillance methods such as gastroenteritis or rashes among patients and employees, insects and varmints, humidity and temperature abnormalities, or product defects. Areas with high-risk patients, high risk procedures, and high volume should command special attention from IC. Examples of such areas include the operating room, intensive care units, emergency departments, interventional radiology, and cardiac procedure areas.

IC must collaborate with many other critical departments, such as environmental safety, education, emergency preparedness, and pharmacy. An appreciation of the literature and the standards of practice put forth by each professional discipline will aid in the development of infection prevention approaches.

EXTERNAL PARTNERSHIPS

IC has a direct partnership with the community public health department. At most facilities, the IC department is charged with the notification of reportable diseases. In community outbreaks or disasters, public health and IC work side by side to protect the public's health. Depending on the facility's mission the IC department may be directly involved and collaborate with the public health department for community outreach programs, such as health fairs or educational campaigns. Bioterrorism or emergency preparedness collaborations occur more recently at state and local levels. Relationships with other hospitals, surgical centers, long-term care facilities, and other service providers within the community provide two-way feedback regarding patients' HAI acquisition.

COMPLIANCE ISSUES

The IC department must evaluate many compliance standards or regulations. They may be mandatory such as the OSHA bloodborne pathogen standard; others, such as the CDC's infection prevention guidelines, are not legally required but recommended for good practice. Even when not specifically mandated, guidelines such as the CDC's recommendations often are held as a standard of care and therefore should be carefully evaluated. Failure to adopt recommended practices may place the institution at risk if adverse events occur and are legally pursued. However, different agencies may have conflicting recommendations, or some recommendations may not be based on sound epidemiologic or medical principles (i.e., evidence based). When these situations occur, IC personnel should evaluate the literature and studies cited for the recommendations to propose the best practices for patients and employees thru its governance (such as the IC committee). Professional organizations that have standards for the prevention of HAIs include APIC and SHEA in the United States and CHICA in Canada, as well as the Infection Control Nurses Association in the United Kingdom and the Asia Pacific Society for Infection Control. (Additionally, specialty care organizations such as the Association of Operating Room Nurses, American Society for Gastrointestinal Endoscopy, Society of Gastroenterology Nurses and Associates, the Association for Vascular Access, and the Intravenous Nurses Society have standards or guidelines on preventing infection.) Governmental and nongovernmental regulatory agencies that promote recommendations include JCAHO, CDC, OSHA, CMS, Food and Drug Administrations, Agency for Healthcare Research and Quality, the National Quality Forum, and state and local governments including health departments.

In the past decade, agency requirements for demonstrating the implementation of evidence-based practices and measures that prevent harm have proliferated. Although these requirements may have imposed a considerably increased data burden for hospitals that do not use electronic records systems, the requirements have forced the deployment of improved processes that are expected to result in improved care or health outcomes. For example, before the CMS requirement of timely surgical prophylactic antibiotic delivery, on-time delivery was occurring at an average rate of 56% [37] despite the fact that the literature to support this practice is more than 15 years old [30]. For example, prior to the CMS requirement of collecting and reporting appropriate timing of surgical prophylaxis, appropriate prophylaxis was only occuring at rate of 56%. Despite the fact that the literature to support this practice is more than 15 years old [30], it took regulatory mandates to improve compliance.

INTERVENTION IMPLEMENTATION

The goal of preventing HAIs is accomplished by intervention implementation. The improvement should be chosen [38] using surveillance data; reviewing high-risk, high-volume, problem-prone procedures and processes; and evaluating current regulatory and practice standards. Worthy projects, process owners, and collaborators should be objectively evaluated for readiness to change current practices. According to the principles of change leadership, people will not make needed sacrifices but will hold onto the status quo and resist new strategies without a sense of urgency or need to change [39]. When leaders of areas that need improvement are satisfied with the current performance, the IC team should seek change by first creating an uncomfortable feeling with the status quo. Dissatisfaction with the present condition is essential to instill the motivation for change. Alternatively, IC personnel should find a project that demonstrates the need for improved practices or outcome to partners and key leaders.

Once the project has been selected, IC and the process owners should use an improvement model that is consistent with its organizational model. Different improvement methodologies have advantages and disadvantages; however, ensuring that team members understand the tools and use a systematic method for evaluating the problem and implementing a solution is more important than the superiority of the model. At a minimum, the model should call for the multidisciplinary team to establish a goal and a target for success and determine the measurement component that will demonstrate the project's effectiveness.

EVALUATION OF INTERVENTIONS

An intervention and its evaluation should be designed concurrently. The evaluation should include whether the project was successful as determined by the original goal and target established by the team. It also should include a cost analysis that compares the cost of the intervention with the savings associated with avoided HAIs. Intervention costs should include the time of the intervention team members, the development of the education program, the time of staff required to complete the education, and engineering control such as products and equipment retrofitting.

When an improvement project implements multiple interventions at the same time, the interventions cannot be individually assessed for effectiveness. However, this should not preclude the evaluation of the intervention as a package (most HAI prevention interventions are multifactorial). Often improvements are seen initially, but the success begins to fade over time because the intervention change was not firmly rooted in a new manner of performance. In other words, there was a regression to the old processes [39]. Therefore, continued assessment of the intervention should be incorporated.

The define-measure-analyze-improve-control (DMAIC) improvement model of Six Sigma recognizes the need for a formal process for monitoring the improvement and for developing a response plan if the improvement deteriorates. In most intervention projects, IC should continue to track the HAI rates (outcome measure) while the clinical areas quantify the process measures. For example, IC should monitor central venous catheter-associated bloodstream infection (CVC-BSI) rates while the intensive care unit staff monitors the percentage of femoral lines or the percentage of CVCs placed using maximal barrier precautions. When the process measures are carefully chosen, their monitoring is critical because they have a direct relationship with the desired outcome [40]. In most instances, the process measures worsen before the outcome measure is affected. By tracking the process, the healthcare team can intervene before an adverse HAI outcome occurs.

CONCLUSION

The components to a successful IC program include clearly defined governance, knowledgeable personnel, and a plan for improving HAI rates and infection prevention practices. A predetermined plan guides activities and facilitates the IC team to stay focused on goals without getting unnecessarily sidetracked to other projects or "flavor of the month" campaigns. Positive relationships with the hospital personnel and external agency representatives will directly influence the IC's ability to meet its mission to prevent HAIs in patients, employees, and visitors and to achieve that prevention in a cost-effective manner.

REFERENCES

1. Scheckler WE, Brimhall D, Buck AS, et al. Requirements for infrastructure and essential activities of infection control and epidemiology in hospitals: A concensus panel report. *Am J Infect Control* 1998;26:47–60.

2. Pittet D. Infection control and quality health care in the new millennium. *Am J Infect Control* 2005;33:258–267.

3. Stone PW, Hedblom EC, Murphy DM, Miller SB. The economic impact of infection control: Making the business case for increased infection control resources. *Am J Infect Control* 2005;33:542–547.

4. Garcia R, Barnard B, Kennedy V. The fifth evolutionary era in infection control: Interventional epidemiology. *Am J Infect Control* 2000;28:30–43.

5. Horan-Murphy E, Barnard B, Chenoweth C, et al. APIC/CHICA-Canada infection control and epidemiology: Professional and practice standards. *Am J Infect Control* 1999;27:47–51.

6. Arias KM. Surveillance. In: *APIC text of infection control and epidemiology*. 2nd ed. Washington DC: Association for Professionals in Infection Control and Epidemiology. 2005; 3.1–3.18.

7. Haley RW. The development of infection surveillance and control programs. In Bennett JV, Brachman PS, eds. *Hospital Infections*. 4th ed. Philadelphia: Lippincott–Raven, 1998: 53–64.

8. Haley RW. The scientific basis for using surveillance and risk factor data to reduce nosocomial infection rates. *J Hosp Infect* 1995;30S:3–14.

9. Haley RW, Culver DH, White JW, et al. The efficacy of surveillance and control programs in prevention nosocomial infections in U.S. hospitals. *Am J Epidemiol* 1985; 121:182–205.

10. Horan TC, Lee TB. Surveillance. Into the next millennium. *Am J Infect Control* 1997;25:73–76.

11. Friedman C. Infection Control and Prevention Programs. In: Carrico R, ed. *APIC text of infection control and epidemiology*. 2nd ed. Washington: Association of Professionals in Infection Control and Epidemiology, 2005.

12. Joint Commission on Accreditation of Healthcare Organizations (JCAHO). *2006 Comprehensive accreditation manual for hospitals: The official handbook* (CAMH). Oakbrook Terrace, Illinois: Joint Commission on Accreditation of Healthcare Organizations.

13. Deery HG, Sexton DJ. How to get paid for healthcare epidemiology. In: Lautenbach E, Woeltje KF, eds. *SHEA practical handbook for healthcare epidemiologist*. 2nd ed. Thorofare, NJ: SLACK, Inc, 2004.

14. Becoming Certified. Certification Board of Infection Control and Epidemiology, Inc. 2005 (http://www.cbic.org/Becoming_Certified.asp).

15. O'Boyle C, Jackson M, Henly SJ. Staffing requirements for infection control programs in US health care facilities: Delphi project. *Am J Infect Control* 2002;30:321–333.

16. Soule BM. From vision to reality: Strategic agility in complex times. *Am J Infect Control* 2002;30:107–119.

17. Pottinger JM, Herwaldt LA, Perl TM. Basics of surveillance—An overview. *Infect Control Hosp Epidemiol* 1997;18:513–527.

18. Beck-Sague C, Jarvis WR, Martone WJ. Outbreak investigations. *Infect Control Hosp Epidemiol* 1997;18:138–145.

19. Gaynes RP. Surveillance of nosocomial infections: A fundamental ingredient for quality. *Infect Control Hosp Epidemiol* 1997;18:475–478.

20. Stamm WE, Weinstein RA, Dixon RE. Comparison of endemic and epidemic nosocomial infections. *Am J Med* 1981;70:393–397.

21. CDC. Immunization of health-care workers: Recommendations of the Advisory Committee on Immunization Practices (ACIP) and the Hospital Infection Control Practices Advisory Committee (HICPAC). *MMWR* 1997; 46 (RR-18).

22. Bolyard EA, Tablan OC, Williams WW, et al. Guideline for infection control in health care personnel, 1998. *Am J Infect Control* 1998;26:289–354.

23. Panlilio AL, Cardo DM, Grohskopf LA, et al. Updated U.S. Public Health Service guidelines for the management of occupational exposures to HIV and recommendations for postexposure prophylaxis. *MMWR* 2005;54 (RR-9); 1–17.

24. Kohn LT, Corrigan JM, and Donaldson MS, eds. *To err is human: Building a safer health system.* Washington: National Academies Press, 2000.

25. Murphy DM. Patient safety. In: Corrico R, ed. *APIC text of infection control and epidemiology.* 2nd ed. Washington DC: Association for Professionals in Infection Control and Epidemiology. 2005.

26. JCAHO requirement: The Joint Commission announces the 2007 national patient safety goals and requirements. *Joint Commission Perspectives* 2006; 2(7): 1–31.

27. Personal communication with Peter B. Angood, M.D. May 24, 2006.

28. Bratzler DW, Hunt DR. The surgical infection prevention and surgical care improvement projects: National initiatives to improve outcomes for patients having surgery. *Clin Infect Dis* 2006;43:322–330.

29. Dellinger EP, Hausmann SM, Bratzler DW, et al. Hospitals collaborate to decrease surgical site infections. *Am J Surg* 2005;190:9–15.

30. Classen DC, Evans RS, Pestotnik SL, et al. The timing of prophylactic administration of antibiotics and the risk of surgical-wound infection. *N Engl J Med* 1992;326:281–286.

31. Alexander JW, Fischer JE, Boyajian M, et al. The influence of hair-removal methods on wound infections. *Arch Surg* 1983;118:347–352.

32. Masterson TM, Rodeheaver GT, Morgan FR, Edlich FR. Bacteriologic evaluation of electric clippers for surgical hair removal. *Am J Surg* 1984;148:301–302.

33. Sellick JA Jr., Stelmach M, Mylotte MJ. Surveillance of surgical wound infections following open heart surgery. *Infect Control Hosp Epidemiol* 1991;12:591–596.

34. Ko W, Lazenby WD, Zelano JA, et al. Effects of shaving methods and intraoperative irrigation on suppurative mediastinitis after bypass operations. *Ann Thorac Surg* 1992;53:301–305.

35. Furnary AP, Zerr KJ, Grunkemeier GL, et al. Continuous intravenous insulin infusion reduces the incidence of deep sternal wound infection in diabetic patients after cardiac surgical procedures. *Ann Thorac Surg* 1999;67:352–360.

36. Latham RL, Lancaster AD, Covington JF, et al. The association of diabetes and glucose with surgical-site infections among cardiothoracic surgery patients. *Infect Control Hosp Epidemiol* 2001;22:607–612.

37. Bratzler DW, Houck PM, Richards C, et al. Use of antimicrobial prophylaxis for major surgery: Baseline results from the National Surgical Infection Prevention Project. *Arch Surg* 2005;140:174–182.

38. Murphy DM. From expert data collector to interventionists: Changing the focus for infection control professionals. *Am J Infect Control* 2002;30:120–132.

39. Kotter JP. *Leading change.* Boston: Harvard Business School Press, 1996.

40. Baker OG. Process surveillance: An epidemiological challenge for all heath care organizations. *Am J Infect Control* 1997;25:96–101.

Surveillance of Healthcare-Associated Infections

6

Mary L. Andrus, Teresa C. Horan, and Robert P. Gaynes

DEFINITION OF SURVEILLANCE

Surveillance is "the ongoing, systematic collection, analysis, and interpretation of health data essential to the planning, implementation, and evaluation of public health practice, closely integrated with the timely dissemination of these data to those who need to know" [1]. A healthcare-associated infection (HAI) surveillance system may be sentinel event based, population based, or both. A sentinel infection is one that clearly indicates a failure in the hospital's efforts to prevent HAIs and, in theory, requires individual investigation [2,3]. For example, blood transfusion from a source-patient already identified as a hepatitis carrier should always prompt investigation because it clearly indicates a failure of a hospital's safeguards. Denominator data usually are not collected in sentinel event-based surveillance. Sentinel event-based surveillance will identify only the most serious problems and should not be the only surveillance system in the hospital. Population-based surveillance (i.e., surveillance of patients with similar risks) requires both a numerator (i.e., HAI) and denominator (i.e., number of patients or days of exposure to the risk).

The findings and conclusions in this chapter have not been formally disseminated by the Centers for Disease Control and Prevention and should not be construed to represent any agency determination or policy.

HISTORICAL PERSPECTIVE

Since the first edition of this book, there has been a great deal of discussion and debate among professionals over the desirability of continuing routine surveillance, argued by some to be too personnel intensive in an era of constrained hospital budgets. As this discussion continues, an account of the development of concepts and techniques of surveillance should be considered. Many of these techniques were developed to meet emerging problems, and the basic concept of surveillance has been found effective in reducing HAI risk. Knowledge of the historical reasons for these developments may help improve the efficiency and effectiveness of surveillance without discarding well-conceived approaches that remain effective.

The use of surveillance methods to control HAIs dates back at least to the classic work of Dr. Ignaz Semmelweis in Vienna in the 1840s [4]. Although the Semmelweis story is best remembered as the first demonstration of person-to-person spread of puerperal sepsis and of the effectiveness of hand washing with an antiseptic solution, an equally important achievement was Semmelweis' rigorous approach to the collection, analysis, and use of surveillance data. In contrast, the concurrent work of Dr. Oliver Wendell Holmes on the same subject in the United States was based primarily on the traditional anecdotal case-study approach of clinical medicine.

Semmelweis' investigation constitutes an amazingly contemporary example of the effective use of surveillance in addressing a widespread HAI problem. When he assumed the directorship of the obstetric service at the Vienna Lying-in Hospital in 1847, the apparent risk of maternal mortality had been at high levels for >20 years. The eminent clinicians of the day, in fact, considered the risks to be no more than the expected endemic occurrence that could not be influenced. Semmelweis first undertook a retrospective investigation of maternal mortality and set up a prospective surveillance system to monitor the problem and, later, the effects of control measures. The initial results of his retrospective study of annual hospital mortality showed clearly that the maternal mortality level, which he measured by calculating yearly mortality rates, had increased tenfold following the introduction in the 1820s of the new anatomic school of pathology, which used autopsy as its primary teaching tool. Based on the use of ward-specific mortality, Semmelweis calculated that the risk of death on the ward used for teaching medical students was at least four times higher than that on the ward used for teaching midwifery students. After the septic death of his mentor suggested the presence of a transmissible agent, Semmelweis used the findings from his retrospective surveillance study to implicate the practices of the medical students. After observing their daily routines, he surmised that students might be transferring pathogens from cadavers to the parturient women and that washing hands with a chlorine solution might prevent this transmission. Subsequently, his prospective surveillance data documented a dramatic reduction in maternal mortality immediately following the institution of mandatory hand washing before entering the labor room.

Apparently, due to his abrasive manner, lack of diplomacy, and inability to organize his statistical data into a concise and convincing report, Semmelweis failed to win over his clinical colleagues to his discovery. Within 2 years, he was dismissed from the staff of the hospital, and his successor gradually allowed the strict hand-washing measures to decline. In the absence of continuing surveillance, the epidemic promptly resumed and lasted well into the early part of the 20th century, its severity and means of prevention apparently unappreciated by several more generations of clinicians.

This story illustrates one of the main impediments to infection control today: In the absence of careful epidemiologic data and a diplomatic presentation, clinicians, who are oriented almost entirely toward the treatment of individual patients, often fail to appreciate the severity of the HAI pathogen transmission problem and sometimes resist control measures. It also points out the utility of surveillance in identifying problems and developing and applying control measures. From a methodologic viewpoint, Semmelweis' efforts encompassed almost all aspects of the modern surveillance approach: retrospective collection of data to confirm the presence of a problem; analysis of the data to localize the risks in time, place, and person; controlled comparisons of high- and low-risk groups to identify risk factors; formulation and application of control measures; and prospective surveillance to monitor the problem, evaluate the implemented control measures, and detect future recurrences. The main shortcoming of his approach was in not diplomatically educating his powerful colleagues with a careful report of his findings.

Despite Semmelweis' historical model, the modern era of HAI surveillance grew more from mid-20th century experience. The importance of surveillance for disease control in general arose in the effort to control tropical diseases among troops stationed in the Pacific Theater in World War II. At the end of the war, most of the epidemiologists of the "Malaria Control in War Areas Unit" were transferred to a civilian facility to apply their surveillance and control strategies to the control of malaria in the southern United States. Located in Atlanta, near the endemic areas, the unit was first named the Communicable Diseases Center and later became the Centers for Disease Control and Prevention (CDC). Since the large number of reports of malaria indicated the disease to be widespread, a surveillance system was immediately set up to define the problem. However, as investigators examined each reported case, they found virtually all of the reports had errors in diagnosis. Thus, the mere activity of surveillance "eradicated" the malaria epidemic in the United States [5].

Because of this and similar successes, when the pandemic of staphylococcal infections swept the nation's hospitals in the mid-1950s, CDC staff members were quick to apply the concepts of surveillance to the problem. When asked to assist in investigating a staphylococcal epidemic in a particular hospital, these early investigators often met strong resistance from clinicians and hospital administrators convinced that no unusual infection problems were present in their hospitals. In instances when CDC staff members were able to continue the investigations, the collection and reporting of surveillance data regularly changed those attitudes to strong concern over the documented problems and eagerness to apply control measures. These initial investigations thus confirmed a nationwide staphylococcal epidemic and led the CDC to sponsor several national conferences to discuss the problem [5].

By the early 1980s, some critics were questioning the effectiveness and cost benefit of routine HAI surveillance, although a growing number of hospitals were increasing their surveillance efforts rather than cutting them back [6]. Surveillance was, and remains, a time-consuming activity requiring about 40 to 50% of the time of an infection control professional (ICP) [7]. The inability of some hospitals to establish an adequate number of ICP positions (at least one full-time equivalent per 250 beds) has been a major contributor to disenchantment within the infection control profession.

Several factors have influenced contemporary practices favoring robust surveillance activities in infection control programs. First, the results of the Study on the Efficacy of Nosocomial Infection Control (SENIC) project strongly substantiated the importance of surveillance along with control measures to reduce HAI rates and provided the scientific basis for surveillance of HAIs [8–10]. The conclusion was that hospitals that are effective in reducing their HAI rates have an organized, routine, hospitalwide surveillance system. Second, the requirements of the Joint Commission on Accreditation of Healthcare Organizations (JCAHO, formerly JCAH) have legitimized the need for personnel to perform surveillance [11,12]. Third, the surveillance practices developed in infection control have begun to influence other aspects of the hospital's quality monitoring and improvement activities. The strategies of targeting surveillance to reduce specific endemic problems and monitoring to assess the intervention's effectiveness were incorporated into JCAHO's 1994 infection control standards for accreditation and were applied to hospital quality-assurance programs to reduce noninfectious complications [13,14]. The increasing pressure to continually improve quality is certain to broaden the use of surveillance to aid in the prevention of HAIs [15].

GOALS OF SURVEILLANCE

A hospital should have clear goals for doing surveillance. These goals must be reviewed and updated frequently to address new HAI risks in changing patient populations, such as the introduction of new high-risk medical interventions, changing pathogens and their resistance to antibiotics, and other emerging problems. The collection and analysis of surveillance data must be performed in conjunction with a prevention strategy. It is vital to identify and state objectives of surveillance *before* designing a surveillance program and starting it.

Reducing HAI Rates Within a Hospital

The most important goal of surveillance is to reduce the risks of acquiring HAIs. To achieve this goal, specific objectives for surveillance must be defined based on how the data are to be used and the availability of financial and personnel resources for surveillance [7,8]. Objectives for surveillance can be either outcome or process oriented or both. Outcome objectives are aimed at reducing HAI risk and their associated costs. By using comparative HAI rate analysis and providing feedback to patient-care personnel, outcome data are useful in demonstrating where gaps in HAI prevention activities exist. Process monitors, on the other hand, help to identify delivery of care problems that can have an effect on patient outcomes. Examples of process monitors are observing and evaluating patient-care practices, monitoring equipment and the environment, and providing education. Much of the time spent performing surveillance should be devoted to monitoring patient-care

process objectives because policy seldom equals practice. However, these activities are of limited value without clearly stating outcome objectives. While HAI surveillance has other legitimate purposes, the ultimate goal is to use this process objective to achieve the outcome objective: decreases in HAI rates, morbidity, mortality, and cost.

Establishing Endemic Rates

Surveillance data should be used to quantify baseline rates of endemic HAIs. This measurement provides hospitals with knowledge of the ongoing HAI risk in hospitalized patients. Most HAIs, perhaps 90 to 95%, are endemic (i.e., not part of recognized outbreaks) [16]. Thus, the main purpose for surveillance activities should be to lower the endemic HAI rate rather than identify outbreaks, and many hospital ICPs report that their presence on the wards may be sufficient to influence HAI rates [17]. However, the mere act of collecting data does not usually influence HAI risk appreciably unless it is linked with a prevention strategy. Otherwise, surveillance is no more than "bean counting," an expensive exercise without focus that today's hospitals can ill afford and that ICPs will ultimately find dissatisfying.

Identifying Outbreaks

Once endemic HAI rates have been established, ICPs and hospital epidemiologists may be able to recognize deviations from the baseline that sometimes indicate infection outbreaks. This surveillance benefit must be balanced with the relatively time-consuming task of ongoing data collection because only a small proportion of HAIs, perhaps 5 to 10%, occur in outbreaks [14]. Moreover, HAI outbreaks often are brought to the attention of ICPs by astute clinicians or laboratory personnel much more quickly than by the analysis of routine HAI surveillance data. This lack of timeliness often limits the use of routine HAI surveillance in identifying outbreaks in a hospital.

Convincing Medical Personnel

Convincing hospital personnel to adopt recommended preventive practices is one of the most difficult tasks of an infection control program. Familiarity with the scientific literature on hospital epidemiology and infection control is effective in influencing behavior only if the hospital personnel believe the information is relevant to the specific situation in question. Studies in the literature may not address the many varied situations encountered in a particular hospital. Using information on one's own hospital to influence personnel is one of the most effective means to address a problem and apply the recommended techniques to prevent HAIs. If surveillance data are analyzed appropriately and presented routinely in a skillful manner, medical personnel usually come to rely on them for guidance. The feedback of such information often is quite effective in influencing behavior of healthcare workers to adopt recommended preventive practices [9]. A team approach with ICPs working with clinicians from a variety of disciplines is particularly effective.

Evaluating Control Measures

After a problem has been identified through surveillance data and control measures have been instituted, continued surveillance is needed to ensure that the problem is under control. By continual monitoring, some control measures that seemed rational can be shown to be ineffective. For example, the use of daily meatal care to prevent nosocomial urinary tract infections (UTIs) seemed appropriate but did not control infection [18]. Even after the initial success of control measures, breakdowns in applying them can occur, requiring a constant vigil including the continued collection of surveillance data.

Satisfying Accrediting and Regulatory Agency Surveyors

Satisfying the requirements of accrediting organizations, such as JCAHO, is a very common use of HAI surveillance data but one of the least justifiable. The collection of surveillance data merely to satisfy a surveyor who visits a hospital once every three years (or occasionally more often) is a largely unproductive use of resources. JCAHO also changed its requirements to avoid this task-oriented process of collecting data as unproductive when it altered its standards in 1990. Hospitals are now required to use HAI surveillance in a directed manner to initiate specific interventions designed to lower the risk of HAIs in patients [11]. JCAHO's Agenda for Change has motivated hospitals to use HAI surveillance for its originally intended purpose: to change the outcome of patient care by reducing HAI risk.

Defending Malpractice Claims Previously

One concern about the collection of HAI surveillance data has been that it would create a record that could be used against the hospital in a malpractice claim related to an HAI. A strong surveillance component in an infection control program will demonstrate, however, that a hospital is attempting to detect problems rather than conceal them (see Chapter 17). Additionally, the records of infection control committees are considered privileged in most states and are not discoverable in civil court proceedings. Therefore, surveillance often is helpful in defending against malpractice claims, and it is rarely, if ever, a hindrance.

Comparing Hospitals' HAI Rates

Traditionally, HAI surveillance has been recommended solely for gaining understanding of and reducing HAI rates within individual hospitals. The idea of comparing HAI rates among hospitals, though often suggested by administrators and quality-assurance supervisors, has generally been discouraged by infection control physicians and practitioners. They argue that the mix of intrinsic HAI risk of the patients in different hospitals renders differences among the hospital rates virtually uninterpretable. Studies performed by CDC, however, have suggested that interhospital comparisons can be useful in reducing HAI risk [19,20] if the rates are specific to a particular site of HAI (e.g., UTI) and control for variations in the distributions of the major risk factor(s) for that type of infection (e.g., duration of indwelling urinary catheterization). Conversely, using a single number to express a hospital's overall HAI rate falls short as a valid measure largely because suitable overall risk adjusters for infections of all types are lacking [20–23]. *Therefore, a hospital's overall HAI rate, as presently derived, should not be used for interhospital comparisons.*

Public Reporting of HAI Rates

Many state and national initiatives to mandate or induce healthcare organizations to publicly disclose information regarding institutional and physician performance are underway. Mandatory public reporting of healthcare performance is intended to enable stakeholders, including consumers, to make more informed decisions about healthcare choices and has taken several forms such as report cards and honor rolls. As of this writing, 13 states require hospitals to report publicly their HAI rates [24]. The methods of surveillance and reporting have differed from state to state. In an effort to provide guidance and to establish more uniformity, the CDC's Healthcare Infection Control Practices Advisory Committee (HICPAC) issued a guidance document on public reporting of HAIs in 2005 [25]. Presently the evidence on the merits and limitations of using an HAI public reporting system as a means to reduce HAIs is insufficient. The HICPAC guidance is intended to assist policymakers, program planners, consumer advocacy organizations, and others tasked with designing and implementing HAI public reporting systems. Challenges for meaningful interpretation of publicly reported HAI rates include accuracy in identifying HAIs, risk adjustment to account for varying degrees of risk among the sampled patient population, and the method of expression of the HAI rates that can range from complicated indices to single and perhaps overly simplistic rates intended to measure a facility's experience. HICPAC has made no recommendation for or against mandatory public reporting of HAI rates. Some investigators have recommended that efforts should be directed instead to creating acceptably accurate, objective measures of quality of care and of outcomes, such as process and/or surrogate measures that all healthcare facilities can use [26]. Process measures assess the delivery of care rather than the outcomes. These measures can be useful when their link to beneficial or adverse outcomes is well established.

For example, appropriate delivery of perioperative antibiotic prophylaxis is a case in point of a process measure that emerged from decades of research [27]. Surrogate measures are objective indicators of readily ascertained events that are sufficiently correlated with HAIs to provide useful information about the actual institutional HAI rate [28]. For example, the surgical site infection (SSI) rates following coronary artery bypass, Cesarean section, or breast surgery appear to correlate closely with the proportion of patients who receive extended courses of inpatient antibiotics and is a useful indicator of a hospital's SSI outcomes for those procedures [29].

METHODS OF SURVEILLANCE

Collecting the Data

Definition of Events to Be Surveyed

Carefully defining those events to be surveyed is important as an initial step in developing a HAI surveillance system. Applying accepted definitions systematically in the data-collection process is another key step. In attempting to understand the relationship between UTI and urinary catheterization, for example, it is necessary first to define or establish criteria to decide what will be called a UTI and what will be considered urinary catheterization. Once the event to be surveyed has been defined as concisely and precisely as possible and the criteria for determining its occurrence have been established, then these definitions and criteria are applied systematically and uniformly henceforth. Ideally, all members of the population at risk for the infection would be systematically monitored for the presence or absence of the criteria elements that define the infection being surveyed.

The CDC has published guidelines for determining the presence and classification of HAIs [30]. These guidelines are not rigorous definitions of disease but serve as practical, operational HAI surveillance definitions for most hospitals regardless of their size or medical sophistication. The exact definitions to be used in surveillance in individual hospitals are not as critical as having the infection control committee obtain the concurrence of key hospital staff members who will be applying them. Such widespread advance agreement is necessary to avoid later having the results of surveillance disqualified by disagreements over the definitions.

Role of the ICP

A variety of methods of collecting HAI data has been described [31–33]. In general, the most satisfactory and practical method employs a person (or persons), often called the ICP, whose job description includes collecting and analyzing surveillance data. Details of the qualifications, functions, and responsibilities of the ICP are described elsewhere (see Chapter 5). The ICP reports prevention and surveillance information to the infection control committee and should work directly with the committee chairperson or the hospital epidemiologist. The traditional choice of a nurse to fill this position has been primarily based on the person's professional training and ability to interact primarily with other healthcare personnel in the data-collection process. Experience has shown, however, that persons other than nurses can function well in this position, particularly in the surveillance process. The original studies of surveillance, conducted by CDC in the 1970s, indicated that one full-time-equivalent ICP could conduct surveillance for approximately 250 acute-care hospital beds and have sufficient remaining time for other infection control duties and responsibilities [10]. In recent years, however, as the average length of a patient's hospital stay has decreased and patients' severity of illness has increased, the ICP's job has become more demanding, requiring an increase in infection control resources. ICPs continue to set priorities for the use of their time in ways that will maximize their impact on infection risks.

Minimal Data to Collect About Infections

The precise information collected in conjunction with each HAI depends on the surveillance objective and may vary according to the institution, service, site of infection, or causative agent. Certain essential identifying data, however, can be recommended: the patient's name, age, gender, hospital identification number, ward or location within the hospital, service, and date of admission; the date of onset of the infection; the site of infection; the organism(s) isolated in culture studies; and the antimicrobial susceptibility pattern of the organisms isolated. Additional information should be collected only if it will be analyzed and used by the hospital. Some institutions may wish to include the primary diagnoses of the infected patient, an assessment of the severity of underlying illness(es), the name(s) of the attending physician(s) or other staff who attended the patient, whether the patient was exposed (before the onset of the HAI) to therapies that may predispose to infection (e.g., surgery; antimicrobials, steroids, or immunosuppressive therapy; or instrumentation), what antimicrobial agents were used to treat the infection, and some assessment of mortality related to the HAI. It is important to record the presence or absence of particular risk factors (e.g., the use of invasive devices such as urinary catheters for UTIs, ventilators for pneumonias, and central line catheters for primary bacteremia).

Denominators

The methods for collecting the denominators for HAI rate determination have been controversial and have sometimes been the most labor-intensive aspect of generating HAI rates [29]. Historically, the common denominator was the number of patients admitted to or discharged from the hospital or a particular ward or service [17]. These totals served as a crude estimate of the number of patients at HAI risk. Another denominator used was *patient-days* rather than admissions or discharges. Patient-day denominators are derived by summing the number of days that all patients stayed in the hospital during the surveillance period. Since the patient-day denominator includes length of stay, the resulting HAI rates are at least partially adjusted for differences among patients' lengths of stay. Admissions, discharges, and patient-days can be for the hospital as a whole and for individual patient-care units. These data can be obtained either electronically or in a written monthly report from the hospital medical records department or business office. However, these denominators fail to take into account differences in patient risks for HAIs, such as exposures to certain invasive devices. Calculation of overall rates using these denominators is not recommended [22].

Another method is to collect a record on every patient at HAI risk rather than on only infected patients and to use summary denominator data for rate calculation. As hospitals have become more computerized, this has become easier and more common. In this method, the record contains the risk factors for individual patients (e.g., each patient undergoing a surgical procedure), and then the information about any subsequent HAI is added to the patient's record when detected. Computerization usually is necessary to manage these detailed records. An ICP can use a computerized patient database and computer software to calculate HAI rates, including denominators for whatever time period and patient population selected. While entering data on all patients at risk might seem more time-consuming than other methods, it is preferable for priority-directed surveillance projects, such as generating surgeon-specific SSI rates by risk index category or device-associated infection surveillance by specific nursing care unit. This method offers ICPs more flexibility in the types of rates that can be generated. A full database enables them to calculate rates by any risk factor or combination of risk factors. This alternative is made even more attractive by the ability to "download" denominator records from other hospital software. For example, the records of all operations can be downloaded periodically from the operating room database. As HAI surveillance becomes increasingly automated and directed toward specific prevention objectives, detailed denominators on individual patients at risk are expected to be employed more often (See Chapter 9).

Identifying Sources of Infection Data

To ensure the most complete enumeration of HAIs, ICPs seek a variety of infection information sources from both within and outside the hospital [17]. These active techniques of case finding are used in almost all hospitals and are strongly preferred to passive techniques. The active techniques allow more complete detection of "cases" and provide for the ICP to visit the patient-care areas regularly, interact with and provide consultation to the medical and nursing staffs, and gain firsthand awareness of HAI

problems. Passive techniques include asking physicians or staff nurses to fill out infection report forms or relying solely on reviews of computerized microbiology reports. The usefulness of passive techniques is limited by their inaccuracy in routine detection of HAIs. Hospitals relying on passive techniques typically find extremely low HAI rates, but these usually are due to underreporting rather than good patient-care practice [17]. While the use of administrative data (e.g., billing codes) can be a useful screening tool, this approach also has major shortcomings as a single methodology for identifying infections [34]. The actual collection of HAI data is typically accomplished by a combination of manual and electronic surveillance techniques. The ICP often has electronic access to demographic information, microbiology and pharmacy reports, and sometimes radiology dictation summaries. Many of the data elements used to satisfy the criteria for HAIs, however, are found in the patient chart or by consultation with physicians or nursing or respiratory therapy staff.

The Microbiology Laboratory

Of all case-finding methods, one of the most useful is the periodic (usually daily) review of microbiology laboratory reports. Data-mining computer applications also may be used to identify microorganisms of special significance to the patient population requiring specific infection prevention measures. A review of microbiology results may be performed each morning before patient-care unit rounds, so any new or potential HAIs can be identified at that time. Such review requires that the ICP understand the infectious and epidemiologic potential of various microorganisms; such knowledge might be achieved through laboratory training or a basic infection prevention and control course and should be reinforced by periodic continuing education. However, a review of microbiology laboratory reports alone is not sufficient for the identification of HAIs because (1) cultures are not obtained for all infections or may be handled incorrectly, (2) some infectious agents (e.g., viruses) will not be identified in many hospital laboratories, and (3) for some types of infections (e.g., SSIs and pneumonia), the identification of a potential pathogen from a culture specimen does not mean that infection is present and such infections require clinical detection and verification (see Chapter 10).

Patient-Care Area Rounds

Periodic (preferably daily) patient-care rounds should be included as an integral part of an effective surveillance program. The purposes of such rounds are to identify new HAIs and to follow up previously identified HAIs. New HAIs may be identified outright by physicians or nurses working in the area visited and by review of patient records, temperature records, patients having high-risk procedures (e.g., surgery, central line insertion, intubation and mechanical ventilation, indwelling urinary catheters), and patients in isolation or receiving antimicrobial therapy. Visiting the patient-care unit also may allow direct assessment of the patient and documentation of visible HAIs. The added value of patient-care rounds is the opportunity for the ICP to interact directly with patient-care staff and initiate measures that could prevent HAIs in the future.

Postdischarge Follow-Up

With the progressive reduction in the average length of patient stay in U.S. hospitals, an increasing percentage of some HAIs, most notably SSIs, become manifest after hospital discharge. The percentage of SSIs that becomes apparent after discharge ranges from 20 to 60% [35–41], and at least one study has shown the presence of a strong selection bias in rates based only on in-hospital surveillance. Since the average postoperative length of stay of surgical patients influences the probability that SSIs will be recognized while the patient is in the hospital, this variable must be taken into account when analyzing and evaluating a hospital's SSI rate.

Multihospital analyses of SSI rates in the SENIC project used length of stay as a covariate in multiple regression analyses [10]; others have suggested using the incidence density (i.e., patient-days in the denominator of the SSI rates) [42]. Choice of postdischarge surveillance method is controversial and problematic. Many ICPs follow up with postcard inquiries or telephone calls to the surgeon 21 to 30 days after the date of the operation to determine whether an SSI occurred [39–42]. Though this creates additional work for the surveillance staff, the amount of work may be commensurate with the gain in completeness and accuracy of the SSI rates. Patients themselves are rarely contacted and questioned about signs and symptoms of SSI following selected operative procedures, but the reliability of this information is questionable. Postdischarge antibiotic exposure also may be a resource-efficient adjunct for surveillance of SSIs after discharge [43].

Other Sources

Additional infection information may be obtained through a periodic review of radiology, pharmacy, and laboratory reports; records of personnel health clinic visits; and autopsy reports. The exclusive use of other methods of infection data collection, such as reviewing patients' medical records after discharge or the use of infection report forms filled out by attending physicians or floor nurses, is less satisfactory from the standpoint of infection control. Reviewing patients' medical records after discharge results in a failure to apply indicated infection control precautions and may result in excessive morbidity or mortality among patients or hospital personnel. The use of infection report forms filled out by attending physicians or floor nurses has been used in a number of hospitals, but it suffers from the lack of systematic application of standard definitions and criteria for detecting HAIs and from variation in the thorough reporting of HAIs.

Consolidating and Tabulating Data

Consolidating the HAI data in ways that make them more understandable helps users identify potentially important relationships or patterns of infection that may not be apparent from the raw data on data collection forms. The most effective analyses of surveillance data may take many forms depending on the objective being addressed by the surveillance. For routine, total hospital surveillance, ICPs often simply analyze HAI data in single-variable frequency tables (e.g., number of HAIs by hospital location, body site, or pathogen) and two-way cross-tabulations (e.g., a line listing with the number of HAIs by body site and by pathogen for each patient-care unit), and tally antimicrobial susceptibility patterns for each pathogen by HAI site. In recent years, however, more imaginative analyses have been done, including three-way rate tables (e.g., pathogen by site by patient-care unit), four-way rate tables (e.g., susceptibility patterns by pathogen by site by care unit), and more complex cross-tabulations. Usually these tabulations are performed for subsets of the patients, such as those on a particular service or the patients of a specific surgeon. To do these adequately requires a computer to analyze the patient databases.

Although beginning surveillance personnel should first master the standard frequency and cross-tabulation routines mentioned previously, more experienced ICPs can try more creative ways of organizing the infection data. The basic purpose of tabulating the HAIs is to gain a new understanding of when, where, and in whom the HAIs are occurring. One of the most frequent mistakes made when the raw data are organized is to make initial tabulations hastily and proceed with calculating rates without pausing to examine the data. It often is useful to read over the original listings and the simple tabulations for an initial synthesis of the data that can suggest the need for additional tabulations, graphs, and listings. For example, finding an increased rate of bacteremia in surgical patients might call for a tabulation of bacteremia for each surgical subspecialty or for each surgical ward and surgical intensive care unit and for comparisons with similar rates from previous months or for the same months the previous year. This process of exploration of the data has no rigid rules; what is right is that which works!

Calculating Rates

Definition of Rate

After the initial tabulations of the HAIs have been completed, the infection control staff should have a strong indication of where HAI problems might be occurring. Since these initial analyses are based solely on examination of the overall number of HAIs (numerator data), further analysis involving the calculation of rates is necessary to develop stronger evidence.

A *rate* is an expression of the probability of occurrence of some particular event, and it has the form $k(x/y)$, where

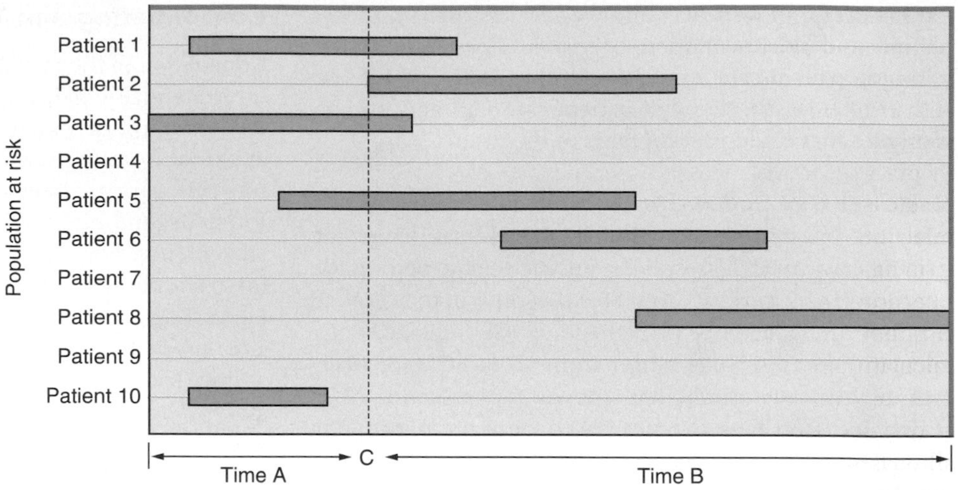

Figure 6-1 Incidence of infection is three during either time A or B (three new cases were added during each time period); *prevalence* of infection during time A is 40% and during B, 60% (four cases and six cases respectively, occur in each period of time; and *point prevalence* of infection at time C is 30% (at that point in time, three cases exist).

x, the numerator, equals the number of times an event has occurred during a specific time interval; *y*, the denominator, equals a population from which those experiencing the event were derived during the same time interval; and *k* equals a round number (100, 1,000, 10,000, 100,000, and so on) called a *base*. The base used depends on the magnitude of *x*/*y*, and it is selected to permit the rate to be expressed as a convenient whole number. For example, if five HAIs were found among 100 patients in a given month, the value of *x*/*y* would be 0.05 HAIs per patient per month; to express the rate as a convenient whole number, *x*/*y* would be multiplied by the base number 100, giving five HAIs per 100 patients per month. If 50 HAIs were found among 10,000 patients in a month, the base number 1,000 would be used to express the rate as 5 HAIs per 1,000 patients per month. It is important to emphasize that in determining a rate, both the time interval and the population must be specified, and these must apply to both the numerator (*x*) and the denominator (*y*) of the rate expression. A practical way of generating a rate is to enter the denominator data, obtained in the data collection stage, below the appropriate numerator figures in the frequency and cross-tables of infections tabulated earlier. From these numerators (indicating the numbers of HAI) and their denominators (indicating the numbers of patients, or patient-days, at HAI risk), HAI rates can be calculated. Alternatively, currently available computer software can display the numerator and denominator and calculate the rate automatically from a database containing all patients at risk and the associated HAIs that occurred.

Types of Rates

Three specific kinds of rates—prevalence, incidence, and attack rate—are fundamental tools of epidemiology and, as such, should be familiar to infection control personnel. *Prevalence* is the number of episodes of the disease found to be *active* within a defined population either during a specified period (period prevalence) or at a specified point in time (point prevalence). These concepts are discussed further in a later section of this chapter. *Incidence* is the number of *new* episodes of disease that occur in a defined population during a specified time period. The incidence rate is obtained by dividing the number of new episodes by the number of people in the population at risk during the specified time period. In Figure 6-1, which portrays the infection status of 10 hospitalized patients, the incidence of infection during either time period A or B, for example, would be three, since three new infections began among the 10 patients in each time period. Assuming that period A was 1 month and period B was 3 months, the incidence rates would be three infections per 10 patients at risk (30%) per month in period A and 10% per month in period B (i.e., exactly equivalent to 30% per 3 months).

An *attack rate* is a special kind of incidence rate. It is usually expressed as a percentage (i.e., *k* = 100 in the rate expression), and it is used almost exclusively for describing outbreaks where particular populations are exposed for limited periods of time (e.g., in common-source outbreaks). Since the duration of an outbreak is reasonably short, the period of time to which the rate refers is not stated explicitly but is assumed. This is what distinguishes an attack rate from an incidence rate when the period of time is always stated. If 100 infants in a newborn nursery, for example, were exposed to a contaminated lot of infant formula over a 3-week period, and if 14 of the infants developed a characteristic illness believed to be caused by the contaminated formula, the attack rate for those infants exposed to the formula would be 14%. Note that the incidence rate would be 14 cases per 100 infants per 3 weeks, preferably expressed as 4.67 cases per 100 infants per week.

Choice of Numerator and Denominator

Basically two types of incidence rates can be calculated: The infection ratio is the number of infections divided by the number of patients at risk during the specified period, and the infection proportion is the number of patients with ≥ 1 infections divided by the number of patients at risk during the period. Since approximately 18% of patients with HAIs have >1 infection, the infection ratio is usually nearly 1.27 times larger than the infection proportion [44]. In practice, most ICPs have found the infection ratio to be far easier to obtain than and equally as useful as the infection proportion; consequently, the commonly used term *infection rate* has come to refer specifically to the infection ratio. Nevertheless, when presenting results, it is important to specify which method has been used for calculating the rate.

Another approach is to use the number of patient-days at risk during the period of surveillance (i.e., the sum of all days spent by all patients in the specified area during the time period covered) for the denominator in a rate calculation. This rate is referred to as the *incidence density*. To get an idea of how the two types of rates compare, rates based on the number of patient-days (R) usually are smaller than those based on admissions or discharges (r) by a factor approximately equal to the average length of stay of the patients (k), that is:

$$R = k \times r$$

For example, if the HAI rate were five HAIs per 100 admissions per month and the patients' average length of stay was 10 days, one would expect to find a rate of approximately five HAIs per 1,000 patient-days. The incidence density is useful primarily in two situations: (1) when the infection rate is a linear function of the length of time a patient is exposed to a risk factor (e.g., indwelling urinary or intravenous catheter) and (2) when the duration of follow-up will influence the measured infection rate (e.g., SSI rates when no postdischarge surveillance is done). The relative merits of the alternative ways of controlling for differences in length of stay, including using the incidence density, performing postdischarge surveillance of surgical patients, and using multivariate analytic methods to control for length of stay, are yet to be clearly defined.

The denominator must reflect the appropriate population at risk as precisely as possible. In determining the attack rate of SSIs among patients on the urology service, for example, only those urology patients who actually undergo a surgical procedure that results in a wound capable of being infected should be included in the denominator. Practical difficulties in obtaining such refined denominators, however, often dictate the use of a less precise, summary denominator (e.g., the total number of admissions or discharges from the urology service during the appropriate period).

In the CDC's National Nosocomial Infections Surveillance (NNIS) system, hospitals that performed surveillance in intensive care units (ICUs) used device-days (e.g., ventilator-days or central line [CL]-days) as the denominator data [45]. The use of device-days may seem like a subtle change from patients, but the choice of denominator was critical for purposes of interhospital comparison. This is more fully illustrated by the distribution of several rates for hospital ICUs (Figure 6-2). The top histogram of this figure shows the number of central-line-associated bloodstream infections (CLABSIs) per 100 patients, the middle histogram shows the number of central line-days divided by patient-days (i.e., central line-utilization), and the bottom histogram shows CLABSIs per 1,000 central line-days. For hospital unit A, the rate on the top histogram, which uses the number of patients as the denominator, was nearly five times higher than the median. However, the middle histogram shows that hospital unit A had the highest central line-utilization rate; that is, $>80\%$ of patient-days were also central line-days. Using central line-days as the denominator of the rate helps to take into account this high utilization of central lines. Hospital unit A's CLABSIs rate was slightly lower than the median (bottom histogram). Although hospital unit A was no longer an outlier, its high central line-use may need to be reviewed for appropriateness. On the other hand, for hospital unit B, the CLABSIs rate (top histogram) was near the median, and its central line-use (middle histogram) was low. When its rate was calculated using central line-days as the denominator, it was quite high, suggesting the need to review central line placement and maintenance practices.

Analyzing the Results

Comparing Patient Groups

Analysis implies careful examination of the body of tabulated data in an attempt to determine the nature and relationship of its component parts. This includes comparing current HAI rates to determine whether significant differences exist among different groups of patients. Suppose, for instance, that both the gynecology and general surgery services had 8 catheter-associated UTIs during a given month; however, during the same month, 20 patients who had indwelling catheters were discharged from the gynecology service and 100 other patients were discharged from the general surgery service. Thus, the rates for gynecology and general surgery patients are 40% and 8%, respectively. Determining whether the difference observed between these infection rates is significant (i.e., higher than what we would expect by random or chance occurrence alone, if indeed no real difference exists) requires the use of a statistical process known as *significance testing*.

Several tests of significance (e.g., the chi-square test, Fisher's exact test for cross-tables, or Student's t-test for comparison of sample means) should be familiar to epidemiologists and ICPs (see Chapter 8). Currently available software packages for computers make even the most sophisticated statistical testing procedures very accessible to all infection control departments [26,42]. In the preceding example, the difference between the observed infection rates (40% versus 8%) is highly significant at $p < 0.001$, according to the Fisher's exact test. This means

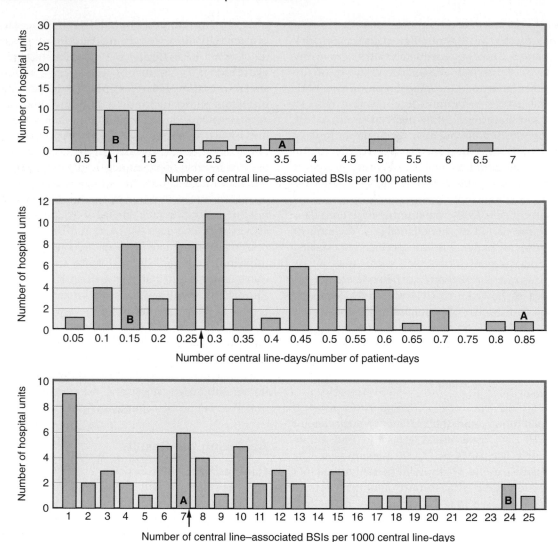

Figure 6-2 Comparison of the distribution of bloodstream infection (BSI) rates (patient based and central line based) and central line utilization in combined coronary and medical intensive care units, National Nosocomial Infections Surveillance (NNIS) System, October 1986–December 1990. A and B represent individual hospital ICU rates. Arrows indicate the median [20].

that a difference as large as or larger than that observed would be expected to occur by chance alone less than 1 time in 1,000. Thus, it is very likely that there is a real difference between the infection rates on the two services, and further investigation is indicated to explain why such a difference exists. If the ICP wants to compare the hospital HAI rates to that of other hospitals, such comparisons can be made only when comparison data that are risk stratified and risk adjusted using the same definitions and protocols are available [43].

Comparing Rates Over Time

Another type of analysis involves the comparison of current HAI rates with previous rates within the same patient care area or population to determine whether significant changes have occurred over time. Current rates and those of preceding periods can be visually inspected

in tabular form, or the rates can be plotted on a graph to detect changes of potential importance. Potentially important deviations from baseline rates then should be tested for statistical significance (see Chapter 8), and further investigation should be undertaken if indicated (see Chapter 7). Although it is convenient to compare rates each month, caution is needed when the denominator of a rate is small. This may be particularly true when examining SSI rates. Tests of significance must often be performed when the estimate of a surgeon's SSI rate is unstable due to a small number of procedures performed.

Identifying Clusters

Screening to identify clusters of similar strains or specific patterns of antimicrobial susceptibility is another potentially valuable analytic tool for detecting outbreaks, especially when it is applied to particular pathogens on specific wards or in particular geographic areas. Pulsed-field gel electrophoresis or other molecular techniques applied to microorganisms can have additional value in identifying clusters (See Chapter 10).

Analyzing Surveillance Data

Analysis of surveillance data must not be limited to HAI rates. Most ICPs are familiar with analyzing the numerator data, specifically the numbers and types of HAIs and their associated pathogens, but an analysis of the denominator data alone can be extremely revealing. For example, if an ICP determines that a hospital's utilization of central lines in ICUs is high compared with that in another hospital ICUs (see hospital unit A in the middle panel of Figure 6-2), a review of appropriateness of device use may be needed. Also, after SSI rates have been assessed, useful information can be obtained by further exploring the distribution of risk factors in each of the risk index categories. For example, while a surgeon with more than the expected number of herniorrhaphy operations in the higher SSI index categories may be operating on more high-risk patients, he or she also may be consistently exceeding the 75th percentile for the duration of surgery for the herniorrhaphy procedure, thus increasing the patients' risk of SSI. The question must be asked, "Are patients unnecessarily being placed at risk of an HAI?" Because examination of appropriateness of medical care and device use is of major interest to performance improvement personnel [21,46,48,49], ICPs may find areas for collaboration with their performance improvement colleagues.

Interpretating the Results

Many consider interpretation of the data to be the final step in analysis; it is the intellectual process by which meaning is ascribed to the tabulated and analyzed body of information. The interpretation may vary from no significant change in the HAI rates to the detection of a serious endemic problem or outbreak in the hospital. Often, however, more information, particularly that obtained through further investigation directed at problem areas identified by the analysis of the surveillance data, will be necessary for the final interpretation of the data. Additional uses of other information collected through surveillance, such as the time of onset of HAI, are described in Chapters 5 and 7.

Reporting the Data

The tabulated data, or at least their analyses and interpretations, should come to the attention of those people in the hospital who can take appropriate actions. A periodic report containing the tabulated data and the analytic results and their interpretations should routinely be submitted to the infection control committee and maintained on record in the hospital. Weekly or even daily reports may be necessary during outbreak or unusual situations. It is inefficient to include a line listing of HAIs in this report. When the analysis yields tables that contain insufficient data to justify inclusion in the report, the tables should be retained and a summary table released whenever sufficient data have accumulated.

The data should be displayed in graphic form to provide clinicians and/or administrators with visual evidence of the existence of a problem and the need to take preventive action. Simple, creative graphics are particularly effective. The ICP should not assume that those individuals have the time or epidemiologic expertise to interpret the data without clearly presented graphics and narratives. The availability of computer software for infection control allows graphic analyses to be performed efficiently and accurately.

In the reporting phase and throughout the surveillance process, measures should be taken to ensure the privacy of the information collected on patients and hospital staff members. For example, the ICP should keep all surveillance forms that list patients by name under very tight security, including a locked filing cabinet or other secure storage. Reports should not mention patients or staff members by name unless there is a good reason for doing so, and the distribution of the reports should be limited to those who need to know. The infection control committee should establish a policy on information privacy, including specific procedures for handling records or reports that identify patients or staff members (e.g., surgeon-specific SSI rates or laboratory data implicating an employee as a human disseminator of an outbreak organism).

PREVALENCE

Definition

Prevalence is a count of the number of all episodes of active disease (existing and new) during a specific period. The prevalence rate is the number of active disease episodes divided by the number of patients at risk for disease during the period. When the period used for the calculation is relatively long, such as a month or more, the measurement is called *period prevalence*. In Figure 6-1, the period prevalence rate of infection during Time A would be 4/10, or 40%, and during Time B, 6/10 or 60%. When the period of time used for the calculation is relatively short, such as ≤1 day, the measurement is called *point prevalence* (i.e., the number of all currently active episodes of disease, old and new, at a given instant in time). The difference between point and period prevalence is arbitrary; an interval that is considered a point on one time scale may become a period on a different time scale.

The Prevalence Survey

The prevalence survey, as applied to HAIs, consists of a systematic study of a defined population for evidence of

HAI at a given point in time; such a survey derives the point prevalence rate for the population. Typically, after a short period of training to standardize definitions and methods, a team of surveyors visits every patient in the hospital on a single day and detects all active HAIs by studying the medical records and examining patients or discussing patients with the clinical staff when necessary. When there are more patients than the survey team can visit in one day, the prevalence study is conducted over several days with care taken to ensure that each patient is visited only once.

If the object is to obtain the prevalence rate of *infections* (the usual procedure), then those infections that have resolved before the day of the visit are not counted. The point prevalence rate then is calculated by dividing the number of infections active on the day of the visit by the number of beds visited and multiplying by an appropriate base number (usually 100). If, on the other hand, the object is to obtain the point prevalence rate of *infected patients*, then all patients with currently active or resolved infections contracted during the current hospitalization are counted. The point prevalence rate is calculated by dividing the number of infected patients by the number of beds visited and multiplying by the appropriate base number. To be consistent with the usual way of defining the incidence rate (i.e., the infection ratio), prevalence surveys should be designed to measure the point prevalence rate of infections.

The relative magnitudes of these various measures are complicated but can be deduced from the fundamental relationship between prevalence and incidence [50]:

$$\text{Prevalence} \approx \text{Incidence} \times \text{Duration}$$

From this general relationship, it is apparent that prevalence rates (both point and period) are always higher than the comparable incidence rates, and the longer the duration of the infections, the greater the difference will become. As explained in the earlier discussion of the two types of incidence rates, the infection ratio is always higher than the infection proportion measured on the same population as long as some patients develop >1 infection. In contrast, the prevalence rate of infections is always lower than the prevalence rate of infected patients because the duration of an infected patient's hospitalization is almost always longer than the duration of the active infection. Interestingly, point and period prevalence rates measured on the same population are usually approximately the same although, due to the larger number of patients studied in a period prevalence survey, estimates of period prevalence are usually more precise than those of point prevalence.

In general, the most useful measure to derive from surveillance is the incidence rate because it provides an estimate of the risk of HAI uncluttered by differences in the durations of various HAIs. The main reason that prevalence rates have been used is simply that a point prevalence survey requires much less effort and can be completed much more rapidly than the ongoing, daily surveillance needed to obtain incidence rates. Point prevalence surveys

have two main disadvantages: First, due to the influence of the duration of infections, the prevalence rate overestimates patients' risk of acquiring infection; second, except in the largest hospitals, the number of patients included in a point prevalence survey (i.e., the number of beds) is usually too small to obtain precise enough estimates of rates to detect important differences (e.g., a difference between the BSI rates on medicine and surgery wards) with statistical significance. Because of these limitations, prevalence surveys are generally useful primarily when a "quick and dirty" estimate is needed and time or resources to obtain a more useful measure of the incidence are insufficient [51,52].

Uses of Prevalence Surveys

Secular Trends

Repeated prevalence surveys in the same institution have been used to document secular trends in the epidemiology of HAIs and to demonstrate effectiveness of infection control measures [51,54]. Prevalence studies in large hospitals have shown shifts in the predominant pathogens associated with HAIs and in the patterns of antimicrobial use for hospitalized patients [55]. However, limitations in the numbers of patients studied and variations in the types of prevalence rates determined in the various surveys have complicated the interpretation of these results. In general, incidence rates derived from ongoing surveillance, although more time-consuming, are much better for detecting and examining secular trends. Prevalence rates should not be compared with incidence rates.

Estimation of Surveillance Accuracy

Prevalence surveys have been used to evaluate a hospital's ongoing surveillance system [56,57]. Typically, a survey team, using the same standard definitions used for routine surveillance by the ICP, visits all patients in the hospital to detect all active HAIs. By comparing the HAIs identified during the prevalence survey with those detected by the routine surveillance system and under the assumption that the survey team correctly detected all active HAIs, an estimate of the percentage of true HAIs detected by the routine surveillance system is derived. Although this percentage approximates the sensitivity of routine surveillance (i.e., the probability that the routine surveillance system will detect a true HAI), the statistic has been referred to as an *efficiency factor* since the difficulty of reliably determining whether HAIs are active at the time of the prevalence survey introduces some error into the assessment [57]. Because the efficiency factor approximates the sensitivity, it can be used to correct the monthly routine estimates of the incidence rates for the degree of under ascertainment.

One of the weaknesses of this application in past studies has been the failure to estimate the specificity of routine HAI surveillance in addition to its sensitivity (efficiency). Specificity is the probability of correctly classifying a patient as uninfected, and it reflects how often the ICP records an HAI when one was not really present. Unfortunately, the specificity of case finding by ICPs in estimating incidence rates in routine surveillance has not been thoroughly studied [58–60]. The process of correcting incidence rates with the efficiency factor assumes that specificity is a perfect 1.0. Corrections for lower levels of specificity would give lower estimates of the incidence rates.

Estimation of Incidence from Prevalence

Modified prevalence surveys can be used to derive a crude approximation of the incidence rates that would have been obtained from continuous surveillance [61]. In this use, surveys are performed at regular intervals (e.g., weekly) that must be considerably less than the average duration of the stay of infected patients. Only HAIs that began since the preceding survey are tabulated. The denominator of the rates should include the number of admissions during the interval plus the census at the start of the period. Obviously, the shorter the interval between prevalence surveys, the more closely the final estimate approximates the true incidence rate. For modified prevalence surveys, some loss in completeness, accuracy, and timeliness in detecting HAIs, as compared to the results of surveillance studies, must be weighed against the potential benefit from a smaller time commitment to case finding.

Other Uses

Perhaps the best uses of prevalence studies are to make valuable estimates of antimicrobial usage patterns, to evaluate the adherence to proper isolation practices, and to monitor practices related to high risk procedures, such as use of intravenous or urinary catheters [55,62,63]. In one study, investigators used sequential prevalence surveys to estimate the impact of their infection control program on the HAI risk [51].

Finally, a single institution has pooled data across prevalence surveys conducted over multiple years to understand the epidemiology of HAIs in a subset of their patient population for the purpose of designing specific prevention interventions [64].

PRIORITY-DIRECTED SURVEILLANCE

Since the mid-1980s, the trend has been away from continuously monitoring all patients for all HAIs in all parts of a healthcare facility ("facilitywide" or "comprehensive" surveillance) in favor of an approach that targets specific patient-care areas, infection sites, infections with certain organisms, or patient-care processes ("priority-directed" surveillance). When the level of effort is matched with the seriousness of the HAI problem, the method is called "surveillance by objective" [65]. Although such targeting was initially motivated by the need to reduce the amount of personnel time devoted to surveillance in hospitals

with inadequately staffed programs, this approach has proven beneficial in reducing HAI rates in certain high-risk patients [66–68].

Unit-Directed Surveillance

Many hospitals have sought to maximize the use of personnel time by directing surveillance toward HAIs in patient-care areas with the highest HAI risk (e.g., ICUs, oncology units). For example, in one hospital, the HAI rate in the ICU was three times higher than in general medical-surgical patients [69]. ICUs tend to house patients who are most susceptible to HAIs—that is, the patients most likely to have suppressed immune systems, to be undergoing invasive diagnostic or therapeutic procedures, or to be receiving intensive nursing and medical care with the attendant risk of person-to-person pathogen spread. Focusing scarce resources on a few relatively small units has the advantages of greatly simplifying the surveillance effort and of preventing HAIs in the patients with the highest risks and greatest likelihood of sustaining severe and life-threatening HAIs.

Another patient-care area that should be considered for unit-directed surveillance is the high-risk nursery (HRN). Neonates in the HRN are highly susceptible to HAIs. Host and environmental factors unique to patients in this unit contribute to the high HAI risk (e.g., low birth weight). BSIs are among the most common HAIs in all birth weight groups, this frequency differing dramatically from that in adult patients with HAIs and should be a major focus for prevention [70]. The NNIS system used the unit-directed surveillance method in its ICU and HRN Surveillance Components [70–72].

Site-Directed Surveillance

Site-directed surveillance focuses on detecting one or more specific types of HAI (e.g., BSI) occurring among either all hospitalized patients or some subset of patients, such as those with certain devices (e.g., central lines), who have undergone certain procedures (e.g., hemodialysis), and/or are treated in certain patient-care areas (e.g., ICU). The latter example represents a combination with the unit-directed approach. The CDC's National Healthcare Safety Network (NHSN) uses this combined approach in its device-associated and procedure-associated modules [73]. In those modules, the facility chooses each month which device-associated HAI in which patient-care area and/or which procedure-associated HAI (SSI or postprocedure pneumonia) to monitor following which procedure.

Surgical Site Infections

Surveillance of SSIs is an important part of a prevention program. Unit-directed surveillance is ineffective for SSIs because these HAIs may not manifest clinically while the patient is on a particular unit. For priority-directed

SSI surveillance, all patients undergoing operations are enrolled in a surveillance registry at the time of the operation, and information on several key risk factors are recorded at that time. The risk factors most likely to be useful in the analysis are the wound classification, type and duration of the operation, and a measure of the severity of the patient's underlying disease, such as the number of underlying diagnoses or the physical status classification of the American Society of Anesthesiologists (ASA) [74–76]. Patients are visited regularly during hospitalization by the ICP to detect SSIs. Attempts should be made to follow up all, or a subset, of the patients for SSIs occurring after discharge [35,36].

The tabulation process should be conducted monthly and should involve three steps. First, each patient is assigned to an intrinsic infection risk category by using a multivariate risk-factor scale. Second, the SSI rate is calculated for the patients in *each* category of the intrinsic infection risk category—not just for clean wounds or low-risk categories. Third, two reports are compiled, one displaying each surgeon's category-specific monthly rates over time (e.g., over 1 or 2 years), and a second comparing the category-specific rates of each surgeon with those of his or her colleagues, for the service overall, and possibly an SSI rate aggregated from other hospitals [20]. Finally, the reports are given to the chief of the surgical service to distribute among and discuss with the practicing surgeons. With this plan, the surveillance time devoted to SSIs would be directed toward the surveillance effort shown to be the most effective in reducing the problem [10,35,77].

Pneumonia

A surveillance plan targeted outside ICUs and toward specific prevention objectives for healthcare-associated pneumonia (HAP) should be used. The development of HAP in ventilated patients has been the subject of much investigation and controversy. Although clinical criteria together with cultures of sputum or tracheal specimens may be sensitive for bacterial pathogens, they are nonspecific in patients with mechanically assisted ventilation [78,79]. Consensus recommendations for standardization methods to diagnose pneumonia in clinical research studies of ventilator-associated pneumonia have been proposed [80–82]. However, these approaches are generally not applicable to the surveillance setting. Further studies are needed to help in the diagnosis of this common clinical entity in the nonresearch setting.

For HAP in inpatients who are not on ventilators, the first consideration is to differentiate pneumonia among surgical and medical patients. The vast majority of preventable episodes of pneumonia among surgical patients are postoperative pulmonary infections representing progression of the usual atelectasis syndrome most commonly following operations of the chest and upper abdomen. In contrast, most preventable pneumonias among adult medical patients are hypostatic infections related to the failure to frequently turn patients with diminished levels of consciousness.

On pediatric and newborn services, the most serious preventable pneumonias follow person-to-person spread of HAIs with viruses (e.g., respiratory syncytial virus. Postoperative pneumonias can be detected with little additional effort if surgical patients are already being monitored for SSIs. Analysis of these rates can be performed for each type of operative procedure or by surgeon. Reports of these analyses then should be discussed just as the SSI rates are (see "Surgical Site Infections").

The ICP also should identify patient-care areas where patients with strokes, drug overdoses, and other high risks for hypostatic pneumonia are congregated. In such areas, all patients at high risk should be followed regularly to detect all episodes of pneumonia. The pneumonia rates among these patients should be regularly reported to the charge nurses of the specified nursing units, and continuing in-service education on the importance of frequently turning these patients and providing pulmonary assistance to prevent pneumonia should be provided.

The ICP should regularly visit units caring for infants or children at high risk for pneumonia from respiratory syncytial virus and similar agents to monitor informally the frequency of upper respiratory infections among patients and employees, especially in the fall and winter months [83]. When these infections become evident, virology studies should be done immediately to detect the presence of viruses. When such pathogens are found, the staff members should be warned of the imminent danger and instructed in meticulous contact precautions to use for infected patients and employees [84]. Approaches to other types of HAP (e.g., Legionnaires' disease or influenza) are described in the revised CDC Guideline for the Prevention of Nosocomial Pneumonia [84].

Bloodstream Infections

While BSIs comprise only about 10 to 15% of all HAIs, their morbidity, mortality, and increasing frequency demand a high degree of surveillance effort [8,85]. However, one must control for a single, major risk factor before rate calculation becomes meaningful, that is, exposure to an intravascular device. Any device-associated BSI should be examined for correctable errors in patient management (e.g., failing to use all protective barriers when inserting the line, failing to change the site of intravenous catheters frequently enough, or improperly sterilizing arterial pressure-monitoring devices). Such errors must be corrected. Calculation of a CVC-BSI rate using central line-days is useful for monitoring endemic problems that may be corrected by changes in policies, practices, or selection of equipment [20].

Urinary Tract Infections

Many ICPs invest little time in the surveillance of UTIs since they are generally of less consequence to the patient than are other HAIs. This relative inattention remains controversial because overall, UTIs remain the most frequent HAIs [86]. Surveillance efforts should be directed to identifying hospital areas where patient-care personnel are not properly managing urinary catheters or other urinary instrumentations. Then catheter-associated UTI rates (stratified or adjusted by categories of the duration of urinary catheterization) on different patient-care areas could be calculated. If rates are higher than desired, an assessment of the indications for inserting and discontinuing catheters and the techniques of aseptically caring for them should be done. By periodically reporting how the UTI rates of the different areas compared, practices could be improved in those areas with consistently higher rates. Alternatively, the infection control staff could annually conduct a 1-month prevalence study of UTIs and catheter care practices. This amount of effort would be commensurate with the magnitude of the problem and would reinforce prevention at least on a yearly basis.

Other Infections

Since HAIs at body sites other than those mentioned are comparatively rare, little time should be spent on their surveillance [20]. Instead, the ICP should depend on other hospital departments to recognize the rare outbreaks of unusual infections and to recognize common factors that might tie the patients together, such as a single unusual organism, spatial clustering, or a relationship with some diagnostic or therapeutic device. For example, the employee health service should maintain surveillance to detect problems of *Mycobacterium tuberculosis* transmission to employees; the director of the newborn nursery should notify the ICP of clusters of staphylococcal pyoderma; and staff who work in the microbiology laboratory should be alert to clusters of unusual pathogens. Only when a suspicious cluster or relationship is found would a more detailed investigation involving the calculation of rates be undertaken. The level of effort is commensurate with the magnitude of the problems, but the efforts are likely to detect problems if they occur. ICPs must remain alert to such problems regardless of which priority-directed surveillance approach is employed.

SURVEILLANCE BY OBJECTIVE

While unit-directed surveillance is efficient and effective for high-risk areas (e.g., ICUs), this approach is less practical when dealing with other patient-care areas of the hospital. An alternative approach, referred to as *surveillance by objective*, matches the level of surveillance effort to the seriousness of the HAI problem [8,9]. Instead of focusing on geographic areas, this priority-directed approach focuses on the types of HAIs to be prevented and assigns levels of effort commensurate to the relative seriousness of the problems.

The first prerequisite of this approach is to establish priority rankings based on the relative seriousness of the different types of HAIs. Two possible parameters for setting these priorities are compared in Table 6-1. In the past, the main parameter had been simply the relative frequency of the different types of HAIs. If this measure were used, UTI would be given the highest priority followed by SSI with pneumonia; primary BSI would receive a lower priority just ahead of a large number of relatively rare infections at other sites [86].

An alternative parameter that appears to be a better measure of the relative seriousness of the various types of HAIs is the total hospital cost attributable to each of the HAIs [87]. This measure reflects both the relative frequency of the HAIs and the relative degree of morbidity as expressed by the costs of the extra days and extra ancillary services necessary to treat the HAIs. By this criterion, BSI

TABLE 6-1
COMPARISON OF THE RELATIVE FREQUENCY OF THE MAJOR TYPES OF NOSOCOMIAL INFECTIONS AND ATTRIBUTABLE COSTS OF HAI

Type of Infection	Percent of all Nosocomial Infections[a]	Mean Attributable Costs[b]	Range Minimum	Range Maximum
Surgical wound infection	22	$25,546	1783	134,602
Pneumonia	15	9,969[c]	7904[c]	12,034[c]
Urinary tract infection	32	1,006	650	1361
Bacteremia	14	36,441	1822	107,156
Other	17	NA		
Total (all sites)	100			

[a]See [86] for data source.
[b]See [87] for source of data.
[c]Ventilator-associated pneumonia (VAP).

would constitute the most serious problem followed by SSI with ventilator-associated pneumonia and UTI in third and fourth places, respectively (see Table 6-1).

HAIs have a substantial impact on patient outcomes in the hospital setting. With trends in healthcare toward shorter hospital stays, increasing the use of invasive devices, increasing the rates of antibiotic resistance, and rising public interest in decreasing HAI-related morbidity and mortality, surveillance activities will require more time and expertise than in the past. Resources for infection surveillance and prevention have not increased proportionally with these demands. Maintaining successful features of traditional surveillance systems, adopting novel surveillance strategies such as using surrogate measures for HAI rates, and employing new approaches to collecting and using information with new technologies such as the Internet will make healthcare surveillance an even better tool for prevention.

REFERENCES

1. Centers for Disease Control. *CDC surveillance update*. Atlanta: Centers for Disease Control, 1988.
2. Scheckler WE. Continuous quality improvement in a hospital system: implications for hospital epidemiology. *Infect Control Hospital Epidemiol* 1992;13:288–292.
3. Seligman PJ, Frazier TM. Surveillance: the sentinel health event approach. In: Halperin W, Baker EL, ed. New York: van Nostrand Reinhold; 1992:16–25.
4. Semmelweis IP. *The etiology, the concept and the prophylaxis of childbed fever*. Leipzig: CA. Hartleben; 1861.
5. Hughes JM. Nosocomial infection surveillance in the United States: Historical perspective. *Infect Control* 1987;8:450.
6. Haley RW, Morgan WM, Culver DH, White JW, Emori TG, Mosser J, et al. Hospital infection control: recent progress and opportunities under prospective payment. *Am J Infect Control* 1985;13(3):97–103.
7. Nguyen GT, Proctor SWE, Sinkowitz-Cochran RL, Garrett DO, Jarvis WR. Status of infection surveillance and control programs in the United States, 1992–1996. Association for Professionals in Infection Control and Epidemiology, Inc. *Am J Infect Control* 2000; 28:392–400.
8. Haley RW. Surveillance by objectives: a priority-directed approach to the surveillance of nosocomial infection. *Am J Infect Control* 1985;13:78–85.
9. Haley RW. *Managing hospital nosocomial control for cost-effectiveness*. Chicago: American Hospital Publishing; 1986.
10. Haley RW, Culver DH, Morgan WM, Emori TG, Munn VP, et al. The efficacy of infection surveillance and control programs in preventing nosocomial infections in U.S. hospitals. *Am J Epidemiol* 1985;121:182–205.
11. Joint Commission on Accreditation of Healthcare Organizations. *2005 Critical access hospitals: surveillance, prevention and control of infection*. Oak Brook, IL: Joint Commission Resources; 2005.
12. Joint Commission on Accreditation of Hospitals. *Accreditation Manual for Hospitals, 1976*. Chicago: Joint Commission on Accreditation of Hospitals; 1976.
13. Lynch P. Jackson M. Monitoring: Surveillance for nosocomial infections and uses for assessing quality of care. *Am J Infect Control* 1985;12:161–65.
14. Massanari RM, Wilkerson KI, Swartzendruber S. Designing surveillance for noninfectious outcomes of medical care. *Infect Control Hosp Epidemiol* 1995;16:419–426.
15. Gastmeier P. Nosocomial infection surveillance and control policies. *Curr Opin Infect Dis* 2004; 295:295–301.
16. Stamm WE, Weinstein RA, Dixon RE. Comparison of endemic and epidemic nosocomial infections. *Am J Med* 1981;70:393–397.
17. Emori TG, Haley RW, Garner JS. Techniques and uses of nosocomial infection surveillance in U.S. hospitals, 1976–1977. *Am J Med* 1981;70:933–940.
18. Stamm WE. Catheter-associated urinary tract infections: epidemiology, pathogenesis, and prevention. *Am J Med* 1991;91:65S–71S.
19. Culver DH, Horan TC, Gaynes RP, Martone WJ, Jarvis WR, Emori TG, et al. Surgical wound infection rates by wound class, operation, and risk index. in U.S. hospitals. 1986–90. *Am J Med* 1991;91:152S–157S.
20. National Nosocomial Infections Surveillance System. Nosocomial infection rates for interhospital comparison: limitations and possible solutions. *Infect Control Hosp Epidemiol* 1991;12:609–621.
21. Chassin MR, et al. Does inappropriate use explain geographic variations in the use of health care services? A study of three procedures. *JAMA* 1987;258:2533–2539.
22. Haley RW. JCAHO Infection control indicators, parts 1 and 2. *Infect Control Hosp Epidemiol* 1990;11:545–548.
23. Larson E. A comparison of methods for surveillance of nosocomial infections. *Infect Control* 1980;1:377–381.
24. Mandatory public reporting of healthcare-associated infections [online] 2006 (accessed 2006 August 26) Available from URL: http://www.apic.org/Content/NavigationMenu/ GovernmentAdvocacy/MandatoryReporting/state_legislation/ state_legislation.htm
25. McKibben L, Horan TC, Tokars JI, Fowler G, Cardo DM, Pearson ML, et al. Guidance on public reporting of healthcare-associated infections: recommendations of the Healthcare Infection Control Practices Advisory Committee. *Am J Infect Control*. 2005;33; 217–26.
26. Tokars JI, Richards C, Andrus M, Klevens M, Curtis A, Horan T, et al. The changing face of surveillance for health care-associated infections. *Clin Infect Dis* 2004;39:1347–52.
27. Burke JP. Maximizing appropriate antibiotic prophylaxis for surgical patients: an update from LDS Hospital, Salt Lake City. *Clin Infect Dis* 2001;33:S78–83.
28. Gaynes R, Platt R. Monitoring patient safety in health care: building the case for surrogate measures. *Jt Comm J Qual Patient Saf* 2006;32:95–101.
29. Yokoe DS, Shapiro M, Simchen E, Platt R. Use of antibiotic exposure to detect postoperative infections. *Infect Control Hosp Epidemiol* 1998;19:317–22.
30. Horan TC, Gaynes RP. Surveillance of nosocomial infections. In: Mayhall CG, ed. *Hospital epidemiology and infection control*, 3rd ed. Philadelphia: Lippincott Williams & Wilkins; 2004; pp 1659–1702.
31. Centers for Disease Control. *Outline for surveillance and control of nosocomial infections*. Atlanta: Centers for Disease Control; 1972.
32. Abrutyn E, Talbot GH. Surveillance strategies: a primer. *Infect Control* 1987;8:459–464.
33. Altemeir WA. *Manual on the control of infection in surgical patients*. Philadelphia: Lippincott; 1976:29–30.
34. Platt R, Yokoe DS, Sands KE. Automated methods for surveillance of surgical site infections. *Emerg Infect Dis* 2001;7:212–216.
35. Condon RE, Haley RW, Lee JT, Meakins JL. Does infection control control infection? *Arch Surg* 1988;123:250–54.
36. Sheretz JR, Garabaldi RA, Kaiser AB, et. al. Consensus paper on the surveillance of surgical wound infections. *Infect Control Hosp Epid* 1992;13:599–605.
37. Manian FA, Meyer L. Comprehensive surveillance of surgical wound infections in outpatient and inpatient surgery. *Infect Control Hosp Epid* 1990;11(10):515–520.
38. Reimar K, Gleed C, Nicolle LE. Impact of postdischarge infections in surgical wound infection rates. *Infect Control* 1987;8(6):237–240.
39. Weigelt JA, Dryer D, Haley RW. The necessity and efficiency of wound surveillance after discharge. *Arch surg* 1992;152:77–82.
40. Zoutman D. surgical wound infections occurring in day surgery patients. *Am J Infect Control* 1990;18(4):277–281.
41. Holtz TH, Wenzel RP. Postdischarge surveillance for nosocomial wound infection: A brief review and commentary. *Infect Control Hosp Epidemiol* 1992;20:206–13.

42. Mertens R, Jans B, Kurz X. A computerized nationwide network for nosocomial infection surveillance in Belgium. *Infect Control Hosp Epidemiol* 1994;15:171–179.

43. Yokoe DS, Platt R. Surveillance for surgical site infections: The uses of antibiotic exposure. to detect postoperative infections. *Infect Control Hosp Epidemiol* 1998;19:317–22.

44. Haley RW, Hooton TM, Culver DH, Stanley RC, Emori TG, Hardison CD, et al., Nosocomial infections in U.S. hospitals 1975–76: estimated nationwide frequency by selected characteristics of patients. *Am J Med* 1981;70(4):947–959.

45. Emori TG, Culver DH, Horan TC, et al. National Nosocomial Infections Surveillance System (NNIS): description of surveillance methods. *Am J Infect Control* 1991;19:19–35.

46. Donabedian A. Contributions of epidemiology to quality assessment and monitoring. *Infect Control Hosp Epidemiol* 1990;11:117–21.

47. Edwards JE, Horan TC. Developing and Comparing Infection Rates. In *APIC Text of Infection Control & Epidemiology*. Washington DC: Association for Professionals in Infection Control and Epidemiology, 2005.

48. McGeer A, Crede W, Hierholzer WJ, Jr. Surveillance for quality assessment: II. Surveillance for noninfectious processes: Back to basics. *Infect Control Hosp Epidemiol* 1990;11:36–41.

49. Myers SA, Gleicher N. A successful program to lower caesarean section rates. *New Eng J Med* 1988;319:1511–6.

50. Rhame FS, Sudderth WD. Incidence and prevalence as used in the analysis of the occurrence of nosocomial infections. *Am J Epidemiol* 1981;113:1–10.

51. French GL. Repeated prevalence surveys for monitoring effectiveness of hospital infection control. *Lancet* 1989;2:1021–3.

52. Anderson BM, Ringertz SH, Gullord TP, Hermansen W, Lelek M, Norman BI, et al. A three-year survey of nosocomial and community-acquired infections, antibiotic treatment and rehospitalization in a Norwegian health region. *J Hosp Infect* 2000;44:214–23.

53. Gastmeier P, Kampf G, Wischnewski N, Hauer T, Schulgen G, Schumacher M, et al. Prevalence of nosocomial infections in representative German hospitals. *J Hosp Infect* 1998;38:37–49.

54. Vaque J, Rosello J, Arribas JL. Prevalence of nosocomial infections in Spain: EPINE study 1990–1997. EPINE Working Group. *J Hosp Infect* 1999;43:105–11.

55. McGowan JE, Jr, Finland M. Infection and usage of antibiotics at Boston City Hospital: changes in prevalence during the decade 1964–1973. *J Infect Dis* 1974;130(2):177–182.

56. Febre N, de Medeiros ES, Wey SB, Larrondo M, Silva V. Is the epidemiological surveillance system of nosocomial infections recommended by the American CDC applicable in a Chilean hospital?. *Rev Med Chil* 2001;129:1379–86.

57. Bennett JV, Scheckler WE, Maki DG, Brachman PS. Current National Patterns: United States, In: PS Brachman, TC Eickhoff ed. *Proceedings of the International Conference on Nosocomial Infections*. Chicago: American Hospital Association, 1971.

58. Haley RW, Schaberg DR, McClish KDK, Quade D, Crossley KB, Culver DH et al. The accuracy of retrospective chart review in measuring nosocomial infection rates: results of validation studies in pilot hospitals. *Am J Epidemiol* 1980;111:534–40.

59. Wenzel RP, Osterman CA, Hunting KJ, Gwaltney JM, Jr. Hospital-acquired infections: I. Surveillance in a university hospital. *Am J Epidemiol* 1976;103:251–6.

60. Emori TG, Edwards JR, Culver DH, et al. Accuracy of reporting nosocomial infections in intensive-care-unit patients to the NNIS system: a pilot study. *Infect Control Hosp Epidemiol* 1998;19:308–316.

61. Wenzel RP, Thompson RL, Landry SM, Russell BS, Miller PJ, Ponce de Leon S, Miller GB Jr. Hospital-acquired infections in intensive care unit patients: an overview with emphasis on epidemics. *Infect Control* 1983;4(5):371–5.

62. Scheckler WE, Garner JS, Kaiser AB, Bennett JV. Prevalence of Infections and Antibiotic Usage in Eight Community Hospitals. In: PS Brachman, TC Eickhoff, ed. *Proceedings of the International Conference on Nosocomial Infections*. Chicago: American Hospital Association, 1971.

63. Jepsen OB, Jensen LP, Zimakoff J, Friis H, Bissoonauthsing CN, Kasenally AT, et. al. Prevalence of infections and use of antibiotics among hospitalized patients in Mauritius. A nationwide survey for the planning of a national infection control programme. *J Hosp Infect.* 1993;25:271–8.

64. Eveillard M, Pisante L, Mangeol A, Dolo E, Guet L, Huang M, et al. Specific features of nosocomial infections in the elderly at a general hospital center. 5 surveys of annual prevalence. *Pathol Biol* 1998;46:741–749.

65. Haley RW. Surveillance by objective: a new priority-directed approach to the control of nosocomial infections. *Am J Infect Control* 1985;13:78–89.

66. Centers for Disease Control and Prevention. Reduction in central line-associated bloodstream infections among patients in intensive care units—Pennsylvania, April 2001–2005. *MMWR* 2005;54:1013–1016.

67. Centers for Disease Control and Prevention (CDC). Monitoring hospital-acquired infections to promote patient safety—United States, 1990–1999. *MMWR* 2000;49:149–53.

68. Quality Indicator Study Group. An approach to the evaluation of quality indicators of the outcome of care in hospitalized patients, with a focus on nosocomial infections. *Infect Control Hosp Epidemiol* 1995;16:308–316.

69. Donowitz LG, Wenzel RP, Hoyt JW. High risk of hospital-acquired infections in the ICU patient. *Crit Care Med* 1982;10:355–359.

70. Gaynes RP, Edwards JR, Jarvis WR, Culver DH, Tolson JS, Martone WJ, et al. Nosocomial infections among neonates in high-risk nurseries in the United States. *Pediatrics* 1996;98:357–361.

71. Jarvis WR, Edwards JR, Culver DH, Hughes JM, Horan TC, Emori TG, et al. Nosocomial infections in adult and pediatric intensive care units in the United States 1986–90. *Am J Med* 1991;91 (Suppl. 3B):185S–191S.

72. Horan TC, Gaynes RP. Surveillance of nosocomial infections. In: *Hospital Epidemiology and Infection Control*. Philadelphia: Lippincott Williams & Wilkins, 2004. Table 94.2, p. 1664–1665.

73. National Healthcare Safety Network (NHSN). NHSN Manual: Patient Safety Component Protocol, available from http://www.cdc.gov/ncidod/dhqp/nhsn_members.html.

74. Haley RW. Nosocomial infections in surgical patients. Developing valid measures of intrinsic patient risk. *Am J Med* 1991;91:145S–149S.

75. Haley RW, Culver DH, White JW, Emori TG, Mosser J, Hughes JM, et al. Identifying patients at high risk of surgical wound infection: a simple multivariate index of patient susceptibility and wound contamination. *Am J Epidemiol* 1984;121:206–16.

76. Keats AS. The ASA classification of physical status: a recapitulation. *J Anesthesiol* 1978;49:233–8.

77. Cruse PJE, Foord R. The epidemiology of wound infection: a 10-year prospective study of 62,939 wounds. *Surg Clin North Am* 1980;60:27–3.

78. Fagon JY, Chastre J, Hance AJ, Domart Y, Trouillet JL, Gibert C. Evaluation of clinical judgment in the identification and treatment of nosocomial pneumonia in ventilated patients. *Chest* 1993;103; 547–53.

79. Torres A, Puig de lLa Bellacasa JP, Xaubet A, Gonzalez J, Rodriguez-Roisin R, Jimenez de Anta MT, et al. Diagnostic value of quantitative cultures of bronchoalveolar lavage and telescoping plugged catheter in mechanically ventilated patients with bacterial pneumonia. *Am Rev Resp Dis* 1989;140:306–310.

80. Meduri GU, Chastre J. The standardization of broncho-scopic techniques for ventilator-associated pneumonia. *Chest* 1992;102:557S–563S.

81. Baselshi V, El-Torky M, Coalson S, Griffen J. The standardization of criteria for processing and interpreting laboratory specimens. *Chest* 1992;102:571S–579S.

82. Wunderink RG, Mayhall G, Gibert C. Methodology for clinical investigation of ventilator-assisted pneumonia: epidemiology and therapeutic intervention. *Chest* 1992;102:580S–588S.

83. Goldwater PN, Martin AJ, Ryan B, Morris S, Thompson J, Kok TW, et al. A survey of nosocomial respiratory syncytial viral infections in a children's hospital: occult respiratory infection in patients admitted during an epidemic season. *Infect Control Hosp Epidemiol* 1991;12:231–238.

84. CDC. Guidelines for preventing health-care-associated pneumonia, 2003: recommendations of CDC and the healthcare Infection Control Practices Advisory Committee. *MMWR* 2004;53(No. RR-3).

85. Banerjee S, Emori G, Culver DH, Gaynes RP, Jarvis WR, Horan T, et al. Secular trends in nosocomial bloodstream infections in the United States, 1980–89. *Am J Med* 1991;91:86S–89S.

86. Klevens RM, Edwards JR, Richards CL, Horan TC, Gaynes RP, Pollock DA, Cardo DM. Estimating healthcare-associated infections and deaths in U.S. hospitals 2002. *Public Health Reports* 2007;122:160–166.

87. Stone PW, Braccia D, Larson E. Systematic review of economic analyses of health care-associated infections. *Am J Infect Control* 2005;33:501–509.

Investigating Endemic and Epidemic Healthcare-Associated Infections

7

William R. Jarvis

Although healthcare-facility infection control (IC) programs have been shown to be effective in reducing the healthcare-associated infection (HAI) rate, endemic and/or epidemic infections associated with the delivery of healthcare continue to occur [1]. It has been estimated that only approximately one-third of all HAIs are preventable [2]. However, IC programs at U.S. hospitals prevent only ~6% of these HAIs because of incomplete implementation of recommended control measures [2,3]. The goals of any healthcare facility IC program should be to educate healthcare workers (HCWs) on the recommended measures to prevent and control HAIs; conduct active, prospective HAI surveillance; analyze HAI surveillance data to identify endemic or epidemic infection problems warranting further investigation; conduct epidemiologic investigations to identify the source of these problems; and implement control measures and assess their efficacy in preventing and controlling these problems. The purpose of this chapter is to describe the epidemiology of endemic or epidemic HAIs, discuss criteria for determining whether to investigate endemic or epidemic HAIs, and outline the systematic approach to such investigations.

DEFINING ENDEMIC OR EPIDEMIC HAIs

Endemic infections are defined as sporadic infections that constitute the background rate of infection at the healthcare facility; the rate of such infections usually fluctuates from month to month, but overall is not statistically significantly different from the background rate of these infections (see Chapters 6, 30). Of all HAIs, endemic infections account for the majority of infections and are the focus of most IC activities. The predominant pathogens and sites of endemic infection are somewhat similar at different types of healthcare facilities but do differ based on the mix of patients (including underlying diseases and severity of illness) and types of procedures performed and devices used (see Chapter 30) (Tables 7-1 and 7-2) [4,5]. Endemic infections can change in type (pathogen, site, or both) and/or rate as the result of a variety of factors, including opening or moving to a new facility, introducing a new or expanding existing clinical services or specialties (e.g., bone marrow or organ transplant, neonatal intensive care unit [ICU], surgical or medical subspecialty), introducing new diagnostic methods (e.g., laboratory or radiology), and so on.

Most endemic HAIs result from breaks in aseptic technique, most commonly from person-to-person transmission via transient HCW hand carriage of the colonizing or infecting pathogen. Numerous studies have documented that HCWs often fail to wash their hands before and between contacts with patients [6]. Nevertheless, investigating endemic problems transmitted in this way focuses attention on the importance of general IC recommendations (including identifying and isolating infectious patients, HCW hand hygiene, environmental cleaning and disinfection,

TABLE 7-1

MOST COMMON NOSOCOMIAL PATHOGENS BY SITE AND UNIT, NATIONAL NOSOCOMIAL INFECTIONS SURVEILLANCE, OCTOBER 1986–DECEMBER 1990*

		Component (%)	
Site	Pathogen	Hospital-Wide	Intensive Care Unit
Blood	Coagulase-negative staphylococci	27.9	28.2
	S. aureus	16.5	16.1
	Enterococci	8.3	12.0
	Candida spp	7.8	10.2
	E. coli	5.6	—
	Enterobacter spp	—	5.3
Surgical wound	S. aureus	17.1	11.7
	Enterococci	13.3	15.8
	Coagulase-negative staphylococci	12.6	13.8
	E. coli	9.4	—
	P. aeruginosa	8.2	9.5
	Enterobacter spp	—	10.3
Respiratory tract	P. aeruginosa	16.9	20.8
	S. aureus	16.1	17.1
	Enterobacter spp	10.5	11.1
	S. pneumoniae	6.5	—
	H. influenzae	6.3	—
	Acinetobacter spp	—	6.4
	K. pneumoniae	—	5.6
Urinary tract	E. coli	25.8	17.5
	Enterococci	15.9	13.0
	P. aeruginosa	12.0	11.3
	Candida spp	9.4	25.0
	K. pneumoniae	6.4	—
	Enterobacter spp	—	6.1

E. coli, Escherichia coli; P. aeruginosa, Pseudomonas aeruginosa; S. pneumoniae, Streptococcus pneumoniae; H. influenzae, Haemophilus influenzae; K. pneumoniae, Klebsiella pneumoniae. S. aureus, Staphylococcus aureus.
*Last hospital-wide data reported from NNIS.
Adapted from Jarvis WR, Martone WJ. Predominant pathogens in hospital infections. J Antimicrob Chemother 1991;28:15–19.

TABLE 7-2

DISTRIBUTION OF NOSOCOMIAL INFECTIONS BY DATE, NATIONAL NOSOCOMIAL INFECTIONS SURVEILLANCE, JANUARY 1993–APRIL 1995

Major Site	No. of Infections	Percentage
Urinary tract	7,376	27.2%
Surgical site	5,058	18.7
Pneumonic lungs	4,673	17.3
Primary bloodstream	4,287	15.8
Other	5,700	21.0

Adapted from National Nosocomial Infections Surveillance (NNIS) Semiannual Report, May 1995. Am J Infec Control 1995;23:377–385. Last hospital-wide data published from NNIS.

clusters often are unexpected and involve either an unusual organism or an organism with an unusual antimicrobial susceptibility pattern (see Chapters 9 and 15). Recognition of clusters of common organisms with common antimicrobial susceptibility patterns may be difficult because they merge with the existing endemic infections. Often IC personnel attempt to determine whether a cluster represents an outbreak based on numerator data only. In such a situation, it is difficult if not impossible to determine whether a detected cluster represents an outbreak unless it involves either a very rare organism (e.g., Vibrio cholera diarrhea) or a common organism with an unusual antimicrobial susceptibility pattern (e.g., vancomycin-resistant Staphylococcus aureus).

Determination of an outbreak should not be based on numerator data alone. Although one episode of nosocomial malaria or cholera in a U.S. hospital represents an epidemic, one cannot determine whether a cluster of nosocomial S. aureus bloodstream infections (BSIs) represent an outbreak unless one can calculate and compare the S. aureus BSI rates in the time periods during and before the cluster. Because of the abrupt nature of epidemics and the feeling that most such outbreaks are preventable, in most situations epidemics warrant investigation.

RECOGNIZING ENDEMIC OR EPIDEMIC HAIs

Surveillance is the cornerstone for rapid recognition of endemic or epidemic HAIs (see Chapter 5). In order to detect either endemic or epidemic HAIs, one must have a surveillance method in place to detect such infections. Because the majority of HAIs arise in severely ill patients exposed to invasive devices (e.g., patients in intensive care units) or those undergoing surgical procedures, surveillance for infections in these populations is most important. If no systematic surveillance system is in place, many clusters

and existing guidelines to prevent these infections) and can be associated with a reduction (often transient) in the rate of these infections. Because many endemic infections are preventable, investigation of such problems by the ICP or hospital epidemiologist may be warranted if the rate of endemic infection is gradually increasing at the institution or the rate of these infections is higher than expected, than reported in the literature, or than reported from other similar institutions.

Epidemic infections are defined as the occurrence of infection at a rate statistically significantly higher than the background rate of such infections; recognized infection may not be recognized and if they are recognized, it is impossible to determine whether the cluster identified is endemic or epidemic unless appropriate denominator data are obtained and rates are calculated and compared.

If active prospective surveillance using standard definitions and methodologies is not conducted, it may be necessary to carry out a specific retrospective study to determine the background rate of infection before one can determine whether the infection problem detected or recognized is endemic or epidemic [7–17]. In institutions in which active prospective surveillance is not being conducted in the area, when a cluster is detected, a retrospective study must be undertaken to attempt to reconstruct the current and past rates of such infection in the area. Only then can one differentiate between an endemic and epidemic problem.

The early detection of infection clusters and the determination of whether the cluster identified is endemic or epidemic are most readily done if active surveillance for such infections and calculation of infection rates in the area are part of an ongoing, validated process. Once the cluster is identified, the investigator next determines whether the problem is endemic or epidemic in nature.

Differentiating endemic from epidemic HAIs requires review of how the numerator and denominator are collected, validation of the accuracy of these data, and assessment of whether factors exist that might influence either the numerator or denominator data (i.e., surveillance artifact) (Table 7-3). Care must be taken to ensure that surveillance artifact is not leading to an erroneous conclusion that either the number of HAIs or the HAI rate is increasing. A wide variety of factors that can inflate or deflate the numerator or denominator data can lead to surveillance artifact; they include changes in the definitions used to ascertain HAIs, HAI detection methods—including surveillance or laboratory methods—changes in the populations of patients served, devices used, or procedures performed.

Because surveillance artifact influencing either the numerator or the denominator data can prejudice HAI rate comparisons, it is important that the accuracy of these

data be determined before rate comparisons are made. Although it is tempting to quickly begin comparative epidemiologic studies to ascertain the source and risk factors for infection, it is imperative that sufficient time be taken before embarking on such analyses to ensure the accuracy of the numerator and denominator data used to demonstrate that the HAI rate is increasing. Otherwise, one will be misled and devote precious personnel resources to conducting an investigation of a less urgent, nonemerging or nonimportant problem.

Numerator data often are the first finding that leads to a belief that there is an epidemic. Thus, confirmation of the validity and accuracy of the numerator data is an important first step. To be consistent, the numerator data should be obtained using the same definition over the time periods being compared. For instance, if the ICP has changed the HAI definitions used, it may appear that the HAI rate also changed when it did not; case ascertainment has altered, and reclassification of the HAIs using the "old" surveillance definitions may show no change in the number of HAIs or the HAI rate. Even if the same surveillance definitions are used, for some sites of infection, it may still be necessary to validate the accuracy of the surveillance data.

For instance, if BSIs are being classified by the ICP as primary or secondary BSIs based on microbiology data, but data concerning the presence of a catheter in the patients with BSIs are not being collected, there may be misclassification of BSIs. If a review of the surveillance definitions used for case ascertainment suggests that the sensitivity and/or specificity of the definitions used is low or allows for considerable subjectivity, it may be necessary to validate the accuracy of the case-ascertainment method by having several members of the IC team review each "case" independently and ensure its accuracy.

Because the existence of an outbreak usually cannot be determined by evaluation of the numerator data alone, one needs to be equally precise in ensuring the validity and accuracy of the denominator data that will be used to calculate the HAI rates in the epidemic and pre-epidemic periods. Selection of the denominator to use in calculating HAI rates is critically important. Previous studies have shown that for ICU patients, the duration of a patient's ICU stay, device (e.g., central venous or urinary catheters or mechanical ventilation) exposure and the duration of that exposure, and severity of illness all contribute to the patient's HAI risk [10–13].

Thus, these important confounding variables must be controlled for by using ICU-specific, device-specific denominator data (e.g., the number of urinary catheter days for the surgical ICU) if valid HAI rate comparisons are to be made [8]. Similarly, use of a surgical patient risk index that attempts to control for some of the most important factors determining a surgical patient's infection risk, such as the type and duration of the surgical procedure, severity of illness, and wound class, is essential if valid HAI rate comparisons are to be made in surgical patients [14,15].

TABLE 7-3
SELECTED CONDITIONS THAT CAN RESULT IN SURVEILLANCE ARTIFACT

- Introduction of new infection definitions.
- New infection control practitioner(s).
- Initiation of surveillance in new area or population of patients.
- Introduction of new laboratory tests
- Introduction of new population of patients.
- Increased or decreased frequency of culturing/testing of patients.
- Introduction of new medical procedure (e.g., endoscopy, cardiac surgery).

In most instances, one can determine whether a perceived problem is an endemic or epidemic problem only by comparison of HAI rates during the suspected epidemic and pre-epidemic periods. Care should be taken when comparing the HAI rate at one's own institution with that reported either in the literature or from other institutions. Unless the surveillance methods used (including HAI definitions and case-ascertainment methods), the populations served, the invasive device used, and types and number of procedures performed are similar and the type of denominator data used for rate calculations are the same, it may be misleading to compare one institution's rate with that of another institution. Thus, because of the large number of confounding variables that can influence the numerator, denominator, or HAI rate, one often is safest comparing rates over time at one's own institution. However, even then, one must be cautious in making such comparisons, ensuring that the comparisons include both similar numerator and similar denominator data.

For example, comparison of nosocomial BSI rates in an ICU to which only medical patients are admitted with rates in another unit at that same institution to which both medical and surgical patients are admitted or comparison of nosocomial BSI, UTI, SSI, or pneumonia rates among patients in a medical ICU to rates in patients in surgical ICUs may be misleading. Because both the mix of patients and the devices used can influence HAI rates, controlling for these factors by making comparisons with similar populations and controlling for the duration of patients' stays and devices used is necessary if valid rate comparisons are to be made. These factors are most easily controlled for by making HAI rate comparisons in a particular unit or population within an institution over time.

Differentiating Endemic from Epidemic Infections

No one definition can be used in all situations to differentiate endemic from epidemic infections or define epidemic infections. Depending on the severity of the problem and the administrative and other pressures present, one may be able to precisely and accurately define the numerator and denominator data or perform a "quick and dirty" analysis to determine whether an epidemic is present and an investigation must be initiated. Once one is confident of the validity and accuracy of these data, one is in a position to compare the rate of the infections or other adverse events recognized in the cluster to the background rate of such events and determine whether the cluster is an epidemic or endemic occurrence. If one can confirm the accuracy of the numerator data but not the denominator data, one may be forced to use a less accurate denominator (e.g., the number of patients or the number of patient-days) to calculate the "rate."

It must be realized that depending on the variation in the possible confounding variables, the findings of the comparison of the "epidemic" to "pre-epidemic" rates (i.e.,

statistically significantly higher, lower, or unchanged) may be misleading. Furthermore, it may sometimes be difficult, even given the appropriate numerator and denominator data, to determine whether a cluster of infections is endemic or epidemic. For instance, if an endemic rate of infection continues to rise, at some point it may be considered epidemic in nature if recent experience is compared with suitable remote baseline data. In other situations, the lack of background rate data (e.g., no surveillance conducted, new patient population or new diagnostic test introduced at the facility) may preclude the possibility of making rate comparisons. However, in most situations, it is possible to either determine or estimate the background rate and to decide whether the detected cluster of HAIs represents an epidemic or endemic problem. The recent development of a variety of computer statistical software packages has simplified the calculation and comparison of HAI rates; however, the ease with which it is possible to make such comparisons has further highlighted the importance of ensuring the accuracy and validity of the numerator and denominator data used.

Some researchers have suggested conducting prospective surveillance and using threshold programs to determine when the HAI rate increases above a certain level that warrants further investigation. Such programs were used in the 1970s in the National Nosocomial Infections Surveillance system and were found to be unreliable because of normal variations in the HAI rate at most institutions. Although it may be easy to establish a high HAI rate above which further investigation is indicated, the sensitivity of such a system would be low. To date, it has been impossible to design a sensitive and specific threshold program that would identify all epidemics when they occur yet not also highlight other nonoutbreaks as clusters requiring investigation. It has been equally difficult to develop a sufficiently sensitive and specific threshold program for the detection of clusters requiring further investigation.

More recently, data have been published from national surveillance and other studies providing HAI rate distributions for a variety of groups of patients [8–15]. These data can be used to compare the HAI rate at one's own institution and assist in determining whether the endemic HAI rate is too high and should be investigated or whether the HAI rate documented at the institution is significantly higher than at one's own institution in the past and significantly higher than national averages. These national benchmark data are most useful for evaluating one's endemic HAI rate rather than for determining whether an epidemic is in progress. Despite these data, there are many populations for which there are no published benchmark HAI rates. Furthermore, some of the published benchmark rates have not carefully controlled for intrinsic or extrinsic risk factors. Thus, one often is forced to decide whether to further investigate an epidemic or endemic problem based on the limited data one has at the institutional level.

DECIDING WHEN TO CONDUCT AN INVESTIGATION

Making the decision to conduct an epidemiologic investigation and determining the extent of that investigation depend on a number of factors. These factors differ at the institutional, local health departmental, state health departmental, federal governmental (Centers for Disease Control and Prevention [CDC]), and private consultant levels. In all situations, factors that influence the decision to initiate the investigation include whether the cluster is endemic or epidemic in nature, the morbidity and mortality associated with the infection cluster, and staff availability and expertise.

If a decision is made within the hospital that an investigation is warranted, the necessary staff should be mobilized and the investigation initiated. If the staff's availability or expertise is insufficient to conduct the investigation, hospital personnel can call in a private consultant, the local or state health departments, or the CDC for assistance. Regardless of the outside source, the exact nature and scope of the investigation desired by hospital personnel and what the outside consultant or organization is offering to do should be well defined and outlined before a request for assistance is extended. In addition, because of the changing epidemiology of HAIs and the possible complexity of an investigation, combined epidemiologic and laboratory investigations may be indicated and the capability to perform these investigations should be documented before an invitation is initiated or as soon as the need for such expertise is realized.

At the federal level (Division of Healthcare Quality Promotion, CDC), the decision to initiate an epidemiologic investigation at a healthcare facility is based on the public health importance of the problem, whether the cluster may represent a nationwide problem (e.g., intrinsic product contamination or a serious problem related to a newly introduced medical device), the morbidity and mortality associated with the cluster, the extent to which the investigation may advance knowledge of healthcare epidemiology and infection control, and staff availability [16,17]. Moreover, because combined epidemiologic and laboratory investigations are frequently most useful, the ability to obtain and genetically type the colonizing or infecting isolates associated with the cluster may influence the decision to collaborate in the investigation. Because the CDC is a nonregulatory agency, its collaboration in the investigation requires the approval of and invitation from both the healthcare facility's IC department and administration and the local and/or state health department.

Clusters of infection caused by very unusual organisms, those associated with great morbidity or mortality, and those of epidemiologic importance (introduction of a new multidrug-resistant pathogen) may warrant initiating an investigation without carefully comparing HAI rates in the epidemic and pre-epidemic periods. These clusters include infections caused by very unusual or never previously reported pathogens (i.e., vancomycin-resistant *S. aureus*, *Rhodococcus* or *Nocardia* sp infections in surgery patients), ≥2 infections caused by organisms usually indicative of a carrier (e.g., Group A streptococcus), isolated infections caused by a multidrug-resistant HAI pathogen (e.g., vancomycin-resistant enterococcus, multidrug-resistant *Mycobacterium tuberculosis*) that, if not controlled, could become endemic or dissemination of a clonal organism, which often suggests an eradicable common source [16–26].

Once a cluster is identified and the decision is made to conduct an investigation, the extent of the investigation must be determined. If the cluster is associated with little morbidity and mortality and involves only colonization or infection of a small number of patients, a brief investigation may be performed. In such circumstances, the possible case-patients' medical records are reviewed, a hypothetical mode of transmission is identified, and interventions are implemented. If a full-scale investigation is to be initiated, a systematic approach should be taken (discussed later). In general, it is recommended that cultures of HCWs, products, solutions, or environmental sources be directed by the epidemiologic data.

Documentation of an epidemiologic association between the outbreak and a product, device, or HCW, with subsequent culture confirmation is preferred to widespread culturing of HCWs, solutions, or equipment with the hope that the source will be identified. Widespread culturing of animate or inanimate objects with the object of serendipitously identifying the source is wasteful of the time of both IC and laboratory personnel (see Chapters 10 and 20). On the other hand, if one cannot preserve the area in which the outbreak is taking place and the inanimate environment is going to be cleaned or the product reprocessed, selected cultures should be obtained before the scene of the outbreak is altered. In addition, it may be important to immediately interview HCWs in the area where the outbreak has occurred because practices may change or recall bias may be introduced if these persons are interviewed days or weeks later.

Last, careful consideration should be given to whether the unit/ward/area should be closed or surgery or other procedures discontinued. If a large number of deaths are associated with the outbreak in one area, closing the area may be warranted. However, if such a decision is made, IC personnel should realize the seriousness of the message being sent. Before closing the area, there should be discussion, and a consensus should be developed concerning what criteria must be met before reopening the area. The decisions to close and reopen an area can be made only at the institutional level. Regardless of whether the unit is closed, IC and administrative personnel should ensure that all potentially relevant materials (devices, medications, solutions, etc.) are saved and quarantined for future evaluation.

If there is serious morbidity or a large number of deaths or if many patients are affected, serious consideration should be given to identifying a spokesperson, best coordinated through IC and public relations staff, who will regularly update both appropriate institutional (e.g., staff and patients) and external (e.g., regulatory, governmental, or media) personnel. The spokesperson should present enough information to assure others that an appropriate institutional investigation is being conducted but should not prematurely reveal preliminary information. All public inquiries should be directed to the identified spokesperson to ensure that one voice is being heard and conflicting stories do not emerge. Open and honest communication with the local or national media is preferable to disseminating mis-information or refusing to speak to them.

It should be remembered that state and federal laws require that healthcare facilities notify public health authorities of selected adverse events (see Chapter 18). Because laws differ in each state, IC personnel should consult the law in the state where their healthcare facility is located. Any outbreaks that may have a public health impact at the county, state, or national level should be reported to local, state, or federal health officials. Any outbreaks associated with intrinsically contaminated or defective products (including solutions, blood or blood products, or devices) should be reported to the Food and Drug Administration (FDA) through the Med-Watch Program (1-800-FDA-1088). If such an outbreak involves many healthcare facilities in more than one state, federal public health agencies are responsible for the investigations.

CONDUCTING AN EPIDEMIOLOGIC INVESTIGATION

Saving Critical Materials

The first step in any investigation is to ensure that critically important isolates and/or materials that may be associated with the outbreak are saved. At the first sign of an outbreak, the IC staff should get in touch with the director of the microbiology laboratory and request that any of the infecting organisms from current and past possible "cases" be saved. Laboratory personnel also should be alerted to keep any subsequent isolates of the outbreak strain that may be recovered during the investigation. If this is not done, laboratory confirmation of the subsequent epidemiologic findings in the form of isolate typing will be impossible. In addition, if there is the possibility that an intrinsically or extrinsically contaminated product device may be the source of the outbreak, such solution or devices should be immediately quarantined.

For example, if there is an unusual cluster of BSIs with the same organism(s) in one unit over a short period of time

(1 to 5 days), a contaminated product should be seriously considered; it may be prudent to collect all medications, multidose vials, or solutions from the involved area and immediately move them to an area where they can be preserved and protected. If extrinsic contamination of a product or solution is suspected, it may be useful to have personnel save products or solutions used in the area as the epidemiologic investigation is being conducted so that these solutions/products can be cultured or studied if epidemiologic studies establish an association between them and the adverse outcome.

The Source, the Pathogen, the Host, and the Mode of Transmission

Epidemiologic investigations have similarities and differences. The approach is similar, although the risk factors assessed may be different. For this reason, standardized forms usually are not used in such investigations; instead, the data collected during each epidemiologic investigation is individualized depending on the data available on the pathogen, host, and known or suspected modes of transmission. Although the approach may differ slightly for each investigation initiated, in general, epidemiologists use a fairly standard system (Table 7-4). Four major areas assessed in any epidemiologic investigation include the source(s), the pathogen(s), the host, and the mode of transmission. Factors in these four areas contribute to the outbreak, and modification of ≥ 1 of these elements usually can terminate the outbreak. For infection to occur, sufficient organisms must be present, the host must be susceptible to the organism, and opportunity must exist for the host to have contact with the organism. The goal of the epidemiologic investigation is to determine which of these factors is the most important in causing the outbreak and which can most easily be modified to interrupt transmission.

It is important to understand the pathogen and the ecologic niche the organism prefers. For instance, *Sternotrophomonas maltophilia* or *Burkholderia cepacia* are increasingly common HAI pathogens that often can be traced to water sources [22–24]. *Malassezia* sp are lipid-loving organisms that usually infect patients receiving intralipid. A nosocomial *Malassezia pachydermitis* outbreak among neonates in a neonatal ICU was traced via colonization of the hands of HCWs via colonization of the ears of their dogs [25,26]. *Aspergillus* sp usually infect immunocompromised patients and can be found in soil and air [27,28]. *Acinetobacter* or *Serratia* spp. emerge in situations of high antimicrobial pressure, and the latter organisms have been traced to intrinsic or extrinsic contamination of antiseptics [29,30]. *Legionella* sp are typically associated with water sources and primarily infect immunocompromised hosts [31]. Some salmonella

TABLE 7-4
GENERAL APPROACH TO AN OUTBREAK INVESTIGATION

The preliminary investigation: quick and dirty
- Review existing information
  - Surveillance records
  - Interviews with clinical/laboratory staff
  - Microbiology records
  - Patients' records
- Verify the diagnosis
- Develop tentative case definition (may be broad, i.e., fairly sensitive but not too specific)
  - Microbiologic
  - Other clinical laboratory
    - Hematology
    - Chemistry
    - Other (e.g., toxicology)
  - Radiologic
  - Pathologic
  - Clinical signs/symptoms
  - Other (e.g., skin testing)
  - Combinations of these areas
- Ascertain cases
  - Descriptive epidemiology
    - Establish the nature of the problem (e.g., SSI), population at risk, location, severity of illness, and timeframe
    - Construct the epidemic curve
      - Time
      - Place
      - Person
  - Establish existence of an outbreak
    - Compare rates
    - Exclude surveillance artifact or pseudoepidemic
  - Assess adequacy of control measures
    - Enforce existing control measures
    - Supplement with additional control measures
  - Decide on a course of observation vs. definitive investigation, taking into account
    - Severity of illness
      - Colonization vs. disease
      - Morbidity vs. mortality
    - Effectiveness of control measures
The comprehensive investigation
- Refine the case definition (e.g., increasing specificity)
- Ascertain additional cases
  - Record reviews
  - Surveys
    - Microbiologic
    - Other (e.g., skin testing, antibody testing)
- Refine descriptive epidemiology
- Refine evaluation establishing the existence of an outbreak
- Develop hypotheses
- Test hypotheses—analytical epidemiology
  - Case control vs. cohort studies
  - Retrospective vs. prospective studies
  - Control selection
- Re-evaluate control measures
  - Implement additional measures if warranted
  - Ask whether additional epidemiologic/laboratory studies are needed
- Draw conclusions and formalize recommendations for control
- Continue surveillance for new cases
- Evaluate the effectiveness of implemented control measures
- Write and distribute a comprehensive report

SSI, surgical site infection

and most Group A streptococcus infections are traced to personnel carriers [32,33].

In general, molecular typing of the infecting pathogen can provide valuable information [34] (see Chapter 10). If the infecting organisms are identical (i.e., clonal), the chances are great that there is a common source (e.g., a solution, device, or HCW) and that an epidemiologic investigation can identify the source, the source can be removed, and the outbreak can be terminated. On the other hand, if molecular typing of the infecting organisms shows that they are not identical (i.e., nonclonal), most likely the organism is being introduced from multiple sources and/or transmitted from person to person via HCW hands. An epidemiologic investigation may pinpoint factors increasing the risk of infection (failure to rapidly identify colonized/infected patients and isolate them, failure of HCWs to perform hand hygiene, etc.), but the empiric reinforcement of such practices as isolation of patients and hand hygiene may terminate the outbreak without a more complete investigation. Thus, reviewing the microbiology of the infecting pathogen can provide valuable clues to the likely source of an infection and facilitate generation of hypotheses about that source.

Next, host factors need to be evaluated. For the host to become infected, there must be sufficient numbers of organisms, and the patient must be susceptible to infection. In some instances, host susceptibility is related to age or immunosuppression that is condition specific (e.g., low birthweight neonates), disease specific (e.g., human immunodeficiency virus–infected patients) or condition or medication induced (patients with hematologic malignancy or bone marrow or organ transplant patients). In other instances, the host has become susceptible to colonization or infection because of exposure to medical devices or other surgical or invasive procedures.

The next factor to be considered is the mode of transmission. HAI pathogens may be transmitted by contact (direct, indirect, droplet) or a common source, or it may be airborne (droplet nuclei, skin squamae) or vectorborne (see Chapter 1). Although HAI pathogens can be transmitted by the airborne route (e.g., *Aspergillus* spp, Influenza, *M. tuberculosis*, measles, or varicella-zoster viruses), the majority are passed by contact, usually necessitating transfer of the organisms from an infected or colonized patient to a susceptible patient via transient HCW hand colonization [18,21,26,29,35] or by droplet (<3 feet) spread (e.g., respiratory syncytial viruses or adenoviruses). With most organisms transmitted by contact, the infected or colonized patient is the source; for some organisms, such as VRE, multidrug-resistant *S. aureus*, and respiratory syncytial viruses and rotavirus, the environment may play a role in infection transmission by fomites.

The predominant site of HAI also can help the epidemiologist focus the investigation on the most likely route of transmission. For instance, a cluster of BSIs is most likely related to an intrinsically contaminated common vehicle or extrinsically contaminated solution or device (including transducers) or to lapses in aseptic technique on the part of HCWs during intravascular catheter device manipulation [36]. Nosocomial pneumonia often is traced to contamination of respiratory therapy equipment or person-to-person transmission of infecting pathogens via HCWs hands [37]. Nosocomial UTIs are typically attributed to contamination during urinary tract manipulation, open urinary drainage systems, or the insertion or maintenance of a urinary catheter [38]. SSIs often are traced to sources in the operating room [16,18,32,39,40,42] or, more rarely, to the postoperative ICU [41] or the preoperative ward.

When initiating an investigation, a review of the source, pathogen, host, and mode of transmission can help guide the direction of the epidemiologic investigation. The more that is known about these areas, the more focused the investigation can be. In contrast, the less that is known about these areas (for instance, the first nosocomial outbreak of *Rhodococcus bronchialis* among surgery patients), the broader the scope of the investigation must be at the beginning [18].

Initial "Case" Review

Regardless of whether a brief or detailed epidemiologic study is being carried out, one of the first steps in the investigation of a possible epidemic or outbreak is to review some or all of the medical records of possible case-patients. The purpose of this review is to characterize the population at risk by time, place, and person so that a "case" definition can be developed. If possible, this review should encompass all known possible case-patients. If the number of possible case-patients is large, one may select a sample of them; if either a random or convenience sample is chosen, the reviewer should be aware that bias may thus be introduced and lead to erroneous conclusions.

For infections that have a long incubation period, meaning that the majority of patients experience onset of symptoms after hospital discharge, review of the medical records of only those who are still hospitalized may lead to an underestimation of the extent of the outbreak and may not describe the affected population accurately. Examples of such outbreaks include many insidious postoperative SSIs (caused by, e.g., nontuberculous mycobacteria, *Nocardia* spp, *Rhodococcus* spp), *S. aureus* infections among newborns, and infections with long incubation periods [18,42–44]. In outbreaks with long incubation periods, after the case definition is developed, extensive case-ascertainment is necessary.

Line-Listing

During the initial case review, a detailed line-listing should be developed for each patient (Table 7-5). Data collected should include demographic and clinical data, the date of hospital admission, wards/units admitted to and the dates of admission to and discharge from each ward/unit, underlying diseases, date of onset of infection and/or colonization, and, if the outbreak involves infection, whether colonization with the infecting pathogen preceded the onset of infection and at what site infection was noted. Additional information is collected specific to the site of the infection/colonization. For example, with SSIs, information is collected on the pre-, intra-, and postoperative courses of the case-patients; these data should include whether a patient was admitted to an ICU before the surgery, the date and type of each surgical procedure, the HCWs who took part in the surgery, and exposures specific to the surgical procedure, including the type and timing of administration of prophylactic antimicrobials.

For BSI outbreaks, the types of catheters, their dates of insertion, and the duration of intravascular catheterization and the types of intravenous fluids, medications, and monitors should be documented. The epidemiologist or ICPs should collect adequate information to characterize the population at risk sufficiently so that the type of outbreak (i.e., colonization or disease), population (i.e., patients affected), place (i.e., specific wards, ICUs, or surgical areas), and estimated outbreak period can be defined. Sufficient detail should be collected to establish a case definition, taking care to avoid generating an enormous amount of useless information. The primary purpose of this review is to try to identify common characteristics among the patients so that one can describe the time period of the outbreak, the group of patients at greatest risk, and the affected area(s) of the healthcare facility. In the course of this review, investigators should ensure that the HAIs are real and that neither surveillance nor diagnostic artifact has resulted in the "appearance" of an outbreak.

Case Definition

The next step in the investigation of an outbreak is the development of a case definition. Initially, unless the disease is known or the time or place of exposure is well defined, the case definition should be broad. This tentative case definition can be further refined as more information is obtained during the conduct of the investigation. Each case definition should specify the estimated *time period* of the outbreak, the *place or places* in the healthcare facility where the outbreak is taking place, and the types of *persons* who are becoming case-patients. In outbreaks of a pathogen-specific disease, development of the case definition may be relatively simple, for instance, all neonatal ICU patients from June 2 to August 30, 2007, with blood cultures positive for *M. pachydermitis* [26]. For syndromes for which a direct association with a specific infectious agent cannot be established from the information available (e.g., initial investigations of toxic shock, Legionnaires' disease, or toxic

TABLE 7-5
EXAMPLE OF LINE-LISTING

Case	Age	Sex	Ward	Type of Surgery	Date of Surgery	Operating Room	Parenteral Antibiotic Prophylaxis	Duration of Surgery (min)	Wound Drain	Fever After Surgery (hr)[a]	Date of Wound Inflammation	Culture Date	Culture Site
1	46	F	5NW	TAH, BSO	4/23	A	No	100	No	17	4/29	4/30	Wound
2	77	M	3C	Cholecystectomy choledocholitn-ectomy	5/02	F	No	150	Yes	32	5/04	5/06	Wound
3	47	M	5SW	Laminectomy	5/06	G	No	120	Yes	24	5/09	5/09	Wound
—	—	—	—	—	—	—	—	—	—	—	—	5/08	Blood
—	—	—	—	—	—	—	—	—	—	—	—	5/10	Blood
4	33	F	3C	Lobar resection & pleural stripping	5/08	D	No	120	Yes	17	5/12	5/16	Wound
5	84	F	2SE	Pyelolithotomy	5/14	C	No	60	Yes	36	5/19	5/21	Wound
—	—	—	—	—	—	—	—	—	—	—	—	5/21	Blood
—	—	—	—	—	—	—	—	—	—	—	—	5/24	Blood
6	55	M	3C	Sigmoid resection	5/20	F	No	105	Yes	48	5/23	5/23	Wound
7	22	F	5SW	ORIF ankle	7/06	A	No	150	No	20	7/07	7/08	Wound
8	65	F	5SW	Bunionectomy	7/21	F	No	45	No	18	7/23	7/23	Wound
9	40	F	4SW	Melanoma resection with skin graft	7/21	A	No	145	Yes	99	7/25	7/25	Wound
10	37	F	5NW	TAH, BSO	7/30	A	No	105	No	32	8/01	8/04	Wound

TAH, total abdominal hysterectomy; BSO, bilateral salpingo-oophorectomy; ORIF, open reduction, internal fixation.
[a]Temperature $\geq 101°$F.

exposures), development of the case definition can be more challenging. In these instances, the case definition should include all of the signs and symptoms common to all of the "tentative cases" reviewed.

In addition, the case definition may include combinations of signs and/or symptoms common to the majority of the cases reviewed. One such case definition might be any patient in the surgical ICU from January 5 to March 19, 2007, who had a temperature $>102°F$ and a >20 mm drop in systolic blood pressure together with any one or more of the following signs: a white blood cell count $>25,000$ cells/mm^3, a platelet count $<20,000/mm^3$, a bilirubin level of >5 mg/dL, or splenomegaly. When formulating a case definition, a balance must be drawn between sensitivity and specificity. It may be preferable to have a case definition that is very specific rather than overly sensitive; in this way, one can be more certain that each "case" identified is a true case. Furthermore, in subsequent analytic epidemiologic studies, missed "case-patients" may be included in the control or noncase group and create bias toward not finding differences between the case and control or noncase-patients; thus, any significant differences identified are probably even more significant. Alternatively, one may wish to identify "definite," "probable," or "possible" case-patients; this approach helps ensure that controls do not include possible or probable case-patients and that case-patients are only those patients most likely to be cases for case-control comparisons.

Case Ascertainment

Having established a case definition, the next step is to conduct extensive case ascertainment. In this process, the IC staff try to identify all of the cases that may have arisen. All potential sources of information should be examined for possible case-identifying information. If the case definition is microorganism based, usually a careful review of the existing microbiology records is all that is needed to identify case patients. Reviewing microbiology methods may be necessary to exclude the possibility that the organism might not be identified or that specimens are referred to an outside laboratory.

Thus, case ascertainment in organism-based outbreaks of BSIs, UTIs, or most SSIs is simplified. Nevertheless, one must be aware of the possibility of changes in culturing frequency upon case detection [44]. However, depending on the site of infection, outbreaks where culturing bias (i.e., clinicians are less likely to document the infection by culture) may exist; for example, nosocomial pneumonia (for which a review of radiology reports in addition to microbiology records may be necessary) or SSIs caused by multiple pathogens (when it may be necessary to review the records of all patients undergoing the procedure to identify those with signs or symptoms of SSIs from whom cultures were not taken) may require more extensive and rigorous case ascertainment. During the case-ascertainment process,

all computerized and noncomputerized data sources (including microbiology, radiology, infection control, pharmacy, operating room, surgery, hemodialysis, other invasive procedures, nursing, or patients' medical records) that may facilitate case ascertainment should be considered.

At the same time that case ascertainment is being conducted, one should review an arbitrarily defined preoutbreak period (usually 6 months to 2 years) for the occurrence of the outbreak adverse event. In this way, one can define the background number of such events. This information will be used to calculate the pre-epidemic rate of the adverse event that will be compared to the epidemic period rate to determine whether an outbreak has occurred or is occurring.

The Epidemic Curve (Time)

Using the information obtained from case definition and case ascertainment, an epidemiologic curve (epi curve) should be drawn. This curve depicts the number of case-patients on the vertical axis, or y-axis, and time on the horizontal axis, or x-axis (Figure 7-1). The line-listing information and epi curve can provide data to facilitate generation of hypotheses about the mode of transmission. The time scale used should be shorter than the presumed incubation period of the adverse event because otherwise person-to-person transmission may appear to be common-source transmission. By plotting the time course of the adverse event during the epidemic and pre-epidemic periods, one can compare the occurrence of the adverse event during the epidemic and background periods, identify clusters of the event, and, based on the shape of the epi curve, generate hypotheses about the mode of transmission.

The shape of the epi curve can suggest the possible mode of transmission. If there is an abrupt increase in the number of adverse events over a short time period, the curve suggests a single exposure to a point source of contamination, such as a contaminated product (Figure 7-1a). In contrast, when the epi curve depicts patients over a more prolonged time course, it is most suggestive of person-to-person transmission (Figure 7-1b). In some situations, there may be more than one mode of transmission operating either sequentially or simultaneously (Figure 7-1c). Additional epi curves depicting the dates of culture or possible exposure also may be informative—particularly when the incubation period is long. It also may be useful to draw epi curves with different time intervals (i.e., day, week, month) on the horizontal axis.

Geographic Assessment (Place)

It is useful to closely examine the place of the outbreak to determine whether there is geographic clustering. Use of spot maps may facilitate recognition of clustering of case-patients that is not otherwise obvious. Do all of the case-patients come from one ward or unit? If all the case-patients

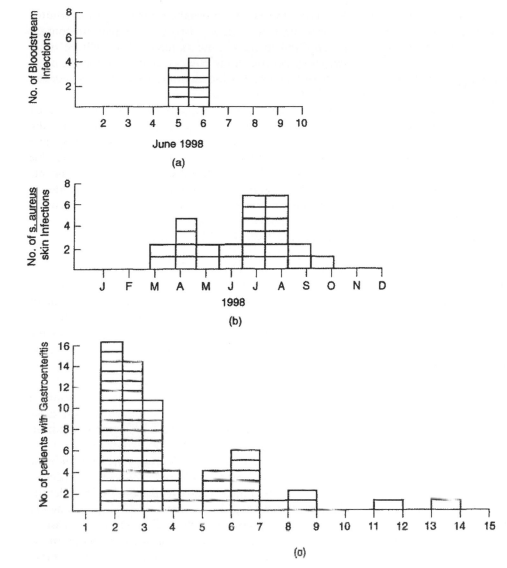

Figure 7-1 Example of epidemic curves. **a:** Distribution of patients with bloodstream infections associated with a contaminated common source medication. **b:** Distribution of patients with *S. aureus* skin infections associated with person-to-person transmissions. **c:** Distribution of patients with gastroenteritis associated with a common contaminated food source followed by patient-to-patient transmission.

are from one ward/unit, one can plot graphically the dates of admission and discharge from that unit (or multiple units) for each case-patient and ask whether there is continuous overlap among the patients. If so, this finding would suggest person-to-person transmission from one colonized or infected patient to the next. If all case-patients have an infection that can be transmitted via the airborne route, is plotting the patients by room location consistent with the ventilation system airflow diagrams or direction of airflow demonstrated by smoke tube? If the case-patients are located in several different wards or units, have they all had common exposure to medications, solutions, devices, procedures, or rooms where a procedure may have been performed? If the outbreak is at one surgical site, have all procedures been performed in one operating room or outpatient surgical suite? Geographically plotting the case-patients by a variety of dates, including those of the time of culture, onset of illness, possible exposures, and so forth, may all be useful.

Host Factors (Person)

Further review of the characteristics of the case patients then is undertaken to try to define the most likely risk factors of infection. What role are specific underlying host factors playing in the outbreak? For instance, are all neonatal ICU patients at risk or only those <1,500 g? Are all surgical patients at risk or only those undergoing cardiac surgery? Are all hematology-oncology patients at risk or only those who have prolonged neutropenia? Each of the case-patients' host characteristics should be reviewed to determine whether there are common features among these patients.

Factors to assess include those intrinsic to the host (i.e., age, gender, race, underlying diseases, and nutritional status) and those extrinsic to the host (e.g., receipt of medications or solutions or environmental exposures—admission to an ICU or procedure room; HCW exposures; exposure to therapeutic measures that might alter host susceptibility, e.g., receipt of antimicrobials; or exposure to invasive procedures or to invasive devices, e.g., central venous or urinary catheters, mechanical ventilation, or arterial pressure monitoring).

Refinement of the Case Definition and Reassessment of the Need for Further Investigation

At this point, the basic elements of the simple epidemiologic investigation are complete. IC should refine the case definition based on the data accumulated. Only the essential elements reflecting the time, place, and persons who have experienced the adverse event should be included. For example, if the line-listing shows that all (or nearly all) of the case-patients are <1,500 g and have stayed in the neonatal ICU for a median of 5 days, the case definition might be modified from that of all neonatal ICU patients to those <1,500 g who stayed in the unit for ≥5 days. Careful addition of patients or deletion of those initially thought to be case-patients who do not fit the case definition should take place. It is imperative that the refined case definition be as precise and accurate as possible because the results of subsequent epidemiologic studies are contingent on this case definition.

If the case definition is in error, it may lead to erroneous conclusions. As mentioned previously, an overly restrictive case definition will exclude true case-patients and diminish the likelihood of finding an association between an exposure and the case-patients. In contrast, an overly inclusive case definition will result in the inclusion of noncase-patients in the case-patient group and may obscure possible associations. In most circumstances, it is preferable to begin the investigation by being overly inclusive and become more restrictive as the investigation proceeds. In some investigations, it may not be possible to divide all patients into case-patient and noncase-patient or control populations. If it has not already been done, one may at this point need to define possible and/or probable case-patients and then perform further analyses including and then excluding these patients in the case-patient group.

Occasionally, the review of the case-patients' medical and microbiology records suggests that there is a cluster of positive cultures but that the patients do not have clinical illness [16]. Such findings should alert one to the possibility of a pseudoepidemic, that is, an apparent cluster of positive cultures that may be false positives or contaminants. In the 1960s and 1970s, such outbreaks most often were associated with cross-contamination in the laboratory during manual processing of cultures. In the 1980s and 1990s, clusters of positive cultures increasingly have been associated with cross-contamination via automated systems [16,17]. Pseudoepidemics have been traced to a variety of sources, including intrinsically or extrinsically contaminated antiseptics or culture media, cross-contamination of cultures during manual or automated processing, or intrinsically or extrinsically contaminated blood collection tubes.

Whenever there is an unusual cluster of positive cultures, particularly if it is an uncommon or environmental organism and the case-patients do not have clinical signs or symptoms indicating HAI, evaluation of the specimen collection and processing methods to exclude a pseudoepidemic should be initiated.

At this point in the investigation, IC personnel may have arrived at the most likely source and mode of transmission of the outbreak. Because of personnel, time, or other constraints, it may be decided to introduce a number of IC interventions thought likely to reduce or interrupt transmission and then discontinue the investigation. If the outbreak is similar to others previously reported, it may be possible simply to implement the previously documented successful IC measures. If this is done, it is imperative that surveillance be maintained for the adverse event so that one can document the effectiveness of the implemented interventions. If the interventions do not reduce (to acceptable levels) or interrupt transmission, it may be necessary to initiate a more comprehensive comparative investigation.

Is Outside Assistance Needed?

If it is decided that a more comprehensive epidemiologic investigation is warranted because the outbreak (a) has not been terminated by the introduced control measures; (b) is unusual, complex, or associated with substantial morbidity or mortality; (c) is of major public health importance; or (d) represents an opportunity to advance our knowledge and/or understanding of healthcare epidemiology, one should re-evaluate whether the personnel, time, and/or expertise are sufficient to conduct the required comprehensive studies. Such investigations may demand a substantial investment in IC, laboratory, and statistical/computer resources. The comprehensive investigation may involve exhaustive evaluation of potential risk factors; a series of several case-control and/or cohort studies; complex analytic techniques, including multivariate analyses and modeling to control for confounding variables; HCW questionnaires, interviews, or observational studies; epidemiologically directed environmental, product, device, and/or HCW cultures; and implementation of interventions and evaluation of the effectiveness of these interventions.

If the adverse event is serious enough to consider a comprehensive investigation, sufficient resources should be dedicated to the investigation to permit the rapid initiation of the study, identification of the source, and introduction of control measures. If healthcare facility IC personnel add the conduct of such an investigation to their ongoing responsibilities, it may mean that the comparative studies will be conducted over several months. By the time the probable source of the outbreak is identified, it is possible either that the device, solution, or source will have been reprocessed or discarded or that the epidemiologically implicated HCW will no longer be colonized with the infecting strain.

If outside advice or assistance is desired, a variety of experts is available including personnel at the local or state health departments, colleagues at other healthcare facilities in the same area, experts at nearby academic centers with an interest in healthcare epidemiology, private consultant epidemiologists, or the CDC. State and local health departments may be able to assist in arranging epidemiologic and/or laboratory support. Healthcare facility administrative and IC personnel or personnel at the state health department can request CDC assistance. In CDC-conducted on-site investigations, both epidemiologic and laboratory support is provided at no cost to the healthcare facility.

Regardless of the outside source of assistance, the investigation should be considered and conducted as a collaborative effort with the healthcare facility personnel. Without the assistance of healthcare facility personnel, a comprehensive investigation cannot be efficiently conducted, and it will be these personnel who will need to implement the recommended control measures. Furthermore, local personnel are likely to be much more knowledgeable about available data sources, local IC and other policies and practices, HCW changes, and the particular control measures that can realistically be successfully implemented at their institution.

The Comprehensive Investigation

The first step in conducting the comprehensive investigation is to review the basic investigation's line-listing, case definition, and case-ascertainment methods to ensure that no shortcuts were taken that may influence the comparative studies. Was the case definition based on a review of all possible cases or just a sample? If sampling was used, was it random sampling, which may be representative of all case-patients, or convenience sampling (i.e., those medical records that were readily available)? Could the case review sampling have biased the case definition? Except in very large outbreaks, it is preferable to review the medical records of all potential case-patients.

Occasionally, it is the small number (often one or two) of patients who are otherwise very similar to the case-patients but who did not have the adverse condition who provide insight into the possible cause of the outbreak. Was the case ascertainment complete? If not, it should be extended and repeated. Does the case ascertainment need to be broadened to a review (and/or contacting) of patients who have been discharged from the hospital or to communicating with IC personnel at nearby hospitals or home care? Was the line-listing extensive enough, or is further review of the case-patient medical records necessary to obtain information on additional exposures or clinical findings? Was the denominator used to calculate the rate of the adverse event and to compare the rates of these events in the epidemic and pre-epidemic periods the correct denominator? If the denominator was not correct, is there

a way to obtain the correct denominator, or must one estimate the denominator?

For example, if the outbreak involves BSIs in the medical ICU but in the initial investigation one had to use either the number of medical ICU patients or the number of patient-days as the denominator, can one obtain the more appropriate denominator, that is, the number of days medical ICU patients spent on central venous catheters? If these data are not available or have not been collected, it may be unrealistic to try to derive them by reviewing the medical records of all medical ICU patients (assuming that the central venous catheter insertion, presence, and removal dates are well documented in the medical records).

However, it would be possible to estimate these denominator data. One could randomly sample time periods during the pre-epidemic and epidemic time periods and, for several days or a week in the pre-epidemic and epidemic periods, determine for all patients in the medical ICU how many had central venous catheters and what proportion of the ICU days those patients were on such catheters. Then one can determine a "central venous catheter use factor" (i.e., the proportion of patient-days spent on central venous catheters times the number of patients in the unit) for each time period. In this way, one can estimate the number of central venous catheter days in the unit during the epidemic and pre-epidemic periods. Such estimation may be necessary when either the necessary data are not available or review of records containing the needed data would be excessively laborious and/or time consuming.

Comparative Epidemiologic Studies

Once one has defined the case, performed comprehensive case ascertainment, developed an extensive line-listing, and drafted epidemic curves, one is ready to develop and test hypothesized risk factors and modes of transmission. This can be done through either a case-control or a cohort study (see Chapters 1 and 8). In a case-control study, all or some of the case-patients are compared with a group of patients who did not experience the adverse event (controls) for exposure to the potential risk factors. In contrast, in a cohort study, such exposures are compared among all the patients in the involved area during the specified period.

Numerous factors influence the decision to conduct a case-control or cohort study including statistical and practical considerations. In a cohort study, one can calculate the relative risk or a quantitative measure of the strength of the association between the exposure and the risk of developing the adverse condition (See Chapter 8). In contrast, in a case-control study, one can estimate the strength of the association between the exposure and the adverse condition only by calculating an odds ratio; one can determine only that case-patients were more likely to be exposed to the factor than were controls. Adverse conditions with a high attack rate lend themselves to cohort studies whereas conditions with low attack rates are better evaluated through a case-control study. If the duration of the outbreak is short and the number of patients in the unit during the outbreak is small, it may be feasible to conduct a cohort study. On the other hand, if the duration of the outbreak is long (months or years) and the number of patients in the involved unit(s) is large (e.g., >100), it may be impractical to conduct a cohort study, and a case-control study may be more realistic. Depending on the duration of the outbreak, the size of the population at risk, and the extent of the data being obtained from the medical records, a case-control study may take days to weeks whereas a cohort study may require weeks to months.

Cohort Study

In a cohort study, all patients in the unit or units of interest or undergoing the particular procedure of interest are evaluated for exposures to the variable(s) of interest. Such a study can be conducted either prospectively or retrospectively. Because case-control studies are easier to perform, take less time, and tend to be more powerful, retrospective cohort studies are less frequently undertaken to evaluate nosocomial endemic or epidemic problems. However, if the case-control study data are insufficient to determine the cause of the outbreak and/or the case-control study has narrowed the population at risk, carrying out a prospective cohort study may be useful.

Case-Control Study

In contrast, in a case-control study, the case-patients are compared with a similar population without the adverse condition. In a case-control study, selection of the controls is critical. Unless it cannot be avoided, historical controls (i.e., patients present in the unit but in the time period before the outbreak) should not be used. Such patients may not have had the same opportunity for exposure and may not be similar to the population affected. Random selection of patients in the same unit at the same time as the case-patients is preferred. If one is concerned that there could be differences in ≥1 factors influencing the types of exposures of case-patients and controls, a small, focused case-control study focusing on these factors can be done before the comprehensive case-control study. For instance, if by examination of the line-listing, one becomes concerned that birthweight (e.g., <1,500 g) and duration of neonatal ICU stay (i.e., >5 days) influenced the types of exposure of the patients, one can first evaluate these two factors. If they are found to be significantly different between case- and control-patients, selection of controls could be limited only to those neonates who weighed <1,500 g and who stayed in the neonatal ICU >5 days.

There are several other methods to control for such confounding variables (matching, stratification, or multivariate analyses). In matching, one selects controls by matching ≥1 factors (e.g., birthweight, duration of stay, severity of illness, underlying disease) with the case-patients. It must be realized that such matching factors cannot be evaluated as potential risk factors. Furthermore, the more factors one wishes to match between case- and control-patients, the more difficult it is to identify controls without reviewing all of their records looking for these factors. It is preferable to randomly select the controls and evaluate the factors under consideration for their strength of association with the adverse condition. Then, if they are found to be statistically significant, they can be controlled for through stratified or multivariate analyses. In contrast, in matched analyses, it is assumed that these factors are not significant without assessing whether the assumption is true.

Several important decisions must be made when conducting a case-control study. The first is whether to include all or a sample of the case-patients. In general, it is best to include all case-patients to increase the power of the study and to avoid introduction of bias. Second, one must decide how to select the controls. To enhance the likelihood of determining the source of the outbreak, controls should have similar opportunity for exposure to the potential risk factors as the case-patients. In other words, they should be selected from the same population (same ward or unit or undergoing the same procedure) as the case-patients and be hospitalized during the same period as the case-patients. Third, once the population of potential controls is identified, one must decide how many controls to select for each case-patient.

The number of controls selected is based on statistical power and practical considerations. If the attack rate is high and the number of case-patients is large, one control per case-patient may be sufficient. If the number of case-patients is small (e.g., <20), one should select 2 to 3 controls per case-patient. The proportional increase in power associated with the selection of >3 controls per case declines markedly, and the proportional increase in power by selecting >4–5 controls usually does not justify the increased volume of work. Last, one must decide how the controls are going to be selected. There are at least two selection methods: random and stratified or proportional sampling.

The random selection of controls is the easiest and most widely used method. With this method, all potential controls are listed and then selected using a random numbers table. Random numbers tables can be found in most statistics books and may be generated by numerous statistical software packages. If one has 500 potential controls and wishes to select 50, one just lists the controls in numerical order from 0 to 500 and then generates 50 random numbers between 1 and 500. Alternative random selection methods include choosing every "nth" control from the list of controls or selecting the patient who came before and/or after the admission or surgery of the case-patient. The random numbers method is preferred because the other methods may introduce bias—all patients are not admitted to a unit randomly and in outbreaks associated with surgery, patients at risk may not undergo surgery at night or on weekends.

If one is concerned about the distribution of some factor among the case-patients, such as admission to one of several ICUs or an SSI that affects patients who have undergone a variety of surgical procedures, one may wish to select controls using the proportional or stratified method. The more factors one is concerned about, the more difficult and tedious it will be to match these factors. To identify a match, one needs to review the characteristics in the control-patients' medical records; this process requires review and discarding of large numbers of controls until the desired factors are identified. In contrast, using the stratified or proportional method, controls are placed into categories based on the variables of concern (e.g., type of surgery, admission into ICU), and then the proportion of controls desired is randomly selected from each category. For example, if in an SSI outbreak 10% of case-patients had cardiac surgery, 20% had neurosurgery, 30% had orthopedic surgery, and 40% had general surgery, the controls would be distributed into categories by the type of surgery they had undergone. Then they would be selected from each surgical category in the same proportion as the case-patients.

Once the case- and control-patients are selected, one can compare the exposures of interest. These exposures should be compared statistically using one of the available statistical software packages. If only one risk factor is statistically significantly different between case- and control-patients, no further epidemiologic analytic studies are necessary. If there are significant differences in 2–3 risk factors, further analysis using stratification may demonstrate which of these factors is the most important. In addition, if case- and control-patients differ significantly in ≥2 factors, multivariate analyses can be performed to identify the independent importance of these factors. For many HAI outbreak investigations, numerous risk factors are identified as significant. Because some of these variables are confounding factors, they are highly correlated with the causative risk factors. Multivariate techniques can be used to try to identify the independent importance of the factors found to have significance in univariate analyses. Multivariate techniques require the close cooperation of the epidemiologist and the statistician for appropriate conduct and interpretation.

Observational Studies

Often outbreaks associated with healthcare facilities are the result of failure by HCWs to fully comply with current recommendations or policies. Therefore, IC personnel should observe HCWs performing the procedures in question to document the adequacy of their understanding and compliance with IC recommendations. Observational studies can help generate hypotheses about the cause of the outbreak, or they can confirm the findings of the epidemiologic studies. For instance, if the comparative analyses have linked transmission of the etiologic agent to a particular product and HCW, observation of this person preparing or manipulating the product may identify how the product was contaminated.

IC personnel should review all written policies associated with the practices in question, interview supervisory staff, and identify any changes in the procedures in question before, during, and after the outbreak. IC personnel should observe the implicated procedures and/or HCWs and directly question the personnel who are performing the implicated procedures. It may be useful to observe HCWs on all shifts and to distribute a questionnaire asking the HCWs about their particular practices. For instance, in questionnaires distributed to them, HCWs often claim to perform hand hygiene before and between contacts with patients, but observational studies usually document that such hand hygiene occurs ~30%–40% of the time [6].

Culture Surveys

Cultures of the environment and/or HCWs should not be performed before the comparative epidemiologic studies are completed. Cultures of the environment may identify the causative agent, but this may represent secondary contamination rather than the source of contamination. Many common HAI pathogens, such as gram-negative organisms and fungi, can be isolated from the environment even in the absence of an outbreak. Similarly, a positive culture from an HCW can represent the source of the outbreak but also may represent secondary contamination from the environment, colonized or infected patients, transient carriage, or carriage of the organism independent of the outbreak. Because identification of an HCW carrier may require removal from work, conclusive epidemiologic data identifying a person as associated with transmission in the outbreak is needed to warrant such action. Random culture surveys of products, the environment, or personnel are costly both in materials and time.

Once the comparative epidemiologic studies have been completed, cultures should be obtained from the epidemiologically implicated sources (products or personnel). At the same time, several other cultures should be carried out on HCWs or products representing controls to avoid the risk of identifying the product or HCW before the investigation is completed and appropriate recommendations can be made. The performance of cultures of only those products or HCWs who are epidemiologically implicated reduces the number of cultures to be obtained, the personnel resources needed to conduct the cultures (they should not be performed by the implicated HCW[s]), and the burden on the laboratory. Cultures of nonsterile areas (e.g., floors, sinks, walls) and other animate or inanimate objects that do not have plausible connections to the outbreak are a waste of valuable resources and may generate uninterpretable data.

If the epidemiologic data identify a source yet the cultures of the person or product do not disclose the causative agent, one should not abandon the hypothesis. The epidemiologic data should always supercede the laboratory data. When low-level contamination of a product occurs, it may require cultures of large numbers of the product to pinpoint the contamination. Furthermore, the cultures of the implicated HCW may give negative results if the colonized site is not cultured or if the HCW shows positive results only intermittently or has treated himself or herself and is no longer culture positive. IC personnel should never vindicate a source that has been identified by a well-designed epidemiologic study even in the absence of culture confirmation.

Because the appropriate method of culturing inanimate and animate objects varies, IC personnel should consult with the microbiologist before such culturing is initiated. For cultures of HCWs' hands, the broth hand-wash method is preferred [45]. For water or dialysate used in hemodialysis, the pour-plate or milepore filter method is preferred [46]. For cultures of the environment when low numbers of organisms are anticipated, the use of premoistened swabs and inoculation into nutrient broth may facilitate recovery of the organism. When investigating outbreaks associated with possible airborne transmission, the use of settle plates or air samplers may expedite recovery of the implicated pathogen [19,20,28,47–52].

Typing of the Outbreak Strain

When the outbreak strains are available from the case-patients and the environment or implicated HCW(s) or products, it is essential that they be saved for potential future studies. Although outbreaks can be clonal (caused by one strain) or nonclonal (caused by multiple strains of one species); typing the outbreak strains can be a vital addition to the epidemiologic study. A wide variety of nonmolecular and molecular typing methods are available for many of the pathogens associated with outbreaks in healthcare facilities (See Chapters 10 and 16) [34]. The finding of clonality among isolates increases the likelihood that the outbreak is caused by a contaminated product or colonized HCW, whereas the finding of a nonclonal outbreak increases the likelihood that the pathogen is being transmitted via HCW hands from one source (patient or environment) to another patient. For this reason, it may be useful to type some outbreak strains, particularly those that are common to the environment, water, or HCW. Such typing may influence the direction of the comparative studies.

Typing methods include biotyping, antimicrobial susceptibility testing, multilocus enzyme electrophoresis, serotyping, phage typing, and a variety of molecular methods, such as plasmid analysis, restriction endonuclease analysis, chromosomal analysis, ribotyping, restriction fragment length polymorphism, or pulsed-field gel electrophoresis. In general, the molecular methods—in particular, pulsed-field gel electrophoresis—have become the most useful for epidemiologic typing [34]. However, the field of molecular typing is evolving rapidly, and polymerase chain reaction–based pulsed-field gel electrophoresis typing and other methods are proving useful for organisms for which previous nonmolecular or molecular typing methods have been deemed inadequate.

Making Recommendations and Evaluating the Efficacy of the Recommendations

Once the epidemiologic and laboratory studies have been completed, one can assess the results and make appropriate recommendations to terminate the outbreak and prevent further transmission. Often these recommendations are based on existing guidelines. Several outbreak investigations have documented that often transmission stems from failure to fully implement IC guideline recommendations, not that the guideline recommendations are inadequate [50–52]. Occasionally, the outbreak investigation identifies a practice needing revision or a contaminated product that should be removed. More often, the investigation finds lapses in aseptic technique that require further HCW education. Thus, it is imperative that once the recommendations are made, follow-up studies be initiated to ensure that there is compliance with the recommendations and that transmission is terminated.

Furthermore, during the investigation, one has the opportunity to improve general IC measures throughout the hospital (even if the outbreak is taking place in only one unit) and to improve methods of documentation of information that would have made the investigation easier. For instance, if, during an investigation of BSIs in ICU patients, it is impossible to determine the dates of central venous catheter insertion and removal, the prospective collection of such data in a standardized manner by ICU staff should be included in the recommendations.

To ensure that the outbreak investigation is conducted efficiently and that hospital HCWs fully implement the recommendations, hospital administrative personnel should be actively involved in the investigation and follow-up. IC personnel should alert hospital administrative staff as soon as the outbreak is detected. IC personnel should update administrative staff during the course of the investigation and then review with them the investigation findings and recommendations. Follow-up meetings with administrative staff should review the adequacy of implementation of the recommendations and determine whether the outbreak has been terminated.

For complex outbreaks that involve a variety of services or are causing significant morbidity or mortality, a task force, which should include administrative staff, should be formed at the beginning of the investigation, and this group should be responsible for monitoring the adequacy of implementation of the recommendations and evaluation of their efficacy. The successful conclusion of any investigation of an endemic or epidemic problem is the documentation through follow-up data that the endemic or epidemic problem has been controlled or terminated by the implemented control measures. Any successful investigation requires the close cooperation of a wide variety of people from many hospital departments. It becomes the responsibility of these people to translate the recommendations into action.

If the investigation is conducted in close collaboration with staff members of other departments, they will in turn help with the implementation and monitoring of the recommendations in their departments. To educate and inform those associated with the outbreak or the investigation, it is important that a report be written at the conclusion of the investigation summarizing the methods used, the results, and the recommendations. This report should be circulated to all of those assisting with the study, all service chiefs or heads of departments where the outbreak took place, and the administrative, risk management, and hospital public relations departments. In this way, all necessary personnel are informed about the findings and recommendations of the investigative team. Feedback of follow-up data to these departmental staff members will help them improve conditions and practices in their departments. Investigations of endemic or epidemic problems should be viewed as collaborative efforts between the IC personnel and other departments. With the cooperation of other departments, a successful outcome is enhanced; without it, success is unlikely.

REFERENCES

1. Haley RW, Culver DH, White JW, et al. The nation-wide nosocomial infection rate: a new need for vital statistics. *Am J Epidemiol* 1985;121:159–167.
2. Haley RW, Culver DH, White JW, et al. The efficacy of infection surveillance and control programs in preventing nosocomial infections in U.S. hospitals. *Am J Epidemiol* 1985;121:182–205.
3. Haley RW, White JW, Culver DH, Hughes JM. The financial incentive for hospitals to prevent nosocomial infections under the prospective payment system: an empirical determination from a nationally representative sample. *JAMA* 1987;257:1611–1614.
4. Jarvis WR, Martone WJ. Predominant pathogens in hospital infections. *J Antimicrob Chemother* 1991;28:15–19.
5. Centers for Disease Control and Prevention. National Nosocomial Infections Surveillance (NNIS) system report, data summary from January 1992 through June 2004, issued October 2004. *Am.J Infect Control* 2004;32:470–485.
6. Jarvis WR. Handwashing: the Semmelweis lesson forgotten? *Lancet* 1994;344:1311–1312.
7. Garner J, Jarvis WR, Emori G, et al. The Centers for Disease Control definitions for nosocomial infections, 1988. *Am J Infect Control* 1988;16:128–140.
8. National Nosocomial Infections Surveillance (NNIS) System. Nosocomial infection rates for interhospital comparison: limitations and possible solutions. *Infect Control Hosp Epidemiol* 1991;12:609–621.
9. Emori TG, Culver DH, Horan TC, et al. National Nosocomial Infections Surveillance System (NNIS): description of methodology and surveillance components. *Am J Infect Control* 1991;19:19–36.
10. Jarvis WR, et al., and the National Nosocomial Infections Surveillance System. Nosocomial infection rates in adult and pediatric intensive care units. *Am J Med* 1991;91:185S–191S.
11. Richards MJ, Edwards JR, Culver DH, Gaynes RP. Nosocomial infections in medical intensive care units in the United States. National Nosocomial Infections Surveillance system. *Crit Care Med* 1999;27:887–892.
12. Richards MJ, Edwards JR, Culver DH, Gaynes RP. Nosocomial infections in pediatric intensive care units in the United States. National Nosocomial Infections Surveillance system. *Pediatrics* 1999;103:e39.
13. Gaynes RP, et al., and the National Nosocomial Infections Surveillance System. Comparison of rates of nosocomial infections in neonatal intensive care units in the United States. *Am J Med* 1991;91:192S–197S.
14. Culver DH, et al., and the National Nosocomial Infections Surveillance System. Surgical wound infection rates by wound class, operative procedure, and patient risk index. *Am J Med* 1991;91:152S–157S.
15. Haley RW, Culver DH, Morgan WM, et al. Identifying patients at high risk of surgical wound infection: a simple multivariate index of patient susceptibility and wound contamination. *Am J Epidemiol* 1985;121:206–215.
16. Jarvis WR, and the Epidemiology Branch, Hospital Infections Program. Nosocomial outbreaks: the Centers for Disease Control's Hospital Infections Program experience, 1980–1990. *Am J Med* 1991;9(3B):101S–106S.
17. Jarvis WR. Hospital Infections Program, Centers for Disease Control and Prevention On-site Outbreak Investigations, 1990–1999. *Semin Infect Control* 2001;1.74–84.
18. Richet HM, Craven PC, Brown JM, et al. *Rhodococcus (Gordona) bronchialis* sternal wound infections following coronary artery bypass graft surgery. *N Engl J Med* 1991;324:104–109.
19. Edlin BR, Tokars JI, Grieco MH, et al. An outbreak of multidrug-resistant tuberculosis among hospitalized patients with the acquired immunodeficiency syndrome: epidemiologic studies and restriction fragment length polymorphism analysis. *N Engl J Med* 1992;326:1514–1522.
20. Jarvis WR. Nosocomial transmission of multidrug-resistant *Mycobacterium tuberculosis*. *Res Microbiol* 1993;144:117–122.
21. Shay DK, Maloney SM, Montecalvo M, et al. Epidemiology and mortality of vancomycin-resistant enterococcal bloodstream infections. *J Infect Dis* 1995;172:993–1000.
22. Villarino ME, Stevens L, Schable B, et al. Epidemic *Xanthomonas maltophilia* infections and colonization in an intensive care unit. *Infect Control Hosp Epidemiol* 1992;13:201–206.
23. Tablan OC, Martone WJ, Doershuk CF, et al. Colonization of the respiratory tract with *Pseudomonas cepacia* of patients with cystic fibrosis: risk factors and outcomes. *Chest* 1987;91:527–533.
24. Mangram A, Jarvis WJ. Nosocomial *Burkholderia cepacia* outbreaks and pseudo-outbreaks. *Infect Control Hosp Epidemiol* 1996;17:718–720.
25. Welbel SF, McNeil M., Pramanik A, et at. Nosocomial *Malassezia pachydermitis* bloodstream infections in a neonatal intensive care unit. *Pediatr Infect Dis J* 1994;13:104–109
26. Chang H, Miller H, Watkins N, et al. An epidemic of *Malassezia pachydermitis* in intensive care nursery associated with health care workers' dogs. *N Eng J of Med* 1998;33:706–711.
27. Richet HM, McNeil MM, Davis BJ, et at. *Aspergillus fumigates* sternal wound infection in patients undergoing open-heart surgery. *Am J Epidemiol* 1992;135:48–58.
28. Buffington J, Reporter R, McNeil MM, et at. An outbreak of invasive aspergillosis among hematology and bone marrow transplant patients at a Los Angeles hospital. *J Pediatr Infect Dis* 1994;13:386–393.
29. Beck-Sague CM, Jarvis WR, Brook JP, et al. Epidemic bacteremia due to *Acinetobacter baumanni* in five intensive care units. *Am J Epidemiol* 1990;132:723–733.
30. Archibald LK, Manning ML, Bell LM, et al. Patient density, nurse-to-patient ratio and nosocomial infection risk in a pediatric cardiac intensive care unit. *Pediatr Infect Dis J* 1997;16:1045–1048.
31. Breiman RD, Fields BS, Sanden G, et al. An outbreak of Legionnaire's disease associated with shower use: possible role of amoebae. *JAMA* 1990;263:924.
32. Mastro TD, Farley TA, Elliot JA, et al. An outbreak of surgical wound infections due to group A *Streptococcus* carried on the scalp. *N Engl J Med* 1990;323:968–972.

33. Cookson ST, Jarvis WR. Nosocomial gastrointestinal infections. In: RP Wenzel, ed. *Prevention and control of nosocomial infections*, 3rd ed. Baltimore, MD: Williams and Wilkins, 1997.

34. Jarvis WR. Usefulness of molecular epidemiology for outbreak investigations. *Infect Control Hosp Epidemiol* 1994;15:500–503.

35. Pertowski CA, Baron RC, Lasker B, et al. Nosocomial outbreak of *Candida albicans* sternal wound infection following cardiac surgery. *J Infect Dis* 1995;172:817–823.

36. Jarvis WR, Cookson ST, Robles B. Prevention of nosocomial bloodstream infections: a national and international priority. *Infect Control Hosp Epidemiol* 1996;17:272–275.

37. Tablan OC, Anderson LJ, Besser R, et al. Guidelines for prevention of healthcare-associated pneumonia, 2003. *MMWR* 2004;53(RR-3):1–36.

38. Wong ED, Hooton TM. *Guideline for prevention of catheter-associated urinary tract infections*. Atlanta: Centers for Disease Control and Prevention, 1981.

39. Berkelman RL, Martin D, Graham DR, et al. Streptococcal wound infections caused by a vaginal carrier. *JAMA* 1982;247(19):2680–2682.

40. Mangram AJ, Horan TC, Pearson ML, et al., and the Hospital Infection Control Practices Advisory Committee. Guideline for prevention of surgical site infection, 1999. *Infect Control Hosp Epi* 1999;20:247–278.

41. Safranek TJ, Jarvis WR, Carson LA, et al. *Mycobacteria chelonae* wound infections after plastic surgery employing contaminated gentian violet skin marking solution. *N Engl J Med* 1987;317:197–201.

42. Lowry PW, Blankenship RJ, Gridley W, et al. A cluster of legionella sternal-wound infections due to postoperative topical exposure to contaminated tap water. *N Engl J Med* 1991;324:109.

43. Nakashima AK, Allen JR, Martone WJ, et al. Epidemic bullous impetigo in a nursery due to a nasal carrier of *Staphylococcus aureus*: role of epidemiology and control measures. *Infect Control* 1984;5(7):326–331.

44. Haley RW, Culver DH, Morgan WM, et al. Increased recognition of infectious diseases in U.S. hospitals through increased use of diagnostic tests, 1970–76. *Am J Epidemiol* 1985;121(2):168–181.

45. Petersen NJ, Collins DE, Marshall JH. A microbiological assay technique for hands. *Health Lab Sci* 1973;10:18–22.

46. Franson MAH, ed. *Standard methods for examination of water and wastewater*. 16th ed. Washington, D.C.: American Public Health Association, 1985.

47. Beck-Sague CM, Dooley SW, Hutton MD, et al. Outbreak of multidrug-resistant tuberculosis among persons with HIV infection in an urban hospital: transmission to staff and patients and control measures. *Am J Med* 1992;268:1280–1286.

48. Edlin BR, Tokars JI, Grieco MH, et al. An outbreak of multidrug-resistant tuberculosis among hospitalized patients with the acquired immunodeficiency syndrome: epidemiologic studies and restriction fragment length polymorphism analysis. *N Engl J Med* 1992;326:1514–1522.

49. Pearson ML, Jereb JA, Frieden TR, et at. Nosocomial transmission of multidrug-resistant *Mycobacterium tuberculosis*: a risk to hospitalized patients and health-care workers. *Ann Intern Med* 1992;117:191–196.

50. Maloney SM, Pearson M, Gordon M, et al. Efficacy of control measures in preventing transmission of multidrug-resistant tuberculosis to patients and healthcare workers. *Ann Intern Med* 1995;122:90–95.

51. Wenger P, Otten J, Breeden A, Orfas D, et al. Control of nosocomial transmission of multidrug-resistant *Mycobacterium tuberculosis* among healthcare workers and HIV-infected patients. *Lancet* 1995;345:235–240.

52. Stroud LA, Tokars JI, Grieco MH, et al. Evaluation of infection control measures in preventing the nosocomial transmission of multidrug-resistant *Mycobacterium tuberculosis* in a New York City hospital. *Infect Control Hosp Epidemiol* 1995;16:141–147.

Epidemiological Methods for Investigating Infections in the Healthcare Setting

8

Ebbing Lautenbach

INTRODUCTION

A sound understanding of the principles and approaches of epidemiology is critical to the study of infectious diseases in the healthcare setting. The urgency of comprehending and applying epidemiological principles is supported by the fact that the incidence and impact of healthcare-acquired infections (HAIs) and antimicrobial resistance have increased markedly since the last edition of this textbook. In addition, the applicability of techniques traditionally reserved for healthcare epidemiology have been recognized as uniquely suited to other emerging issues (e.g., patient safety, bioterrorism, drug use management, quality assessment, technology assessment, product evaluation, and risk management.) [1,2].

The value of epidemiological methods in the study of HAIs has been recognized for some time [3–6]. The ability to accurately quantify new patterns of HAIs, design and carry out rigorous studies to identify factors associated with disease, and devise and evaluate interventions to address emerging issues are vital to the study of HAIs. Indeed, during the past 5 years, there has been a renewed interest and vitality in efforts to explore previously unstudied aspects of epidemiological methods in the study of HAIs and antimicrobial resistance [7–10].

There are two primary goals of this chapter. The first goal is to review basic epidemiologic principles relevant to the study of HAIs including (1) measures of disease frequency, (2) study design, (3) measures of effect, (4) bias, and (5) confounding. The second goal is to discuss in more detail specific current epidemiologic issues in the study of HAIs including (1) quasi-experimental study design, (2) case-crossover study design, (3) control group selection in studies of antimicrobial resistance, (4) definitions of antibiotic exposure, and (5) assessment of mortality as an outcome of infection. The overriding focus of this chapter is discussion of epidemiologic methods applicable to the study of HAIs and antimicrobial resistance. The reader is also directed to numerous published textbooks solely dedicated to general epidemiology, infectious diseases epidemiology, and statistical analysis [11–17].

MEASURES OF DISEASE FREQUENCY

Accurately quantifying the frequency of disease is important for measuring the scope of the problem (i.e., how many people are affected by the disease) and for allowing comparison between different groups (i.e., those with and without a particular risk factor of interest). The most commonly used measures of disease frequency are prevalence and incidence.

Prevalence

Prevalence is defined as the proportion of people with disease at a given point in time (e.g., the proportion of hospitalized patients who have a HAI). This also may be referred to as the "point prevalence."

$$\text{Prevalence} = \frac{\text{Number of diseased individuals}}{\text{Total population}}$$

Prevalence, which is a proportion and has no units, depends on both the incidence (i.e., the number of new episodes that develop) and the disease duration (i.e., how long a diseases lasts once it has developed). The greater the incidence and duration of disease, the higher the resultant prevalence. Prevalence is useful for measuring the burden of disease (i.e., the overall proportion of persons affected by the disease). Because all populations are dynamic, the prevalence may vary depending on when it is measured. If a dynamic population is at steady state (i.e., cases leaving = cases entering), the prevalence will be constant over time.

Incidence

Incidence is defined as the number of new episodes of diseases occurring in a specified period of time. Incidence may be described in several ways. Cumulative incidence is defined as the number of new episodes of disease in a particular time period divided by the total number of disease-free individuals at risk of the disease at the beginning of the time period (e.g., the proportion of patients who develop an HAI during hospitalization).

$$\text{Cumulative incidence} = \frac{\begin{array}{c}\text{Number of new cases}\\ \text{of disease between } t_0 \text{ and } t_1\end{array}}{\begin{array}{c}\text{total disease free individuals}\\ \text{at risk of disease at } t_0\end{array}}$$

The cumulative incidence, like prevalence, is a proportion and thus has no units. To calculate the cumulative incidence, one must have complete follow-up on all individuals so as that their final disposition with regard to the outcome is known. Although this measure describes the total proportion of new episodes occurring in a time period, it does not describe when in the time period they occurred. For the cumulative incidence of HAIs, the period implied is the hospitalization until a first event or until discharge. However, patients do not stay in hospital and remain at risk for exactly the same period of time. Thus, comparing the cumulative incidence of infection among patient groups with differing lengths of stay may be very misleading.

The incidence rate (or incidence density) is defined as the number of new episodes of disease in a specified quantity of person-time of observation among individuals at risk (e.g., the number of HAIs per 1000 hospital days).

$$\text{Incidence} = \frac{\begin{array}{c}\text{Number of new episodes of disease}\\ \text{during given period}\end{array}}{\begin{array}{c}\text{Total person-time of observation among}\\ \text{individuals at risk}\end{array}}$$

The value of this measure can be seen when comparing infection rates in groups that differ in their time at risk (e.g., short-stay patients vs. long-stay patients). When the time at risk in one group is much longer than in another, the incidence rate is the most convenient way to correct for time. This allows one to separate the effect of time (duration of exposure) from the effect of daily risk. Incidence rate usually is restricted to first events (e.g., the first episode of HAI). It is standard to consider only first events because second events are not statistically independent from first events in the same individuals.

Unlike cumulative incidence, the incidence rate does not assume complete follow-up of subjects. However, even when follow-up is complete (and thus cumulative incidence could be calculated), reporting the incidence rate may still be preferable. Cumulative incidence reports only the overall number of new episodes occurring during the period (regardless of whether they occur early or late in the time period). By comparison, the incidence rate, by incorporating the time at risk, accounts for potential difference in time to occurrence of the event.

The assumption in the incidence rate is that all time at risk is equal (e.g., the likelihood of developing a HAI in the first 3 days after hospital admission is the same as the likelihood of developing an infection during days 4 through 6 of hospitalization). If all time periods are not equivalent, the incidence rate may be misleading.

STUDY DESIGN

Various study designs may be chosen when seeking to address a clinical question. These study designs, in order of increasing methodological rigor, include case report, case series, ecologic study, cross-sectional study, case-control study, cohort study, and randomized controlled trial. Randomized controlled trials, case-control studies, and cohort studies are considered analytic studies while the other designs are considered descriptive studies.

Case Report/Case Series

A case report is the clinical description of a single patient (e.g., a single episode of a patient with a bloodstream infection due to fluoroquinolone-resistant *Escherichia coli* (FQREC)). A case series is a report of >1 patient with the disease of interest. In addition to serving as a clinical or therapeutic example, a case report/series can function to generate hypotheses that may then be tested in future analytic studies. The primary limitation of a case report/series is that it describes at most a few patients and may not be generalizable. In addition, because a case report/series does not include a comparison group, one cannot determine which characteristics in the description of the patient(s) are unique to the illness.

Ecologic Study

In an ecologic study, one compares geographic and/or time trends of an illness to trends in risk factors (i.e., a comparison of annual hospital-wide use of fluoroquinolones (FQs) with annual prevalence of FQREC). Ecologic studies often use aggregate data that are routinely collected for other purposes (e.g., antimicrobial susceptibility patterns from a hospital's clinical microbiology laboratory). As a result, one advantage of the ecologic study is that it is often relatively quick and easy to do. Thus, such a study may provide early support for or against a hypothesis. However, one cannot distinguish between various hypotheses that might be consistent with the data. Perhaps most important, ecologic studies do not incorporate patient-level data. With such a study, one knows only that there is a correlation between annual hospital-wide use of FQs and yearly prevalence of FQREC, not that the actual patients infected with FQREC received FQs.

Cross-Sectional Study

A cross-sectional study assesses the status of subjects with regard to the risk factor and disease at the same point in time. A cross-sectional study to investigate FQREC might assess all patients currently hospitalized and whether they have an FQREC infection and whether they are receiving FQs. A cross-sectional study is relatively easy to carry out because all subjects are assessed at only one point in time. As such, this type of study may provide early evidence for or against a hypothesis. A major disadvantage of a cross-sectional study is that it does not capture the concept of elapsed time (i.e., it is not possible to determine whether the risk factor or the outcome came first). Furthermore, a cross-sectional study does not provide information about the transition between health states.

Case-Control Study

To compare the various types of analytic studies (e.g., case-control, cohort, experimental-randomized controlled trial), it is useful to consider the traditional 2 by 2 table (Figure 8-1). While all three study designs seek to investigate the association between a risk factor (or exposure) and an outcome of interest, they differ fundamentally in how patients are enrolled in the study. In a case-control study, patients are entered into the study based on the presence or absence of the outcome (or disease) of interest. These two groups (i.e., those with the disease and those without

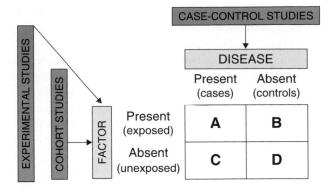

Figure 8-1 Study designs.
Adapted from: Lautenbach E. Epidemiological methods in infection control. In: Lautenbach E. Woeltje K, editors. *Practical Handbook for Healthcare Epidemiologists*. Thorofare, New Jersey: Slack Inc; 2004. (65).

the disease) are then compared to determine if they differ with regard to their presence of risk factors of interest.

A case-control study design, which is always retrospective, is particularly attractive when the outcome being studied is rare because one may enroll all patients with the outcome of interest. As such, this study design is much more efficient than the comparable cohort study in which a group of patients with and without an exposure of interest would need to be followed for a period of time to determine who develops the outcome of interest. Another advantage of the case-control study is that one may study a number of risk factors for the outcome of interest. One limitation of a case-control study is that only one outcome may be studied. Another disadvantage of this approach is that one cannot directly calculate the incidence or relative risk because the investigator fixes the number of cases and controls to be studied.

Of great importance in a case-control study is the process by which cases and controls are selected. Cases may be restricted to any group of diseased individuals. However, they must arise from a theoretical source population so that a diseased person not selected is presumed to have arisen from a different source population. For example, in studying risk factors for nosocomial FQREC infection, the theoretical source population could be considered to be the population of patients hospitalized at the institution. Thus, a patient at that institution with a clinical FQREC isolate would be included as a case. However, a patient with FQREC infection at a different hospital would not be included. Cases also must be chosen in a manner independent of their status with regard to an exposure of interest.

Careful attention also is required when selecting controls. Controls should be representative of the theoretical source population that gave rise to the cases. Thus, if a control were to have developed the disease of interest, the person would have been selected as a case. In the preceding example, controls may be randomly selected from among all non-FQREC infected patients in the hospital.

In investigating the possible association between prior FQ use and FQREC infection, these two groups (i.e., patients with FQREC infection and a random sample of all other hospitalized patients) could be compared to determine what proportion of patients in each group had experienced recent FQ exposure. Finally, like cases, controls must be chosen in a manner independent of their status with regard to an exposure of interest and should not be selected because they have characteristics similar to cases. The selection of controls in case-control studies of antimicrobial resistance will be discussed in more detail in a later section of this chapter.

Cohort Study

Unlike a case-control study, patients are entered into a cohort study based on the presence or absence of an exposure (or risk factor) of interest (Figure 8-1). These two groups (i.e., those with the exposure and those without the exposure) are then compared to determine whether they differ with regard to the development of the outcome of interest. A cohort study may be either prospective or retrospective, which depends on when it is conducted with regard to when the outcome of interest occurs. If patients are identified as exposed or unexposed and then followed forward in time to determine whether they develop the outcome, it is a prospective cohort study. If the study is conducted after all outcomes have already occurred, it is a retrospective cohort study. As an example, one might identify all patients who receive a FQ in the hospital (i.e., the exposed) and compare them to a randomly selected group of patients who do not receive a FQ (i.e., the unexposed). These groups could then be followed forward to determine what proportion of patients in each group develops the outcome of interest (i.e., FQREC infection).

An advantage of a cohort study is that one may study multiple outcomes from a single risk factor or exposure. Also, this study design allows the investigator to calculate an incidence and a relative risk in comparing the two groups. Potential limitations of a cohort study include substantial time and cost requirements due to often prolonged follow-up of subjects. In addition, if the outcome is rare, a large number of subjects will need to be followed to ensure adequate sample size. Finally, the longer the study duration, the more likely subjects will be lost to follow-up, potentially biasing the study results. Some of these limitations are mitigated in a retrospective cohort study because outcomes already have occurred and patients do not need to be followed prospectively.

Randomized Controlled Trial

The randomized controlled trial is very similar to the cohort study (Figure 8-1). However, in a cohort study, patients are enrolled already with or without the exposure of interest. In a randomized controlled trial, the investigator assigns the exposure randomly. This study design provides the most convincing demonstration of causality because patients in both groups should (provided randomization has worked appropriately) be equal with regard to all important variables except the one variable (exposure) manipulated by the investigator. While randomized controlled trials may provide the strongest support for or against an association of interest, they are costly studies, and there may be ethical issues that preclude their conduct. For example, in studying the association between FQ use and FQREC infection, one could not ethically assign patients to receive FQ if they did not require the drug. One alternative to the randomized controlled trial is the quasi-experimental study design, which will be discussed in a later section of this chapter.

MEASURES OF EFFECT

Relative Risk (RR)

The RR (also called the risk ratio) is the ratio of two probabilities: the probability of the outcome among the exposed divided by the probability of the outcome in the unexposed (Figure 8-2). An RR can be calculated from a cohort study or a randomized controlled trial because from these study designs, one can derive population-based rates or proportions. An RR of 1.0 is called the value of no effect, or the null value. An RR = 2.0 means that the exposed subjects were twice as likely to have the outcome of interest as the unexposed subjects. An RR = 0.5 means that the exposed were half as likely to experience the outcome as the unexposed, indicating a protective effect of the exposure.

Odds Ratio (OR)

In a case-control study, subjects are enrolled based on the outcome of interest. One then compares these two groups (i.e., those with the outcome and those without it) to determine what proportion of subjects in each group demonstrates a risk factor of interest. Unlike the cohort study, one cannot directly calculate an RR. What one can calculate in a case-control study is the OR, which is defined as the odds of exposure in subjects with the outcome divided by the odds of exposure in subjects without the outcome (Figure 8-2). An OR = 1.0 is called the value of no effect, or the null value.

As noted, one cannot calculate an RR from a case-control study because this type of study offers no insights into the absolute rates or proportions of disease among subjects. However, in situations in which the disease under study is rare (<10%), the OR derived from a case-control study closely approximates the RR that would have been derived from the comparable cohort study. Figure 8-2 shows how the case-control formula approaches the formula for RR when the rare outcome criterion is met.

		OUTCOME	
		Present (cases)	Absent (controls)
FACTOR	Present (exposed)	A	B
	Absent (not exposed)	C	D

Relative Risk

Risk of disease among exposed = A / (A+B)

Risk of disease among unexposed = C/ (C+D)

$$\text{Relative Risk} = \frac{A / (A+B)}{C / (C+D)}$$

Odds Ratio

Odds of exposure given disease = A / C

Odds of exposure given no disease = B / D

$$\text{Disease Odds Ratio} = \frac{A/C}{B/D} = \frac{AD}{BC}$$

Relationship between relative risk and odds ratio

When disease is rare, B>>A, and D>>>C

$$\text{Relative Risk} = \frac{A / (A+B)}{C / (C+D)} \sim \frac{AD}{BC} = \text{Odds ratio}$$

Figure 8-2 Relative risk and odds ratio.
(Adapted from Lautenbach E. Epidemiological methods in infection control. In: Lautenbach E, Woeltje K, editors. *Practical Handbook for Healthcare Epidemiologists*. Thorofare, New Jersey: Slack Inc; 2004.)

Measures of Strength of Association

p Value

The chi-square test for comparison of two binomial proportions is the most common method of measuring strength of association in a 2 by 2 table. This calculation is identical for all 2 by 2 tables whether or not data were derived from a cohort or case-control study. When the chi-square value has been calculated, the associated probability that the observed difference between binomial proportions could have arisen by chance alone can be looked up. A *p* value of <.05 indicates that an effect at least as extreme as that observed in the study is unlikely to have occurred by chance alone because there is truly no relationship between the exposure and the disease. Although this is the conventional interpretation, there is nothing particularly unique about the 0.05 cutoff for statistical significance. One limitation of the *p* value is that this value reflects both the magnitude of the difference between the groups and the sample size. Consequently, even a small difference between groups (if the sample size is large) may be statistically significant even if it is not clinically important. Conversely, a larger effect that would be clinically important may not be statistically significant if the sample size is small.

95% Confidence Interval

Because of the limitations of the *p* value just noted, it is preferable to report the 95% confidence interval (CI) for a given RR or OR. The 95% CI provides a range within which the true magnitude of the effect (i.e., the RR or the OR) lies with a certain degree of assurance. Observing whether the 95% CI crosses 1.0 (i.e., the value of null effect) provides the same information as the *p* value. If the 95% CI crosses 1.0, the *p* value will almost never be <0.05. The impact of the sample size can be ascertained from the width of the confidence interval. The narrower the confidence interval, the less variability was present in the estimate of the effect, reflecting a larger sample size. The wider the confidence interval, the smaller the sample size. When interpreting results that are not statistically significant, the width of the confidence interval may be helpful. A narrow confidence interval implies that there is most likely no real effect whereas a wide interval suggests the data also are compatible with a true effect and that the sample size was simply inadequate.

BIAS

Bias is the systematic error in the collection or interpretation of data. Types of bias include information bias (i.e., distortion in the estimate of effect due to measurement error or misclassification of subjects on one or more variables) and selection bias (i.e., distortion in the estimate of effect resulting from the manner in which subjects are selected for the study). For example, a common type of information bias in case-control studies is recall bias. One may compare patients with a FQREC infection to a random sample of noninfected controls in an effort to identify risk factors for FQREC infection. If patients with a FQREC infection are aware of their diagnosis, they may be more likely to try to identify possible reasons for experiencing a resistant infection. If this group is more likely to remember recent antibiotic use than are controls, the association between recent antibiotic use and FQREC infection will be spuriously strengthened.

The potential for bias must be addressed when the study is designed because it cannot be corrected during the analysis of the study. Indeed, blinding in randomized controlled trials is a commonly used method to minimize the potential for bias in such studies. In addition to evaluating whether bias may exist, one also must consider the likely impact of the bias on the study results. Bias may be nondifferential (i.e., biasing toward the null hypothesis and making the two groups being compared look artificially similar) or differential (i.e., biasing away from the null hypothesis and making the two groups being compared look artificially dissimilar).

CONFOUNDING

Confounding occurs when the association observed between an exposure and outcome is due, in part, to the effect of some other variable. To be a confounder, a variable must be associated with both the exposure and outcome of interest but cannot be a result of the exposure. Confounding can result in an over- or underestimate of the effect of the exposure of interest. For example, in assessing the association between an FQREC infection and mortality, one must consider underlying severity of illness as a potential confounder. Patients with more severe illness are more likely to develop FQREC infection. In addition, more severe illness also is more likely to result in mortality. Thus, because it is associated with both the exposure and outcome of interest, severity of illness is a potential confounding variable. Unlike bias, a confounding variable may be controlled for in the study analysis. However, to do this, data regarding the presence or absence of the confounder must be collected during the study. Thus, it also is important to consider the potential for confounding variables in the design of the study.

SPECIAL ISSUES IN HEALTHCARE EPIDEMIOLOGY METHODS QUASI-EXPERIMENTAL STUDY DESIGN

In addition to the study designs reviewed previously, the quasi-experimental study is a design frequently employed in healthcare epidemiology investigations [18]. This design also is frequently referred to as a "before-after" or "pre-post intervention" study [19,20]. The goal of a quasi-experimental study is typically to evaluate an intervention without using randomization. The most basic type of quasi-experimental study involves the collection of baseline data, the implementation of an intervention, and the collection of the same data following the intervention. For example, the baseline prevalence of FQREC in a hospital would be calculated, an intervention to improve FQ use would then be instituted, and the prevalence of FQREC again would be measured after a prespecified time period. Many different variations of quasi-experimental studies exist and include (1) institution of multiple pretests (i.e., collection of baseline data on more than one occasion), (2) repeated interventions (i.e., instituting and removing the intervention sequentially), and (3) inclusion of a control group (i.e., a group on which baseline and subsequent data are collected but on which no intervention is implemented) (Table 8-1) [18,21].

Although often employed in evaluations of HAI interventions, critical evaluation of the advantages and disadvantages of quasi-experimental studies has only recently been conducted [18,21]. Indeed, a recent systematic review of four infectious diseases journals found that during a two-year period, 73 articles focusing on infection control and/or antimicrobial resistance used a quasi-experimental study design [18]. Of these articles, only 12 (16%) used a control group, 3 (4%) provided justification for the use of the quasi-experimental study design, and 17 (23%) mentioned at least one of the potential limitations of such a design [18]. More attention has recently been focused on increasing the quality of quasi-experimental study design and conduct to enhance the validity of conclusions

TABLE 8-1
HIERARCHY OF QUASI-EXPERIMENTAL STUDY DESIGNS

A. QUASI-EXPERIMENTAL DESIGNS WITHOUT CONTROL GROUPS

1. One-group pretest-posttest design	O1 X O2
2. One-group pretest-posttest design using a double pretest	O1 O2 X O3
3. One-group pretest-posttest design using a nonequivalent dependent variable	(O1a, O1b) X (O2a, O2b)
4. Removed-treatment design	O1 X O2 O3 remove X O4
5. Repeated-treatment design	O1 X O2 removeX O3 X O4

B. QUASI-EXPERIMENTAL DESIGNS THAT USE CONTROL GROUPS

0. Posttest-only design with nonequivalent groups	X O1 / O2
1. Untreated control group design with dependent pretest and posttest samples	O1a X O2a / O1b X O2b
2. Untreated control group design with dependent pretest and posttest samples and a double pretest	O1a O2a X O3a / O1b O2b O3b
3. Untreated control group design with dependent pretest and posttest samples and switching replications	O1a X O2a O3a / O1b O2b X O3b

*O = Observational Measurement, X = Intervention under study, and time moves from left to right

In general, studies in category B are of higher study design quality than those in category A. Also, as one moves down within each category, the studies become of higher quality e.g. study 5 in category A is of higher study design quality than study 4 etc.

(Adapted from: Harris AD, Lautenbach E, and Perencevich E. 2005. A systematic review of quasi-experimental study designs in the fields of infection control and antibiotic resistance. *Clin Infect Dis* 41:77–82 (18))

drawn regarding effectiveness of interventions in the areas of infection control and antibiotic resistance [18].

The quasi-experimental study design offers several advantages. The study designs available when one wishes to study the impact of an intervention are limited. In general, a well-designed and adequately powered randomized controlled trial provides the strongest evidence for or against the efficacy of an intervention. However, there are several reasons why a randomized controlled trial may not be feasible in the study of infection control interventions. Randomizing individual patients to an intervention of infection control interventions often is not a reasonable approach given the person-to-person transmission of resistant pathogens. One might consider randomizing specific units or floors within one institution to receive the intervention. However, these units are not self-contained, and patients and healthcare workers frequently move from unit to unit. Thus, any effect on reduced transmission/acquisition of new resistant infections noted in the intervention units is also likely to result in some reduction in resistant infections in nonintervention areas (i.e., contamination). This would bias the results toward the null hypothesis (i.e., no effect of the intervention). Similarly, if only certain areas in an institution were randomized to the intervention, enhanced attention to infection control that might be part of an intervention would likely be evident to nonintervention floors, given that many healthcare workers (e.g., physicians, nurses) work in multiple areas. This might result in enhanced infection control practices on nonintervention floors, which would bias the results toward the null. In such a situation, a well-designed quasi-experimental study offers a compelling alternative approach. In addition, this study design is frequently used when it is not ethical to conduct a randomized controlled trial. In addition, when an intervention must be instituted rapidly in response to an emerging issue (e.g., an outbreak), the first priority is to address and resolve the issue. In this instance, it would be unethical to randomize an intervention across patient groups.

Several primary limitations exist in quasi-experimental studies including regression to the mean, uncontrolled confounding, and maturation effects. Implementation of an intervention is often triggered in response to a rise in the rate above the norm [22]. The principle of regression to the mean predicts that these elevated rates will tend to decline even without intervention. This may serve to bias the results of a quasi-experimental study because it may be falsely concluded that an effect is due to the intervention [19,20]. Several approaches may be employed to address this potential limitation. First, incorporating a prolonged baseline period before the intervention permits an evaluation of the natural fluctuation in rates of the outcome over time and permits a more comprehensive assessment of possible regression to the mean. Second, changes in the outcome of interest may be measured at a

control site (e.g., another institution) during the same time period. Finally, the use of segmented regression analysis may assist in addressing possible regression to the mean in that the immediate change in prevalence coincident with the intervention will be assessed as will the change in slope over time [23–25].

Uncontrolled confounding, another potential limitation in quasi-experimental studies, is most likely to occur when variables other than the intervention change over time or differ when comparing the pre- and postintervention periods [19,20]. This limitation can be addressed by measuring known confounders (e.g., hospital census, number of admissions) and controlling for them in analyses. However, not all confounders are known or easily measured (e.g., quality of medical and nursing care). To address this, one may assess a nonequivalent dependent variable to evaluate the possibility that factors other than the intervention influenced the outcome [18,21]. A nonequivalent dependent variable should have similar potential causal and confounding variables as the primary dependent variable except for the effect of the intervention. For example, in assessing the impact of an intervention to limit FQ use on FQREC prevalence, one might consider incidence of catheter-associated bloodstream infections as a nonequivalent dependent variable. While FQREC prevalence and catheter-associated bloodstream infection might both be affected by such factors as patient census, it is unlikely that FQ use specifically would affect the incidence of catheter-associated bloodstream infections.

Maturation effects are related to natural changes that patients experience with the passage of time [19,20]. In addition, cyclical trends (e.g., seasonal variation) may be a threat to the validity of attributing an observed outcome to an intervention. This potential limitation may be addressed through approaches noted earlier including the assessment of a prolonged baseline period, use of control sites, implementation of interventions at different time periods at different sites, and assessment of a nonequivalent dependent variable.

Case-Crossover Study Design

The case-crossover study design also has been increasingly recognized as a useful approach when addressing issues in healthcare epidemiology [26]. In this design, each case serves as her or his own control (i.e., self-matching). For each subject, the exposure status is measured in the "case" time period occurring shortly before the outcome. Then this is compared to the exposure status in one or more earlier "control" time periods. Then, RR are estimated by comparing the frequency of exposure immediately before the case event (the case period) vs. the earlier period (the control period).

This study design offers several advantages. Because cases serve as their own controls, the design adjusts for many of the differences between cases and controls that might confound a traditional case-control study. This study design also is less susceptible to confounding by indication [27]. All retrospective studies relying on patient recollection of exposure data may suffer from recall bias. Another potential advantage of the case-crossover study is that the same person is recalling data from both the control and case time periods since because person serves as his or her own control [27,28].

Several disadvantages of the case-crossover design also exist. An underlying assumption in this design is that confounders are not changing over time in a systematic way; otherwise, this may be a source of confounding [27]. In addition, bias could result from temporal changes in the exposure of interest or through the selection of the control time window [27].

The case-crossover study design is ideally suited to studying brief exposures with immediate and transient effect and acute outcomes with abrupt onset (e.g., motor vehicle accidents, injury) [29,30]. Also, exposures must vary over time within an individual; otherwise, there would be no ability to compare exposed and unexposed periods within the individual. However, it has been suggested that with lengthened exposure assessment windows for both the case and control time periods, case-crossover methods also may be useful for studying exposures with prolonged effects and outcomes with insidious onsets [31–33]. This may be particularly relevant for studying the adverse effects of prolonged drug exposures (e.g., antimicrobials) given the concerns regarding control selection bias and confounding inherent in traditional case-control studies of adverse effects [31].

With regard to healthcare epidemiology specifically, this design has been used successfully to study sharps injuries in healthcare workers [28]. In this study, the case-crossover design was well suited to assess the relationship between brief, transient exposures, such as fatigue or rushing, and the acute event of a sharps injury. Another recent study used a case-crossover approach to study the association between wet, humid weather and the incidence of legionellosis [34]. This approach was useful in controlling for seasonal factors that might confound the relationship between weather and disease occurrence to facilitate the identification of acute weather patterns associated with legionella infection [34].

Control Group Selection in Studies of Antimicrobial Resistance

Many studies have focused on identifying risk factors for antimicrobial resistance. The majority of these studies have been case-control–designed studies. As noted previously, how controls are selected in case-control studies is critical in ensuring the validity of study results. Recent work has highlighted this issue of control group selection specifically for studies of antibiotic resistance [7,35–38].

Historically, two types of control groups have been used in studies of antimicrobial resistant organisms [7]. The first

type of control group is selected from patients who do not harbor the resistant pathogen. The second type of control group is selected from among subjects with a susceptible form of the infection. For example, in a study of risk factors for infection with FQREC in hospitalized patients, the first type of control group would be selected from among the general hospitalized patient population while the second control group would be selected from among those patients with a FQ-susceptible *E. coli* (FQSEC) infection. The choice of control group should be based primarily on the clinical question being asked. While use of this second type of control group has historically been a more common approach, it has recently been demonstrated that the use of this type of control group (e.g., patients infected with the susceptible form of the organism) may result in an overestimate of the association between antimicrobial exposure and resistant infection [37,38]. Using the example of FQREC, the explanation for this finding has been postulated as follows: If the controls are represented by patients with FQSEC infections, it is very unlikely that these patients would have recently received FQs (i.e., the risk factor of interest) because exposure to FQs may have eradicated FQSEC colonization. Thus, the association between FQ use and FQREC would be overestimated [39]. A limitation of using the first type of approach (i.e., using patients without infection as controls), is that, in addition to identifying risk factors for resistance, this approach also identifies risk factors for infection with that organism in general (regardless of whether the infection is resistant or susceptible). Thus, there is no way to distinguish the degree to which a risk factor is associated with the resistance phenotype vs. associate with infecting organism in general [36].

One concern with using the second type of control group (i.e., selecting from all hospitalized patients) is the potential for misclassification bias. Specifically, subjects selected as controls who have never had a clinical culture obtained may in fact harbor unrecognized colonization with the resistant organism under study [35]. Because it is probable that patients colonized with the resistant organism would likely have had greater prior antimicrobial exposure than subjects not colonized, this misclassification would likely result in a bias toward the null (i.e., the cases and controls would appear falsely similar with regard to prior antimicrobial use). Another concern with using the second type of control group and identifying patients who have never had a clinical culture as controls is that differences between cases and controls may reflect the fact that clinical cultures were performed for case-patients but not for controls. Because procurement of cultures is not a random process but is based on clinical characteristics, it is possible that the severity of illness or antibiotic exposure may be greater among cases regardless of the presence of antibiotic-resistant infection [7]. One potential approach would be to limit eligible controls to those patients for whom at least one clinical culture has been performed and does not reveal the resistant organism of interest. Such a negative culture would suggest that the patient is likely not colonized with the resistant organism. However, recent work has demonstrated that using clinical cultures to identify eligible controls leads to the selection of a control group with a higher co-morbidity score and greater exposure to antibiotics compared with a control group for which clinical cultures were not performed [35].

One proposed approach to addressing the difficulties in control group selection in studies of antimicrobial resistance is the case-case-control study design [36,40–42]. In this design, two case-control studies effectively are performed. In the first study, cases are defined as those patients harboring the resistant organism while controls are those patients without the pathogen of interest. In the second study, cases are instead defined as those patients harboring the susceptible bacteria while controls, similar to those in the first approach, are those patients without the pathogen of interest [36]. These two separate studies are then carried out with risk factors from the two studies compared qualitatively. This approach allows for the comparison of risk factors identified from the two studies to indicate the relative contribution of the resistant infection over and above simply having the susceptible infection. A potential limitation in this approach is the difficulty in matching for potential confounders because of the use of only one control group [36]. Because there are two different case groups, case variables (e.g., duration of hospitalization, patient location) cannot be used for matching. In addition, the qualitative comparison of results from the two studies in this design leaves open the question as to how much of a difference in results is meaningful.

Definitions of Antibiotic Exposure

Many studies have sought to uncover risk factors for infection or colonization with resistant organisms [10,43]. Elucidating such risk factors is essential to inform interventions designed to curb further emergence of resistance. Past studies have particularly focused on antimicrobial use as a risk factor because it can be modified in the clinical setting [44,45]. However, the approaches used to define prior antibiotic exposure vary considerably across studies [7]. More important, only recently have attempts been made to identify the impact of differences in these approaches on study conclusions.

A recent study investigated methods used in past studies to describe the extent of prior antibiotic use (e.g., exposure yes/no vs. duration of exposure) and the impact of using different methods on study conclusions [46]. A systematic review of all studies investigating risk factors for extended-spectrum β-lactamase-producing E. coli and Klebsiella species (ESBL-EK) was conducted. Among the 25 included studies, prior antibiotic use was defined as a categorical variable in 18 studies, four studies defined prior antibiotic exposure as a continuous variable, and

three studies included both a categorical and a continuous variable to describe prior antibiotic exposure. Only one paper provided an explicit justification for its choice of variable to describe prior antibiotic exposure. The authors then re-analyzed a dataset from a prior ESBL-EK risk factor study [47], developing two separate multivariable models, one in which prior antibiotic use was described as a categorical variable (e.g., exposure yes/no) and one in which antibiotic use was described as a continuous variable (e.g., antibiotic days). Results of the two multivariable models using different methodological approaches differed substantially. Specifically, third-generation cephalosporin use was a risk factor for ESBL-EK when antibiotic use was described as a continuous variable but not when antibiotic use was described as a categorical variable [46].

These results suggest that describing prior antibiotic use as a categorical variable may mask significant associations between prior antibiotic use and resistance. For example, when the categorical variable is used, a subject who received only one day of an antibiotic would be considered identical to a subject who received 30 days of the same antibiotic. However, the risk of resistance is almost certainly not the same in these two individuals. Describing prior antibiotic use as a continuous variable allows for a more detailed characterization of the association between length of exposure and resistance. Recent work in the medical statistics literature emphasizes that the use of cutpoints can result in misinterpretation of data and that dichotomizing continuous variables reduces analytic power and makes it impossible to detect nonlinear relationships [48]. Indeed, the relationship between prior antimicrobial use and resistance may not be linear (i.e., the risk of resistance may not increase at a constant rate with increasing antimicrobial exposure). It is possible that the risk of resistance does not increase substantially until a certain amount of antimicrobial exposure has been attained (e.g., a "lower threshold"). A more precise characterization of this "lower threshold" would serve to better inform antibiotic use strategies.

Another issue regarding defining prior antimicrobial use centers around how specific agents are grouped. For example, antibiotic use could be classified by agent (e.g., cefazolin), class (e.g., cephalosporins), or spectrum of activity (e.g., gram-negative). Antibiotics are frequently grouped together in classes even though individual agents within the class may differ significantly [49], and such categorizations may mask important associations. It is unknown whether using different categorization schemes results in different conclusions regarding the association between antibiotic use and resistance. A recent study explored these issues, focusing on ESBL-EK as a model [50]. In a systematic review, 20 studies of risk factors for ESBL-EK that met inclusion criteria revealed tremendous variability in how prior antibiotic use was categorized. Categorization of prior antibiotic use was defined in terms of the specific agents, drug class, and often a combination of both. No study justified its choice of categorization method. There also was marked variability across studies with regard to which specific antibiotics or antibiotic classes were assessed. As expected, a majority of the studies ($n = 16$) specifically investigated the use of β-lactam antibiotics as risk factors for ESBL-EK. A variable number of studies also examined the association between the use of other antibiotics and ESBL-EK infection: aminoglycosides (9 studies), FQs (10 studies), and trimethoprim-sulfamethoxazole (7 studies). In a reanalysis of data from a prior study of risk factors for ESBL-EK [47], two separate multivariable models of risk factors for ESBL-EK were constructed, one with prior antibiotic use categorized by class and the other with prior antibiotic use categorized by spectrum of activity [50]. The results of these multivariable models differed substantially. Recent work has reported similar findings when focusing on risk factors for carbapenem-resistant *Pseudomonas aeruingosa* [51].

Another final important issue is how remote antibiotic use is assessed. A recent systematic review of studies investigating risk factors for ESBL-EK (noted earlier) [46] found that the time window during which antibiotic use was reviewed ranged from 48 hours to one year before the resistant infection. Furthermore, studies often did not explicitly state how far back in time prior antibiotic use was assessed [46].

Assessment of Mortality as an Outcome of Infection

Studies have increasingly focused on more clearly identifying the impact of HAIs and antimicrobial resistance [52]. These studies seek to identify risk factors for negative outcomes such as mortality, increased cost, and prolonged length of hospital stay. Increasing attention has recently been paid to potential methodological issues in assessing the relationship between an antimicrobial-resistant infection and mortality [7,52]. One important issue is the need to control for severity of illness. An oft-noted risk factor for resistant infection is greater underlying severity of illness. However, severity of illness also is a predictor of mortality. These characteristics suggest that severity of illness is likely to be an important confounder in the association between resistant infection and mortality (i.e., severity of illness is associated with both the exposure and outcome of interest). Several measures assess severity of illness including the Acute Physiology and Chronic Health Evaluation (APACHE) II score [53], and the McCabe-Jackson Score [54]. It is important to note that no severity of illness score has been developed or validated specifically to predict outcome in patients with infection. Regardless of the measure used, it is critical to assess the score and control for it in studies assessing the impact of resistant infection on mortality.

It is important to carefully consider when severity of illness is assessed [55]. The vast majority of studies

have assessed severity of illness at the time the infection is diagnosed (i.e., when the culture is initially drawn). However, the culture is generally obtained because of clinical suspicion of infection, suggesting that infection has already progressed at some time point before the culture was obtained. Because infection will typically also lead to a more severe illness, it is likely that severity of illness measured on the day the culture is obtained is more accurately an intermediate variable (e.g., infection leads to a more severe illness, which then ultimately leads to death). Controlling for an intermediate variable in this way usually causes an underestimate of the effect of the exposure of interest on the outcome [56]. To avoid this issue, it has been suggested that severity of illness be assessed at least 48 hours before the date the culture was obtained to provide a more reasonable assessment of the patient's underlying severity of illness rather than the severity of illness caused by the infection itself [55]. Interpreting the results of studies that control for severity of illness on the day the culture is obtained should be interpreted with caution because they may represent an underestimate of the true association between resistant infection and mortality [55].

Length of stay in the hospital before infection also is an important potential confounder in the association between resistance and mortality. Increased length of stay is a risk factor for resistant infection and is a risk factor for negative clinical outcomes [7]. A recent study assessing mortality associated with *E. coli* bacteremia first compared patients with *E. coli* bacteremia to unmatched controls without bacteremia and then compared them to patients without *E. coli* bacteremia but matched by prior length of hospital stay [57]. The authors found similar associations between *E. coli* bacteremia and mortality regardless of whether matching was used [57]. Although these results suggest little impact of controlling (through matching) for length of stay, the results should be interpreted with caution because the prior length of stay in the patient groups was relatively short (median 6 days) [7].

Similar to the preceding discussion, the choice of control group also is relevant in studies of outcomes [55]. Of note, because studies addressing outcomes related to infection are primarily cohort studies, "controls" in these studies are more appropriately referred to as the "unexposed" or "reference" group. As in case-control studies of antibiotic resistance, there are effectively two choices for a reference group. In the first, patients with a resistant infection (e.g., FQREC) are compared with patients with the susceptible counterpart (e.g., FQSEC). In the second type of control group, patients with a resistant infection (e.g., FQREC) are compared to patients with no infection. Although either approach is valid, each addresses slightly different clinical questions. In the first, the result provides an assessment of the added impact of harboring a resistant infection vs. a susceptible infection. In the second, the impact of having a resistant infection vs. no infection is ascertained. It has been demonstrated that the latter type of comparison typically results in a higher estimate of the impact of resistance on mortality [58,59].

A final issue with regard to assessment of mortality as an outcome is how mortality is defined. Crude in-hospital mortality has been the most common measure of mortality likely because it is the least subjective in its assessment. However, this definition of mortality fails to distinguish those patients in which infection clearly resulted in death as opposed to those in which infection occurred but was likely unrelated to mortality (e.g., infection occurs several weeks before death). Some studies have proposed approaches to categorizing the outcome of mortality relative to how likely it is to have been a result of infection. One approach would be to assign an arbitrary time period after the infection (e.g., one week) beyond which the occurrence of mortality would be assumed to be independent of the infection. Another approach has proposed categories designed to assess *attributable mortality* as an outcome [47,60–62]. In this definition, the possible outcomes are classified as follows: (1) *mortality directly attributable to infection*: death during hospitalization in the setting of clinical evidence of active infection and a positive culture result, (2) *mortality indirectly attributable to infection*: failure or further compromise of an organ system due to infection and death occurring during hospitalization as a result of organ failure, (3) *mortality unrelated to infection*: death occurring during hospitalization after an episode of infection but due to causes independent of the infectious process, and (4) *survival*: patient discharged alive from the hospital. The proportion of deaths directly and indirectly attributable to infection define the attributable mortality. While this approach may more appropriately designate mortality as attributable to infection, many of the criteria remain quite subjective. Of note, recent studies using both this approach and crude in-hospital mortality as outcomes found no substantive differences in final study results [63,64].

SUMMARY

To best respond to the increasingly complicated field of HAIs and antimicrobial resistance, a strong understanding of epidemiologic principles and approaches is essential. This chapter has reviewed basic principles of epidemiology and a number of more specific topics with particular relevance to HAIs and antimicrobial resistance. While a resurgence in the study of epidemiological methodology in HAIs has occurred in recent years, this field of inquiry must continue to expand in the future. Only by providing the most rigorously derived evidence can we hope to devise and implement successful strategies to limit future infections in the healthcare setting.

REFERENCES

1. Scheckler WE. Healthcare epidemiology is the paradigm for patient safety. *Infect Control Hosp Epidemiol* 2002;23:47–51.
2. Gerberding JL. Hospital-onset infections: a patient safety issue. *Ann Intern Med* 2002;137:665–670.
3. Haley RW, Quade D, Freeman HE, Bennett JV. Study on the efficacy of nosocomial infection control (SENIC Project). Summary of study design. *Am J Epidemiol* 1980;111:472–485.
4. Haley RW, Schaberg DR, McClish DK, et al. The accuracy of retrospective chart review in measuring nosocomial infection rates: results of validation studies in pilot hospitals. *Am J Epidemiol* 1980;111:516–533.
5. Freeman J, McGowan JE Jr. Methodologic issues in hospital epidemiology. I. Rates, case-finding, and interpretation. *Rev Infect Dis* 1981;3:658–667.
6. Freeman J, McGowan JE Jr. Methodologic issues in hospital epidemiology. II. Time and accuracy in estimation. *Rev Infect Dis* 1981;3:668–677.
7. D'Agata EM. Methodologic issues of case-control studies: a review of established and newly recognized limitations. *Infect Control Hosp Epidemiol* 2005;26:338–341.
8. Paterson DL. Looking for risk factors for the acquisition of antibiotic resistance: a 21st century approach. *Clin Infect Dis* 2002;34:1564–1567.
9. Schwaber MJ, De-Medina T, Carmeli Y. Epidemiological interpretation of antibiotic resistance studies—what are we missing? *Nat Rev Microbiol* 2004;2:979–983.
10. Harbarth S, Samore M. Antimicrobial resistance determinants and future control. *Emerg Inf Dis* 2005;11:794–801.
11. Agresti A. *Categorical data analysis*. New York: Wiley Interscience, 2002.
12. Hennekens CH, Buring JE, Mayrent SL. *Epidemiology in medicine*. 1st ed. Philadelphia: Lippincott Williams & Wilkins, 1987.
13. Hosmer DW, Lemeshow SL. *Applied logistic regression*. 2nd ed. New York: Wiley Interscience, 2000.
14. Kleinbaum DG, Kupper LL, Morgenstern H. *Epidemiologic research: principles and quantitative methods*. New York: Van Nostrand Reinhold, 1982.
15. Nelson KE, Williams CM, Graham NMH. *Infectious disease epidemiology: theory and practice*. New York: Aspen Publishers, 2000.
16. Rothman KJ, Greenland S. *Modern epidemiology*. Philadelphia: Lippincott Williams & Wilkins, 1998.
17. Thomas JC, Weber DJ. *Epidemiologic methods for the study of infectious diseases*. Oxford: Oxford University Press, 2001.
18. Harris AD, Lautenbach E, Perencevich E. A systematic review of quasi-experimental study designs in the fields of infection control and antibiotic resistance. *Clin Infect Dis* 2005;41:77–82.
19. Shadish WR, Cook TD, Campbell DT. *Experimental and quasi-experimental designs for generalized causal inference*. Boston: Houghton Mifflin Company, 2002.
20. Cook TD, Campbell DT. *Quasi-experimentation: design and analysis issues for field settings*. Chicago: Rand McNally Publishing, 1979.
21. Harris AD, Bradham DD, Baumgarten M, et al. The use and interpretation of quasi-experimental studies in infectious diseases. *Clin Infect Dis* 2004;38:1586–1591.
22. Morton V, Torgerson DJ. Effect of regression to the mean on decision making in health care. *BMJ* 2003;326:1083–1084.
23. Ramsay CR, Matowe L, Grilli R, et al. Interrupted time series designs in health technology assessment: lessons from two systematic reviews of behavior change strategies. *Int J Technol Assess Health Care* 2003;19:613–623.
24. Wagner AK, Soumerai SB, Zhang F, Ross-Degnan D. Segmented regression analysis of interrupted time series studies in medication use research. *J Clin Pharm Ther* 2002;27:299–309.
25. Matowe LK LC, Crivera C, Korth-Bradley JM. Interrupted time series analysis in clinical research. *Ann Pharmacother* 2003;37:1110–1116.
26. Maclure M. The case-crossover design: a method for studying transient effects on the risk of acute events. *Am J Epidemiol* 1991;133:144–153.
27. Schneeweiss S, Sturmer T, Maclure M. Case-crossover and case-time-control designs as alternatives in pharmacoepidemiologic research. *Pharmacoepidemiol Drug Saf* 1997;6 (suppl 3):S51–S59.
28. Fisman DN, Harris AD, Sorock GS, Mittleman MA. Sharps-related injuries in health care workers: a case-crossover study. *Am J Med* 2003;114:688–694.

29. Sorock GS, Lombardi DA, Hauser RB, et al. A case-crossover study of occupational traumatic hand injury: methods and initial findings. *Am J Ind Med* 2001;39:171–179.

30. Redelmeier DA, Tibshirani RJ. Association between cellular-telephone calls and motor vehicle collisions. *N Engl J Med* 1997;336:453–458.

31. Wang PS, Schneeweiss S, Glynn RJ, et al. Use of the case-crossover design to study prolonged drug exposures and insidious outcomes. *Ann Epidemiol* 2004;14:296–303.

32. Dixon KE. A comparison of case-crossover and case-control designs in a study of risk factors for hemorrhagic fever with renal syndrome. *Epidemiology* 1997;8:243–246.

33. Suissa S. The case-time-control design. *Epidemiology* 1995;6: 248–253.

34. Fisman DN, Lim S, Wellenius GA, et al. It's not the heat, it's the humidity: wet weather increases legionellosis risk in the greater Philadelphia metropolitan area. *J Infect Dis* 2005;192:2066–2073.

35. Harris AD, Carmeli Y, Samore MH, et al. Impact of severity of illness bias and control group misclassification bias in case-control studies of antimicrobial-resistant organisms. *Infect Control Hosp Epidemiol* 2005;26:342–345.

36. Kaye KS, Harris AD, Samore M, Carmeli Y. The case-case-control study design: addressing the limitations of risk factor studies for antimicrobial resistance. *Infect Control Hosp Epidemiol* 2005;26:346–351.

37. Harris AD, Karchmer TB, Carmeli Y, Samore MH. Methodological principles of case-control studies that anlayzed risk factors for antibiotic resistance: a systematic review. *Clin Infect Dis* 2001; 32:1055–1061.

38. Harris AD, Samore MH, Lipsitch M, et al. Control-group selection importance in studies of antimicrobial resistance: examples applied to *Pseudomonas aeruginosa*, *Enterococci*, and *Escherichia coli*. *Clin Infect Dis* 2002;34:1558–1563.

39. Carmeli Y, Samore MH, Huskins C. The association between antecedent vancomycin treatment and hospital-acquired vancomycin-resistant enterococci. *Arch Intern Med* 1999;159: 2461–2468.

40. Kaye KS, Harris AD, Gold H, Carmeli Y. Risk factors for recovery of ampicillin-sulbactam-resistant *Escherichia coli* in hospitalized patients. *Antimicrob Agents Chemother* 2000;44:1004–1009.

41. Harris AD, Smith D, Johnson JA, et al. Risk factors for imipenem-resistant *Pseudomonas aeruginosa* among hospitalized patients. *Clin Infect Dis* 2002;34:340–345.

42. Harris AD, Perencevich E, Roghmann MC, et al. Risk factors for piperacillin-tazobactam-resistant *Pseudomonas aeruginosa* among hospitalized patients. *Antimicrob Agents Chemother* 2002;46:854–858.

43. Livermore DM. Can better prescribing turn the tide of resistance? *Nat Rev Microbiol* 2004;2:73–78.

44. Patterson JE. Antibiotic utilization: is there an effect on antimicrobial resistance? *Chest* 2001;119 (suppl 2):426S–430S.

45. Safdar N, Maki DG. The commonality of risk factors for nosocomial colonization and infection with antimicrobial-resistant Staphylococcus aureus, enterococcus, gram-negative bacilli, Clostridium difficile, and Candida. *Ann Intern Med* 2002;136:834–844.

46. Hyle EP, Bilker WB, Gasink LB, Lautenbach E. Impact of different methods of describing extent of prior antibiotic exposure on the association between antibiotic use and resistance. *16th Annual Meeting of the Society for Healthcare Epidemiology of America (SHEA)*, 2006 March 18–21; Chicago, IL, 2006.

47. Lautenbach E, Patel JB, Bilker WB, et al. Extended-spectrum β-lactamase-producing *Escherichia coli* and *Klebsiella pneumoniae*: risk factors for infection and impact of resistance on outcomes. *Clin Infect Dis* 2001;32:1162–1171.

48. Royston P, Altman D, Sauerbrei W. Dichotomizing continuous predictors in multiple regression: a bad idea. *Stat Med* 2006;25:127–141.

49. Donskey CJ. The role of the intestinal tract as a reservoir and source for transmission of nosocomial pathogens. *Clin Infect Dis* 2004;39:219–226.

50. MacAdam H, Zaoutis TE, Gasink LB, Bilker WB, Lautenbach E. Investigating the association between antibiotic use and antibiotic resistance: Impact of different methods of categorizing prior antibiotic use. *International Journal of Antimicrobial Agents*; 2006; 28:325–32.

51. Gasink LB, Bilker WB, Zaoutis TE, Lautenbach E. Impact of different methods of classification of prior antibiotic use in the assessment of risk factors for carbapenem resistant *Pseudomonas aeruginosa*. *American Journal of Infection Control* (in press).

52. Cosgrove SE. The relationship between antimicrobial resistance and patient outcomes: mortality, length of hospital stay, and health care costs. *Clin Infect Dis* 2006;42 (suppl 2):S82–S89.

53. Knaus WA, Drapier EA, Wagner DP, Zimmerman JE. APACHE II: A severity of disease classification system. *Crit Care Med* 1985;13:818–829.

54. McCabe WR, Jackson GG. Gram-negative bacteremia. I. Etiology and ecology. *Arch Intern Med* 1962;110:847–855.

55. Cosgrove SE, Carmeli Y. The impact of antimicrobial resistance on health and economic outcomes. *Clin Infect Dis* 2003;36:1433–1437.

56. Robins JM. The control of confounding by intermediate variables. *Stat Med* 1989;8:679–701.

57. Blot S, De Bacquer D, Hoste E, et al. Influence of matching for exposure time on estimates of attributable mortality caused by nosocomial bacteremia in critically ill patients. *Infect Control Hosp Epidemiol* 2005;26:352–356.

58. Engemann JJ, Carmeli Y, Cosgrove SE, et al. Adverse clinical and economic outcomes attributable to methicillin resistance among patients with *Staphylococcus aureus* surgical site infection. *Clin Infect Dis* 2003;36:592–598.

59. Kaye KS, Engemann JJ, Mozaffari E, Carmeli Y. Reference group choice and antibiotic resistance outcomes. *Emerg Inf Dis* 2004;10:1125–1128.

60. Noskin GA, Peterson LR, Warren JR. *Enterococcus faecium* and *Enterococcus faecalis* bacteremia: acquisition and outcome. *Clin Infect Dis* 1995;20:296–301.

61. Lautenbach E, Schuster MG, Bilker WB, Brennan PJ. The role of chloramphenicol in the treatment of bloodstream infection due to vancomycin-resistant *Enterococcus*. *Clin Infect Dis* 1998;27:1259–1265.

62. Weinstein MP, Murphy JR, Reller LB, Lichtenstein KA. The clinical significance of positive blood cultures: A comprehensive analysis of 500 episodes of bacteremia and fungemia in adults. II. Clinical observations, with special reference to factors influencing prognosis. *Rev Infect Dis* 1983;5:54–70.

63. Lautenbach E, Metlay JP, Bilker WB, et al. Association between fluoroquinolone resistance and mortality in *Escherichia coli* and *Klebsiella pneumoniae* infections: Role of inadequate empiric antimicrobial therapy. *Clin Infect Dis* 2005;41:923–929.

64. Hyle EP, Lipworth AD, Zaoutis TE, et al. Impact of inadequate initial antimicrobial therapy on mortality in infections due to extended-spectrum beta-lactamase-producing enterobacteriaceae: variability by site of infection. *Arch Intern Med* 2005;165:1375–1380.

Use of Computerized Systems in Healthcare Epidemiology

9

Keith F. Woeltje

INTRODUCTION

Computers have become ubiquitous in modern society. Children's toys contain more raw computing power than was present on the Apollo spacecraft that carried men to the moon. Not surprising, computers have become essential tools in healthcare epidemiology. Nevertheless, their use in this setting varies widely; their uses will be reviewed in this chapter.

PERSONAL COMPUTERS

Hardware

Personal computers (PCs) started as machines built by geeky enthusiasts in the 1970s but became widely commercially available in the 1980s. In the first years of the 21st century, computers have become commodity items. PC prices have fallen steadily while computing power has increased exponentially. Until a few years ago, considerable thought had to be given to buying a personal computer in balancing price, capability, and upgradeability. Now, even the most inexpensive PCs available at large electronics stores can readily handle basic computer needs.

Hospitals or universities may have recommended (or required) minimum standards for PCs purchased for work use and may even have specified that computers be purchased from certain vendors. As a general rule, spending money on more memory (RAM) rather than a slightly faster processor is a better investment. Because more and more training materials (and software) are now being distributed on DVDs, a DVD drive should be considered essential (and it is now uncommon to find a computer sold without one). Also essential is the ability to connect to a local network. This is typically via a direct Ethernet cable connection but may, in some settings, be done wirelessly. Unless the user will be storing many multimedia files (e.g., photos and video), most data and reports generated by an infection control (IC) program does not use a lot of hard drive space, so a massive hard drive is typically not high on the priority list. Being able to write to optical media (such as a CD-R or DVD-R) is a nice feature for sharing and archiving data.

The most important decision in choosing computer hardware is based on determining what operating system one wants to use. The operating system (OS) is computer software that controls the actual workings of the hardware (e.g., displaying the information on a screen, taking input from a keyboard). Other software is written to work with the OS; software written to run on one OS will not run on another OS. However, some software may have different versions that run on different OSs. If someone needs a particular program and that program is only available for one OS, this will dictate what OS to choose.

Currently, different versions of Microsoft Windows taken together are the most commonly used OS. The newest version, Windows Vista, should be available by the time this text is printed. Microsoft Windows runs on computer hardware from a wide variety of vendors. Because it is the most commonly used OS, many computer programs are available only in versions that run on Microsoft Windows. Another OS is Macintosh OS X; it will run only on computer hardware made by Apple Computer. Some computer programs that are made for Microsoft Windows also have different versions that run on Macintosh OS X. Recent changes in Apple Macintosh hardware allows users in certain circumstances also to run the Microsoft Windows OS, potentially allowing users to run programs written for both OSs on their machines.

Linux (**www.linux.org**) is another OS; it originally was used primarily by computer enthusiasts and information technology (IT) professionals. Initially, it was used particularly for servers (computers attached to a network that provides services to other computers, e.g., storing files or sending out Web pages). However, Linux has made some inroads as a desktop OS in some large companies, especially outside of North America. Linux is an example of "open-source software," which is developed as a collaborative effort of programmers around the world. Open-source software is typically available free of charge with any associated cost being for the cost of the media or for technical support, not the software itself. Another key characteristic of open-source software is that the source code (the text of the program written by the programmers) also is available, so that end-users can make or commission modifications in the program if they choose. Linux comes in a bewildering variety of versions (termed "distributions" or, more commonly, "distros") that vary primarily as to the software that comes along with the OS (**www.distrowatch.com**). Linux runs on a wide variety of computer hardware.

Basic Software

A computer and its OS alone would not be able to accomplish very much. Additional software is needed to perform basic tasks, such as word processing. Although stand-alone programs of productivity software are available, they typically are obtained in suites with all components somewhat integrated, allowing consistency of use across programs. Microsoft Office has become the most commonly used office suite, but a variety of competitors exist, including the free, open-source, OpenOffice.org (**www.openoffice.org**). Most institutions prefer to have all employees use the same program for ease of interchanging information, but most of these programs can convert between the most common formats.

Word processing software (e.g., Microsoft Word or Corel's Word Perfect) is the cornerstone of computer productivity software. It allows letters, reports, and so on to be easily edited and formatted for distribution. Presentation software (e.g., Microsoft PowerPoint, Apple Keynote) assists with the development of attractive "slide shows" (although actual physical slides are rarely used

now with the increasing use of digital projectors). The most common error with this software is the temptation to include excessive special effects, to have distracting backgrounds, and to include too much information on one slide. Presentation software also can be easily used to lay out posters for display at scientific meetings.

Spreadsheet software (e.g., Microsoft Excel, OpenOffice .org Math) is designed primarily to manipulate numbers, not text. Spreadsheets are extremely useful to healthcare epidemiologists for calculating rates and doing basic statistics. The column and row structure of spreadsheets also allows them to be used as simple databases, such as a line-listing for an outbreak investigation. Spreadsheet software also can make graphs for visualization of data. These graphs can then be imported into a word processing document or slide presentation for distribution to others.

Desktop relational database software (e.g., Microsoft Access, FileMaker) is not included in many basic editions of office suite software but may be available in more extended or "professional" editions. Although in some respects more difficult to use than other desktop computer productivity software, database software can offer healthcare epidemiologists significant advantages over other methods of storing data, such as using spreadsheet software. For example, if blood culture data are being stored as part of a study, if a given blood culture has > 1 organism, then in a spreadsheet either a number of columns need to be included (e.g., "organism_1," "organisms_2") if data from a given culture are all to be included on one row, or a number of separate rows need to be used to record the information from a single culture. Both alternatives may introduce difficulties in subsequent data retrieval and analysis. A relational database, however, would allow the information to be structured in a manner that avoids these issues.

Because most office productivity software can be used at a basic level without any special training, the benefits of formal training are frequently underappreciated. Various levels of training classes may be offered by larger organizations or may be available at local community colleges. On-line training or structured textbooks provide additional alternatives. The time and expense spent on training will be returned many times in productivity gains. In particular, database software requires some training to use it appropriately. An excellent introduction to databases at a conceptual level (and not tied to any particular program) is *Database Design for Mere Mortals* [1].

NETWORKED COMPUTERS

Although a stand-alone PC can bring a huge productivity boost to a healthcare epidemiology/IC office, the potential utility of the computer increases significantly when it is networked to other computers. The PC then is no longer limited to data that have been entered by hand or files brought to it on some form of solid media. Instead, the PC can now share information with other computers at high speeds. The more computers that are networked together, the more valuable the network, termed "Metcalf's Law" [2].

Internet

The Internet is really a network of computer networks [3]. Precursors to the Internet began as a research project in the late 1960s sponsored by the U.S. Department of Defense's Advanced Research Project Agency. The Internet as we know it started on January 1, 1983 [4]. The Internet has grown exponentially in the intervening decades. Research is underway for the next generation Internet, termed "Internet2" (**www.internet2.edu/**).

World Wide Web

For many people, the World Wide Web ("the Web") is synonymous with the Internet. The World Wide Web started in 1990 as a research project at the European Organization for Nuclear Research (CERN) [5]. The purpose of the Web is to provide access to on-line documents (Web pages), including an easy mechanism for one page to refer to another. These pages can be viewed with software called Web browsers. Since its inception, the Web has grown beyond simple text to include images and multimedia presentations and allow downloads of files of various types. For healthcare epidemiologists, the Web provides a wealth of resources. An example is the Supercourse, a Web-based set of lectures in epidemiology (available at **www.pitt.edu/~super1/**). Many professional organizations have Web sites that provide news, guidelines, and links to other resources for both members and nonmembers. Examples include the Society for Healthcare Epidemiology of America (SHEA, **www.shea-online.org**), the Association of Professionals in Infection Control and Epidemiology (APIC, **www.apic.org**), the Community and Hospital Infection Control Association—Canada (CHICA—Canada, **www.chica.org**), the Hospital Infection Society (HIS, **www.his.org.uk**), and the International Federation of Infection Control (IFIC, **www.theific.org**). Government organizations such as the Centers for Disease Control and Prevention (CDC, **www.cdc.gov**) provide a wealth of resources including guidelines, information on specific diseases and outbreaks, and reference materials. State and local health departments also may have Web sites that provide valuable information on local issues. The Web also provides easy access to information from companies regarding their products. Literature searches of the U.S. National Library of Medicine's MEDLINE database also can be conducted on the Web using the PubMed system (**www.pubmed.gov**). Some hospitals and other organizations block or severely limit access of employees to the Web. Healthcare epidemiology/IC programs can make a strong argument for having relatively unfettered Web access to do their jobs correctly.

E-mail

Electronic mail, or e-mail, is probably even more popular than the World Wide Web in terms of total numbers of users. Sending files as attachments in an e-mail has become a preferred method of sending data from one person to another. In addition, e-mail can serve as a means to alert healthcare epidemiologists to significant issues in a timely fashion. Organizations (e.g., SHEA and APIC) send e-mail alerts to their members when warranted. Healthcare professionals also can sign up for alerts and updates on terrorism and emergency response from the CDC at **www.bt.cdc.gov/clinregistry/index.asp**. In addition, the CDC's Division of Healthcare Quality Promotion has a Rapid Notification System for Healthcare Professionals that sends out e-mail alerts related to outbreaks and product recalls. The sign-up page is at **www2a.cdc.gov/ncidod/hip/rns/hip_rns_subscribe.html**. Alternatively, one can send an e-mail message to LISTSERV @CDC.GOV with a blank subject line and the text "subscribe HIP-RNS" (without the quotes) in the message.

E-mail "list-serv" software allows e-mail to be sent to many persons by sending an e-mail to a particular e-mail address. This facilitates group discussions via e-mail. Popular e-mail groups for healthcare epidemiologists include ProMED-mail (sign up at **www.promedmail.org/**), which is sponsored by the International Infectious Diseases Society, and the Emerging Infections Network (request sign-up information from **ein@uiowa.edu**), which is sponsored by the Infectious Diseases Society of America and the CDC. Because of the rise of unsolicited commercial e-mails (termed "spam"), many institutions have "spam filters" in place to reduce the influx of these nuisance messages. Unfortunately, these filters may filter out legitimate e-mail. List-serv e-mails, in particular, may be filtered out as "bulk e-mail." Local IT personnel should be consulted to determine what steps are needed to ensure that desired e-mail reaches the recipient.

SPECIALIZED SOFTWARE

An IC program could be quite productive and organized using only the software contained in an office suite. To go beyond basic data analysis requires substantial effort to set up formulas on a spreadsheet. Even with such effort, some advanced data analysis would simply not be possible. Advanced needs require specialized software.

General Statistical Software

For more extensive analysis than can be done with a spreadsheet, a healthcare epidemiologist could use general-purpose statistical software. A wide range of programs exists, from basic statistical packages included with some statistics texts to expensive, very complex programs that can perform even the most esoteric analysis. Widely used statistics packages include SAS, SPSS, and Stata. Many other very capable commercial programs are available. R (**www.r-project.org**) is an open-source general-purpose statistical package. EpiTools (available from **www.epitools.net/**) is a set of tools for use with the R statistical package designed to add functions of use to epidemiologists. Although some of these programs allow for some form of direct data entry, they really are designed to import data that was entered using another program (e.g., a database or spreadsheet). Thus, using these programs for routine healthcare epidemiology use takes some effort. A user who is facile with a given program may choose to do basic analyses in that program. For the most part, these statistical programs are overkill for most IC programs and are used primarily in research settings or by facilities that have dedicated statistical analysts.

Healthcare Epidemiology–Specific Software

A number of software packages have been designed specifically for healthcare epidemiology/IC programs. They allow the user to enter surveillance data (both denominator and numerator data) and will then generate reports and graphs on rates. Popular programs include AICE Millenium and EpiQuest. Some of these programs include the ability to compare a facility's rates with benchmarks from the CDC's National Nosocomial Infections Surveillance (NNIS) System (now known as the National Healthcare Safety Network, or NHSN). Some of these programs also have provisions for importing data directly from available electronic sources. Using these sources will likely require working with hospital IT support services to ensure that data are sent in an appropriate format.

Some healthcare epidemiology–specific software is designed to import essentially all information from available electronic sources. Such programs include Infection Control Assistant, MedMined, QC Pathfinder, and SETNET. Although each of these programs has different features, they tend toward more real-time analysis of electronically available data, such as microbiology results. These programs may detect clusters of antimicrobial-resistant organisms relatively quickly but may be less able to generate surgical site infection (SSI) rate graphs, for example.

The advantage of these specialized IC/healthcare epidemiology software packages is that they are designed with the needs of an infection control practitioner (ICP)/healthcare epidemiologist in mind. Although they are somewhat configurable, they require minimal set up to generate useful information. This narrow specialization also is their downside; if a user needs a specific functionality that is not included in the package, the user must use other software. Vendors are eager to hear what features their users would like to see, but a feature is typically added only if there is substantial interest. A wide variety of options are available, and the features offered by each program continually increases. Each program may have features not offered by any of the others. Facilities interested in such software should determine what features they require, request information from each vendor, and do a careful cost-benefit analysis.

General Epidemiology Software

Some programs occupy a middle ground between the general statistical software packages and the healthcare epidemiology–specific software. They provide more support for data entry and management than general-purpose statistical programs while providing more flexible statistical analysis than most specialty IC/healthcare–epidemiology software packages. The primary downside is the considerable work that would be necessary to set up specific functionality that comes "ready-made" with IC specific software. The benefit is the ability to design in the specific functionality the user desires.

Epi Info

Epi Info (**www.cdc.gov/epiinfo/**) is a program designed and distributed free by the CDC. Early versions of the program were designed to run on Microsoft MS-DOS to assist CDC Epidemiologic Intelligence Service Officers (EISOs) in investigating outbreaks. It was steadily upgraded, and in the late 1990s a version for Microsoft Windows was finally released. Initially named "Epi Info 2000," to distinguish it from the MS-DOS version, the name has subsequently been simplified to "Epi Info" again. Versions for other OSs are not available.

Epi Info does not generate specific reports or graphs designed for healthcare epidemiologists. Rather, it is a collection of tools that can be used in a wide variety of ways, including collecting and analyzing epidemiologic data. Functions are available to design data entry screens. Once designed, data can be entered, stored, and retrieved using the program. Internal data are stored in a relational database, which allows for sophisticated data storage if that is needed. Double data entry (see later Data Entry section) for ensuring data integrity is supported.

Epi Info provides an extensive range of statistical analysis tools. Analysis is not limited to data entered and stored using the software. The program can import and analyze data that have been stored in a number of database and spreadsheet formats. Results also can be displayed in a variety of graphical formats. Advanced statistical analysis, including logistic regression and Kaplan-Meier survival analysis, is available.

In addition to statistical analysis, Epi Info contains modules for nutritional anthropometry, mapping of data using geographic information system (GIS) standards, and even a simple word processor for producing reports. Additional modules can be developed by programmers outside the CDC to extend the program's capabilities. The software allows for data entry on different computers with later merging of the data into one dataset. Overall, Epi Info provides a framework for developing quite sophisticated systems for healthcare epidemiology–data gathering and analysis.

EpiData

EpiData (**www.epidata.dk/**) started as a Windows-friendly data entry program for the older MS-DOS versions of Epi Info. This program has now become EpiData Entry. It enables the user to design data entry screens and then enter and manage data. EpiData Entry supports double data entry. Once entered, the data can be exported in a variety of formats for additional analysis. This includes export into SAS, SPSS, and Stata formats. As such, EpiData Entry is a good companion program to a general statistical package to provide the data entry and management functions the statistical programs lack.

EpiData Analysis is a newer program released in the fall of 2005. It provides additional data management functions beyond those offered by EpiData Entry. It also provides some basic descriptive statistical analysis and graphical functions, including statistical process control (SPC) charts. Although not presently as full featured as Epi Info, additional analysis functions are apparently planned.

Other Software and Resources

Sometimes an epidemiologist just needs to do a quick calculation, such as a 2×2 table. Such a simple task can actually be tedious to do in a full-fledged statistical package. Epi Info has a StatCalc module that is designed for quick calculations; however, it is based on the old MS-DOS version and is not as user friendly as more modern programs. A similar and free program that is designed specifically for Microsoft Windows is EpiCalc 2000, written by Mark Myatt (**www.brixtonhealth.com**; this Web site also contains links to a wide variety of other programs that may be of use to healthcare epidemiologists). For those with ready access to the Internet, the OpenEpi project (**www.openepi.com**) provides epidemiology analysis tools available in any Web browser.

Many more software packages that are of use to healthcare epidemiologists exist than can be described here. Many of the Web pages mentioned provide links to additional resources. A source of many links for statistical analysis is statpages.org/. A quick search using an Internet search engine can yield a wide variety of additional options.

Data Entry and Integrity

In order to use computers for any form of data analysis, the data must first be entered in a form that the computer can access. For a stand-alone computer, this is typically done through keyboard entry. If entering a large amount of data (e.g., transcribing information from paper data collection forms), double data entry can provide a higher level of assurance that the data have been entered correctly. This entails entering every form into two separate copies of the same database (often done by two different people) and then comparing the results to ensure that they are identical. Any discrepancies are resolved by referring back to the original data form. Not all software is capable of allowing for double data entry, but it is a nice feature to use to provide the highest level of data integrity. The EpiData Web site (**www.epidata.dk/documentation.php**) has a variety of publications that describe additional good practices for data management that can be downloaded.

With the increasing use of computers in healthcare facilities, more and more data needed by the healthcare epidemiologist already is available in electronic form. Patient demographics may be available from the admissions office, information on surgical procedures may be available from the operating room scheduling system, and so on. As noted previously, depending on what software is being used, data may need to be converted into a specific format to be imported. A variety of de facto standards exist (e.g., many programs can export and import data in Microsoft Excel format). If data are not already available in a format that can be used directly, frequently the hospital's IT department can write a program to convert the information into a useable format. As electronic medical records [6] become more commonly used, even more information may be available to the healthcare epidemiologist. It will be essential to work with the appropriate committees as an electronic medical record is being implemented at an institution to ensure that important data (e.g., presence of a central venous catheter on a given day) are being captured in a manner that allows for easy data querying and aggregation [7].

For items that are not available electronically, a variety of methods beyond simple paper forms have been used to collect the information. These include using forms that can be scanned in rather than requiring manual keyboarding of the information [8]. Small handheld computers (personal digital assistants, or PDAs) also have been used to collect data at the point of care [9]. Some software for PDAs allows for selecting choices from a variety of options, thus making data entry easier than entering words character by character. Such a system has been used at Barnes-Jewish Corporation (BJC) HealthCare member hospitals to report information to the system IC and Healthcare Epidemiology Consortium [10].

Once data have been entered by whatever means, provisions must be made to prevent data loss. An external means of backing up data should be considered essential. A variety of options are available, including external hard drives, external tape drives (less common as hard drive prices have fallen), and recordable CDs or DVDs. If using a second hard drive, an external drive is preferred to a second internal drive so that an internal component failure (e.g., a short circuit in the power supply) does not damage both drives simultaneously. For networked computers, storage space may be available on their local network; this provides a good alternative to an external hard drive. All back-up systems are useless if not utilized. Users should remember to make backups regularly, or even better, should have software in place that automates the process. Copies of data should be stored in a secure place; for the highest level of security, this could mean an off-site location. Data stored on network drives managed by the institutional IT department are typically backed up on a daily basis.

ELECTRONIC SURVEILLANCE

Computers were first introduced into most hospitals in the form of large main-frame computers used for financial systems; computers were out of reach of most healthcare epidemiologists. When PCs became available, they were quickly adopted for use in IC. Schifman reported in 1985 on the use of custom software at the Tucson Veterans Administration Medical Center (VAMC); microbiology data were entered by hand to generate positive culture rates by ward by site (sputum blood, urine), and the results for each month were compared to the previous 12-month average [11]. The landmark Study of the Efficacy of Infection Control (SENIC) [12] demonstrated the value of surveillance in IC. In addition, 1985 was the year that the first precursor program to Epi Info was released. This convergence of the demonstrated need to do surveillance for HAIs and the increased availability of relatively inexpensive computers and software to assist the process led to the steady integration of computers into hospital IC programs.

For most healthcare facilities, PCs are used to perform retrospective analysis on data that have been entered. Some amount of data may be pulled from a variety of electronic sources, but typically, all of this information constitutes "denominator data" for analysis. "Numerator data" (i.e., which patients actually have HAIs) are typically determined by manual surveillance performed by ICPs. Computers may aid their data entry, but much of the work of detection and recording is still manual. Although this remains largely true today, efforts continue to shift more of this work onto computers. Such shifts require that a substantial amount of data be readily available electronically.

At the most basic level, computers can provide surveillance assistance that is relatively simple but can provide considerable time savings. One such basic assistance is simple aggregation of microbiology data [13]. Many hospitals provide such reports to their IC departments; these reports are generated by the hospital's laboratory systems and either printed or sent electronically to IC.

Some hospitals have been able to provide even more computer assistance. The Later Day Saints (LDS) hospital in Salt Lake City, Utah, developed the Health Evaluation through Logical Processing (HELP) system, a groundbreaking computer support system for clinicians. By applying a variety of rules to available information (e.g., microbiology data, patient date of admission), the HELP system could detect patients likely to have an HAI [14–16]. At Barnes Hospital (now BJC Hospital) in St. Louis, Missouri, the GermWatcher system was developed in the early 1990s [17–19]. Positive microbiology cultures are evaluated by an expert system that ranks them as likely contaminants or not and prioritizes cultures for ICPs (e.g., a sputum culture growing an acid fast bacteria is higher priority than a urine culture with *E. coli*). This assistance allows the ICPs to focus on patients most likely to have significant HAIs and not have to spend time scrutinizing all positive cultures. A data warehouse developed in Chicago that included data from Cook County Hospital and two smaller hospitals was recently described [20]. One goal in developing this system was to facilitate similar computer-assisted surveillance. Other facilities have developed similar systems [21,22].

In addition to the systems that have been developed at large academic medical centers as described, similar capabilities now are available to hospitals that do not have the expertise to build their own systems. Some of the commercial IC software described earlier, such as MedMined, SETNET, QC Pathfinder, and Infection Control Assistant, have components that offer similar surveillance assistance [23–26].

Beyond simple assisted surveillance, efforts have been made to fully automate surveillance for nosocomial bloodstream infections (BSIs). A retrospective evaluation of blood cultures from six hospitals in the Boston area suggested that a simple system of rules applied to microbiology data alone had a sensitivity of 64% and a specificity of 98% [27]. A similar study using data from neonatal intensive care units in six New York City hospitals reported a sensitivity of 79% and a specificity of 96% [28]. In both instances, the negative predictive value was much better than the positive predictive value. This suggests the possibility that although neither system would be capable of fully automated BSI surveillance, both could eliminate patients not likely to have true BSIs, thus aiding ICPs in selecting patients whose charts should be reviewed. A study in two Chicago hospitals evaluated a variety of rule-based approaches to BSI, compared with ICP review, compared with "gold standard" review by physician investigators [29]. The best computer algorithm had a sensitivity of 81% and a specificity of 72%. However, the temporal trends of the computer algorithm over time tended to track well with the reference standard. This suggests that although the automated method may not give a "true" rate, it may be possible to follow trends over time without any active surveillance by an ICP. If rates become unexpectedly high, a specific investigation could be launched.

As with BSIs, efforts have been made to automate a significant portion of the effort required for SSI surveillance. Studies in Boston evaluated use of hospital discharge diagnoses combined with inpatient antibiotic administration data to detect SSIs after cesarean section [30]. A combination of this information had a positive predictive value of 94% with a sensitivity of 59%. This method was later validated for coronary artery bypass graft (CABG) surgery at hospitals in Boston and Israel [31] and at a number of U.S. hospitals for CABG, breast, and cesarean section surgeries [32]. Overall sensitivities in the latter study ranged from 93% to 97%, but positive predictive values were only 20% to 42%. Predictive value was particularly sensitive to antibiotic prescribing practices at the various hospitals. As with some of the BSI approaches mentioned, such methods may still be very valuable by allowing ICPs to narrow their focus to the patients most likely to really have an SSI, thus making surveillance more efficient. The Boston investigators also have reported using similar surveillance methods to detect SSIs in patients after hospital discharge by evaluating health maintenance organization (HMO) data [33]. Given the difficulty of postdischarge surveillance, such methods hold some promise but may be limited by the availability of records. Another approach to assist (but not fully automate) SSI surveillance was instituted in a Paris hospital where computer surveillance for positive cultures from surgical patients was used as a screen [34].

In addition to HAI surveillance, hospital computers can assist with other IC tasks. Many hospitals have systems in place in which patients who are known to be carriers of antimicrobial-resistant organisms, such as methicillin-resistant *Staphylococcus aureus* (MRSA), can be flagged in a hospital computer system. This flag then triggers automatic placement into appropriate isolation precautions if the patient is readmitted. Typically, turning such flags on and off is itself a manual task. However, some automated systems (such as GermWatcher and others) can highlight patients who have positive cultures with such organisms, making it less likely that they will be missed and hence not flagged. Implementation of such a system in Geneva, Switzerland, resulted in significantly more patients being isolated at the time of admission [35]. An even more automated system for ensuring that patients are placed in appropriate isolation was described at Columbia-Presbyterian Medical Center. Automated computer protocols evaluated chest radiograph reports using a natural-language processor. The automated system also evaluated patients for evidence of immunocompromised status by evaluating laboratory data for evidence of human immunodeficiency virus (HIV) infection and pharmacy data for use of medications used only to treat HIV. This automated system was able to identify patients who should have been on isolation but were not [36].

Not all attempts to use computers to assist or automate HAI surveillance have been successful. In particular, the use of electronic hospital claims data alone has been shown to correlate poorly with true HAIs [37–39].

WHAT NOT TO AUTOMATE

Computers have many advantages over older paper systems in areas of data analysis, data sharing, and data backups. However, computers crash and may not always be available, entering data can be time-consuming, and sometimes data sharing can mean multiple copies of the same information that have been changed by different people and are now incompatible. At many hospitals, old paper-based systems continue to work just fine. An example is keeping track of patients with antimicrobial resistant organisms using an index card system. Such a system may be accessed more readily than launching a database program, searching for the patient's entry, and then closing the program. For hospitals that have such older systems, the decision to put the information into electronic format may be a complicated one, especially if a large amount of legacy information will have to entered into the computer. A split system, whereby only new data, or only limited older data, are entered into the computer may be an option if old information only rarely needs to be accessed. Likewise, changes to newer versions of software, or changes to "more automated" versions of processes that are already somewhat computer assisted may lead to changes in work flow that actually make the overall process less efficient. Any decision to "computerize" or upgrade an existing process should be based on a careful analysis of expected benefits and a realistic assessment of the negative aspects of the change. Changes should not be made simply for the sake of change or to have the "latest technology." Unfortunately, in some instances, decisions by software vendors to no longer support older products will force a hospital epidemiology program to upgrade even if there are no real benefits to the process.

CONCLUSIONS

Computers are ubiquitous in modern life, including in healthcare epidemiology. As computers become more powerful and as more information becomes available electronically, healthcare epidemiologists can anticipate an even greater use of automated tools. Still, computers are only tools. At their best, they can perform the tedious portions of surveillance and calculations for us, but it will still take a person to interpret the data and use it to improve patient care.

ACKNOWLEDGMENT

Thanks to Ashleigh Goris for her assistance with this chapter.

REFERENCES

1. Hernandez MJ. Database design for mere mortals. 2nd ed. Reading, MA: Addison-Wesley Professional, 2003.
2. Wikipedia contributors. Metcalfe's law. Wikipedia The Free Encyclopedia, June 1, 2006 (en.wikipedia.org/w/index.php?title=Metcalfe's_law&oldid=56401684) accessed June 27, 2006.
3. Wikipedia contributors. Internet. Wikipedia, The Free Encyclopedia. June 27, 2006 (en.wikipedia.org/w/index.php?title=Internet&oldid=60875572) accessed June 27, 2006.

4. Leiner BM, Cerf VG, Clark DD, et al. A brief history of the Internet, December 10, 2003 (www.isoc.org/internet/history/brief.shtml) accessed May 29, 2006.
5. Connolly D. A little history of the World Wide Web, 2000 (www.w3.org/History.html) accessed May 30, 2006.
6. Dick RS, Steen EB, Detmer DE, eds. The computer-based patient record: an essential technology for health care. Rev. ed. Washington, DC: National Academy Press, 1997.
7. Classen DC, Burke JP. The computer-based patient record: the role of the hospital epidemiologist. *Infect Control Hosp Epidemiol* 1995;16:729–736.
8. Thompson IM. Automated entry of nosocomial infection surveillance data: use of an optical scanning system. *J Hosp Infect* 1999;43(suppl):S275–S278.
9. Farley JE, Srinivasan A, Richards A, et al. Handheld computer surveillance: shoe-leather epidemiology in the "palm" of your hand. *Am J Infect Control* 2005;33:444–449.
10. Murphy DM. From expert data collectors to interventionists: changing the focus for infection control professionals. *Am J Infect Control* 2002;30:120–132.
11. Schifman RB, Palmer RA. Surveillance of nosocomial infections by computer analysis of positive culture rates. *J Clin Microbiol* 1985;21:493–495.
12. Haley RW, Culver DH, White JW, et al. The efficacy of infection surveillance and control programs in preventing nosocomial infections in U.S. hospitals. *Am J Epidemiol* 1985;121:182–205.
13. Burken MI, Zaman AF, Smith FJ. Semi-automated infection control surveillance in a Veterans' Administration medical center. *Infect Control Hosp Epidemiol* 1990;11:410–412.
14. Evans RS, Gardner RM, Bush AR, et al. Development of a computerized infectious disease monitor (CIDM). *Comput Biomed Res* 1985;18:103–113.
15. Evans RS, Larsen RA, Burke JP, et al. Computer surveillance of hospital-acquired infections and antibiotic use. *JAMA* 1986;256:1007–1011.
16. Burke JP, Classen DC, Pestotnik SL, et al. The HELP system and its application to infection control. *J Hosp Infect* 1991;18(suppl A):424–431.
17. Kahn MG, Steib SA, Fraser VJ, Dunagan WC. An expert system for culture-based infection control surveillance. Proceedings—the Annual Symposium on Computer Applications in Medical Care 1993; 171–175.
18. Kahn MG, Steib SA, Dunagan WC, Fraser VJ. Monitoring expert system performance using continuous user feedback. *J Am Med Inform Assoc* 1996;3:216–223.
19. Kahn MG, Bailey TC, Steib SA, et al. Statistical process control methods for expert system performance monitoring. *J Am Med Inform Assoc* 1996;3:258–269.
20. Wisniewski MF, Kieszkowski P, Zagorski BM, et al. Development of a clinical data warehouse for hospital infection control. *J Am Med Inform Assoc* 2003;10:454–462.
21. Pokorny L, Rovira A, Martin-Baranera M, et al. Automatic detection of patients with nosocomial infection by a computer-based surveillance system: a validation study in a general hospital. *Infect Control Hosp Epidemiol* 2006;27:500–503.
22. Leth RA, Moller JK. Surveillance of hospital-acquired infections based on electronic hospital registries. *J Hosp Infect* 2006;62: 71–79.
23. Brossette SE, Sprague AP, Hardin JM, et al. Association rules and data mining in hospital infection control and public health surveillance. *J Am Med Inform Assoc* 1998;5:373–381.
24. Hymel PA, Brossette SE. Data mining-enhanced infection control surveillance: sensitivity and specificity. Abstract, Society for Healthcare Epidemiology of America (SHEA) Annual Meeting, Toronto, Canada. 2001.
25. Wright MO, Perencevich EN, Novak C, et al. Preliminary assessment of an automated surveillance system for infection control. *Infect Control Hosp Epidemiol* 2004;25:325–332.
26. Steinzor N, Pickett S. APIC investigates surveillance technology. *APIC News* 2005;24:12–19.
27. Yokoe DS, Anderson J, Chambers R, et al. Simplified surveillance for nosocomial bloodstream infections. *Infect Control Hosp Epidemiol* 1998;19:657–660.
28. Graham PL III, San Gabriel P, Lutwick S, Haas J, Saiman L. Validation of a multicenter computer-based surveillance system for hospital-acquired bloodstream infections in neonatal intensive care departments. *Am J Infect Control* 2004;32:232–234.
29. Trick WE, Zagorski BM, Tokars JI, et al. Computer algorithms to detect bloodstream infections. *Emerg Infect Dis* 2004;10:1612–1620.
30. Hirschhorn LR, Currier JS, Platt R. Electronic surveillance of antibiotic exposure and coded discharge diagnoses as indicators of postoperative infection and other quality assurance measures. *Infect Control Hosp Epidemiol* 1993;14:21–28.
31. Yokoe DS, Shapiro M, Simchen E, Platt R. Use of antibiotic exposure to detect postoperative infections. *Infect Control Hosp Epidemiol* 1998;19:317–322.
32. Yokoe DS, Noskin GA, Cunningham SM, et al. Enhanced identification of postoperative infections among inpatients. *Emerg Infect Dis* 2004;10:1924–1930.
33. Sands, K., Vineyard, G., and Livingston, J. Efficient identification of postdischarge surgical site infections using automated medical records. *J Infect Dis* 1999;79:434–441.
34. Chalfine A, Cauet D, Lin WC, et al. Highly sensitive and efficient computer-assisted system for routine surveillance of surgical site infections. *Infect Control Hosp Epidemiol* 2006;27:791–793.
35. Pittet D, Safran E, Harbarth S, et al. Automatic alerts for methicillin-resistant Staphylococcus aureus surveillance and control: role of a hospital information system. *Infect Control Hosp Epidemiol* 1996;17:496–502.
36. Knirsch CA, Jain NL, Pablos-Mendez A, et al. Respiratory isolation of tuberculosis patients using clinical guidelines and an automated clinical decision support system. *Infect Control Hosp Epidemiol* 1998;19:94–100.
37. Wright SB, Huskins WC, Dokholyan RS, et al. Administrative databases provide inaccurate data for surveillance of long-term central venous catheter-associated infections. *Infect Control Hosp Epidemiol* 2003;24:946–949.
38. Romano PS, Chan BK, Schembri ME, Rainwater JA. Can administrative data be used to compare postoperative complication rates across hospitals? *Med Care* 2002;10:856–867.
39. Sherman ER, Heydon KH, St John KH, et al. Administrative data fail to accurately identify cases of healthcare-associated infection. *Infect Control Hosp Epidemiol* 2006;27:332–337.

The Role of the Laboratory in Control of Healthcare-Associated Infections*

10

William R. Jarvis

Healthcare-associated infections (HAIs) continue to present a major problem in hospitals today. Because of the importance of this subject, each hospital laboratory has the responsibility of supporting activities related to HAI surveillance, control, and prevention [1,2]. Each laboratory can make major contributions toward infection control as long as the people responsible for infection control or the clinical microbiology laboratory cooperate closely to attack this problem. Often the same people have both of these responsibilities; nearly half of those who chair infection control committees are laboratory personnel [3].

Laboratory personnel attempt to minimize the occurrence of HAIs in the following seven ways: (1) participating in hospitalwide infection control activities, especially those of the hospital infection control committee or service team, (2) recovering and accurately identifying responsible organisms, (3) determining antimicrobial susceptibility of selected HAI pathogens, (4) reporting in timely fashion laboratory data relevant to infection control and participation in HAI surveillance, (5) providing additional studies, when necessary, to establish the similarity or difference

of organisms, (6) providing, on occasion, microbiologic studies of the hospital environment, and (7) training infection control personnel.

Since 1990, improvements in laboratory instrumentation and procedures have provided dramatic aid to infection control efforts in several ways [4]. Among these are techniques for more rapid detection and differentiation of organisms and improved systems of reporting for both patient data and trend analysis. Perhaps the most dramatic advances have come in special procedures for examining ("typing") hospital organisms for similarity or difference; in this area, molecular and other techniques have permitted more definitive examination of a wider range of organisms than was possible before [5,6].

PARTICIPATION IN HOSPITALWIDE INFECTION CONTROL ACTIVITIES

Relationship of the Laboratory to the Infection Control Committee

A clinically oriented member of the laboratory staff can contribute substantially by serving on the infection control committee or service team, as it may be called

---

*This chapter has been slightly revised from the previous edition version authored by John E. McGowan, Jr. and Robert A. Weinstein.

today. Such participation is essential in contributing to a harmonious relationship among clinical, infection control, and microbiology personnel [7].

In the typical hospital, most members of the infection control committee do not have a background in microbiology [8]. Thus, it is of great importance for the representative of the laboratory to provide the microbiologic expertise that is critical to many decisions of the group. This knowledge may be required for assessing the importance of culture data, determining the validity of laboratory techniques used to identify HAIs, and designing and implementing investigations and survey projects.

The diagnostic microbiology laboratory is engaged primarily in the evaluation of cultures related to infection. Because these are crucial data for successful infection control, the laboratory activities should be closely coordinated with the infection control committee. For example, the adequacy of the basic techniques for primary isolation, speciation, and antimicrobial susceptibility testing should be discussed by the microbiologists and the infection control committee. Laboratory resources often are stretched by patient-care requirements, especially in smaller hospitals [9]. Laboratory support for infection control activities must be given with discretion. For example, the use of laboratory resources to assess culture personnel or the environment should never be permitted when the epidemiologic indications are unclear [9].

Major changes in reimbursement methods for U.S. hospitals have occurred as managed care has become popular [10]. In view of these changes, it seems that the laboratory microbiologist can provide an added service to the infection control committee and other hospital committees concerned with infection control. Under managed care and pay for performance, new and intensive attempts will continue to evaluate the validity and usefulness of hospital programs, such as infection control [11]. Techniques for assessment are familiar to clinical microbiology personnel, who routinely have to make similar cost–benefit judgments for laboratory equipment, instruments, and procedures [12]. The insights and methods used for such laboratory activities should be helpful to the infection control team and the various committees (e.g., infection control, quality assurance, pharmacy, and therapeutics) as they review the benefit of their activities and attempt to improve the productivity of the program [13].

Budgetary Considerations

Costs for laboratory procedures that are not related directly to the care of patients (e.g., bacteriologic sampling of personnel or the environment) should be borne by a budget separate from that of the laboratory. To facilitate all of the microbiologic activities necessitated by an outbreak, the laboratory (or the hospital epidemiologist or the infection control committee, depending on the hospital's organizational structure) should have a contingency fund to enable personnel, materials, and space to be temporarily assigned to epidemic aid support [14]. An investigation of an outbreak should not be financed by charging individual patients for cultures taken during the study. This will become less an issue as capitated care becomes more prominent and direct charges to patients for specific services decline.

ACCURATE IDENTIFICATION OF ORGANISMS INVOLVED IN HEALTHCARE-ASSOCIATED INFECTION

Infection control personnel search constantly for evidence that a common organism has spread from patient to patient or from staff to patient. Thus, information permitting the successful tracing of organism movements within the hospital may be of value to the hospital infection control team, whether the positive cultures represent episodes of HAI or indicate colonization of the patient [15]. Although some clinical features of illness provide information about etiology, the main sources for this determination usually are the data provided by the clinical laboratory. Hence, the ability of the laboratory staff to isolate and identify responsible microorganisms is crucial to infection control [16].

The spectrum of organisms causing HAIs has changed dramatically since the mid-1980s [17,18]. Enterobacteriaceae, *Staphylococcus aureus*, *Pseudomonas aeruginosa*, and coagulase-negative staphylococci remain frequently associated with HAIs [2,19]. Among the patterns of special concern are the appearance of fungi and viruses as they become more frequent HAI agents [19]. Fortunately, technologic developments in the laboratory over the same period have continued to increase the efficiency with which HAI organisms can be recognized and recovered [4]. There are three main aspects to this. First, new instruments and devices have become widely available. These permit easier detection of the presence of organisms in blood cultures, identification of organisms, and testing of susceptibility to antimicrobials. Some of these devices are automated, permitting the laboratory to provide these improved services with the same or fewer personnel [20]. Many of the instruments can be cost effective for limited numbers of specimens; as a result, small and large laboratories can now include some of these methods in their programs. Use of these instruments and devices also has led to a more standard approach throughout the United States to the identification and susceptibility testing of HAI pathogens. Thus, most of the organisms causing HAI outbreaks or special endemic problems can be identified in the hospital laboratory.

Second, nonculture tests have permitted identification of HAI agents that would not have been recognized in earlier years [21]. Immunologic and nucleic acid testing methods have added to our ability to recognize viruses and other organisms that are difficult or impossible to grow in culture; some of these are involved in HAI. Amplification techniques, such as the polymerase chain reaction (PCR), and other gene-based methods are making tests for diagnosis of infection or colonization even more sensitive [22,23]. Some of these tests are useful for rapid identification of isolates even if they cannot be characterized by routine biochemical methods [24].

Third, these newer tests and instruments not only permit identification of additional agents but also allow more rapid diagnosis of both new and old pathogens. This speedier testing should provide earlier recognition of outbreaks and more efficient handling of organisms in endemic nosocomial or community-acquired infections [25], which should reduce the likelihood of community-acquired organisms becoming HAIs.

Even with these new technologic developments, certain basic principles of operation remain crucial to producing reliable microbiologic data. Several of these are discussed here.

Collection and Transport of Specimens

Specimen collection, transport, and handling must be of sufficiently high quality to provide valid data [26]. Specimens that are not collected or transported properly may give inaccurate results, even when handled as well as possible once they reach the laboratory. In turn, these inaccurate results may lead to improper clinical decisions by physicians, unnecessary labor by laboratory personnel, and unnecessary patient charges. This is especially true for the newer molecular techniques [27].

The laboratory must monitor specimen handling continually and work closely with both inpatient and ambulatory care units to ensure minimization of the possibility of contaminated specimens. This is necessary to ensure that laboratory information presented to the hospital epidemiologist reports organisms actually associated with the patient's site of culture rather than contaminants.

Certain laboratory findings suggest specific handling errors [1]. For example, a frequent failure to isolate organisms from deep wounds or abscesses of patients who are not on antibiotics or the inability to recover pathogens seen on Gram stain in episodes of presumed anaerobic infections suggests inadequate anaerobic transport media, delay or inappropriate refrigeration of specimens in transit, or use of inadequate techniques for isolating anaerobes. The frequent recovery of three or more different organisms in clean-voided, midstream urine specimens suggests unsatisfactory technique in collecting specimens, a delay in transporting specimens to the laboratory, or a delay in culturing them. The finding of negative cultures from a high percentage of patients with positive smears for bacteria suggests unsatisfactory specimen collection or handling, errors in staining, contaminated reagents, or errors in culture techniques [28].

Specimen collection and handling should be assessed regularly to detect and correct such problems; the frequency with which probable contaminants are isolated from clinical specimens can be a measure of the quality of specimen collection in a specific hospital area. For example, determining frequency of urine specimens with characteristics

that suggest specimen contamination permits wards with high rates to be singled out for evaluation and, if necessary, for in-service education programs instituted by laboratory or infection control personnel. In addition, identifying people who draw blood cultures that frequently contain diphtheroids, coagulase-negative staphylococci, or other probable skin contaminants may permit re-instruction of these personnel in aseptic technique. Periodic review of the relative incidence of false-positive smears for acid-fast bacilli or of specimens with heavy bacterial contamination may highlight problems in sputum collection and processing [26].

Many hospitals record both the time the specimen was collected and the time the laboratory received it so that transport time can be monitored periodically or continuously and the culturing of old specimens avoided. Evaluation of turnaround time has become an important element of laboratory quality assurance [29].

Initial Evaluation of Specimens

Assessing specimens at the time they are received in the laboratory is one of the best ways to evaluate their suitability. For example, microscopic review of Gram stain of sputum specimens remains the best way to determine whether these specimens are contaminated [30]; specimens identified as inadequate are not processed further and do not confuse either clinician or epidemiologist. A new specimen should be requested unless the clinician provides notice of special circumstances (e.g., immunosuppression) that might make it worthwhile to proceed with culture [25].

Culture or smear results for other types of specimens also may suggest contamination at the time of collection. For example, urine specimens with ≥ 3 different organisms present ordinarily suggest contamination in patients without chronic indwelling urine catheters. Such specimens should be held for 2 to 3 days without further processing. The patient's physician should be notified so that unusual clinical situations requiring further identification of the specimen can be recognized. Scoring systems for use in determining acceptable wound, vaginal, cervical, or other specimens also have been described [31]. Application of such criteria ensures that the information generated from the specimens that are processed completely will more likely correlate with true infecting organisms and will reduce unnecessary laboratory costs. Repeat specimen collection should be requested for these inadequate specimens, and additional processing of organisms isolated from poor specimens (e.g., speciation, susceptibility testing) should be delayed or eliminated. The culture report should alert the clinician about the questionable value of the specimen so that results will be used cautiously, if at all, for guidance in diagnosis and therapy.

For specimens from sputum and wounds, reporting the morphologic characteristics of bacteria seen on Gram stain may be misleading if no statement is made regarding the presence or absence of white blood cells. Both sites may be extensively contaminated with skin, oropharyngeal, or intestinal bacterial flora. When organisms are found only in the presence of abundant squamous epithelial cells, it is unlikely that they are the causative agents, and reports of such mixed flora without qualification about the accompanying cells may lead the clinician falsely to assume mixed flora as the cause of the infection. Substantial effort will be conserved and superior information ultimately provided if repeat collection is requested for such specimens.

Microscopy at the time of specimen submission can help other aspects of microbiologic diagnosis. For example, examination on Gram stain for morphology can identify organisms that might be epidemiologically important but not reflected by culture. Thus, presence of a mixed flora on Gram stain of a sputum specimen, when coupled with an aerobic culture yielding only *Hemophilus influenzae*, may indicate possible mixed aerobic–anaerobic infection rather than pneumonia due to *Hemophilus*. Because infection control implications of these two causes may differ, evaluations of this type by the laboratory can be important. Similarly, nonculture methods for identifying the presence of parvovirus B19 (e.g., demonstration by electron microscopy or gene probe) have helped us learn more about this organism as a cause of HAIs [32].

Anaerobic culture of specimens should be limited to (1) those that show leukocytes on Gram stain, (2) those with no evidence of contaminating squamous cells and organisms suggestive of anaerobic species, and (3) specimens from patients whose unusual circumstances suggest the need for anaerobic culture. These limitations result in the reporting of isolates that have a much higher probability of association with infection. The application of sensitive techniques for culturing and identifying anaerobes to specimens containing endogenous flora is costly and produces misleading information [33]. Large numbers of anaerobic organisms are present in the normal flora of skin, oral cavity, and genital and gastrointestinal tracts. Therefore, swabs from superficial portions of skin or mucous membrane lesions, specimens of expectorated sputum, and any materials contaminated with feces should be considered inappropriate for anaerobic culture [33]. Submission for anaerobic culture of such specimens or of specimens from sites that are rarely infected by anaerobes (e.g., urine) suggests the need for in-service education of hospital personnel.

Efforts such as those outlined substantially reduce errors in the diagnosis and use of unnecessary antimicrobial therapy. Such an approach also improves the specificity of infection surveillance data that otherwise might include isolates of questionable etiologic significance.

Identification of Isolates

Once a specimen has been received in the laboratory, it must be processed in a way that maximizes the likelihood of recovering older and newer agents causing HAIs. Often it is difficult to determine the causative

HAI agents. Recovery of an organism does not ensure that it is the causative HAI agent [25]; thus, etiologic diagnosis cannot be made with certainty in many instances. Most episodes today for which the cause is known involve gram-positive cocci or gram-negative aerobic bacilli [17,18]. Most frequent among these gram-negative rods are *Klebsiella, Enterobacter, Pseudomonas, Serratia, Proteus,* or *Escherichia coli* (in approximately that order) (see Chapter 29). More recently, organisms such as *Acinetobacter Flavobacterium, Legionella,* and *Pseudomonas* species other than *P. aeruginosa* have become increasingly prominent.

Anaerobic bacterial organisms (usually found in mixed aerobic–anaerobic infections) have become less frequent in HAIs since the mid-1980s. However, viral agents (e.g., rotavirus), fungi, and parasites, such as *Pneumocystis* and *Toxoplasma*, have been identified as important causes of HAIs [17,18]. This expansion of the list of possible microbial pathogens for hospitalized patients has made it more difficult for both microbiologists and clinicians to deal effectively with HAIs. Effective handling of such problems requires the laboratory staff to keep up with the steadily emerging oganisms important in cross-infection and to implement and maintain culture and other techniques that bring these to light.

Need for Complete Identification

The degree to which organism identification routinely is carried can be important to HAI control efforts. Infection control personnel constantly are searching for evidence that a common organism has spread from patient to patient [4]. The ability to detect such an event is enhanced by identifying the organism at least to the level of species. Reporting of "biotyping" information (i.e., pattern of response to biochemical testing) on occasion can be of value in differentiating organisms that are frequently encountered, but this identification is not needed on a routine basis [16].

In today's environment of cost controls, the value of complete identification of all isolates is questionable [34]. Regardless of the extent to which full identification is conducted, it is important that standard criteria and nomenclature be consistently applied. Otherwise, attack rates for HAIs with various species may identify false problems (e.g., because of previously unreported species or strains) or fail to identify true problems. Furthermore, such surveillance data may not be comparable to data developed in other institutions or in cooperative surveillance programs.

Even more important, incomplete or incorrect identification of organisms may obscure real problems and make retrospective epidemiologic investigation impossible. For example, a report of "*Klebsiella Enterobacter* group" fails to distinguish between two species (*Klebsiella* or *Enterobacter spp.*) that have different epidemiologic patterns of infection within the hospital [35]. Similarly, identifying an isolate as *Burkholderia cepacia* (formerly *Pseudomonas cepacia*), an organism frequently associated with illness or pseudoepidemics caused by contaminated water or other solutions [36], provides more useful epidemiologic information than identifying the organism only as "nonfermenting gram-negative bacillus," in which the strain is lumped with a group of organisms that may not have as characteristic a hospital reservoir.

Because of these considerations, laboratories should maintain the capability to identify gram-negative aerobic bacilli to the genus level. The laboratory also should have the capability to identify organisms to the species level when special or recurring problems in a given institution make such information useful for dealing with HAI problems.

Many hospitals find it advantageous to use commercial, multiple test media for biochemical testing that provide this degree of characterization. Acceptable methods for microbiologic identification procedures are described in detail elsewhere [37]; additional assistance in identifying unusual isolates beyond the stated expertise of an individual laboratory is available from state, national, or private reference laboratories.

Sometimes it is the pattern of susceptibility to antimicrobials that discriminates epidemiologically significant organisms from other apparently similar hospital organisms. For example, many U.S. hospitals encounter HAIs due to *Enterococcus* strains resistant to vancomycin [38]. Such organisms can be the subject of infection control activities only if the laboratory maintains effective and efficient means for their identification [39].

Need for Accuracy and Consistency

Many spurious outbreaks have been traced to inaccurate or inconsistent microbiologic procedures. An "outbreak" of *S. aureus* infection, for example, may be caused by delayed reading of coagulase tests, resulting in misidentification of coagulase-negative organisms as coagulase positive. Unfortunately, most of the available rapid tests identify organisms that are not common HAI pathogens. The challenge, therefore, remains to develop rapid testing methods for the organisms closely associated with HAI (especially staphylococci, enterococci, and gram-negative aerobic bacilli). Recently, such tests for these organisms using rapid selective media or PCR have become available.

Performance characteristics (e.g., sensitivity, specificity, reproducibility) of some of the rapid tests for identification of hospital pathogens are not good [40]. This means that the rapid tests are used only as an adjunct to other testing. Some of these tests tend to *increase* care costs rather than decrease them, and their utility is not clear. Improving test methodology will be essential if tests such as these are to assume a strong role in infection control [41].

The renaming of organisms that result from more precise knowledge of organism relationships also can cause confusion for HAI personnel. For example, the renaming as *Xanthomonas maltophilia* of the emerging nosocomial pathogen formerly called *Pseudomonas maltophilia* gave false

alarm to institutions not used to seeing or dealing with what appeared to be a new intruder [42]. That organism now has again been renamed as *Stenotrophomonas maltophilia*. This constant effort to be more and more precise in taxonomy is less desirable in the era of managed care, and some now question the practice of slavish adherence to taxonomic and nomenclatural changes in the clinical setting [34].

Introduction of New Procedures

The laboratory also must consider whether additional laboratory techniques can make testing results more relevant. For example, cultures of intravenous catheter tips may become positive because of contamination at the time of catheter removal or from the intravascular device becoming contaminated. Several semiquantitative and quantitative methods for culture of intravenous catheters [43] have been shown to be useful in distinguishing between these possibilities (see Chapter 37). Similar claims of usefulness have been made for cultures of other fluids, burn wounds (see Chapter 36), or surgical wounds (see Chapter 35). It is not clear that these special techniques generate useful information.

Quality Control

Just as an effective clinical microbiology laboratory is essential to an effective infection control program, adequate quality control is essential to the practice of good clinical microbiology [31]. Such a quality control program begins with a comprehensive procedure manual that establishes standards for performance, including the definition of acceptable and unacceptable quality of specimens and specimen containers, permissible delay between collection and receipt of the specimen in the laboratory, and times during which specimens are accepted for processing. The action to be taken by workers when specimens are not in accord with these standards also must be defined. These standards should be communicated to clinicians and nurses and to laboratory personnel.

The procedure manual also should cover administrative aspects of laboratory operation related to infection control and employee safety [44]. Minimum standards for identification of isolates, including a list of the equipment and reagents to be monitored and the measures to be made to ensure reproducible and accurate performance, should be provided. The periodic evaluation of skills of all employees, including evening, night, and weekend workers, should be included in the program.

Participating in proficiency testing programs helps the laboratory maintain competence, particularly if proficiency test specimens are submitted to the laboratory in a blinded fashion and are handled by routine procedures [45]. If problems develop with such an evaluation, the identity of the problem specimens should be made known and the personnel challenged to deal with the specimen in a fashion as careful as possible to ensure that the laboratory actually has within its capability the correct handling and identification procedures for the organisms.

In addition to such outcome-oriented projects, periodic review of selected laboratory materials, media, and other equipment should be performed. On occasion, erroneous microbiologic results related to the inadvertent use of contaminated or faulty materials may occur. For example, an epidemic of pseudomeningitis was traced to contamination of funnels and an automated Gram-staining apparatus [46]. Such "pseudo-outbreaks" must be considered when laboratory culture or stain results do not correlate with clinical or epidemiologic findings.

Hospital-supported continuing education is essential for high-quality work in the microbiology laboratory. It is especially important for personnel in smaller hospital laboratories to stay abreast of technologic advances and trends in HAI occurrence and diagnosis [9]. Fortunately, a number of organizations, including the American Society for Microbiology, the Association for Professionals in Infection Control, the Society for Healthcare Epidemiology of America, and the American Society of Clinical Pathologists, provide frequent programs on HAI topics.

ACCURATE CHARACTERIZATION OF ANTIMICROBIAL SUSCEPTIBILITY OF HEALTHCARE-ASSOCIATED INFECTION PATHOGENS

A standardized method of antimicrobial susceptibility testing subject to quality control evaluation is essential in any clinical microbiology laboratory and is equally critical to infection control studies. Occasionally, an epidemiologist suspects that a group of HAIs with organisms of the same species have a common origin. To investigate whether strains in this cluster are common or different, the usual practice is to examine results of speciation, biochemical tests, and the pattern of susceptibility to antimicrobial agents [4]. Often these results answer the question of relationships. Occasionally, additional tests are needed; these are described in a later section of this chapter.

New patterns of antimicrobial resistance have been characteristic of the organisms causing HAIs in the recent past (see Chapters 14, 15, 40). Organisms that had been consistently susceptible to older antimicrobials have developed resistance to these drugs, and some HAI pathogens have developed resistance to new antimicrobials almost as soon as the drugs were marketed [47]. Methicillin-resistant *S. aureus* (see Chapter 14, 40) or coagulase-negative strains are involved in HAIs nationwide [48]. Enterococci have increased in importance as HAI pathogens; some of these strains have become resistant to aminoglycoside and β-lactam drugs that had been the drugs of choice for treatment of serious infection due to this organism. Since the 1990s, strains of enterococci resistant to vancomycin

(see Chapter 14, 40) have become widespread in many healthcare settings [49]. *Enterobacteriaceae*, a common source of HAIs, have developed resistance to some of the newer β-lactam and fluoroquinolone antibiotics. The sequential appearance and persistence of these resistant organisms suggests spread of the resistant organisms within the hospital [35].

Several of these current resistance patterns require new or modified laboratory techniques for detection. For example, detection of vancomycin-resistant *S. aureus* requires several modifications of susceptibility testing techniques and is especially a problem for automated systems of detection [50]. Vancomycin-resistant enterococcal (VRE) strains also require special means for identifying resistance, and for these organisms, automated detection systems are less reliable [49]. Detection of high-level aminoglycoside resistance in enterococci also presents challenges [51]. Detection of resistance to newer cephalosporins, ureidopenicillins, or β-lactamase inhibitor compounds in enterobacteriaceal strains poses special problems as well, although the role of automated testing systems seems more secure [52].

Many laboratories use the Kirby-Bauer disk agar-diffusion method or an equivalent test system for routine testing of antimicrobial susceptibility of bacteria [53]. However, many other laboratories routinely perform a more quantitative evaluation of sensitivity, using broth-dilution or agar-dilution test methods [53]. In addition, tube dilution, E-test, or other methods of establishing minimum inhibitory concentration or susceptibility to "gate" concentrations of antibiotics must be used for testing organisms that have not been standardized for testing by a disk method. The latter include a number of anaerobic bacteria, fungi, or yeasts. Other sources may be consulted for detailed discussion of the performance and quality control of these procedures [37,54].

Some microorganisms can be additionally differentiated by indicating the relative degree to which susceptibility or resistance to antimicrobials is present [4]. This can be done by noting the absolute value of zone size in agar-diffusion testing or by providing assessment of minimum inhibitory concentration. Situations in which this more quantitative information would be useful should be delineated jointly by the laboratory and infection control team.

Selection of Strains for Susceptibility Testing

Applications of susceptibility tests to bacteria that are doubtfully related to infection must be avoided, and the laboratory should establish specific guidelines for the selection of isolates for susceptibility determination. For example, the request for testing of susceptibility should be carefully evaluated when the organisms isolated are endogenous flora present at sites in which they are not normally pathogens. Similarly, testing organisms from mixed culture should be avoided in most instances because of the unclear role of the various isolates [33]. Direct testing of urine and spinal fluid is not essential in most instances. Potential pathogens with well-established susceptibility to antimicrobials (e.g., *Streptococcus pyogenes* to penicillin) should not be tested routinely.

Selection of Drugs for Routine and Special Testing

The laboratory should undertake the selection of drugs for routine testing after consultation with the infection control committee and the pharmacy and therapeutics committee; the chosen agents should reflect both the common usage practices of physicians in the hospital and the spectrum of pathogens that are frequently encountered [55]. Occasionally, testing of susceptibility to certain drugs is performed for epidemiologic purposes; results of such testing may be omitted from routine clinical reporting. Similarly, certain antimicrobials for which the hospital wishes to control usage may be tested but not reported routinely or tested only after consultation.

Different groups of antimicrobials often are used for gram-negative or gram-positive aerobic organisms. Drugs included in each panel should be periodically evaluated and updated. The epidemiologic value of susceptibility patterns may be enhanced by inclusion of certain antibiotics that are not in routine clinical use. Such additional information also can provide valuable taxonomic and quality-control information, but these benefits must be weighed against the extra time and cost required for testing and recording of the additional studies.

For some of the newer HAI pathogens, susceptibility testing methods are not very good. For example, susceptibility testing methods for fungi do not correlate well with clinical outcome [56]. Thus, another challenge is the need to develop susceptibility testing methods for some of the newer organisms closely associated with HAIs, especially gram-negative nonfermentive bacilli, fungi, or viruses.

Quality Control

Consistent and accurate identification of organisms over time is necessary for susceptibility data to be useful for clinical and epidemiologic purposes. In addition, errors in performance of susceptibility tests may result in information that is misleading about therapy. To minimize this possibility, detailed quality control procedures must be maintained for all elements of the susceptibility testing process [53,54]. Special attention must be given to the storage of reagents, control of batch-to-batch variation in media, use of control strains for testing, and monitoring of incubation temperatures and atmosphere. When results of these quality control tests exceed acceptable limits, reports on clinical isolates should be withheld until satisfactory control results are obtained. The reproducibility of susceptibility tests also can be assessed by participation in quality-control programs of groups such as the College of American Pathologists and the

Centers for Disease Control and Prevention (CDC), which periodically distribute unknown specimens for evaluation. Such testing programs focus on clinically and epidemiologically important strains; correct identification assures the laboratory and infection control personnel that the laboratory applies proper techniques and skills.

TIMELY REPORTING OF LABORATORY DATA AND PARTICIPATION IN SURVEILLANCE OF HEALTHCARE-ASSOCIATED INFECTION

To deal with individual problems of HAIs in the hospital as they arise, control measures must be taken as quickly as possible and must be based on accurate assessments of the problems and their causes [4]. Without rapid identification and reporting of the organisms involved, control measures cannot be efficiently designed and implemented.

Laboratory records represent an important tool for infection control professionals (ICPs) [7]. Development of computerized laboratory information systems has progressed rapidly, and this has led to major improvements in several ways that the laboratory can provide infection control information [57].

Surveillance

Laboratory records are an important tool for the surveillance of HAIs [7]. More than 80% of infections defined by other criteria as nosocomial may be identified by review of positive cultures from the microbiology laboratory. Review of laboratory records is the most common method for surveillance of hospital infection carried out in the United States. Therefore, data gathered by ICPs during laboratory visits form an important base to which additional surveillance data from clinical rounds must be added. Both sources must be used to obtain an accurate estimate of the true rate of HAI occurrence in a given hospital (see Chapter 5, 6).

For both endemic and epidemic HAIs, microbiologic and immunologic reports may be the starting point for additional epidemiologic investigations. These investigations often require information about attributes of the patient, the personnel involved in care, and/or the diagnostic and therapeutic procedures provided to the patient. Obtaining these nonlaboratory data usually is easier when the patient is still present in the hospital or at least is fresh in the minds of hospital personnel. Promptly reporting pertinent laboratory results facilitates information retrieval of this type.

Computer programs have been developed to identify clusters of infections with the same organism and susceptibilities that occur at the same time in the same patient care area (ward or service) [58]. Such programs have permitted identification of outbreaks; whether they provide such information in rapid enough fashion to permit the use of control measures remains open to question [59].

The laboratory can indicate only which organisms were present in culture. The epidemiologist or ICP must supplement this information with clinical data to determine whether organisms found in culture indicate infection or colonization [15]. If colonization is present, the identification of organisms in the culture may be of little help to the clinician (but important for infection control). To the epidemiologist, however, both the organisms involved in episodes of exogenous colonization and those of infection are of interest. Either may be evidence of the spread of organisms from one site to another, indicating an area in which control measures may halt transmission. Data used for this purpose must be accurate, which emphasizes the role of continuing quality control studies in the laboratory.

Reporting of Results

To facilitate HAI surveillance of all infections requiring isolation or notification of public health authorities, a copy of positive culture results should be provided to the infection control personnel. Physicians or nurses sometimes are lax about notifying public health authorities of reportable diseases. Isolation of such organisms is reported to health authorities more efficiently if the responsibility for reporting is delegated to the ICP or some other person designated by the infection control committee (see Chapter 5, 6, 12).

Availability of a computerized laboratory information system can make it possible for the laboratory routinely to produce frequent and tailored reports for the ICP (see Chapter 5). For example, such a report is generated at the start of each day at Grady Memorial Hospital [7]. The report lists selected positive cultures and immunologic tests from the previous day sorted by ward in the order in which each practitioner makes daily rounds. The *only* culture results selected and printed on this report are those specified as relevant by the ICP. This maintains a relatively concise report while ensuring that the ICP has access to all information of current interest. The list of results to be selected is changed on a periodic basis to make sure that current needs are addressed (e.g., when the name of an organism has changed or when a new HAI pathogen has arisen at the institution).

Prompt reporting by telephone to both clinicians and infection control personnel is essential when presumptive identification of isolates of nosocomial significance is made; this is the only way to ensure proper treatment of the patient and the application of proper infection control precautions [60]. Occasions for reporting include incidents such as the presumptive identification of certain agents in meningitis, isolation of *Salmonellae* or *Shigellae* spp. from stool specimens, positive smears or cultures of *Mycobacterium tuberculosis* bacilli from any patient or employee, or isolation of *S. aureus* from lesions of a newborn or other nursery patient.

Laboratory studies may provide early warning of the emergence within a hospital of highly infectious microorganisms, multidrug-resistant organisms, or clusters of unusual infections. In some hospitals, laboratory workers may be the first to detect these and other trends of infection. When findings suggest a possible outbreak, notification requires quicker action than a final report because rapid epidemiologic investigations triggered by the first preliminary data from the laboratory often are profitable. The major elements needed in any early warning are the interest and expertise of the laboratory worker in calling results to the attention of infection control colleagues. This may be done by telephone, pager, computer, or e-mail if urgent; if not, discussion during the daily visit of the infection control staff usually suffices.

Such reporting facilitates the efforts of the infection control personnel. At the same time, early warning must not be requested for so many situations that this becomes an unreasonable burden on laboratory personnel. The key is consultation between laboratory and infection control personnel to establish which findings need to be given critical-value status [60].

Laboratory Records

In addition to instituting control measures, infection control workers often need to analyze laboratory data from various periods to try to detect patterns of infection [4]. To assist in this effort, it is helpful if the laboratory can provide an archival summary of organisms on a periodic basis. Data of particular usefulness might include compiled listings of organisms by culture site, date, patient, and ward; a summary of susceptibility testing results for various species of organisms for given time periods might also be helpful. Computer storage and retrieval of all results can aid this process considerably. Some newer laboratory information systems permit downloading of information pertinent to infection control to a desktop computer [59]. Then these data can be used both by the laboratory and in infection control if these departments have a compatible desktop computer. The specific laboratory data that can aid epidemiologic analyses vary from hospital to hospital. The information to be included and the frequency with which such summaries are made should be determined by the people providing and working with the data in each hospital.

Laboratory records should be retained in such a way that they facilitate such retrospective epidemiologic investigations and quality control activities. The source of each specimen, date of collection, patient identification, hospital number, hospital service, ward, and organisms identified in the final report should be recorded. Records of results of antimicrobial sensitivity tests and of any special biochemical or typing reactions also should be kept.

All cultures should be recorded so that results are readily available by date, type of specimen, and pathogens isolated. Culture data on inpatients and outpatients should be maintained separately. Computer storage and retrieval of all results is optimal [59]. These records also can be maintained in simple, inexpensive, and epidemiologically useful bound log books that are kept chronologically for each major type of specimen (e.g., blood, wound, skin, cerebrospinal fluid, urine, stool, sputum). Sole reliance on a filing system of loose laboratory slips is not desirable because specific data are difficult to retrieve and easily lost.

The permanent records of the microbiology laboratory should include dates and other details of any major changes in culturing techniques, tests used, or laboratory procedures. Dates of changes in the criteria for identification and taxonomic designations applied to isolates should be recorded as well.

Retention Period for Records

No analysis of previous data can be made if the records are not available. Thus, it is incumbent on the laboratory staff to maintain the microbiologic records in some accessible format (e.g., computer file, final report sheets, disk or tape storage) for a reasonable period. The length of time such records can be maintained depends on hospital size, laboratory work volume, available storage facilities, and infection control needs. Thus, storage time should be determined by laboratory personnel after consultation with the hospital infection control staff. One author considers 18 months to be a reasonable minimum [16]. With computer storage, it may be possible to maintain data for long periods.

Summary Reports for Clinical Use

Development of profiles for susceptibility of frequently tested pathogens to drugs commonly in use can be of considerable assistance in guiding therapy for sepsis of unclear cause and other infections. Testing other organisms (e.g., slow-growing bacteria or organisms requiring special test procedures) may be performed at intervals to develop a profile of their susceptibility. As long as susceptibility patterns can be presumed to remain stable, such testing may be a useful substitute for testing each isolate at the time of recovery.

These summaries of susceptibility patterns should be available to the medical staff on at least an annual basis [7]. In addition to the hospital epidemiologist (see Chapter 2), any or all of the infection control committee, medical staff committees, and quality assurance committee also should receive susceptibility summaries to guide their review of antibiotic use. The use of a laboratory information system to tabulate the data directly or to download the raw data to a desktop computer for calculation of results has eased the burden of performing this task by hand. The laboratory information system also can be used to provide information about proper use of antimicrobial agents [47]. Increasingly, laboratory data can be downloaded from computer files to infection control or other computer systems.

Tabulations that may be of particular use include frequency of susceptibility to individual drugs by site of infection or ward (which may provide guidance to the clinician for empiric therapy of infection before the causative organism has been identified) and tabulation of frequency of susceptibility to individual antimicrobials by pathogen (which may be used to direct therapy after an organism has been identified but before susceptibility tests have been completed) [58].

A list of the relative costs of the currently used antimicrobials may be developed with cooperation of the pharmacy; inclusion of this information with susceptibility summaries may increase the incentive to reduce costs of antimicrobial use [58].

ADDITIONAL STUDIES TO ESTABLISH SIMILARITY OR DIFFERENCE OF ORGANISMS

On occasion, the epidemiologist suspects that a group of HAIs with organisms of the same species have a common origin. Determining the features of the epidemiologic problem or testing certain hypotheses about reservoir or mode of spread may be aided if the laboratory can define whether the individual strains are related or unrelated to each other [4]. To investigate whether strains in this cluster are common or different, the usual initial practice is to examine results of speciation, biochemical tests, and pattern of susceptibility to antimicrobial agents. However, for organisms commonly encountered in the hospital (e.g., *S. aureus* or *Klebsiella*), the general pattern of these results may be similar by chance alone. Conversely, for other organisms (e.g., *P. aeruginosa*), the variation in these characteristics from strain to strain is so small that the tests provide little information about similarity or difference of tested strains. Testing of additional antimicrobials not ordinarily included or of susceptibility to other antibacterial substances (e.g., silver) may differentiate strains in some instances. Many times, however, these tests can show no differences. In these situations, examination ("typing") of additional organism characteristics (markers) can be of great assistance [61].

Although hospital laboratory personnel may not have the facilities to perform specialized typing procedures, they should know which organisms can be typed and which cannot and where specific procedures can be obtained. When epidemiologically important isolates require special typing, it may be necessary to forward them to public health or private reference laboratories. Potentially pathogenic materials should be packaged for air transport in conformance with federal regulations [62].

Methods for Typing of Isolates

A variety of techniques has been used for typing isolates [61]. Selected typing systems of special value in

TABLE 10-1

TYPING SYSTEMS FOR ORGANISMS CAUSING NOSOCOMIAL INFECTION: SOME PHENOTYPIC METHODS AND EXAMPLES OF USE FOR SPECIFIC ORGANISMS

  I. Pattern of susceptibility *to* antimicrobials ("antibiogram")
   Klebsiella [62]
   Legionella [63]
   MRSA [64]
   Pseudomonas aeruginosa [65]
 II. Pattern of susceptibility to heavy metals ("resistotyping")
   MRSA [66]
   Candida albicans [67]
III. Biotyping
   Serratia marcescens [68]
   Enterococci [69]
   Burkholderia cepacia [70]
 IV. Phage susceptibility ("phage typing")
   MRSA [64,71]
  V. Serotyping
   Klebsiella [72]
   Streptococcus agalactiae [73]
   Serratia [74]
   P. aeruginosa [65]
 VI. Bacteriocin production
   Enterobacter [75]
   Serratia [76]
VII. Immunoblotting
   MRSA—Southern blot hybridization after protein electrophoresis [77]
VIII. Multilocus enzyme electrophoresis
   S. agalactiae [73]
   Enterococci [78]
   Coagulase-negative staphylococci [79]

MRSA, methicillin-resistant *Staphylococcus aureus*.

TABLE 10-2

TYPING SYSTEMS FOR ORGANISMS CAUSING NOSOCOMIAL INFECTION: SOME GENOTYPIC METHODS AND EXAMPLES OF USE FOR SPECIFIC ORGANISMS

  I. Plasmid profile analysis ("fingerprinting")
   Serratia marcescens [74]
   Coagulase-negative staphylococci [80]
   Burkholderia cepacia [70]
 II. *Restriction* endonuclease analysis
   A. Restriction endonuclease analysis of plasmids
    MRSA [81] *Streptococcus pyogenes* [82]
   B. Restriction enzyme analysis of chromosomes
    Clostridium difficile [83]
III. Ribotyping
   S. marcescens [68]
   Legionella pneumophila [84]
   MRSA [85]
   Escherichia coil [86]
   B. cepacia [70]
 IV. Pulsed field gel electrophoresis
   Enterococci [69,87]
   L. pneumophila [88]
   MRSA [71,81,89]
   Pseudomonas aeruginosa [90]
   B. cepacia [70]
   Mycobacterium tuberculosis [91]
   A. Contour-clamped homogeneous electric field electrophoresis
   Enterococci [92]
   Candida lusitaniae [93]
  V. Analysis *of* nucleic acid amplification products
   A. DNA typing by repeated PCR assay
    Streptococcus pneumoniae [94]
    Citrobacter [95]
   B. Arbitrary primed PCR
    Acinetobacter [96]
    C. difficile [97]
    M. tuberculosis [98]
    B. cepacia [71]
    L. pneumophila [88]
    Stenotrophomonas maltophilia [99]
   C. Whole-cell repetitive extragenic PCR
    Acinetobacter [100]
   D. Random amplification of polymorphic DNA
    E. coli [86]
    Enterococci [87]
    Enterobacter [101]
    S. maltophilia [102]
    Aspergillus [103]
    Candida albicans [104]
 VI. Nucleotide sequence analysis
   Hepatitis B virus [105]

MRSA, methicillin-resistant *Staphylococcus aureus*; PCR, polymerase chain reaction.

investigating HAI problems are summarized in Tables 10-1 and 10-2. So many typing systems are being used today for so many organisms that only a few examples can be provided in the tables. Several reviews provide detailed descriptions of the procedures used for each [1,61]. Many are beyond the capabilities of the usual clinical laboratory, but a number can be conducted when circumstances dictate.

Although routine typing of all strains is not cost effective, some laboratories store selected isolates for later typing should it prove desirable. Some typing systems monitor changes in characteristics expressed by the microorganism (phenotype; see Table 10-1), and others analyze changes from organism to organism in chromosomal or extrachromosomal genetic elements (genotype; see Table 10-2). Each is considered in turn.

Phenotypic Techniques

A number of organisms involved in HAIs have been differentiated successfully by antimicrobial susceptibility testing. The pattern of resistance or susceptibility to

several different antimicrobials often is referred to as the "antibiogram" of the organism [106]. Test antimicrobials not in routine clinical use can be of assistance here [107]. However, the antibiogram of strains in the same clone can change over time [108]. Susceptibility to various chemicals, especially heavy metals (i.e., resistotyping), also has proved valuable in selected instances [67].

Biotyping is the use of certain characteristic biochemical reactions to identify subgroups of bacteria. Typing schemes using this method have been devised for a variety of bacterial organisms, both anaerobes and aerobes, and found to be useful in infection control investigations. The process can be simplified by automated performance and analysis by use of computerized methods [109]. Unfortunately, the biotype codes generated by many of the commercial identification systems are poorly reproducible [108]. The method is most useful when unusual biotypes characterize the HAI pathogen.

Bacteriophages are viruses that can kill certain bacteria by lysis. Susceptibility to bacteriophages (i.e., phage typing) is a characteristic used for typing a number of organisms of nosocomial importance. The technique has been useful for grouping strains of S. aureus. However, this procedure usually is available only in reference laboratories, and plasmid transfer of phage characteristics apparently can occur, so it has been replaced by genotypic techniques in most situations [72].

Serotyping is a technique used for typing many gram-negative aerobic bacilli, especially Klebsiella pneumoniae isolates [73]. The technique can be helpful for other organisms as well, in both outbreak situations and research investigations. However, when reagents are not readily available or when typing procedures are complex, the techniques are available only in referral laboratories.

Many bacteria produce products that can kill or inhibit the growth of other organisms. Production of such bacteriocins by an organism, or susceptibility of the organism in question to those produced by other bacteria, can be used as a typing tool for a number of organisms. However, the method requires careful use of controls; widespread agreement on standards for reagents and interpretation is unusual. In addition, reproducibility of results is a problem; all strains should be tested at the same time [110]. Thus, the method also has been supplanted in favor of genotypic procedures for most situations.

Electrophoretic typing of proteins results from isolating relevant proteins, separating them by protein agar gel electrophoresis, and staining the gel so that the resulting pattern can be observed. The individual enzymes present in a given organism vary in structure from those present in other organisms; this is reflected in their different mobility when subjected to electrophoresis. Separating these compounds by electrophoresis on a starch gel can provide information on variation in a number of different enzymes at the same time. Such testing is called multilocus enzyme electrophoresis. A variant of this is immunoblotting, in which a nitrocellulose membrane is used as a site for the application of antisera of various sorts.

Genotypic Techniques

Molecular and other, newer techniques have permitted more definitive typing of a wider range of organisms than ever before [61,111,112]. These methods have helped immeasurably in defining mode of spread, reservoirs, and asymptomatic and unsuspected sources of infection [113]. It is now clear that these techniques can provide an epidemiologic picture different from that of prior methods. In many instances, these techniques have supplanted the traditional phenotypic methods [114].

The simplest of these genetic techniques is the analysis of the plasmid profile of a given organism or group of organisms. Most bacterial species carry plasmids, which are extrachromosomal pieces of DNA that encode a variety of genes. After isolation, plasmids are separated by electrophoresis and the pattern (number and size) of the plasmids from different organisms are compared (so-called fingerprinting). Of course, if an organism has few or no plasmids, this technique provides little assistance. In addition, the rapid pace of gain or loss of plasmids by a single organism and the frequent exchange of plasmids between different organisms makes interpretation of this technique difficult [61,115].

Both plasmids and chromosomal DNA can be subdivided further for typing purposes by using restriction endonuclease enzymes that divide the genetic material into smaller fragments. The fragments then can be separated by agar gel electrophoresis and compared as a further fingerprinting step. The bacterial chromosome usually contains some regions that are variable and other regions that are quite similar among different strains of the same species ("conserved"). The regions with different nucleotide sequence result in different patterns in the agarose gel for different organisms. These are known as restriction fragment length polymorphisms. Plasmid evaluation by this method usually is simpler than that for chromosomal DNA. The utility of this technique for analysis of chromosomal elements is subject to confounding by presence of DNA in plasmids and may be difficult to interpret because of the number and variety of patterns produced.

Ribotyping is the use of ribosomal RNA as a probe to detect variations in the DNA sequences associated with ribosomal operons [111]. Although most genes are present in bacteria in single copies, ribosomal operon genes are unique in that they are present in multiple copies. This makes analysis easier. In addition, only a small section of the genome is being examined, so a small number of bands are produced in the analysis. These are easier to analyze than the huge number of fragments that result from analysis of the whole chromosome. However, ribosomal gene patterns are relatively stable within a given species, so the ability to discriminate between or among epidemiologic isolates may be hindered to a certain degree [61].

Pulsed-field gel electrophoresis also begins with lysis of organisms and digestion of their chromosomal DNA with restriction endonucleases [114]. However, the restriction fragments are resolved into a pattern of discrete bands in the gel by switching the direction of current. The number and size of fragments from different organisms then are compared. This alteration of electric field more readily allows resolution of large DNA molecules. The method allows typing of a broad range of bacteria. A hindrance is that there are no standardized criteria for analyzing the fragment patterns; however, consensus approaches are being proposed [114].

A variant of pulsed-field gel electrophoresis is contour-clamped homogeneous electric field electrophoresis. It is used primarily to compare large chromosomal DNA fragments [1]. DNA is separated by subjecting the molecules alternately to perpendicular electric fields. The high-molecular-weight DNA then can be subjected to agarose gel electrophoresis or digested by restriction endonucleases. Bacteria, yeast, and mycobacteria can be studied using this approach.

Amplification techniques like PCR are widely used in characterizing HAI pathogens [116]. Analysis of the products of such amplification can provide information on organism typing. By enhancing the number of target molecules by several logs of concentration, the study of the variability of the individual targets is enhanced. However, specialized equipment and personnel are needed to conduct this procedure, and this is a major problem for many hospitals [117].

Variations using amplification methods are emerging constantly. One is the use of repeated PCR assay aimed at different parts of small sections of a genome. Arbitrary primed PCR assays are variations of the amplification technique using short primers whose nucleotide sequence is not directed at a known genetic site [100]. These result in amplification of unpredictable loci and generate a set of restriction fragments that can be compared for different isolates. Because the discriminatory power of the assay is not clear, interpretation of these tests depends even more strongly than usual on the correlation with epidemiologic data.

There has been a dramatic recent increase in methods and equipment for analyzing the exact nucleotide sequence of microbes. It now is technically possible to compare multiple isolates by sequencing the same genetic site from all [61]. Differences in content and arrangement of nucleotides are being used for epidemiologic typing studies [106]. Further work is needed to define the exact role that such techniques should play in cost-effective epidemiologic analysis.

Choosing Typing Systems

Although the potential benefit of these new techniques for hospital infection control is great, some cautions are needed regarding their use [4,114,118]. Sometimes the new systems for analysis have impeded rather than aided in outbreak investigations. For example, some investigations

produce conflicting results from typing studies carried out by different techniques [72]. Incorrect results also may arise from contamination of reagents, a special concern with use of PCR, with which sensitivity is so great that the chance of contamination is high [119]. Some typing methods provide data of doubtful value or results that are difficult to interpret for a given epidemiologic situation [120]. To improve these, further information is needed to evaluate their validity as a tool for infection control [4]. Some have suggested that in analyzing subgroups of clonal organisms, it is necessary to use at least two typing methods [72,115].

Even if the methods are valid, overinterpretation, or underinterpretation of the results is a potential problem. Typing never proves that organisms are the same [61]. On the other hand, the use of too many individual markers in several typing methods can cause problems as well [121]. For example, use of 20 different antibiotics in typing a series of specimens in which organisms are defined as different if their pattern of susceptibility varies by more than one drug almost guarantees that organisms that actually are part of the outbreak will be identified as different and thus considered unrelated [4].

Results from some typing methods may be redundant; if so, this needs to be discovered so that the less expensive methods can be used. An important question for current investigation should be not whether new tests provide additional discrimination but how much discriminating ability they add to readily available tests [122]. For example, in a study of infections with coagulase-negative staphylococci, antibiogram, biotyping, phage typing, and plasmid profiling all were performed. The antibiogram, selected as the first stage of the scheme because it was the simplest and cheapest test, proved to be the most discriminatory stage, providing 66% of the discriminating ability between strains [123].

A related issue is how often most hospitals really need these newer techniques. Most of them are used for research (detailing routes of transmission or reservoirs of organisms) rather than for acting on outbreaks. For most of the newer molecular testing methods, instruments and reagents are not readily available and have yet to be widely automated [117]. The expertise to perform and interpret the tests is not widespread, and standards are lacking for most assays [117]. In addition, outbreak organisms rarely are all isolated at once, so typing procedures are performed at separate times; the need for control of batch-to-batch variation in media, reagents, phages, and so on is especially crucial with many of these typing procedures. These considerations explain why many newer typing procedures should not be performed in the routine clinical laboratory [117]. Thus, not every laboratory must be able to perform every, or even most, of these tests. The laboratory director must be aware of the available tests, determine which can be performed on-site when needed, and identify referral laboratories (e.g., colleague, state, private) where other methods are available on request.

Storage of Strains

For supplemental tests to be performed, such as those described in the preceding section, the organisms must be available. Thus, a related duty of the clinical laboratory staff is to retain strains that may relate to HAIs for a given period while it is determined whether additional testing is needed. In cooperation with infection control personnel, the laboratory staff should subculture and save epidemiologically important isolates, whether such isolates are from outbreaks or from single instances of unusual or potentially epidemic diseases. Isolates may be conveniently and inexpensively stored by placing a small amount of growth on a blank paper disk that is placed in a 2-ml glass screw-cap vial containing a few granules of silica gel. If the vial is kept tightly closed, isolates may be held up to 6 months; they can then be easily retrieved by placing the disk in broth.

A system for reviewing and periodically discarding these isolates also must be established. How long a storage period is required for this purpose varies from hospital to hospital and should be agreed on between epidemiologist and clinical laboratory director. The technique used to ensure the viability of the organisms (e.g., freezing, lyophilization) should be determined by the laboratory staff after considering the equipment and personnel that are available for this task.

OCCASIONAL MICROBIOLOGIC STUDIES OF HOSPITAL PERSONNEL OR ENVIRONMENT

In some situations, HAIs may result from environmental or personnel sources. In evaluating such episodes, the infection control staff may ask the laboratory staff to process specimens from employees, environmental sources, or hospital equipment (e.g., respiratory therapy machines) as part of the investigation [4]. Such environmental culturing, however, should focus on investigation of documented infections in patients (see Chapters 7, 19) [2]. When such culturing is necessary, its costs should be considered part of the hospitals' infection control program, and charges for the cultures should not be billed to the patients involved in the outbreak.

A few procedures of this type should be done routinely (Table 10-3). Others are elective, performed in association with episodes of patient illness or as part of an educational program. A third group is specifically not recommended. Each is dealt with in turn.

Routine Environmental Sampling

Surveillance cultures of the hospital environment and personnel once were advocated on a routine basis. During the 1970s, studies found these programs to be of minimal

TABLE 10-3
MICROBIOLOGIC STUDIES OF HOSPITAL PERSONNEL AND THE HOSPITAL ENVIRONMENT

Recommended for routine performance

Monitoring sterilization
   Steam sterilizers
   Ethylene oxide sterilizers
   Dry heat sterilizers
   Flash sterilizers (but no standard method)
   Sampling infant formula prepared in the hospital and other
     specific high-risk hospital-prepared products
Monitoring dialysis fluid
Elective environmental monitoring
Surveys to investigate a specific problem of patient infection
Surveys for educational purposes

Procedures not recommended

Routine culture surveys of patients or hospital personnel
Routine culture of commercial products labeled as sterile
Routine testing of antiseptics and disinfectants
Routine culture of blood units
Routine monitoring of disinfection process for respiratory
   therapy equipment

value in infection control; by 1980, most institutions took the approach that routine environmental culturing should be severely limited. Since then, limiting cultures of the environment has become even more imperative because of changes in the economics of healthcare in the United States. Fortunately, further studies have supported this selective approach [124]. Close communication between epidemiologist and microbiologist about the need for such cultures continues to be essential to keep from wasting valuable resources.

In the absence of an epidemic, sampling should be minimal; microbiology and infection control personnel should be firm in not conducting indiscriminate routine microbiologic sampling and testing (see Chapter 7, 19) [2]. However, routine checks on the adequacy of sterilizer function, culture of dialysis infusates and the water used to prepare them, and culture of infant formula and some other products prepared in the hospital may help prevent infections from these sources (Table 10-3).

Monitoring of Sterilization

All steam sterilizers should be checked at least once each week with a suitable live-spore preparation [125]; if sterilization is performed less often, testing should be done on each day that sterilization is done (see Chapters 19, 20). Ethylene oxide gas sterilizers should be checked with each load of items that come into contact with blood or other tissues. In addition, each load in either type of sterilizer should be monitored with a spore test if it contains implantable objects. These implantable objects should not be used until the spore test is reported as negative, usually at 48 hours of incubation. Dry-heat sterilizers should be monitored at least once each month [125].

The process of flash sterilization is used when contaminated items will be needed again in a short period of time. This time requirement makes the use of biologic indicator testing impractical [126]. This means that this method of sterilization is not feasible for items that are to be implanted in patients. Products for monitoring flash sterilization are being evaluated, but no consensus exists for the way they should be used. Likewise, low-temperature sterilization technologies are being developed to replace ethylene oxide use; these include vaporized hydrogen peroxide, gas plasmas, ozone, and chlorine dioxide [127]. Some progress has been made in developing biologic indicators for these newer systems [128], but no consensus yet exists. Developing these standard testing systems should remain a high priority.

All sterilizers should be equipped with time–temperature recorders to provide evidence of adequate exposure for each load. However, evidence that a sterilizing temperature has been held for an adequate time does not prove that sterilization took place; the temperature is measured at the outlet valve and does not reflect whether adequate sterilization occurred within dense volumes of fluid or large, dense, fabric-wrapped packs. The use of chemical monitors (e.g., test tapes or heat-sensitive color indicators) within the autoclave is recommended for the outside of each package sterilized [125]. This provides an indication that a sterilizing temperature may have been reached, although such monitors do not show whether there was an adequate duration of exposure. Therefore, additional monitoring systems are required, which ordinarily involve the laboratory: Biologic monitoring with spore strips generally has been accepted as the most effective way to determine successful sterilization (see Chapters 19, 20).

Microorganisms chosen for spore strip tests are more resistant to sterilization than are most naturally occurring pathogens. The test organisms are provided in relatively high concentrations to ensure a margin of safety. The spores may be provided either in impregnated filter paper strips or in solution in glass ampules. For steam sterilization, the thermophile *Bacillus stearothermophilus* is used, and for ethylene oxide and dry-heat sterilizers, *Bacillus subtilis* (var. *niger*) is used. Both species frequently are incorporated simultaneously in the test strips, and these can be used to test for adequate sterilization with either procedure.

Most spore strip preparations are packaged in envelopes that contain one or two test strips and a control strip. The test strips are packaged in separate envelopes and are removed and sterilized at the time other material is processed. Subsequently, the test strips and control strip are cultured by placing the strips in tubes of tryptic-digest casein-soy (TS) broth that are incubated at 37°C (99°F) for

B. subtilis and 56°C (133°F) for *B. stearothermophilus*. It is not necessary to culture a positive control strip for each test; if strips are obtained from a single lot, only 10% of the positive control strips need be tested.

Spore solutions are prepared in sealed glass ampules for testing the adequacy of sterilization fluids. These ampules should be incubated at 56°C (133°F) in a water bath. If there is no change in the indicator by 7 days, the test is reported as negative. Alternatively, the fluid may be inoculated with a test culture, which may be subcultured after autoclaving.

Other types of spore preparations are commercially available and require different handling. In each case, the manufacturer's directions should be followed closely.

Test strips or spore solutions should always be placed in the center of the specimen to be tested, never on an open shelf in the autoclave. The center of a pack located near the bottom front exhaust valve will be exposed for the least adequate duration and temperature of sterilization and thus provides the best location for a test measurement. Testing the sterilization of fluids is accomplished by placing an ampule containing a spore solution in the largest vessel.

Use of ampules containing spore solutions is not appropriate for checking sterilization of microbiologic culture media because these media do not require the duration of exposure that is required for sterilization of material known to contain large populations of bacteria. Heating bacteriologic culture media to a temperature sufficient to ensure the sterilization of a test strip or spore ampule results in damage to the medium through overheating.

The likelihood of cross-contamination can be reduced by minimizing the handling of the strip after sterilization. Test strips can be removed from their envelopes and placed in sterile glass tubes before sterilization. The tube then is sterilized with the screw-cap removed or with other closures permeable to steam in place. After sterilization, the tube is sent to the laboratory, where the nutrient broth is added.

The handling of spore strips in the laboratory requires considerable care to prevent secondary contamination. The transfer should be made in a laminar-flow cabinet if available using sterile forceps and scissors. The forceps and scissors are common sources of contamination, which may be insufficiently sterilized by flaming or wiping with alcohol. Alcohol may contain viable spores that might not be killed by flaming, and flaming may be insufficient to heat instruments to a temperature that destroys viable spores. Care should be taken not to cross-contaminate the sterilized spore strips with the control strips.

Condensation on the cover of a 56°C (133°F) water bath may cause contamination of the caps and closures of tubes. A heating block may be used to avoid this, or the bath may be left uncovered; the latter makes it necessary to provide a reservoir to maintain the water level because the evaporation rate is high at this temperature. Uninoculated culture media should be incubated at 35°C (95°F) or at

56°C (133°F) to ensure that contamination does not yield false-positive reports.

Gram staining and subculturing should be performed to detect secondary contamination of test cultures. If organisms other than gram-positive bacilli are observed, the test should be repeated and reported as "possible laboratory contamination, test being repeated."

Whenever positive results are obtained, the sterilizers should be checked immediately for proper use and function. Careful examination must be made of thermometer and pressure gauge readings, and recent time and temperature records must be reviewed. If any deficiency is observed or if the repeat sterility test still results in growth, engineering personnel and experts in autoclave maintenance and function should be consulted promptly. Objects other than those used for implants do not need to be recalled at this point unless defects are discovered in the sterilizer or its use; if spore tests remain positive after proper use of the sterilizer is documented, the machine should be removed from service until the defects are corrected (see Chapter 20).

Sampling of Infant Formula and Other Food Products Prepared in the Hospital

Few hospitals still prepare their own infant formula. However, infant formula prepared in the hospital kitchen should be monitored on a weekly basis [129]. A guideline for interpreting culture suggests that <25 organisms per milliliter be present and that no virulent bacteria, such as *Salmonella* or *Shigella spp.*, be present [129]. The guideline is an arbitrary one, however, and should be a matter of local preference.

On occasion, other food products prepared in hospitals are considered as potential sources for HAI. Extensive guidelines for appropriate culture techniques have been developed [130] and should be consulted as necessary.

Culture of Blood Components

The American Association of Blood Banks [131] does not recommend routine sterility culturing of transfusion components. Likewise, surveillance bacterial cultures are not recommended for specific transfusion practices (e.g., exchange transfusions for neonates) [132].

Culture of Dialysis Fluid

The water used for preparing dialysis fluid should be tested by colony count at least once per month. Guidelines of the Association for Advancement of Medical Instrumentation [133] specify that the water used to prepare dialysis fluid and water used to rinse and reprocess dialyzers should contain <200 viable organisms per milliliter, and the dialysate <2,000 colony-forming units (cfu) per milliliter. Defined methods for such testing vary from one regulatory body to the next; in general, the correlation between the specified levels and occurrence of patient disease is poor. Counts obtained vary markedly with media and conditions of incubation [134] (see Chapter 24).

Periodic Sampling of Disinfected Equipment

Any article that makes direct contact with the vascular system or tissue other than unbroken skin should be sterile. Whenever possible, steam or gas sterilization should be applied. If chemical disinfection or pasteurization, rather than sterilization, is used on equipment such as cystoscopes, other endoscopes, or anesthesia equipment, some authorities recommend (and some require) that periodic microbiologic sampling be done to ensure the absence of pathogens after processing. Methods and equipment for testing have been specified [134].

The frequency of sampling such disinfected devices depends on any evidence that HAIs are associated with their use and an assessment by the infection control committee of the adequacy of standards for control of contamination of such equipment. There is little agreement on which items of this type should be tested or how often. If such a monitoring program is begun, it may be possible to cut back the frequency of culturing after a period of time in which cultures are negative as long as no changes are made in equipment and techniques used.

Infections have resulted from contamination of transplant materials such as bone marrow during processing [135]. Thus, on occasion, local or regional regulations require routine culture of transplant organs or tissues (e.g., eye, bone, allografts, porcine heart valves), laminar flow hoods, or pharmacy admixture solutions.

Elective Environmental Monitoring

A wide variety of items and substances can be responsible for cross-infection. Thus, environmental surveys may be useful during the investigation of specific problems within a hospital and should be instituted in response to, and specifically address, epidemiologic findings [4]. For example, microbiologic assessment of foods may be needed during investigation of suspected foodborne illness in the hospital setting [136]. Elective culturing programs may also be instituted in association with educational efforts.

Support for Investigation of Specific Problems of Healthcare-Associated Infections

These must be dealt with as rapidly as possible [4] (see Chapter 7). This means that the laboratory may face exceptional demands for service at the beginning of and throughout an epidemic period [16]. Advance preparation for such situations makes response easier in the time of need. The laboratory personnel should prepare contingency plans for the types of outbreaks that have occurred most frequently in the past in the hospital so that they are ready to deal with these exceptional requests in a smooth fashion.

Investigation of an HAI outbreak may require isolation and identification of isolates in specimens not only from patients but also from personnel who might be colonized with the outbreak strain and from environmental objects that might be similarly contaminated [4]. Such activity may require the laboratory staff to process and evaluate large numbers of cultures, and special techniques may be necessary to accomplish such projects. For example, reliable detection of colonization with VRE requires the use of selective media such as Enterococcosel broth [137]. The laboratory staff and the infection control team can process this work efficiently by carefully assessing the sites to be cultured and determining which culture media and techniques will be used.

A detailed description of suitable culture techniques for every possible vehicle of cross-infection is beyond the space allocation and practical scope of this chapter. The interested reader is referred to detailed protocols available for culture survey of hemodialysis equipment, dialysis fluid, intravascular devices, air cultures, and environmental and medical device surfaces, blood bank products, and water for *Legionella spp.* [134]. The development of selective media and techniques for culture of environmental objects continues to evolve as new potential reservoirs and vectors of HAI have been recognized [16]. The infection control worker and laboratorian must be familiar with the general aspects of culture procedures discussed in the following sections, but they should not obtain or process such cultures unless surveillance of infections in patients specifically implicates these items as potential HAI sources.

Because standard methods for the microbiologic evaluation of such culture procedures do not exist or are of doubtful validity, considerable expense may be incurred in producing information that is worthless or misleading. Requests for such cultures, therefore, should be approached with caution, and the infection control staff should be clear regarding how the culture results will affect patient care or epidemiologic control measures before undertaking such tasks [4]. Specific areas of support are considered in turn.

Culture of Blood Products After a Transfusion Reaction

Bacteria present in blood components can cause a septic transfusion reaction [138]. Fortunately, this is a very rare occurrence. Such reactions usually are due to endotoxin produced by organisms that can grow in the cold. If a transfusion reaction is suspected by clinical signs, the transfusion should be halted immediately and the unit examined. If further evaluation of the signs, symptoms, and clinical course of the patient then suggests bacterial contamination of the blood product, cultures of the suspect component(s) may be indicated at various temperatures [131,134]. It also is desirable to collect blood culture specimens by venipuncture from the patient and from all intravenous solutions in use for that patient.

Cultures of Parenteral Fluids and Intravascular Therapy Equipment

The investigation of bacteremia associated with parenteral therapy may require investigation of the needle, hub or catheter, portions of the administration set, the fluid being administered, and portions of the cap or closure provided with the fluid [134,139] (see Chapter 37). Blood culture specimens should be collected simultaneously from the patient. It is especially important to keep careful track of lot numbers, which should be recorded on the patient's chart and on all subsequent laboratory records.

Needles and catheters must be submitted separately from the hubs and other portions of the administration set that may have been exposed to superficial contamination. If portions of the administration set are suspected, these must be received properly capped to exclude spurious contamination. The bottle and administration set should remain connected and be placed in a plastic bag to minimize contamination during delivery to the laboratory.

The standard method for culture of catheters and needles has been the semiquantitative method in which the catheter tip is rolled across a plate containing solid media. Some authors suggest flushing the inside with nutrient broth or a quantitative sonication method for culture of the catheter instead of (or in addition to) a semiquantitative culture [140]. Substitution of hub cultures and cultures of the skin around the insertion point has been suggested as an alternative sample not requiring removal of the catheter [141]. Quantitative cultures are time-consuming and are a drain on personnel resources; the need to use them rather than the more efficient semiquantitative methods has not been demonstrated [140].

Methods for Culturing Hands and Skin

Several methods are suitable for culture of hands [134]. The simplest is to take a sterile swab, moisten it with sterile saline or a culture broth appropriate to skin organisms (brain–heart infusion broth is one), and then swab the palmar surface of the hand or hands. A rapid and simple way to obtain these cultures also is provided by pressing the subject's palm gently on a large culture plate containing a suitable agar medium (or a Rodac plate; see the section on culture of floors and other surfaces). When a more quantitative estimate of the organisms present is desired, 50 ml of culture broth can be poured into a sterile container or plastic bag. The person to be cultured is asked to rub hands together in the broth for 30 seconds. An estimate of cfu per milliliter can be obtained [142]. A bag-wash method has been found to enhance recovery of yeasts from hands of healthcare workers (HCWs) [143].

In contrast to these simple methods, sampling of hands associated with testing of antiseptics or disinfectants is a more complicated process and requires special techniques [144].

On occasion, monitoring antibiotic-resistant organisms has involved investigation of the skin of patients or HCWs as potential sources of resistant organisms. However, quantitative culturing of skin or gastrointestinal tract seldom is indicated [15]. To quantify skin microflora, several methods have been developed [134].

Methods for Culturing Tubes and Containers

Cultures of external surfaces or internal cavities (e.g., tubes and containers) may be conducted by a swab–rinse technique [134].

Sampling of Respiratory Therapy Equipment

Disinfection of respiratory therapy and anesthesia equipment is discussed in Chapter 21. In situations of high endemic or epidemic levels of occurrence of nosocomial respiratory infections, sampling respiratory therapy apparatus may be of value [145,146].

Sampling of Air

Airborne spread of nosocomial bacterial or viral infection is known to occur [147] but is probably uncommon; air sampling should be required infrequently [148]. Common recent indications for use of this technique in healthcare settings include monitoring production areas for pharmaceuticals in operating rooms, and in investigating suspected episodes of airborne infection [149]. Air sampling may be performed with either settling plates or more sophisticated equipment [134,150].

Particles suspended in hospital air vary greatly in size and in the number of microorganisms they contain. The average diameter of airborne microbial particles in ward air is approximately 13 µm, but 7% are <4 µm in size and 30% are >18 µm. Particles with a mean size of 13 µm settle at a rate of approximately 1 foot/minute. Because the surface of a standard 100-mm Petri dish represents an area of approximately 1/15 square foot and assuming that the air in the study area contains particles of average size, an open Petri dish in still air will sample microbial particles from nearly 1 cubic foot of air during 15 minutes of exposure [151].

Although this is an inexpensive way to evaluate airborne microbial contamination, quantitative results may correlate poorly with those obtained with mechanical, volumetric air samplers because of variation in particle size and unknown influences of air turbulence. Under low-humidity conditions, droplet nuclei of approximately 3 µm can remain suspended indefinitely and can be collected only with high-velocity, volumetric air samplers.

A slit sampler is suitable for many precise air sampling applications [149]. Brain–heart infusion or tryptic soy agar (TSA) media should be used in the sampling plates. A staged sampler [150] should be needed only when there is some reason to determine the size distribution of the particles, which should be an extremely infrequent event in most U.S. hospitals. Efficient vacuum sources must be used for both samplers, and the rate of flow of air must be properly calibrated to ensure accurate results.

The total number of airborne microbial particles is not measured precisely by observing growth after impaction on an agar plate because an airborne microbial particle may contain more than one viable cell. Air-sampling techniques in which volumetric samples are taken by bubbling air through collection fluid break up airborne particulate matter and better reflect the total number of organisms than air samplers that impinge contaminated particles on agar.

Culture of Floors and Other Surfaces

Methods for sampling floors and other surfaces have been described in detail [134]. Standards for acceptable levels of contamination of floors and bedside tables as sampled by the Rodac plate technique have been suggested by a committee of the American Public Health Association [152]. There is no evidence, however, that any particular level of contamination is directly correlated with an increased risk of infection, and such standards probably are useful only in assessing the adequacy of house-cleaning procedures.

Sampling Water and Ice

Water that meets U.S. Public Health Service standards for drinking water frequently contains up to 1 million or more microorganisms per milliliter, and some of these organisms are potential pathogens. Ice also can contain organisms that can pose a threat of infection, especially in patients with compromised host defenses. However, correlation of levels of microorganisms with occurrence of patient illness has been rare.

Samples of water or melted ice can be obtained by collection in a sterile container. If chlorine is present, it can be inactivated by thiosulfate. The specimen is cultured by passing large quantities through a 0.45-µm (or 0.22-µm) Millipore filter and culturing the filter in broth or directly on agar. More than 4 colonies per 100 ml is considered abnormal by this test [151].

When transmission of *Legionella* infection occurs in the hospital setting, culture of water is recommended. Guidelines for such cultures have been proposed [153].

Developing Selective Media for Surveys

To reduce the workload in the laboratory and to expedite the processing of specimens, selective survey media should be used whenever possible for culturing specimens during outbreak investigations. Susceptibility data on known or suspected epidemic strains may be used to identify an appropriate selective medium for use in surveys of the animate and inanimate environment of the hospital. Once the implicated organism is isolated and tested on appropriate media containing ≥1 antibiotics to which it is resistant, the media can be used to exclude numerous bacteria unrelated to the outbreak. This may accelerate the detection of contaminated equipment or infected patients. Pretesting of the media is essential because of possible synergy or antagonism between the added antimicrobials or between these drugs and the media; such interactions could cause inhibition of growth of the epidemic strain or failure to inhibit growth of nonimplicated organisms.

Other selective media also may be useful. For example, cetrimide medium may be helpful in selectively isolating *P. aeruginosa* from contaminated material or mixed cultures. Similarly, tetrathionate broth is an excellent medium for selective pre-enrichment of *Salmonella spp.* cultures. Mueller-Hinton agar containing sorbitol, a pH indicator, and antibiotics (vancomycin, colistin, and nystatin) provides selective differentiation of *Serratia* spp. Many epidemic strains of *S. aureus* are resistant to mercuric chloride, and the incorporation of small amounts of this compound in TSA can be helpful in inhibiting nonepidemic strains of *S. aureus, Staphylococcus epidermidis,* and most gramnegative organisms except *Pseudomonas spp.*

Vancomycin-resistant strains of enterococci have become a problem in many U.S. hospitals; agar containing small concentrations of vancomycin have been of use in investigating hospital problems due to these strains [39,137]. The resistance of epidemic microorganisms to heavy metals, dyes, disinfectants, and other antimicrobial substances also may be used to identify and construct selective media for surveys.

Surveys for Educational Purposes

Sampling techniques that are not directly related to epidemiologic surveys may prove useful in educational programs; visible evidence of contamination of hands, clothing, equipment, and surfaces may serve to teach the need for effective aseptic technique and sanitation.

Sampling That Is Not Recommended

Routine Culture Surveys of Patients and Personnel

Routine culturing of patients or hospital personnel is not recommended (see Chapter 7). Surveys may be useful during investigation of specific problems within a hospital and should be instituted in response to, and specifically address, epidemiologic findings.

Routine Culture of Commercial Products

Although commercial patient-care items that are labeled sterile (e.g., intravascular catheters and fluids) occasionally have been contaminated with viable organisms that can cause patient disease, routine sampling of these items is not recommended because the low frequency of contamination makes it difficult (because of the large number of specimens that would have to be taken) and expensive to perform adequate sterility testing.

Routine Testing of Antiseptics and Disinfectants

In-use testing of antiseptics and disinfectants should not be a routine procedure for hospital microbiology laboratories [134]. No consensus is available about the optimal methods for such testing against many organisms, including viruses [154]. If contamination of commercial products

sold as sterile is suspected, infection control personnel should be notified and the nearest office of the U.S. Food and Drug Administration contacted immediately [151]. State regulations may require immediate notification of state health authorities as well.

Random Culture of Blood Units

The American Association of Blood Banks [131] does not recommend random culture of blood units to ensure sterility.

Routine Monitoring of Disinfection Process for Respiratory Therapy Equipment

Guidelines from the CDC advise to "not routinely perform surveillance cultures of patients or of equipment or devices used for respiratory therapy, pulmonary function testing, or delivery of inhalation anaesthesia" [146].

TEACHING MICROBIOLOGIC ASPECTS OF HEALTHCARE-ASSOCIATED INFECTION TO INFECTION CONTROL PERSONNEL

The people responsible for infection control usually are not trained in clinical laboratory procedures. Because the key to success in infection control efforts is communication, it is necessary that all involved speak the same language. For this purpose, training infection control personnel in the language of the clinical laboratory microbiologist is important. Training many infection control personnel in microbiology is inadequate or out of date. The goal of such teaching is not necessarily to make the infection control staff accomplished laboratory workers but to familiarize them with the procedures and practices of the laboratory, the microorganisms involved in HAIs, the validity of test procedures used in identifying these pathogens, and the strengths and weaknesses of the resulting data.

Similarly, it is important for the microbiologist to learn some of the concepts of infection control, because few laboratory directors or technologists have adequate grounding in epidemiology or infection control. Especially important is exposure to techniques used for measuring frequency of infection and the concept of colonization versus infection.

Such joint efforts permit ready communication between the two groups of colleagues. Teaching of this type can be done in a formal fashion but also is effective when included as part of the day-to-day informal contacts between the infection control staff and laboratory personnel (see Chapter 2).

REFERENCES

1. Mahayni R, Zervos M. The clinical laboratory's role in hospital infection control. *Laboratory Medicine* 1994;25:642–647.

2. Emori TG, Gaynes RP: An overview of nosocomial infections, including the role of the microbiology laboratory. *Clin Microbiol Rev* 1993;6:428–442.

3. Schifman RB. *ASCP check sample—microbiology: Surveillance for nosocomial infections: The laboratory component.* Skokie, IL: American Society *of* Clinical Pathologists, 1989.

4. McGowan JE Jr, Metchock BG. Basic microbiologic support for hospital epidemiology. *Infect Control Hosp Epidemiol* 1996;17:298–303.

5. Sadler HS, Hollis RJ, Pfaller MA. The use of molecular techniques in the epidemiology and control of infectious diseases. *Clin Lab Med* 1995;15:407–431.

6. Arbeit R. Laboratory procedures for the epidemiologic analysis of microorganisms. In: P. Murray, E. Baron. J. Jorgensen, et al., eds. *Manual of clinical microbiology.* 8th ed. Washington, DC: American Society for Microbiology, 2003.

7. McGowan JE Jr. Communication with hospital staff. In: Balows A, Hausler WJ Jr, Herrmann KL, et al., eds. *Manual of clinical microbiology.* 5th ed. Washington, DC: American Society for Microbiology, 1991:151–158.

8. Wiblin RT, Wenzel RP. The infection control committee. *Infect Control Hosp Epidemiol* 1996;17:44–46.

9. Boyce JM. Hospital epidemiology in smaller hospitals. *Infect Control Hosp Epidemiol* 1995;16:600–606.

10. Swartz K, Brennan TA. Integrated healthcare, capitated payment, and quality: The role of regulation. *Ann Intern Med* 1996;124:224–228.

11. Simmons BP, Parry MF, Williams M, et al. The new era of hospital epidemiology: What you need to succeed. *Clin Infect Dis* 1996;22:550–553.

12. Scott DR. Influence of managed care and health maintenance organizations on the clinical microbiology laboratory. *Diagn Microbiol Infect Dis* 1995;23:17–21.

13. McGowan JE Jr, MacLowry JD. Addressing regulatory issues in the clinical microbiology laboratory. In: Murray PR, Baron EJ, Pfaller MA, et al., eds. *Manual of clinical microbiology.* 6th ed. Washington, DC: American Society for Microbiology, 1995:67–74.

14. McGowan JE Jr, Metchock B. Infection control epidemiology and clinical microbiology. In: Murray PR, Baron EJ, Pfaller MA, et al., eds. *Manual of clinical microbiology.* 6th ed. Washington, DC: American Society for Microbiology, 1995.

15. Greene JN. The microbiology of colonization, including techniques for assessing and measuring colonization. *Infect Control Hosp Epidemiol* 1996;17:114–118.

16. Goldmann DA. New microbiologic techniques for hospital epidemiology. *Eur J Clin Microbiol* 1987;6:344–347.

17. National Nosocomial Infections Surveillance (NNIS) System Report, data summary from January 1992 through June 2004, issued October. *Am J Infect Control* 2004;32:470–485.

18. Vincent J-L, Bihari DJ, Suter PM, et al. The prevalence of nosocomial infection in intensive care units in Europe: Results of the European Prevalence of Infection in Intensive Care (EPIC) study. *JAMA* 1995;274:639–644.

19. Jenkins SG. Evaluation of new technology in the clinical microbiology laboratory. *Diagn Microbiol Infect Dis* 1995;23:53–60.

20. Relman DA. The identification of uncultured microbial pathogens. *J Infect Dis* 1993;168:1–8.

21. Haynes KA, Westerneng TJ. Rapid identification of *Candida albicans, C. glabrata, C. parapsilosis* and *C. krusei* by species-specific PCR of large subunit ribosomal DNA. *J Med Microbiol* 1996;44:390–396.

22. Grundy JE, Ehrnst A, Einsele H, et al. A three-center European external quality control study of PCR for detection of cytomegalovirus DNA in blood. *J Clin Microbiol* 1996;34:1166–1170.

23. Thanos M, Schonian G, Meyer W, et al. Rapid identification of *Candida* species by DNA fingerprinting with PCR. *J Clin Microbiol* 1996;34:615–621.

24. Kiehn TE, Ellner PD, Budzko D. Role of the microbiology laboratory in care of the immunosuppressed patient. *Rev Infect Dis* 1989;11(Suppl 7):S1706–S1710.

25. Wilson ML. General principles of specimen collection and transport. *Clin Infect Dis* 1996;22:766–777.

26. Farkas DH, Kaul KL, Wiedbrauk DL, et al. Specimen collection and storage for diagnostic molecular pathology investigation. *Arch Pathol Lab Med* 1996;120:591–596.

27. Morris AJ, Tanner DC, Reller LB. Rejection criteria for endotracheal aspirates from adults. *J Clin Microbiol* 1993;31:1027–1029.

28. Valenstein P. Laboratory turnaround time. *Am J Clin Pathol* 1996;105:676–688.

29. Flournoy DJ, Beal LM, Smith MD. What constitutes an adequate sputum specimen? *Laboratory Medicine* 1994;25:456–459.

30. Baron EJ. Quality management and the clinical microbiology laboratory. *Diagn Microbiol Infect Dis* 1995;23:23–34.

31. Dowell SF, Torok TJ, Thorp JA, et al. Parvovirus B19 infection in hospital workers: Community or hospital acquisition? *J Infect Dis* 1995;172:1076–1079.

32. Washington JA II. Effective use of the microbiology laboratory. *J Antimicrob Chemother* 1988;22(Suppl A):101–112.

33. Wegner DL. Resolved: That taxonomy should be more medically relevant. *Clinical Microbiology Newsletter* 1996;18:121–128.

34. Weinstein RW. Enterobacteriaceae. In: Mayhall CG, ed. *Infection control and hospital epidemiology.* Baltimore: Williams & Wilkins, 1996.

35. Hamill RJ, Houston ED, Georghiou PR, et al. An outbreak of *Burkholderia* (formerly *Pseudomonas*) *cepacia* respiratory tract colonization and infection associated with nebulized albuterol therapy. *Ann Intern Med* 1995;122:762–766.

36. P. Murray, E. Baron. J. Jorgensen, M. Pfaller, et al., eds. *Manual of clinical microbiology.* 8th ed. Washington, DC: American Society for Microbiology, 2003.

37. Gordts B, Van Landuyt H, Ieven M, et al. Vancomycin-resistant enterococci colonizing the intestinal tracts of hospitalized patients. *J Clin Microbiol* 1995;33:2842–2846.

38. Barton AL, Doern GV. Selective media for detecting gastrointestinal carriage of vancomycin-resistant enterococci. *Diagn Microbiol Infect Dis* 1995;23:119–122.

39. Perkins MD, Mirrett S, Reller LB. Rapid bacterial antigen detection is not clinically useful. *J Clin Microbiol* 1995;33:1486–1491.

40. Robinson A. Rationale for cost-effective laboratory medicine. *Clin Microbiol Rev* 1994;7:185–199.

41. Marshall WF, Keating MR, Anhalt JP, et al. *Xanthomonas maltophilia*: An emerging nosocomial pathogen. *Mayo Clin Proc* 1989;64:1097–1104.

42. Schmitt SK, Knapp C, Hall GS, et al. Impact of chlorhexidine-silver sulfadiazine-impregnated central venous catheters on in vitro quantitation of catheter-associated bacteria. *J Clin Microbiol* 1996;34:508–511.

43. August MJ, Hindler JA, Huber TW, et al. *Cumitech 3A: Quality control and quality assurance practices in clinical microbiology.* Washington, DC: American Society for Microbiology, 1990.

44. Richardson H, Wood D, Whitby J, et al. Quality improvement of diagnostic microbiology through a peer-group proficiency testing program. *Arch Pathol Lab Med* 1996;120:445–455.

45. Southern PM Jr, Colvin DD. Pseudomeningitis again: Association with cytocentrifuge funnel and Gram-stain reagent contamination. *Arch Pathol Lab Med* 1996;120:456–458.

46. McGowan JE Jr. Antibiotic-resistant bacteria and healthcare systems: Four steps for effective response. *Infect Control Hosp Epidemiol* 1995;18:67–70.

47. Casewell MW. New threats to the control of methicillin-resistant *Staphylococcus aureus*. *J Hosp Infect* 1995;30(Suppl):465–471.

48. Jett B, Free L, Sahm DE. Factors influencing the Vitek gram-positive susceptibility system's detection of *vanB*-encoded vancomycin resistance among enterococci. *J Clin Microbiol* 1996;34:701–706.

49. Centers for Disease Control and Prevention. *Staphylococcus aureus* with reduced susceptibility to vancomycin—United States, 1997. *MMWR* 1997;46:765–766.

50. Swenson JM, Ferraro MJ, Sahm DF, et al. Multilaboratory evaluation of screening methods for detection of high-level aminoglycoside resistance in enterococci. *J Clin Microbiol* 1995;33:3008–3018.

51. Washington JA II, Knapp CC, Sanders CC. Accuracy of microdilution and the AutoMicrobic system in detection of beta-lactam resistance in gram-negative bacterial mutants with derepressed beta-lactamase. *Rev Infect Dis* 1988;10:824–829.

52. Sahm DF, Neumann MA, Thornsberry C, et al. *Cumitech 25: Current concepts and approaches to antimicrobial agent susceptibility testing.* Washington, DC: American Society for Microbiology, 1988.

53. National Committee for Clinical Laboratory Standards. *Performance standards for antimicrobial susceptibility testing: Sixth informational supplement* (M100-S6). Villanova, PA: NCCLS, 1995.

54. Jorgensen JH. Selection of antimicrobial agents for routine testing in a clinical microbiology laboratory. *Diagn Microbiol Infect Dis* 1993;16:245–249.

55. Ghannoum MA, Rex JH, Galgiani JN. Susceptibility testing of fungi: Current status of correlation of in vitro data with clinical outcome. *J Clin Microbiol* 1996;34:489–495.

56. Desseau RB, Steenberg P. Computerized surveillance in clinical microbiology with time series analysis. *J Clin Microbiol* 1993;31:857–860.

57. Stratton CW VI, Ratner H, Johnston PE, et al. Focused microbiologic surveillance by specific hospital unit: Practical application and clinical utility. *Clin Ther* 1993;15(Suppl A):12–20.

58. Wenzel RP, Streed SA. Surveillance and use of computers in hospital infection control. *J Hosp Infect* 1989;13:217–229.

59. Lundberg GD. Critical (panic) value notification: An established laboratory practice policy (parameter). *JAMA* 1990;263:709.

60. Maslow JN, Mulligan ME, Arbeit RD. Molecular epidemiology: Application of contemporary techniques to the typing of microorganisms. *Clin Infect Dis* 1993;17:153–164.

61. Shea YR. Specimen collection and transport. In: Isenberg HD, ed. *Volume I: Clinical microbiology procedures handbook.* Washington, DC: American Society for Microbiology, 1992:1.1.1.–30.

62. Venezia RA, Scarano FJ, Preston KE, et al. Molecular epidemiology of an SHV-5 extended-spectrum β-lactamase in Enterobacteriaceae isolated from infants in a neonatal intensive care unit. *Clin Infect Dis* 1995;21:915–923.

63. Vickers RM, Stout JE, Tompkins LS, et al. Cefamandole-susceptible strains of *Legionella pneumophila* serogroup 1: Implications for diagnosis and utility as an epidemiologic marker. *J Clin Microbiol* 1992;30:537–539.

64. Bannatyne RM, Wells BA, MacMillan SA, et al. A cluster of MRSA: The little outbreak that wasn't. *Infect Control Hosp Epidemiol* 1995;16:380.

65. Holder IA, Volpel K, Ronald G, et al. Studies on multiple *Pseudomonas aeruginosa* isolates from individual burn patients by RFLP, O antigen serotyping, and antibiogram analysis. *Burns* 1995;21:441–444.

66. Rossney AS, Coleman DC, Keane CT. Evaluation of an antibiogram-resistogram typing scheme for methicillin-resistant *Staphylococcus aureus*. *J Med Microbiol* 1994;41:441–447.

67. Hunter PR. Discrimination of strains of *Candida albicans* isolated from deep and superficial sites by resistotyping. *Mycoses* 1995;38:37–40.

68. Chetoui H, Delhalle E, Osterrieth P, et al. Ribotyping for use in studying molecular epidemiology of *Serratia marcescens:* Comparison with biotyping. *J Clin Microbiol* 1995;33:2637–2642.

69. Kuhn I, Burman LG, Haeggman S, et al. Biochemical fingerprinting compared with ribotyping and pulsed-field gel electrophoresis of DNA for epidemiological typing of enterococci. *J Clin Microbiol* 1995;33:2812–2817.

70. Ouchi K, Abe M, Karita M, et al. Analysis of strains of *Burkholderia* (*Pseudomonas*) *cepacia* isolated in a nosocomial outbreak by biochemical and genomic typing. *J Clin Microbiol* 1996;33:2353–2357.

71. Jorgensen M, Givney R, Pegler M, et al. Typing multidrug-resistant *Staphylococcus aureus:* Conflicting epidemiological data produced by genotypic and phenotypic means clarified by phylogenetic analysis. *J Clin Microbiol* 1996;34:398–403.

72. Trautmann M, Cross AS, Reich G, et al. Evaluation of a competitive ELISA method for the determination of *Klebsiella* O antigens. *J Med Microbiol* 1996;44:44–51.

73. Quentin R, Huet H, Wang F-S, et al. Characterization of *Streptococcus agalactiae* strains by multilocus enzyme genotype and serotype: Identification of multiple virulent clone families that cause invasive neonatal disease. *J Clin Microbiol* 1995;33:2576–2581.

74. Bonten MJM, Gaillard CA, van Tiel FH, et al. A typical case of cross-acquisition? The importance of genotypic characterization of bacterial strains. *Infect Control Hosp Epidemiol* 1995;16:415–416.

75. Gaston MA, Strickland MA, Ayling-Smith BA, et al. Epidemiological typing of *Enterobacter aerogenes*. *J Clin Microbiol* 1989;27:564–565.

76. Larose P, Picard B, Thibault M, et al. Nosocomial *Serratia marcescens* individualized by five typing methods in a regional hospital. *J Hosp Infect* 1990;15:167–172.

77. Kreiswirth BN, Lutwick SM, Chapnick EK, et al. Tracing the spread of methicillin-resistant *Staphylococcus aureus* by Southern blot hybridization using gene-specific probes of *mec* and *Tn554*. *Microbial Drug Resistance* 1995;1:307–313.

78. Tomayko JF, Murray BE. Analysis of *Enterococcus faecalis* isolates from intercontinental sources by multilocus enzyme electrophoresis and pulsed-field gel electrophoresis. *J Clin Microbiol* 1995;33:2903–2907.

79. Tan TQ, Musser JM, Shulman RJ, et al. Molecular epidemiology of coagulase-negative *Staphylococcus* blood isolates from neonates with persistent bacteremia and children with central venous catheter infections. *J Infect Dis* 1994;169:1393–1397.

80. Camargo LFA, Strabelli TMV, Ribeiro FG, et al. Epidemiologic investigation of an outbreak of coagulase-negative *Staphylococcus* primary bacteremia in a newborn intensive care unit. *Infect Control Hosp Epidemiol* 1995;16:595–596.

81. Liu PY-F, Shi Z-Y, Lau Y-J, et al. Use of restriction endonuclease analysis of plasmids and pulsed-field gel electrophoresis to investigate outbreaks of methicillin-resistant *Staphylococcus aureus* infection. *Clin Infect Dis* 1996;22:86–90.

82. Jamieson FB, Green K, Low DE, et al. A cluster of surgical wound infections due to unrelated strains of group A streptococci. *Infect Control Hosp Epidemiol* 1993;14:265–267.

83. Samore MH, Bettin KM, DeGirolami PC, et al. Wide diversity of *Clostridium difficile* types at a tertiary referral hospital. *J Infect Dis* 1994;170:615–621.

84. Schoonmaker D, Heimberger T, Birkhead G. Comparison of ribotyping and restriction enzyme analysis using pulsed-field gel electrophoresis for distinguishing *Legionella pneumophila* isolates obtained during a nosocomial outbreak. *J Clin Microbiol* 1992;30:1491–1498.

85. Nath SK, Shea B, Jackson S, et al. Ribotyping of nosocomial methicillin-resistant *Staphylococcus aureus* isolates from a Canadian hospital. *Infect Control Hosp Epidemiol* 1995;16:717–724.

86. Bingen E, Bedu A, Brahimi N, et al. Use of molecular analysis in pathophysiological investigation of late-onset neonatal *Escherichia coli* meningitis. *J Clin Microbiol* 1995;33:3074–3076.

87. Barbier N, Saulnier P, Chachaty E, et al. Random amplified polymorphic DNA typing versus pulsed-field gel electrophoresis for epidemiological typing of vancomycin-resistant enterococci. *J Clin Microbiol* 1996;34:1096–1099.

88. Pruckler JM, Mermel LA, Benson RF, et al. Comparison of *Legionella pneumophila* isolates by arbitrary primed PCR and pulsed-field gel electrophoresis: Analysis from seven epidemic investigations. *J Clin Microbiol* 1995;33:2872–2875.

89. Cookson BD, Aparicio P, Deplano A, et al. Inter-centre comparison of pulsed-field gel electrophoresis for the typing of methicillin-resistant *Staphylococcus aureus*. *J Med Microbiol* 1996;44:179–184.

90. Talon D, Cailleaux V, Thouverez M, et al. Discriminatory power and usefulness of pulsed-field gel electrophoresis in epidemiological studies of *Pseudomonas aeruginosa*. *J Hosp Infect* 1996;32:135–145.

91. Bendall RP, Drobniewski FA, Jayasena SD, et al. Restriction fragment length polymorphism analysis rules out cross-infection among renal patients with tuberculosis. *J Hosp Infect* 1995;30:51–56.

92. Donabedian S, Chow JW, Shlaes DM, et al. DNA hybridization and contour-clamped homogeneous electric field electrophoresis for identification of enterococci to the species level. *J Clin Microbiol* 1995;33:141–145.

93. King D, Rhine-Chalberg J, Pfaller MA, et al. Comparison of four DNA-based methods for strain delineation of *Candida lusitaniae*. *J Clin Microbiol* 1995;33:1467–1470.

94. van Belkum A, Sluijter M, de Groot R, et al. Novel BOX repeat PCR assay for high-resolution typing of *Streptococcus pneumoniae* strains. *J Clin Microbiol* 1996;34:1176–1179.

95. Harvey BS, Koeuth T, Versalovic J, et al. Vertical transmission of *Citrobacter diversus* documented by DNA fingerprinting. *Infect Control Hosp Epidemiol* 1995;16:564–569.

96. Siau H, Yuen KY, Wong SSY, et al. The epidemiology of *Acinetobacter* infections in Hong Kong. *J Med Microbiol* 1996;44:340–347.

97. Collier MC, Stock F, DeGirolami PC, et al. Comparison of PCR-based approaches to molecular epidemiologic analysis of *Clostridium difficile*. *J Clin Microbiol* 1996;34:1153–1157.

98. Cockerill FR, Williams DE, Eisenach KD, et al. Prospective evaluation of the utility of molecular techniques for diagnosing nosocomial transmission of multidrug-resistant tuberculosis. *Mayo Clin Proc* 1996;71:221–229.

99. van Belkum A, van Leeuwen W, Kluytmans J, et al. Molecular nosocomial epidemiology: High speed typing of microbial pathogens by arbitrary primed polymerase chain reaction assays. *Infect Control Hosp Epidemiol* 1995;16:658–666.

100. Snelling AM, Gerner-Smidt P, Hawkey PM, et al. Validation of use of whole-cell repetitive extragenic palindromic sequence-based PCR (REP-PCR) for typing strains belonging to the *Acinetobacter calcoaceticus–Acinetobacter baumanii* complex and application of the method to the investigation of a hospital outbreak. *J Clin Microbiol* 1996;34:1193–1202.

101. Davin-Regli A, Saux P, Bollet C, et al. Investigation of outbreaks of *Enterobacter aerogenes* colonisation and infection in intensive care units by random amplification of polymorphic DNA. *J Med Microbiol* 1996;44:89–98.

102. Davin-Regli A, Bollet C, Auffray JP, et al. Use of random amplified polymorphic DNA for epidemiological typing of *Stenotrophomonas maltophilia*. *J Hosp Infect* 1996;32:39–50.

103. Leenders A, van Belkum A, Janssen S, et al. Molecular epidemiology of apparent outbreak of invasive aspergillosis in a hematology ward. *J Clin Microbiol* 1996;34:345–351.

104. Robert F, Lebreton F, Bougnoux ME, et al. Use of random amplified polymorphic DNA as a typing method for *Candida albicans* in epidemiological surveillance of a burn unit. *J Clin Microbiol* 1995;33:2366–2371.

105. Roll M, Norder H, Magnius LO, et al. Nosocomial spread of hepatitis B virus (HBV) in a hemodialysis unit confirmed by HBV DNA sequencing. *J Hosp Infect* 1995;30:57–63.

106. Graham DR, Dixon RE, Hughes JM, et al. Disk diffusion antimicrobial susceptibility testing for clinical and epidemiologic purposes. *Am J Infect Control* 1985;13:241–249.

107. Farmer JJ III. Conventional typing methods. *J Hosp Infect* 1988;11(Suppl A):309–314.

108. Mollby R, Kuhn I, Katouli M. Computerised biochemical fingerprinting: A new tool for typing of bacteria. *Rev Med Microbiol* 1993;4:231–234.

109. Pfaller MA. Typing methods for epidemiological investigation. In: P. Murray, E. Baron. J. Jorgensen, et al., eds. *Manual of Clinical Microbiology*. 8th ed. Washington, DC: American Society for Microbiology, 2003.

110. Bingen EH, Denamur E, Elion J. Use of ribotyping in epidemiological surveillance of nosocomial outbreaks. *Clin Microbiol Rev* 1994;7:311–327.

111. Miller JM. Molecular technology for hospital epidemiology. *Diagn Microbiol Infect Dis* 1993;16:153–157.

112. Jarvis WR. Usefulness of molecular epidemiology for outbreak investigations. *Infect Control Hosp Epidemiol* 1994;15:500–503.

113. Tenover FC, Arbett RD, Goering RV, et al. Interpreting chromosomal DNA restriction patterns produced by pulsed-field gel electrophoresis: Criteria for bacterial strain typing. *J Clin Microbiol* 1995;33:2233–2239.

114. Noble WC, Howell SA. Labile antibiotic resistance in *Staphylococcus aureus*. *J Hosp Infect* 1995;31:135–141.

115. van Belkum A. DNA fingerprinting of medically important microorganisms by use of PCR. *Clin Microbiol Rev* 1994;7:174–184.

116. Holzman D. Progress toward practical DNA-based infectious disease diagnostics. *ASM News* 1995;61:329–330.

117. Acceptability of the "bar code doctor." *Lancet* 1996;347:555–556.

118. McHugh TD, Ramsay ARC, James EA, et al. Pitfalls of PCR: Misdiagnosis of cerebral nocardia infection. *Lancet* 1995;346:1436.

119. Pfaller MA. Epidemiology of fungal infections: The promise of molecular typing. *Clin Infect Dis* 1995;20:1535–1539.

120. Fredricks DN, Reiman DA. Sequence-based identification of microbial pathogens: A reconsideration of Koch's postulates. *Clin Microbiol Rev* 1996;9:18–33.

121. Hunter PR. Reproducibility and indices of discriminatory power of microbial typing methods. *J Clin Microbiol* 1990;28:1903–1905.

122. Ludlam HA, Noble WC, Marples RR, et at. The evaluation of a typing scheme for coagulase-negative staphylococci suitable for epidemiological studies. *J Med Microbiol* 1989;30:161–165.

123. Rutala WA, Weber DJ. Environmental interventions to control nosocomial infections. *Infect Control Hosp Epidemiol* 1995;16:442–443.

124. Rutala WA. Antisepsis, disinfection, and sterilization in hospitals and related institutions. In: P. Murray, E. Baron. J. Jorgensen, et al., eds. *Manual of clinical microbiology*. 8th ed. Washington, DC: American Society for Microbiology, 2003.

125. Garner J, Favero M. Guidelines for the prevention and control of nosocomial infections: Guideline for handwashing and hospital environmental control. *Am J Infect Control* 1985;14:110–129.

126. Rutala WA, Weber DJ. Low-temperature sterilization technologies: Do we need to redefine "sterilization?" *Infect Control Hosp Epidemiol* 1996;17:87–91.

127. Wright AM, Hoxey EV, Soper CJ, et al. Biological indicators for low temperature steam and formaldehyde sterilization: Investigation of the effect of change in temperature and formaldehyde concentration on spores of *Bacillus stearothermophilus* NCIMB 8224. *J Appl Bacteriol* 1996;80:259–265.

128. Sehulster L, Chinn RY, HICPAC. Guidelines for environmental infection control in health-care facilities: Recommendations of CDC and the Healthcare Infection Control Practices Advisory Committee (HICPAC). *MMWR Recomm Rep.* 6;52(RR-10):1–42.

129. Centers for Disease Control guidelines for hospital environmental control: Microbiologic surveillance of the environment and of personnel in the hospital. *Infect Control* 1981;2:145.

130. Bryan FL. Procedures to use during outbreaks of foodborne disease. In: Murray PR, Baron EJ, Pfaller MA, et al. eds. *Manual of clinical microbiology*. 6th ed. Washington, DC: American Society for Microbiology, 1995:229–236.

131. American Association of Blood Banks. *Technical manual.* 11th ed. Arlington, VA: AABB, 1993.

132. Pillay T, Pillay DG, Hoosen AA, et al. Utility of surveillance bacterial cultures in neonatal exchange blood transfusions. *J Hosp Infect* 1995;31:67–71.

133. Association for Advancement of Medical Instrumentation. *Hemodialysis systems.* ANSI/AAMI RD5-1992. Arlington, VA: AAMI, 1992.

134. Gilchrist MJR. Epidemiologic and infection control microbiology. In: Isenberg HD, ed. *Clinical microbiology procedures handbook.* 2nd ed. Washington, DC: American Society for Microbiology, 1992:11.1.1–11.1.3.

135. Smith D, Bradley SJ, Scott GM. Bacterial contamination of autologous bone marrow during processing. *J Hosp Infect* 1996;33:71–76.

136. Barrie D. The provision of food and catering services in hospital. *J Hosp Infect* 1996;33:13–32.

137. Landman D, Quale JM, Oydna E, et al. Comparison of five selective media for identifying fecal carriage of vancomycin-resistant enterococci. *J Clin Microbiol* 1996;34:751–752.

138. Centers for Disease Control and Prevention. Red blood cell transfusions contaminated with Yersinia enterocolitica—United States, 1991–1996, and initiation of a national study to detect bacteria-associated transfusion reactions. *MMWR* 1997;46(24):553–555.

139. Goetz AM, Rihs JD, Chow JW, et al. An outbreak of infusion-related *Klebsiella pneumoniae* bacteremia in a liver transplantation unit. *Clin Infect Dis* 1995;21:1501–1503.

140. Reimer LG. Catheter-related infections and blood cultures. *Clin Lab Med* 1994;14:51–58.

141. Whitman ED, Boatman AM, Haun WE, et al. Comparison of diagnostic specimens and methods to evaluate infected venous access ports. *Am J Surg* 1995;170:665–670.

142. Horn WA, Larson EL, McGinley KJ, et al. Microbial flora on the hands of healthcare personnel: Differences in composition and antibacterial resistance. *Infect Control Hosp Epidemiol* 1988;9:189–193.

143. Strasbaugh LJ, Sewell DL, Tjoelker RC, et at. Comparison of three methods for recovery of yeasts from hands of health-care workers. *J Clin Microbiol* 1996;34:471–473.

144. Larson E, Rotter ML. Handwashing: Are experimental models a substitute for clinical trials? Two viewpoints. *Infect Control Hosp Epidemiol* 1990;11:63–66.

145. Cobben NAM, Drent M, Jonkers M, et al. Outbreak of severe *Pseudomonas aeruginosa* respiratory infections due to contaminated nebulizers. *J Hosp Infect* 1996;33:63–70.

146. Tablan OC, Anderson LJ, Besser R, et al. Guidelines for preventing healthcare–associated pneumonia, 2003: Recommendations of CDC and the Healthcare Infection Control Practices Advisory Committee. *MMWR* 2004;53(RR03):1–36.

147. Gundermann KD. Spread of microorganisms by air-conditioning systems: Especially in hospitals. *Ann N Y Acad Sci* 1980;353:209.

148. Humphreys H. Microbes in the air: When to count! (The role of air sampling in hospitals). *J Med Microbiol* 1992;37:81–82.

149. Benbough JE, Bennett AM, Parks SR. Determination of the collection efficiency of a microbial air sampler. *J Appl Bacteriol* 1993;74:170–173.

150. Groschel DH. Air sampling in hospitals. *Ann NY Acad Sci* 1980;353:230.

151. McGowan JE Jr. Changing etiology of nosocomial bacteremia and fungemia and other hospital-acquired infections. *Rev Infect Dis* 1985;7(Suppl 3):S357–S370.

152. Committee on Microbial Contamination of Surfaces, Laboratory Section, American Public Health Association. A comparative microbiological evaluation of floor-cleaning procedures in hospital patient rooms. *Health Lab Sci* 1970;7:3.

153. Ta CA, Stout JE, Yu VL, et al. Comparison of culture methods for monitoring Legionella species in hospital potable water systems and recommendations for standardization. *J Clin Microbiol* 1995;33:2118–2123.

154. Woolwine JD, Gerberding JL. Effect of testing method on apparent activities of antiviral disinfectants and antiseptics. *Antimicrob Agents Chemother* 1995;39:921–923.

The Practice

of Epidemiology

in Community Hospitals

11

William E. Scheckler and August J. Valenti

The methods of epidemiology and infection control are broadly applicable regardless of the size, location, or affiliation of a healthcare facility. The day-to-day practice of healthcare epidemiology in most community hospitals is normally more a matter of developing and implementing policies, educating staff, applying appropriate isolation precautions, and conducting surveillance than engaging in the kind of science common to larger academic centers. Nonetheless, the progressively more visible patient safety movement, which appropriately regards healthcare-associated infections (HAIs) as preventable, adverse events, is forcing small hospitals to pay closer attention to the collection, analysis, and feedback of HAI rates. Over the past several years, regulatory agencies and accrediting bodies have responded to pressures to reduce errors and adverse outcomes in hospitals by introducing more process indicators and outcome measures related to HAIs in their assessment of quality.

Until recently, surprisingly little has been published on infection control practices in the community. Evidence of increasing interest in the state of infection control in community hospitals is reflected by a number of newly published studies examining how these infection control programs are configured and how they are responding to the challenges of resource availability, drug-resistant organisms, and antibiotic stewardship [1].

In 2003, the U.S. not-for-profit community hospitals accounted for 61% of the 4,895 acute care hospitals [2]. As hospitals' bed numbers decrease, the percentage of those hospitals classified as rural markedly increases. Overall, 44% of the 4,895 hospitals were classified as rural. Of these rural hospitals, 74% had ≤99 beds. This chapter has been added to this text to help the hospitals that are not major teaching and academic centers and that are not governmentally owned (e.g., Veteran's Administration hospitals). As has been noted, there is a paucity of data from these hospitals in the area of studies of infectious diseases, HAI prevention, and control [3–6]. Fortunately, National Nosocomial Infections Surveillance (NNIS) system of the Centers for Disease Control and Prevention's (CDC) has always included a number of such community hospitals. The NNIS was merged into the National Healthcare Safety Network (NHSN) in January 2006. This new Web-based system should make access to data entry and analysis for all community hospitals more accessible and useful. Before 2006, the >2,300 hospitals <100 beds could not participate in NNIS. This chapter has been designed for both these smaller hospitals and the larger community institutions in the hope that HAIs can be better prevented and patient care safety improved.

To help target some key issues, we have made extensive use of a collaborative set of evidence-based recommendations published in February 1998 [7] as the major reference for our chapter. We also will display the thoughts of our colleagues in hospital epidemiology who shared their top issues and key frustrations with us in a survey provided at the March 2006 Society for Healthcare Epidemiology of America (SHEA) meeting in Chicago and at the May 2006 statewide Wisconsin Association of Professionals in Infection Control and Epidemiology (APIC) meeting. The results of these "convenience sample" surveys are consistent with our own experiences and what we identified in visits to hospitals around the country in the last 5 years.

The survey results are of interest. They should encourage the Joint Commission on Accreditation of Healthcare Organizations (JCAHO) to think further about how to make a culture of safety, which must include a team of experts in HAI prevention and control, an absolute requirement and responsibility of the hospital administration and leadership (Table 11-1). Lack of time, an increasing scope of work, a frequent paucity of administration-provided resources, and sense of value highlight the results. A few quotes from the Wisconsin data are relevant. A common thread in the era of pandemic influenza and bioterrorism preparedness concerns the lack of time (hours, staff, or both): "I have the desire to be proactive rather than always reactive, but there is not enough time…." The frustration with lack of administration support is articulated best from two quite different hospitals. From a 600 bed hospital: "The Infection Control Department is perceived as a thorn in their [administration's] side instead of an important component of healthcare" and from a 100 bed facility: "Infection control has always been seen as a [cost center] rather than an income-producing department."

Our informal surveys underscore some of the findings published in a formal survey conducted among Volunteer Hospitals of America (VHA) hospitals in various regions of the country by Christenson et al. [8]. These authors conducted a demographic survey of 31 hospitals ranging in size from <50 beds to >500 beds to assess the staffing, structure, and functions of infection control departments in participating hospitals. Participants were asked to conduct observational studies of compliance with process measures, such as hand-hygiene practices, ventilator-associated pneumonia rates, and catheter-related bloodstream and urinary infections. A third of the participants reported levels of infection control staffing below the level of 1 infection control professional (ICP) per 100 occupied beds. Only one hospital reported data entry and analytic support within the infection control department. The results of the process observations showed variability in compliance with evidence-based strategies for preventing HAIs.

Sustained compliance with best practices frequently requires repeated educational interventions, and one can expect varying degrees of availability of trained ICPs performing these interventions to impact results. As Christenson et al. note, the size of the study imposes limitations on the conclusions one can draw but it is hoped that such studies will encourage broader examinations of infection control practices and contribute to evidence-based practices aimed at better control of HAIs globally. Clearly, more study is needed to examine whether there is a correlation between staffing and compliance with evidence-based practices and, ultimately, outcomes.

Good surveillance and infection control activities reduce multidrug-resistant organism rates in acute care hospitals, yet two recent surveys of Canadian hospitals (where antibiotic-resistant organisms are less a problem than in the United States, but are, nonetheless, on the rise) revealed that effective surveillance and control activities are not in place in many Canadian hospitals [9–11]. In 2000, a survey of 72% of Canadian hospitals with >80 acute care beds revealed that there was less than 1 ICP per 250 beds in 42% of hospitals, and only 60% of infection control programs had physicians or doctoral professionals with infection control training. Surgical site infection (SSI) rates were provided to surgeons in only 37% of hospitals. A follow-up study indicated that surveillance and control activities in acute care hospitals in Canada are being performed in roughly two-thirds of the 120 hospitals responding to a survey.

TABLE 11-1

THE TOP ISSUES AND FRUSTRATIONS OF INFECTION PREVENTION AND CONTROL TEAM MEMBERS IN 2006

Top Issues	Top Frustrations
1. Collecting, interpreting, and using HAI infection surveillance data.	1. Need to find enough time to do multiple tasks and the ability to usefully and appropriately prioritize those tasks. Dealing with the ever-increasing scope of work.
2. Getting healthcare workers (HCWs), especially nurses and doctors, to consistently use evidence-based guidelines, especially for isolation and hand hygiene.	2. Lack of administrative understanding, support, and buy-in of the central role of HAI prevention and control as the paradigm for patient safety.
3. Having the problem of multidrug-resistant organisms and the need for appropriate antibiotic use and surgical prophylaxis.	3. The ability and willingness of the HCWs, including both doctors and nurses, to use policies correctly and understand the benefits of those policies for their patients.
4. Trying to use and keep up with new evidence and guidelines to create useful and up-to-date policies, procedures, and care measures which the HCWs will understand and use.	
5. Addressing the increasing need for both old and new disease reporting, planning for new crises and potential outbreaks and still doing the preceding 1–4.	

(Source: 94 responses from hospital epidemiologists and infection control professionals at the March 2006 SHEA meeting and the May 2006 Wisconsin APIC Chapters Meeting.)

The reasons that infection control programs in many community hospitals are struggling to implement best practices are complex and certainly worthy of further study. We propose a number of recommendations that we hope will be useful to small hospitals facing these challenges. The authors' extensive background and experience will be used to fill in the gaps where the scientific evidence is sketchy or nonexistent because of a lack of studies.

Most of the top issues in Table 11-1 are discussed in detail in other chapters of this book. Scheckler et al. have articulated the principal goals for infection control and epidemiology [7]:

- Protect patient.
- Protect HCWs, visitors, and others in the healthcare environment.
- Accomplish these two goals in a cost-effective manner, whenever possible.

They also note both the value and necessity of measuring the effectiveness of the procedures, policies, and programs put in place to accomplish the three goals. Most hospital epidemiologists agree that, as with medications, conducting prospective, controlled trials of a current procedure compared with a newer procedure is optimal. The outcome of most interest, of course, is the HAI rate targeted by the procedure. Rarely can studies like the medication studies using a double blind controlled method be done. Complicating HAI studies further is that outbreak situations and endemic situations may not show the same results in separate studies because the underlying issues may be different. At times, these realities lead to a conflict in recommendations [12–14].

We recommend a careful review of this article by our epidemiologist and ICP colleagues in community hospitals [7]. Our careful review of the article indicates that the discussion and the 23 recommendations are still useful. Since the publication of this paper in 1998, additional studies have supported and increased the evidence supporting these recommendations.

KEY ISSUES IN COMMUNITY HOSPITALS

Adequate HAI Prevention and Control Team: Who, How Much Time, and How Many

Anyone who has even the most modest knowledge of healthcare expenditures knows that the crunch is on and has been for a number of years. The 1999 Institute of Medicine report, "To Err Is Human" [15] brought the concept of patient safety, or lack of it, to the forefront of public discourse. Lost in this report, however, was the long-standing paradigm of HAI prevention; it was barely mentioned. A subsequent paper showed the value of infection control in the safety push [16]. As our colleagues indicate, lack of time and support are their principal challenges. The complexity of modern healthcare has made simple calculations of the full-time equivalent (FTE) size of the HAI prevention and control team difficult. Scheckler et al. did not use a number. A recent process by the APIC [17] suggested the number of one ICP per 100 beds based on consensus. The literature has no recommendations correlating bed size or discharges with hours needed for a physician hospital epidemiologist.

Our recommendations, which follow, are based on our own extensive experience, our review of the literature, and the reality of increased needs to review renovation and new building projects and to plan for bioterrorism events and/or new influenza epidemics.

Recommendations

1. For every 100 staffed beds in an acute care hospital, there should be at least one FTE trained ICP and 4 hours of a paid physician hospital epidemiologist.
2. The smallest hospital should have the services of an ICP for at least 8 hours a week (20% time), which should include some time—at least 3 days a week—at the hospital. Likewise, a physician hospital epidemiologist should be accessible to even the smallest institution by e-mail and telephone and should be paid for the time spent consulting.
3. Adequate computer equipment, Internet access, and time for continuing education are essential for the ICPs *no matter what the size of the hospital.*
4. With acute care hospitals of ≥200 staffed beds, one FTE of staff support—secretarial and/or medical record specialist—must be available.

These recommendations are, in the view of the authors, bare-bone essentials. Ample evidence indicates that a proactive HAI prevention team can substantially help reduce adverse events in the patients the hospital serves. The critical issue is making the administrative decision makers aware of the literature/evidence.

Administrative Understanding and Support

JACHO attempted in its 2006 requirements for HAI prevention and control and patient safety to require that the administrative authorities of the hospital—chief executive offices (CEO) and board—support the staff and resources to do the job. The fact that these requirements appear to have made little impact in our surveys and our experience with many hospitals suggests that they are either too new to be effective or that they are low on the JACHO surveyors' priority list.

Recommendations

1. Every acute care hospital must have in place a budget plan for HAI prevention and control. This plan should include the ICP and hospital epidemiologist positions and time required per our four recommendations noted in the preceding section.

2. JACHO must articulate and enforce its new requirement concerning hospital administrative responsibility in the area of HAI prevention and control as an integral part of patient safety.
3. Patient safety activities and quality improvement initiatives in a hospital must not replace the necessary roles of ICPs and hospital epidemiologists but should use their methods and expertise. The 40 years of experience in HAI control and the science base developed should not be replaced by the newest fad.

Changing Human Behavior

Hand hygiene is essential before and after contact with a patient or his or her immediate environment whether using gloves or not. One hospital used the "Clean In, Clean Out" sign in every patient room. However, multiple studies since the CDC's landmark Healthcare Infection Control Practices Advisory Committee (HICPAC) Hand Hygiene Guidelines was released [18] have shown only modest compliance with this intervention, which has proven effective since the time of Semmelweis. All HCWs seem better at hand hygiene after rather than before seeing a patient. Nurses tend to be much better than doctors. And, most surprisingly, nonsurgical primary care physicians and intensivists are better than their surgical colleagues [19].

Isolation guidelines from the CDC's HICPAC are due to be formally released in late 2006. A recent additional Federal Office of Management and Budget review has substantially encumbered the final review process for HICPAC guidelines, even after HICPAC vetted all public comments and expert review and approved a final guideline. This additional step appears to have doubled the time it takes to update or generate a guideline from two to four years. This, in our opinion, is both regrettable and totally unnecessary given the expertise of HICPAC.

However, a long-standing concern of ICPs and hospital epidemiologists is the almost cavalier attitude of some nurses and physicians toward isolation precautions. The apparent lack of understanding regarding the rationale for careful hand hygiene and the use of personal protective equipment (PPE) by those involved in direct patient care frustrates the infection control community. The recent severe acute respiratory syndrome (SARS) outbreak should have demonstrated to all HCWs the value of appropriate use of PPE.

Recommendations

1. One effective way to measure the success of hand-hygiene implementation is by direct observation of the hospital medical and nursing staff use of the CDC HICPAC Hand Hygiene Guidelines with direct feedback to the units and types of staff on their percentage use of appropriate hand hygiene.
2. Select an alcohol hand rub (foam or gel) that is most acceptable to staff in trials.

3. Authorize all HCWs to ask for a "time out" to review missed opportunities for the proper use of PPE in patient isolation situations.
4. Enable the admitting and/or supervising nurse on a unit to put a new patient in isolation if the patient's admitting diagnosis or condition warrants.
5. Whenever possible, use a "forcing function" or engineering control rather than human behavioral change to implement a new policy.
6. Establish a culture of accountability for clinicians on all units/wards. It is the responsibility of clinicians and chiefs/directors of wards/units, rather than only infection control, to ensure compliance with infection control recommendations.

Control of Resistant Organisms

No matter what the setting or size of a hospital, the problem of multidrug-resistant pathogen infection is a major preoccupation for ICPs and has led to calls for action from many quarters. Data comparing percentages of nosocomial *Staphylococcus aureus* infections with Methicillin-resistant *Staphylococcus aureus* in NNIS hospitals with <200 beds to those with >200 beds between 1992 and 2002 demonstrates that smaller hospitals, formerly behind larger hospitals in their percentage of MRSA HAIs, have caught up with larger hospitals [20]. There is a need for more study of resistance rates in the community healthcare setting; however, most studies of the epidemiology and control of resistant organisms have come from large, academic centers. Diekema et al. conducted a survey of >400 U.S. hospitals and found that antimicrobial resistance rates were strongly associated with the size, geographic location, and academic affiliation of hospitals [21].

Hospitals, especially those with intensive care units (ICUs), and long-term care facilities are important epicenters and repositories of resistance. Increasing rates of community onset MRSA (CO-MRSA) also are having an impact on hospitals as CO-MRSA strains are recognized as causes of HAI infections as well [22]. Unfortunately, many centers, discouraged by the increase in MRSA and the cost of control, relaxed previously recommended infection control practices in the recent past. In contrast, some northern European countries adopted national, comprehensive programs resulting in impressive control of resistant organisms.

Cost and safety issues surround these infections: increased morbidity and mortality, more expensive and limited treatment options, longer hospital stays, patient dissatisfaction, the cost and inconvenience of precautions, litigation, and adverse publicity for healthcare facilities (especially where drug resistance is publicly reported and/or considered a measure of quality) and are an increasing reality in today's consumer-driven patient safety movement.

With the identification of vancomycin-resistant *S. aureus* (VRSA), CO-MRSA, more virulent strains of *Clostridium difficile* (CDAD), increased recognition of extended-spectrum beta-lactamase-resistant organisms, fungal resistance, multidrug-resistant *M. tuberculosis*, to name some of the most concerning organisms, it is imperative that community hospitals have a complete understanding of the resistance patterns in their institutions, their affiliates, and their region. Similarly, they must keep up with developing recommendations for controlling these infections even if such infections have not yet affected them.

While antibiotic resistance is a daunting problem, a substantial body of literature demonstrates that these organisms can be successfully controlled with multidisciplinary efforts that include active surveillance cultures, contact or barrier precautions, careful environmental cleaning, effective antimicrobial stewardship, and strict compliance with evidence-based hand-hygiene practices. The degree to which control measures should be adopted universally, particularly in regions with low prevalence rates of resistance, is one of the issues surrounding the debate among experts over developing guidelines for managing resistance. This can confuse and deter smaller hospitals that are attempting to determine and implement best practices for identification and control of these organisms.

Recommendations

In 2003, the Society for Healthcare Epidemiology of America published an extensive review of the literature and guidelines for the control of MRSA and Vancomycin-resistant enterococcus (VRE) [9]. It is widely known that the publication of this guideline during the simultaneous development of draft guidelines by HICPAC sparked a vigorous debate among experts as to how to interpret and apply the best science to control these organisms. Most hospitals must decide what they will take from each of the guidelines to develop strategies for preventing the dissemination of resistance. Both guidelines should be studied carefully. The recently released CDC HICPAC Multidrug Resistant Organism (MDRO) Guideline recommends that if a hospital's rate of infection with these pathogens is not decreasing, it should implement more aggressive measures, including active surveillance cultures. We present an approach to managing MRSA and VRE adopted by the MaineHealth® Infection Control Consortium in the Appendix to this chapter.

The most salient difference between the two guidelines is the screen and isolate or "search and destroy" practice [13]. The SHEA guidelines recommend aggressive use of active surveillance cultures to identify patients colonized with these organisms (because routine clinical cultures do not detect the colonized reservoir) and placing those patients on contact precautions. To date, the HICPAC draft guidelines favor a graduated approach with increased intensity of control activities in settings where baseline measures fail to decrease transmission rates. A major argument used by those who find the SHEA document too rigorous is that

many studies used multiple interventions and are unable to weigh the strength of any single intervention or combination of interventions (an argument never made with any of the other CDC HICPAC guidelines, although this is also true of them). However, Muto et al. vigorously defend the SHEA approach of active surveillance cultures and contact isolation, citing the success of northern European countries and Western Australia in controlling these infections. They contrast this with the failure of standard precautions and failure to control these organisms in other areas of Europe and Australia where a less aggressive approach is used [23,24]. In European countries, the delivery of medical care differs from that in U.S. healthcare facilities for whom these guidelines are intended. In countries and institutions where an aggressive approach, such as that recommended in the SHEA guidelines, has been adopted, however, impressive control of MRSA and VRE have been achieved.

The implications of these guidelines for community hospitals are significant. As Strausbaugh et al. [13] note, neither guideline addresses in a more comprehensive sense the goal of these control efforts. In addition, neither guideline currently considers how resources should be allocated for control programs—an issue of great importance to community hospitals without research dollars to divert to such endeavors.

Translating the science coming out of larger academic centers into practice at the level of smaller, nonteaching hospitals is complicated by a lack of understanding of which interventions are most effective and an imprecise understanding of the epidemiology of these organisms outside of large hospitals. Some experts argue that it is better to direct efforts and resources at reducing SSIs and device-related HAIs as a means to control resistance rather than to implement the type of "search and destroy" strategies that have been successful in Europe. Indeed, the former approach is gaining momentum as a result of national quality efforts toward implementing proven methods of reducing such infections by encouraging the utilization of "bundles" of evidence-based best practices for prevention [13]. However, it is far from clear that this will be an adequate national strategy for decreasing rates of MRSA and VRE in the United States and in community hospitals.

West et al. recently published a paper on the effect of targeted surveillance cultures of high-risk populations for control of MRSA in a community hospital system [25]. They acknowledged the workload and expense associated with universal surveillance cultures and the reluctance of administrations to accept such efforts. They used the SHEA guidelines for isolation of patients colonized or infected with MRSA and achieved reductions in MRSA in a cost-effective manner. Patients infected with MRSA had been placed in isolation since 1988, but infection rates remained stable despite the additional measure of screening nares specimens from patients in the ICU, a practice initiated in 2001. Only after active surveillance cultures targeted high-risk patients throughout the hospital was a significant reduction in MRSA infection rates realized. However, Huang et al. have documented the impact of routine screening cultures and isolating colonized patients in ICUs on hospitalwide MRSA bacteremia. They achieved a 40% reduction in MRSA-BSIs in non-ICU patients and a 67% reduction hospitalwide. Using interrupted time-series design for their analysis of 9 years of data, they determined that the statistically significant factor in bringing about these reductions was active surveillance cultures with subsequent placement of patients on contact precautions in the ICU. Typical multiple interventions, such as the introduction of alcohol gels, a handwashing campaign, and maximal sterile barrier precautions for insertion of central lines, did not have significant impact on the rates [26].

Resistant Gram-Negative Organisms

The size, location, and services of a hospital also can conceivably impact the risk for acquisition of these organisms. Extended-spectrum and AmpC beta-lactamase-producing bacteria are important HAIs, and *Pseudomonas aeurignosa* resistance to quinolones, imipenem, and third-generation cephalosporins; *Enterobacter* resistance to third-generation cephalosporins; and multidrug-resistant *Acinetobacter* are on the rise worldwide [27].

The National Committee for Clinical Laboratory Standards (NCCLS) issued its guideline in 1999 to help laboratories identify extended-spectrum beta-lactamase-producing *Klebsiella* species and *Escherichia coli*[28]. Despite current recommendations, not all clinical microbiology laboratories routinely identify extended-spectrum beta-lactamase (ESBL)-producing organisms (ESBL-producing organisms). Surveys looking at the ability of clinical laboratories to detect ESBLs identified a serious gap in this regard [29,30]. Community hospital outbreaks are well described [31,32].

Risk factors for acquiring these organisms are similar to those for the acquisition of other HAI gram-negative organisms: indwelling catheters, increased severity of illness, urgent abdominal surgery, ventilator use, and prolonged hospital stay. Lautenbach et al. found patients infected with pathogens with ESBLs had a greater cumulative antibiotic exposure than did controls; total antibiotic exposure was the only independent predictor of infections with these organisms [33]. Their study suggested that curbing the use of all classes of antibiotics used against gram-negative organisms may be important. Control measures should focus on limiting contact transmission of resistant isolates and controlling antibiotic use. Although more study is needed, some have suggested implementing infection control measures for pathogens with ESBLs similar to those used to control MRSA and VRE [9].

Recommendations for the control of ESBL-producing and other multidrug-resistant gram-negative organisms of epidemiologic importance follow. We prefer an aggressive approach to control these organisms until scientific evidence suggests that less aggressive measures are adequate. Harris et al. have published an excellent summary and analysis of the data on active surveillance cultures to identify colonized patients and whether they should be placed on contact precautions [27]. They provide a framework for decision making and recommendations for future investigations. Hospital epidemiologists must determine what is best in their institutions. The following recommendations have been adapted from Paterson and Yu for pathogens producing ESBLs; however, some of these recommendations also could be applied to control other highly resistant gram-negative organisms of epidemiologic importance [34].

1. Laboratories should follow NCCLS guidelines for detecting ESBL-producing organisms among all isolates of *Klebsiella pneumoniae* or *E. coli* and should report these to clinicians and infection control personnel.
2. Proper hand hygiene, gloves, and gowns should be employed when caring for infected or colonized patients.
3. Clinical and laboratory staff, patients, and their visitors should be educated about these organisms.
4. Affected patients should be isolated or cohorted, and HCW staffing assignments should minimize the potential for cross-transmission.
5. Antibiotic controls, especially of extended-spectrum cephalosporins, should be instituted.
6. Consider periodic rectal and urine cultures of patients in ICUs to identify carriers. In some institutions, active surveillance cultures is used only in outbreak situations [27].
7. Inform receiving units or other facilities of infected or colonized patients.
8. Because carriage can persist for months, previously colonized or infected patients should be regarded as colonized until proven otherwise and medical records should be flagged to indicate status at readmission.
9. Colonized or infected patients may be admitted to nursing homes where they should be placed in single rooms with private bathrooms. The use of common areas by colonized patients should be considered on an individual basis.

Although competent antibiotic stewardship and infection control programs are of demonstrable efficacy in reducing the spread of resistance, overall use of antibiotics, and cost, such expertise may not be available to the smaller community hospital due to lack of monetary or human resources [35,36]. In many hospitals, antimicrobial stewardship is a coresponsibility of infection control, the pharmacy and therapeutics committee, and clinicians. The proportional influence of infection control compared with optimization of antibiotic use on the reduction of HAIs due to resistant organisms seems to depend, to some extent, on the organism and mode of transmission [37,38]. Horizontally transmitted organisms, such as MRSA, VRE, or *C. difficile*, seem more amenable to infection control measures whereas resistance arising from the endogenous flora of patients receiving antibiotics, such as ESBL-producing organisms, requires more emphasis on antibiotic controls. Choosing the most appropriate antibiotic, dose, and duration of therapy based on the proper collection and interpretation of cultures; using an up-to-date clinical microbiology laboratory; treating infection rather than colonization; and limiting the use of certain agents should be part of an overall strategy to reduce resistance in all hospitals [39]. A concurrent review of antibiotic use by specialists along with computer-assisted antibiotic decision support can be extremely helpful in controlling the spread of resistance [40]. Such programs require a substantial commitment of resources by a hospital but can result in cultural changes, reduced costs, and lower rates of bacterial resistance [41]. Promoting infection control and antimicrobial stewardship in all hospitals should be priorities in a national strategy to combat resistance.

The community hospital must be considered in the context of its "trade routes," which provide opportunities for the dissemination of resistance (Figure 11-1). Antimicrobial resistance is commonly a *regional* problem, involving >1 facility in a geographic area. A recent study of the epidemiology of MRSA and VRE among hospitals in Iowa (ranging from ~86 to >858 beds in diverse geographic regions of the state) uncovered differences in the epidemiology of these two organisms; these findings have important implications for their control [42]. For instance, they found that VRE and MRSA shared some risk factors for acquisition as well as some significant differences in that MRSA was endemic in rural hospitals (rural location and hospital size of <200 beds were significant risk factors for MRSA infection) while hospitalization at a smaller hospital had a negative correlation with VRE infection. The

authors present compelling evidence of the importance of understanding the regional epidemiology of resistance and identifying reservoirs of these organisms.

Thinking regionally also has been of benefit in controlling VRE and MRSA within a geographic area. A landmark investigation in 32 healthcare facilities in the Siouxland region of South Dakota, Iowa, and Nebraska reported by Ostrowsky et al. demonstrated that control of VRE could be accomplished in a regional healthcare system by performing active surveillance cultures to detect colonization in high-risk patients and using contact precautions for colonized and infected patients [43]. This study demonstrates the efficacy of using evidence-based guidelines in all healthcare facilities in a region.

Cooperative partnerships among centers can improve efforts at controlling multidrug-resistant pathogens and other important HAIs. Kaye et al. recently reported on the work of the Duke Infection Control Outreach Network [44]. They used a standardized approach to surveillance, provided frequent feedback, and followed uniform policies using CDC guidelines at 12 hospitals in their network. They achieved a reduction in bloodstream infections, nosocomial MRSA infections, ventilator-associated pneumonia, and blood borne pathogen exposures among employees. Kaye et al. estimated remarkable economic benefits. As of this writing, their 32 hospital consortium continues to report reductions in these areas and in catheter-associated urinary tract infections on their Web site (**www.dicon.mc.duke.edu/**). There are other examples of successful regional approaches to multidrug-resistant organisms [45].

Our own experience is with a 13-facility infection control consortium sponsored by MaineHealth® that is modeled on the successful outcomes of the Barnes Jewish Hospital Infection Control and Hospital Epidemiology Consortium in the St. Louis area, from which we received valuable support in developing our group [46]. The increased cooperation among the MaineHealth® Infection Control Consortium participants, which include very small rural hospitals and larger hospitals (200 to 600 beds), home care agencies, long-term care facilities, a rehabilitation hospital, and so on has been a positive and productive experience to date. The group is sharing expertise, data, and policies on the control of multidrug-resistant organisms and providing member institutions with evidence-based algorithms and standard approaches to regional problems such as CDAD, VRE, MRSA and vaccination strategies. Clinicians and others can link to a single Web site for updated guidelines, policies, and patient educational resources. Regional standardization of policies and shared educational documents contribute to the confidence of clinicians, administrators, and patients.

Burdens of Expanded Work

Planning for a bioterrorism event, dealing with the possibility of the admission of a SARS patient returning

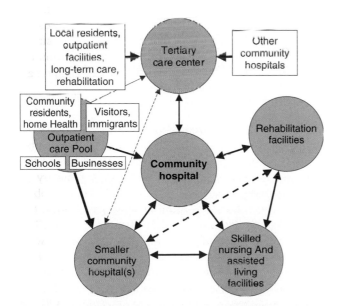

Figure 11-1 Relationships among diverse healthcare facilities in the community setting—routes for the spread of antibiotic resistance.

from Asia, and finally having to plan for "the next" pandemic of influenza have sequentially added new work to an already stressed infection control program. It is not the function of this chapter to replicate what is well covered in other parts of this text. Suffice it to say that these issues are an important part of the field of healthcare epidemiology in community hospitals. They also require close collaboration with local and state public health authorities. The need for an expanded review of the infection control issues and risks in hospital renovation and building projects has also taken on a new urgency in recent years. More work means more time needed. These issues illustrate in a profound way the reality of interdependence as new challenges unfold even as this book is published.

Requirements for Infrastructure and Essential Activities of Infection Control and Epidemiology in Hospitals [6]

The recommendations of the "essentials" are so relevant to this chapter that we repeat them here with permission. When possible, the panel used an evidence-based approach. Recommendations therefore are categorized in Table 11-2, using a modification of the scheme developed by the Clinical Affairs Committee of the Infectious Diseases Society of America and the CDC HICPAC classification scheme.

TABLE 11-2
RECOMMENDATION CATEGORIES

I. Strongly recommended	Strongly recommended for implementation based on
	■ Evidence from at least one properly randomized, controlled trial.
	■ Evidence from at least one well-designed clinical trial without randomization.
	■ Evidence from cohort or case-control analytical studies (preferably from more than one center).
	■ Evidence from multiple time-series studies.
II. Recommended	Recommended for implementation based on
	■ Published clinical experience or descriptive studies.
	■ Reports of expert committees.
	■ Opinions of respected authorities.
III. Recommended when required by government rules or regulations	

Functions

Managing Critical Data and Information

Recommendation 1: Surveillance of HAIs must be performed (Category I). The surveillance process should incorporate at least the following elements:

- Identification and description of the problem or event to be studied.
- Definition of the population at risk.
- Selection of the appropriate methods of measurement, including statistical tools and risk stratifications.
- Identification and description of data sources and data collection personnel and methods.
- Definition of numerators and denominators.
- Preparation and distribution of reports to appropriate groups.
- Selection of specific events to be monitored, which should be guided by validated, nationally available benchmarks appropriately adjusted for patient risks so that meaningful comparisons can be made.

Recommendation 2: Surveillance data must be analyzed appropriately and used to monitor and improve infection control and healthcare outcomes (Category I).

Recommendation 3: Clinical performance and assessment indicators used to support external comparative measurements should meet the criteria delineated by SHEA and APIC (Category II).

Specifically, these indicators and their analyses must address the following parameters:

- Relation to outcome or process.
- Ability to measure variation in quality.
- Definition of numerators and denominators.
- Reliability, completeness, and feasibility of data collection.
- Appropriate risk adjustment.
- Comparability of populations; severity and case-mix adjustments for external comparison.
- Training required for indicator implementation.
- Applicable benchmarks of standards of care.

Setting and Recommending Policies and Procedures

Recommendation 4: Written infection prevention and control policies and procedures must be established, implemented, maintained, and updated periodically (Categories II and III).

- The policies and procedures should be scientifically valid.
- The policies and procedures should be reviewed for practicality and cost.
- The policies and procedures should lead to improved prevention or improved patient outcomes.

Recommendation 5: Policies and procedures should be monitored periodically for performance (Categories II and III).

Compliance with Regulations, Guidelines, and Accreditation Requirements

Recommendation 6: Healthcare facilities should use infection control personnel to assist in maintaining compliance with relevant regulatory and accreditation requirements (Category II).

Recommendation 7: Infection control personnel should have appropriate access to medical or other relevant records and to staff members who can provide information on the adequacy of the institution's compliance with regard to regulations, standards, and guidelines (Category II).

Recommendation 8: The infection control program should collaborate with and provide liaison to appropriate local and state health departments for reporting communicable diseases and related conditions and to assist with control of infectious diseases (Categories II and III).

Employee Health

Recommendation 9: Infection control program personnel should work collaboratively with the facility's employee health program personnel (Category II).

- The infection control program should review and approve all policies and procedures developed in the employee health program that relate to the transmission of infections in the hospital.
- Infection control personnel should be available to the employee health program for consultation regarding infectious disease concerns.

Recommendation 10: At the time of employment, all facility personnel should be evaluated by the employee health program for conditions relating to communicable diseases (Categories II and III).

The evaluation should include the following:

- Medical history, including immunization status and assessment for conditions that may predispose personnel to acquiring or transmitting communicable diseases.
- Tuberculin skin testing or QuantiFeron Gold testing.
- Serologic screening for vaccine-preventable diseases if indicated.
- Medical examinations that are indicated by the preceding evaluation.

Recommendation 11: Appropriate employees or other HCWs should have periodic medical evaluations to assess for new conditions related to infectious diseases that may have an impact on patient care, the employee, or other HCWs, which should include review of immunization and tuberculin skin-test or QuantiFeron Gold status if appropriate (Categories II and III).

- All facilities should maintain confidential medical records on all HCWs.

- The employee health program should have the capability to track employee immunization and tuberculin skin-test or QuantiFeron test status.

Recommendation 12: Employees must be offered appropriate immunizations for communicable diseases (Categories I and III).

- Immunizations should be based on regulatory requirements and recommendations of an advisory committee on immunization practices for HCWs.

Recommendation 13: The employee health program should develop policies and procedures for evaluating ill employees, including the assessment of disease communicability, indications for work restrictions, and management of employees who have been exposed to infectious diseases including postexposure prophylaxis and work restrictions (Category I).

Intervening Directly to Prevent Transmission of Infectious Diseases

Recommendation 14: All healthcare facilities must have the capacity to identify the occurrence of outbreaks or clusters of infectious diseases (Category I).

- Infection control personnel should review microbiology records regularly to identify unusual clusters or a greater-than-usual incidence of certain species or strains of microorganisms.
- In patient areas of the healthcare facility in which active prospective surveillance is not conducted, infection control programs should maintain regular contact with clinical, medical, and nursing staff to ascertain the occurrence of disease clusters or outbreaks, to assist in maintaining and monitoring infection control procedures, and to provide consultation as required.

Recommendation 15: All healthcare facilities must have access to the services of personnel who are trained and experienced in conducting outbreak investigations (Category II).

Recommendation 16: When an outbreak occurs, the infection control team must have adequate resources and authority to ensure a comprehensive and timely investigation and the implementation of appropriate control measures (Category II).

Education and Training of Healthcare Workers

Recommendation 17: Healthcare facilities must provide ongoing educational programs in infection prevention and control to HCWs (Categories II and III).

- Infection control personnel with knowledge of epidemiology and infectious diseases should be active participants in planning and implementing the educational programs.

Recommendation 18: Educational programs should be evaluated periodically for effectiveness, and attendance should be monitored (Categories II and III).

- Educational programs should meet the needs of the group or department to which they are given and must provide learning experiences for people with a wide range of educational backgrounds and work responsibilities.

Resources

Personnel

Recommendation 19: The personnel and supporting resources, including secretarial services, available to the hospital epidemiology and infection control program should be proportional to the size, complexity, and estimated risk of the population served by the institution (Category II).

Recommendation 20: All hospitals should have the continuing services of trained hospital epidemiologist(s) and ICP(s) (Category I).

Recommendation 21: ICPs should be encouraged to obtain certification in infection control (Category II).

Nonpersonnel

Recommendation 22: Each healthcare facility should provide or make available in a timely fashion sufficient office space and equipment, statistical and computer support, and clinical microbiology and pathology laboratory services to support the HAI surveillance, prevention, and control program of the institution (Category II).

Recommendation 23: Resources should be provided for continuing professional education of hospital epidemiologist(s) and ICP(s) (Category II).

CONCLUSIONS

Despite the historical primacy of infection control among hospital quality and safety initiatives—and its documented efficacy—today's infection control programs that are still trying to manage the traditional duties of surveillance, outbreak management, and education are now asked to include an increasing number of responsibilities. Moreover, they are or soon will be under increased pressure generated by the consumer-driven movement toward public reporting of HAIs—a movement that is not always grounded in good science. The modern infection control program must maintain its standards in an environment of cost-cutting and competition for resources with diverse quality initiatives. Some ICPs are leading these efforts, but others are struggling to find a place at the table.

Community hospitals, particularly rural facilities, are not always able to attract professionals with infection control expertise or interest, and even when these professionals are available, hospital administrators may be unable or reluctant to provide appropriate support for them so they can accomplish their traditional responsibilities in addition to investigating process breakdowns or working on the cultural changes necessary for the adoption of evidence-based practices. It could be argued that cultural and policy changes are more easily brought about in smaller institutions, but a number of factors other than size influence these processes in our experience. The wise epidemiologist weighs systems problems against ignorance or more culpable explanations for resistance to adopting practices of proven efficacy such as hand hygiene.

How, then, is the institution to find creative solutions to the challenges of infection control in the community? Partnering with other institutions to form regional infection control and quality consortia gives small hospitals an opportunity to share resources and expertise with larger hospitals in addition to providing academicians with new opportunities for scientific study. In return, academic hospital epidemiologists should consider how they can support their community-based colleagues in developing scientific studies that will lead to the development of evidence-based practices suitable to the populations they serve.

Working with public health authorities in identifying and managing outbreaks or controlling regional infectious problems can benefit both the private and the public sectors. Infection control working groups, which bring public health and private professionals together for regular discussion of common concerns, afford another opportunity to share expertise and resources. A number of states have found such cooperation gratifying and effective.

Community-based infection control professionals must take a greater role in educating their colleagues, administrators, government, and the public about the importance, causes, and metrics of HAIs. ICPs must convey the validity and utility of sound epidemiologic methodology to those involved in developing the public reporting of HAIs. It is increasingly important to the well-being of patients that those who manage community hospitals appreciate the efficacy of infection control programs. If community-based ICPs and hospital epidemiologists wish to continue their leading role as patient safety advocates, they must be willing to educate a wider audience on the evolution, methodology, and value of healthcare epidemiology. They also must be ready to discuss the impact of their recommendations on the resources of their facilities and the community at large.

There is hope that the recent surge of interest in reducing the number of HAIs—part of the overall focus on patient safety—will lead to increased resources to control HAIs, implementation of evidence-based practices, improved monitoring of outcomes, and a better understanding of how to address the global issue of antibiotic resistance. It is our hope that these efforts will benefit the large number of patients in U.S. community hospitals and elsewhere.

APPENDIX

MAINEHEALTH® INFECTION CONTROL CONSORTIUM GUIDELINES FOR THE MANAGEMENT OF MRSA AND VRE

Consistent use of standard precautions remains the basis for preventing the spread of infection in all facilities. In addition to standard precautions, transmission-based precautions for "organisms of epidemiological significance" remain important once an organism has been identified. This document seeks to lay the foundation for the basics of care. In certain circumstances, it may be necessary to exceed the basic guidelines, and that decision is the prerogative of any individual institution. In addition, as new guidelines and information are published, it will be necessary to alter or update this document after review and approval by the Consortium DRO Committee.

Prevention is the first principle in the management of drug-resistant organisms (DROs). A DRO prevention and control strategy incorporates evidence-based infection control practices, antibiotic stewardship, laboratory support, and active surveillance. Active surveillance cultures are believed to be essential to the identification of the pool of colonized patients that may be missed by only monitoring results of clinical cultures. Early identification of colonized patients and prompt institution of precautions is necessary to decrease transmission [9,46–79].

The description of what constitutes "contact precautions" remains gray in the literature as draft recommendations from the CDC appear to recommend mandatory gloving and gowning for entry into the room. The previously published CDC guidelines call for anticipation of the likelihood of contact with the patient or his or her environment and the decision of whether personal protective equipment (PPE) is needed [9,53,66,80–88]. We have chosen to include both at this time, as some institutions are following the older guidelines and others are following the recently released CDC MDRO guidelines (which are similar to the SHEA guidelines with regard to mandatory gowns and gloves).

There is a lack of information in the literature regarding the discontinuation of precautions and "clearance" of multidrug-resistant organisms. A number of studies examined the duration of colonization and found it could persist for months to years. Several articles reported varying degrees of success with decolonization protocols. Some Maine institutions have adopted a "once a MDRO, always a MDRO" policy. Others require several screening cultures from various sites for clearance. The subgroup felt that in consideration of the risk factors for MDRO, acquisition was the place to start deciding which patients were likely to remain positive and decrease unnecessary

expense and the emotional impact of active surveillance cultures. After an extensive review, we have proposed a set of exclusion criteria and then standardized the sites and number of cultures required to "prove" culture-negative status. Standardizing the criteria for clearance culturing and the sites/method of culturing will benefit all patients but especially those patients that move between institutions [49,93–107].

We also researched the utilization of precaution gowns and gloves for visitors. We found varying requirements in the literature. After careful review, we believe that the chain of transmission falls primarily on the actions of HCWs as they move from patient to patient, not on the actions of visitors, who are there only to see their loved one. We currently do not support the requirement of the routine use of gowns and gloves for visitors; rather, we would emphasize the need for family education regarding hand hygiene with the caveat that if the family members are likely to soil their clothing because of participation in nursing type care of the patient, gowning and/or gloving may be appropriate [13,108,109].

After review and discussion, the following guidelines are presented as current "best practice."

RECOMMENDATIONS FOR ACUTE CARE MANAGEMENT OF MRSA AND VRE

A. Standard Precautions
   1. Standard Precautions will be the basic practice for all patients before or after diagnosis of colonization or infection with an MDRO.
   2. Institution of contact or MDRO precautions are addressed later in this document.
B. Active Surveillance Cultures of Patients with Known History of DROs
   1. Patients with a known history of MRSA should not be screened for MRSA.
   2. Patients with a known history of VRE should not be screened for VRE.
C. Active Surveillance Cultures of Patients with Unknown History of DROs
   1. Culture high risk populations (to be defined by each facility).
      a. Groups that may be considered "high risk" include patient's from long-term care or physical rehabilitation units, dialysis patients, transfers with extended stays in acute care facilities, and patients with chronic conditions.
   2. Obtain culture within 48 hours of admission.
   3. Repeat active surveillance cultures once a week at a predetermined day/time identified by each unit/facility. Repeat screening of known positives is not necessary.

4. Cultures are to be of the following:
   a. MRSA.
      i. Nares—one swab used to culture both nostrils.
      ii. Groin—one swab used to culture the fold of the skin on each side (an alternative site may be indicated in certain health care settings).
      iii. Open wounds—culture any open area such as a pressure ulcer, diabetic foot ulcer, etc.
   b. VRE.
      i. Perirectal culture using one swab.
      ii. Some studies suggest that patients being screened for *Clostridium difficile* who also are VRE positive contribute to environmental contamination and transmission. Consideration may be given to a program that includes testing for both *C. difficile* and VRE in patients with diarrhea.
5. Pooling of specimens decreases the sensitivity of MRSA detection compared with processing each swab separately therefore, pooling is not recommended.

D. Patients Who Are Culture Positive or Have a History of a Positive Culture
1. Place patient on Contact Precautions* upon every admission or at identification of positive culture.
2. Utilize contact precautions
   a. Gloves—wear upon entry into room.
   b. Gowns—wear upon entry into room as recommended by the draft 2004 CDC Guidelines. Current SHEA and previous CDC guidelines recommend utilization if in contact with the patient or environment.
   c. Masks—wear only when transmission by droplets is suspected or according to Standard Precautions based on nature of patient care activity.
3. Decolonization—no recommendation is made to routinely attempt decolonize. Decision to attempt decolonization should be made within a facility in consultation with the infection control department.
4. Patients should be placed in a private room or may be cohorted with another/other patient(s) who has/have the same organism in any location on the body (i.e., VRE with VRE or MRSA with MRSA or MRSA/VRE with another patient with MRSA/VRE) and no other active infection.
5. Family and visitors to patients on Contact Precautions need to be instructed in the importance of hand hygiene upon entering and leaving the patient's room. Additionally they should be instructed to refrain from visiting other patients or entering patient care locations (i.e., on-unit kitchenettes, solariums). Visitors who may be at risk of clothing or skin contamination from blood or body fluids due to type of activity they may be providing should be instructed in the use of gowns and gloves. Visitors without this type of exposure do not routinely need to wear gowns or gloves.

E. Discontinuation of Precautions for Patients with MDROs of MRSA or VRE Across the Healthcare Continuum
1. Although patients may test negative, multiple studies indicate that it is likely that colonization is only temporarily undetectable and recolonization is expected.
2. The routine testing of previously positive patients for discontinuation of precautions should be discouraged. In the unlikely case that the patient passes *all* of the following exclusion criteria, screening may be indicated:
   a. Not hospitalized (defined as 8-hour or longer stay in an acute care facility) within the last 6 months.
   b. Not treated with antibiotic therapy, including intranasal mupirocin, within the last 6 months.
   c. Not admitted to or treated at a long-term care or rehabilitation facility in the last 6 months.
   d. Currently has no indwelling lines which include but is not limited to PICC, tunneled, peripheral, central, arterial or dialysis type devices.
   e. Has not undergone any invasive procedure within the last 6 months.
3. Screen as follows.
   a. For MRSA clearance.
      i. Obtain three sets of screening cultures from the following sites
         (1) Nares—one swab used to culture both nostrils.
         (2) Groin—one swab used to culture the fold of the skin on each side (an alternative site may be indicated in certain healthcare settings).
         (3) Any open wound—such as a pressure ulcer, diabetic foot ulcer.
         (4) Original site of MRSA if known. If from sterile site must have had at least one culture that is negative.
      ii. Obtain cultures × 3 no closer than 72 hours (*Could say daily—there are no data from CDC showing the advantage of any approach. Three on one day or on three separate consecutive days would be acceptable. Really no data for making this recommendation*) apart per CDC recommendations.
   b. For VRE clearance
      i. Obtain perirectal culture × 3 no closer than 7 days (*Same as above—this approach leaves patients in isolation for 21 days—Really not necessary*) apart per CDC recommendations.

---

*The CDC HICPAC MDRO Guideline recommends "enhanced contact precautions" for drug-resistant organisms. Some facilities have elected to create a category of precautions to address this that includes Enhanced Contact Precautions, Contact Precautions Plus, or MDRO Precautions. Regardless of the nomenclature, the basic precaution requirements remain the same.

c. Alert laboratory of the screening nature of testing and of the specific organisms being screened for.

REFERENCES

1. Valenti AJ. Towns, gowns, and gloves: The status of infection control in community hospitals. *Infect Control Hosp Epidemiol* 2006; 27:225–227.
2. *AHA Hospital Statistics, 2005.* Chicago, IL: Health Forum LLC, 2005: 11–25.
3. Scheckler WE. Hospital epidemiology and infection control in small hospitals. In: Mayhall C. G. *Hospital epidemiology and infection control.* 3rd ed. Philadelphia: Lippincott Williams and Wilkins, 2004.
4. Scheckler WE, Bobula JA, Beamsley MB, Hadden ST. Bloodstream infections in a community hospital: A 25-year follow-up. *Infect Control Hosp Epidemiol* 2003;24:936–941.
5. Samore MH, Bateman K, Alder SC, et al. Clinical decision support and appropriateness of antimicrobial prescribing: A randomized trial. *JAMA* 2005;294:2305–2314.
6. Stevenson KB, Searle K, Stoddard GJ, Samore MH. Methhicillin-resistant Staphlococcus aureus and vancomycin-resistant entero-cocci in rural communities, western United States. *Emerg Infect Dis* 2005;11:895–903.
7. Scheckler WE, Brimhall D, Buck AS, et al. Requirements for infrastructure and essential activities of infection control and epidemiology in hospitals: A consensus panel report. *Infect Control Hosp Epidemiol* 1998;19:114–124.
8. Christenson M, Hitt JA, Abbott G, et al. Improving patient safety: Resource availability and application for reducing the incidence of healthcare-associated infection. *Infect Control Hosp Epidemiol* 2006;27:245–251.
9. Muto CA, Jernigan JA, Ostrowsky BE, et al. SHEA guideline for preventing nosocomial transmission of multidrug-resistant strains of Staphylococcus aureus and Enterococcus. *Infect Control Hosp Epidemiol* 2003;24:362–386.
10. Zoutman DE, Ford BD, Bryce E, et al. The state of infection surveillance and control in Canadian acute care hospitals. *Am J Infect Control* 2003;31:266–273.
11. Zoutman DE, Ford BD, Canadian Hospital Epidemiology Committee and Canadian Nosocomial Infection Surveillance Program, Health Canada. The relationship between hospital infection surveillance and control activities and antibiotic-resistant pathogen rates. *Am J Infect Control* 2005;33:1–5.
12. Jackson M, Jarvis WR, and Scheckler WE. HICPAC/SHEA—Conflicting guidelines: What is the standard of care? *Amer J Infect Control* 2004;32:504–511.
13. Strausbaugh LJ, Siegel JD, Weinstein RA. Preventing transmission of multidrug-resistant bacteria in health-care settings: A tale of two guidelines. *Clin Infect Dis* 2006;42:828–835.
14. Muto CA. Why are antibiotic-resistant nosocomial infections spiraling out of control? *Infec Control Hosp Epidem* 2005;26:10–12.
15. Kohn LT, Corrigan JM, Donaldson, eds. To err is human: Building a safer health system. Washington, DC: Institute of Medicine, 1999.
16. Scheckler WE. Healthcare epidemiology is the paradigm for patient safety. *Infect Control Hosp Epidemiol* 2002;23:47–51.
17. O'Boyle C, Jackson M, Henly SJ. Staffing requirements for infection control programs in US healthcare facilities: Delphi project. *Am J Infect Control* 2002;30:321–333.
18. Centers for Disease Control and Prevention. Guideline for hand hygiene in health-care settings: Recommendations of the Healthcare Infection Control Practices Advisory Committee and the HICPAC/SHEA/APIC/IDSA Hand Hygiene Task Force. *MMWR* 2002;51(RR-16):1–49.
19. Eckmanns T, Bessert J, Behnke M, et al. Compliance with antiseptic hand rub use in intensive care units: The hawthorne effect. *Infect Control Hosp Epidemiol* 2006;27:931–934.
20. Centers for Disease Control and Prevention. National Nosocomial Infections Surveillance (NNIS) System Report, data summary from January 1992 through June 2003, issued August 2003. *Am J Infect Control* 2003;31:481–498.
21. Diekema DJ, BootsMiller T, Vaughn T, et al. Antimicrobial resistance trends and outbreak frequency in United States hospitals. *Clin Infect Dis* 2004;38:78–85.
22. Davis SL, Rybak MJ, Amjad M, et al. Characteristics of patients with healthcare-associated infection due to SCCmec Type IV methicillin-resistant Staphylococcus aureus. *Infect Control Hosp Epidemiol* 2006;27:1025–1031.
23. Muto CA, Jarvis WR, Farr BM. Another tale of two guidelines. *Clin Infect Dis* 2006;43:796–797.
24. Farr BM. Doing the right thing (and figuring out what that is). *Infect Control Hosp Epidemiol* 2006;27:999–1003.
25. West TE, Guerry RN, Hiott M, et al. The effect of targeted surveillance for control of methicillin-resistant Staphylococcus aureus in a community hospital system. *Infect Control Hosp Epidemiol* 2006; 27:233–238.
26. Huang SS, Yokoe DS, Hinrichsen VL, et al. Impact of routine intensive care unit surveillance cultures and resultant barrier precautions on hospital-wide methicillin-resistant Staphylococcus aureus bacteremia. *Clin Infect Dis* 2006;43:971–978.
27. Harris AD, McGregor JC, Furuno JP. What infection control interventions should be undertaken to control multidrug-resistant gram-negative bacteria? *Clin Infect Dis* 2006;43:S57–S61.
28. Hanson ND. Performance standards for antimicrobial susceptibility testing: NCCLS approved standard M100-S9. Wayne, PA: National Committee for Clinical Laboratory Standards, 1999.
29. Steward CD, Wallace D, Hubert SK, et al. Ability of laboratories to detect emerging antimicrobial resistance in nosocomial pathogens: A survey of project ICARE laboratories *Diagn Microbiol Infect Dis* 2000; 38:59–67.
30. Tenover FC, Mohammed JM, Gorton T, Dembeck ZF. Detection and reporting of extended-spectrum β-lactamase (ESBL) producing organisms in Connecticut. *Clin Infect Dis.* 1998; 27:1064.
31. Quale JM, Landman D, Bradford PA, et al. Molecular epidemiology of a citywide outbreak of extended-spectrum beta-lactamase-producing Klebsiella pneumonia infection. *Clin Infect Dis* 2002;35:834–831.
32. Rahal JJ, Urban C, Segal-Maurer S. Nosocomial antibiotic resistance in multiple gram-negative species: Experience at one hospital with squeezing the resistance balloon at multiple sites. *Clin Infect Dis* 2002;34:499–503.
33. Lautenbach E, Patel JB, Bilker WB, et al. Extended-spectrum beta-lactamase-producing Escherichia coli and Klebsiella pneumonia: Risk factors for infection and impact of resistance on outcomes. *Clin Infect Dis* 2001;32:1162–1171
34. Paterson DL, Yu VL. Editorial response: Extended-spectrum β-lactamases: A call for improved detection and control. *Clin Infect Dis* 1999;29:1419–1422.
35. Fraser G, Stogsdill P, Owens RC. Antimicrobial stewardship initiatives: A programmatic approach to optimizing antimicrobial use. In: Owens RC, Ambrose PG, Nightingale CH, eds. *Antibiotic optimization: Concepts and strategies in clinical practice.* New York: Marcel Dekker, 2005:261–326.
36. Philmon C, Smith T, Williamson S, Goodman E. Controlling use of antimicrobials in a community teaching hospital. *Infect Control Hosp Epidemiol* 2006;27:239–244.
37. Sefton AM. Mechanisms of antimicrobial resistance: Their clinical relevance in the new millennium *Drugs.* 2002;62:557–566.
38. Rice LB. Controlling antibiotic resistance in the ICU: Different bacteria, different strategies. *Cleve Clin J Med* 2003;70:793–800.
39. Centers for Disease Control and Prevention. Campaign to Prevent Antimicrobial Resistance in Healthcare Settings: Why a campaign? Atlanta: CDIC, 2001. (www.cdc.gov/drugresistance/healthcare/problem.htm)
40. Burke JP and Mehta R. Role of computer-assisted programs in optimizing the use of antimicrobial agents In: Owens RC, Ambrose PG, Nightingale CH, eds. *Antibiotic optimization: concepts and strategies in clinical practice.* New York: Marcel Dekker, 2005:261–326.
41. Bantar C, Sartori B, Vesco E, et al. A hospitalwide intervention program to optimize the quality of antibiotic use: Impact on prescribing practice, antibiotic consumption, cost savings, and bacterial resistance. *Clin Infect Dis* 2003;37:180–186.

42. Polgreen, PM, Beekmann SE, Chen YY, et al. Epidemiology of methicillin-resistant *Staphylococcus aureus* and vancomycin-resistant *Enterococcus* in a rural state. *Infect Control Hosp Epidemiol* 2006;27:252–256.

43. Ostrowsky BE, Trick WE, Sohn AH, et al. Control of vancomycin-resitant *Enterococcus* in health care facilities in a region. *N Engl J Med* 2001;344:1427–1433.

44. Kaye KS, Engemann JJ, Fulmer EM, et al. Favorable impact of an infection control network on nosocomial infection rates in community hospitals. *Infect Control Hosp Epidemiol* 2006;27:228–232.

45. Nicolle LE, Dyck B, Thompson G, et al. Regional dissemination and control of epidemic methicillin-resistant Staphylococcus aureus: Manitoba Chapter of CHICA-Canada. *Infect Control Hosp Epidemiol* 1999:20:202–205.

46. Murphy DM. From expert data collectors to interventionists: Changing the focus for infection control professionals. *Am J Infect Control* 2002;30:120–132.

47. Goldman DA, Weinstein RA, Wenzel RP, et al. Strategies to prevent and control the emergence and spread of microorganisms in a hospital: A challenge to hospital leadership. *JAMA* 1996; 273(3):234–40.

48. Chaix C, Durand-Zaleski I, Alberti C, Brun-Buisson C. Control of endemic methicillin-resistant *Staphylococcus aureus*: A cost benefit analysis in an intensive care unit. *JAMA* 1999;282:1745–1751.

49. Muto, CA. Methicillin-resistant *Staphylococcus aureus* control: We didn't start the fire, but it's time to put it out. *Infect Control Hosp Epidemiol* 2006:27:111–113.

50. Arnold MS, Dempsey JM, Fishman M, et al. The best hospital practices for controlling methicillin-resistant *Staphylococcus aureus*: On the cutting edge. *Infect Control Hosp Epidemiol* 2001;23:69–76.

51. Kearns AM, Pitt TL, Cookson BD. Screening for methicillin-resistant *Staphylococcus aureus*: Which anatomical sites to culture. *J Hosp Infect Soc* 2005:351–352.

52. Simor AE, Ofner-Agostini M, Paton S, et al. Clinical and epidemiologic features of methicillin-resistant *Staphylococcus aureus* in elderly hospitalized patients. *Infect Control Hosp Epidemiol* 2005:838–841.

53. Atta, MG, Eustace JA, Song X, et al. Outpatient vancomycin use and vancomycin-resistant enterococcal colonization in maintenance dialysis patients. *Kidney International* 2001;9:718–724.

54. Wernitz MH, Swidsinski S, Weist K, et al. Effectiveness of a hospital-wide selective screening programme for methicillin-resistant *Staphylococcus aureus* (MRSA) carriers at hospital admission to prevent hospital-acquired MRSA infections. *Clin Microbiol and Infect* 2005;11:457–465.

55. Van Gemert-Pijnen J, Hendriz MF, van der Palen J, Schellens PJ. Performance of methicillin-resistant *Staphylococcus aureus* protocols in Dutch hospitals. *Am J Infect Control* 2005;33:377–384.

56. Hainsworth T. Draft guideline on treatment and prevention of MRSA. *Nursing Times* 2005;101:26–27.

57. Khoury J, Jones M, Grim A, et al. Eradication of methicillin-resistant *Staphylococcus aureus* from a neonatal intensive care unit by active surveillance and aggressive infection control measures. *Infect Control Hosp Epidemiol* 2005;26:594–597.

58. Eveillard M, Lancien E, Barnaud G, et al. Impact of screening for MRSA carriers at hospital admission on risk-adjusted indicators according to the imported MRSA colonization pressure. *J Hosp Infect* 2005;59:254–258.

59. McDonald LC, Hageman JC. Vancomycin intermediate and resistant *Staphylococcus aureus*: What the nephrologist needs to know. *Nephrology News & Issues* 2004;18:63–64.

60. Lucet JC, Grenet K, Armand-Lefevre L, et al. High prevalence of carriage of MRSA at hospital admission in elderly patients: Implication for infection control strategies. *Infect Control Hosp Epidemiol* 2005;26:121–126.

61. Lee TA, Hacek DM, Stroupe KT, et al. Three surveillance strategies for vancomycin-resistant enterococci in hospitalized patients: Detection of colonization efficiency and a cost effectiveness model. *Infect Contrl Hosp Epidemiol* 2005;26:39–46.

62. Furuno JP, Harris AD, Wright MO, et al. Prediction rules to identify patients with MRSA and VRE upon hospital admission. *Am J Infect Control* 2004;32:436–440.

63. Cheng AC, Harrington G, Russo P, et al. Rate of nosocomial transmission of vancomycin-resistant enterococci from isolated patients. *Intern Med J* 2004;34:510–512.

64. Axon RN, Engemann JJ, Butcher J, et al. Control of nosocomial acquisition of vancomycin-resistant enterococci through active surveillance of hemodialysis patients. *Infect Control Hosp Epidemiol* 2004;25:436–438.

65. Hachem R, Graviss L, Hanna H, et al. Impact of surveillance for VRE on controlling a bloodstream outbreak among patients with hematologic malignancy. *Infect Control Hosp Epidemiol* 2004;25:391–394.

66. Perenveich EN, Fisman DN, Lipsitch M, et al. Projected benefits of active surveillance for vancomycin-resistant enterococci in intensive care units. *Clin Infect Dis* 2004;38:1108–1115.

67. Harris AD, Nemoy L, Johnson JA, et al. Co-carriage rates of VRE and ESBL producing bacteria among a cohort of intensive care unit patients: Implication for an active surveillance program. *Infect Control Hosp Epidemiol* 2004;25:105–108.

68. Jernigan JA, Clemence MA, Stott GA, et al. Control of methicillin-resistant *Staphylococcus aureus* at a university hospital: One decade later. *Infect Control Hosp Epidemiol* 1995;16:686–696.

69. Dall'Antonia M, Coen PG, Wilkis M, et al. Competition between methicillin-sensitive and resistant Staphyloccus aureus in the anterior nares. *J Hosp Infect* 2005;61:62–67.

70. Asensio A, Guerrero A, Quereda C, et al. Colonization and infection with MRSA associated factors and eradication. *Infect Control Hosp Epidemiol* 1996;17:20–28.

71. Pan A, Carnevale G, Colombini P, et al. Trends in methiciliin-resisitant *Staphylococcus aureus* (MRSA) bloodstream infections: Effect of the MRSA "search and isolate" strategy in a hospital in Italy with hyperendemic MRSA. *Infect Control Hosp Epidemiol* 2005;26:127–133.

72. Farr BM. Prevention and control of methicillin-resistant *Staphylococcus aureus* infections. *Current Opinion in Infectious Diseases* 2004;17:317–322.

73. Lucet JC, Paoletti X, Lolom I, et al. Successful long term program for controlling methicillin-resistant *Staphylococccus aureus* in intensive care units. *Intensive Care Med* 2005;31:1051–1057.

74. Weinstein RA. Antibioitic resistance in hospitals and intensive care units: The problem and potential solutions. *Semin Respir & Criti Care Med* 2003;24:113–120.

75. Bissett L. Controlling the risk of MRSA infection: Screening and isolating patients. *Brit J Nurs* 2005;14:386–390.

76. Tomic V, Svetina Sorli P, Trinkaus D, et al. Comprehensive strategy to prevent nosocomial spread of methicillin-resistant *Staphylococcus aureus* in a highly endemic setting. *Arch Intern Med* 2004;164:2038–2043.

77. Evans RS, Lloyd JF, Abouzelof RH, et al. System-wide surveillance for clinical encounters by patients previously identified with MRSA and VRE. *Medinfo* 2004;11:212–216.

78. Salgado CK, Farr BM. What proportion of hospital patients colonized with methicillin-resistant *Staphylococcus aureus* are identified by clinical microbiological cultures? *Infect Control Hosp Epidemiol* 2006;27:116–121.

79. Eveillard M, de Lassence A, Lancien E, et al. Evaluation of a strategy of screening multiple anatomical sites for methicillin-resistant *Staphylococcus aureus* at admission to a teaching hospital. *Infect Control Hosp Epidemiol* 2006;27:181–184.

80. Shlaes DM, Gerding DN, John, JF, et al. Society for Healthcare Epidemiology of America and Infection Diseases Society of America Joint Committee on the Prevention of Antimicrobial Resistance: Guidelines for the prevention of antimicrobial resistance in hospitals. *Infect Control Hosp Epidemiol* 1997;18:275–291.

81. Macini EM, Bonten MJM. Vancomycin-resistant enterococci: Consequences for therapy and infection control. *Clin Microbiol Infect* 2005 (Supplement 4):43–56.

82. Tokars JI, Gehr T, Jarvis WR, et al. Vancomycin-resistant enterococci colonization in patients in seven hemodialysis centers. *Kidney International* 2001;60:1511–1516.

83. Panhotra BR, Saxena AK, AL-Mulhim AS. Contamination of patients' files in intensive care units: An indication of strict handwashing after entering case notes. *Am J Infect Control* 2005;33:398–401.

84. Mascini Em, Bonten MJ. Johnston P, Norrish AR, Brammar T, et al. Reducing methicillin-resistant *Staphylococcus aureus* (MRSA)

patient exposure by infection control measures. *Ann Coll Surg Engl* 2005;87:123–125.

85. Faria NA, Oliveria DC, Westh H, et al. Epidemiology of emerging methicillin-resistant *Staphyloccus aureus* (MRSA) in Denmark: A nationwide study in a country with low prevalence of MRSA infection. *J Clin Microbiol* 2005;43:1836–1842.

86. Ott M, Shen J, Sherwood S. Evidence-based practice for control of methicillin-resistant *Staphyloccus aureus*. AORN Journal 2005;81:361–372.

87. Cepeda JA, Whithouse T, Cooper B, et al. Isolation of patients in single rooms or cohorts to reduce spread of MRSA in intensive-care units: Prospective two center study. *Lancet* 354:295–304.

88. Grant J, Ramman-Haddad L, Dendukuri N, Libman MD. The role of gowns in preventing nosocomial transmission of methicillin-resistant *Staphylococcus aureus* (MRSA): Gown use in MRSA control. *Infect Control Hosp Epidemiol* 2006;27:191–194.

89. Grmek-Kosnik I, Ihan, A, Dermota U, et al. Evaluation of separate vs pooled swab cultures, different media, broth enrichment and anatomical site of screening for the detection of methicillin-resistant *Staphylococcus aureus* from clinical specimens. *J Hosp Infect* 2005;61:155–161.

90. Kniehl E, Becker A, Forster DH. Bed, bath and beyond: Pitfalls in prompt eradication of methicillin-resistant *Staphylococcus aureus* carrier status in healthcare workers. *J Hosp Infect* 2005;59:180–187.

91. Maslow JN, Brecher S, Gunn J, et al. Variation and persistence of methicillin resistant *Staphylococcus aureus* strains among individual patients over extended periods of time. *Eur J Clin Microbiol Infect Dis* 1995;14:282–290.

92. Vivoni AM, Santos KR, de-Oliveria MP, et al. Mupirocin for controlling methicillin-resistant *Staphylococcus aureua*: Lessons from a decade of use at a university hospital. *Infect Control Hosp Epidemiol* 2005;26:662–667.

93. Yale discontinuation of contact precautions IC policy (www.med.yale.edu/ynhh/infection/guidelines/MRSA/discontinue.html).

94. Brigham and Women's Hospital. A program to remove patients from unnecessary contact precaution.

95. AMEDD, Army. Discontinuation of contact precautions: Criteria for removing from contact precautions for MRSA: Criteria for removing patient from contact precautions for VRE.

96. Australian Infection Control Association. Multi-resistant organisms screening and clearance recommendations.

97. Franklin Memorial Hospital. MRSA screening policy.

98. Maine Medical Center. Discontinuation of infection control precautions policy.

99. Sanford MD, Widmer AF, Bale MJ, et al. Efficient detection and long-term persistence of the carriage of methicillin-resistant *Staphylococcus aureus*. *Clin Infect Dis* 1994;19:1123–1128.

100. Gould IM. The clinical significance of methicillin-resistant *Staphyloccus aureus*. *J Hosp Infect* 2005;61:277–282.

101. Kampf G. What should be done with nasal *Staphylococcus aureus* carriers? *J Hosp Infect* 2005;61(4)353–4.

102. Harbarth S, Liassine N, Dharan S, et al. Risk factors for persistent carriage of methicillin-resistant *Staphyloccus aureus*. *Clin Infect Dis* 2000;31:1380–1385.

103. Johns Hopkins Division of Infectious Diseases Antibiotic Guide. Resistance in *S. aureus*: Epidemiology and control of gram-positive infections. (www.hopkins-abguide.org).

104. Romance L, Nicolle L, Ross J, Law B. An outbreak of methicillin-resistant *Staphylococcus aureus* in a pediatric hospital—How it got away and how we caught it. *Can J Infect Control* 1991;6:11–13.

105. Vriens MR, Blok HE, Gigengack-Baars AC, et al. Methicillin-resistant *Staphylococcus aureus* carriage among patients after hospital discharge. *Infect Control Hosp Epidemiol* 2005;25:629–633.

106. Sandri AM, Dalarosa MG, DeAlcantara LR, et al. Reduction in incidence of nosocomial methicillin-resistant *Staphylococcus aureus* (MRSA) infection in an intensive care unit: Role of treatment with mupirocin ointment and chlorahexidine baths for nasal carriers of MRSA. *Infect Control Hosp Epidemiol* 2006;27:185–187.

107. Humphrey H. Implementing guidelines for the control and prevention of methicillin-resistant *Staphylococcus aureus* and vancomycin-resistant enterococci: How valid are international comparisons of success? *J Hosp Infect* 2006;62:133–135.

108. University of Virginia Health System. *The problem pathogen partnership* (www.healthsystem.virginia.edu/internet/PPP).

109. Calfee DP, Durbin LJ, Germanson TP, et al. Spread of methicillin resistant staphylococcus aureus (MRSA) among household contact of individual with nosocomially acquired MRSA. *Infect Control Hosp Epidemiol* 2003;24:422–426.

The Role

of Professional

and Regulatory Organizations

in Infection Control

Barbara M. Soule

INTRODUCTION

In the late 1950s and early 1960s, an epidemic of a new, virulent, antibiotic-resistant strain of *Staphylococcus aureus* infections swept through U.S. hospitals. There were rapid and dramatic increases in infections in newborns and obstetrical and surgical patients. Up to 25% of newborn infants developed superficial pyodermas or more serious deep infections and about 1% of healthy postpartum mothers died of *S. aureus* sepsis [1].

These infections highlighted the deficiencies in care practices for patients and focused the attention of healthcare providers on healthcare-associated infections (HAIs) [2]. Two influential national agencies came forward to assist hospitals in their efforts to prevent HAIs [3]. The collaboration between healthcare professionals, public health, governmental, and trade organizations established ties that shaped the early evolution of infection prevention and control programs (IC) and forged relationships that continue today.

This chapter describes the context, role, and influence of regulatory, voluntary, public, and professional entities on the practices and outcomes of IC and hospital epidemiology. A case-study illustrates the interplay among the entities using the development and implementation of hand hygiene evidence-based practices in healthcare.

EARLY HISTORY

The Centers for Disease Control (now the Centers for Disease Control and Prevention [CDC]) and the American Hospital Association (AHA) were the first to partner with healthcare organizations and professionals engaged in IC. During the height of the staphylococcal epidemic, the CDC created a small unit of epidemiologists to provide assistance to hospitals struggling to understand and contain HAIs [1]. The CDC hosted the first national Conference on the Prevention of Hospital-Acquired Staphylococcal disease in 1958 [4], published guidance on isolation techniques for hospitals [5] and began training nurses who were filling the new role of infection control nurse in 1968 [6]. In 1965, the CDC sponsored a pilot study of six community hospitals to evaluate the epidemiology of HAIs in nonuniversity hospitals [6,7]. This initial work evolved into the National Nosocomial Infections Surveillance (NNIS) system (now the National Healthcare Safety Network) (NHSN), the only national HAI database in the United States [8,9]. The CDC remains the primary governmental partner for infection control professionals (ICPs) and hospital epidemiologists.

In the late 1950s and early 60s, the AHA recognized the need to disseminate advice for controlling HAIs to its member hospitals [3,10,11]. They recommended that hospitals establish a committee on HAIs; create an HAI surveillance and reporting system; use strict aseptic practices in surgeries, delivery rooms, and nurseries; minimize the use of antibiotics; and identify which infections occurred in the hospital and the community. These recommendations served as early guidelines for IC programs. Later, reports and technical briefings addressed evolving issues such as Human Immunodeficiency Virus (HIV)/Acquired Immune Deficiency Syndrome (AIDS) and hepatitis B virus (HBV) [12,13]. The AHA established The Advisory Committee on Infections within Hospitals that evolved into the Technical Panel on Infections within Hospitals and remained in existence until 1995. Today, the AHA continues to advocate for IC issues through its state hospital associations.

The CDC, AHA, and others helped drive the IC agenda. By 1976, nearly 90% of hospitals were performing HAI surveillance and had an infection control committee, and close to half had an infection control nurse at least part-time [14]. Interestingly, there were no regulations or standards for IC at that time, so early IC efforts occurred voluntarily in hospitals [6].

As questions arose about the effectiveness and value of IC, the CDC performed a nationwide study over a 10-year period. The Study on the Efficacy of Nosocomial Infection Control (SENIC) project provided strong evidence that effective IC programs with specific surveillance, reporting, and staffing components could demonstrate a decrease in HAIs [15]. Through the decades, the CDC and the AHA have maintained the prominence of the prevention and control of HAIs on their agenda by sponsoring studies, programs, advocacy, and evidence-based guidelines to assist the field in defining the epidemiology of HAIs and using scientific practices to reduce HAI risk.

VOLUNTARY AND REGULATORY STANDARD-SETTING ORGANIZATIONS: INFLUENCE ON INFECTION PREVENTION AND CONTROL

External evaluation and controls of health services involve setting standards against which organizational operations and programs can be measured. Florence Nightingale developed early standards for IC in her efforts to control the patient's environment, improve sanitation, and reduce infections during the Crimean War in the mid-1800s [16]. Today, some standards, such as those from the National Quality Forum [17] and the Agency for Healthcare Research

and Quality (AHRQ) [18], are voluntary and developed by consensus. They are used by organizations for professional self-examination and determination of competence in program activities and outcomes. Other standards are used to determine reimbursement for care services. Those developed by the Joint Commission (JC) [19] and the American Osteopathic Association (AOA) [20] are voluntary whereas those from the Centers for Medicare and Medicaid Services (CMS) [21] are mandatory and required for healthcare licensure and/or payment. Regulatory standards, such as those from the Occupational Safety and Health Administration (OSHA) [22] or the Federal Drug Administration (FDA) [23] are promulgated based on federal and/or state statutes that delegate standard setting, interpretation, and oversight to a specific federal or state agency.

Three key steps characterize the external evaluation process [24]. First, formal standards are created and adopted to define a set of performance expectations for the programs that participate. Second, the standards are audited externally to determine the degree of compliance by the organization. Both Cruse and Haley recognized the positive effect of assessing surgical site infections (SSIs) using an external observer (the ICP and physician) and providing incidence data and trends on the SSI rates to the surgeons [1,25]. Accreditation and regulatory agencies also conduct both scheduled and unannounced surveys to monitor compliance with their standards and to respond to complaints. Third, rewards or sanctions are designated depending on the degree of compliance with the standards. This might include awarding, withholding, or revoking accreditation or licensure or issuing citations or fines and recommendations for improvement in care provided.

Many standard-setting organizations influence IC practices. Although it is not possible to discuss all in detail, a summary is provided in Table 12-1. Four that have been particularly important are covered here.

The Joint Commission (JC)

The JC is a voluntary, nongovernmental, not-for-profit organization that is a coalition of several major healthcare organizations. Historically, its standards originated from the American College of Surgeons' (ACS) Minimum Standards for Hospitals based on Ernest Codman's outcome-based monitoring system [26]. Codman's system was to track each patient to determine whether the treatment was effective and, if not, to determine why, so that subsequent patients could be treated more effectively. Onsite hospital inspections using these standards were begun in 1918 by the ACS and in 1953 by the JCAH (now JC). In 1965, Congress passed the Social Security Amendment with a provision that JCAH-accredited hospitals were "deemed" to be in compliance with the Medicare Conditions of

TABLE 12-1
ORGANIZATION REFERENCES AND WEB SITES

Organization	Site	Description
Quality		
Agency for Healthcare Research and Quality (AHRQ)	**www.ahrq.gov**	Contains quality and patient safety guidelines and literature
American Health Quality Association	**www.ahqa.org/pub/inside**	Reference documents for quality
American Society for Quality (ASQ) Quality Institute for Healthcare	**qihc.asq.org/**	Reference documents for quality
CDC Division of Healthcare Quality Promotion (DHQP)	**www.cdc.gov/ncidod/dhqp /about.html**	Guidelines and associated recommended measures
Institute for Healthcare Improvement (IHI)	**www.ihi.org/IHI/**	Guidance documents for implementing evidence-based practices
Institute of Medicine (IOM)	**www.iom.edu/**	Overviews of medical errors and national quality progress
National Association for Healthcare Quality (NAHQ)	**www.nahq.org/**	Reference documents for quality
National Committee for Quality Assurance	**www.ncqa.org/**	Quality standards for health plans
National Initiative for Children's Healthcare Quality	**www.nichq.org/nichq**	Quality measures specific to children
National Quality Forum (NQF)	**www.qualityforum.org**	National voluntary consensus measures for a variety of conditions, including HAI
The Leapfrog Group	**www.leapfroggroup.org/**	Publicly reported quality and patient safety measures
Infection control		
Association for Professionals in Infection Control and Epidemiology	**www.apic.org**	Resources for epidemiology, including guidelines
Center for Infectious Diseases Research and Policy University of Minnesota	**www.cidrap.umn.edu**	Resources for epidemiology, including guidelines
Centers for Disease Control and Prevention (CDC)	**www.cdc.gov**	Resources for epidemiology, including guidelines
Infectious Diseases Society of America (IDSA)	**www.idsociety.org**	Resources for epidemiology, including guidelines
National Foundation for Infectious Diseases (NFID)	**www.nfid.org**	Resources for infectious diseases
Society for Healthcare Epidemiology of America (SHEA)	**www.shea-online.org**	Resources for epidemiology, including guidelines
World Health Organization (WHO)	**www.who.int/en/**	Resources for epidemiology and current data on outbreaks
Patient safety		
Agency for Healthcare Research and Quality (AHRQ)	**www.ahrq.gov/qual:**	Quality and patient safety information; patient safety network
American Hospital Association (AHA)	**www.aha.org**	Resources for hospitals
American Society for Healthcare Risk Management (ASHRM)	**www.ashrm.org/ashrm/index.jsp**	Resources for risk management
American Society for Health-System Pharmacists (ASHP)	**www.ashp.org/patient-safety/index.cfm**	Resources for patient safety related to medication
Anesthesia Patient Safety Foundation	**www.apsf.org/**	Resources for patient safety related to anesthesia
Association of Operating Room Nurses (AORN) Patient Safety Center	**www.patientsafetyfirst.org/**	Resources for patient safety
ECRI (formerly the Emergency Care Research Institute)	**www.ecri.org/**	Resources for patient safety
Emergency Medicine Patient Safety Foundation	**www.empsf.org/**	Resources relative to emergency medicine
IHI-Patient Safety Center	**www.ihi.org**	Resources for patient safety
Joint Commission International Center for Patient Safety	**www.jcipatientsafety.org**	Resources for patient safety
National Patient Safety Agency, United Kingdom	**www.npsa.nhs.uk**	International resources for patient safety
National Patient Safety Foundation (NPSF)	**www.npsf.org**	Resources for patient safety

(continued)

TABLE 12-1
(CONTINUED)

Organization	Site	Description
NQF Patient Safety Taxonomy	www.qualityforum.org/ txsafetytaxonomybrief	Voluntary national measures for a variety of medical conditions
Partnership for Patient Safety		Resources for patient safety
Patient Safety Institute	www.ptsafety.org/	Resources for patient safety
Premier Safety Institute	www.premierinc.com	Resources on patient and healthcare worker safety topics
U. S. National Institute of Health; U.S. National Library of Medicine Patient Safety	www.nlm.nih.gov	MedLine Plus site for patient safety literature
U.S. Department of Defense Patient Safety Program	patientsafety.satx.disa.mil/	Resources for patient safety
U.S. Quality Interagency Coordination Task Force (Quic)	www.quic.gov/report/toc.htm	Resources for quality
Veterans Health Administration National Center for Patient Safety (NCPS)	www.patientsafety.gov/	Resources for patient safety

Regulatory

Center for Medicare and Medicaid Services (CMS)	www.cms.hhs.gov	Promulgates Conditions of Participation for inclusion in Medicare and Medicaid programs; Web site publicly displays quality comparative data for hospitals
Environmental Protection Agency (EPA)	www.epa.gov	Regulates air and water discharges, disinfectants used on surfaces
Federal Drug Administration (FDA)	www.fda.gov	Regulates single-use medical devices, antiseptics, and disinfectants used on medical devices
Federal Register	www.gpoaccess.gov	Searchable site of agency regulations
Library of Congress		Searchable site of U.S. legislation
National Fire Protection Association (NFPA)	www.nfpa.org/index.asp	Sets codes/regulations to reduce fire hazards
National Institute for Occupational Safety and Health (NIOSH, CDC)	www.cdc.gov/niosh/homepage.html	Conducts research and makes recommendations regarding prevention of HCW injuries
Nuclear Regulatory Commission	www.nrc.gov	Regulates nuclear devices and materials used in laboratories, patient testing
Occupational Safety and Health Administration (OSHA)	www.osha.gov	Regulates worker health including bloodborne pathogens, respirator use
U. S. Department of Transportation	www.dot.gov/index.cfm	Regulates transportation of waste
U.S. Government Accountability Office (GAO)	www.gao.gov/	Critiques of regulations, agencies
U.S. Regulations	www.regulations.gov/fdmspublic/ component/main	Searchable site of all U.S. regulations

Accreditation

American Osteopathic Association (AOA)	www.osteopathic.org/	Alternative to JCAHO for "deemed" status
Joint Commission on Accreditation of Healthcare Organizations (JCAHO)	www.jointcommission.org/	Standards for hospitals, long-term care, ambulatory, behavioral, home health, office-based surgery, and other settings

Consumer

Americans Mad and Angry	www.americansmadandangry.org/	Consumer stories regarding medical errors, including HAIs
Consumer's Union	www.consumersunion.org/	Campaign to require public reporting of HAIs
Consumers Advancing Patient Safety (CAPS)	patientsafety.satx.disa.mil/	Tips for consumers
Federation of State Medical Boards	www.docinfo.org	Quality information on doctors
Healthgrades	www.healthgrades.com	Public comparison of mortality rates for various conditions abstracted from administrative data sets
Patient guard	www.patientguard.com/protect.html	Tips to protect patients
Public citizen	www.citizen.org/pressroom	Information on hospitals and doctors
Reduce infection deaths	www.hospitalinfection.org/	Consumer stories regarding HAIs

Participation and could receive Medicare and Medicaid funds [27].

The JC published the first standards for IC in 1976 [28]. When the standards were published, some professionals noted the lack of a substantive body of scientific information to indicate whether, if followed, they would reduce HAIs [3]. The most recent standards have added requirements for risk assessment, evaluation of goals and strategies, assessment of IC data, and evidence of performance improvement efforts [19]. The infection control standards apply to all healthcare settings surveyed by the JC including hospitals; long-term care, home health, behavioral health, and ambulatory settings; laboratories; office-based surgeries; and others. The fourth iteration of IC standards became effective in 2005 after development with the input of an expert panel of infection control and epidemiology professionals from a variety of professional organizations [19].

American Osteopathic Association (AOA)

The AOA was founded in 1897 to advance the tenets of osteopathic medicine and provide support for doctors of osteopathy medicine [20]. The organization serves >50, 000 physician members, providing education, research, and guidance on providing cost effective and ethical care. The AOA serves as the accrediting agency for all osteopathic medical colleges and healthcare facilities using a voluntary process.

For organizations not inclined to participate in the JC or AOA surveys, an alternative is to rely on the annual state surveys from the state health department for determining entitlement to Medicare and Medicaid reimbursement.

Centers for Medicare and Medicaid Services (CMS)

The CMS (formerly the Health Care Financing Administration [HCFA]) was established in 1977 by the U.S. Department of Health and Human Services (DHHS). This federal agency is responsible for administering and enforcing the Medicare and Medicaid reimbursement programs.

The CMS generates infection control standards under its Conditions of Participation (CoP) [21] for hospitals and long-term care and home care agencies. In contrast to the JC and AOA voluntary standards, those from CMS are mandatory for continued participation/reimbursement from Medicare and Medicaid. The regulations require the hospital to develop, implement, and maintain an IC program for the prevention, control, and investigation of HAIs [21]. The JC standards and the CMS CoP for IC are similar but not identical. When differences exist and healthcare organizations voluntarily participate in JC accreditation, the organization must adhere to both sets of standards.

Occupational Health and Safety Administration (OSHA)

OSHA is a governmental agency organized under the U.S. Department of Labor [22]. Its mission is to ensure the safety and health of U.S. workers by setting and enforcing standards; providing training, outreach, and education; establishing partnerships; and encouraging continual improvement in workplace safety and health [22]. In 1991, OSHA issued the Bloodborne Pathogens Standard (BBP) to protect healthcare workers (HCWs) from exposures and subsequent infections [29]. Under the general Duty Clause of the standard, employers are required to provide a work environment "free from recognized hazards that are causing or are likely to cause death or serious physical harm to his employees" [29]. The BBP Standard has been well integrated into IC programs and healthcare organizations with policies, education and training, administrative controls, and safe practices. In January 2001, OSHA revised the BBP standard in conformance with the requirements of the federal Needlestick Safety and Prevention Act of 2000 [30], requiring healthcare organizations to redefine engineering controls to include safer medical devices and systems in concert with the users of the devices and to involve frontline HCWs in device evaluation and selection. A subsequent study in one hospital indicated significant decreases in sharps injuries [31]. The influence of these two OSHA standards has had a positive effect on reducing HCW infections in the United States. Some states (called "state-plan states") have retained authority for occupational safety standards; the state can exceed but not lessen protections required by federal OSHA.

Other Standard-Setting Organizations

Many other organizations issue standards that affect IC in some way. These include the Environmental Protection Agency (EPA) standards for the disposal and transportation of medical waste and a registry of liquid chemical products used for surface disinfection and sterilization in hospitals [32]. The FDA regulates antiseptics and medical devices through the Safe Medical Device Act, the reuse of single-use devices, the safety of the blood supply, and most food safety [23]. The Government Accountability Office (GAO) has published standards for the minimum elements of an IC program with a focus on economic issues [33]. Recently, the National Fire Protection Association (NFPA) participated with ICPs and others in a lengthy debate about the placement of alcohol-based hand hygiene products in egress corridors of facilities [34]. This is later described further. These and other organizations are listed in Table 12-1.

INFECTION CONTROL HEALTH POLICY: THE ROLE OF SCIENCE AND POLITICS

The public health policy process is complex. It reflects the heterogeneity of participants, their pluralistic interests, and the policy process itself. Policy formulation and adoption do not occur in a vacuum, nor do they occur in an orderly manner [35]. The public, interest groups, government agencies, and policy makers bring to bear their personal, political, ideological, and cultural values as they determine which policies they will consider, support, or oppose [36]. Not all HAI issues become candidates for public policy. The subject must generate anxiety or dissatisfaction or be perceived as a problem by the public or the policy makers [37]. Those that involve personal fear, urgency, or threats are more likely to reach the policy agenda. Some issues describe actual risks; others escalate public fear through sensationalism or misperceptions based on lack of scientific knowledge. Often, the process reflects a combination of these elements.

In the 1980s, HIV/AIDS first became a policy issue due to public fear and uncertainty regarding its transmission, the persons affected by it, and the lack of adequate information about it [38,39]. Medical waste disposal then became a related policy issue. Medical waste had rarely been demonstrated to pose a risk of human disease if managed in a reasonable manner [40], yet the advent of AIDS intensified the fear about transmission of HIV from used hospital supplies, hospitals, or clinics, which reached policy discussion [40]. The potential for an avian influenza pandemic has found a place on the policy agenda because of the anxiety, scientific uncertainty, and alarm it has generated about potential morbidity and mortality. On the other hand, significant matters (e.g., antimicrobial resistance, immunizations, and device-related infections) have until recently been largely managed by the health professionals without becoming politically charged health policy issues.

Health issues must be articulated to attract the attention of policy makers. Some problems are difficult to quantify because of their "invisible" nature [37]. One strategy to gain attention is to collect and share data that characterize the magnitude of a problem; another is to publicize unfortunate events. Infections among the homeless, immigrants, or other politically underpowered populations are largely left to health professionals to manage. In contrast, the increasing availability of HAI data has amplified visibility and resulted in increased public awareness and concern. Consumer groups have successfully articulated the need for mandatory public reporting of HAI data and lobbied state legislatures to enact HAI reporting statutes (Table 12-1). Infection control societies, the CDC, and others have joined the conversation, and the media have kept the issue before the public.

Both science and politics contribute to health policy formulation. Science is essential but often not sufficient. It contributes a relatively impartial and rational aspect to policy making, but political factors, such as economics, social values, and public perception, may be more powerful in policy determination [36]. The 2005 update of the CDC Tuberculosis (TB) Guidelines involved extensive negotiations and lobbying between ICPs, agencies such as the CDC and its National Institute for Occupational Safety and Health (NIOSH) to focus on science to determine respiratory policies for TB protection [41]. The revised CDC's Hospital Infection Control Practices Advisory Committee (HICPAC) Guidelines on Isolation have been in development for several years while professionals debated the science, politics, and costs of managing multidrug-resistant organisms (MDROs) in healthcare organizations [42]. The balance between the forces that determine the infection prevention agenda is a continuing challenge.

THE ERA OF PARTNERSHIPS: CONSENSUS, AND COLLABORATION

Patient Safety and Quality Organizations

In 1999, the landmark Institute of Medicine (IOM) report, *To ERR Is Human*, generated intense media, policy, and provider discussion about the safety of U.S. healthcare and its impact on morbidity, mortality, and cost of medical errors [43]. A subsequent report in 2001, *Crossing the Quality Chasm*, discussed the necessary redesign of the healthcare system to improve patient safety [44]. Finally, the third report, *Leadership by Example: Coordinating Government Roles in Improving Healthcare Quality*, not only discussed immunization but also estimated that >40,000 lives could be saved annually through wider implementation of CDC guidelines [45].

Such reports have led to the development of numerous patient safety and quality organizations and have spurred the development of various pay-for-performance quality programs and large state and national collaboratives designed to improve healthcare quality and prevent HAIs. As with regulatory agencies, it is not possible to discuss all patient safety and quality organizations; therefore, several will be highlighted.

The Agency for Healthcare Research and Quality (AHRQ)

Previously known as the Agency for Healthcare Policy and Research (AHCPR), AHRQ, as it is known today, arose out of the Healthcare Research and Quality Act of 1999 [18]. As such, it is the lead federal agency on quality-of-care research with responsibility to coordinate all federal quality improvement efforts and health services research. It is organized under the U.S. Department of Health and Human Services, and, through its 12 evidence-based practice centers, it supports scientific quality research and maintains the National Guideline Clearinghouse, a Web site devoted to collecting and organizing various evidence-based practice guidelines developed by other agencies and professional societies [46]. Through its web site, the AHRQ provides inpatient quality indicators that can be abstracted from administrative data in order to assist hospitals to identify problem areas that need further improvement [18]. In addition, AHRQ's patient safety indicators include postoperative sepsis, wound dehiscence, and selected infections [18]. In a compendium of quality recommendations published by AHRQ, 28% of recommendations are infection-control related, and 5 of 11 "clear opportunities for improvement," including the use of full barriers for central venous catheter insertion and appropriate use of surgical prophylaxis, are infection related [47]. Using patient safety indicator data, Zhan identified excess charges, mortality, and length of stay associated with various infection indicators [48]. The AHRQ Web site contains numerous free resources that can be used for improvement efforts, including information for consumers.

National Quality Forum (NQF)

The NQF is a public-private not-for-profit partnership composed of approximately 170 organizations that was established in 1999 as part of the President's Commission on Quality [17]. Its goal is to standardize healthcare performance measures that can be used to compare healthcare across the United States. This includes voluntary measures for inpatient and outpatient settings, standardization of patient safety taxonomy, and incorporation of evidence-based recommendations [17]. The first set of 39 measures included SSI prophylaxis, immunizations for selected conditions, and device-associated HAIs

In early 2006, the NQF named a steering team that will develop by February 2007 national voluntary consensus standards for reporting HAIs [17]. The steering team will receive reports from six technical advisory panels including experts on intravascular catheters and bloodstream infections (BSIs), urinary tract infections (UTIs), ventilator-associated pneumonia (VAP), SSIs, pediatric infections, and reporting and implementation [17]. Many of the NQF measures have been subsequently adopted by CMS and JC as hospital performance measures.

The Institute for Healthcare Improvement (IHI)

The IHI is a not-for-profit organization founded in 1991 with the goal to improve the quality of healthcare delivered to patients around the world [49]. In January, 2005, the IHI initiated a nationwide voluntary collaborative, the Save 100,000 Lives campaign, with the goal of reducing healthcare-related deaths by 100,000 in 18 months [49]. Three of six campaign initiatives involve reducing HAIs through implementation of ventilator and central line "bundles" (groups of evidence-based practices shown to reduce infection risk) and appropriate SSI prophylaxis. To date, >3000 hospitals have voluntarily signed on to participate in one or more campaign initiatives. The campaign provides access to best practices sharing and frequent conference calls and tracks progress on its Web site countdown [49]. In addition to information regarding the Save 100,000 lives campaign, the Web site provides many other resources designed to improve quality of care.

Table 12-2 lists selected consensus documents that influence IC and HAI prevention practices.

Evidence-Based Practices

Evidence-based practices are defined as practices supported by some level of scientific review, which can range from scales using a weighted scheme (e.g., the CDC methodology that gives the highest weight to randomized, controlled clinical trials) to expert consensus. The AHRQ National Guideline Clearinghouse provides descriptions of different evidence rating techniques [46].

For IC, the most widely used evidence-based guidelines originate from the CDC's Healthcare Infection Control Practices Advisory Committee (HICPAC) [50] (Table 12-3), the Association for Professionals in Infection Control and Epidemiology (APIC) [51], and the Society for Healthcare Epidemiology of America (SHEA) [52], which all use a weighted rating scale for evidence determination.

HICPAC consists of 14 members serving overlapping four-year terms and nonvoting liaisons from APIC, SHEA, CMS, and other representatives as necessary [53]. The committee advises the CDC on needed guideline updates and drafts new guidelines as necessary. All meetings are open to the public, and draft guidelines are published in the Federal Register in order to solicit additional broad input before finalization [53]. The final step includes peer review through the Office of Management and Budget (OMB).

In contrast, professional society guidelines often are developed by committees with deep experience in infection control and healthcare epidemiology with final approval by SHEA's board of directors.

THE INFLUENCE OF PROFESSIONAL ORGANIZATIONS ON INFECTION CONTROL AND HEALTHCARE EPIDEMIOLOGY PRACTICE

The Association for Professionals in Infection Control and Epidemiology (APIC)

The APIC [51] was founded in 1972 as the first U.S. professional organization dedicated to reducing HAIs [54]. The organization is composed of >10,000 ICPs and healthcare epidemiologists who manage IC programs in multiple healthcare settings throughout the world [51]. In 1978, APIC emphasized the need for trained ICPs [55] and encouraged professionals to use epidemiological principles and methods to address infection, quality, and risk issues [56], and more recently, patient safety challenges [56]. APIC publishes a comprehensive text of IC [57] and professional and practice standards [58]. The Certification Board of Infection Control (CBIC), established by APIC in 1980, offers certifying examinations for ICPs and epidemiologists [59]. A major focus of

TABLE 12-2
SELECTED CONSENSUS DOCUMENTS FOR INFECTION PREVENTION AND CONTROL

Document/Guideline	Author(s) or Publisher(s)
Management of outbreaks of methicillin-resistant *Staphylococcus aureus* infection in the neonatal intensive care unit: a consensus statement	Gerber SI, et al. *Infect Control Hosp Epidemiol* 2006;27:139–145.
Multisociety guideline for reprocessing flexible gastrointestinal endoscopes	Nelson D. et al. *Dis Colon Rectum* 2004;47(4):413–20 (**www.shea-online.org/Assets/files/position_papers/SHEA_endoscopes.pdf**) accessed February 2006.
Infection control, recommendations for patients with cystic fibrosis: microbiology, important pathogens, and infection control practices to prevent patient-to-patient transmission.	Saiman L. et al. and the Cystic Fibrosis Foundation. *Infect Control Hosp Epidemiol* 2003;24:S6–S52.
Anthrax as a biological weapon, 2002: updated recommendations for management	Inglesby TV et al. *JAMA* 2002;287:2236–2252.
National Institutes of Health Consensus Development Conference Statement Management of Hepatitis C, 2002 June 10–12, 2002	NIH. *Consens State Sci Statements* 2002;19:1–46 National Institutes of Health (**consensus.nih.gov/2002/2002HepatitisC2002116html.htm**) accessed April 2006.
Requirements for infrastructure and essential activities of infection control and epidemiology in out-of-hospital settings: a consensus panel report	Friedman C. et al. *Am J Infect Contrl* 1999;27:418–430.
Global Consensus Conference: Final recommendations	*Am J Infect Contrl* 1999;27:503–513.
Requirements for infrastructure and essential activities of infection control and epidemiology in hospitals: a consensus panel report	Scheckler WE et al. *Infect Control Hosp Epidemiol* 1998;19:114–124.
Methicillin-resistant *Staphylococcus aureus* outbreak: a consensus panel's definition and management guidelines	Wenzel RP et al. *Am J Infect Control* 1998;2:102–10.
Society for Healthcare Epidemiology of America and Infectious Diseases Society of America Joint Committee on the Prevention of Antimicrobial Resistance: guidelines for the prevention of antimicrobial resistance in hospitals	Shlaes DM et al. *Infect Control Hosp Epidemiol* 1997;18:275–291.
Infectious disease testing for blood transfusions. NIH Consensus Development Panel on Infectious Disease Testing for Blood Transfusions	*JAMA* 1995;274:1374–1379.

APIC is to translate the HAI science and guideline recommendations into practice.

The Society of Healthcare Epidemiology of America (SHEA)

In 1980, a group of physicians, mainly specialists in infectious diseases, founded the SHEA [60]. This professional organization is dedicated to developing and applying the science of healthcare epidemiology to the study and improvement of HAIs and other adverse outcomes. One of the organization's goals is to translate knowledge into effective policy and practice [52]. SHEA has approximately 2000 members with a large international membership component. SHEA changed its name to substitute "Healthcare" for "Hospital" in recognition that the skills of healthcare epidemiologists should be applied to the broader context of healthcare in areas beyond IC and settings outside of the hospital. Later, SHEA expanded its membership to include ICPs. A major focus of SHEA is to develop and disseminate the science on which IC practices are designed.

SHEA and APIC have both actively and successfully advocated for sensible and pragmatic IC policies and the resources necessary to sustain an active program. Both organizations publish position papers, consensus documents (Table 12-2), scientific research studies in peer-reviewed journals, and thoughtful articles about the state of the art and policy issues for the field. The associations create or endorse guidelines from other organizations, such as the Infectious Diseases Society of America (IDSA) or the Institute of Healthcare Improvement (IHI), to add strength to recommendations that promote best practices. Both APIC and SHEA proactively educate their members and engage lawmakers, regulatory agencies, the CDC, and others in the development of infection control regulations and standards, as well as the response to emerging issues. Their participation in developing the CDC HICPAC guidelines (Table 12-3) is invaluable. SHEA, APIC, and the CDC have worked together on a number of projects, for example, the Communications Network, which is designed to quickly and efficiently disseminate critical IC information to their members [61]. These efforts have greatly influenced IC practice and policies.

TABLE 12-3

CENTERS FOR DISEASE CONTROL AND PREVENTION HICPAC GUIDELINES, GUIDANCE AND RECOMMENDATIONS (WWW.CDC.GOV/NCIDOD/DHQP /HICPAC_PUBS.HTML)

Year	Document
2007	Guidelines for Isolation Practices (Pending)
2007	Guideline on Disinfection and Sterilization (Pending)
2006	Management of Multi-Resistent Organisms in Healthcare Settings
2006	Influenza Vaccination of Health-Care Personnel
2005	Guidance on Public Reporting of Healthcare-Associated Infections
2004	Guidelines for Preventing Healthcare Associated Pneumonia
2003	Guidelines for Environmental Infection Control in Health-Care Facilities
2003	Recommendations for Using Smallpox Vaccine in a Pre-Event Vaccination Program
2002	Guidelines for Preventing Intravascular Device-Related Infections
2002	Guideline for Hand Hygiene in Healthcare Settings
1999	Guideline for the Prevention of Surgical Site Infections
1998	Guideline for Infection Control in Healthcare Personnel
1997	Immunization of Health Care Workers
1995	Recommendations for Preventing the Spread of Vancomycin Resistance

The Interplay and Influence of Professionals and Agencies on Practice: Hand Hygiene: A Case Study

Efforts to increase hand hygiene compliance illustrate the interplay between various guidelines, accreditation standards, professional societies, and regulatory bodies.

Hand hygiene has been recognized since the time of Ignaz Semmelweis to be one of the most important interventions to prevent the transmission of infections among patients. Although the evidence to support hand hygiene practices has been known for >150 years, actual compliance has been poor, ranging from 5%–81% [62], prompting the CDC in its Hand Hygiene Guideline to recommend the broad use of alcohol-based hand rubs (ABHR) in an effort to increase compliance and thus reduce HAIs [62]. APIC and SHEA quickly embraced the guidelines.

Shortly after publication, questions were raised about whether the use of ABHR would be compliant with OSHA Bloodborne Pathogens Standard [63], which required "hand washing" after exposure to blood or other potentially infectious material (OPIM) [63]. In March 2003, OSHA issued a standard interpretation [64], noting that ABHR would be appropriate when no actual contact with blood or OPIM had occurred but that soap and running water would still be required when actual exposure had taken

place [64]. This was just the tip of the iceberg in terms of regulatory interplay.

In 2004, the JC added compliance with the CDC IA, IB, and IC Hand Hygiene recommendations to its National Patient Safety Goals [65]. This elevated CDC's voluntary guidelines to the level of a national standard of care because most U.S. healthcare inpatient facilities are accredited by JC.

The next hurdle to overcome related to ABHR dispenser placement; CMS requires adherence to the national Life Safety Code as part of Medicare/Medicaid conditions of participation [21]. It was not until April 15, 2004, that professional societies acting in conjunction with the American Institute of Architects (AIA) [66], the American Society for Healthcare Engineering (ASHE) [67], the EPA [32], the FDA [23], JC [65], and the CDC collaborated with CMS to adopt a temporary interim amendment to the 2000 edition of the National Fire Protection Life Safety Code that would allow ABHR dispensers to be placed in egress corridors under certain specified conditions [68]. Finally, in late 2005, the NFPA adopted the 2006 Life Safety Code after approval by the International Code Council, settling the issue of dispenser placement [68].

That is still not the end of the story of interagency cooperation and collaboration. The World Health Organization's Global Patient Safety Challenge for 2005–2006 addresses HAI reduction through its "Clean Care Is Safer Care" program focusing international attention on improving hand hygiene, including the use of ABHR when appropriate [69,70].

Finally, IHI has recently adopted the improving hand hygiene challenge, developing support tools in collaboration with CDC, APIC, and SHEA to improve implementation of CDC evidence-based recommendations in healthcare facilities [71]. The campaign goal is to galvanize healthcare facilities to implement recommendations with the same enthusiasm with which they participated in the Save 100,000 Lives campaign.

CONCLUSIONS

A wide variety of regulatory, accrediting, and not-for-profit state, national, and international collaborating partners are now paying attention to HAIs and working with the CDC and IC professional societies to prevent infections in patients and healthcare workers. As never before, ICPs, epidemiologists, and standard-setting and advisory groups have the ground support to be able to reduce HAI to the irreducible minimum.

REFERENCES

1. Haley, RW. *Managing hospital infection control for cost effectiveness: a strategy for reducing infectious complications.* Chicago: American Hospital Association Publishing, 1986.

2. Nahamias AJ, Eickhoff TC. Staphylococcal infection in hospitals: recent developments in epidemiologic and laboratory investigation. *N Engl J Med* 1961;265:74–81, 120–128, 177–182.

3. Eickhoff TC. Standards for hospital infection control. *Ann Intern Med* 1978;89:829–831.

4. American Hospital Association: Prevention and control of *Staphylococcus* infections in hospitals. In U.S. Public Health Service-Communicable Disease Center and National Academy of Sciences-National Research Council: *Proceedings of the National Conference on Hospital-Acquired Staphylococcal Disease*, Atlanta, GA, 1958, Communicable Disease Center.

5. No authors. Centers for Disease Control (CDC). *Isolation techniques for use in hospitals*. 2nd ed. U.S. Dept. Health, Education, and Welfare, 1975.

6. Garner JS, Emori TG. Nosocomial infection surveillance and control programs. In: Lennette EH, ed. *Manual of clinical microbiology*. 4th ed. Washington: American Society for Microbiology, 1985:105–109.

7. Eickhoff TC, Brachman PS, Bennett JV, Brown J. Surveillance of nosocomial infections in community hospitals. I. Surveillance methods, effectiveness and initial results. *J Infect Dis* 1969;120:305–317.

8. Hughes JM. Nosocomial infection surveillance in the United States: historical perspective. *Infect Control* 1987;8(11): 450–453.

9. Tokars JI, Richards C, Andrus M, et.al. The changing face of surveillance for health care-associated infections. *Clin Infect Dis.* 2004;39(9):1347–1352.

10. American Hospital Association (AHA): Prevention and control of *Staphylococcus* infection in hospitals. In: *Proceedings of the national conference on hospital-acquired* Staphylococcal *disease*. Atlanta, GA: U.S. Public Health Service Communicable Disease Center and National Academy of Sciences–National Research Council, 1958.

11. No authors. *Infection control in the hospital*. Chicago: American Hospital Association, 1968.

12. No authors. Special report: a hospital-wide approach to AIDS-recommendations of the advisory committee on infections within hospitals Chicago: American Hospital Association, 1987.

13. Technical Panel on Infections within Hospitals. Technical briefing on management of health care workers infected with human immunodeficiency virus (HIC) and hepatitis B virus (HBV). Chicago: American Hospital Association, 1991.

14. Haley RW, Schachtman RH. The emergence of infection surveillance and control programs in U.S, hospitals: an assessment, 1976. *Am J Epidemiol* 1980;111:574–591.

15. Haley, RW, Culver DH, White JW, et al. The efficacy of infection surveillance and control programs in prevention nosocomial infections in U.S. hospitals. *Am J Epidemiol.* 1985;121: 182–205.

16. Nightingale F. *Notes on nursing*. New York: D Appleton & Co., 1860.

17. National Quality Forum (NQF). *A national framework for healthcare quality measurement and reporting*. Washington, DC: NQF, 2002.

18. Agency for Healthcare Research and Quality (AHRQ) (www.ahrq .gov/qual/) accessed May 2006.

19. Joint Commission. Surveillance prevention and control of infection. *Comprehensive accreditation manual for hospitals: the official handbook (CAMH)*. Oakbrook Terrace, IL: Joint Commission Resources, 2007.

20. American Osteopathic Association (AOA) (www.osteopathic.org/) accessed May 2006.

21. Center for Medicare and Medicaid Services (CMS). *State operations manual* (www.cms.hhs.gov/manuals/downloads/som107c08.pdf) accessed May 2006.

22. Occupational Safety and Health Administration (OSHA) (www .osha.gov/) accessed May 2006.

23. Federal Drug Administration (FDA) (www.fda.gov/) accessed May 2006.

24. Jackson MM. Setting standards. In: Wenzel, RP, ed. *Assessing quality health care: perspectives for clinicians*. Baltimore: Williams & Wilkins, 1992, 65–84.

25. Cruse PJE. Surgical wound sepsis. *Can Med Assoc J* 1970;111: 563–557.

26. Roberts JS, Coale JG, Redman RR. A history of the Joint Commission on Accreditation of Hospitals. *JAMA* 1987;258: 936–940.

27. 20 C.F.R. §§ 1861(e), 1865(a).

28. No authors. *Accreditation manual for hospitals*. Chicago: Joint Commission on Accreditation of Hospitals, 1976.

29. Occupational Safety and Health Administration. Occupational exposure to bloodborne pathogens. Final rule. *Fed Register* 1991 Dec 6;56:64004–64182 (29 CFR.1910.1030).

30. Pub L No. 106–430, 114 Stat 1901 *Needlestick Safety and Prevention Act*, Nov. 6, 2000.

31. Sohn S, Eagan J, Sepkowitz KA, Zuccotti G. Effect of implementing safety-engineered devices on percutaneous injury epidemiology. *Infect Control Hosp Epidemiol* 2004;25:532–535.

32. Environmental Protection Agency (EPA) (www.epa.gov/) accessed May 2006.

33. General Accountability Office (GAO) (www.gao.gov/) accessed May 2006.

34. National Fire Protection Association (NFPA) (www.nfpa.org/) accessed May 2006.

35. Weissert CS, Weissert WG. *Governing health: the politic of health policy*. 2nd ed. Baltimore: The Johns Hopkins University Press, 2002.

36. Lindblom, CE. Woodhouse, E.J. *The policy making process*. 3rd ed. Englewood Cliffs, NJ: Prentice-Hall, 1993

37. Anderson JE, *Public policy making: An introduction*. Boston: Houghton Mifflin, 1990.

38. Shilts R. *And the band played on: Politics, people, and the AIDs epidemic*. New York: St. Martins Press, 1987.

39. Eisenberg L. The genesis of fear: AIDS and the public's response to science. *Law, Med, and Health Care* 1986;14:243–240.

40. Rutala WA, Odette RL, Samsa GP. Management of infectious waste by U.S. hospitals. *J Am Med A* 1989;262;1635–1640.

41. Guidelines for preventing the transmission of *Mycobacterium tuberculosis* in health-care settings, 2005 Recommendations and Reports. *MMWR;* 2005/54(RR17):1–141.

42. 69 FR 33034, June 14, 2004.

43. Institute of Medicine: *To err is human* (www.iom.edu/CMS/8089 /5575.aspx) accessed May 2006.

44. Institute of Medicine. *Crossing the quality chasm: a new health system for the 21st century* (www.iom.edu/CMS/8089/5432.aspx) accessed May 2006.

45. Institute of Medicine. *Leadership by example: coordinating government roles in improving healthcare quality* (www.iom.edu/CMS/ 3809/4623/4309.aspx) accessed May 2006.

46. National Guidelines Clearinghouse (www.guideline.gov/) accessed May 2006.

47. Shojania LG, Duncan BW, McDonald KM, Wachter RM, eds. *Agency for healthcare research and quality: making healthcare safer: A critical analysis of patient safety practices. AHRQ publication 01-E058 2001* (www.ahrq.gov/clinic/ptsafety/index.html#toc) accessed May 2006.

48. Zhan C, Miller MR. Excess length of stay, charges, and mortality attributable to medical injuries during hospitalization. *J Am Med A* 2003;290:1917–1929.

49. Institute for Healthcare Improvement (www.ihi.org/ihi) accessed May 2006.

50. Centers for Disease Control and Prevention: Healthcare Infection Control Advisory Committee (HICPAC) (www.cdc.gov/ncidod/ dhqp/hicpac_pubs.html) accessed May 2006.

51. Association for Professionals in Infection Control and Epidemiology (APIC) (www.apic.org/AM/Template.cfm?Section=Home) accessed May 2006.

52. Society for Healthcare Epidemiology of America (SHEA). (www.shea-online.org/) accessed May 2006.

53. CDC Healthcare Infection Control Advisory Committee Charter (www.cdc.gov/ncidod/dhqp/hicpac_charter.html) accessed May 2006.

54. Russell B. The Association for Professionals in Infection Control and Epidemiology, Inc. *Infect Control Hosp Epidemiol.* 9, September 1995;16:522–525.

55. Association for Practitioners in Infection Control (APIC). APIC position paper 1978. *APIC Journal* 1978;6:9.

56. Association for Practitioners in Infection Control. APIC position paper 1985. *Am J Infect Control* 1986;14:36A–38A.

57. Association for Professionals in Infection Control. APIC text of infection control and epidemiology, 2005 ed. (www.APIC.org) accessed May, 2006.

58. Horan-Murphy E, Barnard B, Chenoweth C, et al. APIC/CHICA-Canada Infection Control and Epidemiology: Professional and Practice Standards. Association for Professionals in Infection Control and Epidemiology, Inc, and the Community and Hospital Infection Control Association-Canada. *Am J Infect Control* 1999;27:42–51.

59. Certification Board of Infection Control and Epidemiology, Inc. (CBIC) (www.CBIC.org) accessed 2006.

60. Goldmann DA. Why SHEA? *Am J Infect Control* 1983;4:444–467.

61. Communications Network (APIC, SHEA, CDC) (www.CommNetwork@apic.org) accessed May 2006.

62. Guideline for hand hygiene in healthcare settings. *MMWR.* 2002;51(RR-16):1–44.

63. Occupational Safety and Health Administration. 29 CFR 1910.1030(d)(2).

64. Occupational Safety and Health Administration. Acceptable use of antiseptic-hand cleansers for bloodborne pathogen decontamination and as an appropriate handwashing practice. (www.osha.gov) accessed May 2006.

65. JC National patient safety goals. (www.jointcommission.org/Standards/NationalPatientSafetyGoals/) accessed May 2006.

66. American Institute of Architects (AIA) (www.aia.org/) accessed May 2006.

67. American Society for Healthcare Engineering (ASHE) (www.ashe.org/ashe/index.jsp) accessed May 2006.

68. National Fire Protection Association (NFPA). Life safety code amendment TAI 00 1 (101) (www.nfpa.org/search.asp?query=ABHR) accessed May 2006.

69. World Health Organization. *Clean care is safer care* (www.who.int/patientsafety/challenge/en) accessed May 2006.

70. Who Guidelines on Hand Hygiene in Health Care (Advanced Draft) 2006 www.who.int/patient accessed April 2007.

71. Institute for Healthcare Improvement. *How-to guide: improving hand hygiene* (www.ihi.org/IHI/Topics/CriticalCare/IntensiveCare/Tools/HowtoGuideImprovingHandHygiene.htm) accessed May 2006.

Antimicrobial Stewardship: Programmatic Efforts to Optimize Antimicrobial Use

Robert C. Owens, Jr.

INTRODUCTION

Microbes account for 90% of the 10^{14} cells in the human body [1]. Thus, it should not be surprising that the well-known benefits of antimicrobials must be balanced with an appreciation of their unintended effects on beneficial microbiota and the evolution of resistance. In essence, of use antimicrobials is a double-edged sword. Their life-saving benefits and disease-modifying effects can be nothing short of miraculous; however, the opposing edge of the sword can be just as sharp. Examples include serious patient harm in the form of adverse drug events (e.g., hepatotoxicity, torsades de pointes, anaphylaxis, renal failure), development of potentially life-threatening *Clostridium difficile*-associated disease (CDAD), and the emergence of resistance [2,3]. While the first two can occur during therapy and are more tangible to the practicing clinician, the emergence of resistance often occurs late and may be less obvious.

It has been said that those who move forward without taking a moment to look back are doomed to repeat history. In 1956, noted microbiologist Ernest Jawetz wrote:

On the whole, the position of antimicrobial agents in medical therapy is highly satisfactory. The majority of bacterial infections can be cured simply, effectively, and cheaply. The mortality and morbidity from bacterial diseases has fallen so low that they are no longer among the important unsolved problems of medicine. These accomplishments are widely known and appreciated . . . [4]

He goes on to state the intentions of his paper: *"the author wishes to call attention to the abuse of antibiotics, its causes and results . . ."* [4]. In the current antimicrobial era, some 50-plus years after these initially optimistic observations were made, an increasing number of infections are not easily treated, morbidity and mortality are appreciable, and many infectious diseases have become unsolved problems of modern medicine. The theme of Jawetz's latter plea remains a challenge facing many infectious diseases experts today, calling attention to the abuse of antibiotics and its causes and results.

In fact, published data note that many prescribers today still do not fully value the importance of preserving these therapeutic resources. Twenty-five million pounds of antibiotics are produced yearly for human consumption and are administered to 30–50% of hospitalized patients with nonhospitalized Americans receiving 160 million courses [5]. Yet data suggest that as much as 50% of all antimicrobial use is inappropriate. Stewarding these precious resources has become a priority for many organizations, including the Infectious Diseases Society of America (IDSA), the Society of Healthcare Epidemiology of America (SHEA), the Society of Infectious Diseases Pharmacists, the Alliance for the Prudent Use of Antimicrobials, the Centers for Disease Control and Prevention (CDC), and the World Health Organization. In fact, joint guidelines endorsed by multiple societies recently have been published that reiterate the need for proactive, programmatic efforts to optimize the use of antimicrobials in healthcare settings [6].

Since the initial work of Finland and McGowan, a variety of interventional strategies has been shown to reduce unnecessary antimicrobial use, to optimize the dose and duration, and to minimize the collateral adverse effects of their use [7–9]. Most studies have evaluated the impact of interventions on inpatient antimicrobial use and, to a lesser degree, outpatient antimicrobial use. This chapter shall reinforce why the judicious use of antimicrobials is essential and the implementation (including potential barriers) of an institutional approach is necessary to optimizing antimicrobial use. It shall also discuss the collaborative nature of these programs with infection control and prevention programs and the microbiology laboratory.

RATIONALE FOR OPTIMIZING ANTIMICROBIAL USE

Antimicrobial Resistance

Optimizing antimicrobial use through appropriate selection, dosing, and duration can be viewed as a strategy to minimize the development of resistance among clinically important pathogens [10]. Factors promoting resistance are complex, numerous, and extend beyond the use of antimicrobial agents in humans; as such, it is not surprising that they do not allow for a prompt resolution [11]. Although antimicrobial resistance has been present on this earth since the days of the primordial soup, its practical onset began in the 1920s with the observation that Pfeiffer's bacillus (now *Haemophilus influenzae*) showed a natural resistance to penicillin before its introduction for human use [12]. With the introduction of Gerhard Domagk's sulfa drugs in the 1930s, strains of *Neisseria gonorrhea* and *Streptococcus pneumonae* were noted to have developed so-called "insensitivity" [12]. Observations from the laboratory moved to the clinic in the 1940s shortly after the introduction of penicillin for the treatment of human infections. The miracle drug, penicillin, while initially effective for the treatment of *Staphylococcus aureus* bloodstream infection (BSI), began to fail to treat infections caused by penicillinase-elaborating strains as reported in *Time* magazine on May 15, 1944.

Important to this discussion is the fact that studies have established a strong relationship between antimicrobial use and resistance. Levy et al. developed a biologic model that showed a clear relationship between antimicrobial use and

the selection of resistance in humans [13]. Additionally, supportive data can be gleaned from *in vitro* investigations, ecologic studies correlating drug exposure with resistance, controlled trials in which patients with prior use of antimicrobials were more likely to be colonized or infected with resistant bacteria, or prospective studies in which drug use was associated with the development of resistant flora [13–15]. With many pharmaceutical companies no longer supporting anti-infective development and fewer new chemical entities being identified, we, now more than ever, should be concerned about the consequences of antimicrobial resistance [16].

Data from surveillance studies demonstrate that for community-acquired respiratory pathogens, resistance among *S. pneumoniae* or *H. influenzae* can be an obstacle in selecting and dosing the ideal regimen [17,18]. For healthcare-associated infections (HAIs), resistance is an important impediment to treating patients with the correct antimicrobial and dose in a timely fashion. The effects of selecting the wrong antimicrobial and at the incorrect dose have measurable effects on patient outcomes as highlighted by several recent studies [19,20]. Thus, an important value provided by a programmatic approach dedicated to the oversight of antimicrobial use and employed by the healthcare system is to "quarterback" and operationalize efforts to maximize the benefits of antimicrobials. Antimicrobial stewardship programs (ASPs) are able to drive the multidisciplinary development of locally customized disease-based guidelines, protocols, and order sets and to provide real-time human and, where available, computerized decision support in addition to their day-to-day interventions.

Patient Safety

Whether being used appropriately or inappropriately, antimicrobials have the potential for causing serious harm to patients. For example, macrolides, ketolides, or fluoroquinolones are associated with QT interval prolongation; macrolides or ketolides are associated with metabolic liability in the form of cytochrome P450 3A4 inhibition; trimethoprim-sulfamethoxazole is associated with Stevens-Johnson Syndrome; and β-lactams are best known for hypersensitivity reactions [3,21,22] while all antimicrobials are associated with CDAD [23]. Disturbingly, the rate and severity of CDAD is increasing and our traditional treatment options appear to be less effective [24,25]. The potential harm caused by antimicrobials should incentivize even the most temerarious clinicians not to casually prescribe antimicrobials in the setting of a nonbacterial infection or to stop therapy in a timely manner and carefully monitor patients off antimicrobials [2]. In addition, antimicrobials are unique and unlike any other drug class. One can develop an infection due to a resistant pathogen without ever having received the particular antimicrobial it is resistant to; hence, antimicrobials are considered societal drugs because their use has societal consequences [26].

PROGRAMS TO OPTIMIZE ANTIMICROBIAL USE

Hospital-Based ASPs

A variety of studies has evaluated the impact of interventions on antimicrobial use in healthcare systems. These studies have been conducted using a wide range of resources, methodologies, interventions (often multiple), and outcome measures (usually considering cost, antimicrobial consumption, patient safety, and less frequently resistance). The culmination of these studies was considered and led to a guidance document developed jointly by IDSA and SHEA to provide the framework for developing, implementing, and monitoring the impact of ASPs [6].

IDSA/SHEA Guidelines for Developing an Institutional Program to Enhance Antimicrobial Stewardship

An effective ASP is financially self-supporting and is aligned with patient safety goals [8,27–33]. For these reasons, there should be no excuse for an institution not to have a formal program dedicated to improving the quality of antimicrobial use. Realizing that institutions vary in size and type of specialty services offered, the ASP should be customized accordingly.

Interventional Strategy

Two major interventional styles have evolved over recent years. The first is *prospective audit and feedback* ("back-end" program). This entails obtaining a daily (or every-other-day for smaller hospitals) list of patients receiving antimicrobials and determining interventions such as pharmacodynamic dosage adjustment, streamlining the deescalation and identification of redundant therapy based on culture and susceptibility results, parenteral-to-oral conversions, drug interaction identification, guideline/protocol compliance, and recommendation of more cost-effective treatments (Figure 13-1). Recommendations are provided to the prescriber in either written form or by direct conversation. Written forms of communication usually take place on nonpermanent forms placed in the patients' medical record that are removed at discharge. This allows flexibility in what can be written and allows the ASP team member to communicate educational messages effectively and to provide citations or references on why the intervention is being recommended. The benefits of this type of program are its customizability to smaller- [29] or larger-size healthcare facilities [9,27]; it avoids taking away the prescriber's autonomy, which also increases productive "educational" dialogue; and it circumvents the potential for delays in initiating timely antimicrobial therapy since the antimicrobial already is prescribed. The downside is that recommendations are optional (although there are ways to correct repeated unaccepted recommendations by communicating

with either the department chief or an institutional committee [e.g., medical executive committee, pharmacy and therapeutics committee, patient safety committee]). Our program at Maine Medical Center (MMC) has employed this primary strategy for >5 years [8,27,33], and others have operated for longer periods of time [28].

The second chief strategy is a *preauthorization* or "front-end" program that restricts most antimicrobials to an approval process. A team member carries a pager or telephone and receives approval requests for restricted antimicrobials. At the time of interaction, the antimicrobial either is justified and approved, or an alternative recommendation is given. The University of Pennsylvania [34,35], The University of Pittsburgh [36], and others [37] have used preauthorization as their primary strategy for several years. The benefits of this strategy include the ability to funnel all initial antimicrobial prescribing through experts versed in antimicrobial therapy and the typical demonstration of these programs for immediate and significant cost savings. The potential downsides to this strategy include the loss of prescriptive autonomy that may lead to "gaming the system" [38] and the fostering of potentially adversarial relationships (if not properly implemented with buy-in from important and opinionated prescribers), the potential for delaying initial therapy, time- and resource-intensive plans (usually 7-days per week with contingency plans for night coverage), and the necessity to make decisions when the least amount of information is known about the actual infection (culture and antimicrobial susceptibility results are not available for 2–3 days and the quality of information relayed to the ASP team member by prescriber can be variable [39]).

In reality, although ASPs may lean toward one of the two primary strategies, overlap often exists. For example, the program at Maine Medical Center, while relying primarily on prospective audit and feedback, does incorporate a limited number of antimicrobials that require approval [8]. One of the most valuable aspects of an ASP is the institutionwide responsibility for overseeing the use of antimicrobials. Although in moderate-size or larger hospitals, an infectious diseases (ID) physician consultation service, ID pharmacist, and infection control department often are present and co-exist or collaborate on specific areas of interest, responsibility at the institutional level for antimicrobial stewardship usually is not assigned. An administratively supported ASP aligns resources from these various specialties and assigns responsibility to them.

Team Members

The IDSA/SHEA guidelines for developing an institutional program to enhance antimicrobial stewardship are very clear about the following: the ASP is directed or codirected by the two core team members, an ID physician and an ID-trained pharmacist, both receiving remuneration for their time. The pharmacist should have formal training in ID or

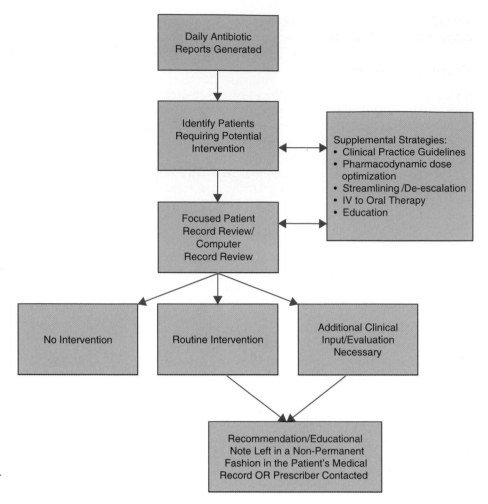

Figure 13-1 Concurrent review program workflow diagram.

be knowledgeable in the appropriate use of antimicrobials with training being made available to maintain competency. Other team members optimally include a dedicated computer information support specialist, microbiologist, and an infection control professional/hospital epidemiologist. Figure 13-2 illustrates an optimal schematic for collaboration and partnership that Maine Medical Center uses and was adapted from previous models [40]. Administrative and committee support (e.g., pharmacy and therapeutics committee) is critical. The particular interventional philosophy, responsibilities, remuneration, and reporting measures should be discussed in advance of implementation to address expectations and resources. Effective communication between the ASP, administration, and an appropriate committee should be maintained to facilitate dialogue over time as the healthcare environment continues to change.

PROSPECTIVE AUDIT AND FEEDBACK AND PREAUTHORIZATION STUDIES

Prospective Audit and Feedback Strategy

Fraser et al. [27] designed a prospective randomized controlled study of interventions for targeted antimicrobials in hospitalized patients. The team included a part-time ID physician and a PharmD with antimicrobial expertise. The intervention group (N = 141) received suggestions (written or verbally) whereas the control group did not (N = 111). Controlling for severity of illness between groups, outcomes were similar with respect to clinical and microbiologic response to therapy, adverse events, inpatient mortality, or readmission rates. Interventions included change to oral therapy (31%), regimen or dosing changes (42%), stopping therapy (10%), or ordering additional laboratory tests (18%); 85% of the suggestions were instituted. Multiple logistic regression models identified randomization to the intervention group as the sole predictor of lower antimicrobial expenditures. A conservative annualized reduction in antimicrobial expenditures of $97,500 was realized. The intervention group also showed a trend toward reduced mean length of stay compared to the controls (20 days versus 24 days, respectively). Fifty percent of patients receiving targeted regimens had their treatment refined on the third day of therapy resulting in narrower spectrum therapy and lower antimicrobial costs; most important, reducing antimicrobial use did not adversely impact patient outcomes. This study later was used as a platform to implement an ASP that is more

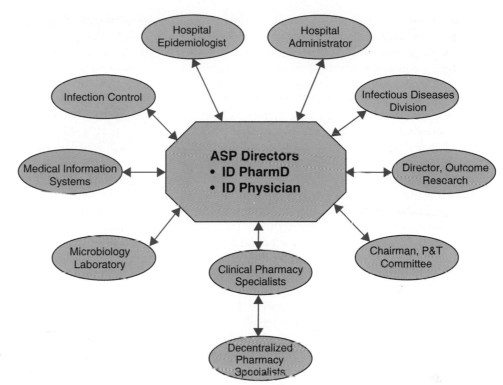

Figure 13-2 Multidisciplinary involvement and core team members.

robust in types of activities and numbers of patients served by the program. The team currently includes a part-time ID physician (2 hours per day, 5 days per week) and a full-time ID PharmD. Close collaboration exists with the Department of Epidemiology and Infection Prevention, the ID division, the pharmacy, administration, the patient safety officer, and the pharmacy and therapeutics committee.

Srinivasan et al. studied the impact of an antimicrobial management program on antimicrobial expenditures at Johns Hopkins Hospital. Before the introduction of a comprehensive ASP, the hospital used a closed formulary system and employed prior approval requirements for several antimicrobials. The ASP consisted of a hospital-funded ID physician, ID PharmD, and data analyst. The team concurrently reviewed antimicrobial therapy in all areas of the hospital except pediatrics and oncology. Their interventions included a survey and the use of institution-specific guidelines, concurrent antimicrobial review, and educational sessions. A "knowledge, attitude, and beliefs" survey was used to determine awareness of antimicrobial use and resistance and sense deficiencies in knowledge that could lead to targeted education among house staff [41]. Interestingly, only 18% viewed the program as an obstacle to patient care and 70% wanted additional feedback on antimicrobial choices. Hospital guidelines were published and updated annually. Antimicrobial therapy interventions occurred before culture and susceptibility results were available only when actively solicited or when called for prior authorization of an antimicrobial agent. For

all others, interventions were suggested at the time the microbiologic data became available. Compliance with suggested recommendations by the ASP was 79%. Costs for antimicrobial agents for the covered areas decreased by 6.4% the first year and 2.2% the second year. Assuming a steady inflation rate of 4.5%, savings translated to $224,753 and $413,998 for fiscal years 2002 and 2003, respectively.

Bantar et al. demonstrated the impact of their ASP's interventional component on antimicrobial use, cost savings, and antimicrobial resistance [42]. The ASP consisted of an ID physician, two pharmacists, a microbiologist and laboratory technologist, an internal medicine physician, and a computer systems analyst. In six-month periods, four consecutive intervention strategies were unveiled. During the first six months, an optional antibiotic order form (ID diagnosis, pertinent epidemiologic data) was introduced and baseline data were collected (i.e., bacterial resistance, antibiotic use, prescribing practice, HAI, and crude mortality rates). In the second period, an "initial intervention" period consisted of transforming the optional order form to a compulsory form and providing feedback to clinicians based on a review of the data collected in the first period. In the third period, called the "education" period, clinicians were verbally engaged with each new antimicrobial order by members of the multidisciplinary team. The fourth or "active control" period was similar to the third period, but the ASP team member modified prescriptions if necessary. During the four periods, no antimicrobial agent was restricted. To estimate the rates of use of a particular drug in relation to other drugs, an index was calculated (e.g., rate of cefepime use to that for third-generation cephalosporins—ceftriaxone and ceftazidime—equaled cefepime/consumption of ceftriaxone and ceftazidime × 100). Consumption data were measured in defined daily doses (DDD). The program periods were associated with declining cost savings as time advanced (periods 2, 3, and 4 were associated with a reduction of $261,955, $57,245, and $12,881, respectively). Comparing antibiotic order forms from period 1 (voluntary form and pre-intervention, N = 450) with period 4 (mandatory form with active intervention, N = 349), the ASP identified an increase in microbiologically based treatment intent (27% versus 62.8%, respectively, $P < 0.0001$). The team intervened on twenty-seven percent of the period 4 antibiotic order forms. Of the interventions, either the dose or duration (not specified) was reduced in 11.5%, 47% involved streamlining therapy to a narrower choice, and 86.1% was associated with cost reduction. HAI impact (e.g., length of hospitalization and mortality; only length of stay was impacted significantly [$P = 0.04$]). The increased rate of cefepime use relative to third-generation cephalosporins was associated with declining third-generation cephalosporin resistance rates among *Proteus mirabilis* or *Enterobacter cloacae* but not to *E. coli* or *K. pneumoniae*. The increased rate of aminopenicillin/sulbactam use relative to the third-generation cephalosporins in conjunction with a sustained reduction in vancomycin use was associated with a reduction in MRSA rates. In addition, *P. aeruginosa* resistance rates to carbapenems declined to 0% and were strongly associated with the reduction in carbapenem consumption.

The particular study by Bantar et al. is different than others in that it used a staggered approach to implementation. Although the cost reduction appeared to dwindle significantly in each newly introduced period, one cannot ignore the cumulative impact of the overall impact on cost. In addition, the final period offers a comprehensive mechanism for long-standing success and serves as a template to introduce other initiatives as deemed necessary. Part of the success related to reduction in resistance rates noted by this program is related to the high rate of carbapenem or ceftriaxone use and the "seldom" ordered cefepime or aminopenicillin/sulbactam in conjunction with the types of problem pathogens noted at their hospital (e.g., ampC phenotypes and carbapenem-resistant *P. aeruginosa*). Penicillin-based inhibitor combinations or cefepime have been noted to more often favorably impact the environment, in contrast to high usage rates of carbapenem or third-generation cephalosporin [9,43,44].

Another study demonstrated the impact of a multidisciplinary ASP using a blend of interventions including minimal formulary restrictions, comprehensive education (e.g., direct communication, antibiograms, peer feedback every six months), rounding with medical teams, and

introduction of guidelines (appropriate initial empirical therapy, transitional therapy, duration of therapy) [31]. All adult patients admitted to the medicine service were consecutively evaluated before the introduction of the program (N = 500 patients) and postimplementation. Using defined daily dose (DDD) data and hospital expenditure data, is study showed a 36% reduction in overall antimicrobial use ($P < 0.001$), intravenous antimicrobial use (46%, $P < 0.01$), or overall expenditures (53%, $P = 0.001$) without compromising the quality of patient care (determined by inpatient survival, clinical improvement/cure, duration of hospitalization, and readmission rates ≤ 30 days). These benefits were sustained for the four-year period evaluated.

Carling et al. [28] evaluated their ASP over a 7-year period. It consists of a physician (one-quarter time support) and PharmD (full-time support), both with specialty training in ID. Antimicrobial consumption was measured by using DDD/1000 patient-days for targeted antimicrobial agents. This program operated 8 hours per day and 5 days per week, and during this time, new orders are typically evaluated within 4 hours of their entry. Orders falling outside the 8-hour day are reviewed as a priority the next time the PharmD is on duty. Informal written notes are generated when the team identifies a problematic regimen and then is placed in the patient's chart. "Academic detailing" also occurs between the PharmD and the prescribing clinicians to supplement the written recommendations. They evaluated their impact on vancomycin-resistant enterococcus (VRE), methicillin-resistant *Staphylococcus aureus* (MRSA), and CDAC by means of internal benchmarking and externally benchmarking themselves with similar hospitals within the CDC's National Nosocomial Infections Surveillance (NNIS) system. Over the 7 years, a 22% reduction in parenteral broadspectrum antibiotics occurred ($P < 0.0001$) during which time was a 15% increase in the acuity of their patient population observed. Reductions in HAIs caused by *C. difficile* ($P = 0.002$) or resistant enterobacteriaceae ($P = 0.02$) were reported. MRSA rates remained unaffected.

A smaller hospital (120-bed community hospital) also has successfully implemented an ASP using a prospective audit and feedback strategy [29]. The ASP involved an ID physician, a clinical pharmacist, and representatives from infection control and the microbiology laboratory. The ID physician was involved approximately 8–12 hours per week. Antimicrobial therapy was reviewed three days a week in patients receiving targeted drugs or prolonged durations of therapy. Recommendations were conveyed using a form that was temporarily placed in the patient's chart and by telephone, if necessary. During the first year, 488 recommendations were made with a 69% acceptance rate; antimicrobial expenditures were reduced by 19%, saving an estimated $177,000. Common interventions were the discontinuation of redundant antimicrobial therapy, the discontinuation of treatment due to inappropriate use or excessive duration, the transition from intravenous to oral therapy, or the substitution or addition of an antibiotic to the regimen.

Preauthorization Strategy

White et al. [37] implemented an ASP restricting the use of antimicrobials based on cost and/or spectra of activity. A 24-hour per day, 7-day per week on-call system was established via a dedicated pager that clinicians would call to receive approval for restricted agents. In their quasi-experimental study, patients in the preimplementation period were similar to the post implementation period in severity of illness. Outcome measures that were not statistically significant between groups were survival ($P = 0.49$), infection-related length of stay for BSI ($P > 0.05$) or, more important, time to administration of the antimicrobial ($P > 0.05$). Benefits received in the post-ASP implementation group were improved susceptibilities to a number of bug-drug combinations, primarily involving nonfermenting Gram-negative rods or enterobacteriaceae, significant reduction in the use of a number of broadspectrum agents, and a significant reduction in annualized antimicrobial costs ($803,910) and costs per patient-day ($18 to $14.4).

Various well-conducted studies at the University of Pennsylvania over the last two decades have contributed to our current knowledge of ASPs in general [40]. Gross et al. [34] initially employed a dedicated beeper schedule for weekdays during normal business hours that was covered by an antimicrobial management team (AMT) member (an ID PharmD or ID physician). Second-year ID fellows covered evenings and weekends. At night, restricted drugs were released pending next morning follow-up. Taking advantage of their existing program. The AMT evaluated interventions performed by the ID fellows versus those made by the ID PharmD and/or ID physician. They concluded that interventions performed by the veteran ASP team members (ID PharmD and/or ID physician) were more cost effective and resulted in narrower spectrum therapy compared with interventions made by ID fellows. Based on the results of their study, the ID fellows have been more fully incorporated into their ASP and work with the PharmD and ID physician more directly. The AMT also have published their intranet/Internet resource list of restricted antimicrobials and guidelines on a Web site that can be accessed, at least in part, by others (**www.uphs.upenn.edu/bugdrug**). In addition to the preauthorization method for active interventions. The AMT also work closely with the hospital epidemiologist, are involved in establishing guidelines for antimicrobial use and dosing, are proactively involved in the antimicrobial formulary, work closely with the pharmacy and therapeutics committee, provide education, and continuously evaluate antimicrobial consumption trends [40].

Potential Barriers

The literature reports some pitfalls that some programs have experienced. Delays in the approval for a necessary antimicrobial agent can be detrimental to critically ill patients who need initial broadspectrum antimicrobial therapy. White et al. showed no delay in the administration of antimicrobial agents before or after the introduction of its program; however, approval times and time to antibiotic administration must be monitored as a process measure [37]. The perception of threatened autonomy can be a significant impediment to the efficacy of the program. The experience of LaRocco et al. [29] and the author [8] using the prospective audit and feedback strategy with few restricted antimicrobials promotes education at the point of intervention, neutralizing negative emotions. Thus, regardless of approach, constant communication with frontline prescribers and education are vital. The concept of *gaming the system* cannot be ignored and is a function of human nature. One program reported an HAI outbreak following introduction of its ASP [38]. A 30% relative increase in HAI documentation in the medical record occurred (HAI incidence increased from 11 to 14.3 per 1000 patient-care days, $P < 0.05$) [38]. After further investigation into this counterintuitive finding, the HAI outbreak was termed a "pseudo-outbreak." Clinicians were required to document infection in the medical record to justify antimicrobial use; thus, more clinicians were documenting infections in an attempt to use particular restricted antimicrobials.

The perception that ASPs are solely financially driven also can be an impediment. However, the guidelines of the IDSA/SHEA and other authorities endorse these programs not based on the potential for cost savings but as a means to improve patient safety and to reduce the selective pressure exerted by unnecessary antimicrobial use that facilitates the evolution of antimicrobial resistance. Typically, as a side effect of interventions to optimize antimicrobial use to improve efficacy and reduce resistance, a cost saving is observed that financially justifies the program. Administrators need to be cognizant of this when helping to develop ASPs. Program funding can be a barrier for some institutions, but as mentioned in SHEA/IDSA guidelines and as numerous studies in the area of ASPs point out, ASPs typically pay for themselves as a side effect of their existence.

SUPPLEMENTAL PROGRAMS TO THE PRIMARY ASP STRATEGY

Formulary Interventions

A survey of teaching hospitals suggests that 80% of them limit prescriber access to antibiotics using a variety of mechanisms [45]. Formulary restriction is the most direct way to influence antimicrobial use and is central to the primary *preauthorization* ASP strategy. Most hospitals, regardless of having an ASP, employ this strategy by limiting access to the numbers of antimicrobial drugs within a class. This limitation is a passive intervention strategy, whereas enforcement through ASPs using either *preauthorization* or *prospective audit and feedback* strategies shifts the ASP strategy to an active intervention.

Careful selection of drugs within a class involves an in-depth analysis of not only the basics (efficacy, safety, and cost) but also should include an evaluation of resistance-evoking potential when possible as well as a pharmacodynamic evaluation of the drug. A benefit of having an ASP allows this process to be centralized, and working closely with the pharmacy and therapeutics committee helps to establish an optimal formulary stocked with the best drugs for the given institution. The cost evaluation should extend beyond purchase prices, although leveraging contracts is a useful tool [46]. An important factor is that the overall cost of care should be considered when an antimicrobial is evaluated, but this is not always done because of the compartmentalization of costs within an institution (also referred to as the "silo" mentality). For example, although 8–10 fold more expensive than intravenous vancomycin in purchase cost, the use of oral linezolid has been shown to decrease the length of stay and improve discharge dynamics for patients with MRSA infections [47–50]. This is particularly financially appealing for institutions from the perceptions of those operating at maximal census (because bed costs far outweigh drug costs) and with high MRSA rates and of, the infection control of reduced transmission dynamics when length of stay is shortened, and, most important, of the patient who can be at home rather than hospitalized. In the Maine Medical Center's institution, ASP, working with the care coordination and infection control departments, has taken advantage of efficiently transitioning the patient after becoming clinically stable to an oral MRSA therapy, such as linezolid and, in some cases, minocycline. The purposes of this transition is to reduce the barrier to discharge posed by home intravenous therapy arrangement or skilled nursing facility placement if solely for administering intravenous vancomycin [33].

Practical, evidence-based examples of preferentially replacing drugs with increased resistance-evoking potential (e.g., ceftazidime) with a member of the same class exist, but these examples have demonstrated a reduced ability to select for resistance (e.g., cefepime) [8,9,42,51]. A number of studies of hospitals still characterized by high third-generation cephalosporin use have demonstrated that the replacement of third generation cephalosporins with either cefepime or piperacillin/tazobactam is an effective strategy (particularly in concert with infection control interventions) to minimize the selective pressure that facilitates the appearance of problematic β-lactamases (e.g., AmpC enzymes, extended spectrum β-lactamases) or VRE [9,52–54]. The contrast between vancomycin and

daptomycin is another example that highlights the point that not all drugs are created equal in their potential to select for antimicrobial resistance. Less high-level vancomycin-resistant *S. aureus* strains have been reported than daptomycin nonsusceptible *S. aureus* strains. The difference is that vancomycin has been used for severely ill patients with BSIs, endocarditis, or meningitis, for > 3 decades. As many [6] daptomycin-resistant strains were selected during therapy in a single trial [55]. Also, it has been observed that linezolid resistance can occur more readily in enterococci than in staphylococci [56]. However, staphylococcal resistance to linezolid remains low after six years of use. Nuances related to the propensity for the antimicrobial to become resistant to the pathogens of interest within a particular institution's patient population should be considered from a formulary perspective, and monitoring the drug's susceptibility performance in a perpetual manner is an important component of an ASP working directly with the hospital epidemiologist and the microbiology laboratory [57].

Finally, determining when an antimicrobial may fit into order sets and guidelines and how its use will be monitored completes a comprehensive evaluation of how the antimicrobial will be most effectively used within the institution. For follow-up of an antimicrobial's use in the institution, the support of the pharmacy and therapeutics committee is vital because it provides a mechanism to report back inappropriate use of the drug and has the power (in many facilities) to be an effective countermeasure to correcting inappropriate use by intervening.

The ASP's involvement in the antimicrobial formulary is not limited to drug evaluations but should work periodically with the pharmacy to evaluate pricing contracts, which can be complicated and may fluctuate. Having someone with an expertise in antimicrobials working with the pharmacy buyer can greatly improve the institutional purchase costs and ensure that the hospital/healthcare system is receiving competitive pricing. Also, frequent communication with the pharmacy buyer has been a requisite over the last several years due to antimicrobial shortages. The ASP can facilitate preparation for shortages when advanced notice is given can be helpful to maintain par levels of necessary drugs, can provide insight into alternative drugs that will likely be used in their place, and can communicate these shortages with alternatives to the prescribers. In fact, an ongoing nationwide shortage of piperacillin/tazobactam has periodically challenged the Maine Medical Center, which developed a product that can be easily substituted. The combination product (cefepime combined with metronidazole in the same mini bag) can be given as a single administered product due to its stability and compatibility in combination, is administered on average two fewer times per day (cefepime and metronidazole can be given every 12 hours for most infections), and is approximately 30% less expensive than piperacillin/tazobactam [58]. Because MMC has an institutionally supported ASP, it was able to creatively dedicate resources to an idea that both is beneficial to patients and cost effective.

Pharmacodynamic Dose Optimization

Dose optimization interventions are likely to be one of the most common interventions by an ASP. Although formerly viewed as a means to efficiently trim excess drug exposure secondary to renal dysfunction, the modern application of pharmacodynamic principles is important to maximize drug exposure for organisms with elevated minimum inhibitory concentrations (MICs), patients with excess body mass indices, and for closed-space or otherwise difficult to penetrate sites of infection (e.g., meningitis, endocarditis, pneumonia, and bone and joint infections). A recent paper provides a more in-depth review of the subject and serves as a primer for all ASPs that are incorporating optimal dosing strategies [59]. Although MMC approached its program with the thought that many patients would receive downward dose adjustments for renal impairment, what we found was a significant proportion of patients requiring increased drug exposure [8,33]. Other examples of pharmacodynamic dose-optimization include regimens intended to more effectively treat higher MIC pathogens such as continuous or "prolonged" infusion of short half-life β-lactams (e.g., piperacillin/tazobactam, cefepime, meropenem), and extended-interval aminoglycoside dosing. As previously mentioned, MMC has exploited the fact that metronidazole with its prolonged half-life (~10 hours) and active metabolite can be given every 12 hours instead of every 6–8 hours for non-*C. difficile*, noncentral nervous system infections. As mentioned, MMC has created a clinical program that integrates cefepime and metronidazole into a single administration product that can be infused twice daily, mimicking the spectrum of activity provided by piperacillin/tazobactam [58].

Educational Efforts

The first step in any process leading to change are the development of pertinent information and its dissemination. Early attempts at influencing prescribing behaviors relied heavily on educational efforts: It was simplistically believed that the reason physicians frequently inappropriately prescribed antibiotics was that they were "therapeutically undereducated" [60]. The assumption was that the misuse of antibiotics was more often the result of insufficient information rather than inappropriate behavior.

Over the years that MMC has taught antibiotic principles and specifics of therapy, it has been impressed by the intense interest of both physicians in training and established practitioners in learning more about antibiotics. Equally as impressive is the *laissez-faire* and even fatalistic attitude toward retaining and applying lessons learned in these educational sessions. Without direct application to current patients, prescribers often refer to antibiotics as "alphabet soup" and "impossible to understand." These impressions are supported in the literature. Although a supplemental cornerstone to any ASP, educational efforts when applied alone are the least effective and certainly the shortest lasting way to affect prescriber behaviors. Active intervention that is supplemented by education is a synergistic method for changing behavior.

Computer-Assisted Decision Support Programs

Direct computer-based physician order entry (CPOE) is rapidly becoming the standard of care and has been adopted as one of the Leapfrog initiatives to avoid medication errors and improve the quality of care [33]. Computer-assisted decision support programs have been designed to provide real-time integrated patient and institutional data including culture and antimicrobial susceptibility results, laboratory measures of organ function, allergy history, drug interactions, cumulative or customized location-specific antimicrobial susceptibility data, and cost information. These programs provide therapeutic choices for clinicians and allow for the incorporation of clinical judgment by overriding suggestions. Autonomy is preserved while ensuring that important variables in the choice of antimicrobial therapy are considered.

Almost all published data on the effect of computer-assisted decision support programs on antibiotic use are from researchers at the Later Day Saints Hospital in Salt Lake City, Utah. The approach of these studies has been associated with reductions in antibiotic doses, inappropriate orders, costs, treatment duration, and associated adverse drug events [61–63]. This degree of computer sophistication is not universally available but has been made available through a variety of commercial systems [64,65]. MMC has used its own CPOE system to design a logic-based algorithm to optimize the treatment of pneumonia (community, healthcare, and hospital acquired). A recent randomized control trial of clinical decision support on the appropriateness of antimicrobial prescribing demonstrated improved appropriateness and reduced overall use of antimicrobials for respiratory tract infections [66]. In this rural outpatient setting, hand-held personal digital assistants (PDAs) and paper forms of decision support supplemented the prescribing decision and choice of therapy. Patient-specific data had to be entered into the PDA, which provided a logic-based recommendation that was measurably useful in the prescribing process.

Adaptation of Locally Customized Published Guidelines

National guidelines by the IDSA and SHEA are available and are useful to construct clinical pathways locally for a variety of infections. In some instances as when sufficient time has passed between the publication of national guidelines and the change of the disease process, there should be a mechanism to develop updated evidence-based guidelines. A good example of this is the management of CDAD. Being one of the first identified institutions in North America with a hypervirulent strain (BI/NAP1) of *C. difficile*, MMC saw the clinical and prescribing impact almost immediately. Shortly thereafter, the center intervened by developing consensus among feuding specialties on the proper approach to managing CDAD and created guidelines, a clinical pathway, and a follow-up order set, all of which could be accessed on its intranet site and/or in its CPOE system [23]. From the identification of the BI/NAP1 strain of *C. difficile* to its proper management, the ASP in conjunction with Maine Medical Center's department of epidemiology and infection prevention, environmental services, and administration, it spearheaded an institutional approach to managing this high morbidity-associated infection. MMC also evaluated and reported the impact of the CDAD guidelines that supplemented active interventions made by its ASP on the use of nonevidence-based treatment strategies and demonstrated a significant improvement in the treatment variability of this infection [67].

TGuidelines published by the American Thoracic Society and the IDSA for the management of healthcare-associated, ventilator-associated, or hospital-acquired pneumonia suggest a very broad spectrum approach for the empiric treatment of these infections because of the high probability of mortality associated with inadequate therapy. In addition, these guideline recommend shortened durations of therapy. From these recommendations, we developed a consensus and published a locally customized (per our susceptibility patterns) guideline and continue to meet monthly to discuss the tracking of process measures. One difficulty with simply creating and making guidelines available to clinicians is that compliance is voluntary, and we have found that without active follow-up, clinicians fall back on old habits. Thus, one benefit of having an ASP is having the resources to provide active intervention in the intensive care unit (ICU) from whether it is recommending streamlining/deescalation when culture and susceptibility results are known to stopping antimicrobial therapy at day 7–8 instead of the traditional 14 or more days.

Process and Outcome Measurements

The IDSA/SHEA guidelines for developing an institutional program to enhance antimicrobial stewardship recommend that outcomes be measured [6]. This guideline is one reason for having a data system and an information specialist assist the ASP members in quantifying their impact. Without this support, the ASP team members could spend more time justifying their positions and measuring outcomes than on the actual day-to-day functioning of the

program and evaluating antimicrobial therapy, which is the team's primary purpose. Antimicrobial consumption can be measured for targeted (or all) antimicrobials. Using antimicrobial expenditure data has significant limitations but is helpful in evaluating where money is being spent. A more meaningful measure of antimicrobial consumption is the use of DDD data; standardized definitions are available at www.whocc.no/atcddd/. Converting grams of antibiotic used to DDD per 1000/patient-days allows for a useful internal and external benchmark of antimicrobial consumption. Other measures include antimicrobial days of therapy. Regardless of mechanism chosen, establishing a baseline of antimicrobial use before implementing a program allows the team to track the progress of interventions on use over time. These measures also can be used to quantify the impact of parenteral to oral conversions. In addition, periodically reporting to the pharmacy and therapeutics committee or other committee structure allows other clinicians and administrators to be aware of both the successes and the challenges the ASP has faced.

OPTIMIZING OUTPATIENT ANTIMICROBIAL USE

Although a departure from the institutional approach to programmatically addressing antimicrobial stewardship, discussing the importance of antimicrobial stewardship in the outpatient setting is worthwhile. More casual prescribing of antimicrobials, patient demand, and managed care constraints have plagued the optimal use of antimicrobials in this venue. Many times the prescription of an antimicrobial is issued under less than scientific circumstances and with less information available. Unfortunately, what Jawetz [4] reported in the 1950s it is still true today.

> He (the physician) is under great pressure to prescribe the "newest," "best," "broadest," antibiotic preparation, prescribe it for any complaint whatever, quickly, and preferably without worrying too much about specific etiologic diagnosis or proper indication of the drug. The pressures come from several main sources: (a) In lay magazines and newspapers patients read exaggerated, uncritical, and often misleading claims made for newly discovered drugs. "Scientists announce new potent weapon against colds." "Antibiotic cures and prevents many infections." "New drug saves lives." Most of these accounts are quite meaningless, yet patients proceed to demand the new, marvelous drug from their doctors. The physician may be embarrassed to admit that he knows nothing of this supposed discovery (many doctors find it necessary to read medical news in *Time, Reader's Digest* and similar media to cope with their patients' pseudo-knowledge), or, he may prefer not into lengthy explanations as to why he thinks little of the new drug. It may be simpler and quicker to yield to the patient's insistent demand, and prescribe.

> So have we made any progress?

To Treat or Not to Treat

National guidelines for the management of a variety of upper respiratory tract infections (URTIs) provide objective criteria for when to prescribe antimicrobials [68]. Optimizing treatment begins with this question, "Does the patient need antibiotics?" In both pediatric and adult practices, the patient often extracts the unnecessary antibiotic prescription from the time-strapped clinician. Additionally, national guidelines for the diagnosis and treatment of URTIs provide basic tenants for the treatment of these infections, but clinicians unfortunately appear to frequently ignore them. In a study of two private practices, 71% of pediatricians indicated that a parent had requested an unwarranted antibiotic at least four times within the previous month [69]. In 35% of these instances, the pediatrician admitted prescribing an antibiotic. In 61% of instances, the parent requested a different antibiotic than that selected by the prescriber.

In addition, a *laissez-faire* attitude regarding national treatment guidelines for diagnosing and treating infection exists. In a study conducted by the CDC, pediatricians and family practitioners were evaluated for self-reported versus actual practice regarding antimicrobial use for URTIs [70]. While 97% agreed that the overuse of antimicrobials is a chief factor driving antimicrobial resistance and 83% believed that they should consider selective pressure for antimicrobial resistance when deciding to prescribe antibiotics for URTIs, a large contingent ignored basic tenants of judicious antimicrobial use. For example, 69% considered purulent rhinitis diagnostic for sinusitis, 86% prescribed antimicrobials for bronchitis regardless of the duration of cough, and 42% prescribed antimicrobials for the common cold [70]. In addition, family practitioners were more likely than pediatricians to omit the requirement for prolonged symptoms to diagnose and treat sinusitis (4 versus 10 days, respectively) and to omit laboratory testing for pharyngitis (27% versus 14%, respectively) [70].

Outpatient Interventions to Improve Antimicrobial Use

Several studies have demonstrated successful outcomes in outpatients including a decrease in overall antimicrobial use and improvement in the appropriateness of therapy. Several methods have been used to effect change including education, consensus guidelines, data feedback, medical information system reminders, financial disincentives, and the use of opinion leaders [71–73]. Most of the literature evaluating the impact of interventions on antimicrobial use has occurred in the acute care inpatient setting and may not be generalizable to the outpatient venue. With that said, there is an increasing body of literature is evaluating the impact of multiple educational strategies aimed at both the prescriber and the patient.

Razon et al. [74] conducted a one-day seminar on the diagnosis and prudent use of antimicrobials for the treatment of URTIs in children. Using a quasi-experimental study design to determine the impact of the educational intervention, the researchers determined that the appropriateness of treatment improved for both otitis media (OR 1.8, $p < 0.01$) and pharyngitis (OR 1.35, $p < 0.01$) [74]. In addition, overall antimicrobial use for otitis media and URTI decreased from ($p < 0.05$) [74]. No change in appropriateness or antimicrobial use was noted for sinusitis, however.

A statewide educational intervention performed by the Wisconsin Antibiotic Resistance Network (WARN) used a two-pronged approach. On one hand, clinicians were targeted recipients of education at professional conferences, meetings, grand rounds, satellite conferences and multiple mailings and CD-ROM presentations were distributed. On the other hand, the public was educated by means of multilingual brochures and posters, tear-off sheets, coloring sheets, stickers, magnets, and handouts. These educational means were distributed statewide to clinics, pharmacies, childcare facilities, managed care organizations, and community groups. In addition, mass media events included radio and television advertisements. Minnesota was used as the control state. Postintervention (in 2002), Wisconsin clinicians perceived a significant decline in the number of requests by patients for antimicrobials (50% in 1999 to 30%; $p < 0.001$) and in requests by parents for their children (25% in 1999 to 20%; $p = 0.004$) [75]. Decisions of clinicians in Wisconsin to treat with antimicrobials were less influenced by nonpredictive clinical findings (purulent nasal discharge, $p = 0.044$; productive cough, $p = 0.010$) [75]. For both states in the post intervention period, treatment scenarios involving viral respiratory illnesses in adults were less likely to include antimicrobials; however, the same scenario in pediatric patients was only lower in Wisconsin.

In a somewhat similar intervention, Rubin et al. [76] evaluated their efforts to improve antimicrobial prescribing for URTIs in a rural community. They used patient education materials, a media campaign, a small group session conducted with physicians, and a treatment algorithm for URTIs. Although Medicaid claims data and community pharmacy data demonstrated a reduction in the rate of antimicrobial prescriptions, a third data-source (using medical record review) did not support a reduction in diagnosis-specific rate of antimicrobial use. All three data sources did, however, demonstrate a reduction in macrolide use. In a similar rural community, clinical decision support (on paper and handheld computers) to aid clinicians in the diagnosis and management of acute respiratory tract infections plus a communitywide educational intervention was compared with a communitywide educational intervention alone [77]. The communitywide educational intervention with clinical decision support demonstrated a reduction in overall antimicrobial use and increased the appropriateness of therapy.

Changing prescribing behaviors is one thing; maintaining those changes is another. As aids to sustaining any process improvement effect, mechanisms available to inpatient facilities (e.g., point-of-use information reminders and computerized decision support as well as formal ASPs) are needed to sustain outcome measures. As Samuel Johnson said >200 years ago, "Men more frequently need to be reminded than informed." The long-term effectiveness of this strategy has been demonstrated in hospitals [8,9], but the optimal method to sustain initial efforts in the community remains unclear. Of the tested outpatient strategies, combining clinical decision support tools in addition to education appears to provide the most promising opportunity for sustainable antimicrobial stewardship. Perhaps as a result of many of the state and local educational interventions, a study conducted by the CDC documented a significant decline in antimicrobial use in the pediatric population between 1989–1990 and 1999–2000 [78].

CONCLUSIONS

The problem of increasing antimicrobial resistance—due in part to suboptimal antimicrobial use coupled with the fact that a growing number of pharmaceutical companies have abandoned anti-infective research and development—has resulted in a growing public health crisis. Because of their intensity of antimicrobial use, both institutional and community settings are target-rich environments for proactive interventions to improve antimicrobial stewardship. Various studies have concluded that programmatic means to steward the use of antimicrobials optimizes patient safety, addresses antimicrobial resistance, reduces unnecessary antimicrobial use and, as a side effect, minimizes direct and indirect costs to the healthcare system. The IDSA/SHEA guidelines for developing an institutional program to enhance antimicrobial stewardship serve as a starting place for institutions considering adopting an ASP. Finally, Calvin Kunin, MD, once stated "there are simply too many physicians prescribing antibiotics casually . . . The issues need to be presented forcefully to the medical community and the public. Third-party payers must get the message that these programs [antimicrobial stewardship] can save lives as well as money" [79].

REFERENCES

1. Schiff GD, Wisniewski M, Bult J, et al. Improving inpatient antibiotic prescribing: Insights from participation in a national collaborative. *Jt Comm J Qual Improv* 2001;27:387–402.
2. McDonald LC, Killgore GE, Thompson A, et al. An epidemic, toxin gene-variant strain of *Clostridium difficile*. *N Engl J Med* 2005;353:2433–41.
3. Owens RC Jr. QT prolongation with antimicrobial agents: Understanding the significance. *Drugs* 2004;64:1091–124.
4. Jawetz E. Antimicrobial chemotherapy. *Anhu Rev Microbiol* 1956;10:85–114.
5. Wenzel RP, Edmond MB. Managing antibiotic resistance. *N Engl J Med* 2000;343:1961–63.
6. Dellit TH, Owens RC Jr, McGowan JEJ, et al. Infectious Diseases Society of America and the Society for Healthcare Epidemiology of America: Guidelines for developing an institutional program to enhance antimicrobial stewardship. *Clin Infect Dis* 2007; in press.
7. Davey P, Brown E, Fenelon L, et al. Interventions to improve antibiotic prescribing practices for hospital inpatients. *Cochrane Database Syst Rev* 2005; CD003543.
8. Owens RC Jr., Fraser GL, Stogsdill P. Antimicrobial stewardship programs as a means to optimize antimicrobial use: Insights from the Society of Infectious Diseases Pharmacists. *Pharmacotherapy* 2004;24:896–908.
9. Owens RC Jr., Rice L. Hospital-based strategies for combating resistance. *Clin Infect Dis* 2006;42 (suppl 4):S173–81.
10. Glowacki RC, Schwartz DN, Itokazu GS, et al. Antibiotic combinations with redundant antimicrobial spectra: Clinical epidemiology and pilot intervention of computer-assisted surveillance. *Clin Infect Dis* 2003;37:59–64.
11. McGowan JE Jr. Do intensive hospital antibiotic control programs prevent the spread of antibiotic resistance? *Infect Control Hosp Epidemiol* 1994;15:478–83.
12. Moberg CL, Rene Dubos: A harbinger of microbial resistance to antibiotics. *Microb Drug Resist* 1996;2:287–97.
13. Levy SB, FitzGerald GB, Macone AB. Changes in intestinal flora of farm personnel after introduction of a tetracycline-supplemented feed on a farm. *N Engl J Med* 1976;295:583–88.
14. Bell DM. Promoting appropriate antimicrobial drug use: Perspective from the Centers for Disease Control and Prevention. *Clin Infect Dis* 2001;33 (suppl 3):S245–50.
15. Dinubile MJ, Friedland I, Chan CY, et al. Bowel colonization with resistant gram-negative bacilli after antimicrobial therapy of intra-abdominal infections: Observations from two randomized comparative clinical trials of ertapenem therapy. *Eur J Clin Microbiol Infect Dis* 2005;24:443–49.
16. Projan SJ. Why is big Pharma getting out of antibacterial drug discovery? *Curr Opin Microbiol* 2003;6:427–30.
17. Pottumarthy S, Fritsche TR, Jones RN. Comparative activity of oral and parenteral cephalosporins tested against multidrug-resistant *Streptococcus pneumoniae*: Report from the SENTRY Antimicrobial Surveillance Program (1997–2003). *Diagn Microbiol Infect Dis* 2005;51:147–50.
18. Sader HS, Fritsche TR, Mutnick AH, Jones RN. Contemporary evaluation of the *in vitro* activity and spectrum of cefdinir compared with other orally administered antimicrobials tested against common respiratory tract pathogens (2000–2002). *Diagn Microbiol Infect Dis* 2003;47:515–25.
19. Osmon S, Ward S, Fraser VJ, Kollef MH. Hospital mortality for patients with bacteremia due to *Staphylococcus aureus* or *Pseudomonas aeruginosa*. *Chest* 2004;125:607–16.
20. Kollef MH. Inadequate antimicrobial treatment: An important determinant of outcome for hospitalized patients. *Clin Infect Dis* 2000;31 (suppl 4):S131–38.
21. Owens RC Jr., Ambrose PG. Antimicrobial safety: Focus on fluoroquinolones. *Clin Infect Dis* 2005;41 (suppl 2):S144–57.
22. Owens RC Jr., Nolin TD. Antimicrobial-associated QT interval prolongation: Pointes of interest. *Clin Infect Dis* 2006;43:1603–11.
23. Owens RC. Clostridium difficile-associated disease: An emerging threat to patient safety: Insights from the Society of Infectious Diseases Pharmacists. *Pharmacotherapy* 2006;26:299–311.
24. Pepin J, Valiquette L, Alary ME, et al. *Clostridium difficile*-associated diarrhea in a region of Quebec from 1991 to 2003: A changing pattern of disease severity. *CMAJ* 2004;171:466–72.
25. Pepin J, Routhier S, Gagnon S, Brazeau I. Management and outcomes of a first recurrence of *Clostridium difficile*-associated disease in Quebec, Canada. *Clin Infect Dis* 2006;42:758–64.
26. Sarkar P, Gould IM. Antimicrobial agents are societal drugs: How should this influence prescribing? *Drugs* 2006;66:893–901.
27. Fraser GL, Stogsdill P, Dickens JD Jr., et al. Antibiotic optimization: An evaluation of patient safety and economic outcomes. *Arch Intern Med* 1997;157:1689–94.
28. Carling P, Fung T, Killion A, et al. Favorable impact of a multidisciplinary antibiotic management program conducted during 7 years. *Infect Control Hosp Epidemiol* 2003;24:699–706.
29. LaRocco A Jr. Concurrent antibiotic review programs—A role for infectious diseases specialists at small community hospitals. *Clin Infect Dis* 2003;37:742–43.

30. Ansari F, Gray K, Nathwani D, et al. Outcomes of an intervention to improve hospital antibiotic prescribing: Interrupted time series with segmented regression analysis. *J Antimicrob Chemother* 2003;52:842–48.

31. Ruttimann S, Keck B, Hartmeier C, et al. Long-term antibiotic cost savings from a comprehensive intervention program in a medical department of a university-affiliated teaching hospital. *Clin Infect Dis* 2004;38:348–56.

32. Lutters M, Harbarth S, Janssens JP, et al. Effect of a comprehensive, multidisciplinary, educational program on the use of antibiotics in a geriatric university hospital. *J Am Geriatr Soc* 2004;52:112–16.

33. Fraser GL, Stogsdill P, Owens RC Jr. Antimicrobial stewardship initiatives: A programmatic approach to optimizing antimicrobial use. In: Owens RC Jr, Ambrose PG, Nightingale CH, eds. *Antibiotic Optimization: Concepts and Strategies in Clinical Practice*. New York: Marcel Dekker, 2005:261–326.

34. Gross R, Morgan AS, Kinky DE, et al. Impact of a hospital-based antimicrobial management program on clinical and economic outcomes. *Clin Infect Dis* 2001;33:289–95.

35. John JF Jr., Fishman NO. Programmatic role of the infectious diseases physician in controlling antimicrobial costs in the hospital. *Clin Infect Dis* 1997;24:471–85.

36. Paterson DL. The role of antimicrobial management programs in optimizing antibiotic prescribing within hospitals. *Clin Infect Dis* 2006;42 (suppl 2):S90–95.

37. White AC Jr., Atmar RL, Wilson J, et al. Effects of requiring prior authorization for selected antimicrobials: Expenditures, susceptibilities, and clinical outcomes. *Clin Infect Dis* 1997;25:230–39.

38. Calfee DP, Brooks J, Zirk NM, et al. A pseudo-outbreak of nosocomial infections associated with the introduction of an antibiotic management programme. *J Hosp Infect* 2003;55:26–32.

39. Linkin DR, Paris S, Fishman NO, et al. Inaccurate communications in telephone calls to an antimicrobial stewardship program. *Infect Control Hosp Epidemiol* 2006;27:688–94.

40. Fishman N. Antimicrobial stewardship. *Am J Med* 2006;119:S53–61.

41. Srinivasan A, Song X, Richards A, et al. A survey of knowledge, attitudes, and beliefs of house staff physicians from various specialties concerning antimicrobial use and resistance. *Arch Intern Med* 2004;164:1451–56.

42. Bantar C, Sartori B, Vesco E, et al. A hospitalwide intervention program to optimize the quality of antibiotic use: Impact on prescribing practice, antibiotic consumption, cost savings, and bacterial resistance. *Clin Infect Dis* 2003;37:180–86.

43. Harris AD, Smith D, Johnson JA, et al. Risk factors for imipenem-resistant *Pseudomonas aeruginosa* among hospitalized patients. *Clin Infect Dis* 2002;34:340–45.

44. Georges B, Conil JM, Dubouix A, et al. Risk of emergence of *Pseudomonas aeruginosa* resistance to beta-lactam antibiotics in intensive care units. *Crit Care Med* 2006;34:1636–41.

45. Lesar TS, Briceland LL. Survey of antibiotic control policies in university-affiliated teaching institutions. *Ann Pharmacother* 1996;30:31–34.

46. Scott RD, Solomon SL, Cordell R, et al. Measuring the attributable costs of resistant infections in hospital settings. In: Owens RC Jr, Ambrose PG, Nightingale CH, eds. *Antibiotic optimization: Concepts and strategies in clinical practice*. New York: Marcel Dekker, 2005:141–79.

47. Parodi S, Rhew DC, Goetz MB. Early switch and early discharge opportunities in intravenous vancomycin treatment of suspected methicillin-resistant staphylococcal species infections. *J Manag Care Pharm* 2003;9:317–26.

48. Itani KM, Weigelt J, Li JZ, Duttagupta S. Linezolid reduces length of stay and duration of intravenous treatment compared with vancomycin for complicated skin and soft tissue infections due to suspected or proven methicillin-resistant *Staphylococcus aureus* (MRSA). *Int J Antimicrob Agents* 2005;26:442–48.

49. Li Z, Willke RJ, Pinto LA, et al. Comparison of length of hospital stay for patients with known or suspected methicillin-resistant Staphylococcus species infections treated with linezolid or vancomycin: A randomized, multicenter trial. *Pharmacotherapy* 2001;21:263–74.

50. McKinnon PS, Sorensen SV, Liu LZ, Itani KM. Impact of linezolid on economic outcomes and determinants of cost in a clinical trial evaluating patients with MRSA complicated skin and soft-tissue infections. *Ann Pharmacother* 2006;40:1017–23.

51. Owens RC Jr., Ambrose PG, Quintiliani R. Ceftazidime to cefepime formulary switch: Pharmacodynamic and pharmacoeconomic rationale. *Conn Med* 1997;61:225–27.

52. Lautenbach E, LaRosa LA, Marr AM, et al. Changes in the prevalence of vancomycin-resistant enterococci in response to antimicrobial formulary interventions: Impact of progressive restrictions on use of vancomycin and third-generation cephalosporins. *Clin Infect Dis* 2003;36:440–46.

53. Lipworth AD, Hyle EP, Fishman NO, et al. Limiting the emergence of extended-spectrum Beta-lactamase-producing enterobacteriaceae: Influence of patient population characteristics on the response to antimicrobial formulary interventions. *Infect Control Hosp Epidemiol* 2006;27:279–86.

54. Owens RC Jr, Ambrose PG, Jones RN. The antimicrobial formulary: Reevaluating parenteral cephalosporins in the context of emerging resistance. In: Owens RC Jr, Ambrose PG, Nightingale CH, eds. *Antibiotic Optimization: Concepts and Strategies in Clinical Practice*. New York: Marcel Dekker, 2005:383–430.

55. Fowler VG Jr., Boucher HW, Corey GR, et al. Daptomycin versus standard therapy for bacteremia and endocarditis caused by *Staphylococcus aureus*. *N Engl J Med* 2006;355:653–65.

56. Pai MP, Rodvold KA, Schreckenberger PC, et al. Risk factors associated with the development of infection with linezolid- and vancomycin-resistant Enterococcus faecium. *Clin Infect Dis* 2002;35:1269–72.

57. Valenti AJ. The role of infection control and hospital epidemiology in the optimization of antibiotic use. In: Owens RC Jr, Ambrose PG, Nightingale CH, eds. *Antibiotic Optimization: Concepts and Strategies in Clinical Practice*. New York: Marcel Dekker, 2005:209–59.

58. Nolin TD, Lambert DA, Owens RC Jr. Stability of cefepime and metronidazole prepared for simplified administration as a single product. *Diagn Microbiol Infect Dis* 2006;56:179–84.

59. Ambrose PG, Bhavnani SM, Rubino CM, et al. Pharmacokinetics-pharmacodynamics of antimicrobial therapy: It's not just for mice anymore. *Clin Infect Dis* 2007;44:79–86.

60. Melmon KL, Blaschke TF. The undereducated physician's therapeutic decisions. *N Engl J Med* 1983;308:1473–74.

61. Evans RS, Pestotnik SL, Classen DC, Burke JP. Evaluation of a computer-assisted antibiotic-dose monitor. *Ann Pharmacother* 1999;33:1026–31.

62. Pestotnik SL, Classen DC, Evans RS, Burke JP. Implementing antibiotic practice guidelines through computer-assisted decision support: Clinical and financial outcomes. *Ann Intern Med* 1996;124:884–90.

63. Evans RS, Pestotnik SL, Classen DC, et al. A computer-assisted management program for antibiotics and other antiinfective agents. *N Engl J Med* 1998;338:232–38.

64. Pestotnik SL. Expert clinical decision support systems to enhance antimicrobial stewardship programs. Insights from the society of infectious diseases pharmacists. *Pharmacotherapy* 2005;25:1116–25.

65. Burke JP, Mehta RR. Role of computer-assisted programs in optimizing the use of antimicrobial agents. In: Owens RC Jr, Ambrose PG, Nightingale CH, eds. *Antibiotic Optimization: Concepts and Strategies in Clinical Practice*. New York: Marcel Dekker, 2005:327–52.

66. Samore MH, Bateman K, Alder SC, et al. Clinical decision support and appropriateness of antimicrobial prescribing: A randomized trial. *JAMA* 2005;294:2305–14.

67. Owens RC Jr., Loew B, Soni S, Suissa S. Impact of interventions on non-evidence based treatment strategies during an outbreak of *Clostridium difficile*-associated disease due to BI/NAP1. Abstract 687. In: *Program and abstracts of the 44th Annual Infectious Diseases Society of America*. Toronto, Ontario, CA. 2006:60.

68. Rosenfeld RM, Culpepper L, Doyle KJ, et al. Clinical practice guideline: Otitis media with effusion. *Otolaryngol Head Neck Surg* 2004;130:S95–118.

69. Palmer DA, Bauchner H. Parents' and physicians' views on antibiotics. *Pediatrics* 1997;99:E6.

70. Watson RL, Dowell SF, Jayaraman M, et al. Antimicrobial use for pediatric upper respiratory infections: Reported practice, actual practice, and parent beliefs. *Pediatrics* 1999;104:1251–57.

71. Greco PJ, Eisenberg JM. Changing physicians' practices. *N Engl J Med* 1993;329:1271–73

72. Soumerai SB, Avorn J. Principles of educational outreach ("academic detailing") to improve clinical decision making. *JAMA* 1990;263:549–56.

73. Davey P, Brown E, Fenelon L, et al. Systematic review of antimicrobial drug prescribing in hospitals. *Emerg Infect Dis* 2006;12:211–16.

74. Razon Y, Ashkenazi S, Cohen A, et al. Effect of educational intervention on antibiotic prescription practices for upper respiratory infections in children: A multicentre study. *J Antimicrob Chemother* 2005;56:937–40.

75. Kiang KM, Kieke BA, Como-Sabetti K, et al. Clinician knowledge and beliefs after statewide program to promote appropriate antimicrobial drug use. *Emerg Infect Dis* 2005;11:904–11.

76. Rubin MA, Bateman K, Alder S, et al. A multifaceted intervention to improve antimicrobial prescribing for upper respiratory tract infections in a small rural community. *Clin Infect Dis* 2005;40:546–53.

77. Samore MH, Bateman K, Alder SC, et al. Clinical decision support and appropriateness of antimicrobial prescribing: A randomized trial. *JAMA* 2005;294:2305–14.

78. McCaig LF, Besser RE, Hughes JM. Trends in antimicrobial prescribing rates for children and adolescents. *JAMA* 2002;287:3096–102.

79. Kunin CM. Antibiotic armageddon. *Clin Infect Dis* 1997;25:240–41.

14

Multiply Drug-Resistant Pathogens: Epidemiology and Control

Michael Lin, Robert A. Weinstein, and Mary K. Hayden

OVERVIEW

Since the introduction of penicillin in the 1940s, hospitals have been witness to a continual battle between our antibiotic armamentarium and the organisms that colonize and infect our patients. The promise that each antibiotic discovery brings has been tempered by the eventual emergence of organisms resistant to the drug. The lag between introduction of a new antibiotic and emergence of resistant bacteria is variable; widespread resistance to penicillin was seen in *Staphylococcus aureus* within 5 years of introduction of the antibiotic, but vancomycin resistance in this same pathogen was not observed until vancomycin had been in clinical use for over 30 years. At other times, resistance has occurred even before the clinical use of a specific antibiotic; for example, sulfonamide and aminoglycoside resistance can be found in gram-negative bacilli isolated long before our use of these compounds. Such disparities have led to a controversy over whether antibiotic use/abuse or other host and environmental factors are most responsible for the increasing prevalence of antibiotic-resistant pathogens (ARP) in the community and in hospitals. Nevertheless, it appears to be conventional wisdom that our antibiotic choices seldom remain more than a very few drugs ahead of the resistant strains. Furthermore, the same organisms that acquire resistance to one antibiotic are more likely to acquire resistance to multiple antimicrobials [1].

Although antibiotic resistance has emerged in the community, the hospital remains an epicenter for colonization and infection by ARPs, due to three forces [2]. First, potent broad-spectrum antimicrobial consumption is, by necessity, high in hospitals given the acuity of illness seen. Such "antibiotic pressure" directly or indirectly provides a driving force for selecting and maintaining organisms that are able to evolve or acquire mechanisms of resistance. Second, hospitals provide a convenient meeting ground for patients to acquire ARPs from reservoirs such as other patients, the environment, shared equipment, and hospital personnel. Third, the average patient in the hospital is more debilitated and immune compromised than ever before as more routine medical care for healthier patients has shifted to the outpatient setting.

Over the past 50 years, various resistant bacteria have risen to prominence in the hospital setting (Figure 14-1). In the early 1960s, penicillin-resistant *S. aureus* became

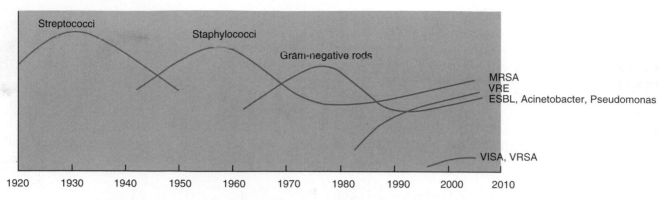

Figure 14-1 Schematic representation of emerging healthcare-associated infections over time. MRSA, methicillin-resistant *Staphylococcus aureus*; VRE, vancomycin-resistant enterococci; VISA, vancomycin-intermediate *S. aureus*; VRSA, vancomycin-resistant *S. aureus*; ESBL, extended-s β-lactamase-producing Enterobacteriaceae; Acinetobacter, multidrug-resistant *Acinetobacter baumannii*; Pseudomonas, multidrug-resistant *Pseudomonas aeruginosa*. Adapted from Herwaldt LA, Wenzel RP. Dynamics of hospital-acquired infections [372].

epidemic and ultimately widespread. Subsequent attempts to treat resistant *S. aureus* infections with methicillin were soon thwarted by the emergence of methicillin resistance (MRSA). In the 1970s, vancomycin became available for treatment of infections due to gram-positive cocci, and gram-negative bacilli such as *Pseudomonas aeruginosa* and *Enterobacteriaceae* became dominant healthcare-associated infection (HAI) pathogens. By the 1980s, introduction of broadspectrum antimicrobials, particularly advanced-generation cephalosporins, provided better treatment options for gram-negative bacteria. This advantage was short-lived; soon, large families of β-lactamases that mediate resistance to the newer cephalosporins were described in *Enterobacteriaceae*. During the same time, the proportion of hospital *S. aureus* isolates resistant to methicillin increased steadily, and vancomycin-resistant enterococci (VRE) surfaced. Other pathogens of low virulence, such as yeast, methicillin-resistant coagulase-negative staphylococci, and *Corynebacterium jeikeium*, also became significant HAI pathogens (Figure 14-1). A common feature of these microbes is their multidrug resistance. The 1990s witnessed staphylococcal and pseudomonal resistance to the new fluoroquinolone antibiotics, and imipenem resistance in Enterobacteriaceae. In the past decade, hospitals identified strains of *Acinetobacter baumannii*, *P. aeruginosa*, *Klebsiella pneumoniae*, and *Enterococcus faecium* resistant to virtually all available antimicrobial agents, and high-level vancomycin resistance was reported in *S. aureus*.

The specter of panresistant "superbugs" with little to no reasonable antimicrobial treatment has raised concern that, at least for some infections, we are effectively entering a postantibiotic age [3]. Understanding the forces that promote increasing antibiotic resistance is the basis of hospital infection control efforts. In this chapter, we review the epidemiology of multidrug-resistant pathogens in hospitals and discuss prevention and control strategies.

DEFINITIONS

Describing a pathogen is as "resistant" usually refers to loss of susceptibility to key drugs that are normally used in treatment. The key drug may be either a first-line antimicrobial that is preferred for treatment of a specific organism because of superior efficacy or low toxicity (e.g., oxacillin for *S. aureus*) or an antimicrobial to which resistance may be a marker for broader no-susceptibility (e.g., ceftazidime resistance in *K. pneumoniae* suggesting production of an extended-spectrum β-lactamase [ESBL]). Traditionally, antibiotic resistance has been defined phenotypically (i.e., by an ability of the microbe to grow in a high concentration of the antibiotic of interest). However, resistance can be expressed in a heterogeneous manner by a population of bacterial cells, which can make phenotypic detection difficult or unreliable. This phenomenon is seen in methicillin-resistant staphylococci; laboratories have developed numerous modifications of traditional susceptibility testing methods to optimize the sensitivity of phenotypic resistance detection. Testing directly for the gene that encodes resistance, *mecA* in this example, may allow more accurate and rapid classification of resistant strains. There are other reasons to consider moving toward a genetic definition of resistance: recent data suggest that the epidemiology, and potentially the control, of pathogens that have similar resistance phenotypes but different genetically encoded mechanisms of resistance may not be the same [4]. For example, a study of carbapenem-resistant *P. aeruginosa* found that in the subset of patients admitted to hospitals, those infected with metallo-β-lactamase–producing strains were different than patients infected with porin-deficient strains with respect to preceding antibiotic exposure, presence and type of co-morbid illness, and invasiveness of infection [5].

From the standpoint of the hospital clinical microbiology laboratory, there are other pitfalls in defining resistance. Newer generations of automated antimicrobial susceptibility systems (e.g., VITEK® 2, bioMérieux, Durham, NC) have the ability to detect susceptibility to multiple common antimicrobials via fluorescence-based methods. Common limitations to such systems include failing to detect resistance in certain antimicrobial classes, particularly those that are expressed heterogenously or that require induction for optimal expression, such as β-lactams and vancomycin [6]. Both automated and manual susceptibility testing methods (e.g., the Kirby-Bauer disk method) may yield inaccurate results due to device or operator-dependent errors, such as use of outdated or incorrectly placed antimicrobial disks, variations in bacterial inoculum, and incorrect agar depth or pH. There often is a lag between emergence of resistance and the general availability of an accurate method for its detection. Examples of this problem include detection of vancomycin resistance in enterococci [7,8] and staphylococci [9,10], carbapenem resistance in *K. pneumoniae* [11,12], and ESBL production in *Enterobacteriaceae* [13]. ESBLs are particularly difficult to detect; different ESBLs have different affinities for third-generation cephalosporins and may be misclassified as susceptible, depending on the substrate used. Sometimes, instead of the development of a new method, the resistance breakpoint is lowered to improve a test's sensitivity for detection of decreased susceptibility to an antibiotic [14].

Although there is no standard definition for "multiple resistance" or "multidrug resistance," one definition used is resistance to ≥ 2 unrelated antibiotics to which an organism is normally considered susceptible [15]. For example, *Mycobacterium tuberculosis* is multiply resistant when it is not susceptible to isoniazid and rifampin. In practice, the term may also commonly refer to an organism that is susceptible to only one or two remaining antimicrobial classes. "Multidrug resistance," when used in the context of *A. baumannii*, usually refers to strains that are susceptible only to one or two antimicrobials, such as carbapenems and colistin. While in most instances, multidrug resistance refers to resistance acquired or evolved by a microbe, some bacterial species of epidemiologic concern, such as *Steontrophomonas maltophilia* and *Burkholderia cepacia*, are intrinsically resistant to multiple classes of antibiotics. The strict definitions of "multidrug resistance" change depending on the context of the organism discussed; clarifying such definitions is mainly important for the purposes of investigation and publication and less so for clinical practice.

Determining whether resistant organisms are hospital acquired or community acquired can be problematic because patients may be asymptomatically colonized when they enter the hospital. For example, 15% to 25% of patients colonized or infected with aminoglycoside-resistant gram-negative bacilli and as many as 50% of patients who appear to acquire cefazolin-resistant Enterobacteriaceae after surgery have brought these strains into the hospital [16,17]. Molecular markers may help in distinguishing between hospital and community strains of organisms [18,19]. MRSA, when acquired in the community, usually carries

a virulence factor Panton-Valentine leukocidin that can be detected with polymer chain reaction (PCR) or other laboratory tests. Nevertheless, even these markers lose their utility when typically community-acquired MRSA assimilates into the hospital ecology [20].

As medical care of patients becomes shifted into hospital-related facilities, such as nursing homes, dialysis centers, and infusion clinics, these environments become reservoirs for multidrug-resistant organisms. Such "healthcare-associated" infections currently are grouped with community-acquired infections for the purposes of surveillance, but the ecology and resistance patterns of these associated pathogens are more similar to nosocomial than traditional community-acquired organisms [21].

In addition to the difficulties in defining hospital acquisition, there often is the question of whether the patient has clinical disease (infection) due to the resistant strain or is merely colonized. This distinction is relevant mainly for organisms isolated from nonsterile sites, such as the respiratory tract or an open ulcer. ARP colonization is an important epidemiologic problem because it increases the reservoir of resistant bacteria (Figure 14-2) and often is a precursor to clinical disease [22].

MECHANISMS AND GENETICS OF RESISTANCE

At least 17 classes of antimicrobials have been developed to treat bacterial infections [23]. Each class has been countered by one or more mechanisms of resistance over the years (Table 14-1). Furthermore, under selective pressure and for other unknown reasons, bacteria frequently aggregate several mechanisms to confer broad resistance to multiple classes of antimicrobials.

The genetics by which antimicrobial resistance develops in particular organisms have broad implications for the ecology of resistance and success of control measures. Whether or not resistance genes exist on chromosomes or mobile genetic elements dictates how quickly resistance genotypes can be acquired or spread and how successfully restrictions in antimicrobial use can directly or indirectly control spread.

Chromosomal antimicrobial resistance usually is the result of spontaneous mutation and natural selection of strains that survive under the antimicrobial selection pressure. For some antimicrobials, such as rifampin, a single-point mutation is all that is needed for resistance. For other antimicrobials, such as fluoroquinolones, a stepwise progression of low-level to high-level resistance usually takes place through sequential mutations [24]. Conditions that favor spontaneous chromosomal mutation include an overwhelming number of organisms (increasing the likelihood of a favorable mutation), incomplete or ineffective antimicrobial therapy (allowing mutants to survive), and a relatively small number of mutations needed

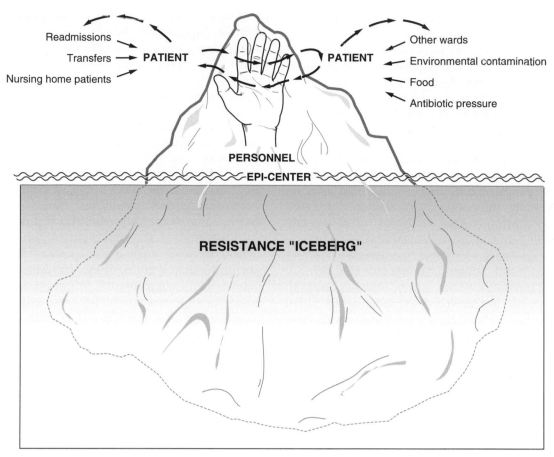

Figure 14-2 The dynamics of nosocomial resistance: resistance iceberg [15]. Adapted with permission from R.A. Weinstein, and S.A. Kabins, Strategies for prevention and control of multiple drug-resistant nosocomial infection. *Am J Med* 1981;70:449.

TABLE 14-1

KEY RESISTANCE PROBLEMS OF SELECT HEALTHCARE-ASSOCIATED INFECTION PATHOGENS

Organism	Key Resistances	Additional Resistances
Staphylococcus aureus	Methicillin (all β–lactams), vancomycin	Penicillin, macrolides, tetracyclines, clindamycin, fluoroquinolones
Coagulase-negative staphylococci	Methicillin (all β-lactams)	Penicillin, macrolides, tetracyclines, clindamycin, fluoroquinolones
Enterococcus faecium, Enterococcus faecalis	Vancomycin, ampicillin, aminoglycosides	Cephalosporins, clindamycin, fluoroquinolones, trimethoprim-sulfamethoxazole
Corynebacterium jeikeium	Cephalosporins, penicillins, aminoglycosides, fluoroquinolones	Macrolides, tetracyclines
Enterobacteriaceae	Cephalosporins, fluoroquinolones, aminoglycosides, carbapenems	Penicillins, trimethoprim-sulfamethoxazole
Pseudomonas aeruginosa	Antipseudomonal cephalosporins, antipseudomonal penicillins, aminoglycosides, fluoroquinolones, carbapenems	Other β-lactams, trimethoprim-sulfamethoxazole, tetracycline
Acinetobacter baumannii	Sulbactam, carbapenems, aminoglycosides	Cephalosporins, penicillins, trimethoprim-sulfamethoxazole. Fluoroquinolones
Steontrophomonas maltophilia	Trimethoprim-sulfamethoxazole, ticarcillin-clavulanate	Carbapenems, cephalosporins, penicillins, aminoglycosides, fluoroquinolones
Burkholderia cepacia	Trimethoprim-sulfamethoxazole, carbapenems, fluoroquinolones	Cephalosporins, penicillins, aminoglycosides, tetracyclines

for resistance. Examples of chromosomal mutation as the dominant factor in *de novo* resistance include multidrug-resistant *M. tuberculosis*, fluoroquinolone-resistant bacteria (although this may be changing), and drug-resistant viruses such as human immunodeficiency virus (HIV) [25]. The chromosomal location of a gene makes it more difficult to spread horizontally between different strains or species, although naked DNA can be transferred from one organism to another through the process of transformation. *S. pneumoniae*, like all streptococci, are naturally transformable; it is likely that the origins of penicillin resistance lie in acquisition of chromosomal genes that encode low-affinity penicillin-binding proteins from other commensal streptococcal species [26].

Resistance genes also may reside on mobile genetic elements—chromosomal or extrachromosomal—that allow for interstrain or interspecies spread [27]. Resistance genes usually are located in gene cassettes, which are carried by integrons and transposons (which are functionally similar vectors that differ in the types of recombination genes). The permutations of mobile elements are vast: integrons are found alone or inside transposons; both integrons and transposons often are carried by plasmids and bacteriophages [28]. Such variations allow for gene shuffling and provide bacteria with vast capacity to adapt to changing environments or antimicrobial pressure. Importantly, mobile elements frequently carry multiple resistance mutations simultaneously, allowing for broad resistance to be conferred quickly from one bacterial species to another. Such a situation exists among *Enterobacteriaceae*, which can acquire ESBLs via plasmids and multiple resistances (such as trimethoprim, aminoglycoside, and fluoroquinolone resistance) via integrons that may reside on the same plasmids [29,30].

SPECIFIC RESISTANCES AND INCIDENCE

Several disturbing trends in resistance have been observed over the years (Figure 14-1) (Table 14-1). A surge in aminoglycoside resistance was a chief concern in the 1970s and 1980s, particularly in nosocomial *Enterobacteriaceae* or *P. aeruginosa*. Resistance levels vary considerably between geographic regions; for example, gentamicin resistance in *P. aeruginosa* ranged from 15.8% in North America to 28.3% in Europe and 38.2% in Latin America from 1997–2000 [31]. Since the 1980s, the availability of second-generation cephalosporins (e.g., cefoxitin and cefuroxime), third-generation cephalosporins (e.g., ceftriaxone and ceftazidime), and β-lactam-β-lactamase inhibitor combination agents (e.g., piperacillin-tazobactam) has highlighted an additional set of resistances in gram-negative bacilli. For instance, *Enterobacter* spp. initially were considered susceptible to cephalosporins but frequently developed resistance during therapy. The culprit was spontaneous de-repression of an intrinsic chromosomal β-lactamase [32]. Further

discovery of a family of plasmid-mediated ESBLs conferring broad resistance to various penicillins and cephalosporins has made many gram negatives, such as *Escherichia coli* and *Klebsiella* spp., difficult to control without turning to "antibiotics of last resort" such as carbapenems. ESBLs evolved by point mutations from common, older plasmid-borne enzymes and are transferable to bacteria that do not have the intrinsic chromosomal resistance. ESBL-producing *K. pneumoniae* represented the fastest growing resistant pathogen monitored in the CDC's National Nosocomial Infections Surveillance (NNIS) system in 2003, reaching 20.6% overall resistance (up 47% compared to the five years prior) [33].

Because carbapenems are some of the broadest spectrum antimicrobials available and because they are critical in treating ESBL-producing bacteria and other highly resistant gram-negative organisms such as *A. baumannii*, the increases seen over the years in carbapenem resistance have been sobering. Carbapenem resistance is mediated by various mechanisms, such as loss of the outer membrane protein OprD, production of carbapenemases, or up-regulation of the efflux system MexEF-OprN [34]. Analysis of NNIS data from 1998 to 2004 reveals that while carbapenem resistance in *Enterobacter* spp. remained low (0.70%), the prevalence of imipenem resistance in *P. aeruginosa* was 19% (increased from 11.1% in the late 1980s) [33,35]. Carbapenem-resistance in *A. baumannii* is especially concerning because some hospital strains are virtually pan-resistant to conventional classes of drugs.

The prevalence of trimethoprim and sulfonamide resistance in gram-negative bacteria remains a concern primarily in outpatient settings where oral trimethoprim alone or trimethoprim sulfamethoxazole (TMP-SMX) combination often is prescribed empirically for the treatment of urinary tract infections (UTIs). Resistance to trimethoprim is mediated via alterations in the target enzyme dihidrofolate reductase [36] while resistance to sulfonamides is mediated by alterations in its target enzyme dihydropteroate synthase [37]. These resistance genes often are linked to other resistance genes on integrons, allowing for efficient spread and indirect selective pressure from associated antibiotics. For example, in Sweden, one hospital found rising rates of TMP-SMX resistance in its *E. coli* isolates despite concomitant decreases in the overall use of the drug, likely because antibiotic selective pressure favored the other genes that were linked on the same integron [38]. In general, TMP-SMX resistance rates in *E. coli* are variable, depending on the region of the United States, from 7% in the Eastern states to 32% in the Western states [39]. In one center, which saw a rise in TMP-SMX resistance in *E. coli* of 8.1% to 15.8% between 1992 and 1999, resistance was associated with prior TMP-SMX use [40].

Methicillin resistance has been a major concern in staphylococci since the 1980s. In 63 NNIS hospitals from 1974 to 1981, the percentage of *S. aureus* infections resistant to methicillin increased modestly from 2.4% to 5%, due primarily to epidemics in four large teaching institutions [41]. In 1992, the pooled percentage of resistance had risen to 32.1%, and in 2004, to 53% [33,42]. Methicillin resistance in nosocomial *S. aureus* and coagulase-negative staphylococci is endemic in most U.S. hospitals.

Fluoroquinolones target enzymes responsible for bacterial DNA replication, such as DNA gyrase and topoisomerase, giving them broad efficacy against many gram-negative organisms and some gram-positive organisms [43]. Since the 1980s, their potency and oral bioavailability have made their use widespread in treatment of infections (particularly pulmonary, urinary, and gastrointestinal) and in prophylaxis (e.g., in neutropenic patients). Widespread increases in fluoroquinolone resistance have been reported in many bacteria, in particular *Enterobacteriaceae*, *P. aeruginosa*, *S. pneumoniae*, and *S. aureus* [44–47]. In the United States, 93% of MRSA [48] and nearly 30% of nosocomial *P. aeruginosa* [33] were resistant to ciprofloxacin in 2003. While most of this resistance is likely selected for in humans, the use of fluoroquinolones as growth promoters in food animals may play a greater role in driving resistance than previously suspected [49–51].

HOST FACTORS PREDISPOSING TO COLONIZATION OR INFECTION WITH ANTIBIOTIC-RESISTANT ORGANISMS

A number of patient risk factors have been associated with acquisition of ARPs (Table 14-2). Our epidemiologic understanding of these factors remains limited because most studies have been retrospective due to practical restraints, limiting the covariates to more easily obtainable data, such as antimicrobial use. Many of the identified factors are undoubtedly linked and may serve as indirect markers of more difficult-to-measure covariates such as frequency of patient-to-staff contact. It also is important to recognize that risk factors may differ, depending on whether epidemic vs. endemic periods are being studied and whether the ARP is isolated during episodes of colonization vs. infection.

Recently, attention has been directed at other methodologic issues that may lead to biased estimates of risk for antibiotic resistance [52]. First, results of case-control designs, used extensively in studying the risk of acquiring ARPs, are influenced by how the control group is selected. In many studies, control groups are selected either from patients in the population who are uninfected or from patients who carry the antibiotic-susceptible form of the bacterium of interest [53]. Use of either control group may result in slightly differing estimates of risk. When resistant cases are compared to uninfected controls, risk factors for acquisition of both the susceptible and the resistant phenotype of the organism may be identified [53]. If, instead, controls are selected that are already colonized or infected with the susceptible form of the organism, the odds of

TABLE 14-2	
EXAMPLES OF HOST FACTORS ASSOCIATED WITH HEALTHCARE-ASSOCIATED COLONIZATION OR INFECTION BY AN ANTIMICROBIAL-RESISTANT ORGANISM IN SELECTED CASE-CONTROL STUDIES	

Factor	Reference
More frequently identified	
Duration of hospital or ICU stay (adjusted or matched in many studies)	[55–57]
Prior antimicrobials	[23,57,65,180,205,289,373–383]
Intensive care unit	[57,374,383]
Invasive devices or procedures	[374,378]
central venous catheter	[180,375]
endotracheal intubation	[375,382]
urinary catheter	[289]
nasogastric tube	[376,384]
Underlying comorbidities	[65,180,289,375]
Prior colonization or infection with resistant organism	[65,385]
Prior hospitalization or residence in long-term care facility	[55,56,205]
Risk factors less frequently identified	
Age	[56,383]
Sex	[205,375,376]
Chemotherapy	[386]
Endoscopy	[386]
Surgery (or number of operations)	[56]
Proximity to other patients	[180]

association between certain variables and acquisition may be overestimated [54]. An alternative study design, "case-case-control," uses both types of controls and two separate case-control analyses within a single study in order to differentiate risk factors associated with acquisition of the susceptible and resistant phenotypes of the organism [53].

A second important methodologic principle is adjustment for time at risk [52]. Not surprisingly, duration of hospital stay (and specifically, "time at risk" before the index colonization or infection) often is identified as a significant risk factor [55–57]. In case-control studies that identify risk factors for antibiotic resistance, time at risk needs to be accounted for via multivariate analysis or by matching cases and controls [52].

A third methodologic principle that has been identified as important is adjustment for co-morbid conditions [52]. A systematic review of 37 published studies carried out by Harris et al. found that while the majority (73%) adjusted appropriately for co-morbid illness, only 11 studies (30%) adjusted for patient time at risk [52].

A final methodologic concern is the analysis of aggregated antibiotic use data to estimate patient-level risk of acquiring an antibiotic-resistant organism [58]. Analysis of aggregated data may not accurately reflect the risk of exposure to an individual patient because population studies do not link individual outcomes to individual exposures [58]. Population studies are useful in allowing the measurement of the total effect of an exposure.

Despite the concerns about study designs and analyses, there is a striking commonality of risk factors for colonization or infection with pathogens such as antimicrobial-resistant S. aureus, Enterococcus spp., and gram-negative bacilli [59]. These risk factors include advanced age; underlying diseases and severity of illness; inter-institutional transfer of the patient, especially from a nursing home; prolonged hospitalization; gastrointestinal surgery or transplantation; exposure to invasive devices of all types, especially central venous catheters; and exposure to antibiotics, especially cephalosporins [59]. Other risk factors are identified in Table 14-3.

Of the risk factors listed, the role of antimicrobials in promoting resistant organisms has attracted much attention in the literature, perhaps because of its potential for modification, compared to some other risk factors. Although it appears intuitively that rising antimicrobial consumption would promote increases in resistance, the relationship between antimicrobials and resistance at the patient level and population level remains unclear. Thus, it is often difficult for hospitals to decide between diverse antimicrobial stewardship strategies, such as reducing all classes of antimicrobial use, targeting specific antimicrobial classes, or rotating available antibiotics.

For some pathogens, the selective pressure of antimicrobials in an individual patient may promote the growth of resistant strains of organisms that arise by spontaneous mutation. Organisms susceptible to de novo resistance, such as HIV or M. tuberculosis, are those that can acquire resistant traits through single or relatively few point mutations, thus making such an occurrence a statistical probability in the setting of high numbers of organisms. Similarly, fluoroquinolone or rifampin resistance can develop spontaneously in S. aureus through relatively small numbers of mutations. In such settings, simultaneous treatment with multiple antimicrobials to avoid treatment failure is a cornerstone of preventing resistance, echoing the philosophy of "hit hard and hit early" advised by Paul Ehrlich in the early twentieth century [60].

In contrast, for many important ARPs, such as MRSA and VRE, resistance is mediated by complex genes that would unlikely occur spontaneously in any individual patient. In such instances, development of resistance involves horizontal acquisition of either resistant organisms themselves or genetic vectors such as plasmids carrying resistance genes. Furthermore, in contrast to obligate pathogens such as M. tuberculosis, many important ARPs such as enterococci colonize the gut or skin, allowing opportunities for indirect exposure to the selective pressures of antimicrobials intended for other pathogens.

These important differences explain why the use of antimicrobials may lead to a rise in the prevalence of ARPs on a population level through a variety of indirect mechanisms [61]. For VRE, use of cephalosporins

TABLE 14-3

RELATIVE IMPORTANCE OF SELECTED FACTORS IN THE EMERGENCE OF SOME MULTIDRUG RESISTANT ORGANISMS WITHIN HOSPITALS[a]

Multidrug-Resistant Organism, Defined by Key Resistance Marker	Patient-to-Patient Transmission Via Contaminated Healthcare Worker Hands	Environment-to-Patient Via Contaminated Healthcare Worker Hands	Colonized Healthcare Worker Directly to Patient	Airborne Transmission	Endogenous Selection by Antibiotic Pressure
Methicillin-resistant Staphylococcus aureus	+++	+/++	+	+/−	+
Vancomycin-resistant enterococcus	+++	++	−	−	++
Extended-spectrum β-lactamase producing Enterobacteriaceae	+++	+	−	−	+++
Imipenem-resistant Pseudomonas aeruginosa	+	+	+	−	+++
Imipenem-resistant Acinetobacter baumannii	+++	+++	−	−	++

[a]The relative importance is an indication of the need to address each factor in control measures for specific resistant pathogens.

eliminates competitive gut flora, promoting opportunities for horizontal acquisition of the organism [62]. Furthermore, use of anti-anaerobic drugs appears to facilitate fecal excretion of resistant enterococci, leading to further opportunities for transmission [63]. On an ecologic level, the emergence of VRE in the 1980s was likely due to the accelerating use of vancomycin during that decade [64]. However, although many classes of antibiotics have been associated with emergence of VRE, prior receipt of vancomycin by an individual patient appears to have minimal effect on the risk of VRE acquisition once VRE have become established in a patient population.

SOURCES OF RESISTANT STRAINS

The source of most resistant strains in hospitals appears to be other colonized/infected patients [15,67–69]. Because the normal oropharyngeal and intestinal flora of hospital patients may be displaced by multiply resistant enteric bacteria and *P. aeruginosa* (urine, perineum, and wounds may be similarly affected), there are often many colonized patients for each patient with recognized infection, the so-called "iceberg effect" (Figure 14-2) [70,71]. This shift in flora often occurs within a very few days of hospital admission and affects the older, generally sicker or more debilitated patients. The importance of various risk factors (e.g., specific exposures vs. more hands-on care in general) and the pathophysiology of this shift (e.g., possible changes in membrane receptors or ligands, antibiotic suppression of normal flora, potential contribution of biofilm formation on devices such as nasogastric and endotracheal tubes) are not well delineated [72–75]. In our experience, some of this shift in endemic strains may result from emergence of low-count community-acquired flora in the face of antibiotic exposure rather than from true nosocomial acquisition [76].

It is important to realize that multidrug-resistant bacteria can be recovered from the normal, intact skin of patients [68,77–79] and from body fluids, secretions, and wounds. While the perineal or inguinal areas of patients usually are most heavily contaminated, the axillae, trunk, arms, and hands also are frequently colonized [80]. Pathogens most often found at these sites are *A. baumannii.*, staphylococcal spp., and enterococcal spp., perhaps in part because these pathogens are more resistant to desiccation compared to other bacteria [80–82]. In one study, VRE was cultured from the antecubital fossae of 29% of ventilated patients studied in a medical ICU [68]. These findings have implications for control strategies aimed at these pathogens, which are addressed later in this chapter.

Personnel have been documented sources of resistant gram-positive strains, such as MRSA [83–86] and even coagulase-negative staphylococci [87]. However, personnel carriage of resistant gram-negative bacilli (other than transient hand carriage described in the following section) appears to be very unusual. Exceptions include outbreaks

reportedly traced to carriers of *Acinetobacter* spp., *Citrobacter* spp., or *Proteus* spp. *Acinetobacter* spp., one of the few gram-negative bacilli that may be among normal skin flora, was noted in one outbreak to recur periodically despite disinfection of the apparent environmental reservoirs. The outbreak ultimately was traced to the colonized hands of a respiratory therapy technician who had dermatitis and apparently contaminated respiratory therapy equipment while assembling it [88]. There also have been clusters of *Citrobacter* spp. infections of the central nervous system in neonates [89,90] traced to hand carriage by nurses and an outbreak of *Proteus mirabilis* infections in newborns traced to a nurse who was a chronic carrier [91]. In another study, endemic *P. aeruginosa* infection was maintained in a neonatal ICU by persistent carriage on HCWs hands; artificial fingernails or nail wraps were both risk factors for hand colonization in this study [92].

Food-borne contamination with multiply resistant gram-negative bacilli has been cited in several investigations [41,93] and has been incriminated particularly in oncology units [94]. Despite the potential importance of these observations, however, the overall role of food in introducing resistant strains into the general hospital remains unclear.

Environmental sources and reservoirs of resistant strains have been a recurrent problem, especially when patient-care equipment becomes contaminated. Extensive outbreaks of UTIs (and respiratory tract, perineal, or intestinal colonization) may result when urine-measuring devices, contaminated by enteric bacilli or *P. aeruginosa*, are shared by many patients [95,96]. MRSA contamination of ultrasonic nebulizer filters was linked to an outbreak of infection and colonization on a head and neck surgical ward [97], and electronic thermometers contaminated with VRE were implicated as vehicles of transmission in an outbreak in a medical-surgical ICU [98].

Finally, there has been perennial concern about contamination of many areas of the inanimate environment with which patients do not have direct contact, such as flowerpots and sink traps [99–101]. Despite sometimes heavy contamination, these sites usually have not been implicated epidemiologically in the spread of bacteria in hospitals. However, for high-risk immunocompromised patients, especially those who have the opportunity for environmental exposures (e.g., the debilitated oncology patient who sits at the sink to wash), strains from sink surfaces have been linked to patient colonization and infection [94].

Contamination of inanimate environmental surfaces that are touched by HCWs may be a more important source of at least some multidrug resistant bacteria in hospitals. This has been studied most carefully for VRE. In one report, HCWs were shown to transfer VRE from contaminated sites in a patient's room—such as a blood pressure cuff, bed rail, or soap dispenser—to clean sites in the room or on a patient's skin via their hands or gloves during routine patient care activities in 10.6% of opportunities [102].

Similarly, HCWs were found to contaminate their gloves with MRSA by touching only environmental sites in patient rooms; although subsequent transfer of MRSA was not evaluated in this study, it is likely to occur [103].

MODES OF TRANSMISSION

The most important way that ARPs are spread in the hospital is from an infected/colonized patient to a susceptible patient via transient carriage on hands of HCWs (Table 14-3). Such spread contributes to the iceberg of colonized patients and greatly increases the source and reservoir of ARPs in the hospital (Figure 14-2). While much of the evidence incriminating HCW hands is circumstantial and based on finding resistant bacteria colonizing or contaminating HCW hands, both experimental and mathematical models and observational studies in patient care settings have demonstrated that HCWs can transfer pathogens from their hands or gloves to patients' skin or devices [102,104–108]. Moreover, the weight of experience, dating back to the successful introduction of hand-hygiene as a control measure by Semmelweis, strongly supports this concept. Indexes of hands-on exposure to personnel used in a few studies to quantitate patients' risk have provided an additional measure.

The contribution of transfer of pathogens from contaminated environmental surfaces to patients via HCW hands is receiving renewed attention, as noted [102]. Given the lower colony counts typically found at environmental sites compared to patient sites [68] for most pathogens, this route of transmission appears to be less important than transfer from patient to patient (Table 14-3).

HCWs who are persistently colonized with ARPs sometimes can transfer these pathogens directly to patients (Table 14-3) [92,109]. This is particularly important for MRSA and may be underappreciated in settings where MRSA is endemic and cross-transmission is frequent [109].

Common-source spread of ARPs has been noted primarily in outbreak settings. The attention of the medical community (and newspaper and journal editors) often is attracted to such epidemics because of striking features, such as large numbers of patients infected with very resistant bacteria, unusual breaks in techniques or protocols, or contaminated commercial products. Perhaps more common than such "extravaganzas" are the ongoing episodes of limited cross-infection due to contamination of shared patient-care equipment (e.g., urine or other measuring containers and other environmental reservoirs), which probably account for a significant portion of endemic infections [110].

Airborne spread of ARPs has been documented rarely. For MRSA, the most recent experience suggests that airborne spread is uncommon [86]. Similar increases in MRSA acquisition rates during outbreaks of severe acute respiratory syndrome (SARS) in two geographically separate hospitals raised the concern that there may have been an interaction between the SARS coronavirus and MRSA that led to efficient airborne transmission of MRSA from colonized to noncolonized patients [111]. It seems more likely that the increases noted were due to a failure of HCWs to change gloves and gowns and to cleanse their hands reliably between patients [112,113].

For gram-negative bacilli, there was concern in one hospital that contamination in a 16-story chute-hydropulping waste disposal system led to airborne dispersal and transmission of *Pseudomonas* spp. and enteric bacilli [114]. Waste pulp in the chute had 108 colony-forming units (cfu) per gram; air samples from hallways connecting the chute and nursing units had >150 cfu per cubic foot of air. After closing the chute, air counts fell by >75%, and the incidence of nosocomial gram-negative BSIs fell by >65%. However, this experience appears unique.

Various insect vectors, such as flies and cockroaches, are probably unimportant in the transmission of ARPs in most U.S. hospitals.

EPIDEMICS

The events leading to any nosocomial epidemic are probably multifactorial. In most outbreaks of multiply drug-resistant bacteria, precipitating events have not been well elucidated. Factors that could increase person-to-person spread include poor aseptic practices, as in crowded units or when the nurse-to-patient ratio becomes too low. Spread from the environment is facilitated by poor housekeeping practices that lead to reservoirs of resistant organisms within the hospital as when contaminated urine is allowed to remain in urine-measuring or testing devices. Excessive use of antibiotics may increase the selective pressure for ARPs.

Certain chance events may precipitate outbreaks, such as contamination of a commercial product, admission of a patient who is a heavy shedder of ARPs [115], or acquisition of resistance by a bacterial species that is adept at colonization or unusually resistant to disinfection. Also, advances in medical technology, such as transplantation, dialysis, and new prosthetic devices, create additional epidemic risks.

Particular hospital areas, especially intensive care, burn, and neurosurgical units are prone to outbreaks. These areas house acutely ill patients who are subjected to many invasive procedures and often are exposed to multiple antibiotics under circumstances in which adherence to asepsis may be reduced in the rush of crisis care. We have found that multiply resistant bacteria may breed in such units, or epicenters (Figure 14-2) [95]. As colonized patients are transferred to other areas of the hospital, they may leave a trail of resistance.

OUTBREAKS DUE TO PLASMIDS AND OTHER MOBILE GENETIC ELEMENTS

Most reported outbreaks have been due to epidemic spread of single strains. Application of newer molecular laboratory techniques to investigation of ARPs in hospitals has allowed the recognition of outbreaks caused by mobile genetic elements, such as integrons, plasmids, and transposons. While horizontal gene transfer due to these elements is important in the dissemination of antibiotic resistance in gram-positive bacteria [116–118], the rapid spread of resistance in this manner is recognized more often in gram-negative species. Several plasmid outbreaks have been described in which a resistance plasmid has caused either simultaneous or sequential resistance to occur in epidemic fashion in different species or genera [119,120]. Mobile genetic resistance elements have been found to spread throughout a city, a region, and even an entire country [5,121–124].

The epidemiology of most of these outbreaks, specifically the reservoirs for the resistance elements, time and place of transfer of genetic material, and pressures involved, has been largely speculative [125–127]. Transfer can occur in the gastrointestinal tract, on skin, in urine, or in the environment (e.g., in urine containers) and may be facilitated by antimicrobial therapy [128,129]. Moreover, relatively avirulent bacterial strains may serve as reservoirs for resistance. For example, gentamicin resistance in *Staphylococcus epidermidis* or *S. aureus* may be mediated by identical plasmids that can pass between these two species *in vitro* and on human skin [130]. Because clonal dissemination or clustering is identified in many integron and plasmid outbreaks, it appears that cross-transmission plays a major role in their dissemination [5,124,131,132].

Outbreaks due to plasmids or integrons may be difficult to detect [131] but should be sought through surveillance for the occurrence of multiple species or genera with identical or very similar multiple drug (or even just key drug) resistance patterns [131]. If available, characterization of the genetic element by PCR, restriction endonuclease digestion, or DNA sequencing could facilitate detection. Once recognized, epidemics due to transferrable genetic elements are at present controlled much like single-strain outbreaks (see the following Control section). More extensive epidemiologic investigation of resistance elements is required to determine the most effective control measures.

OTHER MULTIPLE STRAIN OUTBREAKS

Occasionally, common sources may become contaminated with several bacterial sps., leading to outbreaks of otherwise unrelated strains. For example, one multiple-strain outbreak of orthopedic wound infections was traced to a common bucket used to mix cast material. The bucket was not routinely disinfected and contained a variety of contaminants that probably were inoculated into wounds during application of casts. An unusual series of outbreaks of postoperative infection due to multiple organisms at seven different hospitals was linked to exposure to propofol, an anesthetic agent with a lipid-based vehicle that is able to support the rapid growth of a variety of microorganisms

at room temperature [133]. Apparently, lapses in aseptic technique by anesthesia personnel at/near the time of surgery resulted in extrinsic contamination of syringes or vials containing this agent. Such outbreaks may go unrecognized unless one strain predominates or the strains or epidemiologic circumstances are very unusual.

CONTROL

Control of antibiotic resistance is important primarily because resistance limits treatment options, sometimes to less effective or more toxic therapies. Delayed or ineffective treatment may underlie the reported increases in morbidity and mortality associated with infection due to several multidrug-resistant bacteria [134–139]. Excess cost or length of stay also has been found to be associated with infection due to these pathogens, especially MRSA, suggesting that control may result in cost savings for hospitals [134,140,141].

The past decade has yielded a large body of knowledge related to the epidemiology of multidrug-resistant bacteria in hospitals. Molecular epidemiologic studies have discriminated those pathogens that disseminate primarily by clonal expansion and that therefore should be more effectively eradicated by interruption of cross-transmission [117] from those that arise mainly by mutation and selection of patients' endogenous flora, and that therefore might better be controlled by relieving antibiotic pressure [142,143]. Mathematical models of transmission have allowed predictions about the effectiveness of various interventions that would be difficult or impractical to study in large clinical trials [19,144–147]. Study design and analysis have become more rigorous, providing better information about the effects of infection control measures [52–54].

Nevertheless, it is clear that there is still much we do not know. Many of the published reports of successful control of nosocomial ARPs, especially MRSA and VRE, have important limitations. First, many were conducted during epidemics while the majority of hospitals confronting these pathogens now face endemic resistance; the epidemiology of the problem and the effectiveness of control measures may be different in these two settings. Second, most studies implemented multiple interventions either simultaneously or sequentially, making it impossible to determine which were linked to the outcome. This information is especially important in controlling resistance in endemic settings; because of the long-term investment required and the potential for adverse outcomes related to some interventions [148–150], it is essential that we implement only measures that are both necessary and sufficient to achieve control. Third, while research methodologies have improved, few intervention trials have used optimal study designs (e.g., randomized cluster or cross-over). Most of the information available to us comes from quasi-experimental studies that may have failed to take into account stochastic or secular changes, that did not adequately control for bias or confounding, or that may have had very short periods of follow-up [151]. Fourth, in studies of infection control interventions that required the active participation of HCWs in a clinical setting, such as studies of the effect of contact isolation on acquisition of colonization by a ARPs, compliance monitoring was rarely performed. Studies that did monitor compliance often found it to be poor, raising questions about the validity of the causal inferences made by the authors. Finally, the reason for the success of isolation interventions is not known (i.e., whether the outcome is related to improved hand hygiene—a positive, intended effect—or to fewer HCW contacts with colonized or infected patients—an unintended effect with potentially negative consequences) [148–150].

The lack of definitive information has resulted in a divergence of opinion in the infection control community about the interventions that should be endorsed [152–154]. Although we believe that additional research in this area is needed to attempt to resolve the controversies, we feel strongly that we must work now with the information available toward controlling ARPs in hospitals. This is particularly important because of increasing pressure from the lay public and legislatures who will otherwise mandate our response to the problem [155,156].

It is likely that various combinations of control measures are effective and that success or failure depends on the epidemiology of the problem (e.g., monoclonal outbreak vs. polyclonal endemicity, the population affected, the intensity of care required, and the degree of compliance with individual measures that constitute the intervention). We suggest a multifaceted, flexible approach to the control of ARPs in acute care hospitals. Some potential components to include in such a program are discussed next.

Education

Antibiotic resistance is a problem for the entire healthcare community, not just for infection control practitioners All hospital personnel should be educated to recognize the deleterious effects of antibiotic resistance and their role in controlling it. Several studies have demonstrated that physicians tend to perceive antibiotic resistance as less important in their own institutions than nationally even if they have access to information showing that local rates of resistance are high [157,158]. Mandatory education sessions should emphasize local data and response and should be tailored to clinicians' areas of interest; frequent reminders such as posters with simple messages or educational alerts may be effective adjunctive educational measures [157].

Support of Hospital Leaders

Hospital administration should support efforts to control antibiotic resistance by providing adequate funding for an effective infection control program and by incorporating infection control into the objectives of the organization's patient and occupational safety programs [159]. In addition, senior hospital leadership, including department heads and other opinion leaders, should be recruited to conspicuously promote these objectives and to model good behavior (e.g., strict adherence to hand hygiene) [80,160–163]. Finally, there is evidence on several levels that coordination of efforts regionally and even nationally [164–168] may result in substantial and durable reductions in ARPs. These collaborations should be sought when feasible (e.g., in integrated healthcare systems).

Prevention of Infection

Although the strength of evidence in support of some infection control interventions is debated, there is consensus on the effectiveness of bundling preventive measures that have been effective individually, combined with monitoring and feedback, to significantly reduce or eliminate device-related or surgical-site infections (SSIs) [169–172]. Reducing infection rates not only would decrease individual patients' risk of morbidity from ARPs but also should result in reduced antibiotic prescribing, thereby lessening antibiotic pressure selective for ecologic resistance. Preventing infection is a key strategy in the current CDC 12-step campaign to prevent antimicrobial resistance in hospitalized adults (Table 14-4) [173].

Passive Surveillance

Surveillance of clinical laboratory results should be maintained to detect clusters of resistant bacteria (≥ 2 patients with similarly resistant organisms) so that cross-infection or important environmental reservoirs can be identified

TABLE 14-4
CAMPAIGN TO PREVENT ANTIMICROBIAL RESISTANCE, 12-STEP PROGRAM FOR HOSPITALIZED ADULTS, 2002

Strategy: Prevent infection
    Step 1: Vaccinate
    Step 2: Get the catheters out
Strategy: Diagnose and treat infection effectively
    Step 3: Target the pathogen
    Step 4: Access the experts
Strategy: Use antimicrobials wisely
    Step 5: Practice antimicrobial control
    Step 6: Use local data
    Step 7: Treat infection, not contamination
    Step 8: Treat infection, not colonization
    Step 9: Know when to say "no" to vancomycin
    Step 10: Stop treatment when infection is cured or unlikely
Strategy: Prevent transmission
    Step 11: Isolate the pathogen
    Step 12: Break the chain of contagion

and controlled. Stratification of clinical isolate antibiotic susceptibility results by hospital unit may detect unit-specific trends in bacterial incidence or antibiotic resistance that would otherwise be masked [174,175]. For example, the emergence of multiply-resistant *P. aeruginosa* in the burn and medical intensive care units (ICUs) of one hospital was apparent when antibiograms from these areas were analyzed separately, although resistance in *P. aeruginosa* hospitalwide was stable during the same period [176]. Use of molecular epidemiologic tools, such as pulsed-field gel electrophoresis, can enhance standard laboratory surveillance efforts and reveal relationships between isolates that are not otherwise obvious [177]. Other laboratory-based surveillance strategies include screening stools submitted for *Clostridium difficile* toxin and testing for the presence of VRE or MRSA [178,179]. In two separate studies, this approach appeared to be complementary to focused active surveillance for these pathogens. If supported by the hospital and laboratory information systems, electronic alerts that notify admitting personnel of patients who were colonized/infected with a resistant pathogen on a previous admission can help expedite isolation of patients [180,181].

Spurious changes in resistance frequencies may result if unreliable or inconsistent methods are used to create, record, and analyze susceptibility data [182]. For example, inclusion in a report of multiple isolates of MRSA from a single patient might be incorrectly interpreted as a cluster of infections. Guidelines to avoid these kinds of problems when analyzing and presenting cumulative susceptibility test data have been published [183].

Hand Hygiene

Because most cross-transmission of pathogens in hospitals occurs from patient to patient via contaminated HCWs' hands (Figure 14-1) (Table 14-3), promotion of hand hygiene is an essential component of any policy to prevent spread of ARPs. Strategies for successful promotion of hand hygiene in hospitals have included education; observation and feedback; engineering changes (extra sinks, well-stocked hygiene supplies); posters, cartoons, and other visual reminders; administrative sanctions or rewards; and avoidance of excessive workload and understaffing [184,185]. Alcohol-based handrubs are the most efficacious agents for reducing the number of bacteria on HCWs' hands [80,186], and their introduction to a healthcare facility may improve hand hygiene adherence [187,188]. The consistently suboptimal or transient improvements wrought by behavioral interventions suggest that technological innovations, such as "killer gloves" that generate antimicrobial ClO_2 may hold the most promise for progress in this area [189].

Contact Precautions and Active Surveillance

Numerous studies have evaluated the effects of contact precautions alone or with other interventions, such as active surveillance cultures, on the control of ARPs during outbreak and endemic periods; most of the published studies have evaluated the effect of these measures on acquisition of VRE or MRSA [164,166,180,181,190–193]. Few studies have evaluated the individual components of this approach (i.e., identifying an at-risk patient; obtaining a specimen for culture [or, more recently, PCR]; testing the specimen for the ARP; providing the nurse or physician with the result; placing the patient in a private room or cohorting the patient with other carriers; posting signs indicating that the patient is in isolation; stocking the patient's room with isolation supplies; requiring visitors and HCWs who care for the patient to wear gloves and gowns; enforcing strict hand hygiene; and providing for adequate environmental hygiene, including waste removal). Which of these components is critical for successful control may not be obvious. During a 3-month period, we obtained daily surveillance cultures from patients to evaluate *S. aureus* cross-transmission in a medical ICU where this pathogen was endemic; however, HCWs were not informed of culture results, and patients were not isolated [194]. Despite ongoing admission of MRSA-positive patients and stable, only moderate rates of hand hygiene adherence, we did not detect a single instance of methicillin-susceptible *S. aureus* or MRSA cross-acquisition. This experience, although very short term, suggested that the act of obtaining surveillance cultures per se may be a critical part of control efforts.

Gloves, a key element of both standard and contact precautions, have been found to be highly effective in preventing contamination of HCWs' hands during routine care activities that require touching a patient or the patient's immediate environment [107,108]. Wearing gloves for all patient encounters (universal gloving) was a major component of a successful program to control MRSA in a surgical ICU; in a different study, requiring HCWs to wear gloves for contact with any patient body substance was associated with a decreased incidence of *C. difficile* diarrhea compared to wards where gloves were not required [195]. Gloves are not a substitute for hand hygiene; small tears or defects may result in inapparent soiling of hands, and hands can become contaminated when gloves are removed. In addition, cross-transmission of ARPs is facilitated if HCWs fail to remove gloves between patients.

Wearing a clean cover gown when caring for patients who are infected/colonized with ARPs can prevent contamination of HCWs' clothing; whether ARPs can be transferred from contaminated clothing to patients is not known. The requirement to gown was cited as a key component in a successful multimodal control of an outbreak of VRE [191]. Three prospective evaluations of the added benefits of gowns compared to gloves alone to prevent VRE transmission yielded conflicting results [196–198]. In one study in which gowns did not demonstrate additional benefit, gown use was associated with increased compliance with infection control procedures [198]. Gowns likely provide the most benefit when worn to care for patients who are shedding large numbers of resistant bacteria in urine, stool, secretions or drainage or who are carrying ARPs that are known to contaminate and survive in the hospital environment (e.g., antibiotic-resistant *A. baumannii*, VRE, or MRSA [102,199–201]). Similar logic dictates that wearing a mask may be useful to prevent HCW nasal MRSA colonization during aerosol-generating procedures or when there is evidence of aerosolization from heavily colonized sources (e.g., burn wounds [159]).

Active surveillance cultures have been cited as a key component of a number of interventions that reported control of VRE or MRSA [164,180,192,193,202]. Studies differed in their screening criteria and schedules, sensitivity of laboratory methods used for detection of resistance, and whether patients were isolated pre-emptively or only after return of a positive result. The last factor is particularly important for hospitals that outsource their microbiology work; although in-house PCR assays may provide results within 24 hours, the turnaround time for a VRE screening culture performed at a typical reference laboratory is 3–7 days [203,204]. Nevertheless, identification and isolation of patients whose colonization status would otherwise remain unknown (Figure 14-2) has benefit, especially if adherence to routine infection control measures (e.g., hand hygiene) is poor. A variety of models has been developed to predict carriage of ARPs at the time of hospital admission so that only patients at highest risk can be screened and unnecessary cultures can be minimized [205–208]. Active surveillance cultures may be particularly effective in closed units, such as neonatal or burn ICUs.

While housing patients colonized/infected with ARPs in private rooms is preferred, this commodity is limited in some hospitals, and nosocomial resistance problems have been controlled in multibed settings [209]. When private rooms are not available, patients carrying the same resistant pathogen may be cohorted [146,159]. A recent study of the effect of placing MRSA carriers in private rooms or cohorted bays found no benefit in preventing MRSA acquisition in the ICUs of two hospitals where MRSA was endemic [210], although incomplete screening of patients on admission and low adherence to hand hygiene (21% overall) may have confounded the intervention's effect. On rare occasions, units have been closed to control transmission [168].

Occasionally, HCWs are the source of an outbreak or cluster of infections; this has been demonstrated especially for MRSA [84–86]. Surveillance of HCWs and decolonization of carriers may be necessary to control transmission.

Adherence Monitoring

Adherence to interventions is crucial to the success of infection control measures (e.g., hand hygiene and contact precautions). Based on observational and interventional studies and behavioral models, it is probably unrealistic to expect 100% compliance with any intervention, and the adherence threshold for success of measures such as hand hygiene is not known. Nonetheless, the Joint Commission on Accreditation of Healthcare Organizations expects that hand hygiene adherence should occur with no more than a "sporadic miss." Monitoring and providing feedback of results, especially if immediate, have been shown to improve compliance with infection control procedures in several studies [187,188,211–213]. Direct observation by monitors who are known to the observed worker may yield inaccurate results due to a Hawthorne effect. Alternative methods of adherence monitoring include tracking the use of supplies, such as alcohol hand rub or gowns, although these have not been as accurate as direct observation because they do not ensure that the use of the product was appropriate or that the recommended hand hygiene was performed.

Disinfection and Cleaning of the Environment

Careful attention to cleaning and disinfection of patient rooms may be particularly important for control of ARPs that have been shown to persistently contaminate the inanimate environment in hospitals, such as VRE, antibiotic-resistant *A. baumannii*, or MRSA [201,209,214]. Recent evidence has implicated surfaces contaminated with these pathogens as important sources of cross-transmission; these findings have revitalized interest in environmental "source-control" [102,103,215]. In one recent report, hydrogen peroxide vapor fogging was found to be superior to routine terminal cleaning in eradicating MRSA from environmental surfaces, furniture, and equipment in patient rooms [216]. Another study found that nebulizing a 0.5% solution of a new polymeric guanidine disinfectant, AKACID Plus, for 100 minutes in experimentally contaminated rooms eliminated pathogenic *S. aureus*, *E. coli*, and *P. aeruginosa* from plastic and stainless steel surfaces [217]. In a laboratory evaluation, application of a novel silver-based disinfectant to clean glass surfaces created a film that demonstrated residual bactericidal activity against a variety of pathogens for up to 8 hours and up to five cycles of water rinsing, abrasion, and contamination [218]. Copper surfaces are being evaluated as a means of reducing survival of epidemic MRSA in the hospital environment [219].

Standard methods of environmental decontamination also are undergoing renewed scrutiny. In a study we performed, strict enforcement of routine environmental cleaning procedures was highly effective in controlling VRE over an 11-month period in a medical ICU where this pathogen was endemic. The intervention was associated with less environmental VRE contamination, decreased contamination of HCW hands, and a >3-fold reduction in VRE acquisition by patients [215]. These improvements occurred despite ongoing admission of VRE-colonized patients and only moderate rates of HCW adherence to proper hand hygiene. In our experience, neither extraordinary efforts nor special germicides were needed;

careful adherence to routine procedures, achieved by closely monitoring cleaning personnel, was the key to success.

Decolonization

Decolonization of patients has sometimes been a component of control programs, especially if more routine infection control measures could not be employed or were unsuccessful [209,220]. A majority of studies were of MRSA-colonized patients; attempts were made to eradicate MRSA nasal carriage with topical mupirocin alone or in combination with oral antibiotics or cleansing skin and hair with antimicrobial soap. Commonly observed drawbacks to this approach include frequent recolonization with the same strain and development of mupirocin resistance. A recent Cochrane systematic review of randomized clinical trials of MRSA-decolonization concluded that there is insufficient evidence to support the use of systemic or topical antimicrobial therapy to eradicate nasal or extranasal MRSA [221].

We evaluated an alternative method of patient decolonization in a study of VRE acquisition in an MICU with high-level endemicity. In this 15-month study, patients were cleansed daily with cloths impregnated with 2% chlorhexidine gluconate [222]. This approach, which we termed "source control," was associated with significantly less VRE on patients' skin and a reduction in the incidence of VRE acquisition from 26 to 9 colonizations per 1000 patient-days [222].

Antibiotic Controls

Because antimicrobial consumption appears to drive both the emergence and transmission of multiply resistant organisms, much effort has gone into studying antibiotic management in the hopes of curbing selective pressure. The relationship between antibiotic use and resistance is complex; restriction of an antibiotic may not correlate directly with a reduction in its resistance. For example, there is minimal evidence that limiting vancomycin exposure decreases the risk of VRE acquisition in VRE-free patients [66]. Conversely, restriction of one antibiotic may be associated with a reduction in resistance to another; a 10-fold decrease in fluoroquinolone use was associated with a statistically significant decline in the incidence density and prevalence of MRSA in a recent study in a French hospital [223]. Furthermore, a decrease in one class of antibiotic may be followed by an increase in another class. In 1995, in response to the rising incidence in ESBL-producing *K. pneumoniae*, one hospital reduced the use of cephalosporins through formulary restriction and guideline modifications. An 80% reduction in cephalosporin use led to a 44% reduction in the incidence of ceftazidime-resistant *K. pneumoniae* hospitalwide but at the apparent expense of a 69% increased incidence of imipenem-resistant *P. aeruginosa* [224].

In general, antibiotic control programs should promote good antibiotic stewardship, such as curbing overall antimicrobial consumption and de-escalating or narrowing antimicrobial therapy when appropriate. Consideration also should be given to limiting the use of antibiotics that appear to cause the most "collateral damage" (i.e., are most often associated with the development of ARP colonization/infection, such as fluoroquinolones and cephalosporins) [225,226]. More deliberate approaches to manipulation of antibiotic exposure, such as antibiotic cycling (rotating a predominant antibiotic at time points that are separated by months to years) have been studied in various institutions with mixed results. In the ICU setting, cycling was associated with decreases in ventilator-associated pneumonia, hospital mortality, and incidence of resistant pathogens [227–229]. Unfortunately, several subsequent studies failed to show an effect of cycling on acquisition of resistant gram-negative bacteria [230,231]; in one investigation, cycling appeared to predispose to development of resistance [232].

THRESHOLD FOR INVESTIGATION AND GOALS OF CONTROL PROGRAM

Some organisms always warrant prompt attention because of key resistances. Such bacteria include MRSA, *S. aureus* with reduced susceptibility to glycopeptides, VRE, carbapenem-resistant gram-negative rods, and ESBL-producing *Enterobacteriaceae*. The responses of different hospitals to control of any of these pathogens may differ depending on the perceived risk they pose to their patients; for example, a patient housed in an ICU or transplant ward is more likely to suffer serious morbidity from VRE colonization than is a patient in a rehabilitation facility. The prevalence of a pathogen in the institution also may influence action; isolation of vancomycin-resistant *S. aureus* would evoke a more aggressive response than isolation of MRSA. Resources available to the infection control program are another factor that will shape prevention and control efforts.

Taking these variables into account, hospitals should set goals for control programs aimed at these or other ARPs. First, a hospital should determine which ARPs and units to target. Next, an assessment should be made of the extent of the problem (i.e., rare or occasional episodes of the ARP, one or more ongoing outbreaks, or low- or high-level endemicity). Finally, the hospital should determine whether the goal is eradication of a specific organism, control of an outbreak, or reduction of the number of endemic episodes to the lowest achievable level [152]. Because several studies have shown that inter- and intrahospital transfer of colonized/infected patients is a major source of incident cases, cooperation among wards and institutions that share patients may significantly improve a program's odds of success [59]. We caution against too narrow a focus; close attention to control of a single ARP may result in disregard of another, leading to its uncontrolled dissemination [233].

SPECIFIC ORGANISMS

Staphylococcus aureus

Despite aggressive control efforts, MRSA continues to be one of the most problematic ARPs in the hospital setting. In a survey of U.S. hospitals in 2004, 36% of *S. aureus* clinical isolates were resistant to methicillin, with two-thirds of hospitals reporting increasing incidence of resistance [234]. The situation is even more extreme in ICUs; the CDC's NNIS survey of ICUs reported *S. aureus* to be methicillin-resistant nearly 60% of the time in 2003 [33].

Modern-day methicillin resistance in *S. aureus* did not develop through *de novo* genetic resistance; rather, it is the result of selective expansion of clones carrying resistance genes on a genomic subunit called the staphylococcal cassette chromosome *mec* (SCC*mec*). At least 5 SCC*mec* types (I–V) have been identified, all of which carry an altered penicillin-binding protein (PBP2a) that confers β-lactam resistance.

Buoyed by the selective pressure of increased antimicrobial consumption within hospitals, MRSA has traditionally been isolated within the hospital and associated settings. Such nosocomial MRSA isolates are associated particularly with SCC*mec* types I–III, which often carry genes that confer broad resistance to aminoglycosides, macrolides, lincosamides (e.g., clindamycin), and tetracyclines in addition to β-lactam resistance [235]. However, since its first description in 1998, the prevalence of community-acquired MRSA (CA-MRSA) has increased dramatically in the United States[236,237]. CA-MRSA is predominantly associated with the SCC*mec* type IV, which is a smaller element that retains β-lactam resistance but generally lacks other resistance genes. CA-MRSA isolates also are associated with virulence factors such as PVL, which may predispose affected patients to soft-tissue abscesses or severe disease such as necrotizing fasciitis and necrotizing pneumonia. The presence of a community reservoir of CA-MRSA has now led to a dramatic shift in hospital MRSA ecology with as many as 20% of MRSA-HAIs caused by CA-MRSA strains in some hospitals [20]. Furthermore, these CA-MRSA strains appear to be accumulating resistance to additional antibiotic classes.

Although their isolation is still mostly sporadic, reports of *S. aureus* with intermediate susceptibility (VISA) or resistance (VRSA) to vancomycin have been increasing. The surveillance definition of VISA is an isolate of *S. aureus* with a vancomycin MIC between 8 and 16 μg/mL; VRSA is defined as having a vancomycin MIC ≥32 μg/mL. Nearly all VISA or VRSA strains reported thus far have expressed multidrug resistance, including resistance to methicillin [238]. Both VISA and VRSA present challenges in detection. The most reliable susceptibility testing methods use broth microdilution, commercial vancomycin screening agar (6 μg/mL), or Etest® (AB Biodisk), although some automated systems have been validated for VRSA detection [239]. In order to facilitate more accurate detection of VISA or VRSA, the Clinical Laboratory Standards Institute recently lowered the vancomycin categorical breakpoints for *S. aureus* to 4–8 μg/mL (intermediate susceptibility) and ≥16 μg/mL (resistant); corresponding changes in surveillance definitions are expected to follow [238,240].

VISA infection was first reported in Japan [241] and France [242]; since then, similar strains have been isolated from other parts of the world, including six strains confirmed in the United States with reports of others [238]. The decreased susceptibility to vancomycin seen in VISA strains appears to be related to thickened cell walls, changes in cellular metabolism, and enhanced cell wall turnover; the redundant peptidoglycan in the cell wall serves as a substrate for vancomycin but prevents it from reaching its cytoplasmic membrane target [243].

Because of the rarity of VISA infections, the epidemiology has not been well defined. In a prospective surveillance and nested case-control study conducted in the United States, independent risk factors for infection due to *S. aureus* with reduced susceptibility to vancomycin (vancomycin MIC ≥4 μg/mL) were antecedent vancomycin use and MRSA infection in the previous 2–3 months [244]. Outbreaks and fatal clinical infection due to VISA have been described, indicating that although these strains grow more slowly than MRSA, they maintain similar virulence [245,246].

High-level vancomycin resistance was first reported in *S. aureus* in 2002 [247]. It has since been noted in four other strains, all of which carried the *vanA* gene complex, which was originally identified in VRE [248]. Although all of the strains characterized thus far were identified in the United States and four were identified in the state of Michigan, no epidemiologic links among the cases have been found, and no secondary cases have been detected. All case patients were chronically ill; one had not been exposed to vancomycin for 5 years [249]. It is assumed that each of the VRSA strains independently acquired vancomycin resistance from VRE, probably via gene transfer. Evidence in support of this hypothesis includes successful plasmid-mediated transfer of *vanA* from *E. faecalis* to *S. aureus* in laboratory experiments, and concomitant or recent carriage of VRE by at least 3/6 confirmed VRSA patients [250,251]. Generation of additional *de novo* VRSA strains will likely be affected by the endemicity of VRE.

The main hospital reservoir of resistant staphylococci, like that of susceptible strains, is the anterior nares of patients. Less appreciated is that MRSA often colonizes healthy skin in the axillae, hand, arm, and inguinal areas; touching these sites can lead to contamination of hands or gloves of HCWs [109]. Rectal carriage and colonization of stools also have been described [179,252]. In addition, a broad range of inanimate objects have been found to be contaminated with MRSA in the rooms of colonized/infected patients, and HCWs have been shown to contaminate their gloved hands after touching these sites even when they did not touch the patient [201]. These features point to the primacy of contact precautions as a means of controlling resistant *S. aureus*; in one study, implementation of contact precautions during an outbreak in a neonatal ICU reduced the rate of spread of MRSA from 0.14 to 0.009 transmissions per day [193].

Control of resistant *S. aureus* has been a primary concern for infection control research and practice. For MRSA, accurate laboratory identification, recognition of previously colonized patients at readmission, appropriate isolation of all identified infected/colonized patients, and environmental cleaning and decontamination are effective in decreasing hospital endemicity and outbreaks [151,154,253,254]. Because HCWs who are colonized in the anterior nares or at other sites can sometimes transmit MRSA directly to patients (Table 14-3), a search for personnel sources should be made if these other measures are unsuccessful. HCWs who are epidemiologically linked to spread of MRSA should undergo decolonization and remain on furlough from direct patient care until their cultures are negative; successful treatment regimens have included topical mupirocin alone or in combination with oral antibiotics and antimicrobial soap for bathing [255]. Because the number of patients who are asymptomatically colonized often greatly exceeds the number with known infection, active surveillance cultures may play an important role for MRSA control in some settings [154,254]. Additional measures to control endemic and epidemic MRSA colonization should be tailored to the individual healthcare setting and guided by surveillance data and available resources. How these practices may be affected by the spread of CA-MRSA and vancomycin-resistant species remains unclear.

Enterococcus spp

Since the mid-1980s, enterococci have emerged as significant HAI pathogens, becoming the third most frequent cause of bloodstream infection (BSI) in the United States [256]. Two species, *E. faecalis* and *E. faecium*, account for the vast majority of enterococcal infections. Enterococci are not highly virulent organisms. They cause infections primarily in debilitated or immunocompromised patients, in whom they are associated with significant attributable morbidity, mortality, and increased length of hospital stay [62,257–259].

Enterococci are intrinsically resistant to all cephalosporins, penicillinase-resistant penicillins, and clindamycin. The rise in incidence of enterococci since the 1970s is temporally correlated with increased worldwide use of antimicrobials with little or no antienterococcal activity, particularly cephalosporins [62]. Ampicillin, the preferred therapy for enterococcal infections, can be rendered ineffective in the face of a low-affinity penicillin-binding protein, PBP-5 [260]. Alterations to or overproduction of this protein are responsible for high-level ampicillin resistance in *E. faecium* [261]. Rarely, ampicillin resistance is attributable to β-lactamase production [262].

The spread of vancomycin-resistance among enterococci is a worrisome trend. Such resistance was not described until the late 1980s [263], and now approaches 30% of all U.S. enterococcal infections [33]. Vancomycin resistance is associated primarily with *vanA* or *vanB* gene clusters, which are complex genetic elements frequently found on transferrable plasmids [264]. Vancomycin resistance has never been demonstrated to develop as a *de novo* mutation under antimicrobial pressure [265]; therefore, the first step toward colonization or infection with VRE must be exposure to a resistant enterococcal strain. Most VRE are *E. faecium*; in this species, *vanB* resistance has sometimes been found linked to high-level ampicillin resistance on a large mobile genetic element [266].

Resistance to aminoglycosides, which are used for synergy in treating serious enterococcal infections, ranges in the United States from 30-60% and is more often associated with *E. faecium* [267]. Sporadic reports of resistance to quinupristin-dalfopristin, linezolid, and daptomycin, often the only drugs available to treat VRE, emerged soon after release of each antibiotic [268–271]. The prospect of untreatable enterococcal infection in the future remains.

Antimicrobial pressure is an important risk factor for patient acquisition of vancomycin-resistant enterococci in the hospital. Antecedent use of cephalosporins and antimicrobials with antianaerobic effects has been associated consistently with VRE colonization [62,65]. These data suggest a model in which antimicrobials that are active against endogenous gut flora but inactive against enterococci promote enterococcal colonization and high-level stool shedding [62,63]. In contrast, prior exposure to vancomycin itself does not appear to be a strong risk factor for acquisition of VRE in settings where these strains already are prevalent [65].

In hospitals, VRE usually spread by horizontal transmission of resistant clones on the contaminated HCW's hands; transfer of plasmids or other genetic elements plays a lesser role [117,272]. The number of colonized patients usually is far greater than the number of those who are infected; this "iceberg effect" (Figure 14-2) also plays an important part in the nosocomial dissemination of these pathogens [272].

Strategies for control of epidemic and endemic multidrug-resistant enterococci, in particular VRE, are based on several observations. First, enterococci survive easily on intact patient skin, environmental surfaces, and HCW hands and clothing, providing ample opportunity for horizontal transmission [79,102,107,273]. In epidemic settings, proximity to an index patient has been shown to be an important factor in acquisition of resistant enterococci. In endemic settings, "colonization pressure," or the proportion of VRE-colonized patients, when high, is the most important variable influencing acquisition of VRE [180,274]. Second, in the United States, patients in acute-care hospitals or residing in LTCFs constitute the most important reservoir for resistant enterococci [275]. In Europe, community colonization with VRE is common and probably related to widespread use of the glycopeptide avoparcin in animal farming during the last decades of the twentieth century [276]. The epidemic strains causing infection in European hospitals appear to be different than non-epidemic community strains, however, and may be differentiated from them by detection of the variant *esp* gene, a virulence factor [19]. Third, antibiotic exposure may influence the epidemiology of VRE in at least two ways: by elevating a VRE-negative patient's risk of acquiring VRE and by increasing the density of VRE in the stool of VRE-positive patients, thereby raising the odds of skin or environmental contamination and facilitating cross-transmission [4,66]. Finally, establishment of VRE endemicity, a situation faced by many U.S. hospitals, follows a predictable course from detection of rare and sporadic cases, to monoclonal outbreak, to polyclonal endemicity [272]. Control of VRE is substantially easier if implemented in the earlier stages than in the later ones.

Approaches to control of VRE should highlight contact isolation for known colonized/infected patients and hospital hygiene [215,254,277,278]. Active surveillance cultures to detect VRE colonization may enhance control efforts in both epidemic and endemic situations [164,202,254,279] and might be warranted especially in healthcare settings comprising patients at high risk for serious enterococcal infection, such as transplant, oncology, and ICUs. As with MRSA, accurate and sensitive laboratory identification and recognition of previously colonized patients at readmission are important [280]. In a mathematical model, staff cohorting was shown to be very effective in reducing VRE transmission, even with moderate levels of compliance, but this strategy has not been tested in a clinical setting [146]. In another study, we bathed patients in an ICU daily with 2% chlorhexidine-impregnated cloths and lowered VRE acquisition nearly 3-fold (RR, 0.4), an effect similar to the reduction reported in a study of enhanced infection control measures that used at least seven interventions in an oncology unit [222,281]. No antibiotic regimen has proven useful for intestinal decolonization; early investigations of probiotic approaches to decolonization have shown some promise [282].

Enterobacteriaceae

The Enterobacteriaceae comprise a large group of aerobic, gram-negative bacteria that frequently cause clinically significant infection in hospital patients. In this group, *E. coli*, *Klebsiella* spp. and *Enterobacter* spp. have particular epidemiologic importance by virtue of their tendency to develop broad antibiotic resistance. Other Enterobacteriaceae that may develop multidrug-resistant phenotypes include *Serratia marcescens*, *Citrobacter* spp., *Proteus* spp., *Providencia* spp., and *Morganella* spp. Aminoglycoside resistance also is increasing, but carbapenem resistance remains uncommon in most geographic regions [283].

Antibiotic resistance in *Enterobacteriaceae* has accelerated over the past two decades. Several key resistance phenotypes, each mediated by multiple mechanisms, are particularly problematic; they include resistance to fluoroquinolones, cephalosporins, and carbapenems. The forces driving the increased incidences of the different resistances are interrelated; rising resistance to fluoroquinolones and cephalosporins leads to greater use of carbapenems, providing selective pressure for development of carbapenem resistance. These selective pressures may predispose to the development of panresistance, which has already been described in *K. pneumoniae* [284]. Such a development is sobering because the genetic elements (plasmids and integrons) that confer broad resistance often are mobile and easily transferred from one gram-negative species to another, making their recognition and control difficult [131].

Fluoroquinolone resistance among *Enterobacteriaceae* has increased significantly since their use began in the 1980s. Data from England and Wales reflecting hospital BSIs showed that from 1990 to1999, ciprofloxacin resistance rates for *Enterobacter* spp. and *Klebsiella* spp. rose from 2.1% and 3.5% to 10.9% and 7.1%, respectively [45]. The NNIS survey from 1992 to 2004 reported fluoroquinolone-resistance among *E. coli* to be 7.3% across ICUs with some hospitals reporting rates of resistance in excess of 19% [33]. Increasing trends have been seen in the most common *Enterobacteriaceae*, particularly in HAIs [285]. Multiple chromosomal point mutations affecting topoisomerase targets and cell wall permeability and efflux contribute to the resistance phenotype [286]. Alarmingly, plasmid-mediated fluoroquinolone resistance, which was first identified in 1998, has now been found worldwide. It often is located with an ESBL gene on a class I integron, thus facilitating transfer of both fluoroquinolone and cephalosporin resistance among *Enterobacteriaceae* [25,287].

Resistance to third-generation cephalosporins in *Enterobacteriaceae* often is conferred through plasmid-mediated ESBLs. These have been identified primarily in *E. coli* and *Klebsiella* spp., but they are known to exist in other species such as *Enterobacter*, *Serratia*, *Citrobacter*, and *Proteus*. In Europe, overall rates of *Klebsiella* spp.–producing ESBLs reached 13.6% in 2004, compared to 4.4% in the United States [283]. In Latin America, 45.4% of *Klebsiella* spp. isolates appear to harbor ESBLs [288]. In U.S. ICUs, as many as 20% of *Klebsiella* spp. (representing a 5-year increase of 47%) may express the ESBL phenotype [33].

The epidemiology of ESBL-producing species HAIs appears to be evolving [289]. In the past, nosocomial ESBL epidemics in the United States and Europe were generally due to clonal dissemination of *Klebsiella* spp. and *E. coli*, usually containing TEM or SHV genotypes, or to plasmid outbreaks. More recently, ESBL-producing *Enterobacteriaceae*, primarily *E. coli* strains carrying a CTX-M genotype, have been described in community settings in patients without prior hospital contact [121,290,291]. The expansion of ESBL resistance into the community presents challenges for prospective identification of colonized patients upon admission and infection control.

Broad penicillin and cephalosporin-resistance in some *Enterobacteriaceae* is conferred by chromosomal AmpC β-lactamases. Chromosomal mutations leading to AmpC β-lactamase hyperproduction are seen in *Enterobacter* spp., *Citrobacter* spp., *Serratia* spp., *Providencia* spp., and *Morganella* spp. Plasmid-encoded AmpC resistance also has disseminated into *Klebsiella* spp. and *Proteus* spp. In the United States and Europe, approximately 14% of *Enterobacter* spp. express the hyperproducing phenotype. While AmpC-producing bacterial isolates are resistant to β-lactamase inhibitors such as clavulanate, ESBL-producing isolates usually are susceptible, allowing for discrimination during surveillance. However, in strains that produce multiple β-lactamases, differentiation may not be possible without more detailed molecular evaluation.

Predictably, carbapenem resistance through diverse mechanisms has developed in areas where it has been heavily used to combat ESBL epidemics. It has been associated with up-regulation of AmpC β-lactamase and altered membrane porins in *K. pneumoniae* and *Enterobacter cloacae* [292,293]. A variety of β-lactamases active against carbapenems also has been described in *Enterobacteriaceae* [294,295], including a plasmid-associated KPC-type β-lactamase that is now endemic in the northeast United States [296].

Laboratory detection of ESBLs and KPC-type β-lactamases can be difficult because bacteria producing either enzyme can appear falsely susceptible when tested using routine methods [297,298]. Recommendations for optimal detection have been published [12,240].

Resistant *Enterobacteriaceae* may asymptomatically colonize the gastrointestinal, urinary or respiratory tracts, and chronically colonized patients often are a source for large numbers of cross-infections [299,300]. Some *Enterobacteriaceae*, such as *Serratia* spp., survive well in the wet inanimate environment. There have been several outbreaks described in which devices or equipment contaminated with resistant *S. marcescens*, notably ventilators or graduated cylinders used to measure urine, led to epidemics of UTI, peritonitis, or pneumonia [300]. Such evidence suggests that contact precautions and environmental decontamination are important for epidemic control.

The optimal means for control of resistant *Enterobacteriaceae* depend on which bacterial genus and mechanism of resistance are involved. ESBL-producing *K. pneumoniae* often cause clonal outbreaks, emphasizing the importance of contact precautions as a control measure. Hyperproduction of chromosomal AmpC β-lactamase, such as is seen in *E. cloacae*, is probably best controlled by reducing selective pressure by cephalosporins. However, it is important to realize that resistance to third-generation cephalosporins in bacterial genera that encode chromosomal AmpC also can be due to plasmid-mediated ESBLs, in which case cross-transmission may be the more important force in an outbreak or cluster of infections [124]. Complex situations such as an increase in phenotypic resistance

encoded by various genetic mechanisms among different bacterial genera (e.g., ceftazidime-resistance due to diverse chromosomal or plasmid-encoded β-lactamases in different strains of *Enterobacteriaceae* [an "allodemic"]) may be most effectively controlled by reducing antibiotic selective pressure [301].

Molecular studies suggest that plasmids and integrons encoding resistance to several classes of antibiotics play a dominant role in horizontal transmission of genetic information among different strains and species of *Enterobacteriaceae* [29,302,303]. Spread of integrons appears to be facilitated by antimicrobial pressure and cross-contamination [302]. Future efforts to slow the spread of multidrug-resistant *Enterobacteriaceae* will likely involve as yet undiscovered methods for detecting and combating integron dissemination.

Pseudomonas aeruginosa

P. aeruginosa has intrinsic resistance to many available antibiotics. It contains multiple efflux pumps, including MexAB-OprM and MexXY-OprM, that remove a heterogeneous group of antimicrobials from its intracellular space, including β-lactams, fluoroquinolones, macrolides, sulfonamides, tetracycline, and trimethoprim [304]. It also carries an inducible chromosomal AmpC β-lactamase that complements the efflux system to confer further β-lactam resistance [305]. Importantly, *P. aeruginosa* has shown the ability to acquire resistance to all traditionally effective agents, such as antipseudomonal penicillins, third- and fourth-generation cephalosporins, aminoglycosides, fluoroquinolones, and carbapenems.

Multiple mechanisms contribute to resistance [34]. Fluoroquinolone resistance is mediated by mutations to target genes for DNA gyrase (*gyrA*) and topoisomerase IV (*parC*) [306]. Stepwise derepression (and subsequent overproduction) of AmpC β-lactamase allows for increasing resistance to most antipseudomonal β-lactam agents, such as piperacillin, ceftazidime, and cefepime, although carbapenems are unaffected by this mechanism [307]. Up-regulation of specific efflux pumps can increase resistance to most β-lactams, meropenem (but not imipenem), fluoroquinolones, and aminoglycosides [304]. Pan-aminoglycoside resistance occurs via aminoglycoside-modifying enzymes coupled with increased efflux and decreased membrane permeability [308]. Imipenem resistance appears to be particularly associated with loss of a membrane porin, OprD [309]. Sequential acquisition of mutations is facilitated by a subset of *P. aeruginosa* "hypermutators" [310], well described in cystic fibrosis patients although perhaps more rare in ICUs [311], that have the propensity to develop genetic changes, such that virtual panresistance can occur with a small group of mutations, such as increased efflux, loss of OprD, and aminoglycoside impermeability.

In addition to chromosomal mutation, integrons have been described in epidemic spread of panresistance in

P. aeruginosa. Metallo-β-lactamases, such as VIM, IMP, and SPM, which confer resistance to carbapenems, often are linked with aminoglycoside acetyltransferases (AAC) and other resistance genes and have led to HAI outbreaks of panresistant *P. aeruginosa* [312–314].

Prevalence of multidrug resistance in *Pseudomonas aeruginosa* (defined as resistant to ≥ 3 antimicrobial classes) has increased in the United States, from 7.2% in 2001 to 9.9% in 2003 [315]. Dramatic increases in multidrug-resistant phenotypes have been seen in South America, particularly Brazil, where prevalence reached 35% in 2001 [316]. These population statistics do not capture the particularly high burden of multidrug-resistant *P. aeruginosa* that exists in many ICUs, burn, and cystic fibrosis units.

Within the hospital environment, *P. aeruginosa* is ubiquitous in animate and inanimate reservoirs [317]. It can be cultured from almost any wet surface including water faucets [318,319], patient-related equipment [320], and containers of fluid such as distilled water [321] and dialysate [322]. Furthermore, patient gastrointestinal colonization serves as an important reservoir for endogenous infection and a source of horizontal transmission to other patients. While epidemics are well-described secondary to contaminated environmental sources, the dynamics between the endogenous and exogenous reservoirs that contribute to endemic colonization and infection in the hospital setting are less clear. Recent evidence suggests that periods of endemicity, characterized by polyclonal infection, are promoted by patients who are colonized on admission. In these patients, exposure to antimicrobial pressure then becomes a risk factor for clinical infection. While some studies suggest gastrointestinal and respiratory colonization to be the most important source for endemic HAIs [323], other studies suggest important contribution from environmental sources [324,325]. Control of multidrug-resistant *P. aeruginosa* ultimately requires a multifaceted approach with hospital hygiene to prevent horizontal transmission from exogenous sources and control of antimicrobial pressure to prevent endogenous infection [317].

Acinetobacter spp

Acinetobacter spp., including the highly resistant *A. baumannii*, have emerged as important HAI pathogens particularly in ICUs among patients with impaired host defenses. *Acinetobacter* spp. are most commonly seen in pulmonary and BSIs followed by wound and UTIs [326].

The incidence of *Acinetobacter* spp. nosocomial bloodstream infection has been estimated at 1.5% in the United States [327]; however, because of the epidemic nature of *Acinetobacter* outbreaks, true incidence varies widely between continents and medical centers. In some New York City hospitals, approximately 10% of all gram negative isolates were reported as *A. baumannii* in 2000 [328].

Acinetobacter spp. have shown a remarkable propensity to develop wide antimicrobial resistance with some species almost completely resistant to Federal Drug Administration–approved antimicrobial agents [329]. Resistance mechanisms such as chromosomal, integron, and plasmid-mediated β-lactamases (including penicillinases, metalloenzymes, and oxacillinases), porin protein mutations, and target site mutations confer resistance to major antimicrobials such as ceftazidime, aminoglycosides, fluoroquinolones, ampicillin-sulbactam, and imipenem [330, 331]. A few remaining older agents (colistin) and newer agents (tigecycline) have been used to treat multidrug resistant *Acinetobacter* with some success [332,333].

The ability of *Acinetobacter* spp. to survive on dry, inanimate surfaces for long periods of time [82,334] suggests that the hospital environment serves as a reservoir for multidrug-resistant strains to persist during epidemics. Although several *Acinetobacter* spp. are common constituents of healthy human skin flora, *A. baumannii* is rarely found except on the skin of hospital patients during outbreaks, and transiently on HCW hands or other skin [334,335]. It is likely that animate and inanimate vectors have led to numerous hospital outbreaks, which are usually clonal or oligoclonal in nature [330]. Interhospital spread of multidrug-resistant *Acinetobacter* clones has been reported [336].

Successful control of epidemics due to multidrug-resistant *Acinetobacter* has been achieved primarily through attention to basic infection control measures coupled with careful environmental disinfection and vector control. In 1991, an outbreak of *A. baumannii* susceptible to only polymyxins and sulbactam occurred at a New York hospital, primarily in the surgical ICU [330]. Cultures of both environmental and HCW hands yielded growth of multidrug-resistant *A. baumannii*. Methods used to control the epidemic included thorough cleaning and surveillance of the entire affected unit, increased enforcement of hospital HCW hand hygiene, and cohorting of colonized/infected patients (and their nurses when possible). The use of imipenem also was restricted. This multifaceted strategy resulted in eradication of multidrug-resistant *A. baumannii* for more than five years. Similar approaches have been successful in control of outbreaks in other centers [337,338].

Coagulase-Negative Staphylococci (CNS)

Multiply-resistant coagulase negative staphylococci have become endemic in hospitals across the world. Greater than 70% of all CNS isolates are resistant to methicillin [339]. Furthermore, despite their relative avirulence, CNS are routinely one of the most common causes of BSIs in the hospital, especially in patients with central venous catheters. CNS infections often are associated with prosthetic implanted devices such as joints, heart valves, and neurosurgical shunts [340]; the rising use of such therapies portends a significant burden of CNS infection in the future.

Glycopeptide resistance has been noted sporadically in *Staphylococcus haemolyticus* and *Staphylococcus epidermidis*.

In Europe, where the glycopeptide teicoplanin is used, teicoplanin resistance across intermediate and highly resistant ranges has been detected [341]. Over the same period, however, vancomycin has remained effective with only sporadic reports of resistance described [342]. The mechanisms of CNS vancomycin resistance remain ill-defined but are probably related to cell wall changes similar to that employed by vancomycin-intermediate *S. aureus* [343]. This mechanism can appear *de novo* during therapy and appears unrelated to *vanA*- or *vanB*-mediated vancomycin resistance seen in VRE.

High levels of patient colonization with methicillin-resistant-CNS in the hospital have rendered control measures ineffective. Resistant CNS are present in low numbers on the skin of patients and emerge in the hospital as predominant flora and potential pathogens, especially under antimicrobial selection [344,345]. Prevention of infection associated with catheter and prosthetic devices by adhering to aseptic strategies remains important. Colonized surgeons have been implicated as sources of staphylococcal postoperative infections, suggesting the need to consider this mode of transmission when postoperative infection rates exceed expected norms [346].

Corynebacterium jeikeium

Corynebacterium jeikeium, in contrast to other *Corynebacterium* spp., is notable for its intrinsic resistance to a wide variety of antimicrobials, including β-lactams, aminoglycosides, macrolides, tetracycline, and quinolones; vancomycin most often is used for treatment [347]. *C. jeikeium* is a cause of HAI, particularly among patients with malignancies, neutropenia, and intravenous catheters or who are exposed to broadspectrum antimicrobials [348].

Like most diphtheroids, *C. jeikeium* commonly colonizes the skin of hospital patients [349,350]. *C. jeikeium* is endemic in hospitals, and different strains likely are transferred horizontally between patients [351]. Control of endemic infection with *C. jeikeium*, like control of CNS, depends in large part on good aseptic technique to prevent perioperative or device-related infections.

Steontrophomonas maltophilia

S. maltophilia is a multidrug-resistant organism that has had increasing importance in causing a variety of infections, particularly pneumonia and BSI, in immunocompromised and critically ill patients [326]. It is ubiquitous in the environment, being found in water, soil, and plants. In the hospital, S. *maltophilia* has been isolated from a variety of aqueous reservoirs and equipment, including tap water [352], chlorhexidine disinfectant diluted with contaminated deionized water [353], and components of mechanical ventilators [354].

S. *maltophilia* carry multiple mechanisms for broad antimicrobial resistance, including efflux pumps, selective membrane porins, and β-lactamases, that provide protection against extended-spectrum penicillins, cephalosporins, aminoglycosides, carbapenems, and fluoroquinolones [355,356]. Although trimethoprim-sulfamethoxazole remains the first choice in treatment, resistance to this agent has emerged, from 2% in Canada and Latin America to 10% in Europe [326].

Control of S. *maltophilia*, like other ubiquitous environmental organisms, rests primarily on identifying common sources during epidemics and maintaining optimal hospital hygiene. In one carefully controlled study, prior receipt of imipenem did not appear to be a strong risk factor for acquiring S. *maltophilia* infection [357].

Burkholderia cepacia

B. cepacia is widely distributed in the environment; it is particularly suited to growing in liquid reservoirs and on moist surfaces [358]. Outbreaks have been traced to nutritionally deficient and biologically hostile sources, including tap water; deionized water; intrinsically and extrinsically contaminated dilute, aqueous benzalkonium chloride; povidone-iodine; or nebulized solution in respiratory equipment [359]. Community and hospital-acquired *B. cepacia* infections have been well described in cystic fibrosis patients, in whom both colonization and infection are associated with increased mortality [360]. Nosocomial transmission of *B. cepacia* between cystic fibrosis patients has been documented through person-to-person contact [361] and via shared respiratory equipment [362]. Besides infecting cystic fibrosis patients, *B. cepacia* is an opportunist, causing respiratory, urinary, and BSIs in critically ill patients.

B. cepacia is intrinsically resistant to aminoglycosides, anti-pseudomonal penicillins, and polymyxins [363]. Much of the intrinsic resistance may be attributed to decreased membrane permeability [364], presence of efflux pumps [365], and an inducible chromosomal β-lactamase [366].

Control of *B. cepacia* epidemics usually involves identifying a common source if one is present, ideally through a case-control or cohort investigation [359]. Cohorting of colonized patients and contact precautions may prevent horizontal spread [367], although this strategy has been studied mainly among cystic fibrosis patients [368]. It is noteworthy that although many common-source outbreaks have resulted in true clinical infections with *B. cepacia*, pseudo-outbreaks also have been described. In one such investigation, multiple positive blood cultures detected in a hospital were the result of contaminated povidone-iodine used in the phlebotomy process rather than true BSIs [369].

FUTURE CHALLENGES

The ingenious ways in which microorganisms learn to evade our antimicrobial pharmacopeia will no doubt continue to astound, and at times confound, and perplex us. As the pressures on our antimicrobial armamentarium increase and as our patients are subjected to more invasive procedures and immunosuppressive regimens, we can anticipate greater resistance and more problems with the traditionally avirulent normal flora.

Unfortunately, our control of resistant strains has advanced little since the singular contribution of Semmelweis. Moreover, we still have trouble encouraging and motivating personnel to follow the most basic concepts in asepsis. Given this reality, success in the future may hinge on development of new technologies such as less infection-prone devices; novel products for intestinal decolonization; topical agents with persistent bactericidal activity that can be applied to patients' skin, to environmental surfaces, or to HCW hands, gloves, or clothing; and computer order entry systems that facilitate antimicrobial stewardship [189,222,282,370]. In the meantime, we should not abandon our efforts to improve HCW use of hand hygiene products, because changes in behavior are possible but occur only after years of sustained effort.

We also need to use advances in molecular microbiology, modeling, and statistics to obtain a better understanding of the epidemiology of ARP HAIs, not only in single-strain outbreaks but also in the endemic setting and in outbreaks due to plasmids and other transmissible genetic elements [117,131,301,371]. As we increase our understanding of bacterial and host factors that control colonization with normal flora and lead to overgrowth of resistant bacteria, new approaches may emerge for preventing colonization with HAI pathogens, blocking adherence of unwanted resistant strains or transmission of resistance elements, or preventing progression from colonization to infection.

For now, we believe the key is not to delay in applying the strategies available to us and not to apply measures in too piecemeal a fashion lest control always lag behind resistance. The growing interchange of resistant bacteria among LTCFs, acute care hospitals, and community populations emphasizes the need for concerted control effort [370].

REFERENCES

1. Levy SB. Multidrug resistance—a sign of the times. *N Engl J Med* 1998;338:1376–1378.
2. Weinstein RA. Nosocomial infection update. *Emerg Infect Dis* 1998;4:416–420.
3. Cohen ML. Epidemiology of drug resistance: implications for a post-antimicrobial era. *Science* 1992;257:1050–1055.
4. Paterson DL. Looking for risk factors for the acquisition of antibiotic resistance: a 21st-century approach. *Clin Infect Dis* 2002;34:1564–1567.
5. Laupland KB, Parkins MD, Church DL, et al. Population-based epidemiological study of infections caused by carbapenem-resistant *Pseudomonas aeruginosa* in the Calgary Health Region: importance of metallo-beta-lactamase (MBL)-producing strains. *J Infect Dis* 2005;192:1606–1612.
6. Joyanes P, del Carmen Conejo M, et al. Evaluation of the VITEK 2 system for the identification and susceptibility testing of three species of nonfermenting gram-negative rods frequently isolated from clinical samples. *J Clin Microbiol* 2001;39:3247–3253.
7. Tenover FC, Swenson JM, O'Hara CM, Stocker SA. Ability of commercial and reference antimicrobial susceptibility testing methods to detect vancomycin resistance in enterococci. *J Clin Microbiol* 1995;33:1524–1527.
8. Endtz HP, Van Den Braak N, Van Belkum A, et al. Comparison of eight methods to detect vancomycin resistance in enterococci. *J Clin Microbiol* 1998;36:592–594.
9. Liu C, Chambers HF. *Staphylococcus aureus* with heterogeneous resistance to vancomycin: epidemiology, clinical significance, and critical assessment of diagnostic methods. *Antimicrob Agents Chemother* 2003;47:3040–3045.
10. Tenover FC, Weigel LM, Appelbaum PC, et al. Vancomycin-resistant *Staphylococcus aureus* isolate from a patient in Pennsylvania. *Antimicrob Agents Chemother* 2004;48:275–1280.
11. Giakkoupi P, Tzouvelekis LS, Daikos GL, et al. Discrepancies and interpretation problems in susceptibility testing of VIM-1-producing *Klebsiella pneumoniae* isolates. *J Clin Microbiol* 2005;43:494–496.
12. Landman D, Salvani JK, Bratu S, Quale J. Evaluation of techniques for detection of carbapenem-resistant *Klebsiella pneumoniae* in stool surveillance cultures. *J Clin Microbiol* 2005;43:5639–5641.
13. Pfaller MA, Segreti J. Overview of the epidemiological profile and laboratory detection of extended-spectrum beta-lactamases. *Clin Infect Dis* 2006;42:S153–S163.
14. Hanberger H, Nilsson LE, Claesson B, et al. New species-related MIC breakpoints for early detection of development of resistance among gram-negative bacteria in Swedish intensive care units. *J Antimicrob Chemother* 1999;44:611–619.
15. Weinstein RA, Kabins SA. Strategies for prevention and control of multiple drug-resistant nosocomial infection. *Am J Med* 1981;70:449–454.
16. Flynn DM, Weinstein RA, Nathan C, Gaston MA, Kabins SA. Patients' endogenous flora as the source of "nosocomial" Enterobacter in cardiac surgery. *J Infect Dis* 1987;156:363–368.
17. Olson B, Weinstein RA, Nathan C, Chamberlin W, Kabins SA. Occult aminoglycoside resistance in *Pseudomonas aeruginosa*: epidemiology and implications for therapy and control. *J Infect Dis* 1985;152:769–774.
18. Fey PD, Said-Salim B, Rupp ME, Hinrichs SH, et al. Comparative molecular analysis of community- or hospital-acquired methicillin-resistant *Staphylococcus aureus*. *Antimicrob Agents Chemother* 2003;47:196–203.
19. Willems RJ, Homan W, Top J, et al. Variant esp gene as a marker of a distinct genetic lineage of vancomycin-resistant *Enterococcus faecium* spreading in hospitals. *Lancet* 2001;357:853–855.
20. Seybold U, Kourbatova EV, Johnson JG, et al. Emergence of community-associated methicillin-resistant *Staphylococcus aureus* USA300 genotype as a major cause of healthcare-associated blood stream infections. *Clin Infect Dis* 2006;42:647–656.
21. Friedman ND, Kaye KS, Stout JE, et al. Healthcare-associated bloodstream infections in adults: a reason to change the accepted definition of community-acquired infections. *Ann Intern Med* 2002;137:791–797.
22. Smith DL, Dushoff J, Perencevich EN, et al. Persistent colonization and the spread of antibiotic resistance in nosocomial pathogens: resistance is a regional problem. *Proc Natl Acad Sci USA* 2004;101:3709–3714.
23. Alanis AJ. Resistance to antibiotics: are we in the post-antibiotic era? *Arch Med Res* 2005;36:697–705.
24. Zhao X, Drlica K. Restricting the selection of antibiotic-resistant mutants: a general strategy derived from fluoroquinolone studies. *Clin Infect Dis* 2001;33:S147–S156.
25. Nordmann P, Poirel L. Emergence of plasmid-mediated resistance to quinolones in Enterobacteriaceae. *J Antimicrob Chemother* 2005;56:463–469.
26. Hakenbeck R, Konig A, Kern I, et al. Acquisition of five high-Mr penicillin-binding protein variants during transfer of high-level beta-lactam resistance from Streptococcus mitis to Streptococcus pneumoniae. *J Bacteriol* 1998;180:1831–1840.
27. O'Brien TF. Emergence, spread, and environmental effect of antimicrobial resistance: how use of an antimicrobial anywhere can increase resistance to any antimicrobial anywhere else. *Clin Infect Dis* 2002;34:S78–S84.

28. Toussaint A, Merlin C. Mobile elements as a combination of functional modules. *Plasmid* 2002;47:26–35.

29. Leverstein-van Hall MA, He MB, AR TD, Paauw A, Fluit AC, Verhoef J. Multidrug resistance among *Enterobacteriaceae* is strongly associated with the presence of integrons and is independent of species or isolate origin. *J Infect Dis* 2003;187:251–259.

30. Villa L, Pezzella C, Tosini F, et al. Multiple-antibiotic resistance mediated by structurally related IncL/M plasmids carrying an extended-spectrum beta-lactamase gene and a class 1 integron. *Antimicrob Agents Chemother* 2000;44:2911–2914.

31. Jones RN, Kirby JT, Beach ML, et al. Geographic variations in activity of broad-spectrum beta-lactams against *Pseudomonas aeruginosa*: summary of the worldwide SENTRY Antimicrobial Surveillance Program (1997–2000). *Diagn Microbiol Infect Dis* 2002;43:239–243.

32. Olson B, Weinstein RA, Nathan C, et al. Broad-spectrum beta-lactam resistance in Enterobacter: Emergence during treatment and mechanisms of resistance. *J Antimicrob Chemother* 1983;11:229.

33. National Nosocomial Infections Surveillance (NNIS) System Report, data summary from January 1992 through June 2004, issued October 2004. *Am J Infect Control* 2004;32:470–485.

34. Livermore DM. Multiple mechanisms of antimicrobial resistance in *Pseudomonas aeruginosa*: our worst nightmare? *Clin Infect Dis* 2002;34:634–640.

35. Gaynes RP, Culver DH. Resistance to imipenem among selected gram-negative bacilli in the United States. *Infect Control Hosp Epidemiol* 1992;13:10–4.

36. Grape M, Sundstrom L, Kronvall G. New dfr2 gene as a single-gene cassette in a class 1 integron from a trimethoprim-resistant *Escherichia coli* isolate. *Microb Drug Resist* 2003;9:317–322.

37. Radstrom P, Swedberg G, Skold O. Genetic analyses of sulfonamide resistance and its dissemination in gram-negative bacteria illustrate new aspects of R plasmid evolution. *Antimicrob Agents Chemother* 1991;35:1840–1848.

38. Grape M, Farra A, Kronvall G, Sundstrom L. Integrons and gene cassettes in clinical isolates of co-trimoxazole-resistant Gram-negative bacteria. *Clin Microbiol Infect* 2005;11:185–192.

39. Talan DA, Stamm WE, Hooton TM, et al. Comparison of ciprofloxacin (7 days) and trimethoprim-sulfamethoxazole (14 days) for acute uncomplicated pyelonephritis pyelonephritis in women: a randomized trial. *JAMA* 2000;283:1583–1590.

40. Brown PD, Freeman A, Foxman B. Prevalence and predictors of trimethoprim-sulfamethoxazole resistance among uropathogenic *Escherichia coli* isolates in Michigan. *Clin Infect Dis* 2002;34:1061–1066.

41. Haley RW, Hightower AW, Khabbaz RF, et al. The emergence of methicillin-resistant *Staphylococcus aureus* infections in United States hospitals: possible role of the house staff-patient transfer circuit. *Ann Intern Med* 1982;97:297–308.

42. Gaynes RP, Culver DH, Horan TC, al. e. Trends in methicillin-resistant *Staphylococcus aureus* in United States hospitals. *Infect Dis Clin Pract* 1993;2:452.

43. Hooper DC. Mechanisms of action of antimicrobials: focus on fluoroquinolones. *Clin Infect Dis* 2001;32:S9–S15.

44. Polk RE, Johnson CK, McClish D, et al. Predicting hospital rates of fluoroquinolone-resistant *Pseudomonas aeruginosa* from fluoroquinolone use in US hospitals and their surrounding communities. *Clin Infect Dis* 2004;39:497–503.

45. Livermore DM, James D, Reacher M, Graham C, et al. Trends in fluoroquinolone (ciprofloxacin) resistance in Enterobacteriaceae from bacteremias, England and Wales, 1990–1999. *Emerg Infect Dis* 2002;8:473–478.

46. Fridkin SK, Hill HA, Volkova NV, et al. Temporal changes in prevalence of antimicrobial resistance in 23 US hospitals. *Emerg Infect Dis* 2002;8:697–701.

47. Goldstein EJ, Garabedian-Ruffalo SM. Widespread use of fluoroquinolones versus emerging resistance in pneumococci. *Clin Infect Dis* 2002;35:1505–1511.

48. Klevens RM, Edwards JR, Tenover FC, et al. Changes in the epidemiology of methicillin-resistant *Staphylococcus aureus* in intensive care units in US hospitals, 1992–2003. *Clin Infect Dis* 2006;42:389–391.

49. Lautenbach E, Fishman NO, Metlay JP, et al. Phenotypic and genotypic characterization of fecal *Escherichia coli* isolates with decreased susceptibility to fluoroquinolones: results from a large hospital-based surveillance initiative. *J Infect Dis* 2006;194:79–85.

50. Johnson JR, Kuskowski MA, Menard M, et al. Similarity between human and chicken *Escherichia coli* isolates in relation to ciprofloxacin resistance. Status. *J Infect Dis* 2006;194:71–78.

51. Collignon P, Angulo FJ. Fluoroquinolone-resistant *Escherichia coli*: food for thought. *J Infect Dis* 2006;194:8–10.

52. Harris AD, Karchmer TB, Carmeli Y, Samore MH. Methodological principles of case-control studies that analyzed risk factors for antibiotic resistance: a systematic review. *Clin Infect Dis* 2001;32:1055–1061.

53. Kaye KS, Harris AD, Samore M, Carmeli Y. The case-case-control study design: addressing the limitations of risk factor studies for antimicrobial resistance. *Infect Control Hosp Epidemiol* 2005;26:346–351.

54. Harris AD, Samore MH, Lipsitch M, et al. Control-group selection importance in studies of antimicrobial resistance: examples applied to *Pseudomonas aeruginosa*, Enterococci, and *Escherichia coli*. *Clin Infect Dis* 2002;34:1558–1563.

55. Suntharam N, Lankford MG, Trick WE, et al. Risk factors for acquisition of vancomycin-resistant enterococci among hematology-oncology patients. *Diagn Microbiol Infect Dis* 2002;43:183–188.

56. Lucet JC, Chevret S, Durand-Zaleski I, et al. Prevalence and risk factors for carriage of methicillin-resistant *Staphylococcus aureus* at admission to the intensive care unit: results of a multicenter study. *Arch Intern Med* 2003;163:181–188.

57. Harris AD, Smith D, Johnson JA, et al. Risk factors for imipenem-resistant *Pseudomonas aeruginosa* among hospitalized patients. *Clin Infect Dis* 2002;34:340–345.

58. Harbarth S, Harris AD, Carmeli Y, Samore MH. Parallel analysis of individual and aggregated data on antibiotic exposure and resistance in gram-negative bacilli. *Clin Infect Dis* 2001;33:1462–1468.

59. Safdar N, Maki DG. The commonality of risk factors for nosocomial colonization and infection with antimicrobial-resistant *Staphylococcus aureus*, enterococcus, gram-negative bacilli, clostridium difficile, and candida. *Ann Intern Med* 2002;136:834–844.

60. Ehrlich P. Chemotherapeutics: scientific principles, methods and results. *Lancet* 1913;ii:445–451.

61. Lipsitch M, Samore MH. Antimicrobial use and antimicrobial resistance: a population perspective. *Emerg Infect Dis* 2002;8:347–354.

62. Rice LB. Emergence of vancomycin-resistant enterococci. *Emerg Infect Dis* 2001;7:183–187.

63. Donskey CJ, Chowdhry TK, Hecker MT, et al. Effect of antibiotic therapy on the density of vancomycin-resistant enterococci in the stool of colonized patients. *N Engl J Med* 2000;343:1925–1932.

64. Kirst HA, Thompson DG, Nicas TI. Historical yearly usage of vancomycin. *Antimicrob Agents Chemother* 1998;42:1303–1304.

65. Carmeli Y, Eliopoulos GM, Samore MH. Antecedent treatment with different antibiotic agents as a risk factor for vancomycin-resistant enterococcus. *Emerg Infect Dis* 2002;8:802–807.

66. Harbarth S, Cosgrove S, Carmeli Y. Effects of antibiotics on nosocomial epidemiology of vancomycin-resistant enterococci. *Antimicrob Agents Chemother* 2002;46:1619–1628.

67. Selden R, Lee S, Wang WL, et al. Nosocomial klebsiella infections: intestinal colonization as a reservoir. *Ann Intern Med* 1971;74:657–664.

68. Bonten MJ, Hayden MK, Nathan C, et al. Epidemiology of colonisation of patients and environment with vancomycin-resistant enterococci. *Lancet* 1996;348:1615–1619.

69. Toltzis P, Hoyen C, Spinner-Block S, et al. Factors that predict preexisting colonization with antibiotic-resistant gram-negative bacilli in patients admitted to a pediatric intensive care unit. *Pediatrics* 1999;103:719–723.

70. Gilmore DS, Schick DG, Montgomerie JZ. *Pseudomonas aeruginosa* and *Klebsiella pneumoniae* on the perinea of males with spinal cord injuries. *J Clin Microbiol* 1982;16:865–867.

71. Montgomerie JZ, Morrow JW. Pseudomonas colonization in patients with spinal cord injury. *Am J Epidemiol* 1978;108:328–336.

72. Fainstein V, Rodriguez V, Turck M, et al. Patterns of oropharyngeal and fecal flora in patients with acute leukemia. *J Infect Dis* 1981;144:10–8.

73. O'Neal PV, Brown N, Munro C. Physiologic factors contributing to a transition in oral immunity among mechanically ventilated adults. *Biol Res Nurs* 2002;3:132–139.

74. Leibovitz A, Baumoehl Y, Steinberg D, Segal R. Biodynamics of biofilm formation on nasogastric tubes in elderly patients. *Isr Med Assoc J* 2005;7:428–430.

75. Safdar N, Crnich CJ, Maki DG. The pathogenesis of ventilator-associated pneumonia: its relevance to developing effective strategies for prevention. *Respir Care* 2005;50:725–741.

76. Flynn DM, Weinstein RA, Kabins SA. Infections with gram-negative bacilli in a cardiac surgery intensive care unit: the relative role of enterobacter. *J Hosp Infect* 1988;11:367–373.

77. Larson EL, McGinley KJ, Foglia AR, et al. Composition and antimicrobic resistance of skin flora in hospitalized and healthy adults. *J Clin Microbiol* 1986;23:604–608.

78. Bayuga S, Zeana C, Sahni J, et al. Prevalence and antimicrobial patterns of *Acinetobacter baumannii* on hands and nares of hospital personnel and patients: the iceberg phenomenon again. *Heart Lung* 2002;31:382–390.

79. Beezhold DW, Slaughter S, Hayden MK, et al. Skin colonization with vancomycin-resistant enterococci among hospitalized patients with bacteremia. *Clin Infect Dis* 1997;24:704–706.

80. Boyce JM, Pittet D. Guideline for hand hygiene in health-care settings: recommendations of the Healthcare Infection Control Practices Advisory Committee and the HIC-PAC/SHEA/APIC/IDSA Hand Hygiene Task Force. *MMWR Recomm Rep* 2002;51(RR-16):1–45.

81. Bonilla HF, Zervos MJ, Kauffman CA. Long-term survival of vancomycin-resistant *Enterococcus faecium* on a contaminated surface. *Infect Control Hosp Epidemiol* 1996;17:770–772.

82. Wendt C, Dietze B, Dietz E, Ruden H. Survival of *Acinetobacter baumannii* on dry surfaces. *J Clin Microbiol* 1997;35:1394–1397.

83. Craven DE, Reed C, Kollisch N, et al. A large outbreak of infections caused by a strain of *Staphylococcus aureus* resistant of oxacillin and aminoglycosides. *Am J Med* 1981;71:53–58.

84. Gaynes R, Marosok R, Mowry-Hanley J, et al. Mediastinitis following coronary artery bypass surgery: a 3-year review. *J Infect Dis* 1991;163:117–121.

85. Boyce JM, Opal SM, Potter-Bynoe G, Medeiros AA. Spread of methicillin-resistant *Staphylococcus aureus* in a hospital after exposure to a healthcare worker with chronic sinusitis. *Clin Infect Dis* 1993;17:496–504.

86. Sheretz RJ, Reagan DR, Hampton KD, et al. A cloud adult: the *Staphylococcus aureus*-virus interaction revisited. *Ann Intern Med* 1996;124:539–547.

87. Boyce JM, Potter-Bynoe G, Opal SM, et al. A common-source outbreak of *Staphylococcus epidermidis* infections among patients undergoing cardiac surgery. *J Infect Dis* 1990;161:493–499.

88. Buxton AE, Anderson RL, Werdegar D, Atlas E. Nosocomial respiratory tract infection and colonization with Acinetobacter calcoaceticus: epidemiologic characteristics. *Am J Med* 1978;65:507–513.

89. Graham DR, Anderson RL, Ariel FE, et al. Epidemic nosocomial meningitis due to *Citrobacter diversus* in neonates. *J Infect Dis* 1981;144:203–209.

90. Parry MF, Hutchinson JH, Brown NA, et al. Gram-negative sepsis in neonates: a nursery outbreak due to hand carriage of *Citrobacter diversus*. *Pediatrics* 1980;65:1105–1109.

91. Burke JP, Ingall D, Klein JO, et al. Proteus mirabilis infections in a hospital nursery traced to a human carrier. *N Engl J Med* 1971;284:115–121.

92. Foca M, Jakob K, Whittier S, et al. Endemic *Pseudomonas aeruginosa* infection in a neonatal intensive care unit. *N Engl J Med* 2000;343:695–700.

93. Shooter RA. Bowel colonization of hospital patients by Pseudomonas aeruginosa and *Escherichia coli*. *Proc R Soc Med* 1971;64:989–990.

94. Griffith SJ, Nathan C, Selander RK, et al. The epidemiology of *Pseudomonas aeruginosa* in oncology patients in a general hospital. *J Infect Dis* 1989;160:1030–1036.

95. Weinstein RA, Kabins SA. Strategies for prevention and control of multiple drug-resistant nosocomial infection. *Am J Med* 1981;70:449.

96. Marrie TJ, Major H, Gurwith M, et al. Prolonged outbreak of nosocomial urinary tract infection with a single strain of *Pseudomonas aeruginosa*. *Can Med Assoc J* 1978;119:593–596.

97. Schultsz C, Meester HH, Kranenburg AM, et al. Ultra-sonic nebulizers as a potential source of methicillin-resistant *Staphylococcus aureus* causing an outbreak in a university tertiary care hospital. *J Hosp Infect* 2003;55:269–275.

98. Livornese LL Jr., Dias S, Samel C, et al. Hospital-acquired infection with vancomycin-resistant *Enterococcus faecium* transmitted by electronic thermometers. *Ann Intern Med* 1992;117:112–116.

99. Feeley TW, Du Moulin GC, Hedley-Whyte J, et al. Aerosol polymyxin and pneumonia in seriously ill patients. *N Engl J Med* 1975;293:471–475.

100. Levin MH, Olson B, Nathan C, et al. Pseudomonas in the sinks in an intensive care unit: relation to patients. *J Clin Pathol* 1984;37:424–427.

101. Perryman FA, Flournoy DJ. Prevalence of gentamicin- and amikacin-resistant bacteria in sink drains. *J Clin Microbiol* 1980;12:79–83.

102. Duckro AN, Blom DW, Lyle EA, et al. Transfer of vancomycin-resistant enterococci via health care worker hands. *Arch Intern Med* 2005;165:302–307.

103. Hardy KJ, Oppenheim BA, Gossain S, et al. A study of the relationship between environmental contamination with methicillin-resistant *Staphylococcus aureus* (MRSA) and patients' acquisition of MRSA. *Infect Control Hosp Epidemiol* 2006;27:127–132.

104. Bauer TM, Ofner E, Just HM, et al. An epidemiological study assessing the relative importance of airborne and direct contact transmission of microorganisms in a medical intensive care unit. *J Hosp Infect* 1990;15:301–309.

105. Salzman TC, Clark JJ, Klemm L. Hand contamination of personnel as a mechanism of cross-infection in nosocomial infections with antibiotic-resistant *Escherichia coli* and Klebsiella-Aerobacter. *Antimicrobial Agents Chemother* (Bethesda) 1967;7:97–100.

106. Knittle MA, Eitzman DV, Baer H. Role of hand contamination of personnel in the epidemiology of gram-negative nosocomial infections. *J Pediatr* 1975;86:433–437.

107. Tenorio AR, Badri SM, Sahgal NB, et al. Effectiveness of gloves in the prevention of hand carriage of vancomycin-resistant enterococcus species by health care workers after patient care. *Clin Infect Dis* 2001;32:826–829.

108. Pittet D, Dharan S, Touveneau S, et al. Bacterial contamination of the hands of hospital staff during routine patient care. *Arch Intern Med* 1999;159:821–826.

109. Boyce JM, Havill NL, Kohan C, et al. Do infection control measures work for methicillin-resistant *Staphylococcus aureus*? *Infect Control Hosp Epidemiol* 2004;25:395–401.

110. Weinstein RA, Nathan C, Gruensfelder R, Kabins SA. Endemic aminoglycoside resistance in gram-negative bacilli: epidemiology and mechanisms. *J Infect Dis* 1980;141:338.

111. Bassetti S, Bischoff WE, Sherertz RJ. Outbreak of methicillin-resistant *Staphylococcus aureus* infection associated with an outbreak of severe acute respiratory syndrome. *Clin Infect Dis* 2005;40:633–635.

112. Poutanen SM, Vearncombe M, McGeer AJ, et al. Nosocomial acquisition of methicillin-resistant *Staphylococcus aureus* during an outbreak of severe acute respiratory syndrome. *Infect Control Hosp Epidemiol* 2005;26:134–137.

113. Yap FH, Gomersall CD, Fung KS, et al. Increase in methicillin-resistant *Staphylococcus aureus* acquisition rate and change in pathogen pattern associated with an outbreak of severe acute respiratory syndrome. *Clin Infect Dis* 2004;39:511–516.

114. Grieble HG, Bird TJ, Nidea HM, et al. Chute-hydropulping waste disposal system: a reservoir of enteric bacilli and Pseudomonas in a modern hospital. *J Infect Dis* 1974;130:602.

115. Gaynes RP, Weinstein RA, Smith J, et al. Control of aminoglycoside resistance by barrier precautions. *Infect Control* 1983;4:221–224.

116. Daum RS, Ito T, Hiramatsu K, et al. A novel methicillin-resistance cassette in community-acquired methicillin-resistant

Staphylococcus aureus isolates of diverse genetic backgrounds. *J Infect Dis* 2002;186:1344–1347.

117. Kim WJ, Weinstein RA, Hayden MK. The changing molecular epidemiology and establishment of endemicity of vancomycin resistance in enterococci at one hospital over a 6-year period. *J Infect Dis* 1999;179:163–171.

118. Naas T, Fortineau N, Snanoudj R, et al. First nosocomial outbreak of vancomycin-resistant *Enterococcus faecium* expressing a VanD-like phenotype associated with a vanA genotype. *J Clin Microbiol* 2005;43:3642–3649.

119. Markowitz SM, Veazey JM Jr., Macrina FL, et al. Sequential outbreaks of infection due to *Klebsiella pneumoniae* in a neonatal intensive care unit: implication of a conjugative R plasmid. *J Infect Dis* 1980;142:106–112.

120. Rubens CE, Farrar WE, McGee ZA, et al. Evolution of a plasmid-mediating resistance to multiple antimicrobial agents during a prolonged epidemic of nosocomial infections. *J Infect Dis* 1981;143:170.

121. Wiener J, Quinn JP, Bradford PA, Multiple antibiotic-resistant *Klebsiella* and *Escherichia coli* in nursing homes. *JAMA* 1999;281:517–523.

122. Giakkoupi P, Xanthaki A, Kanelopoulou M, et al. VIM-1 Metallo-beta-lactamase-producing *Klebsiella pneumoniae* strains in Greek hospitals. *J Clin Microbiol* 2003;41:3893–3896.

123. Corkill JE, Anson JJ, Hart CA. High prevalence of the plasmid-mediated quinolone resistance determinant qnrA in multidrug-resistant *Enterobacteriaceae* from blood cultures in Liverpool, UK. *J Antimicrob Chemother* 2005;56:1115–1117.

124. Bosi C, Davin-Regli A, Bornet C, et al. Most *Enterobacter aerogenes* strains in France belong to a prevalent clone. *J Clin Microbiol* 1999;37:2165–2169.

125. Roe E, Jones RJ, Lowbury EJ. Transfer of anibioic resistanceetween *Pseudomonas aeruginosa*, *Escherichia coli*, and other gram-negative bacilli in rns. *Lancet* 1971;1:149–152.

126. Walsh TR, Toleman MA, Poirel L, Nordmann P. Metallo-beta-lactamases: the quiet before the storm? *Clin Microbiol Rev* 2005;18:306–325.

127. Gootz TD. The forgotten Gram-negative bacilli: what genetic determinants are telling us about the spread of antibiotic resistance. *Biochem Pharmacol* 2006;71:1073–1084.

128. Kruse H, Sorum H. Transfer of multiple drug resistance plasmids between bacteria of diverse origins in natural microenvironments. *Appl Environ Microbiol* 1994;60:4015–4021.

129. Trieu-Cuot P, Derlot E, Courvalin P. Enhanced conjugative transfer of plasmid DNA from *Escherichia coli* to *Staphylococcus aureus* and Listeria monocytogenes. *FEMS Microbiol Lett* 1993;109:19–23.

130. Jaffe HW, Sweeney HM, Nathan C, et al. Identity and interspecific transfer of gentamicin-resistance plasmids in *Staphylococcus aureus* and *Staphylococcu epidermidis*. *J Infect Dis* 1980;141:738–747.

131. Nijssen S, Florijn A, Top J, et al. Unnoticed spread of integron-carrying *Enterobacteriaceae* in intensive care units. *Clin Infect Dis* 2005;41:1–9.

132. Neuwirth C, Siebor E, Lopez J, et al. Outbreak of TEM-24-producing *Enterobacter aerogenes* in an intensive care unit and dissemination of the extended-spectrum beta-lactamase to other members of the family *Enterobacteriaceae*. *J Clin Microbiol* 1996;34:76–79.

133. Bennett SN, McNeil MM, Bland LA, et al. Postoperative infections traced to contamination of an intravenous anesthetic, propofol. *N Engl J Med* 1995;333:147–154.

134. Cosgrove SE, Kaye KS, Eliopoulous GM, Carmeli Y. Health and economic outcomes of the emergence of third-generation cephalosporin resistance in Enterobacter species. *Arch Intern Med* 2002;162:185–190.

135. DiazGranados CA, Zimmer SM, Klein M, Jernigan JA. Comparison of mortality associated with vancomycin-resistant and vancomycin-susceptible enterococcal bloodstream infections: a meta-analysis. *Clin Infect Dis* 2005;41:327–333.

136. Vergis EN, Hayden MK, Chow JW, et al. Determinants of vancomycin resistance and mortality rates in enterococcal bacteremia. a prospective multicenter study. *Ann Intern Med* 2001;135:484–492.

137. Cosgrove SE, Sakoulas G, Perencevich EN, et al. Comparison of mortality associated with methicillin-resistant and methicillin-susceptible *Staphylococcus aureus* bacteremia: a meta-analysis. *Clin Infect Dis* 2003;36:53–59.

138. Cosgrove SE, Qi Y, Kaye KS, et al. The impact of methicillin resistance in *Staphylococcus aureus* bacteremia on patient outcomes: mortality, length of stay, and hospital charges. *Infect Control Hosp Epidemiol* 2005;26:166–174.

139. Engemann JJ, Carmeli Y, Cosgrove SE, et al. Adverse clinical and economic outcomes attributable to methicillin resistance among patients with *Staphylococcus aureus* surgical site infection. *Clin Infect Dis* 2003;36:592–598.

140. Cosgrove SE, Carmeli Y. The impact of antimicrobial resistance on health and economic outcomes. *Clin Infect Dis* 2003;36:1433–1437.

141. Cosgrove SE. The relationship between antimicrobial resistance and patient outcomes: mortality, length of hospital stay, and health care costs. *Clin Infect Dis* 2006;42:S82–S89.

142. Harris A, Torres-Viera C, Venkataraman L, et al. Epidemiology and clinical outcomes of patients with multiresistant *Pseudomonas aeruginosa*. *Clin Infect Dis* 1999;28:1128–1133.

143. Speijer H, Savelkoul PH, Bonten MJ, et al. Application of different genotyping methods for *Pseudomonas aeruginosa* in a setting of endemicity in an intensive care unit. *J Clin Microbiol* 1999;37:3654–661.

144. Pelupessy I, Bonten MJ, Diekmann O. How to assess the relative importance of different colonization routes of pathogens within hospital settings. *Proc Natl Acad Sci USA* 2002;99:5601–5605.

145. Perencevich EN, Hartley DM. Of models and methods: our analytic armamentarium applied to methicillin-resistant *Staphylococcus aureus*. *Infect Control Hosp Epidemiol* 2005;26:594–597.

146. Austin DJ, Bonten MJ, Weinstein RA, et al. Vancomycin-resistant enterococci in intensive-care hospital settings: transmission dynamics, persistence, and the impact of infection control programs. *Proc Natl Acad Sci USA* 1999;96:6908–6913.

147. Bootsma MC, Diekmann O, Bonten MJ. Controlling methicillin-resistant *Staphylococcus aureus*: quantifying the effects of interventions and rapid diagnostic testing. *Proc Natl Acad Sci USA* 2006;103:5620–5625.

148. Kirkland KB, Weinstein JM. Adverse effects of contact isolation. *Lancet* 1999;354:1177–1178.

149. Stelfox HT, Bates DW, Redelmeier DA. Safety of patients isolated for infection control. *Jama* 2003;290:1899–1905.

150. Tarzi S, Kennedy P, Stone S, Evans M. Methicillin-resistant *Staphylococcus aureus*: psychological impact of hospitalization and isolation in an older adult population. *J Hosp Infect* 2001;49:250–254.

151. Cooper BS, Stone SP, Kibbler CC, et al. Isolation measures in the hospital management of methicillin resistant *Staphylococcus aureus* (MRSA): systematic review of the literature. *BMJ* 2004;329:533.

152. Strausbaugh LJ, Siegel JD, Weinstein RA. Preventing transmission of multidrug-resistant bacteria in health care settings: a tale of 2 guidelines. *Clin Infect Dis* 2006;42:828–835.

153. Jackson M, Jarvis WR, Scheckler WE. HICPAC/SHEA—conflicting guidelines: what is the standard of care? *Am J Infect Control* 2004;32:504–511.

154. Coia JE, Duckworth GJ, Edwards DI, et al. Guidelines for the control and prevention of meticillin-resistant *Staphylococcus aureus* (MRSA) in healthcare facilities. *J Hosp Infect* 2006;63:1–44.

155. McCaughey B. Saving lives and the bottom line: hospitals must answer growing pressure to act on homegrown infections. *Mod Healthc* 2006;36:23.

156. MRSA: how politicians are missing the point. *Lancet* 2005;365:1203.

157. Giblin TB, Sinkowitz-Cochran RL, Harris PL, et al. Clinicians' perceptions of the problem of antimicrobial resistance in health care facilities. *Arch Intern Med* 2004;164:1662–1668.

158. Wester CW, Durairaj L, Evans AT, et al. Antibiotic resistance: a survey of physician perceptions. *Arch Intern Med* 2002;162:2210–2216.

159. Siegel J, Strausbaugh, L, Jackson, M., et al. DRAFT guideline for isolation precautions: preventing transmission of infectious agents in healthcare settings. 2004 (www.premierinc.com/safety

/resources/guidelines/downloads/2004-draft-iso-guideline.pdf) accessed June 21, 2006.

160. Goldmann DA, Weinstein RA, Wenzel RP, et al. Strategies to prevent and control the emergence and spread of antimicrobial-resistant microorganisms in hospitals: a challenge to hospital leadership. *JAMA* 1996;275:234–240.

161. Larson EL, Early E, Cloonan P, et al. An organizational climate intervention associated with increased handwashing and decreased nosocomial infections. *Behav Med* 2000;26:14–22.

162. Pittet D, Hugonnet S, Harbarth S, et al. Effectiveness of a hospital-wide programme to improve compliance with hand hygiene: infection control programme. *Lancet* 2000;356:1307–1312.

163. Gawande A. On washing hands. *N Engl J Med* 2004;350:1283–1286.

164. Ostrowsky BE, Trick WE, Sohn AH, et al. Control of vancomycin-resistant enterococcus in health care facilities in a region. *N Engl J Med* 2001;344:1427–1433.

165. Kotilainen P, Routamaa M, Peltonen R, et al. Elimination of epidemic methicillin-resistant *Staphylococcus aureus* from a university hospital and district institutions, Finland. *Emerg Infect Dis* 2003;9:169–175.

166. Nicolle LE, Dyck B, Thompson G, et al. Regional dissemination and control of epidemic methicillin-resistant *Staphylococcus aureus. Infect Control Hosp Epidemiol* 1999;20:202–205.

167. Rosdahl VT, Knudsen AM. The decline of methicillin resistance among Danish *Staphylococcus aureus* strains. *Infect Control Hosp Epidemiol* 1991;12:83–88.

168. Verhoef J, Beaujean D, Blok H, et al. A Dutch approach to methicillin-resistant *Staphylococcus aureus. Eur J Clin Microbiol Infect Dis* 1999;18:461–466.

169. O'Grady NP, Alexander M, Dellinger EP, et al. Guidelines for the prevention of intravascular catheter-related infections. *MMWR Recomm Rep* 2002;51(RR-10):1–29.

170. Mangram AJ, Horan TC, Pearson ML, et al. Guideline for prevention of surgical site infection, 1999. *Infect Control Hosp Epidemiol* 1999;20:250–278.

171. Berenholtz SM, Pronovost PJ, Lipsett PA, et al. Eliminating catheter-related bloodstream infections in the intensive care unit. *Crit Care Med* 2004;32:2014–2020.

172. Reduction in central line-associated bloodstream infections among patients in intensive care units—Pennsylvania, April 2001–March 2005. *MMWR Morb Mortal Wkly Rep* 2005;54:1013–1016.

173. CDC Campaign to Prevent Antimicrobial Resistance in Health-care Settings. www.cdc.gov/drugresistance/healthcare accesssed June 14, 2006.

174. Bryce EA, Smith JA. Focused microbiological surveillance and gram-negative beta-lactamase–mediated resistance in an intensive care unit. *Infect Control Hosp Epidemiol* 1995;16:331–334.

175. Stratton CW, Ratner H, Johnston PE, Schaffner W. Focused microbiologic surveillance by specific hospital unit as a sensitive means of defining antimicrobial resistance problems. *Diagn Microbiol Infect Dis* 1992;15:11S–18S.

176. Stratton CW, Ratner H, Johnston PE. Focused microbiologic surveillance by specific hospital unit as a sensitive means of defining antimicrobial resistance problems. *Diagn Microbiol Infect Dis* 1992;15:11S.

177. Bodnar UR, Noskin GA, Suriano T, et al. Use of in-house studies of molecular epidemiology and full species identification for controlling spread of vancomycin-resistant *Enterococcus faecalis* isolates. *J Clin Microbiol* 1996;34:2129–2132.

178. Hacek DM, Bednarz P, Noskin GA, et al. Yield of vancomycin-resistant enterococci and multidrug-resistant *Enterobacteriaceae* from stools submitted for Clostridium difficile testing compared to results from a focused surveillance program. *J Clin Microbiol* 2001;39:1152–1154.

179. Boyce JM, Havill NL, Maria B. Frequency and possible infection control implications of gastrointestinal colonization with methicillin-resistant *Staphylococcus aureus. J Clin Microbiol* 2005;43:5992–5995.

180. Byers KE, Anglim AM, Anneski CJ, et al. A hospital epidemic of vancomycin-resistant Enterococcus: risk factors and control. *Infect Control Hosp Epidemiol* 2001;22:140–147.

181. Harbarth S, Martin Y, Rohner P, et al. Effect of delayed infection control measures on a hospital outbreak of methicillin-resistant *Staphylococcus aureus. J Hosp Infect* 2000;46:43–49.

182. Shannon KP, French GL. Antibiotic resistance: effect of different criteria for classifying isolates as duplicates on apparent resistance frequencies. *J Antimicrob Chemother* 2002;49:201–204.

183. Hindler J, Evangelista, AT, Jenkins, SG, et al. *Analysis and presentation of cumulative antimicrobial susceptibility test data; approved guideline.* Wayne, PA: Clincial Laboratory Standards Institute; 2005.

184. *WHO guidelines on hand hygiene in health care* (advanced draft). World Health Organization, 2006.

185. Larson EL. APIC guideline for handwashing and hand antisepsis in health care settings. *Am J Infect Control* 1995;23:251–269.

186. Boyce J. Scientific basis for handwashing with alcohol and other waterless antispetic agents. In: Rutala W, ed. *Disinfection, sterilization and antisepsis: principles and practices in healthcare facilities.* Washington, DC: Association for Professionals in Infection Control and Epidemiology, Inc., 2001, 140–151.

187. Harbarth S, Pittet D, Grady L, et al. Interventional study to evaluate the impact of an alcohol-based hand gel in improving hand hygiene compliance. *Pediatr Infect Dis J* 2002;21:489–495.

188. Hugonnet S, Perneger TV, Pittet D. Alcohol-based handrub improves compliance with hand hygiene in intensive care units. *Arch Intern Med* 2002;162:1037–1043.

189. Barza M. Efficacy and tolerability of ClO2-generating gloves. *Clin Infect Dis* 2004;38:857–863.

190. Faoagali JL, Thong ML, Grant D. Ten years' experience with methicillin-resistant *Staphylococcus aureus* in a large Australian hospital. *J Hosp Infect* 1992;20:113–119.

191. Boyce JM, Mermel LA, Zervos MJ, et al. Controlling vancomycin-resistant enterococci. *Infect Control Hosp Epidemiol* 1995;16:634–637.

192. Haley RW, Cushion NB, Tenover FC, et al. Eradication of endemic methicillin-resistant *Staphylococcus aureus* infections from a neonatal intensive care unit. *J Infect Dis* 1995;171:614.

193. Jernigan JA, Titus MG, Groschel DH, et al. Effectiveness of contact isolation during a hospital outbreak of methicillin-resistant *Staphylococcus aureus. Am J Epidemiol* 1996;143:496–504.

194. Nijssen S, Bonten MJ, Weinstein RA. Are active microbiological surveillance and subsequent isolation needed to prevent the spread of methicillin-resistant *Staphylococcus aureus? Clin Infect Dis* 2005;40:405–409.

195. Johnson S, Gerding DN, Olson MM, et al. Prospective, controlled study of vinyl glove use to interrupt Clostridium difficile nosocomial transmission. *Am J Med* 1990;88:137–140.

196. Puzniak LA, Leet T, Mayfield J, et al. To gown or not to gown: the effect on acquisition of vancomycin-resistant enterococci. *Clin Infect Dis* 2002;35:18–25.

197. Srinivasan A, Song X, Ross T, et al. A prospective study to determine whether cover gowns in addition to gloves decrease nosocomial transmission of vancomycin-resistant enterococci in an intensive care unit. *Infect Control Hosp Epidemiol* 2002;23:424–428.

198. Slaughter S, Hayden MK, Nathan C, et al. A comparison of the effect of universal use of gloves and gowns with that of glove use alone on acquisition of vancomycin-resistant enterococci in a medical intensive care unit. *Ann Intern Med* 1996;125:448–456.

199. Bhalla A, Pultz NJ, Gries DM, et al. Acquisition of nosocomial pathogens on hands after contact with environmental surfaces near hospitalized patients. *Infect Control Hosp Epidemiol* 2004;25:164–167.

200. Jawad A, Seifert H, Snelling AM, et al. Survival of *Acinetobacter baumannii* on dry surfaces: comparison of outbreak and sporadic isolates. *J Clin Microbiol* 1998;36:1938–1941.

201. Boyce JM, Potter-Bynoe G, Chenevert C, King T. Environmental contamination due to methicillin-resistant *Staphylococcus aureus*: possible infection control implications. *Infect Control Hosp Epidemiol* 1997;18:622–627.

202. Calfee DP, Giannetta ET, Durbin LJ, et al. Control of endemic vancomycin-resistant Enterococcus among inpatients at a university hospital. *Clin Infect Dis* 2003;37:326–332.

203. Harbarth S, Masuet-Aumatell C, Schrenzel J, et al. Evaluation of rapid screening and pre-emptive contact isolation for

detecting and controlling methicillin-resistant *Staphylococcus aureus* in critical care: an interventional cohort study. *Crit Care* 2006;10:R25.

204. Bacterial culture, screen for vancomycin-resistant enterococcus. In Cypress, CA: Focus Diagnostics Reference Laboratory, 2006.

205. Furuno JP, McGregor JC, Harris AD, et al. Identifying groups at high risk for carriage of antibiotic-resistant bacteria. *Arch Intern Med* 2006;166:580–585.

206. Sax H, Harbarth S, Gavazzi G, et al. Prevalence and prediction of previously unknown MRSA carriage on admission to a geriatric hospital. *Age Ageing* 2005;34:456–462.

207. Harbarth S, Sax H, Fankhauser-Rodriguez C, et al. Evaluating the probability of previously unknown carriage of MRSA at hospital admission. *Am J Med* 2006;119:275 e15–e23.

208. Tacconelli E. New strategies to identify patients harbouring antibiotic-resistant bacteria at hospital admission. *Clin Microbiol Infect* 2006;12:102–109.

209. Wilks M, Wilson A, Warwick S, et al. Control of an outbreak of multidrug-resistant *Acinetobacter baumannii*-calcoaceticus colonization and infection in an intensive care unit (ICU) without closing the ICU or placing patients in isolation. *Infection Control and Hospital Epidemiology* 2006;27:654–658.

210. Cepeda JA, Whitehouse T, Cooper B, et al. Isolation of patients in single rooms or cohorts to reduce spread of MRSA in intensive-care units: prospective two-centre study. *Lancet* 2005;365:295–304.

211. Tibballs J. Teaching hospital medical staff to handwash. *Med J Aust* 1996;164:395–398.

212. Rosenthal VD, McCormick RD, Guzman S, et al. Effect of education and performance feedback on handwashing: the benefit of administrative support in Argentinean hospitals. *Am J Infect Control* 2003;31:85–92.

213. Cromer AL, Hutsell SO, Latham SC, et al. Impact of implementing a method of feedback and accountability related to contact precautions compliance. *Am J Infect Control* 2004;32:451–455.

214. Rampling A, Wiseman S, Davis L, et al. Evidence that hospital hygiene is important in the control of methicillin-resistant *Staphylococcus aureus*. *J Hosp Infect* 2001;49:109–116.

215. Hayden MK, Bonten MJ, Blom DW, et al. Reduction in acquisition of vancomycin-resistant enterococcus after enforcement of routine environmental cleaning measures. *Clin Infect Dis* 2006;42:1552–1560.

216. French GL, Otter JA, Shannon KP, et al. Tackling contamination of the hospital environment by methicillin-resistant *Staphylococcus aureus* (MRSA): a comparison between conventional terminal cleaning and hydrogen peroxide vapour decontamination. *J Hosp Infect* 2004;57:31–37.

217. Kratzer C, Tobudic S, Assadian O, et al. Validation of AKACID plus as a room disinfectant in the hospital setting. *Appl Environ Microbiol* 2006;72:3826–3831.

218. Brady MJ, Lisay CM, Yurkovetskiy AV, Sawan SP. Persistent silver disinfectant for the environmental control of pathogenic bacteria. *Am J Infect Control* 2003;31:208–214.

219. Noyce JO, Michels H, Keevil CW. Potential use of copper surfaces to reduce survival of epidemic meticillin-resistant *Staphylococcus aureus* in the healthcare environment. *J Hosp Infect* 2006;63:289–297.

220. Maraha B, van Halteren J, Verzijl JM, et al. Decolonization of methicillin-resistant *Staphylococcus aureus* using oral vancomycin and topical mupirocin. *Clin Microbiol Infect* 2002;8:671–675.

221. Loeb M, Main C, Walker-Dilks C, Eady A. Antimicrobial drugs for treating methicillin-resistant Staphylcoccus aureus colonization (Cochrane Review). In: New York: John Wiley, 2004.

222. Vernon MO, Hayden MK, Trick WE, et al. Chlorhexidine gluconate to cleanse patients in a medical intensive care unit: the effectiveness of source control to reduce the bioburden of vancomycin-resistant enterococci. *Arch Intern Med* 2006;166:306–312.

223. Charbonneau P, Parienti JJ, Thibon P, et al. Fluoroquinolone use and methicillin-resistant *Staphylococcus aureus* isolation rates in hospitalized patients: a quasi experimental study. *Clin Infect Dis* 2006;42:778–784.

224. Rahal JJ, Urban C, Horn D, et al. Class restriction of cephalosporin use to control total cephalosporin resistance in nosocomial Klebsiella. *JAMA* 1998;280:1233–1237.

225. Paterson DL. "Collateral damage" from cephalosporin or quinolone antibiotic therapy. *Clin Infect Dis* 2004;38:S341–S345.

226. Livermore DM. Minimising antibiotic resistance. *Lancet Infect Dis* 2005;5:450–459.

227. Kollef MH, Ward S, Sherman G, et al. Inadequate treatment of nosocomial infections is associated with certain empiric antibiotic choices. *Crit Care Med* 2000;28:3456–3464.

228. Gruson D, Hilbert G, Vargas F, et al. Rotation and restricted use of antibiotics in a medical intensive care unit: impact on the incidence of ventilator-associated pneumonia caused by antibiotic-resistant gram-negative bacteria. *Am J Respir Crit Care Med* 2000;162:837–843.

229. Raymond DP, Pelletier SJ, Crabtree TD, et al. Impact of a rotating empiric antibiotic schedule on infectious mortality in an intensive care unit. *Crit Care Med* 2001;29:1101–1108.

230. Warren DK, Hill HA, Merz LR, et al. Cycling empirical antimicrobial agents to prevent emergence of antimicrobial-resistant Gram-negative bacteria among intensive care unit patients. *Crit Care Med* 2004;32:2450–2456.

231. Martinez JA, Nicolas JM, Marco F, et al. Comparison of antimicrobial cycling and mixing strategies in two medical intensive care units. *Crit Care Med* 2006;34:329–336.

232. van Loon HJ, Vriens MR, Fluit AC, et al. Antibiotic rotation and development of gram-negative antibiotic resistance. *Am J Respir Crit Care Med* 2005;171:480–487.

233. Bartley PB, Schooneveldt JM, Looke DF, Morton A, et al. The relationship of a clonal outbreak of *Enterococcus faecium* vanA to methicillin-resistant *Staphylococcus aureus* incidence in an Australian hospital. *J Hosp Infect* 2001;48:43–54.

234. Diekema DJ, BootsMiller BJ, Vaughn TE, et al. Antimicrobial resistance trends and outbreak frequency in United States hospitals. *Clin Infect Dis* 2004;38:78–85.

235. Deresinski S. Methicillin-resistant *Staphylococcus aureus*: an evolutionary, epidemiologic, and therapeutic odyssey. *Clin Infect Dis* 2005;40:562–573.

236. Daum RS. Community-acquired methicillin-resistant *Staphylococcus aureus* infections. *Pediatr Infect Dis J* 1998;17:745–746.

237. Naimi TS, LeDell KH, Como-Sabetti K, et al. Comparison of community- and healthcare-associated methicillin-resistant *Staphylococcus aureus* infection. *JAMA* 2003;290:2976–2984.

238. Fridkin SK. Vancomycin-intermediate and -resistant *Staphylococcus aureus*: what the infectious disease specialist needs to know. *Clin Infect Dis* 2001;32:108–115.

239. Tenover FC, Lancaster MV, Hill BC, et al. Characterization of staphylococci with reduced susceptibilities to vancomycin and other glycopeptides. *J Clin Microbiol* 1998;36:1020–1027.

240. Institute CLS. Performance standards for antimicrobial susceptibility testing; sixteenth informational supplement. In Wayne, PA: Clinical Laboratory Standards Institute, 2006.

241. Hiramatsu K, Hanaki H, Ino T, et al. Methicillin-resistant *Staphylococcus aureus* clinical strain with reduced vancomycin susceptibility. *J Antimicrob Chemother* 1997;40:135–136.

242. Ploy MC, Grelaud C, Martin C, et al. First clinical isolate of vancomycin-intermediate *Staphylococcus aureus* in a French hospital. *Lancet* 1998;351:1212.

243. Sakoulas G, Eliopoulos GM, Moellering RC Jr., et al. Accessory gene regulator (agr) locus in geographically diverse *Staphylococcus aureus* isolates with reduced susceptibility to vancomycin. *Antimicrob Agents Chemother* 2002;46:1492–1502.

244. Fridkin SK, Hageman J, McDougal LK, et al. Epidemiological and microbiological characterization of infections caused by *Staphylococcus aureus* with reduced susceptibility to vancomycin, United States, 1997–2001. *Clin Infect Dis* 2003;36:429–439.

245. Rotun SS, McMath V, Schoonmaker DJ, et al. *Staphylococcus aureus* with reduced susceptibility to vancomycin isolated from a patient with fatal bacteremia. *Emerg Infect Dis* 1999;5:147–149.

246. de Lassence A, Hidri N, Timsit J-F, et al. Control and outcome of a large outbreak of colonization and infection with glycopeptide-intermediate *Staphylococcus aureus* in an intensive care unit. *Clin Infect Dis* 2006;42:170–178.

247. Chang S, Sievert DM, Hageman JC, et al. Infection with vancomycin-resistant *Staphylococcus aureus* containing the vanA resistance gene. *N Engl J Med* 2003;348:1342–1347.

248. Appelbaum PC. MRSA—the tip of the iceberg. *Clinical Microbiology and Infection* 2006;12:3–10.

249. Whitener CJ, Park SY, Browne FA, et al. Vancomycin-resistant *Staphylococcus aureus* in the absence of vancomycin exposure. *Clin Infect Dis* 2004;38:1049–1055.

250. Noble WC, Virani Z, Cree RGA. Co-transfer of vancomycin and other resistance genes from *Enterococcus faecalis* NCTC 12201 to *Staphylococcus aureus*. *FEMS Microbiology Letters* 1992;93:195.

251. Appelbaum PC. The emergence of vancomycin-intermediate and vancomycin-resistant *Staphylococcus aureus*. *Clin Microbiol Infect* 2006;12:16–23.

252. Squier C, Rihs JD, Risa KJ, et al. *Staphylococcus aureus* rectal carriage and its association with infections in patients in a surgical intensive care unit and a liver transplant unit. *Infect Control Hosp Epidemiol* 2002;23:495–501.

253. Loveday HP, Pellowe CM, Jones SR, Pratt RJ. A systematic review of the evidence for interventions for the prevention and control of meticillin-resistant *Staphylococcus aureus* (1996–2004): report to the Joint MRSA Working Party (Subgroup A). *J Hosp Infect* 2006;63:45–70.

254. Muto CA, Jernigan JA, Ostrowsky BE, et al. SHEA guideline for preventing nosocomial transmission of multidrug-resistant strains of *Staphylococcus aureus* and enterococcus. Infection control and hospital epidemiology. *Infect Control Hosp Epidemiol* 2003;24:362–386.

255. Boyce JM. MRSA patients: proven methods to treat colonization and infection. *J Hosp Infect* 2001;48:S9–S14.

256. Wisplinghoff H, Bischoff T, Tallent SM, et al. Nosocomial bloodstream infections in US hospitals: analysis of 24,179 cases from a prospective nationwide surveillance study. *Clin Infect Dis* 2004;39:309–317.

257. Quale J, Landman D, Atwood E, et al. Experience with a hospital-wide outbreak of vancomycin-resistant enterococci. *Am J Infect Control* 1996;24:372–379.

258. Edmond MB, Ober JF, Dawson JD, et al. Vancomycin resistant enterococcal bacteremia: natural history and attributable mortality. *Clin Infect Dis* 1996;23:1234–1239.

259. Lodise TP, McKinnon PS, Tam VH, Rybak MJ. Clinical outcomes for patients with bacteremia caused by vancomycin-resistant enterococcus in a level 1 trauma center. *Clin Infect Dis* 2002;34:922–929.

260. Fontana R, Cerini R, Longoni P, ed. Identification of a streptococcal penicillin-binding protein that reacts very slowly with penicillin. *J Bacteriol* 1983;155:1343–1350.

261. Zorzi W, Zhou XY, Dardenne O, et al. Structure of the low-affinity penicillin-binding protein 5 PBP5fm in wild-type and highly penicillin-resistant strains of *Enterococcus faecium*. *J Bacteriol* 1996;178:4948–4957.

262. Rice LB, Marshall SH. Evidence of incorporation of the chromosomal beta-lactamase gene of *Enterococcus faecalis* CH19 into a transposon derived from staphylococci. *Antimicrob Agents Chemother* 1992;36:1843–1846.

263. Leclercq R, Derlot E, Duval J, Courvalin P. Plasmid-mediated resistance to vancomycin and teicoplanin in *Enterococcus faecium*. *N Engl J Med* 1988;319:157–161.

264. Gold HS. Vancomycin-resistant enterococci: mechanisms and clinical observations. *Clin Infect Dis* 2001;33:210–219.

265. Evers S, Casadewall B, Charles M, et al. Evolution of structure and substrate specificity in D-alanine: D-alanine ligases and related enzymes. *J Mol Evol* 1996;42:706–712.

266. Hanrahan J, Hoyen C, Rice LB. Geographic distribution of a large mobile element that transfers ampicillin and vancomycin resistance between *Enterococcus faecium* strains. *Antimicrob Agents Chemother* 2000;44:1349–1351.

267. Jones RN. Resistance patterns among nosocomial pathogens: trends over the past few years. *Chest* 2001;119:397S–404S.

268. Livermore DM. Quinupristin/dalfopristin and linezolid: where, when, which and whether to use? *J Antimicrob Chemother* 2000;46:347–350.

269. Pai MP, Rodvold KA, Schreckenberger PC, et al. Risk factors associated with the development of infection with linezolid- and vancomycin-resistant *Enterococcus faecium*. *Clin Infect Dis* 2002;35:1269–1272.

270. Munoz-Price LS, Lolans K, Quinn JP. Emergence of resistance to daptomycin during treatment of vancomycin-resistant *Enterococcus faecalis* infection. *Clin Infect Dis* 2005;41:565–566.

271. Rahim S, Pillai SK, Gold HS, et al. Linezolid-resistant, vancomycin-resistant *Enterococcus faecium* infection in patients without prior exposure to linezolid. *Clin Infect Dis* 2003;36:E146–E148.

272. Hayden MK. Insights into the epidemiology and control of infection with vancomycin-resistant enterococci. *Clin Infect Dis* 2000;31:1058–1065.

273. Noskin GA, Stosor V, Cooper I, Peterson LR. Recovery of vancomycin-resistant enterococci on fingertips and environmental surfaces. *Infect Control Hosp Epidemiol* 1995;16:577–581.

274. Bonten MJ, Slaughter S, Ambergen AW, et al. The role of "colonization pressure" in the spread of vancomycin-resistant enterococci: an important infection control variable. *Arch Intern Med* 1998;158:1127–1132.

275. Elizaga ML, Weinstein RA, Hayden MK. Patients in long-term care facilities: a reservoir for vancomycin-resistant enterococci. *Clin Infect Dis* 2002;34:441–446.

276. Leavis HL, Willems RJ, Top J, et al. Epidemic and nonepidemic multidrug-resistant *Enterococcus faecium*. *Emerg Infect Dis* 2003;9:1108–1115.

277. Recommendations for preventing the spread of vancomycin resistance. *MMWR Recomm Rep* 1995;44(RR-12):1–13.

278. Cookson BD, Macrae MB, Barrett SP, et al. Guidelines for the control of glycopeptide-resistant enterococci in hospitals. *J Hosp Infect* 2006;62:6–21.

279. Mascini EM, Troelstra A, Beitsma M, et al. Genotyping and preemptive isolation to control an outbreak of vancomycin-resistant *Enterococcus faecium*. *Clin Infect Dis* 2006;42:739–746.

280. D'Agata EM, Gautam S, Green WK, Tang YW. High rate of false-negative results of the rectal swab culture method in detection of gastrointestinal colonization with vancomycin–resistant enterococci. *Clin Infect Dis* 2002;34:167–172.

281. Montecalvo MA, Jarvis WR, Uman J, et al. Infection-control measures reduce transmission of vancomycin-resistant enterococci in an endemic setting. *Ann Intern Med* 1999;131:269–272.

282. Donskey CJ, Hoyen CK, Das SM, et al. Effect of oral Bacillus coagulans administration on the density of vancomycin-resistant enterococci in the stool of colonized mice. *Lett Appl Microbiol* 2001;33:84–88.

283. Goossens H, Grabein B. Prevalence and antimicrobial susceptibility data for extended-spectrum beta-lactamase- and AmpC-producing Enterobacteriaceae from the MYSTIC Program in Europe and the United States (1997–2004). *Diagn Microbiol Infect Dis* 2005;53:257–264.

284. Miriagou V, Tzelepi E, Daikos GL, et al. Panresistance in VIM-1-producing *Klebsiella pneumoniae*. *J Antimicrob Chemother* 2005;55:810–811.

285. Lautenbach E, Strom BL, Nachamkin I, et al. Longitudinal trends in fluoroquinolone resistance among Enterobacteriaceae isolates from inpatients and outpatients, 1989–2000: differences in the emergence and epidemiology of resistance across organisms. *Clin Infect Dis* 2004;38:655–662.

286. Everett MJ, Jin YF, Ricci V, Piddock LJ. Contributions of individual mechanisms to fluoroquinolone resistance in 36 *Escherichia coli* strains isolated from humans and animals. *Antimicrob Agents Chemother* 1996;40:2380–2386.

287. Martinez-Martinez L, Pascual A, Jacoby GA. Quinolone resistance from a transferable plasmid. *Lancet* 1998;351:797–799.

288. Winokur PL, Canton R, Casellas JM, et al. Variations in the prevalence of strains expressing an extended-spectrum beta-lactamase phenotype and characterization of isolates from Europe, the Americas, and the Western Pacific region. *Clin Infect Dis* 2001;32:S94–S103.

289. Rodriguez-Bano J, Paterson DL. A change in the epidemiology of infections due to extended-spectrum beta-lactamase-producing organisms. *Clin Infect Dis* 2006;42:935–937.

290. Ben-Ami R, Schwaber MJ, Navon-Venezia S, et al. Influx of extended-spectrum beta-lactamase-producing Enterobacteriaceae into the hospital. *Clin Infect Dis* 2006;42:925–934.

291. Rodriguez-Bano J, Navarro MD, Romero L, et al. Epidemiology and clinical features of infections caused by extended-spectrum beta-lactamase-producing *Escherichia coli* in nonhospitalized patients. *J Clin Microbiol* 2004;42:1089–1094.

292. Bradford PA, Urban C, Mariano N, et al. Imipenem resistance in *Klebsiella pneumoniae* is associated with the combination of

ACT-1, a plasmid-mediated AmpC beta-lactamase, and the foss of an outer membrane protein. *Antimicrob Agents Chemother* 1997;41:563–569.

293. Raimondi A, Traverso A, Nikaido H. Imipenem- and meropenem-resistant mutants of *Enterobacter cloacae* and Proteus rettgeri lack porins. *Antimicrob Agents Chemother* 1991;35:1174–1180.

294. Queenan AM, Torres-Viera C, Gold HS, et al. SME-type carbapenem-hydrolyzing class A beta-lactamases from geographically diverse *Serratia marcescens* strains. *Antimicrob Agents Chemother* 2000;44:3035–3039.

295. Rasmussen BA, Bush K, Keeney D, et al. Characterization of IMI-1 beta-lactamase, a class A carbapenem-hydrolyzing enzyme from *Enterobacter cloacae*. *Antimicrob Agents Chemother* 1996;40:2080–2086.

296. Bradford PA, Bratu S, Urban C, et al. Emergence of carbapenem-resistant Klebsiella species possessing the class A carbapenem-hydrolyzing KPC-2 and inhibitor-resistant TEM-30 beta-lactamases in New York City. *Clin Infect Dis* 2004;39:55–60.

297. Paterson DL, Bonomo RA. Extended-spectrum beta-lactamases: a clinical update. *Clin Microbiol Rev* 2005;18:657–686.

298. Bratu S, Mooty M, Nichani S, et al. Emergence of KPC-possessing *Klebsiella pneumoniae* in Brooklyn, New York: epidemiology and recommendations for detection. *Antimicrob Agents Chemother* 2005;49:3018–3020.

299. Schaberg DR, Alford RH, Anderson R, et al. An outbreak of nosocomial infection due to multiply resistant *Serratia marcescens*: Evidence of interhospital spread. *J Infect Dis* 1976;134:181.

300. Gaynes RP, Weinstein RA, Smith J, et al. Control of aminoglycoside resistance by barrier precautions. *Infect Control* 1983;4:221.

301. Baquero F, Coque TM, Canton R. Allodemics. *Lancet Infect Dis* 2002;2(10):591–592.

302. Nijssen S, Florijn A, Top J, et al. Unnoticed spread of integron-carrying *Enterobacteriaceae* in intensive care units. *Clin Infect Dis* 2005;41:1–9.

303. Norrby SR. Integrons: adding another threat to the use of antibiotic therapy. *Clin Infect Dis* 2005;41:10–11.

304. Poole K. Multidrug efflux pumps and antimicrobial resistance in *Pseudomonas aeruginosa* and related organisms. *J Mol Microbiol Biotechnol* 2001;3:255–264.

305. Masuda N, Sakagawa E, Ohya S, et al. Contribution of the MexX-MexY-oprM efflux system to intrinsic resistance in *Pseudomonas aeruginosa*. *Antimicrob Agents Chemother* 2000;44:2242–2246.

306. Jalal S, Ciofu O, Hoiby N, et al. Molecular mechanisms of fluoroquinolone resistance in *Pseudomonas aeruginosa* isolates from cystic fibrosis patients. *Antimicrob Agents Chemother* 2000;44:710–712.

307. Juan C, Moya B, Perez JL, Oliver A. Stepwise upregulation of the *Pseudomonas aeruginosa* chromosomal cephalosporinase conferring high-level {beta}-lactam resistance involves three AmpD homologues. *Antimicrob Agents Chemother* 2006;50:1780–1787.

308. Poole K. Aminoglycoside resistance in *Pseudomonas aeruginosa*. *Antimicrob Agents Chemother* 2005;49:479–487.

309. Quale J, Bratu S, Gupta J, Landman D. Interplay of efflux system, ampC, and oprD expression in carbapenem resistance of *Pseudomonas aeruginosa* clinical isolates. *Antimicrob Agents Chemother* 2006;50:1633–1641.

310. Cirz RT, Romesberg FE. Induction and inhibition of ciprofloxacin resistance-conferring mutations in hypermutator bacteria. *Antimicrob Agents Chemother* 2006;50:220–225.

311. Gutierrez O, Juan C, Perez JL, Oliver A. Lack of association between hypermutation and antibiotic resistance development in *Pseudomonas aeruginosa* isolates from intensive care unit patients. *Antimicrob Agents Chemother* 2004;48:3573–3575.

312. Lolans K, Queenan AM, Bush K, et al. First nosocomial outbreak of *Pseudomonas aeruginosa* producing an integron-borne metallo-beta-lactamase (VIM-2) in the United States. *Antimicrob Agents Chemother* 2005;49:3538–3540.

313. Gibb AP, Tribuddharat C, Moore RA, et al. Nosocomial outbreak of carbapenem-resistant *Pseudomonas aeruginosa* with a new bla(IMP) allele, bla(IMP-7). *Antimicrob Agents Chemother* 2002;46:255–258.

314. Senda K, Arakawa Y, Nakashima K, et al. Multifocal outbreaks of metallo-beta-lactamase-producing *Pseudomonas aeruginosa* resistant to broad-spectrum beta-lactams, including carbapenems. *Antimicrob Agents Chemother* 1996;40:349–353.

315. Karlowsky JA, Jones ME, Thornsberry C, et al. Stable antimicrobial susceptibility rates for clinical isolates of *Pseudomonas aeruginosa* from the 2001–2003 tracking resistance in the United States today surveillance studies. *Clin Infect Dis* 2005;40:S89–S98.

316. Tognim MC, Andrade SS, Silbert S, et al. Resistance trends of Acinetobacter spp. in Latin America and characterization of international dissemination of multi-drug resistant strains: five-year report of the SENTRY Antimicrobial Surveillance Program. *Int J Infect Dis* 2004;8:284–291.

317. Bonten MJ, Weinstein RA. Transmission pathways of *Pseudomonas aeruginosa* in intensive care units: don't go near the water. *Crit Care Med* 2002;30:2384–2385.

318. Reuter S, Sigge A, Wiedeck H, Trautmann M. Analysis of transmission pathways of *Pseudomonas aeruginosa* between patients and tap water outlets. *Crit Care Med* 2002;30:2222–2228.

319. Bert F, Maubec E, Bruneau B, et al. Multi-resistant *Pseudomonas aeruginosa* outbreak associated with contaminated tap water in a neurosurgery intensive care unit. *J Hosp Infect* 1998;39:53–62.

320. Cobben NA, Drent M, Jonkers M, et al. Outbreak of severe *Pseudomonas aeruginosa* respiratory infections due to contaminated nebulizers. *J Hosp Infect* 1996;33:63–70.

321. Favero MS, Carson LA, Bond WW, Petersen NJ. *Pseudomonas aeruginosa*: growth in distilled water from hospitals. *Science* 1971;173:836–838.

322. Lonnemann G. When good water goes bad: how it happens, clinical consequences and possible solutions. *Blood Purif* 2004;22:124–129.

323. Bonten MJ, Bergmans DC, Speijer H, Stobberingh EE. Characteristics of polyclonal endemicity of *Pseudomonas aeruginosa* colonization in intensive care units. Implications for infection control. *Am J Respir Crit Care Med* 1999;160:1212–1219.

324. Bertrand X, Thouverez M, Talon D, et al. Endemicity, molecular diversity and colonisation routes of *Pseudomonas aeruginosa* in intensive care units. *Intensive Care Med* 2001;27:1263–1268.

325. Valles J, Mariscal D, Cortes P, et al. Patterns of colonization by *Pseudomonas aeruginosa* in intubated patients: a 3-year prospective study of 1,607 isolates using pulsed-field gel electrophoresis with implications for prevention of ventilator-associated pneumonia. *Intensive Care Med* 2004;30:1768–1775.

326. Gales AC, Jones RN, Forward KR, et al. Emerging importance of multidrug-resistant Acinetobacter species and *Stenotrophomonas maltophilia* as pathogens in seriously ill patients: geographic patterns, epidemiological features, and trends in the SENTRY Antimicrobial Surveillance Program (1997–1999). *Clin Infect Dis* 2001;32:S104–S113.

327. Wisplinghoff H, Edmond MB, Pfaller MA, et al. Nosocomial bloodstream infections caused by Acinetobacter species in United States hospitals: clinical features, molecular epidemiology, and antimicrobial susceptibility. *Clin Infect Dis* 2000;31:690–697.

328. Quale J, Bratu S, Landman D, Heddurshetti R. Molecular epidemiology and mechanisms of carbapenem resistance in *Acinetobacter baumannii* endemic in New York City. *Clin Infect Dis* 2003;37:214–220.

329. Mahgoub S, Ahmed J, Glatt AE. Completely resistant *Acinetobacter baumannii* strains. *Infect Control Hosp Epidemiol* 2002;23:477–479.

330. Urban C, Segal-Maurer S, Rahal JJ. Considerations in control and treatment of nosocomial infections due to multidrug-resistant *Acinetobacter baumannii*. *Clin Infect Dis* 2003;36:1268–1274.

331. Jain R, Danziger LH. Multidrug-resistant Acinetobacter infections: an emerging challenge to clinicians. *Ann Pharmacother* 2004;38:1449–1459.

332. Falagas ME, Kasiakou SK. Colistin: the revival of polymyxins for the management of multidrug-resistant gram-negative bacterial infections. *Clin Infect Dis* 2005;40:1333–1341.

333. Livermore DM. Tigecycline: what is it, and where should it be used? *J Antimicrob Chemother* 2005;56:611–614.

334. Wagenvoort JH, Joosten EJ. An outbreak *Acinetobacter baumannii* that mimics MRSA in its environmental longevity. *J Hosp Infect* 2002;52:226–227.

335. Seifert H, Dijkshoorn L, Gerner-Smidt P, et al. Distribution of Acinetobacter species on human skin: comparison of phenotypic and genotypic identification methods. *J Clin Microbiol* 1997;35:2819–2825.

336. Manikal VM, Landman D, Saurina G, et al. Endemic carbapenem-resistant Acinetobacter species in Brooklyn, New York: citywide prevalence, interinstitutional spread, and relation to antibiotic usage. Clin Infect Dis 2000;31:101–106.

337. Aygun G, Demirkiran O, Utku T, et al. Environmental contamination during a carbapenem-resistant Acinetobacter baumannii outbreak in an intensive care unit. J Hosp Infect 2002;52:259–262.

338. Pimentel JD, Low J, Styles K, et al. Control of an outbreak of multi-drug-resistant Acinetobacter baumannii in an intensive care unit and a surgical ward. J Hosp Infect 2005;59:249–253.

339. Diekema DJ, Pfaller MA, Schmitz FJ, et al. Survey of infections due to Staphylococcus species: frequency of occurrence and antimicrobial susceptibility of isolates collected in the United States, Canada, Latin America, Europe, and the Western Pacific region for the SENTRY Antimicrobial Surveillance Program, 1997–1999. Clin Infect Dis 2001;32:S114–S132.

340. Huebner J, Goldmann DA. Coagulase-negative staphylococci: role as pathogens. Annu Rev Med 1999;50:223–236.

341. Biavasco F, Vignaroli C, Varaldo PE. Glycopeptide resistance in coagulase-negative staphylococci. Eur J Clin Microbiol Infect Dis 2000;19:403–417.

342. Schwalbe RS, Stapleton JT, Gilligan PH. Emergence of vancomycin resistance in coagulase-negative staphylococci. N Engl J Med 1987;316:927–931.

343. Sieradzki K, Villari P, Tomasz A. Decreased susceptibilities to teicoplanin and vancomycin among coagulase-negative methicillin-resistant clinical isolates of staphylococci. Antimicrob Agents Chemother 1998;42:100–107.

344. Kernodle DS, Barg NL, Kaiser AB. Low level colonization of hospitalized patients with methicillin-resistant coagulase-negative staphylococci and emergence of the organisms during surgical antimicrobial prophylaxis. Antimicrob Agents Chemother 1988;32:202–208.

345. Weinstein RA, Kabins SA, Nathan C, et al. Gentamicin-resistant staphylococci as hospital flora: epidemiology and resistance plasmids. J Infect Dis 1982;145:374–382.

346. Boyce JM, Potter-Bynoe G, Opal SM, et al. A common-source outbreak of Staphylococcu epidermidis infections among patients undergoing cardiac surgery. J Infect Dis 1990;161:493.

347. Johnson AP, Warner M, Malnick H, Livermore DM. Activity of the oxazolidinones AZD2563 and linezolid against Corynebacterium jeikeium and other Corynebacterium spp. J Antimicrob Chemother 2003;51:745–747.

348. Rozdzinski E, Kern W, Schmeiser T, Kurrle E. Corynebacterium jeikeium bacteremia at a tertiary care center. Infection 1991;19:201–204.

349. Gill VJ, Manning C, Lamson M. et al. Antibiotic-resistant group JK bacteria in hospitals. J Clin Microbiol 1981;13:472.

350. Stamm WE, L.S. T, K.F. W, al. e. Infection due to Corynebacterium species in marrow transplant patients. Ann Intern Med 1979;91:167.

351. Pitcher D, Johnson A, Allerberger F, et al. An investigation of nosocomial infection with Corynebacterium jeikeium in surgical patients using a ribosomal RNA gene probe. Eur J Clin Microbiol Infect Dis 1990;9:643–648.

352. Verweij PE, Meis JF, Christmann V, et al. Nosocomial outbreak of colonization and infection with Stenotrophomonas maltophilia in preterm infants associated with contaminated tap water. Epidemiol Infect 1998;120:251–256.

353. Wishart MM, Riley TV. Infection with Pseudomonas maltophilia hospital outbreak due to contaminated disinfectant. Med J Aust 1976;2:710–712.

354. Rogues AM, Maugein J, Allery A, et al. Electronic ventilator temperature sensors as a potential source of respiratory tract colonization with Stenotrophomonas maltophilia. J Hosp Infect 2001;49:289–292.

355. Zhang L, Li XZ, Poole K. Multiple antibiotic resistance in Stenotrophomonas maltophilia: involvement of a multidrug efflux system. Antimicrob Agents Chemother 2000;44:287–293.

356. Crowder MW, Walsh TR, Banovic L, et al. Overexpression, purification, and characterization of the cloned metallo-beta-lactamase L1 from Stenotrophomonas maltophilia. Antimicrob Agents Chemother 1998;42:921–926.

357. Carmeli Y, Samore MH. Comparison of treatment with imipenem vs. ceftazidime as a predisposing factor for nosocomial acquisition of Stenotrophomonas maltophilia: a historical cohort study. Clin Infect Dis 1997;24:1131–1134.

358. Jarvis WR, Olson D, Tablan O, Martone WJ. The epidemiology of nosocomial Pseudomonas cepacia infections: endemic infections. Eur J Epidemiol 1987;3:233–236.

359. Mangram A, Jarvis WR. Nosocomial Burkholderia cepacia outbreaks and pseudo-outbreaks. Infect Control Hosp Epidemiol 1996;17:718–720.

360. Tablan OC, Martone WJ, Doershuk CF, et al. Colonization of the respiratory tract with Pseudomonas cepacia in cystic fibrosis: risk factors and outcomes. Chest 1987;91:527–532.

361. LiPuma JJ, Dasen SE, Nielson DW, et al. Person-to-person transmission of Pseudomonas cepacia between patients with cystic fibrosis. Lancet 1990;336:1094–1096.

362. Burdge DR, Nakielna EM, Noble MA. Case-control and vector studies of nosocomial acquisition of Pseudomonas cepacia in adult patients with cystic fibrosis. Infect Control Hosp Epidemiol 1993;14:127–130.

363. Bonacorsi S, Fitoussi F, Lhopital S, Bingen E. Comparative in vitro activities of meropenem, imipenem, temocillin, piperacillin, and ceftazidime in combination with tobramycin, rifampin, or ciprofloxacin against Burkholderia cepacia isolates from patients with cystic fibrosis. Antimicrob Agents Chemother 1999;43:213–217.

364. Parr TR Jr., Moore RA, Moore LV, Hancock RE. Role of porins in intrinsic antibiotic resistance of Pseudomonas cepacia. Antimicrob Agents Chemother 1987;31:121–123.

365. Burns JL, Wadsworth CD, Barry JJ, Goodall CP. Nucleotide sequence analysis of a gene from Burkholderia (Pseudomonas) cepacia encoding an outer membrane lipoprotein involved in multiple antibiotic resistance. Antimicrob Agents Chemother 1996;40:307–313.

366. Prince A, Wood MS, Cacalano GS, Chin NX. Isolation and characterization of a penicillinase from Pseudomonas cepacia 249. Antimicrob Agents Chemother 1988;32:838–843.

367. Siddiqui AH, Mulligan ME, Mahenthiralingam E, et al. An episodic outbreak of genetically related Burkholderia cepacia among non-cystic fibrosis patients at a university hospital. Infect Control Hosp Epidemiol 2001;22:419–422.

368. LiPuma JJ. Burkholderia cepacia: management issues and new insights. Clin Chest Med 1998;19:473–486, vi.

369. Berkelman RL, Lewin S, Allen JR, et al. Pseudobacteremia attributed to contamination of povidone-iodine with Pseudomonas cepacia. Ann Intern Med 1981;95:32–36.

370. Evans RS, Pestotnik SL, Classen DC, et al. A computer-assisted management program for antibiotics and other antiinfective agents. N Engl J Med 1998;338:232–238.

371. Bonten MJ, Austin DJ, Lipsitch M. Understanding the spread of antibiotic resistant pathogens in hospitals: mathematical models as tools for control. Clin Infect Dis 2001;33:1739–1746.

372. Murray P, Baron E, Pfaller M. Manual of clinical microbiology. In: 6th ed. Washington, DC: American Society of Microbiology Press, 1995:172.

373. Weber SG, Gold HS, Hooper DC, et al. Fluoroquinolones and the risk for methicillin-resistant Staphylococcus aureus in hospitalized patients. Emerg Infect Dis 2003;9:1415–1422.

374. Aloush V, Navon-Venezia S, Seigman-Igra Y, et al. Multidrug-resistant Pseudomonas aeruginosa: risk factors and clinical impact. Antimicrob Agents Chemother 2006;50:43–48.

375. Abbo A, Navon-Venezia S, Hammer-Muntz O, et al. Multidrug-resistant Acinetobacter baumannii. Emerg Infect Dis 2005;11:22–29.

376. Pena C, Gudiol C, Tubau F, et al. Risk-factors for acquisition of extended-spectrum beta-lactamase-producing Escherichia coli among hospitalised patients. Clin Microbiol Infect 2006;12:279–284.

377. Lautenbach E, Patel JB, Bilker WB, et al. Extended-spectrum beta-lactamase-producing Escherichia coli and Klebsiella pneumoniae: risk factors for infection and impact of resistance on outcomes. Clin Infect Dis 2001;32:1162–1171.

378. Garcia-Garmendia JL, Ortiz-Leyba C, Garnacho-Montero J, et al. Risk factors for Acinetobacter baumannii nosocomial bacteremia in critically ill patients: a cohort study. Clin Infect Dis 2001;33:939–946.

379. Kaye KS, Cosgrove S, Harris A, et al. Risk factors for emergence of resistance to broad-spectrum cephalosporins among Enterobacter spp. *Antimicrob Agents Chemother* 2001;45:2628–2630.

380. D'Agata EM, Venkataraman L, DeGirolami P, et al. Colonization with broad-spectrum cephalosporin-resistant gram-negative bacilli in intensive care units during a nonoutbreak period: prevalence, risk factors, and rate of infection. *Crit Care Med* 1999;27:1090–1095.

381. Nouer SA, Nucci M, de-Oliveira MP, et al. Risk factors for acquisition of multidrug-resistant *Pseudomonas aeruginosa* producing SPM metallo-beta-lactamase. *Antimicrob Agents Chemother* 2005;49:3663–3667.

382. Graffunder EM, Preston KE, Evans AM, Venezia RA. Risk factors associated with extended-spectrum beta-lactamase-producing organisms at a tertiary care hospital. *J Antimicrob Chemother* 2005;56:139–145.

383. Furuno JP, Perencevich EN, Johnson JA, et al. Methicillin-resistant *Staphylococcus aureus* and vancomycin-resistant Enterococci co-colonization. *Emerg Infect Dis* 2005;11:1539–1544.

384. Toubes E, Singh K, Yin D, et al. Risk factors for antibiotic-resistant infection and treatment outcomes among hospitalized patients transferred from long-term care facilities: does antimicrobial choice make a difference? *Clin Infect Dis* 2003;36:724–730.

385. Edmond MB, Ober JF, Weinbaum DL. Vancomycin-resistant *Enterococcus faecium* bacteremia: risk factors for infection. *Clin. Inf. Dis.* 1995;20:1126.

386. von Baum H, Ober JF, Wendt C, et al. Antibiotic-resistant bloodstream infections in hospitalized patients: specific risk factors in a high-risk population? *Infection* 2005;33:320–326.

Molecular Biology of Resistance

15

Fred C. Tenover and John E. McGowan, Jr.

A BRIEF HISTORY OF RESISTANCE MECHANISMS AND THE DISCOVERY OF GENE TRANSFER

The development of antimicrobial agents active against a wide array of microbial pathogens in the 1940s and 1950s enabled physicians to begin to turn the tide against a variety of infectious scourges. However, since the early 1970s, the development and spread of bacterial strains that are resistant to these drugs has emerged as a global problem [1–5]. The development of resistance to antimicrobial agents was not anticipated as a serious problem in the beginning of the antimicrobial era because it was assumed that the only mechanism of resistance was likely to be random mutations leading to altered target sites that would prevent the binding of the drug [6]. However, beginning with the discovery in 1940 of penicillinase (an enzyme that hydrolyzes penicillin, destroying its antibacterial properties), first in *Escherichia coli* [7] and then in *Staphylococcus aureus* [8], it became clear that other mechanisms of resistance were likely to be found. Subsequently, active efflux of drugs [9,10], modification of drug target sites [11], and other mechanisms to inactivate drugs chemically [12] have all been found to mediate resistance to various antimicrobial agents.

In the 1950s, the remarkable finding that multiply-resistant strains of *Shigella* were able to transfer the resistance phenotype to other bacterial strains during cell-to-cell mating experiments [13] dramatically changed our understanding of the molecular basis of antimicrobial resistance. Resistance was linked to the presence of extrachromosomal DNA called *plasmids*. Subsequently,

plasmids have been found in most clinically important bacterial pathogens [14,15].

In the 1960s, bacterial viruses were noted to move antimicrobial resistance genes between strains of staphylococci in a process called transduction [16]. In some instances, it appeared that entire plasmids could be moved from one strain of *S. aureus* to another, enhancing the ability of resistance genes to disseminate. In the 1970s, the recognition of transposable elements, often containing antimicrobial resistance genes, that could move from plasmids to bacteriophage [17] or from plasmids to chromosomal locations independent of the usual DNA recombination mechanisms [18] added another dimension to the ability of resistance genes to move among bacteria. This novel mechanism of mobilizing genes among bacterial cells indicated that the likelihood of widespread gene dissemination was high, particularly in environments where antibiotics were present in high concentrations to offer an advantage to those organisms that possessed a resistance mechanism.

The 1980s saw the discovery of another unique genetic element, the integron [19]. Integrons are mobile DNA elements that encode enzymes capable of inserting resistance gene cassettes into a stable DNA backbone that can be located either on a plasmid or the chromosome of an organism. The pool of gene cassettes in nature contains a variety of resistance determinants, ranging from aminoglycoside resistance genes to β-lactamase genes [19]. Integrons allow the accumulation and transmission of constellations of resistance determinants within and among diverse species of bacteria. As many as five different resistance genes may be accumulated together in a single integron. Integrons have played a major role in the development and spread of multidrug resistance among isolates of *Enterobacteriaceae* in Europe [21] and the United States [22].

In the 1990s, another unique element, the chromosomal cassette, was described [23]. Similar to integrons, these large elements, common in staphylococci, are the repository of the *mecA* element that mediates oxacillin resistance [24]. Five variants of the *mecA* cassette, called the staphylococcal cassette chromosome *mec* (SCC*mec*), have been described [25,26]. The most recently described cassettes, types IV and V, are widely disseminated among community-associated strains of methicillin-resistant *Staphylococcus aureus* (MRSA) [25,27].

Our understanding of the various mechanisms of antimicrobial resistance has grown tremendously as has our knowledge of the ways by which genes move among bacteria in a variety of healthcare environments. Both the mechanisms of antimicrobial resistance and the modes of resistance gene dissemination in bacteria are reviewed next.

MECHANISMS OF RESISTANCE

Intrinsic Resistance

Some bacteria are intrinsically resistant to antimicrobial agents because they either lack the target site for that drug or the drug is unable to transit through the organism's cell wall or membrane to reach its site of action [28]. For example, most enterococci are resistant to low levels of aminoglycosides because the drug cannot penetrate the organism's peptidoglycan layer to reach the ribosomes. Only in the presence of cell wall–active agents, such as penicillin or vancomycin, can aminoglycosides reach their site of action [29]. Intrinsic resistance also includes chromosomally encoded enzymes, such as β-lactamases, that are characteristic of some bacterial species. The AmpC enzyme of *Enterobacter cloacae*, which when induced can mediate resistance to extended-spectrum cephalosporins and cephamycins (such as cefoxitin and cefotetan) is an example of such an enzyme [30].

Acquired Resistance

Bacteria that are by nature susceptible to an antimicrobial agent may become resistant by chromosomal mutation or by the acquisition of new genetic material [28]. For example, point mutations that occur in the chromosomal *rpsL* gene that encodes a ribosomal protein found in *E. coli* [31] and *Mycobacterium tuberculosis* [32] may result in an amino acid change that prevents the binding of streptomycin to the ribosome, resulting in resistance.

The acquisition of new resistance genes carried on plasmids, transposable elements, integrons, and other cassettes, usually results in the synthesis of new proteins in the cell. The known modes of plasmid- and transposon-encoded resistance mechanisms include enzymatically inactivating the antimicrobial agent, altering the target

sites for the antimicrobial agent, blocking the transport of the agent into the bacterial cell, enhancing the efflux of the antimicrobial agent out of the cell, and bypassing the metabolic steps inhibited by the antimicrobial agent [28] (Table 15-1). Multiple resistance mechanisms may be encoded on a single plasmid, transposon, integron, or cassette. In addition, organisms may harbor >1 mechanism of resistance for a single class of drugs. Examples of resistance mechanisms for several classes of antimicrobial agents are described in the following sections.

Resistance to β-Lactam Drugs

β-lactam drugs include penicillins, cephalosporins, monobactams, carbapenems, and a variety of other related compounds [30]. Plasmid-mediated resistance to β-lactam agents most often is a result of β-lactamases, that is, enzymes that hydrolyze the β-lactam ring, deactivating the drug. The number of different β-lactamases described from gram-negative and gram-positive organisms exceeds 400 [33] and can be divided into several different classes based on chemical structure, substrate profile, isoelectric point, and amino acid sequence [34]. Point mutations in the structural genes of β-lactamases, such as in bla_{TEM}, bla_{SHV}, and bla_{CTX-M} may result in amino acid alterations that extend the spectrum of drugs that can be inactivated [35]. Such enzymes are deemed extended-spectrum β-lactamases, or ESBLs. In addition, spontaneous mutations that result in changes in the porins of the organism's outer membrane can enhance resistance to ceftazidime [36], or loss of porins can result in resistance to carbapenems [37]. In the early 2000s, carbapenem resistance mediated by a Class A β-lactamase, designated KPC-1, emerged in the United States [38]. *Klebsiella pneumoniae* isolates harboring KPC-1 and the related β-lactamases KPC-2 and KPC-3 emerged and spread in several geographic areas, particularly in New York City [39, 40]. Similar β-lactamases have been recognized elsewhere in the United States and abroad [41]. Carbapenem resistance also can be mediated by the Class B, metallo-beta-lactamases, which includes the enzymes SPM-1, VIM-1, IMP-1, and other related enzymes that are widely disseminated among *Pseudomonas aeruginosa*, *Acinetobacter* species, and other gram-negative organisms [42].

Resistance to β-lactam drugs among bacterial isolates also can be mediated by changes in the organism's penicillin binding proteins (PBPs) (i.e., those proteins involved in cell wall synthesis). Mutations in the genes that encode the PBPs, or the creation of mosaic PBP genes through the acquisition of DNA fragments from related organisms, result in PBPs with reduced affinity for β-lactam agents. These mechanisms of PBP remodeling, together with changes in several other non-PBP loci, are responsible for the dramatic increase in penicillin resistance seen in *Streptococcus pneumoniae* in the early 1990s [43]. Additional mutations in PBP genes result in higher levels of cefotaxime and ceftriaxone resistance [44]. The formation of mosaic

TABLE 15-1

EXAMPLES OF BACTERIAL MECHANISMS OF ANTIMICROBIAL RESISTANCE

Antimicrobial Class	Example	Mechanism	Organisms
Aminoglycosides	Gentamicin	Drug modification	Enterobacteriaceae
			Pseudomonas spp.
			Enterococci
			Staphylococci
	Amikacin	Reduced permeability	Pseudomonas spp.
β-lactam drugs	Penicillin	β-lactamase	Staphylococci
			Enterococci
			Enterobacteriaceae
			Pseudomonas spp.
			Gonococci
		Altered cell wall	Pneumococci
			Meningococci
Fluoroquinolones	Ciprofloxacin	Altered DNA gyrase	Staphylococci
			Pseudomonas spp.
			Enterobacteriaceae
Glycopeptides	Vancomycin	Altered DNA ligase	Enterococci
Macrolides	Erythromycin	RNA methylase	Staphylococci
			Pneumococci
			Streptococci
Tetracyclines	Doxycycline	Drug efflux	Streptococci
			Enterobacteriaceae
			Staphylococci
			Pseudomonas spp.
Trimethoprim	Trimethoprim	Altered enzymes	Enterobacteriaceae
			Pseudomonas spp.

Adapted from Neu HC. Overview of mechanisms of bacterial resistance. *Diagn Microbiol Infect Dis* 1989;12:109S–116S.

PBP genes through acquisition of DNA via transformation has been reported in both *S. pneumoniae* and *Neisseria meningitidis* [45].

Resistance to Erythromycin and Other Macrolides

Erythromycin resistance in bacteria may be mediated by several different mechanisms. These include efflux mechanisms, such as the *msr*(A) pump of staphylococci and the *mef* genes of *S. pneumoniae* and streptococci, and modification of the drug binding sites in rRNA [46]. Methylation of the 23S RNA of the 50S ribosome unit typically occurs at a specific adenine residue in multiple gram-positive organisms, leading to resistance not only to macrolides but also to lincosamides (e.g., clindamycin), and streptogramin B-type drugs. The *erm* genes (for erythromycin rRNA methylase) constitute a family of resistance determinants that have been isolated from many gram-positive species, including staphylococci, streptococci, actinomycetes, and a variety of anaerobes; gram-negative organisms, including *Haemophilus* spp., members of the *Enterobacteriaceae*, and several genera of gram-negative anaerobes; and *Mycobacterium* spp. [46]. Erythromycin resistance also can be the result of esterification or phosphorylation of the drug.

Aminoglycoside Resistance

Aminoglycoside resistance is common in both gram-positive and gram negative organisms and usually is the result of phosphorylation, acetylation, or adenylylation of the antimicrobial agent by plasmid- or transposon-encoded enzymes [12]. The nucleotide sequence diversity among the genes that encode the three subclasses of enzymes is higher than would be expected for genes that diverged in recent times, suggesting that although most of the genes share a common ancestral sequence, divergence occurred long ago, well before the clinical use of antimicrobial agents, making these genes a particularly old group. The enzymes are located at the inner membrane of bacterial cells, and the modified aminoglycoside blocks the transport of the antibiotic into the cell, keeping it from its site of action on the ribosome. Recently, a novel mutation of the *aac6'Ib* enzyme, designated *aac6'Ib-cr* was reported [47]. This subtle change in amino acid sequence enable the enzyme to acetylate ciprofloxacin and several other fluoroquinolones leading to low-level resistance to these agents. The ability of one enzyme to modify two highly divergent classes of antimicrobial agents leading to resistance is very unusual.

Reduced permeability of the cell envelope, which can occur by spontaneous mutation of the genes that encode the cells' porins, changes in the ribosomal target site, or active efflux of drugs out of the cell also contributes to resistance, particularly in gram-negative organisms [9–11].

Tetracycline Resistance

Tetracycline resistance is widespread among gram-positive and gram-negative bacterial species and can be the result of drug efflux, ribosomal protection, or permeability changes [48,49]. Several tetracycline resistance determinants, such as the *tet*(M) gene, which mediates resistance to tetracycline, doxycycline, and minocycline, are widely distributed in species as diverse as *Enterococcus faecalis*, *Neisseria gonorrhoeae*, *Mycoplasma pneumoniae*, and *B. fragilis* [49]. This resistance gene and a number of other tetracycline resistance genes are commonly found on transposable elements, often linked together with determinants for resistance to chloramphenicol or macrolides in gram-positive organisms.

Glycopeptide Resistance

Vancomycin is the glycopeptide most commonly used to treat gram-positive healthcare-associated bacterial infections, such as MRSA, ampicillin-resistant enterococcal infections, and *Clostridium difficile* infections. Resistance in enterococci is mediated by a series of plasmid- and transposon-encoded genes that produce altered DNA ligases that result in a cell wall structure that does not bind the drug [50]. The novel ligases, designated as *vanA*, *vanB*, *vanD*, and *vanG*, are acquired genes, while *vanC* and *vanE* are intrinsic to several species of enterococci. The latter loci typically mediate only low-level resistance among *Enterococcus gallinarum* and *Enterococcus casseliflavus* isolates and are chromosomally mediated traits.

In 2002, the transfer in nature of the *vanA* operon from a vancomycin-resistant *E. faecalis* donor to an MRSA recipient was reported from the State of Michigan [51]. The vancomycin mimimum inhibitory concentration (MIC) for the resulting vancomycin-resistant *S. aureus* (VRSA) isolate was 1024 µg/ml, which is 1000 times the normal vancomycin MIC for *S. aureus* (i.e., 1 µg/ml). Molecular studies by Weigel et al. indicated that the *vanA* operon entered the recipient MRSA strain on an enterococcal plasmid (likely by conjugation), and the plasmid was maintained in the MRSA cell just long enough for the *vanA*-containing transposon Tn*1546* to transfer to a smaller staphylococcal plasmid already present in the MRSA strain [52]. The transfer of the *vanA* operon on Tn*1546* to the MRSA plasmid resulted in the new VRSA isolate. Subsequently, six other VRSA isolates have been documented in the United States, and each contained the *vanA* resistance gene [53, 54, CDC unpublished data]. However, the latter VRSA isolates contained a variety of plasmids, and not all of the isolates demonstrated high vancomycin MICs. The lower vancomycin MIC of the Pennsylvania VRSA (32 µ/ml) strain was attributed to plasmid instability [55].

Low-level resistance to vancomycin also has been reported in *S. aureus* mediated by thickened cell walls that contain thousands of copies of the D-ala-D-ala dipeptide, which is the binding site for vancomycin, and changes in cellular metabolic pathways [56,57]. These organisms, designated as vancomycin-intermediate *S. aureus* (VISA) strains because the vancomycin MICs were in the intermediate range according to Clinical and Laboratory Standards documents [58], were first reported in 1997 [59] and have been reported subsequently from the United States and around the world [60–62]. In some isolates, the changes in cell wall structure and metabolic pathways led to decreased susceptibility to vancomycin, but the changes could not be detected by routine susceptibility testing methods [63]. Population analysis revealed subpopulations that are resistant to vancomycin, and these subpopulations likely lead to clinical failure. Such strains are referred to as "vancomycin-heteroresistant" VISA or hVISA for short [63].

Fluoroquinolone Resistance

Resistance to the fluoroquinolones frequently is mediated by point mutations in either the *gyrA* and *gyrB* genes and/or the analogous *parC* and *parE* loci, which decrease binding of the fluoroquinolones to the target enzymes, DNA gyrase, and topoisomerase IV [64]. Fluoroquinolone resistance is increasing in many species worldwide [65,66]. Plasmid-mediated resistance to the fluoroquinolones, which tends to be low-level, was first reported in 1998 [67]. The gene, designated *qnrA*, is one of a family of small proteins that mediates fluoroquinolone resistance in gram-negative bacteria. Other *qnr* genes, including *qnrB*, have been detected in bacteria in association with *aac6'Ib-cr* aminoglycoside/ciprofloxacin resistance determinant [47,68].

Trimethoprim and Sulfonamide Resistance

Bacteria can recruit and use novel enzymes to bypass inhibited metabolic pathways to avoid killing by several antimicrobial agents. This is the mechanism of resistance used by bacteria to circumvent the action of trimethoprim [69] and sulfonamides [70]. This mechanism is based on plasmid- or transposon-encoded enzymes that substitute for the chromosomal enzymes normally inhibited by these drugs. Sulfonamides work through competitive inhibition of the enzyme dihydropteroate synthetase. The plasmid-coded enzyme bypassing this inhibition is smaller and more heat sensitive and a thousand times as much sulfonamide is required to inhibit it as is needed to inhibit the chromosomal enzyme. Similarly, some bacterial strains resistant to high levels of trimethoprim, an agent that inhibits dihydrofolate reductase, contain a plasmid-mediated gene coding for a new, trimethoprim-resistant dihydrofolate reductase. In each of these instances, the plasmids provide a mechanism whereby products vital to the bacterial cell can be synthesized and the inhibiting effect of the drug bypassed.

Resistance to Multiple Antimicrobial Agents

Resistance to multiple classes of antimicrobial agents, such as chloramphenicol, tetracycline, and fluoroquinolones, in both gram-negative and gram-positive bacterial organisms often is due to efflux of the drugs out of the bacterial cell [9,10]. There are several genetic determinants that mediate such resistance, including *marA*, *mexAB-oprD*, and *norA* [71]. Many multiresistant organisms previously were thought to have permeability barriers that limited the access of drugs to their sites of action. These are now known to contain effective efflux pumps that direct the drug out of the cell before it reaches its internal site of action [9,10]. Of course, solitary resistance to chloramphenicol, tetracycline, or the fluoroquinolones also is seen, although this is often mediated by mechanisms other than efflux.

Antimicrobial Resistance in M. tuberculosis

Resistance to anti-mycobacterial agents, such as isoniazid, rifampin, streptomycin, and ethambutol, often is associated with point mutations in critical genes, including *katG*, *rpoB*, *rpsL*, and *embB* [72–74]. However, a sizeable percentage of resistant strains do not contain mutations in these loci, indicating that there is still much to learn about resistance mechanisms, particularly in *Mycobacterium tuberculosis*. Novel DNA sequencing strategies, such as pyrosequencing, allow detection of mutations associated with resistance in organisms directly from sputum samples or from positive mycobacterial broth culture vials [73,74].

DISSEMINATION OF RESISTANCE GENES IN NATURE

Bacteria can exchange genetic information by means of transformation, transduction, and conjugation [75,76]. Resistance determinants can be encoded on an organism's chromosome or on the plasmids, bacteriophages, transposons, or integrons harbored in the cell, all of which may be moved from cell to cell by transformation, transduction, or conjugation. Thus, there is a multitude of pathways by which resistance genes move from one organism to another. Each of the various genetic elements that harbor resistance determinants has unique features.

Plasmids

Plasmids are self-replicating, extrachromosomal segments of DNA that can be found in many species of bacteria and yeast. Plasmids usually are circular and range in size from 2 to 400 kilobases [15]. The number of proteins encoded on plasmids can be substantial, with larger plasmids (∼300 kilobases) encoding 50 to 75 proteins. The proteins may include enzymes involved in antimicrobial

resistance, virulence, or the molecular machinery for plasmid transfer, in addition to those proteins required for plasmid maintenance. Plasmids usually can be acquired or lost by bacteria without affecting basic cellular functions because most of the genetic information necessary for metabolism and growth of the bacterial cell is located on the chromosome. For some plasmids, no phenotypic properties are known, and they are deemed "cryptic."

Plasmids are categorized by their ability to transfer themselves to other organisms. Those that are self-transmissible from one bacterial cell to another are termed "conjugative" [15]. When a gram-negative bacterial cell contains a conjugative plasmid, a proteinaceous appendage called a "pilus" is synthesized on the outside of the cell; this, together with other plasmid-mediated proteins, enables cell-to-cell transmission of the plasmid DNA. Conjugative plasmids of gram-positive bacteria do not use pili for conjugation; rather, direct cell-to-cell contact is required. In some instances, this is facilitated by plasmid-coded proteins (pheromones) that enhance clumping of donor and recipient cells [77]. Both staphylococci and enterococci have been shown to contain conjugal plasmids.

Nonconjugative plasmids often are smaller in size than conjugative plasmids. Some nonconjugative plasmids can still be transferred to recipient organisms by a process called mobilization in which a co-resident, nonconjugative plasmid takes advantage of the transfer of a conjugative one present in the same cell. In addition, nonconjugative and conjugative plasmids also may be transmitted by bacterial virus vectors through transduction. In this process, plasmid DNA instead of phage DNA is packaged in the viral protein coat and, on infection of a suitable recipient cell, the plasmid DNA is released and begins replication in the new host. Because transduction requires that the plasmid DNA be packaged in the protein coat of a bacteriophage, the amount of plasmid DNA that can be transduced is limited to approximately the size of the phage genome. This process operates much more efficiently for the smaller nonconjugative plasmids and appears to be an important mechanism of plasmid exchange in *S. aureus*. In gram-negative bacilli and streptococci, conjugation and mobilization seem to be the most common means of transfer. Direct uptake of both conjugative and nonconjugative plasmid DNA by a recipient cell also can occur through transformation. However, even in those naturally transformable species, this mode of plasmid transfer probably is uncommon.

Transposons and Insertion Sequences

A transposon is a segment of DNA that can move as an intact unit from one replicating DNA unit (replicon) to another by mechanisms other than those used in generalized recombination [75]. These sequences can "jump" from plasmid to plasmid, plasmid to bacteriophage, plasmid to chromosome, or the reverse using a "transposase" enzyme that is

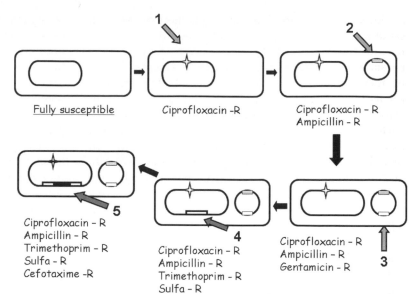

Figure 15-1 A schematic diagram showing the stepwise acquisition of antimicrobial resistance genes by *Escherichia coli*, beginning with (1) a chromosomal mutation in *gyrA* that results in ciprofloxacin resistance (star), followed by (2) acquisition of a plasmid containing a *bla*$_{TEM-1}$ ampicillin resistance gene, followed by (3) insertion of a transposon containing a *aac*[3]-I gentamicin resistance genes into the plasmid, followed by (4) insertion of an integron with sulfa and trimethoprim resistance (*sul*I and *dhfr*I genes, respectively) into the chromosome, and finally (5) insertion of a *bla*$_{CTXM-2}$ cefotaxime resistance gene on a cassette into the integron backbone.

encoded in the element. Transposons encoding–resistance genes to a variety of antimicrobial agents have been described. In theory, any plasmid could gain a transposon if DNA containing the transposon were to coexist in a cell long enough for transposition to occur. Transposons also promote a variety of rearrangements of DNA in adjoining regions, including deletions, inversions, and duplications. Some transposons, particularly those in gram-positive organism, such as enterococci, are conjugative and promote their own transfer from the chromosome of the donor cell to that of the recipient [75,76]. Such elements also have been recognized in *S. pneumoniae* [78]. Simpler genetic structures, called insertion sequences, do not contain antimicrobial resistance determinants but promote gene rearrangements and can modify the expression of resistance genes by inserting strong promoter elements upstream of open reading frames.

Integrons

Integrons are mobile DNA elements that contain "hot spots" of recombination where a variety of antimicrobial resistance gene cassettes can insert, mediated by an integrase enzyme [19]. The gene cassettes must contain a key 59-base-pair region at their termini to be recognized by the integrase enzyme. The gene cassettes do not contain their own promoters, and thus expression depends on insertion into the integron in the appropriate orientation downstream from a promoter element [19]. The cassettes appear to undergo integration and excision as covalently closed circular molecules. Large, complex integrons with as many as five resistance genes have been detected on plasmids in enteric organisms [20,21]. The proximity of the cassette to the integron's promoter has a major effect on expression, with those genes that are proximal to the promoter showing strong and consistent

expression and those that are distal showing low-level or no expression.

Development of Multiresistant Organisms

Multiresistant organism can develop over time by the successive acquisition of mutations and resistance genes using a number of different mechanisms (Figure 15-1). These may include spontaneous mutation, acquisition of plasmids and transposons, and insertion of gene cassettes into integrons. Dissemination of epidemic plasmids in closed populations (sometimes referred to as "plasmid outbreaks") continues to plague hospitals as demonstrated by Neuwirth et al., who noted dissemination of an ESBL-producing strain of *Enterobacter aerogenes* in their hospital followed by transfer of the β-lactamase-encoding plasmid to other species of *Enterobacteriaceae* [79]. Rubens et al. demonstrate how a gentamicin-resistance determinant originally present on a small nonconjugative plasmid was transposed onto a larger, self-transferable plasmid [18]. Once on the conjugative element, the resistance was efficiently transferred among a variety of genera in the hospital. This process provided a mechanism to assemble new resistance determinants on a preexisting plasmid and appears to be one way that multiresistance plasmids can develop.

ENVIRONMENTAL CONDITIONS THAT FAVOR THE DEVELOPMENT OF RESISTANT ORGANISMS—SELECTIVE PRESSURE

Resistant organisms, particularly those that develop through spontaneous mutation, usually will not survive unless there is an advantage to maintaining the resistance phenotype. The environment in many healthcare institutions (hospitals, long-term care facilities, dialysis centers, etc.) is rich with antimicrobial agents that are hostile to antimicrobial-susceptible organisms [80]. Thus, resistant organisms have a survival advantage in this environment. In genetic terms, the presence of antimicrobial agents in the environment is the "selective pressure" that favors the development and spread of resistant strains of bacteria. However, selective pressures are not unique to healthcare institutions. To control the spread of resistant organisms, the selective pressures provided by both hospital and community must be considered [80].

THE HEALTHCARE ENVIRONMENT

The most frequently encountered healthcare-associated pathogens, staphylococci, enterococci, and gram-negative bacilli [81], all have demonstrated the ability to acquire and disseminate resistance genes. Intensive use of antimicrobial agents exerts a selective pressure favoring those organisms that have acquired resistance determinants through mutation or genetic exchange. Even organisms that develop low-level resistance may survive long enough to acquire additional mutations or resistance genes that facilitate long-term survival [82]. Antimicrobial therapy alters or eliminates the normal bacterial flora found in many niches of the human body, which can enhance colonization of skin or other sites with resistant strains because the innate defense provided by the presence of normal flora is gone. This, in turn, likely contributes to enhanced gene transfer among organisms, particularly in the gastrointestinal tract. Plasmid transfer, in particular, often is observed in aqueous reservoirs peculiar to the hospital environment, such as urinary catheter collection bags. Conditions that enhance transfer of plasmids also favor the transmission of transposons and integrons, further increasing the dissemination of resistance genes [76]. Immunocompromised patients who are receiving antimicrobial agents and who are hospitalized for prolonged periods provide a reservoir for resistant organisms [80]. Antimicrobial agents typically find their way into the general inanimate environment of healthcare facilities, which also contributes to the selective advantage obtained by plasmid- or integron-containing organisms. Thus, the healthcare environment is conducive to the development and spread of resistant bacteria.

The Community Environment

The use and sometimes misuse [83] of antimicrobial agents in the community contributes to the selective pressure that results in healthcare-associated pathogens because the gene pools for the organisms are the same [84]. Selective pressures outside of the hospital, including the use of antimicrobial agents in humans, particularly in children for respiratory infections [85], in animals both therapeutically and as growth promoters, in fish (aqua-culture), and on

vegetables [1–4], suggests that the development of resistant strains can and does occur virtually everywhere. The development and spread of plasmid-mediated ampicillin-resistant *Haemophilus influenzae* [86] in the 1970s, multiresistant pneumococci in the 1970s and 1980s [87], and the descriptions of multiply resistant *Salmonella* [88] and *Shigella* [89] provided convincing evidence that problems with resistant organisms are not confined to the hospital. The two locations often come together, as when patients from nursing homes who harbor MRSA are transferred to acute care community hospitals where the patients serve as a nidus for the spread of the pathogen [90].

EPIDEMIOLOGIC STUDIES OF BACTERIAL RESISTANCE

To study the epidemiology of antimicrobial-resistant bacteria, it is imperative to have strain typing methods that are both discriminatory and reproducible [91]. When an outbreak of a resistant strain is suspected in a healthcare system, several techniques can be used to confirm that the isolates are clonal (i.e., derived from a common parent). Biochemical patterns and antimicrobial susceptibility test results can provide initial clues to strain identity, but more definitive information, as provided by pulsed-field gel electrophoresis (PFGE) patterns, repetitive element polymerase chain reaction (rep-PCR) typing, multiple locus variable number tandem repeat assays (MLVA), or multilocus sequence typing (MLST) often are necessary [92].

Pulsed-Field Gel Electrophoresis

Of all of the strain typing methods currently available, PFGE of chromosomal DNA comes the closest to being a universal typing method for bacteria [93]. PFGE uses infrequent cutting restriction endonucleases to cleave the chromosome of an organism into a relatively small number (usually 10 to 25) of fragments (Figure 15-2). The fragments are subjected to electrophoresis through agarose in a special chamber in which the direction of the electrical current is switched frequently according to a preset pattern. This resolves the fragments into discrete patterns that easily can be photographed and analyzed [93]. Interpretive criteria for analyzing restriction fragment banding patterns have been published [93]. This typing method has been validated against epidemiologic data collected during outbreak investigations for a large number of bacterial species.

REP-PCR

REP-PCR uses the repetitive elements present in most bacterial and fungal species to generate banding patterns that can be analyzed in a fashion similar to the banding patterns of PFGE [94–96]. Commercial systems that use

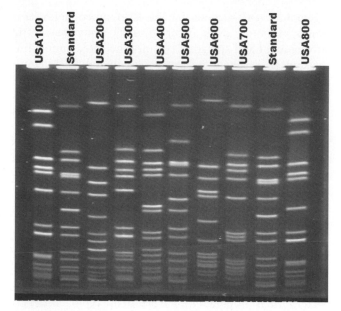

Figure 15-2 Example of pulsed-field gel electrophoresis showing differentiation of eight of the major strain types of methicillin-resistant *Staphylococcus aureus* [104]. Molecular size standards are shown in lanes 2 and 9.

REP-PCR for both strain typing and species identification have been developed [97]. This system yields results that are comparable or slightly less discriminatory than PFGE but with the advantage of much more rapid turnaround time and sophisticated on-line data analysis and reporting [95,96].

MLVA

Analysis of the genomes of a variety of bacterial species has shown that many organisms have chromosomal loci that contain variable numbers of tandem repeats (VNTRs) [98]. The structure and function of the repeats differ widely, but the value of VNTRs for strain typing, particularly for monomorphic species such as *Bacillus anthracis*, is significant. VNTR may represent direct or inverted repeats and may be responsible for antigenic variation or gene regulation. PCR amplification products resulting from the use of specific primers can be analyzed directly for variation in primary nucleotide sequence. Alternatively, variation in the sizes of the PCR products can be assessed by agarose gel or capillary electrophoresis coupled with computer software to facilitate fragment analysis [98]. Multiplex PCR assays can be developed that allow products from multiple loci to be assessed simultaneously [99]. However, when fragment size rather than the actual sequence is used for strain differentiation, the datasets have the limitations of laboratory to laboratory reproducibility inherent in any gel-based technique.

MLVA has been used successfully to type highly monomorphic organisms, such as *B. anthracis* and *Yersinia pestis*, and to differentiate among lineages of common pathogens, such as Shiga-toxin-producing *E. coli, Salmonella typhi,* and *S. aureus* [98]. Initially, the MLVA assay for *B. anthracis* was focused on a single variable repeat region, *vrrA*, which consisted of a series of 12 base pair tandem repeats. The addition of other chromosomal loci and sites on the two virulence plasmids (pXO1 and pXO2) has provided remarkable discrimination among isolates of this highly monomorphic pathogen [100].

MLST

MLST is a DNA sequence-based typing scheme that is primarily used for studying the population biology and structure of bacterial species [92,101]. The principles of MLST are based on an older technique that examined variations in the electrophoresis patterns of multiple enzymes in starch gels, namely multilocus enzyme electrophoresis (MLEE) [102]. In MLEE, various electromorphs were equated with alleles. Similarly, in MLST, isolates are classified based on polymorphisms in the DNA coding sequences of 7 to 10 different metabolic ("housekeeping") genes, where every nucleotide variant in a sequence is considered a unique allele. The set of loci that is sequenced must be identified and validated for each bacterial species [92]. When used for strain typing of isolates associated with outbreaks, the discriminatory power of MLST is typically less than PFGE. However, many pathogenic clones of bacteria are designated using a combination of strain typing methods that often include MLST types, such as pneumococci [103], MRSA [104], and *N. meningitidis* [105].

MLST databases have been established for a variety of organisms and a Web site (**www.mlst.net**) is available to help analyze sequence data generated for a number of bacterial species, ranging from *N. meningitidis* to *S. aureus*. MLST may be useful in some epidemiologic studies, particularly if discriminatory power is enhanced by examining additional loci.

Additional Methods for Laboratory Studies of Resistant Microorganisms

The dissemination of resistance genes occurs on three levels in hospitals. The first level is dissemination of a resistant strain, often on the hands of healthcare workers or through patient contact with environmental reservoirs of resistant organisms. The next level occurs when a resistance plasmid transfers from one organism to another or from one species to another, which amplifies the extent of the problem and makes epidemiologic studies more complex and the outbreak more difficult to control. The third level involves the acquisition of novel resistance genes by the outbreak strain through generalized recombination, transposition, or insertion of resistance gene cassettes into integrons. Examples of this include the acquisition of chloramphenicol resistance by strains of MRSA during an outbreak in a hospital in Seattle [106] or the acquisition of gentamicin-resistance transposons by an epidemic strain of *P. aeruginosa* [107]. Furthermore, spontaneous mutation to a resistant phenotype followed by dissemination of the novel strain also occurs as evidenced by the explosive increase in ciprofloxacin-resistant strains of MRSA reported by Blumberg et al. [108], in which the new resistant strains represented >90% of MRSA isolates over the course of a single year after the introduction of ciprofloxacin in the hospital. Thus, spread of a resistant strain, transfer of plasmids, spontaneous mutation, and genetic exchange in the presence of antibiotic selective pressure are the key factors in the development and spread of resistant organisms in the hospital setting.

CONCLUSIONS

Antimicrobial resistance in bacteria comprises a wide variety of biochemical mechanisms and processes that allow microorganisms to grow in the presence of antimicrobial agents. Bacteria are able to transmit this acquired "knowledge" to other species through transformation, transduction, and conjugation. Specialized structures, including transposons, integrons, and chromosomal cassettes, allow cells to recruit additional genetic information outside of the normal processes of mutation and generalized recombination. The web of genetic exchange in bacteria is very broad and even crosses between gram-positive and gram-negative organisms. Finally, there is no barrier between hospital and the community when it comes to resistant organisms. All bacteria can draw on the same gene pool to find ways to cope with the presence of antibiotics in their environment.

REFERENCES

1. Cohen M. Epidemiology of drug resistance: implications for a post-antimicrobial era. *Science* 1992;257:1050–1055.
2. U.S. Congress, Office of Technology Assessment. *Impacts of antibiotic resistant bacteria*. OTA-H-629. Washington, DC: U.S. Government Printing Office, 1995.
3. American Society for Microbiology. *Report of the ASM task force on antibiotic resistance*. Washington, DC: American Society for Microbiology Press, 1995.
4. Neu HC. The crisis in antibiotic resistance. *Science* 1992;257: 1064–1073.
5. Metlay JP, Powers JH, Dudley MN, et al. Antimicrobial drug resistance, regulation, and research. *Emerg Infect Dis* 2006;12: 183–190.
6. Davies J. Inactivation of antibiotics and the dissemination of resistance genes. *Science* 1994;264:375–382.
7. Abraham EP, Chain E. An enzyme from bacteria able to destroy penicillin. *Nature* 1940;146:837–839.
8. Kirby WMM. Extraction of a highly potent penicillin inactivator from penicillin resistant staphylococci. *Science* 1944;99:452–455.
9. Nikaido H. Prevention of drug access to bacterial targets: permeability barriers and active efflux. *Science* 1994;264:382–388.
10. Poole K. Efflux-mediated antimicrobial resistance. *J Antimicrob Chemother* 2005;56:20–51.
11. Spratt BG. Resistance to antibiotics mediated by target alterations. *Science* 1994;264:388–393.
12. Boehr DD, Moore IF, Wright GD. Aminoglycoside resistance mechanisms. In: White DG, Alekshun MN, McDermott PF, eds.

13. Akiba T, Koyama K, Ishiki Y, et al. On the mechanism of the development of multiple drug resistant clones of *Shigella*. *Japan J Microbiol* 1960;4:219–222.
14. Falkow S. *Infectious multiple drug resistance*. London: Pion Press, 1975.
15. Funnell BE, Phillips GJ, eds. *Plasmid biology*. Washington, D.C.: ASM Press, 2004.
16. Novick RP, Morse SI. In vivo transmission of drug resistance factors between strains of *Staphylococcus aureus*. *J Exp Med* 1967;125: 45–59.
17. Berg DE, Davies J, Allet B, et al. Transposition of R factor genes to bacteriophage. *Proc Natl Acad Sci USA* 1975;72:3628–3632.
18. Rubens CE, McNeil WF, Farrar WE Jr. Transposable plasmid deoxyribonucleic acid sequence in *Pseudomonas aeruginosa* which mediates resistance to gentamicin and four other antimicrobial agents. *J Bacteriol* 1979;139:877–882.
19. Stokes HW, Hall RM. A novel family of potentially mobile DNA elements encoding site-specific gene integration functions: integrons. *Mol Microbiol* 1989;3:1669–1683.
20. Lévesque C, Piche L, Larose C, et al. PCR mapping of integrons reveals several novel combinations of resistance genes. *Antimicrob Agents Chemother* 1995;39:185–191.
21. Leverstein-van Hall MA, Blok HEM, Donders ART, et al. Multidrug resistance among *Enterobacteriaceae* is strongly associated with the presence of integrons and is independent of species or isolate origin. *J Infect Dis* 2003;187:251–259.
22. Rao A, Tenover FC, Boring J, McGowan JE Jr. Class I integron carriage is highly prevalent among antimicrobial resistant isolates of *Escherichia coli* and *Klebsiella* species from U.S. hospitals. *Emerg Infect Dis* 2006;12:1011–1014
23. Katayama Y, Ito T, Hiramatsu K. A new class of genetic element, staphylococcus cassette chromosome mec, encodes methicillin resistance in *Staphylococcus aureus*. *Antimicrob Agents Chemother* 2000;44:1549–1555.
24. Ito T, Katayama Y, Asada K, et al. Structural comparison of three types of staphylococcal cassette chromosome mec integrated in the chromosome in methicillin-resistant *Staphylococcus aureus*. *Antimicrob Agents Chemother* 2001;45:1323–1336.
25. Ma XX, Ito T, Tiensasitorn C, et al. Novel type of staphylococcal cassette chromosome mec identified in community-acquired methicillin-resistant *Staphylococcus aureus* strains. *Antimicrob Agents Chemother* 2002;46:1147–1152.
26. Ito T, Ma XX, Takeuchi F, et al. Novel type V staphylococcal cassette chromosome mec driven by a novel cassette chromosome recombinase, ccrC. *Antimicrob Agents Chemother* 2004;48: 2637–2651.
27. Coombs GW, Pearson JC, O'Brien FG, et al. Methicillin-resistant *Staphylococcus aureus* clones, Western Australia. *Emerg Infect Dis* 2006;12:241–247.
28. Tenover FC. Mechanisms of antimicrobial resistance in bacteria. *Am J Med* 2006;119:S3–S10.
29. Leclercq R, Courvalin P. Enterococcus. In: White DG, Alekshun MN, McDermott PF, eds. Frontiers in Antimicrobial Resistance. A Tribute to Stuart B. Levy. Washington, DC: 2005 ASM Press: 299–313.
30. Livermore DM. β-Lactamases in laboratory and clinical resistance. *Clin Microbiol Rev* 1995;8:557–584.
31. Funatsu G, Wittmann HG. Location and amino acid replacements in protein S12 isolated from *Escherichia coli* mutants resistant to streptomycin. *J Mol Biol* 1972;68:547–450.
32. Nair J, Rouse DA, Bai G-H, et al. The *rpsL* gene and streptomycin resistance in single and multiple drug-resistant strains of *Mycobacterium tuberculosis*. *Mol Microbiol* 1993;10:521–527.
33. www.lahey.org/studies/inc_web.asp.
34. Bush K, Jacoby GA, Medeiros AA. A functional classification scheme for β-lactamases and its correlation with molecular structure. *Antimicrob Agents Chemother* 1995;39:1211–1233.
35. Bradford PA. Extended-spectrum beta-lactamases in the 21st century: characterization, epidemiology, and detection of this important resistance threat. *Clin Microbiol Rev* 2001;14:933–951.
36. Weber DA, Sanders CC, Bakken JS, Quinn JR. A novel chromosomal TEM derivative and alterations in outer membrane

Frontiers in antimicrobial resistance: a tribute to Stuart B. Levy. Washington, DC: ASM Press: 2005,85–100.

proteins together mediate selective ceftazidime resistance in *Escherichia coli. J Infect Dis* 1990;162:460–465.

37. Yigit H, Anderson GJ, Biddle JW, et al. Carbapenem resistance in a clinical isolate of *Enterobacter aerogenes* is associated with decreased expression of OmpF and OmpC analogs. *Antimicrob Agents Chemother* 2002;46:3817–3822.

38. Yigit H, Queenan AM, Anderson GJ, et al. Novel carbapenem-hydrolyzing β-lactamase, KPC-1, from a carbapenem-resistant strain of *Klebsiella pneumoniae. Antimicrob Agents Chemother* 2001; 45:1151–1161.

39. Bradford, P, Bratu S, Urban C, et al. Emergence of carbapenem-resistant *Klebsiella* spp. possessing the class A carbapenem-hydrolyzing KPC-2 and inhibitor resistant TEM-30 beta-lactamases in New York City. *Clin Infect Dis* 2003;39:55–60.

40. Bratu S, Landman D, Haag R, et al. Rapid spread of carbapenem-resistant *Klebsiella pneumoniae* in New York City. *Archives Intern Med* 2005;165:1430–1435.

41. Naas T, Nordmann P, Vedel G, Poyart C. Plasmid-mediated carbapenem-hydrolyzing beta-lactamase KPC in a *Klebsiella pneumoniae* isolate from France. *Antimicrob Agents Chemother* 2005;49: 4423–4424.

42. Walsh TR. The emergence and implications of metallo-beta-lactamases in gram-negative bacteria. *Clin Microbiol Infect* 2005; 11 (suppl 6):2–9.

43. Hakenbeck R, Grebe T, Zahner D, Stock JB. β-lactam resistance in *Streptococcus pneumoniae*: penicillin-binding proteins and non-penicillin-binding proteins. *Mol Microbiol* 1999;33:673–678.

44. Coffey TJ, Daniels M, McDougal LK, et al. Genetic analysis of clinical isolates of *Streptococcus pneumoniae* with high-level resistance to expanded-spectrum cephalosporins. *Antimicrob Agents Chemother* 1995;39:1306–1313.

45. Spratt BG, Dowson CG, Zhang QY, et al. Mosaic genes, hybrid penicillin-binding proteins, and the origins of penicillin resistance in *Neisseria meningitidis* and *Streptococcus pneumoniae.* In: Campisi J, Cunningham D, Inouye M, Riley M, eds. *Perspectives on cellular regulation: from bacteria to cancer.* New York: Wiley-Liss, 1991:73–83.

46. Roberts M, Sutcliffe J. Macrolide, lincosamide, streptogramin, ketolide, and oxazolidinone resistance. In: White DG, Alekshun MN, McDermott PF, eds. *Frontiers in antimicrobial resistance: a tribute to Stuart B. Levy.* Washington, DC: ASM Press, 2005: 66–84.

47. Robicsek A, Strahilevitz J, Jacoby GA, et al. Fluoroquinolone-modifying enzyme: a new adaptation of a common aminoglycoside acetyltransferase. *Nat Med* 2006;12:83–88.

48. Sapunaric FM, Aldema-Ramos M, McMurray LM. Tetracycline resistance, efflux, mutation, and other mechanisms. In: White DG, Alekshun MN, McDermott PF, eds. *Frontiers in antimicrobial resistance: a tribute to Stuart B. Levy.* Washington, DC: ASM Press, 2005:3–18.

49. Roberts M. Tetracycline resistance due to ribosomal protection. In: White DG, Alekshun MN, McDermott PF, eds. *Frontiers in antimicrobial resistance: a tribute to Stuart B. Levy.* Washington, DC: ASM Press, 2005:19–28.

50. Courvalin P. Vancomycin resistance in gram-positive cocci. *Clin Infect Dis* 2006;42 (Suppl 1):S25–S34.

51. Chang S, Sievert DM, Hageman JC, et al. Infection with vancomycin-resistant *Staphylococcus aureus* containing the vanA resistance gene. *N Engl J Med.* 2003;348:1342–1347.

52. Weigel LM, Clewell DB, Gill SR, et al. Genetic analysis of a high-level vancomycin-resistant isolate of *Staphylococcus aureus. Science.* 2003;302:1569–1571.

53. Tenover FC, Weigel LM, Appelbaum PC, et al. Vancomycin-resistant *Staphylococcus aureus* isolate from a patient in Pennsylvania. *Antimicrob Agents Chemother* 2004;48:275–280.

54. Centers for Disease Control and Prevention. Vancomycin-resistant *Staphylococcus aureus*—New York, 2004. *MMWR Morb Mortal Wkly Rep* 2004; 53:322–323.

55. Perichon B, Courvalin P. Heterologous expression of the enterococcal *vanA* operon in methicillin-resistant *Staphylococcus aureus. Antimicrob Agents Chemother* 2004; 48:4281–4285.

56. Hanaki H, Kuwahara-Arai K, Boyle-Vavra S, et al. Activated cell-wall synthesis is associated with vancomycin resistance in methicillin-resistant *Staphylococcus aureus* clinical strains Mu3 and Mu50. *J Antimicrob Chemother* 1998;42:199–209.

57. Cui L, Murakami H, Kuwahara-Arai K, et al. Contribution of a thickened cell wall and its glutamine nonamidated component to the vancomycin resistance expressed by *Staphylococcus aureus* Mu50. *Antimicrob Agents Chemother* 2000;44:2276–2285.

58. Clinical and Laboratory Standards Institute. Performance standards for antimicrobial susceptibility testing; fifteenth informational supplement M100-S16. Wayne, PA: The Committee, 2006.

59. Hiramatsu K, Hanaki H, Ino T, et al. Methicillin-resistant *Staphylococcus aureus* clinical strain with reduced vancomycin susceptibility. *J Antimicrob Chemother* 1997;40:135–136.

60. Fridkin SK. Vancomycin-intermediate and -resistant *Staphylococcus aureus*: what the infectious disease specialist needs to know. *Clin Infect Dis* 2001;32:108–115.

61. Ploy M. C., Grelaud C, Martin C, et al. First clinical isolate of vancomycin-intermediate *Staphylococcus aureus* in a French hospital. *Lancet* 1998;351:1212.

62. Kim M. N., Pai CH, Woo TH, et al. Vancomycin-intermediate *Staphylococcus aureus* in Korea. *J Clin Microbiol* 2000;38: 3879–3891.

63. Hiramatsu K., Aritaka N, Hanaki H, et al. Dissemination in Japanese hospitals of strains of *Staphylococcus aureus* heterogeneously resistant to vancomycin. *Lancet* 1997;350:1670–1673.

64. Jacoby GA. Mechanisms of resistance to quinolones. *Clin Infect Dis* 2005;41 (Suppl 2):S120–S126.

65. Doern GV, Richter SS, Miller A, et al. Antimicrobial resistance among *Streptococcus pneumoniae* in the United States: have we begun to turn the corner on resistance to certain antimicrobial classes? *Clin Infect Dis* 2005;41:139–148.

66. Jones ME, Draghi DC, Thornsberry C, et al. Emerging resistance among bacterial pathogens in the intensive care unit—a European and North American Surveillance study (2000–2002). *Ann Clin Microbiol Antimicrob* 2004;29:3–14.

67. Tran JH, Jacoby GA. Mechanism of plasmid-mediated quinolone resistance. *Proc Natl Acad Sci USA.* 2002;99:5638–5642.

68. Jacoby GA, Walsh KE, Mills DM, et al. *qnrB*, another plasmid-mediated gene for quinolone resistance. *Antimicrob Agents Chemother* 2006;50:1178–1182.

69. Amyes SGB, Towner KJ. Trimethoprim resistance: epidemiology and molecular aspects. *J Med Microbiol* 1990;31:1–19.

70. Wise EM, Abou-Donia MM. Sulfonamide resistance mechanism in *Escherichia coli:* R plasmids can determine sulfonamide-resistant dihydropteroate synthetases. *Proc Natl Acad Sci USA* 1975;72:2621–2626.

71. George AM. Multiple antimicrobial resistance. In: White DG, Alekshun MN, McDermott PF, eds. *Frontiers in antimicrobial resistance: a tribute to Stuart B. Levy.* Washington, DC: ASM Press, 2005:151–164.

72. Finken M, Kirschner P, Meier A, et al. Molecular basis of streptomycin resistance in *Mycobacterium tuberculosis*: alternations of the ribosomal protein A12 and point mutations within a functional 16S ribosomal RNA pseudoknot. *Mol Microbiol* 1993;9: 1239–1246.

73. Arnold C, Westland L, Mowat G, et al. Single-nucleotide polymorphism-based differentiation and drug resistance detection in *Mycobacterium tuberculosis* from isolates or directly from sputum. *Clin Microbiol Infect* 2005;11:122–130.

74. Zhao J-R., Bai Y-J, Wang Y, et al. Development of a pyrosequencing approach for rapid screening of rifampin, isoniazid and ethambutol-resistant *Mycobacterium tuberculosis. Int J Tuberc Lung Dis* 2005;9:328–332.

75. Thomas CM, Nielsen KM. Mechanisms of, and barriers to, horizontal gene transfer between bacteria. *Nat Rev Microbiol* 2005;3:711–721.

76. Frost LS, Leplae R, Summers AO, Toussaint A. Mobile genetic elements: the agents of open source evolution. *Nat Rev Microbiol* 2005;3:722–732.

77. Dunny G, Brown B, Clewell D. Induced cell aggregation and mating in *Streptococcus faecalis*: evidence for a bacterial sex pheromone. *Proc Natl Acad Sci USA* 1978;75:3479–3483.

78. Clewell DB, Gawron-Burke C. Conjugative transposons and dissemination of antibiotic resistance in streptococci. *Ann Rev Microbiol* 1986;40:635–659.

79. Neuwirth C, Siebor E, Lopez J, et al. Outbreak of TEM-24-producing *Enterobacter aerogenes* in an intensive care unit

and dissemination of the extended-spectrum β-lactamase to other members of the family Enterobacteriaceae. *J Clin Microbiol* 1996;34:76–79.

80. Owens RC, Jr, Rice L. Hospital-based strategies for combating resistance. *Clin Infect Dis* 2006;42:S173–181.

81. National Nosocomial Infections Surveillance (NNIS) System Report, data summary from January 1992 through June 2004. *Am J Infect Control* 2004;32:470–485.

82. Baquero F. Low-level antibacterial resistance: a gateway to clinical resistance. *Drug Resistance Updates* 2001;4:93–105.

83. Gonzales R, Sande M. What will it take to stop physicians from prescribing antibiotics in acute bronchitis? *Lancet* 1995;345:665–666.

84. Tenover FC, McGowan JE Jr. Reasons for the emergence of antibiotic resistance. *Am J Med Sci* 1996;311:9–16.

85. McCaig LF, Hughes JM. Trends in antimicrobial drug prescribing among office-based physicians in the United States. *JAMA* 1995;273:214–219.

86. Elwell LP, deGraaff J, Seibert D, et al. Plasmid-linked ampicillin resistance in *Haemophilus influenzae* type b. *Infect Immun* 1975;12:404–410.

87. Klugman K. Pneumococcal resistance to antibiotics. *Clin Microbiol Rev* 1990;3:171–196.

88. Varma JK, Marcus R, Stenzel SA, et al. Highly resistant salmonella Newport—MDR AmpC transmitted through the domestic US food supply: a foodnet case control study of sporadic salmonella Newport infections, 2002–2003. *J Infect Dis* 2006;194:222–230.

89. Sivapalasingam S, Nelson JM, Joyce K, et al. High prevalence of antimicrobial resistance among Shigella isolates in the United States tested by the National Antimicrobial Resistance Monitoring System from 1999 to 2002. *Antimicrob Agents Chemother* 2006;50:49–54.

90. Deresinski, S. 2005. Methicillin-resistant *Staphylococcus aureus*: an evolutionary, epidemiologic, and therapeutic odyssey. *Clin Infect Dis* 40:526–573.

91. Tenover FC, Arbeit RD, Goering RV, and the Molecular Typing Working Group. How to select and interpret molecular strain typing methods for epidemiologic studies of bacterial infections: a review for health care epidemiologists. *Infect Control Hosp Epidemiol* 1997;18:426–439.

92. Molecular methods for bacterial strain typing; proposed guideline. MM 11-P. Wayne, PA: Clinical and Laboratory Standards Institute, 2006.

93. Tenover FC, Arbeit RD, Goering RV, et al. Criteria for interpreting pulsed-field gel electrophoresis patterns. *J Clin Microbiol* 1995;33:2233–2239.

94. Healy M, Huong J, Bittner T, et al. Microbial DNA typing by automated repetitive-sequence-based PCR. *J Clin Microbiol* 2005;43:199–207.

95. Ross TL, Merz WG, Farkosh M, Carroll KC. Comparison of an automated repetitive sequence-based PCR microbial typing system to pulsed-field gel electrophoresis for analysis

of outbreaks of methicillin-resistant *Staphylococcus aureus*. *J Clin Microbiol* 2005;43:5642–5647.

96. Pounder JI, Shutt CK, Schaecher BJ, Woods GL. Clinical evaluation of repetitive sequence-based polymerase chain reaction using the Diversi-Lab System for strain typing of vancomycin-resistant enterococci. *Diagn Microbiol Infect Dis* 2006;54:183–187.

97. Healy M, Reece K, Walton D, et al. Identification to the species level and differentiation between strains of *Aspergillus* clinical isolates by automated repetitive-sequence-based PCR. *J Clin Microbiol* 2004;42:4016–4024.

98. Lindstedt BA. Multiple-locus variable number tandem repeats analysis for genetic fingerprinting of pathogenic bacteria. *Electrophoresis* 2005;26:2567–2582.

99. Sabat A, Krzyszton-Russjan J, Strzalka W, et al. New method for typing *Staphylococcus aureus* strains: multiple-locus variable-number tandem repeat analysis of polymorphism and genetic relationships of clinical isolates. *J Clin Microbiol* 2003;41:1801–1804.

100. Keim P, Price LB, Klevytska AM, et al. Multiple-locus variable-number tandem repeat analysis reveals genetic relationships within *Bacillus anthracis*. *J Bacteriol* 2000;182:2928–2936.

101. Maiden MCJ, Bygraves JA, Feil E, et al. Multilocus sequence typing: a portable approach to the identification of clones within populations of pathogenic microorganisms. *Proc Natl Acad Sci USA* 1998;95:3140–3145.

102. Selander RK, Caugant DA, Ochman H, et al. Methods of multilocus enzyme electrophoresis for bacterial population genetics and systematics. *Appl Environ Microbiol* 1986;51:873–884.

103. McGee L, McDougal L, Zhou J, et al. Nomenclature of major antimicrobial-resistant clones of *Streptococcus pneumoniae* defined by the pneumococcal molecular epidemiology network. *J Clin Microbiol* 2001;39:2565–2571.

104. McDougal LK, Steward CD, Killgore GE, et al. Pulsed-field gel electrophoresis typing of oxacillin-resistant *Staphylococcus aureus* isolates from the United States: establishing a national database. *J Clin Microbiol* 2003;41:5113–5120.

105. Nicolas P, Norheim G, Garnotel E, et al. Molecular epidemiology of *Neisseria meningitidis* isolated in the African Meningitis Belt between 1988 and 2003 shows dominance of sequence type 5 (ST-5) and ST-11 complexes. *J Clin Microbiol* 2005;43:5129–5135.

106. Locksley RM, Cohen ML, Quinn TC, et al. Multiply antibiotic resistant *Staphylococcus aureus*: introduction, transmission, and evolution of nosocomial infection. *Ann Intern Med* 1982;97:317–324.

107. Rubens CE, McNeill WF, Farrar WE. Evolution of multiple antibiotic-resistance plasmids mediated by transposable deoxyribonucleic acid sequences. *J Bacteriol* 1979;140:713–719.

108. Blumberg HM, Rimland D, Carroll DJ, et al. Rapid development of ciprofloxacin resistance in methicillin-susceptible and —resistant *Staphylococcus aureus*. *J Infect Dis* 1991;163:1279–1285.

Economic Evaluation of Healthcare-Associated Infections and Infection Control Interventions

16

Sara E. Cosgrove and Eli N. Perencevich

Organized infection control (IC) programs have expanded in the past decade. However, hospital administrators require more economic justification for maintaining and expanding programs. This is a particular challenge because while it is clear that healthcare-associated infections (HAIs) are costly—$6.5 billion in 2004 dollars in the United States [1]—healthcare administrators do not generally view IC programs as cost-saving because they do not generate revenue for the institution. Thus, hospital epidemiologists and infection control professionals (ICPs) need the tools to prove the worth of the surveillance and interventions that they perform for their healthcare institution.

HAIs are a significant risk to patient safety. Unfortunately, this has not opened the door to improving the resources provided to prevent HAIs. While society would benefit from reduced HAIs, there is currently no direct reimbursement to hospitals for the purpose of IC. This has led to the current situation in which hospitals must make economic decisions about funding IC studies on an individual basis. This situation also has impacted the literature so that most studies describe the hospital perspective of the impact of HAIs (90% of studies) with only 3%

taking a societal perspective [1,2]. As we emphasize here, it is important to complete a business cost analysis from a hospital perspective in order to inform local decisions; however, these such analyses are not useful on a public health level. It has become increasingly important to justify the importance of funding IC activities at a broader level through the completion of cost-effectiveness analyses from the societal perspective.

This chapter will detail important concepts in economic analysis, including types of economic analyses and their strengths, the different perspectives of analyses, and placing monetary values in constant dollar terms. Then it will describe approaches to assess the financial impact of specific HAIs and of control interventions and provide a methodology for developing a cost-effectiveness analysis at a societal level. After completing the necessary review of health economics, it will describe the basic steps needed to complete a business case analysis of a specific IC intervention for an individual institution. While we have attempted to outline important considerations regarding economic measurement of HAIs and related interventions, more detailed texts about design and analysis of economic research are available [3–5].

BASIC ECONOMIC CONCEPTS

This section defines important concepts regarding economic analyses including types of cost analyses, the perspective of the analysis, and discounting and inflating costs.

Types of Economic Analyses

There are four basic types of economic analysis used in health care: cost minimization analysis, cost-effective analysis, cost-utility analysis, and cost-benefit analysis (Table 16-1). Experts have noted that the distinctions between these various forms of analysis are often blurred, yet it is important to consider what is included and not included in each specific analysis so that informed decisions can be made [3]. A recent review of the IC literature found that of 30 publications reporting to be economic analyses, only 8 were cost-effectiveness or cost-consequences analyses. Of note, in the IC and quality improvement literature, there is increasing use of the term business case analysis, which is an extension of a simple cost analysis from a hospital or payer prospective that excludes dollar valuation of human life and morbidity [6,7].

A detailed discussion of performing a business case analysis appears later in this chapter.

Cost-Minimization Analysis

In cost-minimization analyses, the effectiveness of two interventions or products are assumed to be the same (equal efficacy and side effects), and the analysis is aimed at determining which can be delivered least expensively [8]. An example of a cost-minimization analysis in IC is the choice between two brands of nonlatex gloves. In this example, most would just choose the less expensive brand. Note that this type of analysis does not apply to the choice between a brand of latex and a brand of nonlatex gloves, because these can be associated with different levels of health care worker (HCW) satisfaction and also allergic side effects.

Cost-Effectiveness Analysis

In contrast to cost minimization, cost-effectiveness analysis compares interventions or products that have different costs and different effectiveness. If a specific new intervention costs more and is less effective or alternatively costs less and is more effective than an existing intervention, the choice is easy. However, if a new intervention delivers more at increased cost, which occurs frequently in the setting of rapid technologic intervention, the choice often is difficult. In cost-effectiveness analysis, the benefits of an intervention are measured in the most natural unit of comparison, such as lives saved or infections prevented [3]. Programs then are compared in terms of dollars per life-year gained or dollars per infection prevented.

Cost-Utility Analysis

Cost-utility analysis is very similar to cost-effectiveness analysis except that benefits of a specific intervention are adjusted by health preference scores or are utility weighted [3]. Thus, programs are compared in terms of quality-adjusted life years gained (QALY). The rationale of this approach is that it allows the incorporation of disability or side effects associated with the condition being treated or the treatment side effects. For instance, a year spent in an intensive care unit (ICU) would be valued differently by a patient compared to a year spent at home with his or her family. Perhaps four years spent in an ICU would be equal to one year spent healthy, so four years spent in an ICU would equal only one healthy year or rather, one QALY. A good example of a cost-utility analysis (and a cost-effectiveness analysis) in the IC literature is one that studied the use of vancomycin as perioperative prophylaxis during coronary-artery bypass graft surgery [9].

Cost-Benefit Analysis

Cost-benefit analysis is a different form of economic evaluation in that all aspects of the analysis, including the consequences of the intervention, are valued in monetary or dollar terms. If an intervention's benefits measured in dollars exceed its costs, then it is considered worthwhile [4]. The major impediment to the use of cost-benefit analysis in healthcare is the requirement to value human life or health benefits in monetary units, such as a human life-year equaling $200,000. Of note, most economic analyses of IC interventions that claim to be cost-benefit analyses are mislabeled because they do not include a dollar value for the important outcomes of interest (e.g., they do not place a dollar value on a human life or quality of life and do not include dollars saved from saving a life or improving quality of life in the analysis).

TABLE 16-1

DIFFERENTIAL EVALUATION OF OUTCOMES AMONG ECONOMIC ANALYSES

Analysis Type	Valuation of Outcomes	Formulation of Final Reported Outcome
Cost minimization (CMA)	None	Dollars saved
Cost effectiveness (CEA)	Natural units (e.g., infections prevented, life-years saved)	Cost per infection prevented or cost per life year saved
Cost utility (CUA)	Healthy years (quality-adjusted life years-QALYs)	Cost per QALY saved
Cost benefit (CBA)	Monetary units	Net benefit (or loss) in dollars
Business case	Monetary units	Net benefit (or loss) in dollars

Which Type of Analysis is Preferred?

Over the past 10 years, cost-effectiveness analysis and the closely related cost-utility analysis have emerged as the preferred methods for economic evaluation in healthcare [4,7]. Importantly, it is recommended to compare new interventions to a reference case whenever possible using standard units such as cost per lives-saved or QALYs-saved [4]. If an agency wanted to choose between funding a hand-hygiene promotion initiative and a cancer-screening program, it would be difficult to compare cost per infection prevented with cost per cancer detected. However, if the comparison was cost per life-years saved or cost per QALY saved with each program, an informed decision could be reached.

What Is Considered Cost Effective?

A standard threshold for calling a program cost effective is for the intervention to cost less than $50,000/QALY saved; however, some suggest the threshold has increased to $100,000/QALY saved [10]. The World Health Organization recommends that a threshold for calling an intervention cost effective be three times the country's gross domestic product per capita, so this threshold is $94,431 in the United States [11]. Frequently, but incorrectly, researchers will state only that an IC intervention is cost effective or cost beneficial if it is cost saving from a hospital perspective. Most healthcare interventions are not cost saving. A review of all cost-effectiveness analyses published between 1976 and 2002 found only 130/1433

(9%) cost-effectiveness ratios actually saved costs, meaning that they saved lives and money at the same time [12].

Perspective

The economic impact of HAIs and interventions can be assessed from the perspective of society, the hospital, a third-party payer (e.g., a health maintenance organization or the Centers for Medicare and Medicaid Services [CMS]), a government agency (e.g., the Veterans Health Administration [VHA]), or the patient. Studies that examine one perspective can underestimate the full economic effect of an infection or intervention; thus, it is important to recognize the perspective of a study to appropriately interpret its results and to design a study from the perspective of interest (Table 16-2). For instance, outpatient physician visits to treat a surgical site infection (SSI) would be important to include in an analysis for the CMS but would not be included in a typical acute care hospital cost analysis.

The societal perspective is one that incorporates all costs and all health outcomes, regardless of who incurs the costs and who obtains the benefit [4]. Typically, except in instances when a specific organization is funding the analysis, the investigator should choose the societal perspective, which is the broadest and most useful when comparing disparate medical interventions. The U.S. Panel on Cost-Effectiveness in Health and Medicine states that even when a particular analysis is requested from a nonsocietal

TABLE 16-2

EXAMPLES OF COSTS AND OUTCOMES INCLUDED UNDER SEVERAL POTENTIAL ANALYSIS PERSPECTIVES FOR HEALTHCARE-ASSOCIATED INFECTION PREVENTION INTERVENTIONS

Type of Resource	Societal Perspective	Payer Prospective	Hospital Prospective
Hospitalization costs			
Antibiotics	X	X	X
Excess length of stay	X	X	X
Intensive care stay	X	X	X
Intervention costs			
Test costs	X		X
Gown and glove	X		X
Nurse and physician time	X		X
Isolation room	X		X
Outpatient expenses			
Physician visits	X	X	
Antibiotics	X	X	
Home health visits	X	X	
Rehabilitation center stay	X	X	
Patient expenses and outcomes			
Mortality	X		
Morbidity	X		
Infections	X		
Lost wages	X		
Travel expenses	X		

perspective, a complete societal perspective analysis also should be completed [4]. Importantly, a societal perspective analysis will inform broader comparisons of programs and could lead to more equitable distribution of resources to improve public health. It is possible that an analysis from the societal perspective would suggest a different strategy than a more limited perspective [4].

For example, an economic analysis done from a hospital perspective would not include patient morbidity (e.g., reduced functional mobility) and outpatient drug costs (Table 16-2). Thus, a hospital might decide not to fund a SSI prevention program, because it will cost more in implementation and equipment costs than it could recoup through reduced SSI costs, such as in shortening length of stay or decreasing antibiotic costs. However, an insurance company that must pay for additional outpatient physician visits, medications, and home-health visits attributable to the preventable SSIs might want to fund the same SSI prevention program. Of course, neither the hospital nor the insurance company perspective includes patient morbidity, mortality, and other important factors, such as the opportunity cost of lost wages. A societal perspective would include all such factors. It might be that a proper cost-effectiveness analysis of the SSI prevention program showing large cost savings and lives saved from a societal perspective would inform CMS or VHA to fund the program to the entire society's benefit. It is possible that the current lack of societal perspective cost-effectiveness analyses of IC interventions has facilitated the current underfunding of IC programs and the continued incidence of preventable HAIs.

Placing Monetary Values in Constant Dollar Terms

Adjustment for Inflation
When data on costs used in economic analyses come from different years, they should be brought into current year values. For instance, if you wanted to include the cost of a methicillin-resistant *Staphylococcus aureus* (MRSA) bacteremia in a business case analysis for your hospital and you had only an estimate of the cost from 2002, you would need to inflate that amount to current year dollars. The typical method for handling these adjustments is to inflate the dollar amounts using a standard price index (e.g., the Medical Component of the Consumer Price Index) [4,13].

Discounting
It is widely accepted that in economic analyses, all future costs and future health consequences should be stated in terms of their present value [3,4]. The process of converting both future dollars and health outcomes to their present value is called discounting. The U.S. Panel on Cost-Effectiveness in Health and Medicine recommends using a discount rate of both 5% and 3% [4]. For example, if you assume that you will save $10,000 in preventing a MRSA infection next year if you decolonize

a patient with intranasal MRSA colonization this year, using a 3% discount rate, the discounted savings would be $10,000/(1 + 0.03)^n$, or $9,709, where n is the number of years in the future the benefit is accrued.

MEASURING THE ECONOMIC IMPACT OF AN HAI OR INFECTION CONTROL INTERVENTION

Measuring the economic impact of an HAI or an intervention to reduce HAIs is important for two reasons. First, these data can be valuable at the local institutional level. Obtaining data regarding the incidence and attributable cost of an HAI allows an individual institution to understand the financial burden of the HAI, and assessing the impact of an intervention is critical in determining whether it is successful and whether extensions of the interventions should be planned. Second, results regarding costs associated with infection and cost savings associated with interventions provide raw data for use in cost-effectiveness, cost-utility, and cost-benefit analyses. This section describes the design and analysis of studies that quantify the impact of HAIs and that measure the outcomes of IC interventions.

Measuring the Attributable Cost of HAIs

Many studies that aim to define the attributable cost of HAIs have been published. Generally, these studies involve a set of patients who develop the infection of interest and a reference group who do not develop the infection. Outcomes such as attributable mortality, length of hospitalization, and costs are compared for the two groups. These studies are by definition cohort studies because the outcomes of interest (e.g., morbidity, mortality, and cost) occur after the exposure of interest (HAI). Examples of these studies include examinations of the mortality and costs associated with central venous catheter–associated bloodstream infection (CVC-BSI) or MRSA-SSIs [14,15].

Defining Costs
Of critical importance is deciding which "costs" to measure. Potential approaches to evaluating the economic burden of HAIs within an institution include measurement of hospital costs, hospital charges, resources used, and actual reimbursed charges [16]. Hospital costs include daily operating costs (sometimes called fixed costs) that do not vary based on patient volume and the cost of drugs, tests, and other patient care–related activities (sometimes called variable costs), which depend on the number of patients admitted or their length of hospitalization [17]. A hospital must ensure that all of its costs are reimbursed; therefore, it assigns fees to hospital resources that are seen on a patient's bill as charges. Insurance companies, Medicare, and Medicaid will not pay the amount on the bill because they receive discounts; therefore, the

charge on the bill for all patients is greater than the actual hospital costs in order to cover these "losses" [18]. Hospital costs can be a useful outcome measure for an individual hospital because they best reflect the actual economic burden of the hospital. However, while some institutions have implemented complex cost accounting systems that track resources used and assign costs, in most institutions costs are difficult to retrieve [19]. In contrast, hospital charges are less reflective of actual cost but usually are easy to retrieve from administrative databases and are consistent from patient to patient in most settings. Because hospital charges typically overestimate actual cost by 25% to 67%, adjustment using cost-to-charge ratios can be performed [19,20]. Both hospital and departmental cost-to-charge ratios are determined annually based on data submitted to the CMS. Hospital cost-to-charge ratios may be a more accurate measure of costs for a cohort of patients in multiple diagnostic related groups (DRG) while departmental cost-to-charge ratios may be more accurate for a cohort of patients in the same DRG [19,21,22].

Direct measurement of resource utilization through the use of microcosting assesses specifically what services or procedures are used by a patient. However, for comparative purposes, use of resources must be translated into monetary value by multiplying the number of tests by their cost or charge. It is important to note that physician professional fees and costs to the patient in the form of lost work are not captured when assessing only hospital costs or charges. In addition, economic measures of health care are not necessarily set by a market-based pricing system. The costs of care for a specific patient are artificial and arbitrary computations that may vary between sites and at different time periods.

Depending on the perspective of the study, the investigator must determine what proportion of hospital costs are reimbursed by payers. If a portion of the costs of an infection are reimbursed by an insurer, then only the portion not reimbursed should be included in a cost analysis from a hospital perspective [23]. This also is the proper cost estimate of a specific HAI that should end up in the business case analysis discussed later. Hospitals may use different ways to limit costs based on their method of reimbursement. For example, if reimbursement occurs *per diem*, the hospital will focus on reducing costly days of stay, such as ICU or surgery days, rather than the total length of stay; if reimbursement occurs based on the DRG or capitation, total expenses are the focus of cost reduction.

The ratio of the total costs or charges of patients with HAIs compared to those without HAIs within one institution over a relatively short period provides the most generalizable estimate of the magnitude of the economic impact of HAIs. In contrast, absolute values of cost or charge cited in studies should be interpreted with more caution because they may not be applicable beyond the institution in which they were collected. It is important to note that some administrators may view business case analyses with

TABLE 16-3
ATTRIBUTABLE COSTS OF HAIS BASED ON PUBLISHED REPORTS[a]

HAI	Attributable Costs		Range	
	Mean	SD	Minimum	Maximum
Bloodstream infection	36,441	37,078	1,822	107,156
Surgical site infection	25,546	39,875	1,783	134,602
Ventilator-associated pneumonia	9,969	2,920	7,904	12,034
Urinary tract infection	1,006	503	650	1,361

[a]In U.S. Dollars.

skepticism if the cost data used are not from the local institution. Multicenter studies must report measures that are standardized across institutions.

If costs of HAIs cannot be measured within your own institution, it may be necessary to use literature sources for the estimation of the economic impact of specific infections before completing a business case analysis of an intervention. A synthesis of the published literature on the cost of HAIs was published by Stone et al. both for the periods from 1990–2000 and from 2001–2004 [1,24]. Their results were limited by the different methods that costs are estimated in the studies that they evaluated but provide the most complete available data of the costs associated with the most common HAIs (Table 16-3).

Methodologic Issues in Cost Outcomes Studies
Several methodologic issues in the design of these cohort studies merit discussion, including controlling for length of hospitalization before infection, adjusting for underlying severity of illness, and selecting of the reference group.

Adjustment for Length of Hospitalization Before Infection
Adjustment for differences in length of hospital stay before the onset of infection in patients with HAIs and total length of hospital stay of the comparator group who did not develop an HAI is important because there is a direct correlation between length of hospitalization and risk of HAI, cost, length of stay after infection, and mortality. Studies in which no adjustment for the "time at risk" for the development of an HAI has been shown to overestimate the length of hospitalization and costs that are attributable to the HAI by up to twofold [25].

Several methods have been proposed for accurately estimating the extra days spent in the hospital as a result of HAIs and the associated increased costs. At a minimum, patients in the reference group who do not develop an HAI should be hospitalized at least as long as the patients who develop an HAI were hospitalized before acquiring the HAI. This can be accomplished by matching case- and comparator-patients based on length of stay before the HAI or by performing more complicated statistical analyses [25].

Adjustment for Underlying Severity of Illness and Comorbidities

In addition, care must be taken in controlling for pre-HAI illness severity and comorbidity. In studies assessing the impact of HAI, adjustment for underlying illness severity and comorbidities is essential because patients who develop HAIs often have a more severe underlying disease than those who do not, which can independently result in adverse outcomes.

Various methods have been proposed and employed to grade severity of illness, including subjective scores, ICU-data driven measures, or administrative severity scores. However, there is currently no well-validated aggregate illness severity score for infectious disease outcomes. McCabe and Jackson used a simple three-category score to predict mortality in patients with gram-negative bacteremia [26]. This scoring system is widely used but subjective, based completely on the judgment of the individual reviewing the patient record. No objective physiologic data are included, limiting its generalizability from study to study. This system works better as predictor for mortality than as a predictor of morbidity and cost.

Other scores that have been proposed also have significant limitations. The Acute Physiology, Age, and Chronic Health Evaluation (APACHE) score relies heavily on physiologic parameters, the majority of which are collected only in ICU settings, and the score has been validated only to predict mortality in ICU patients [27]. Scoring systems such as the Medical Illness Severity Grouping System (MedisGroup) admission severity group score and the All Patient Refined Diagnosis Related Groups (APR-DRG) that were developed for administrative purposes for risk adjustment have questionable utility in predicting infectious disease outcomes and need further evaluation [28].

The timing of the assessment of underlying disease severity is of significant importance. Severity of illness is strongly influenced by the presence of infection and, therefore, may represent an intermediate variable in the chain of events between the exposure (i.e., the infection) and the outcome of interest if assessed when the patient is actively infected. Because adjustment for an intermediate variable usually causes an underestimation of the effect of the exposure of interest on the outcome, care must be taken to assess severity of illness before (e.g., > 48 hours) the first signs of infection [29]. Results of studies that assign the illness severity score at the time of the infection should be interpreted with caution because they may underestimate the magnitude of the effect that resistance has on outcomes [30].

Aggregate comorbidity measures such as the Charlson Co-morbidity Index [31] or the Chronic Disease Score [32] have been used to summarize patients' underlying comorbidities for the purpose of adjustment in studies examining risk factors and outcomes of patients with HAIs [33–36]. In particular, these scores can be a useful method to summarize the degree of comorbidity when it is not feasible to include all individual comorbidities in an analysis with small numbers of subjects.

The Charlson Comorbidity Index was originally designed as a measure of the risk of one-year mortality attributable to comorbidity in a prospective study of hospitalized patients and has been adapted so that it can be calculated using International Classification of Diseases, Ninth Revision (ICD-9) codes obtained from administrative databases [37]. Commonly, it is used, although not well validated, in HAI risk factor and outcome studies.

The Chronic Disease Score is calculated based on current medication use. It was originally based on outpatient medications and used to predict physician-rated disease status, self-rated health status, hospitalization, and mortality. It has since been modified by investigators to be based on medications prescribed on the day of hospital admission to predict SSI risk and the economic impact of SSI [34,38]. In addition, other investigators have developed and validated new comorbidity risk measures based on the Chronic Disease Score for use in HAI risk-factor studies and infections due to MRSA or vancomycin-resistant enterococci (VRE), although these have not been validated to predict outcomes due to infections [36].

Selection of the Reference Group

The majority of studies assessing HAIs have compared outcomes in patients with the infection of interest to patients without the infection. This design assesses the independent impact of HAI acquisition. However, studies that aim to assess the impact of an HAI caused by a specific organism with a particular antibiotic resistance pattern may have two reference groups, one with infection due to the susceptible organism and one without infection. For example, the outcomes of patients with SSI caused by MRSA can be compared to those with SSI caused by methicillin susceptible *S. aureus* (MSSA) to determine the incremental cost associated with methicillin resistance or can be compared to patients without infection to determine the cost associated with MRSA SSI. The latter type of comparison results in a much higher estimate of adverse events attributable to resistance [15].

Measuring the Economic Impact of Interventions to Reduce HAIs

Optimal decisions concerning IC programs must incorporate the economic impact of the specific interventions. Most of the utility of economic analyses in the area of IC is in convincing hospital administration or public health authorities to fund and support a specific intervention. Unfortunately, the current literature is lacking in high-quality studies, such as randomized controlled trials, that can be used to support the effectiveness and cost effectiveness of specific interventions.

Decision making around infection-control interventions requires the availability of proper cost-effectiveness analyses. Several important papers have outlined the optimal methodologies to use when measuring the economic impact of antimicrobial-resistant pathogens [16,20]. However, a 2005 survey of all infection-control intervention studies published found that 69% used the quasi-experimental design, and only 4% incorporated a cost analysis [39]. From the period January 2001 to June 2004, of the 30 studies claiming to be economic analysis of infection-control interventions, only 5 were proper cost-effectiveness analyses [1]. So few studies have been published that assess the cost effectiveness of interventions that there is a glaring need for proper economic evaluation of most infection-control interventions. Importantly, even in the few studies completed, many have inherent methodologic weaknesses that bias against reporting an infection-control intervention as "cost effective." Following are the strengths and weakness of the basic study designs, which should be used when assessing the effectiveness and cost effectiveness of IC interventions.

Randomized Controlled Trials and Cluster-Randomized Control Trials

IC interventions can be broken down into two basic categories. The first is when the patient who is being intervened on is the same patient who directly benefits from the intervention. An example of this type of intervention is optimal timing of antibiotic prophylaxis to reduce SSI risk [40]. In this example, the person who receives the correct antibiotic(s) at the correct time would be at reduced risk of developing an SSI and no other patients in the hospital would directly benefit from this intervention. Therefore, it can be said that the "unit of analysis" is the individual patient if the purpose is to try to measure the benefit of appropriately timed antibiotic use. In this example, the gold standard study design to evaluate the efficacy and safety is the randomized controlled trial. Even though observational trials, such as cohort studies, can yield similar results to randomized controlled trials, a randomized controlled trial is considered the gold standard for evaluating the efficacy of interventions [41–43].

The second category of IC interventions is one in which the specific IC program is directed at either individual patients or a specific population of patients and a group of patients benefits from the program. An example of this type of intervention is active surveillance culturing for MRSA and isolation of colonized patients in a medical ICU setting. To study these types of programs, a cluster randomized trial may be most useful to adjust for the clustering effect that is inherent in control programs of transmissible infectious diseases [44,45]. Patients impacted by these types of IC programs represent a cluster (e.g., an ICU) exposed to a common environment, care practices, and other patients who are colonized with MRSA. Studies that fail to control for the nonindependence of patient outcomes may overestimate the effectiveness of the intervention. Thus, the "unit of analysis" in this case is the entire ICU if the purpose is to try to measure the benefit of active surveillance in reducing MRSA colonization and infection. Instead of randomizing individual patients, individual ICUs need to be randomized so that multiple hospitals will need to be involved at great economic and time costs. These types of trials are called cluster randomized trials or group randomized trials and are used increasingly by public health officials to study group interventions and individual interventions that have group-level effects [46]. Numerous articles have been written about the specific methodologic and ethical issues in cluster randomized trials [45–49].

Situations in which randomized trials cannot be ethically completed are frequent in hospital epidemiology, such evaluating the costs and effectiveness of an intervention to stop an active outbreak [50,51]. Quasiexperimental studies, also known as pre-post intervention studies, and decision analytic models can be used when it is not feasible to perform randomized controlled trials or cluster-randomized control trials.

Quasiexperimental Studies

Like randomized controlled trials, quasiexperimental studies aim to demonstrate causality between and intervention and an outcome [52]. They differ from randomized trials in that patients are put in the intervention arm and control arm without randomization. As a result, these studies have a potentially lower internal validity in that multiple confounders and biases can affect their quality [53]. Even with these limitations, the quasi-experimental study design has been used with increased frequency in IC research; a 2004 review of the published studies that assessed interventions to reduce HAIs found that 69% used a quasiexperimental design and 23% used a randomized trial [39].

The most basic quasiexperimental design is the one-group pretest and posttest design in which a preintervention period is compared to a postintervention period in the same population. An example of this type of study is one in which MRSA infection rates and associated treatment costs in a medical ICU are measured one month before and one month after an intervention when patients are bathed with chlorhexidine. One would expect MRSA rates and associated costs to fall after the intervention, but because there is only one measurement before and after and no control group, many alternative explanations for the fall in MRSA rates could exist.

There is a variety of suggested improvements in the basic quasiexperimental design. These include adding multiple preintervention and postintervention measurements of rates and costs (e.g., increasing the number of months in which MRSA infection rates and associated treatment costs are measured before and after the intervention), including a nonequivalent control group population (e.g., comparing changes in MRSA rates and costs in the medical ICU to those in a surgical ICU when the intervention has not occurred during the same time period, and removing the intervention (e.g., comparing MRSA rates and costs before the intervention, during the intervention and after the intervention is stopped). A more detailed explanation of options for quasi-experimental study designs can be found elsewhere [52–55].

A recent systematic review of IC and antibiotic stewardship articles published during 2002 and 2003 found that 39/73 studies (53%) used the most basic quasiexperimental study design with single measurements before and after the intervention and no control group [54]. Importantly, studies that assess the cost effectiveness of specific IC interventions using the basic quasiexperimental design should be interpreted with caution.

Decision-Analytic Models and Mathematical Models

Mathematical models are useful tools for evaluating intervention strategies before implementing them in human populations [56–62]. Models allow the use of existing knowledge and data in a rigorous, efficient, and testable manner toward the goal of making medical decisions for the assessed population's greatest benefit. Importantly, clinical trials are expensive, labor intensive, and do not necessarily answer the question adequately for populations with all possible baseline characteristics. Creation and analysis of mathematical models can typically be done more quickly and allow investigation within populations with varying characteristics. Therefore, models can be an ideal way to determine which interventions are most cost effective and when they are most cost effective in preventing the spread of transmissible pathogens, including MRSA or VRE [62–64].

As an example, active surveillance and isolation of patients as a tool to control the spread of resistant organisms in hospitals has been available for years but is implemented only in a minority of hospital ICUs due to perceived costs and lack of definitive clinical trial or other data [65]. Many factors or variables that are related to the population (e.g., size of an ICU, discharge rate), individual patients (e.g., comorbidities, age), or infectious organism being evaluated (e.g., duration of colonization, likelihood of infection) can be individually evaluated with modeling strategies to assess their individual and combined importance in causing the observed outcome. This evaluation is called "sensitivity analysis" and is used in most mathematical and decision models [62,66]. Thus, mathematical models can focus future clinical trials, greatly benefit patients, and optimize the expenditures within the limited budgets of microbiology and IC departments. Given the number and great variety of hospitals and other healthcare institutions that exist, it would be nearly

impossible to perform clinical trials to test the cost effectiveness of all potential IC interventions.

PERFORMING A COST-EFFECTIVENESS ANALYSIS

Plenty of existing works describe the step-by-step completion of a cost-effectiveness analysis [3,5,66]. A complete description of a cost-effectiveness analysis is beyond the scope of this chapter; however, it is important to review the steps typically taken in such an analysis to better interpret the literature for use in your specific clinical or hospital situation. Undertaking a thorough cost-effectiveness analysis is quite complicated and usually is completed with the assistance of a healthcare economist. It is important to contrast the methods and results of a cost-effectiveness analysis to those of the more commonly used business case cost analysis, which we discuss in detail later.

Cost-Effectiveness Analysis Example

The method of completing a cost-effectiveness analysis can be broken down into several steps starting with the clear statement of the problem and the proposed interventions. For example, you may wish to compare several different interventions or strategies for reducing CVC-BSIs. These strategies might include an education program that improves CVC-insertion techniques, use of antibiotic-coated catheters, scheduled replacement of catheters, or elimination of femoral venous site catheters. Inherent in the initial framing of the problem is the determination of the perspective of the analysis, such as hospital or societal perspective.

The second step is then to develop a conceptual model for the infection of interest and the potential interventions [5]. A conceptual model allows the investigator to describe the full range of outcomes and costs that occur with the condition of interest and are potentially impacted by the interventions under study. In our example, patient outcomes attributable to CVC-BSI could include excess length of stay, ICU admission, increased antibiotic exposure, and associated mortality. Costs could include acute care hospital costs, outpatient treatment costs, and lost wages. In many instances, the conceptual framework in a cost-effectiveness analysis is a decision-analytic model in the form of a decision tree (Figure 16-1). Thus, the creation of a decision tree is commonly used to frame the conceptual model and complete the analysis. A decision analysis is not the only methodology available for completing a cost-effectiveness analysis; however, it is now the standard method used because it allows for a sensitivity analysis.

After a framework in the form of a decision tree is completed, the next step is to gather the data necessary to complete the analysis, such as the probability of each outcome and the expected decrease (or increase) in each outcome under each intervention. In our example, it would

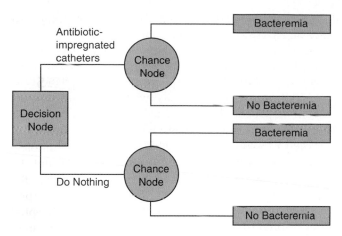

Figure 16-1 Hypothetical decision tree comparing use of antibiotic-impregnated catheters to a "do nothing" strategy in controlling central-venous catheter associate bacteremia.

be important to have an estimate of the daily probability of a CVC-BSI for each day that a CVC is in place. In addition, the probability and length of both excess hospital and ICU stays and mortality associated with BSI would be needed. Most importantly, one would need the proportion of CVC-BSIs prevented under each of the potential interventions and the costs of each intervention.

The data inputs for the decision analytic model can be gathered from existing published literature or from primary data collection using existing hospital administrative or clinical databases. Use of existing literature is important because investigators cannot be expected to complete every possible clinical trial to obtain data for the analysis. Investigators should preferentially use randomized clinical trials, followed by well-designed upper-level quasiexperimental trials and other observational studies [52]. Occasionally, estimates are generated by the use of expert opinion; however, this is typically discouraged and should be carefully examined during the sensitivity analysis.

When all of the necessary outcome probabilities and cost estimates are available, the decision tree can be solved and an estimate of the cost effectiveness of each intervention is completed. Basically, the completed analysis yields a net benefit (benefit of Intervention A minus benefit of Intervention B) and net cost (cost of Intervention A minus cost of Intervention B) of one intervention compared to another alternative intervention. The cost effectiveness is the ratio of net cost to net benefit (e.g., $5,000 per infection prevented, or $15,000 per life saved). In cost-utility analysis, outcomes are presented in QALYs so that the results would be reported in cost per QALY saved (e.g., $2,000 per QALY).

Decision model analysis, like all types of epidemiologic investigation, is associated with uncertainty in the results, particularly when many data inputs are from lower-level studies. It is likely that several input parameters used in the model will be uncertain or have wide confidence intervals.

Importantly, a sensitivity analysis should be performed by varying the model's parameter data and model structure within expected ranges to confirm the model's predictions and assess under what assumptions (e.g., excess length of stay or mortality associated with a CVC-BSI or cost of antibiotic coated catheters) an intervention will be most cost effective in reducing the infections of interest. Sensitivity analyses improve the generalizability of the reported findings so that individual institutions or systems can determine under what conditions the intervention will be cost effective in their own unique hospital or healthcare system.

PERFORMING A BUSINESS CASE ANALYSIS

Given the current reimbursement structure, IC programs often are cost centers, not revenue generating, so they are identified as potential areas for budget cuts [67]. In fact, many IC programs have faced downsizing in recent years [68,69]. Demonstrating value to administrators is increasingly important because health executives are faced with many initiatives and shrinking budgets [70]. To fend off downsizing, IC programs often must complete a business case economic analysis to initiate a new program or justify continuing a program during budget negotiations.

A business case analysis is a type of hospital perspective cost analysis because it typically leaves out patient outcomes. Broadly defined for use in a healthcare improvement intervention, a business case "exists if the entity that invests in the intervention realizes a financial return on its investment in a reasonable time-frame, using a reasonable rate of discounting" [6]. The reasonable return can be through profit, reduction in losses, or cost avoidance. In this instance, the purpose is to look purely at the dollar costs and benefits of an IC intervention or entire program to justify its existence to hospital administrators. The difficulty in making a business case cannot be overlooked because many IC programs lack the economic expertise necessary to complete such an analysis. Anyone considering a business case analysis should contact local institutions' finance administrators for assistance in using the available local cost data.

Often a certain intervention program has been in existence for several years and has kept rates of infections low. If these infections are now rare and no longer perceived as a problem, administrators might want to cut a program focused on controlling the infections, not realizing that the program is highly effective and even cost saving. The same difficulty arises when trying to initiate a new intervention program because it is easy to quantify the costs of a new program but often difficult to estimate the benefits, particularly when very few clinical trials are available to convince administrators and likely even fewer resources to complete studies at your own institution.

One partial solution to facilitate saving an existing program is to examine areas in which the intervention is not in place and compare infection rates in those areas to areas in which the intervention is used. An example would be comparing CVC-BSI rates in a medical ICU where a prevention program exists to those in a surgical ICU that does not have a prevention program. Alternatively, if cost reductions force elimination of a specific program, it would be helpful to stagger the elimination of a program so that as infection rates rise in certain units where an intervention is eliminated, this evidence could be used to re-institute the program.

When an identified problem, new mandate, or new technology leads to the desire to introduce a new IC intervention, it is important to remember that this is the time to collect outcome, cost, and implementation data that will justify this intervention in the future if it faces elimination when the institutional will dissipate. To that end, it often is helpful from an analysis and more importantly from an implementation perspective to roll out a new intervention in a stepwise fashion. This allows comparisons to control populations (wards or ICUs where the intervention has not yet been implemented) using a higher-level quasiexperimental design [52].

Business Case Analysis Example

The steps of a business case analysis parallel those of the cost-effectiveness analysis described earlier. The initial step is framing the problem and developing a hypothesis regarding the potential solutions. For example, you may wish to implement an intervention to reduce SSIs in your hospital. To implement an intervention to reduce these infections, it might be necessary to hire additional staff for your IC department. Thus, you are faced with the task of convincing your hospital administration that the cost of an additional full-time employee (FTE) will be offset by the cost savings through reduced infections, including SSIs.

The next step is to determine the annual cost of the program, in this instance, the salary of an FTE including benefits. This is available from many sources, including your own institutional budgets or available online surveys [71]. For example, an FTE (ICP) might cost $75,000 annually.

You must now determine what costs can be avoided through reduced infections to determine whether the up-front cost of hiring a new ICP can be recouped during a reasonable period of time, usually the current fiscal year. Ideally, you might have data from your own institution that can be analyzed to determine whether SSIs decreased after hiring an ICP. Alternatively, the medical literature must be reviewed to see whether others have published data regarding a similar issue. For example, if 4,000 operations are completed at your institution annually and the current SSI rate is 2%, then 80 SSIs occur per year. If your experience or a literature review suggests that hiring an additional ICP would be expected to reduce SSIs by 25% through additional SSI surveillance including postdischarge surveillance, increased reporting of rates to

surgeons, and improved timing of perioperative antibiotics then an effective ICP would directly prevent 20 SSIs.

After estimating the number of SSIs that could be prevented, the next step is to determine the costs associated with an SSI from your hospital's perspective. If hospital administrative data are readily available, an attributable cost of an SSI could be calculated as described earlier. Alternatively, a literature review might reveal that the average SSI costs $25,000 [1]. At this point, it might be tempting to multiply the expected SSIs prevented, 20, by the estimated costs per SSI and state that hiring an ICP will save $500,000 in SSI costs alone. However, a certain percent of these costs is currently reimbursed by third-party payers. Perhaps at your institution, 75% of costs are reimbursed, so the cost savings from preventing 20 SSI would fall to $125,000. A recent study found that profits on surgical patients fell from $3,288 when there were no complications to $755 when complications occurred [23]. Thus, the hospital still made money when complications occurred but lost a potential profit of approximately $2,500 per complication.

Completing the business case requires taking the estimated cost savings or additional profits and subtracting the costs of the up-front outlay, in this example, the salary and benefits of an ICP. In this example, the total gain to the hospital is estimated to be $50,000. Many IC interventions have multiple benefits. For instance, hand hygiene education that is increased in response to an *Acinetobacter baumannii* outbreak also would be expected to reduce MRSA and VRE infections [72]. To further make the business case for an additional ICP, one could include reduced infections and costs associated with other types of potentially preventable infections that an additional ICP could impact, such as ventilator-associated pneumonia.

Even though a business case analysis does not include the adverse consequences of HAIs, such as patient mortality, hospital administrators do respond to those issues. While patient safety cannot be the whole argument, some calculation of the patient safety improvement associated with the intervention should be included. If mortality associated with an SSI is 5%, preventing 20 SSIs is estimated to prevent one deaths. Additionally, preventing complications, such as SSIs, might be associated with reduced legal costs. These must be included in a proper business case and can influence hospital administration. Thus, a hospitals risk management group should be involved early in any quality improvement program economic analysis.

REFERENCES

1. Stone PW, Braccia D, Larson E. Systematic review of economic analyses of health care–associated infections. *Am J Infect Control.* 2005;33(9):501–509.
2. Mansley EC, McKenna MT. Importance of perspective in economic analyses of cancer screening decisions. *Lancet* 2001;358(9288): 1169–1173.
3. Drummond MF, Sculpher MJ, Torrance GW, et al. *Methods for the economic evaluation of health care programmes.* 3rd. ed. Oxford: Oxford University Press, 2005.

4. Gold MR, Siegel JE, Russell LB, Weinstein MC. *Cost-effectiveness in health and medicine.* 1st ed. New York: Oxford University Press, 1996.

5. Petitti DB. *Meta-Analysis, Decision Analysis, and Cost-Effectiveness Analysis.* 2nd ed. New York: Oxford University Press, 2000.

6. Leatherman S, Berwick D, Iles D, et al. The business case for quality: case studies and an analysis. *Health Aff (Millwood)* 2003;22(2):17–30.

7. Neumann PJ. *Using cost-effectiveness analysis to improve health care.* 1st ed. New York: Oxford University Press, 2005.

8. Stone PW, Hedblom EC, Murphy DM, Miller SB. The economic impact of infection control: making the business case for increased infection control resources. *Am J Infect Control* 2005;33(9):542–547.

9. Zanetti G, Goldie SJ, Platt R. Clinical consequences and cost of limiting use of vancomycin for perioperative prophylaxis: example of coronary artery bypass surgery. *Emerg Infect Dis* 2001;7(5):820–827.

10. Koplan JP, Harpaz R. Shingles vaccine: effective and costly or cost-effective? *Ann Intern Med* 2006;145(5):386–387.

11. World Health Organization. Choosing interventions that are cost effective (WHO-CHOICE) (www.who.int/choice/costs/CER _levels/en/index.html) accessed September 7, 2006.

12. Bell CM, Urbach DR, Ray JG, et al. Bias in published cost effectiveness studies: systematic review. *Bmj* 2006;332(7543):699–703.

13. US Department of Labor Bureau of Labor Statistics. Consumer Price Index. www.bls.gov/cpi/home.htm.

14. Blot SI, Depuydt P, Annemans L, et al. Clinical and economic outcomes in critically ill patients with nosocomial catheter-related bloodstream infections. *Clin Infect Dis* 2005;41(11):1591–1598.

15. Engemann JJ, Carmeli Y, Cosgrove SE, et al. Adverse clinical and economic outcomes attributable to methicillin resistance among patients with Staphylococcus aureus surgical site infection. *Clin Infect Dis* 2003;36(5):592–598.

16. Cosgrove SE, Carmeli Y. The impact of antimicrobial resistance on health and economic outcomes. *Clin Infect Dis* 2003;36(11):1433–1437.

17. Haley RW. Measuring the costs of nosocomial infections: methods for estimating economic burden on the hospital. *Am J Med* 1991;91(suppl 3B):32S–38S.

18. Finkler SA. The distinction between cost and charge. *Ann Intern Med* 1982;96:102–109.

19. Pronovost P, Angus DC. Cost reduction and quality improvement: it takes two to tango. *Crit Care Med* 2000;28(2):581–583.

20. Howard D, Cordell R, McGowan JE Jr, et al. Measuring the economic costs of antimicrobial resistance in hospital settings: summary of the Centers for Disease Control and Prevention–Emory Workshop. *Clin Infect Dis* 2001;33(9):1573–1578.

21. Asby J. *The accuracy of cost measures derived from Medicare cost report data.* Intramural report I-93-01. Washington, DC: Prospective Payment Assessment Commission, 1993.

22. Shwartz M, Young DW, Siegrist R. The ratio of costs to charges: how good a basis for estimating costs? *Inquiry* 1995;32(4):476–481.

23. Dimick JB, Weeks WB, Karia RJ, et al. Who pays for poor surgical quality? Building a business case for quality improvement. *J Am Coll Surg* 2006;202(6):933–937.

24. Stone PW, Larson E, Kawar LN. A systematic audit of economic evidence linking nosocomial infections and infection control interventions: 1990–2000. *Am J Infect Control* 2002;30(3):145–152.

25. Schulgen G, Kropec A, Kappstein I, et al. Estimation of extra hospital stay attributable to nosocomial infections: heterogeneity and timing of events. *J Clin Epidemiol* 2000;53(4):409–417.

26. McCabe W, Jackson G. Gram-negative bacteremia. *Arch Intern Med* 1962;110:847–855.

27. Knaus WA, Draper EA, Wagner DP, Zimmerman JE. APACHE II: a severity of disease classification system. *Crit Care Med* 1985;13(10):818–829.

28. Iezzoni LI. The risks of risk adjustment. *JAMA* 1997;278(19):1600–1607.

29. Robins JM. The control of confounding by intermediate variables. *Stat Med* 1989;8:679–701.

30. Perencevich EN. Excess shock and mortality in staphylococcus aureus related to methicillin resistance. *Clin Infect Dis* 2000;31(5):1311.

31. Charlson ME, Pompei P, Ales KL, MacKenzie CR. A new method of classifying prognostic comorbidity in longitudinal studies: development and validation. *J Chronic Dis* 1987;40(5):373–383.

32. Von Korff M, Wagner EH, Saunders K. A chronic disease score from automated pharmacy data. *J Clin Epidemiol* 1992;45(2):197–203.

33. Batista R, Kaye K, Yokoe DS. Admission-specific chronic disease scores as alternative predictors of surgical site infection for patients undergoing coronary artery bypass graft surgery. *Infect Control Hosp Epidemiol* 2006;27(8):802–808.

34. Kaye KS, Sands K, Donahue JG, et al. Preoperative drug dispensing as predictor of surgical site infection. *Emerg Infect Dis* 2001;7(1):57–65.

35. McGregor JC, Kim PW, Perencevich EN, et al. Utility of the Chronic Disease Score and Charlson Comorbidity Index as comorbidity measures for use in epidemiologic studies of antibiotic-resistant organisms. *Am J Epidemiol* 2005;161(5):483–493.

36. McGregor JC, Perencevich EN, Furuno JP, et al. Comorbidity risk-adjustment measures were developed and validated for studies of antibiotic-resistant infections. *J Clin Epidemiol* 2006;59(12):1266–73.

37. Deyo RA, Cherkin DC, Ciol MA. Adapting a clinical comorbidity index for use with ICD-9-CM administrative databases. *J Clin Epidemiol* 1992;45(6):613–619.

38. Perencevich EN, Sands KE, Cosgrove SE, et al. Health and economic impact of surgical site infections diagnosed after hospital discharge. *Emerg Infect Dis* 2003;9(2):196–203.

39. Larson E. State-of-the-science—2004: time for a "No Excuses/ No Tolerance" (NET) strategy. *Am J Infect Control* 2005;33(9):548–557.

40. Classen DC, Evans RS, Pestotnik SL, et al. The timing of prophylactic administration of antibiotics and the risk of surgical-wound infection. *N Engl J Med* 1992;326(5):281–286.

41. Benson K, Hartz AJ. A comparison of observational studies and randomized, controlled trials. *N Engl J Med* 2000;342(25):1878–1886.

42. Concato J, Shah N, Horwitz RI. Randomized, controlled trials, observational studies, and the hierarchy of research designs. *N Engl J Med* 2000;342(25):1887–1892.

43. Pocock SJ, Elbourne DR. Randomized trials or observational tribulations? *N Engl J Med* 2000;342(25):1907–1909.

44. Hayes RJ, Alexander ND, Bennett S, Cousens SN. Design and analysis issues in cluster-randomized trials of interventions against infectious diseases. *Stat Methods Med Res* 2000;9(2):95–116.

45. Klar N, Donner A. Current and future challenges in the design and analysis of cluster randomization trials. *Stat Med* 2001;20(24):3729–3740.

46. Medical Research Council. *Cluster randomized trials: methodological and ethical considerations,* MRC Clinical Trial Series. London: Medical Research Council, 2002.

47. Bennett S, Parpia T, Hayes R, Cousens S. Methods for the analysis of incidence rates in cluster randomized trials. *Int J Epidemiol* 2002;31(4):839–846.

48. Donner A, Klar N. Pitfalls of and controversies in cluster randomization trials. *Am J Public Health* 2004;94(3):416–422.

49. Elbourne DR, Campbell MK. Extending the CONSORT statement to cluster randomized trials: for discussion. *Stat Med* 2001;20(3):489–496.

50. Muto CA, Giannetta ET, Durbin LJ, et al. Cost-effectiveness of perirectal surveillance cultures for controlling vancomycin-resistant Enterococcus. *Infect Control Hosp Epidemiol* 2002;23(8):429–435.

51. Rao N, Jacobs S, Joyce L. Cost-effective eradication of an outbreak of methicillin—resistant Staphylococcus aureus in a community teaching hospital. *Infect Control Hosp Epidemiol* 1988;9(6):255–260.

52. Harris AD, Bradham DD, Baumgarten M, et al. The use and interpretation of quasi-experimental studies in infectious diseases. *Clin Infect Dis* 2004;38(11):1586–1591.

53. Shadish WR, Cook, T.D., Campbell, D.T. *Experimental and quasi-experimental designs for generalized causal inference.* Boston: Houghton Mifflin, 2002.

54. Harris AD, Lautenbach E, Perencevich E. A systematic review of quasi-experimental study designs in the fields of infection control and antibiotic resistance. *Clin Infect Dis* 2005;41(1):77–82.

55. Shadish WR, Heinsman DT. Experiments versus quasi-experiments: do they yield the same answer? *NIDA Res Monogr* 1997;170:147–164.

56. Austin DJ, Anderson RM. Transmission dynamics of epidemic methicillin-resistant *Staphylococcus aureus* and vancomycin-resistant enterococci in England and Wales. *J Infect Dis* 1999; 179(4):883–891.

57. Austin DJ, Bonten MJ, Weinstein RA, et al. Vancomycin-resistant enterococci in intensive-care hospital settings: transmission dynamics, persistence, and the impact of infection control programs. *Proc Natl Acad Sci USA* 1999;96(12):6908–6913.

58. Austin DJ, Kakehashi M, Anderson RM. The transmission dynamics of antibiotic-resistant bacteria: the relationship between resistance in commensal organisms and antibiotic consumption. *Proc R Soc Lond B Biol Sci* 1997;264(1388): 1629–1638.

59. Austin DJ, Kristinsson KG, Anderson RM. The relationship between the volume of antimicrobial consumption in human communities and the frequency of resistance. *Proc Natl Acad Sci USA* 1999;96(3):1152–1156.

60. Lipsitch M, Cohen T, Cooper B, et al. Transmission dynamics and control of severe acute respiratory syndrome. *Science* 2003;300(5627):1966–1970.

61. Perencevich EN, Fisman DN, Harris AD et al. Benefits of active surveillance for vancomycin resistant enterococcus on admission assessed with a stochastic model (Abstract #1192). Paper presented at 41st Interscience Conference on Antimicrobial Agents and Chemotherapy, September 2001, Chicago, IL.

62. Perencevich EN, Fisman DN, Lipsitch M, et al. Projected benefits of active surveillance for vancomycin-resistant enterococci in intensive care units. *Clin Infect Dis* 2004;38(8):1108–1115.

63. Bootsma MC, Diekmann O, Bonten MJ. Controlling methicillin-resistant *Staphylococcus aureus*: quantifying the effects of interventions and rapid diagnostic testing. *Proc Natl Acad Sci USA* 2006;103(14):5620–5625.

64. Perencevich EN, Hartley DM. Of models and methods: our analytic armamentarium applied to methicillin-resistant Staphylococcus aureus. *Infect Control Hosp Epidemiol* 2005;26(7):594–597.

65. Ostrowsky B, Steinberg JT, Farr B, et al. Reality check: should we try to detect and isolate vancomycin-resistant enterococci patients? *Infect Control Hosp Epidemiol* 2001;22(2):116–119.

66. Hunink M, Glasziou P, Siegel J, et al. *Decision making in health and medicine.* 1st ed. Cambridge, UK: Cambridge University Press, 2001.

67. Murphy DM. From expert data collectors to interventionists: changing the focus for infection control professionals. *Am J Infect Control* 2002;30(2):120–132.

68. Burke JP. Infection control—a problem for patient safety. *N Engl J Med* 2003;348(7):651–656.

69. Calfee DP, Farr BM. Infection control and cost control in the era of managed care. *Infect Control Hosp Epidemiol* 2002;23(7):407–410.

70. Murphy DM, Alvarado CJ, Fawal H. The business of infection control and epidemiology. *Am J Infect Control* 2002;30(2):75–76.

71. 2006 APIC Member Salary and Career Survey (www.apic.org/AM/Template.cfm?Section=Search&section=SecureWrapper&template=/CM/ContentDisplay.cfm&ContentFileID=5981) accessed September 1, 2006.

72. Wright MO, Hebden JN, Harris AD, et al. Aggressive control measures for resistant Acinetobacter baumannii and the impact on acquisition of methicillin-resistant *Staphylococcus aureus* and vancomycin-resistant Enterococcus in a medical intensive care unit. *Infect Control Hosp Epidemiol* 2004;25(2):167–168.

17

Legal Aspects of Healthcare-Associated Infections

Tammy Lundstrom

OVERVIEW

This chapter briefly reviews the basics of medical malpractice as it relates to healthcare-associated infections (HAIs). Then it discusses some of the current legislation that impacts the practice of infection prevention and control and hospital epidemiology. Regulatory agencies and pay-for-performance are discussed elsewhere in this text, so they will not be covered extensively here.

INTRODUCTION

HAIs have received increasing attention since the release of the landmark Institute of Medicine (IOM) report *To Err Is Human*, which highlighted the morbidity and mortality associated with medical errors [1]. HAIs account for an estimated 2 million infections, 90,000 deaths, and $4.5 billion dollars in excess healthcare costs annually [2]. This information has not gone unnoticed by the consumer; a proliferation of consumer Web sites call on regulators, legislators, professional societies, and healthcare organizations themselves to intervene to reduce the incidence of HAIs [3–5]. As of this writing, 15 states through state legislative action have mandated reporting HAIs, 14 of which have mandated public reporting, and most other states have

introduced or are considering such legislation [6]. The Centers for Disease Control and Prevention's (CDC) Healthcare Infection Control Practices Advisory Committee (HICPAC) has issued a guidance document for states considering legislation while concluding that, at the time the document was written, there was not enough evidence to make strong recommendations for or against mandatory public reporting of HAIs [7]. Subsequently, the Association for Professionals in Infection Control and Epidemiology (APIC) and the Society for Healthcare Epidemiology of America (SHEA) issued joint guidance on model legislation [8]. Most legislation introduced after the development of these two documents has incorporated their recommendations.

In 2006, the United States House of Representatives Committee on Energy and Commerce's Subcommittee on Oversight and Investigations held a hearing on HAIs entitled Public Reporting of Hospital-acquired Infection Rates: Empowering Consumers, Saving Lives [9]. After hearing testimony from consumer groups, healthcare organizations, and state collaboratives, the conclusion was that federal legislation is premature and that results from ongoing state efforts may help shape any future federal action.

Although federal action on public reporting of HAIs did not materialize in 2006, many other recent legislative initiatives touch on the practice of infection prevention and control and healthcare epidemiology including privacy laws, the move toward tort (malpractice) reform, public health response to emerging and reemerging pathogens, patient safety legislation, disclosure of adverse events to patients, and changes to Medicare and Medicaid rules, among others. The brief description of each that follows serve as an introduction for those in the infection prevention and control fields.

MEDICAL MALPRACTICE AND HEALTHCARE-ASSOCIATED INFECTION

Despite physician fears of litigation, the landmark Harvard Medical Practice study determined that 3.7% of hospitalizations in New York in 1984 resulted in adverse events, and approximately one-third of these resulted from negligence [10]. Only about 2% of patients suffering negligent injury actually filed malpractice claims [10]. Conversely, less than one-fifth of all claims filed involved negligent injury [10,11]. Nonetheless, there is a strong likelihood that every surgeon will be named in a lawsuit at some time in his or her career [12].

Medical malpractice cases are tried under negligence theory. In a typical medical malpractice case, the plaintiff must prove that the defendant had a duty to the plaintiff, the defendant breached that duty, the breach of duty caused the plaintiff's injury, and the plaintiff actually suffered damages as a result of the breach of duty [13]. Duty usually is established by showing that there is a standard of care that was not followed; this is most frequently shown through the testimony of an expert witness. A national standard of care is frequently sufficient in this era of easy access to information via the Internet, meaning that the expert witness need not come from the same state or area of the country as the defendant but generally is someone with similar background, training, experience, and specialty board certification. Local variation in practice based on facility, service, or equipment differences may still be relevant in some locals [14].

Standards of care also may be established by using evidence-based guidelines, accreditation requirements, federal and state law, and the hospital's own policies and procedures or a combination of them. Thus, when the Joint Commission on Accreditation of Healthcare Facilities [15]. (JCAHO) required hospitals to follow Centers for Disease Control and Prevention (CDC) guidelines for hand hygiene [16], the CDC recommendations look legally more like a national standard of care than the word *guidelines* would lead one to believe. Often an expert witness still is required to authenticate the guideline. In addition, with the proliferation of guidelines from professional societies, experts may interpret evidence differently, leading to inconsistencies between guidelines for the same condition [17]. The defendant could use this to show that there is no professionally agreed upon single standard of care.

As the JCAHO noted, a recent study of obstetric patients found "a six-fold increase in risk of litigation for cases in which there was a deviation from relevant clinical guidelines. Further, one-third of all obstetrical claims analyzed in the study were linked to non-compliant care" [18].

Another legal theory that has been suggested as applicable to medical malpractice is the doctrine of *res ipsa loquiter*, or "the thing speaks for itself." To prevail with this theory, the plaintiff has to prove that (1) the event must be of the kind that ordinarily does not occur in the absence of someone's negligence, (2) it must be caused by an agency or instrumentality within the exclusive control of the defendant, and (3) it must not have been due to any voluntary action or contribution on the part of the plaintiff [19]. This theory is used in circumstances such as surgery on the wrong body part and when the plaintiff underwent surgery and awoke with an injury remote from the surgical site, as in *Ybarra v. Spangard* [19]. It also has been successfully utilized in instances of a retained foreign body after surgery [20].

In a recent case, a plaintiff attempted to use the *res ipsa* doctrine when he developed a *Staphylococcus aureus* surgical site infection following micro lumbar laminectomy [21]. However, the court found that the doctrine did not apply because the infection could have occurred in the absence of anyone's negligence [21]. The plaintiff's expert testified that the infection could have occurred through "(1) foreign object left during surgery; (2) use of non-sterile instruments; (3) non-sterile hands of surgical personnel; (4) other breaks in sterile procedure; (5) post-operative infections of intravenous sites; or (6) presence of the bacteria on the patient's skin" [21]. The expert noted that "intra-operative infections in laminectomy patients occur in 1%–3% of the operations" [21] but had not reviewed the plaintiff's medical records and therefore could not testify that any infection control breaches had actually occurred [21]. In a more recent case, a plaintiff pleading *res ipsa* in a case of staphylococcal infection following cervical surgery lost because she did not present any evidence to show that the infection could not have occurred but for defendant's negligence [22].

Some consumer advocates are promoting the *res ipsa* doctrine for medical malpractice cases involving infection [23]. How courts will respond remains to be seen, but as of this date, the theory has not been very successful.

Recent collaboratives have shown marked reductions in HAIs, particularly catheter-associated bloodstream infection (CA-BSI) or ventilator-associated pneumonia (VAP) when all evidence-based "bundled" practices are followed [24,25]. In fact, some studies have even shown elimination of CA-BSI and/or VAP for many months at a time [25]. However, this example is not equivalent to showing that all such HAIs can be prevented in all patients in all settings, a finding that would make the *res ipsa* doctrine much more likely to yield a successful plaintiff's verdict.

Under theories of *respondeat superior* ("let the master answer") or corporate negligence, the hospital may be held accountable for the actions of its staff and/or physician staff. With *respondeat superior*, the negligent act must be committed in the course of the employee's/physician's duties while acting within the scope of her or his employment. Under corporate negligence, a hospital may be found liable for negligently hiring or retaining its medical or other staff, such as the failure of a hospital to perform background checks on new staff.

It is estimated that medical malpractice costs the U.S. economy $28 billion dollars per year in combined litigation and defensive medicine costs [26]. The JCAHO notes that "there is in fact a fundamental dissonance between the medical liability system and the patient safety movement. The latter depends on the transparency of information on which to base improvement; the former drives such information underground. . . . In sharp contrast to the systems-based orientation of the patient safety movement, tort law targets individual physicians" [27]. The JCAHO offers several suggestions for navigating this patient safety/medical malpractice impasse, including alternative dispute resolution and specialized health courts [27].

INFECTION CONTROL COMMITTEES AND QUALITY PROTECTION STATUTES

Most states have quality protection statutes that shield infection control committee minutes from discovery in the event of a malpractice suit. The theory behind these protective statutes is that investigation and frank discussion for the purpose of quality improvement will be stifled if committee members fear disclosure to plaintiff's attorneys. Infection control committee minutes are protected by the umbrella of quality improvement statues because confidentiality is essential to the functioning of the committee and discussions are aimed at improving the quality of care for subsequent patients.

Hospitals can voluntarily waive quality protection and reveal the results of an investigation if they so desire.

PUBLIC HEALTH EMERGENCIES AND QUARANTINE

Federal statute delegates to the federal government (Department of Health and Human Services [DHHS]) the authority to prevent the introduction of communicable diseases into the Untied States from foreign countries [28]. Infectious diseases covered by federal isolation and quarantine statutes include "cholera, diphtheria, infectious tuberculosis, plague, smallpox, yellow fever, and viral hemorrhagic fevers. Severe acute respiratory syndrome (SARS) was added to this list in April 2003" [28]. In April 2005, executive order added "influenza caused by novel or reemergent influenza

viruses that are causing, or have the potential to cause, a pandemic" to the list [29].

The CDC maintains federal quarantine stations at 18 sites where international travelers arrive [30]. These quarantine stations routinely monitor passengers entering into the United States who are suspected of having a communicable disease; the stations have the authority to temporarily hold planes in order to investigate suspected illness among foreign travelers arriving in the United States. Flight crews are required to notify the quarantine station of ill travelers arriving in the United States aboard inbound flights as soon as illness is detected [30].

In contrast to the federal government, states derive their power to isolate and quarantine under inherent "police power" required to maintain the health, safety, and welfare of its citizens. State laws regarding isolation and quarantine vary considerably.

HIPAA PRIVACY LAWS AND INFECTION CONTROL

The Health Insurance Portability and Accountability Act (HIPAA) of 1996 creates privacy protections for protected health information or information that includes name, date of birth, address, Social Security number, or other information that could be traced back to a single individual [31].

Disclosure of patient health information (PHI) without the authorization of the individual is permitted for purposes including but not limited to: (1) disclosures required by law and (2) "public health activities and purposes" [32]. This includes disclosure to "a public health authority that is authorized by law to collect or receive such information for the purpose of preventing or controlling disease, injury, or disability, including but not limited to, the reporting of disease, injury, vital events . . . , and the conduct of public health surveillance, . . . investigations, and . . . interventions" [32].

"The Privacy Rule permits covered entities to disclose PHI without authorization, to public health authorities or other entities who are legally authorized to receive such reports for the purpose of preventing or controlling disease, injury, or disability. This includes the reporting of disease or injury; reporting vital events (e.g., births or deaths); conducting public health surveillance, investigations, or interventions; reporting child abuse and neglect; and monitoring adverse outcomes related to food (including dietary supplements), drugs, biological products, or medical devices" [33]. The ability to release PHI to public health authorities does not excuse the covered entity from providing an accounting of disclosures to the patient upon request; however, the disclosure accounting may as simple as follows:

Typically, the covered entity must provide the individual with an accounting of each disclosure by date, the PHI disclosed, the identity of the recipient of the PHI, and the purpose of the disclosure. However, where the covered entity has, during the accounting period, made multiple disclosures to the same recipient for the same purpose, the Privacy Rule provides for a simplified means of accounting. In such cases, the covered entity need only identify the recipient of such repetitive disclosures, the purpose of the disclosure, and describe the PHI routinely disclosed. The date of each disclosure need not be tracked. Rather, the accounting may include the date of the first and last such disclosure during the accounting period, and a description of the frequency or periodicity of such disclosures. For example, the vast amount of data exchanged between covered entities and public health authorities is made through ongoing, regular reporting or inspection requirements. A covered healthcare provider routinely may report all episodes of measles it diagnoses to the local public health authority. An accounting of such disclosures to a requesting individual would need to identify the local public health authority receiving the PHI, the PHI disclosed, the purpose of the disclosure (required for communicable disease surveillance), the periodicity (weekly), and the first and last dates of such disclosures during the accounting period (e.g., May 1–June 1, 2003). Thus, the covered entity would not need to annotate each patient's medical record whenever a routine public health disclosure was made [33].

DISCLOSURE OF HAI

The JCAHO, American Medical Association, American Society for Healthcare Risk Management, and many others endorse disclosure of medical errors to patients. The number one contributory factor to sentinel events in the JCAHO database is communication [34]. Consumer groups favor open and honest dialogue when errors occur.

In 2003, the American Hospital Association performed a telephone survey of 500 hospitals with >200 beds to determine hospital attitudes toward disclosure of errors to patients. Of 51% submitting a complete response to the survey, 80% either had a policy on disclosure or was developing one. Of respondents, 65% said they always disclose events that led to serious harm or death, but only 37% said they always disclosure events that lead to short-term harm [35]. In addition, self-admitted disclosure rates were much lower than would have been predicted from rates of adverse events in the published literature. Hospitals were more likely to disclosure nonpreventable than preventable harm [35].

A study using patient and physician focus groups found that physicians thought they should disclose only deviations from the standard of care that caused more than trivial harm, but patients wanted disclosure of more events (deviations from the standard of care, nonpreventable events, poor communication skills, etc.) and wanted *all* events that caused any harm disclosed [36]. A more recent study consisted of a survey of both U.S. and Canadian physicians' attitudes about disclosure. The response rate to the survey was 62%. Responses for U.S.

and Canadian physicians were similar, leading to the conclusion that medical malpractice concerns did not figure into physician attitudes [37]. Ninety-eight percent endorsed disclosure of serious events, and 78% endorsed disclosure of minor harm. Overall, 66% agreed that disclosure reduces malpractice risk [37].

The Veterans Administration (VA) Hospital in Lexington, Kentucky, has practiced active disclosure of adverse events since 1986, including informing the patient about the right to file a malpractice claim. In examining cases filed from 1990–1996 and comparing the Lexington VA with 35 similar VA hospitals that did not practice active disclosure, the authors found no differences in claims filed between disclosing and nondisclosing facilities [38]. However, there is still doubt about how this will translate into the private sector because physicians at the VA cannot be independently sued for malpractice, and veterans can recover without a finding of negligence.

Some states have passed laws that prohibit apologies being used against a physician in a civil action [39,40]. Three states have gone farther—requiring hospitals to disclose adverse events to patients and families in writing [41].

Approximately 21 states have mandatory medical error–reporting systems. Some require reporting of all events including near misses; others require reporting of only serious events. Seven states release incident-specific data [42]. A survey was sent to 203 hospitals; the response rate for chief executive officers (CEOs)/chief organization officers (COOs) was 63%. Most respondents believed that mandatory nonconfidential reporting systems would discourage event reporting within the facility, encourage lawsuits, and have no effect on patient safety. For moderate injuries, respondents from states with confidential reporting systems noted they would be more likely to report than those with nonconfidential systems [42].

The Patient Safety and Quality Improvement Act of 2005 [43] was developed to encourage reporting and analysis of medical errors as recommended by the IOM. Organizations that collect data for the purposes of improving patient safety can apply for designation as a "patient safety organization" (PSO). Data and/or statements prepared by a provider for reporting to a PSO are protected from discovery in a subsequent lawsuit; however, the original source of the information (e.g., medical records) is not [43]. In this way, data prepared for the purpose of submitting to a PSO and then submitted to and analyzed by the PSO would receive similar legal protections as do infection control committees and quality committee proceedings under quality protection statutes. The act directs the DHHS to develop and issue regulations detailing how to implement it [43]. These regulations are still forthcoming.

The American Society for Healthcare Risk Management (ASHRM) Web site contains resources on disclosure of adverse events including a monograph on policy development [44].

HOSPITAL REIMBURSEMENT: THE BUDGET DEFICIT AND RECONCILIATION ACT

Pay-for-performance programs are becoming increasingly common. However, an online recent poll conducted in May 2005 of 2,129 adults age ≥ 18 revealed that 38% of adults favored having health insurance plans pay more to doctors for providing higher quality care. However, 67% said they would be interested in such a program if it helps to lower their costs [45].

In one of the earlier studies of public reporting, those with the lowest scores were most critical of the data validity, and lower scoring facilities had higher levels of performance improvement activities surrounding low-scoring measures upon resurvey [46].

Under the current reimbursement system, in the absence of pay-for-performance programs, hospitals and physicians providing the best evidence-based quality care are paid the same as those whose process and outcomes measures are poor. Although controversy still exists about exact figures and how to best measure them for comparisons, experts agree that HAIs lead to increased morbidity, length of stay, cost, and mortality.

Pay-for-performance programs seek to drive quality improvements. The evidence that prophylactic antibiotics given at the appropriate preoperative time for selective surgical procedures reduce HAIs was known as early as 1992 [47]. However, as of 2005, correct timing of the preoperative antimicrobial dose was only being performed 55.7% of the time [48]. By compensating those who perform at higher levels of quality, payors hope to raise the level of quality in all facilities. On average, patients receive recommended care only 55% of the time, and although per capita spending varies twofold across geographic regions in the United States, this increased cost is not associated with better outcomes [49].

Although public reporting is discussed in another chapter of this text, pay for performance and public reporting go hand in hand because payors want value (high quality and improved outcomes) for dollars spent, consumers want to receive care where quality and safety are better, and healthcare providers want the distinction of being first in quality and patient safety.

The National Quality Forum (NQF) is a public-private partnership of 170 organizations established by the president's commission on quality in 1999. Its goals are twofold: (1) to develop a national strategy for measuring and reporting healthcare quality data and (2) to standardize healthcare performance measures so that comparative data are available across the United States [50]. The NQF has released hospital performance measures from which the Centers for Medicare and Medicaid Services (CMS) has chosen their publicly reported quality data set. The NQF also has released a list of healthcare "never events" and a list of patient safety measures [50]. Most recently, the NQF

charged a steering committee to develop HAI measures suitable for public reporting with the assistance of six technical advisory panels as follows: ventilator-associated pneumonia, bloodstream infection, surgical site infection, urinary tract infection, pediatric HAI measures, and a data integrity and implementation team [50]. The steering team was due to report out its findings for vote by February 2007.

This activity is occurring in the face of the Deficit Reduction Act of 2005 [51]. In fiscal year (FY) 2007, this act requires that CMS expand the starter set of measures from 10 to 22 and impose a 2% reduction in reimbursement for a failure to report data to CMS. It also requires CMS to add measures in 2008 that reflect consensus (e.g., NQF measures). By October 2008 for FY 2009, the DHHS is to consult with CDC to chose two-high volume, high-cost diagnosis-related groups (DRGs) for which the hospital will be reimbursed the simple rather than the complicated DRG rate (reduced reimbursement) if the patient develops an HAI. The two conditions chosen need not be entirely preventable, just *reasonably preventable* if current evidence-based guidelines are followed [51]. In other words, the excess cost of HAI will be borne by the healthcare facility, not the government. The issue for healthcare facilities, of course, is that HAIs may not be preventable even if all evidence-based guidelines are followed all of the time for every patient.

The Federal False Claims Act (FCA) [52], or Whistle-Blower Act, as it is often called, rewards those who uncover fraudulent claims for Medicare reimbursement, for example, by allowing the whistle-blower to sue on behalf of the government and then to collect a percentage of monies recovered in a successful suit from the overcharging party. The whistleblower is to be protected from retaliation [52]. The Deficit Reduction Act will give the states a 10% increase in their share of Medicaid fraud recoveries if they pass state false claims act legislation that is at least as protective as the federal FCA [51]. Finally, all healthcare entities that receive >$5 million in Medicaid funds must educate employees, agents, and contractors about both federal and state whistle-blower acts and provide employees written information on false claims acts and non retaliation policies as well as polices of the institution designed to detect fraud and abuse [51]. These requirements are expected to increase the number of whistle-blower suits filed.

In fact, Erin Brockovich has recently filed one whistle-blower suit on behalf of the federal government (Medicare). In the suit, she alleges that the hospital overcharged Medicare for the excess costs associated with the hospital's medical errors that resulted in additional treatments resulting from the events and increased length of stay [53]. The expenses related to adverse events cited as being charged to Medicare unlawfully include "in-house acquired pressure ulcers, malnutrition, dehydration, fecal impactions, falls, injuries associated with falls, and preventable infections" [54]. If the plaintiff is successful, the results of this lawsuit will have major economic consequences for hospitals and other healthcare facilities.

CONCLUSION

The next few years promise to be active in terms of healthcare law and infection control. The face of infection prevention and control and hospital epidemiology is changing—from attempts to invoke the doctrine of *res ipsa* in HAI suits, to the potential for nonvoluntary quarantine in the event of an influenza or other pandemic, to invoking the FCA whistle-blower statutes against healthcare systems whose patients suffer adverse events, to the continued evolution of pay-for-performance strategies and mandatory HAI reporting legislation. The task of practitioners will be to help shape these changes in a meaningful way that keeps patient safety at the forefront of everything we do.

REFERENCES

1. Institute of Medicine (IOM Report). *To Err Is Human* (www.iom.edu/CMS/8089/5575.aspx) accessed May 2006.
2. Weinstein RA. Nosocomial infection update. *Emerging Infect Dis.* 1998;4:416–20.
3. Committee to Reduce Infection Deaths (www.hospitalinfection.org/) accessed September 2006.
4. Consumers Union (www.consumersunion.org/campaigns/stophospitalinfections/) accessed September 2006.
5. Americans Mad and Angry (The Other AMA) (www.americansmadandangry.org/about-why.php) accessed September 2006.
6. Association for Professionals in Infection Control and Epidemiology State Legislation. (www.apic.org/Content/NavigationMenu/GovernmentAdvocacy/MandatoryReporting /state_legislation/state_legislation.htm) accessed September 2006.
7. Centers for Disease Control and Prevention. Guidance on public reporting of healthcare-associated infections: Recommendations of the Healthcare Infection Control Practices Advisory Committee (www.cdc.gov/ncidod/hip/PublicReportingGuide.pdf) accessed September 2006.
8. Association for Professionals in Infection Control and Epidemiology and Society for Healthcare Epidemiology of America. Model legislation on public reporting of healthcare-associated infections (www.apic.org) accessed June 2006.
9. U.S. Subcommittee on Oversight and Investigations. Public reporting of hospital-acquired infection rates: Empowering consumers, saving lives (energycommerce.house.gov/108/Hearings/03292006hearing1821/hearing.htm#Webcast) accessed September 2006.
10. Brennan TA, Leape LL, Laird N, et al. Incidence of adverse events and negligence to hospitalized patients: Results of the Harvard medical practice study 1. *N Engl J Med* 1991;324:370–76.
11. Studdert DM, Mello MM, Brennan TA. Medical malpractice. *N Engl J Med* 2004;350(3):283–92.
12. Gawande, A. *Complications: A surgeon's notes on an imperfect science.* New York: Metropolitan Books of Henry Holt, 2002. In *Health Care at the Crossroads: Strategies for Improving the Medical Liability System and Preventing Patient Injury* www.jointcommission.org/ accessed September 2006:17.
13. Christie GC, Meeks JE, Pryor ES, Sanders J. Negligence. In: *Cases and Materials on the Law of Torts.* 3rd ed. St. Paul, MN: West, 1997:103.
14. *Primus v. Galgano,* 329 F.3d 236 (1st Cir. 2003).
15. Joint Commission for the Accreditation of Healthcare Organizations. Surveillance prevention and control of infection. In: *2006 Comprehensive accreditation manual for hospital: The official handbook (CAMH).* Oakbrook Terrace, IL: Joint Commission Resources, 2006.
16. Guideline for hand hygiene in healthcare settings. *MMWR* 2002;51(RR-16):1–44.
17. Strausbaugh LJ, Siegel JD, Weinstein RA. Preventing transmission of multidrug-resistant bacteria in healthcare settings: A tale of two guidelines. *Clin Infect Dis* 2006; 42:828–35.
18. Ransom SR, Studdert DM, et al. Reduced medico-legal risk by compliance with obstetrical clinical pathways: A case-control study. *OB/GYN* 2003;101:4. In: *Health care at the crossroads: Strategies for improving the medical liability system and preventing patient injury* (www.jointcommission.org/) accessed September 2006.
19. *Ybarra v. Sangard,* 154 P.2d 687 (1944).
20. *Kambat v. St. Francis,* 89 N.Y.2d 489 (1997).
21. *Neary v. Charleston Area Medical Center, Inc.* Supreme Court of Appeals, West Virginia Civil Action No. 92-C-3717 (1995).
22. *Hoffman v. Pelletier,* 6 A.D.3d 889 (2004).
23. McCughey B. Perspective: The next asbestos. *N.Y. Law Journal* June 6, 2006.
24. Reduction in central-line associated bloodstream infections among patients in intensive care units—Pennsylvania, April 2001–March 2005. *MMWR* 2005;54:1013.
25. Two-year project improves patient safety in hospital ICUs: More than 120 ICUs, 70 hospitals in four states participate. PR Newswire: (www.sev.prnewswire.com/health-care-hospitals/20051013/DETH00513102005-1.html) accessed September 2006.
26. Inglehart J. The malpractice morass: Symbol of societal conflict. *Health Affairs* July/August 2004.
27. Joint Commission on Accreditation of Health Facilities. *Health care at the crossroads: Strategies for improving the medical liability system and preventing patient injury* (www.jointcommission.org/) accessed September 2006.
28. Title 42 United States Code Section 264 (Section 361 of the Public Health Service [PHS] Act (www.cdc.gov/ncidod/dq/lawsand.htm).
29. Department of Health and Human Services. Executive Order April 1, 2005 (www.whitehouse.gov/news/releases/2005/04/20050401-6.html Accessed September 2002).
30. Centers for Disease Control and Prevention. http://www.cdc.gov/ncidod/dq/quarantine_stations.htm. Accessed May 26, 2007.
31. Health Insurance Portability and Accountability Act of 1996 (PL-104-91).
32. 45 CFR §164.512(a), (b)(i).
33. HIPAA privacy rule and public health: Guidance from CDC and the Department of Health and Human Services. *MMWR* 2003;52(S-1):1–12.
34. Joint Commission on Accreditation of Health Facilities. (www.jointcommission.org/) accessed September 2006.
35. American Health and Hospital Association Survey. *Health Affairs* 2003; 22(2):73.
36. Gallagher T, Waterman AD, Ebers AG, et al. Patients' and physicians' attitudes regarding the disclosure of medical errors. *JAMA* 2003;789:1001–07.
37. Gallagher T, Waterman AD, Garbutt JM, et al. US and Canadian physicians' attitudes and experiences regarding disclosing errors to patients. *Arch Intern Med* 2006;166:1605–11.
38. Kraman SS, Hamm G. Risk *Management: Extreme honesty may be the best policy. Ann Intern Med* 1999;131:963–67.
39. Zimmerman R. Doctor's new tool to fight lawsuits: Saying I'm sorry. *Wall Street Journal* May 18, 2004.
40. Zimmerman R. Medical contrition. *Wall Street Journal* May 18, 2004.
41. Liebman CB, Hyman CS. A mediation skills model to manage disclosure of errors and adverse events to patients. *Health Affairs* July/August 2004.
42. Weissman JS, Annas CL, Epstein AM, et al. Erros Reporting and Disclosure Systems: Views From Hospital Leaders. *JAMA* 2005;293:1359–1366.
43. Patient Safety and Quality Improvement Act of 2005. S.544.
44. Disclosure policy: American Society for Healthcare Risk Management (ASHRM) (www.ashrm.org/ashrm/resources/files/DisclosurePart2.Policy.pdf) accessed September 2006.
45. Harris Poll. Public interest in the use of quality metrics in healthcare is mixed—unless it allows them to reduce their health insurance costs. *Wall Street Journal* (http://www.wsj.com/health) accessed June 2006.
46. Hibbard J. Can publicizing hospital quality data improve performance? *Health Affairs* 2003;22:84.

47. Classen DC, Evans RS, Pestotnik SL, et al. The timing of prophylactic antibiotics and the risk of surgical-wound infection. *N Engl J Med* 1992:326:281–86.
48. Bratzler DW, Houck PM, Richards C, et al. Use of antimicrobial prophylaxis for major surgery: Baseline results from the National Surgical Infection Prevention Project. *Arch Surg* 2005;140: 174–82.
49. National Quality Forum. CEO Guide: Pay for Performance 2006. http://38.100.3.36/Search?of=CEO+Guide%3A+Pay+for+ Performance2006&client=default_frontend&proxysheer=default_ frontend&output=xml_no_dth&btnG=Go (or http://www .qualityforum.org/about/) accessed May 25, 2007.
50. National Quality Forum. (www.qualityforum.org) accessed September 2006. (http://www/qualityforum.org/projects/ ongoing/hai/index.asp) accessed May 25, 2007.
51. Deficit Reduction Act of 2005. S.1932 (February 8, 2006). www.acf.hhs.gov/olab/budget/2007/cj2007/Sec3f_cse2007cj.pdf-2006–02.21 accessed May 25, 2007.
52. 32 U.S.C. §3729 et seq.
53. Yi D. Erin Brockovich takes role as plaintiff in Medicare suits. *Los Angeles Times* June 22, 2006.
54. *Brockovich v. Adventist Health*, Superior Court of the State of California for the County of Los Angeles-Central District; Case No: D-57.

Infection Control: A Global View

18

Patricia Lynch, Victor D. Rosenthal, Michael A. Borg, and Sergey R. Eremin

OVERVIEW

History

For centuries, historians and healers have commented about risks for complications associated with healthcare, especially infections. Florence Nightingale began the third edition of *Notes on Hospitals* with "It may be a strange principle to enunciate as the first requirement in a hospital is that it shall do the sick no harm" [1]. As the tools and procedures for care become more sophisticated, however, risk for complications, including healthcare-associated infections (HAI) increases.

Many factors affect infectious diseases: Poverty is a potent amplifier for transmission, morbidity, and mortality of all infections, including HAIs. Wars, homelessness due to poverty and persecution, emergence of new and old deadly and debilitating diseases, global travel and interdependence, economics, and politics all affect transmission and outcomes: Infectious diseases are the second most common cause of death in the world [2]. In the face of such uneven distribution of vital resources, the threat of global epidemics, terrorism with biological weapons and the sheer magnitude of the task, it is easy to feel discouraged about the potential for infection control (IC). There is much more to the story, though, and great cause for optimism.

There are now many well-coordinated global health initiatives, and the benefits of them are apparent in the lives of the recipients and the donors, who have gained skills and experiences of great value. Until recently, there had been no global initiatives to reduce the frequency of HAI, but that picture is slowly changing.

ESTABLISHING PREVENTION OF HAIs AS A GLOBAL PRIORITY

In all countries, resources for national priorities are allocated by governments; healthcare must compete for funding with other major goals, such as education, infrastructure, and the military. Results for building roads, schools, and military are highly visible and often healthcare, being less visible, is a lower priority. Even when it is a priority, the fraction of the health budget that is allocated to prevention of HAIs often is tiny and insufficient. In an ideal world, health issues that have the potential to affect many countries would be addressed globally, and resources would be allocated equitably, recognizing that improvements in global health are not isolated: All benefit indirectly and, in the case of epidemic diseases, many benefit directly.

HAIs are associated with significant patient morbidity and attributable mortality and with increased healthcare costs. Studies conducted in U.S. hospitals have shown that an integrated IC program, including targeted outcome surveillance of device-associated infections (DAIs), can reduce the incidence of HAIs by as much as 32% and lead to reduced healthcare costs [3].

There is a large body of literature which has shown that HAIs are one of the major causes of patient morbidity and mortality in industrialized countries [4,5]. DAIs, such as ventilator-associated pneumonia (VAP) [6–8], central venous catheter-associated bloodstream infection (CVC-BSI) [9–12] and catheter-associated urinary tract infection (CA-UTI) [13] have the greatest challenge to hospital safety and quality healthcare in intensive care unit (ICU) patients.

Prospective targeted epidemiological surveillance of HAIs has been standardized by the Centers for Disease Control and Prevention's (CDC) National Nosocomial Infections Surveillance (NNIS) system, providing definitions for DAIs [14–16]. Targeted surveillance and calculation of DAI rates of infection per 1,000 invasive device-days allows benchmarking with other different institutions in the same or even different countries and facilitates detection and improvement of institutional problems because the specific risk factor is included in the rate calculation.

Global Agenda for IC Research: Research Priorities Project

For many years, lack of any research agenda for the field of infection control was a limitation. In the last 20 years, the field of infection prevention and control has extended beyond the boundaries of HAIs to include all venues where health care is delivered and both patients and care providers. There are still many unanswered fundamental research questions in the areas of infection surveillance, prevention, control, and HAI epidemiology. The lack of an organized and thoughtful research agenda for the future limits the focus to small questions, promotes continued fragmentation, and often wastes valuable resources. An initial research agenda that addresses these newer segments and provides a framework for answering fundamental questions was funded and completed by The Research Foundation for Prevention of Complications Associated with Health Care (formerly APIC Research Foundation) in 2000. These priorities provide a framework for addressing HAI prevention.

The Research Priorities Project [17] used a four-round iterative (Delphi) process with 50 international experts who ultimately identified 21 high-ranked research priorities, which could be condensed into subject areas:

1. Measuring the financial impact of complications and the cost effectiveness of interventions.
2. Studies related to improved antibiotic usage and management of antibiotic resistance.
3. Improving compliance with practices known to be beneficial, especially hand hygiene, appropriate staffing in healthcare institutions, and other proven components of infection prevention and control programs.
4. Surveillance for infectious and noninfectious complications across the spectrum of inpatient and outpatient care delivery.
5. Assessment of prevention strategies at specific sites such as VAP.
6. Preventing occupational transmission of bloodborne pathogens.
7. Creation of regional networks to provide support and information, improve practices, and reduce the steep learning curve more efficiently and economically.

These issues will be addressed in the remainder of the chapter. Although timely in 2,000, currently the priorities would have to include response to biological threats through human intervention ("bioterrorism"), reduction of healthcare-associated transmission of epidemic respiratory diseases such as influenza, and supporting development of early IC programs where they are needed.

Characteristics of Healthcare Facilities

Hospitals and clinics around the world reflect the economic realities of their locations. Any country may have all three tiers represented.

■ In the lowest tier, which is the most common facility at present, adequate supplies of clean water, sterile instruments and supplies for contact with normally sterile body sites, and clean equipment and supplies for contact with mucous membranes and non-intact skin are not available. Adequate hand hygiene is impossible. In these hospitals, patients often share beds and supplies, and families provide much food and care, especially for children. Standards for quality and accreditation do not exist. These facilities rarely have IC information, do not have IC programs, and frequently have HAI outbreaks. Patients and their families often are required to provide care materials, such as syringes, surgical gowns, and medications. Employee training is highly variable and often minimal. Transfusion and injection safety is uncommon and in some regions, transmission of human immunodeficiency virus (HIV) and hepatitis is more frequently related to health care than other means [18].

■ The second tier is the most rapidly growing segment, reflecting economic improvement in much of the world. The hospitals have access to clean water and have sterilizers and cleaning processes, but often availability of sterile or high-level disinfected instruments and supplies is variable. Employees have more training, IC information is available, and occasionally a formal IC program exists with responsibilities assigned to a committee and individuals. Patients are housed in large wards and ICUs. Injection and transfusion safety is variable. Standards for quality are higher and increasing and, in some instances, are measured. Hand hygiene is possible with handwashing or alcohol rubs.

■ The highest tier represents a tiny fraction of hospitals in the world. These facilities, both inpatient and clinics, have single-use sterile instruments and supplies, adequate reprocessing techniques, and abundant clean water. Accreditation processes exist, and most facilities have formal IC programs with committees. Certification of individual knowledge and practices exists and often is required. Complex surveillance systems demonstrate transmission of infectious agents among the patients, particularly in ICUs. Outbreaks of HAIs are rare and quickly recognized. Interestingly, compliance with recommendations for hand hygiene, presurgical antibiotic prophylaxis, and insertion and maintenance of invasive devices, such as central vascular lines and ventilators, is poor, at least by industrial standards such as those for car manufacture or airline maintenance.

Persistent Global Infection Prevention Problems

Global IC efforts are weakened by several factors, the most important of which is inadequate attention and promotion by national and international agencies dedicated to health improvement. Other major issues include poverty and lack of commitment by hospitals, governments, and their ministries of health. Furthermore, the professional societies of physicians, nurses, and laboratorians are not effectively engaged in infection prevention, and many nations have either weak or non existent IC societies.

Global IC is strengthened by factors that unify practitioners and optimize effort, adequate funding and infrastructure, and strong focus. Examples of improvement include the fact that the World Health Organization (WHO) finally has a global health initiative related to HAI prevention and that more than half of all manuscript submissions to the major English-language IC journals are from authors outside the United States, Canada, and the United Kingdom.

LACK OF GLOBAL PLANNING RELATED TO HAIs

The magnitude and scope of the problem of HAIs and the difficulty of gaining improvement have been consistently underestimated by public health agencies. Some examples of global planning have occurred: Severe acute respiratory syndrome (SARS) in 2003 resulted in rapid mobilization of WHO resources coordinated with experts, laboratories, and pharmaceutical research from many national agencies around the world: Tracking and containment of spread was quite successful.

EPIDEMIC RESPIRATORY INFECTIONS

One of the major lessons of SARS received very little attention even in countries with highly developed healthcare facilities: Approximately 40% of SARS infections were acquired in healthcare facilities, presumably reflecting the "normal" transmission rate for similar respiratory pathogens, such as influenza. Transmission of SARS and other epidemic respiratory infections is amplified, not reduced, in healthcare facilities. Massive planning to reduce infection and mortality from H5N1 (Avian) influenza has not recognized the pivotal relationship of healthcare facilities to transmission.

UNSAFE INJECTION AND TRANSFUSION PRACTICES

As part of the Year 2,000 Global Burden of Disease study, investigators quantified the death and disability from injection-associated infections with hepatitis B virus (HBV), hepatitis C virus (HCV), and HIV [18]. They modeled the fraction attributable to healthcare injections in the year 2000 on the basis of the annual number of injections, the proportion of injections administered with reused equipment, the probability of transmission following percutaneous exposure, the prevalence of active infection, the prevalence of immunity, and the total incidence. In 2000, persons in the study regions (countries in the lower 80% of economic strata) received an average of 3.4 injections per year, 39.3% of which were given with reused equipment. In 2000, contaminated injections caused an estimated 21 million HBV infections, 2 million HCV infections, and 260,000 HIV infections, accounting for 32%, 40%, and 5%, respectively, of new infections in that year. This constitutes one of the greatest infection prevention challenges.

HOSPITAL-ACQUIRED NEONATAL INFECTIONS IN DEVELOPING COUNTRIES

Babies born in hospitals in developing countries are at increased risk of neonatal infections because of poor intrapartum and postnatal IC practices. In a major review, reported rates of neonatal infections were 3–20 times higher than those reported for hospital-born babies in industrialized countries [19]. Neonatal infections are estimated to cause 1.6 million annual deaths, or 40% of all neonatal deaths, in developing countries [20]. Neonatal deaths account for more than one-third of the global burden of child mortality [21]. Neonatal mortality rates (deaths in the first 28 days of life) are as high as 40–50 per 1,000 live births in many of the poorest parts of the world. Infections are the major cause of neonatal deaths in developing countries.

WHO: CLEAN CARE IS SAFER CARE: GLOBAL PATIENT SAFETY CHALLENGE

A hopeful sign related to hand hygiene is "Clean Care Is Safer Care," the first global challenge of the WHO World Alliance for Patient Safety [22]. In October 2004, the World Alliance for Patient Safety was formed, focusing first on prevention of HAIs through a combination of initiatives that include mobilizing patients and patient safety organizations, generating teaching tools, directing and conducting research, developing a taxonomy of definitions and data management methods, and coordinating international efforts on future solutions. The intent is to engage all countries in infection prevention.

Countries will be invited to adopt this challenge for their own healthcare systems with the following main principles [23]:

- Formally assessing the scale and nature of HAIs within their healthcare system.
- Adopting an internationally recognized approach to surveillance of the problems so that current baseline incidence of HAI can be established and change can be monitored.
- Conducting an analysis of the root causes of the problem with particular emphasis on "systems thinking."
- Developing solutions to improve safety and reduce risk by focusing on five action areas in particular: (1) hand hygiene, particularly use of alcohol hand rubs, (2) blood safety, (3) injection practices and immunization, (4) water, basic sanitation, and waste management, and (5) clinical procedures.
- Relying on evidence-based best practice in all aspects of addressing the challenge.
- Fully engaging patients and service users as well as healthcare professionals in improvement and action plans.
- Ensuring the sustainability of all action beyond the initial two-year challenge period.

Pittet and Donaldson [22] state the vision of the World Alliance for Patient Safety: "to catalyse commitment by all players—policy makers, frontline staff, patients and managers—to make 'Clean care is safer care' an everyday reality in all countries and everywhere healthcare is provided."

ANTIBIOTIC RESISTANCE AND APPROPRIATE ANTIBIOTIC USE

Antimicrobial resistance poses a particular challenge to developing countries where 45% of deaths are due to infectious diseases [23]. Albeit sparse, available information indicates that the problem is more pronounced in low-resource nations. The SENTRY Antimicrobial Surveillance Program identified the highest prevalence of methicillin-resistant *Staphylococcus aureus* (MRSA) in its collaborating centers within the Far East and Latin America [24] whereas data from the Antibiotic Resistance Surveillance & Control in the Mediterranean Region (ARMed) project (**www.slh.gov.mt/armed**) has shown significantly greater multiresistance in *S. aureus* and *E. coli* within the south and east of the Mediterranean when compared with the more affluent European countries that form the northern border of this region. Studies have proposed a link, at least partial, between antimicrobial use and resistance [25], and it is generally accepted that a pragmatic approach aimed at encouraging good antibiotic prescribing practices should be adopted within healthcare institutions [26].

The axiom describing improper antibiotic prescribing in hospitals as "too many patients receiving unnecessary broadspectrum antibiotics by the wrong route, in the wrong dose and for too long" appears to be particularly relevant in developing countries. Such practices may stem from lack of knowledge of local antibiotic resistance epidemiology as result of inadequate laboratory support, which subsequently influences prescribers to use broadspectrum combinations that offer a stronger psychological reassurance. The situation is compounded by poor quality control of drug production with no guarantee that the indicated amount and type of active ingredient is actually present in the formulation being dispensed or for that matter whether the product being supplied is indeed genuine. Developing nations have reported major problems from counterfeit antibiotics, which either contain little or no active ingredient or in which excipients are adulterated [27]. These drugs proliferate despite the efforts of the regulatory local agencies that often do not possess the necessary analytic capabilities to detect these fakes.

There is good evidence that antibiotic stewardship programs have been successful in modifying antimicrobial prescribing practices, resulting in most instances in reduction of use [28]. Unfortunately, such programs often are lacking in developing countries. Data from ARMed have shown that in even centers with relatively established IC programs and infrastructure, antibiotic policy development, and prescriber feedback of resistance epidemiology often is lacking. Even when these initiatives are in place, sociocultural elements may pose considerable obstacles to progress. Misconceptions may be present among prescribers who feel that personal experience is more relevant than evidence-based recommendations. In the community, patients may choose to self-prescribe and buy over the counter to avoid a doctor's fee or because access to medical advice is too difficult to obtain. Interventions that have been long accepted in Western countries, including prescriber audit and antibiotic restriction, are difficult to implement, especially among senior physicians who possess a high level of influence at both healthcare institution and national levels. Educational opportunities may be limited and the influence of pharmaceutical companies on prescribing decision making is significant. Donations of considerable quantities of antibiotics to healthcare institutions are common practices that often introduce a prescribing bias because the choice of drug would be influenced not on what is microbiologically indicated but on what is easily available (or least expensive).

In the light of these challenges, an integrated approach aimed at improving antibiotic stewardship both within hospitals and in the community is paramount in efforts to reduce HAIs. The WHO has identified, through its Global Strategy for Containment of Antimicrobial Resistance, several areas of intervention to reduce the burden of antimicrobial resistance. The starting point of any strategy needs to focus on training key individuals

TABLE 18-1
KEY RECOMMENDATIONS OF THE WHO GLOBAL STRATEGY FOR CONTAINMENT OF ANTIMICROBIAL RESISTANCE

1. Educate all groups of prescribers and dispensers (including drug sellers) in the importance of appropriate antimicrobial use and containment of antimicrobial resistance.
2. Promote targeted undergraduate and postgraduate educational programs for all health care workers, veterinarians, prescribers and dispensers on accurate diagnosis and management of common infections.
3. Encourage prescribers and dispensers to educate patients on antimicrobial use and the importance of adherence to prescribed treatments.
4. Improve antimicrobial use by supervision and support of clinical practices, especially diagnostic and treatment strategies.
5. Monitor prescribing and dispensing practices and utilize peer group or external standard comparisons to provide feedback and endorsement of appropriate antimicrobial prescribing.
6. Encourage development and use of guidelines and treatment algorithms to foster appropriate use of antimicrobials.
7. Empower formulary managers to limit antimicrobial use to the prescription of an appropriate range of selected antimicrobials.
8. Link professional registration requirements for prescribers and dispensers to requirements for training and continuing education.
9. Establish effective hospital therapeutics committees with responsibility for oversight of antimicrobial use in hospitals.
10. Develop and regularly update guidelines for antimicrobial treatment, prophylaxis, and hospital antimicrobial formularies.
11. Monitor antimicrobial usage, including quantity and patterns of use, and feed back results to prescribers.
12. Ensure on-site availability of microbiology laboratory services which are appropriately matched to the level of the hospital (e.g., secondary, tertiary).
13. Ensure performance and quality assurance of appropriate diagnostic tests, bacterial identification, antimicrobial susceptibility tests of key pathogens, and timely and relevant reporting of results.
14. Ensure that laboratory data are recorded (preferably on a database) and are used to produce clinically and epidemiologically useful surveillance reports of resistance patterns among common pathogens and infections in a timely manner and feed back to prescribers and the infection control programme.
15. Make the containment of antimicrobial resistance a national priority through the creation of a national intersectoral task force to raise awareness about antimicrobial resistance, organize data collection, and allocate resources to promote the implementation of interventions to contain resistance including appropriate utilization of antimicrobial drugs, control and prevention of infection, and research activities.

and allocating resources for effective surveillance, IC, and therapeutic support. Even in the background of limited resources, educational interventions centered on teaching healthcare professionals, especially physicians, and developing and disseminating guidelines will yield good results and improve antibiotic use in healthcare institutions (Table 18-1).

Antimicrobial Resistance in Europe

The European continent provides an interesting multifaceted picture of the epidemiology of multidrug-resistance and its consequences. Data on MRSA produced by the European Antimicrobial Resistance Surveillance System (EARSS) database immediately identifies a consistent north–south shift in prevalence. The north of the continent, especially the Scandinavian countries and Holland, are characterized by very low prevalence of MRSA, in some instances practically nonexistent. Central European countries, including Germany, Poland, and Austria, have intermediate prevalence rates with around 10% of *S. aureus* bacteremias being methicillin resistant. Most, if not all, of the Mediterranean countries exhibit extremely high MRSA infection rates with up to 50% of *S. aureus* isolates being resistant. The United Kingdom and some Eastern European countries (such as

Romania) also follow this pattern. The high MRSA prevalence in the Mediterranean is not restricted only to the European countries of this region. Recent data from the ARMed project has confirmed that MRSA is a major challenge for all of the countries bordering this sea. MRSA proportions >50% have been reported from Turkey, Egypt, and Jordan [29].

It also is apparent that the problem continues to get worse. The most recent EARSS report documents a continued increase in antimicrobial resistance in Spain, Croatia, the United Kingdom, and Italy[EARSS] [3]. Even in the lower prevalence countries, such as Germany, MRSA bacteremia rates have increased almost 20% from its 8.5% level at the beginning of the EARSS study. The Netherlands still maintains a low MRSA rate of 1.1%; however, even this is four times higher than its 1999 rate. There have been some success stories, most notably in Slovenia and France, but they are few and far between, and it is apparent that the struggle against MRSA in most of Europe is one of containment and damage limitation.

The recent emergence of community-acquired MRSA infection in a number of European countries, particularly France, in young, previously healthy adults admitted with severe necrotizing cellulitis or pneumonia increases the importance of controlling MRSA transmission. The community-acquired strains of MRSA are distinct from those causing HAIs and often are found to carry the Panton Valentine leucocidin (PVL) gene [30]. Gould et al. have estimated that MRSA costs the National Health Service of the United Kingdom in excess of £500 million every year while Dancer et al. have calculated extra costs as a result of MRSA infection in a British hospital to range from $3,000 to $30,000 per case [31].

IC Systems in the Former Soviet Union (FSU)

Most developing countries are facing similar problems, but there is a huge geopolitical space in which the situation with IC has several distinctive features. This is the former Soviet Union (FSU: Russia, Ukraine, Belarus, Central Asia, Caucasus, the Baltic states) and, to less extent, its former satellites in Eastern and Southern Europe. These countries have substantial economic, political, and cultural differences, but they share one critical aspect of hospital IC, which is its regulatory framework. In the FSU, HAIs were (and in some countries still are) included in the regulatory purview of an external body (the so-called Sanitary Epidemiologic Service [SES]). This bureau of classically trained epidemiologists and hygienists was responsible for gathering data on infectious diseases and taking corrective, historically authoritarian action. The requirements of SES concerning hospitals were regulated by outdated documents that paid most attention to hospital hygiene, virtually ignoring importance of patient-care practices as major risk factors. Until recently, punitive fines and outdated practices were the norm in IC, and some tension between SES and clinicians remains in many facilities. Although SES continues to wield its power, however, it is currently engaged in a reassessment of hospital epidemiology and IC, realizing that the focal point of IC efforts should be within healthcare facilities themselves.

In addition to a punitive regulatory environment, a historical reluctance to impart potentially embarrassing information coupled with problems in classification and diagnosis still prevents obtaining meaningful HAI surveillance data or national rate estimates. Recently conducted prospective prevalence studies based on the modern internationally recognized technologies (the most reliable data come from the Baltic states, Russia, Kyrgyzstan, and Georgia) have shown that the significance of various infections in most FSU countries (as in many other countries with limited resources) differs from that in the developed countries. Proportion of UTIs, BSIs, and lower respiratory infections rates usually are lower, given relatively low use of invasive devices. At the same time, where reliable data exist, HAI rates often are higher than in the West. Data obtained in most parts of the FSU show that surgical site infections (SSIs) are 2–5 times more frequent compared to NNIS and European surveillance data, which may be partially explained by inadequate antimicrobial prophylaxis and technical and IC deficiencies. For example, Latvia and Lithuania reported overall HAI prevalence rates of 5.6% [32] and 9.2% [33]. Georgia and Russia reported overall SSI incidence rates of 14.7% [34] and 9.5% [35], and Kyrgyzstan reported an overall SSI prevalence rate of 20.2% [36].

The antimicrobial resistance rates, especially MRSA, extended-spectrum beta lactamase (ESBL) producing gram-negatives, or vancomycin-resistant enterococci (VRE), are lower than in most developed countries, but they are increasing, and, taking into account the lack of restrictive antibiotic policies, it is predictable that such rates will increase in the near future.

SURVEILLANCE

Outcome Surveillance

Outcome surveillance is the measurement of the rates and consequences of HAIs, including but not limited to, the following few variables: HAI rates, mortality, extra length of stay, attributable cost, and resistance rates. Development of IC programs in industrialized countries has been supported by outcome surveillance data. Baseline epidemiology should include the previously mentioned activities to plan specific targeted interventions, the most relevant one being the HAI rate.

Outcome surveillance allows evaluation of the cost-effectiveness of specific IC interventions. Such methods also are used to analyze case-control studies to identify risk factors and determine extra cost and mortality. In summary, outcome surveillance is the infrastructure for HAI management. Outcome surveillance of DAI [37,38] has become an integral feature of IC and quality assurance in the industrialized countries since risk adjustment by device use and duration of stay provides a more precise estimate of risk.

Standards for institutional surveillance have been adopted in the United States [37], UK [39], Australia [40], Canada [41], and Germany [42] among other countries. These industrialized countries report HAI rates as DAI per 1,000 device days, allowing them to further analyze the impact of specific risk factors and guide their targeted interventions.

Developing countries more frequently report percentage (cases over discharges or admissions) of HAIs [43–68] (Table 18-2).

Risk of infection is higher among seriously ill patients who often have several indwelling devices, thus the higher infection rates in ICUs. Because the denominator of number of device-days is unknown, it is impossible to compare rates among the hospitals, and the rates are less useful for secular trend comparisons within the same hospital.

Sometimes the HAI rate is reported as number of infections per 1,000 patient-days [43–46,49–53,56–59,66,

TABLE 18-2

OVERALL HEALTHCARE-ASSOCIATED INFECTION RATES IN FACILITIES FROM COUNTRIES DEFINED AS LOW INCOME BY THE WORLD BANK REPORTED AS CRUDE RATES: PROPORTION INFECTED OVER PATIENTS DISCHARGED OR ADMITTED TO THE UNITS AND REPORTED AS PROPORTION INFECTED PER 1,000 PATIENT-DAYS IN THE UNIT OR HOSPITAL

Country	Type of Study/Unit	Type of HAI	HAI Rate (%)	Year	Reference
Argentina	Multicenter adult ICU	Overall	27.0	2003	[43]
Brazil	Multicenter newborn ICU	Overall	28.1	2004	[44]
Brazil	Multicenter adult ICU	Overall	29.6	2006	[45]
Brazil	Newborn ICU	Overall	50.7	2002	[46]
Chile	Hospitalwide	Overall	14.0	2001	[47]
China	Hospitalwide	Overall	3.04	2005	[48]
Colombia	Newborn ICU	Overall	5.3	2005	[49]
Colombia	Multicenter adult ICU	Overall	12.2	2006	[50]
Croatia	Adult ICU	Overall	7.0	2006	[51]
Egypt	Pediatric ICU	Overall	23.0	2005	[52]
India	Multicenter adult ICU	Overall	12.3	2005	[53]
Mexico	Hospitalwide	Overall	21.0	2002	[54]
Mexico	Multicenter adult ICU	Overall	23.2	2000	[55]
Mexico	Multicenter adult ICU	Overall	24.4	2006	[56]
Morocco	Adult medical ICU	Overall	19.3	2005	[57]
Peru	Multicenter adult ICU	Overall	11.2	2005	[58]
Philippines	Adult ICU	Overall	19.1	2006	[59]
Saudi Arabia	Multicenter hospitalwide	Overall	2.8	2004	[60]
Saudi Arabia	Hospitalwide maternity hospital	Overall	4.0	2002	[61]
Saudi Arabia	Hospitalwide	Overall	8.5	2002	[62]
Saudi Arabia	Adult ICU	Overall	19.8	2002	[62]
Saudi Arabia	Newborn ICU	Overall	35.8	2002	[62]
Tanzania	Multicenter hospitalwide	Overall	14.8	2003	[63]
Tanzania	Adult medical ICU	Overall	40.0	2003	[63]
Turkey	Adult ICU	Overall	12.5	2000	[64]
Turkey	Adult ICU	Overall	33.0	2003	[65]
Turkey	Multicenter adult ICU	Overall	20.5	2005	[66]
Turkey	Multicenter adult ICU	Overall	48.7	2004	[67]
Turkey	Neurology ICU	Overall	88.9	2005	[68]
INICC	Multicenter adult ICU	Overall	14.7	2005	[155]
Argentina	Multicenter adult ICU	Overall	90.0 per 1,000 patient-days	2003	[43]
Brazil	Multicenter adult ICU	Overall	30.6 per 1,000 patient-days	2006	[45]
Brazil	Multicenter newborn ICU	Overall	24.9 per 1,000 patient-days	2004	[44]
Brazil	Newborn ICU	Overall	62.0 per 1,000 patient days	2002	[46]
Colombia	Newborn ICU	Overall	6.2 per 1,000 patient-days	2005	[49]
Colombia	Multicenter adult ICU	Overall	18.2 per 1,000 patient-days	2006	[50]
Croatia	Adult ICU	Overall	25.6 per 1,000 patient-days	2006	[51]
Egypt	Pediatric ICU	Overall	40.0 per 1,000 patient-days	2005	[52]
India	Multicenter adult ICU	Overall	21.4 per 1,000 patient-days	2005	[53]
India	Hospitalwide	Overall	36.2 per 1,000 patient-days	2004	[69]
Mexico	Multicenter adult ICU	Overall	39.0 per 1,000 patient-days	2006	[56]
Morocco	Adult medical ICU	Overall	20.4 per 1,000 patient-days	2005	[57]
Peru	Multicenter adult ICU	Overall	25.3 per 1,000 patient-days	2005	[58]
Philippines	Adult ICU	Overall	27.5 per 1,000 patient-days	2006	[59]
Turkey	Multicenter adult ICU	Overall	48.4 per 1,000 patient-days	2005	[70]
Turkey	Neurology ICU	Overall	84.2 per 1,000 patient-days	2005	[66]
INICC[a]	Multicenter adult ICU	Overall	22.5 per 1,000 patient-days	2005	[155]

[a]International Nosocomial Infection Control Consortium.

69,70], but again, the rates may not be compared because of the lack of appropriate denominators.

Device-days were reported in the following recent studies, and infection rates were calculated by number of infections per 1,000 device-days [44,45,50–53,56–59, 66,71–76] (Table 18-3).

Rates of DAI in developing countries were far higher than reported by the NNIS system: The overall rate of CVC-BSI in the International Nosocomial Infection Control Consortium (INICC) medical–surgical ICUs, 12.5 per 1,000 CVC days, is nearly fourfold higher than the 3.4 per 1,000 CVC-days reported for comparable U.S. ICUs; the

TABLE 18-3

DEVICE-ASSOCIATED INFECTIONS REPORTED BY HOSPITALS FROM COUNTRIES DEFINED AS LOW INCOME BY THE WORLD BANK

Country	Type of Study/Unit	Type of HAI	HAI Rate	Year	Reference
Argentina	Multicenter adult ICU	IVD-BSI[a]	30.3 per 1,000 central line days	2004	[71]
Brazil	Multicenter adult ICU	IVD-BSI	9.2 per 1,000 central line days	2006	[45]
Brazil	Multicenter newborn ICU	IVD-BSI	17.3 to 34.9 per 1,000 central line days	2004	[44]
Colombia	Multicenter adult ICU	IVD-BSI	11.3 per 1,000 central line days	2006	[50]
Croatia	Adult ICU	IVD-BSI	8.3 per 1,000 central line days	2006	[51]
Egypt	Pediatric ICU	IVD-BSI	18.7 per 1,000 central line days	2005	[52]
India	Multicenter adult ICU	IVD-BSI	11.1 per 1,000 central line days	2005	[53]
Mexico	Multicenter adult ICU	IVD-BSI	23.1 per 1,000 central line days	2006	[56]
Mexico	Pediatric ward	IVD-BSI	26.0 per 1,000 central line days	2001	[72]
Morocco	Adult medical ICU	IVD-BSI	5.8 per 1,000 central line days	2005	[57]
Peru	Multicenter adult ICU	IVD-BSI	7.8 per 1,000 central line days	2005	[58]
Philippines	Adult ICU	IVD-BSI	8.6 per 1,000 central line days	2006	[59]
Turkey	Hospitalwide	IVD-BSI	9.2 per 1,000 central line days	2004	[73]
Turkey	Multicenter adult ICU	IVD-BSI	24.5 per 1,000 central line days	2005	[66]
Saudi Arabia	Pediatric ICU	IVD-BSI	20.0 per 1,000 central line days	2006	[74]
INICC	Multicenter adult ICU	IVD-BSI	13.0 per 1,000 central line days	2005	[155]
Argentina	Multicenter adult ICU	VAP[b]	46.3 per 1,000 ventilator-days	2004	[71]
Brazil	Multicenter adult ICU	VAP	21.2 per 1,000 ventilator-days	2006	[45]
Brazil	Multicenter newborn ICU	VAP	7.0 to 9.2 per 1,000 ventilator-days	2004	[44]
China	Adult ICU	VAP	32.4 per 1,000 ventilator-days	2004	[75]
Colombia	Multicenter adult ICU	VAP	10.0 per 1,000 ventilator-days	2006	[50]
Croatia	Adult ICU	VAP	47.8 per 1,000 ventilator-days	2006	[51]
Egypt	Pediatric ICU	VAP	10.9 per 1,000 ventilator-days	2005	[52]
India	Multicenter adult ICU	VAP	38.1 per 1,000 ventilator-days	2005	[53]
Mexico	Multicenter adult ICU	VAP	21.8 per 1,000 ventilator-days	2006	[56]
Mexico	Pediatric ward	VAP	28.0 per 1,000 ventilator-days	2001	[72]
Morocco	Adult ICU	VAP	48.1 per 1,000 ventilator-days	2005	[57]
Peru	Multicenter adult ICU	VAP	33.3 per 1,000 ventilator-days	2005	[58]
Philippines	Adult ICU	VAP	22.7 per 1,000 ventilator-days	2006	[59]
Saudi Arabia	Pediatric ICU	VAP	8.9 per 1,000 ventilator-days	2004	[76]
Turkey	Multicenter adult ICU	VAP	24.6 per 1,000 ventilator-days	2005	[66]
INICC[c]	Multicenter adult ICU	VAP	24.6 per 1,000 ventilator-days	2005	[155]
Argentina	Multicenter adult ICU	CAUTI[d]	18.5 per 1,000 device-days	2004	[71]
Brazil	Multicenter adult ICU	CAUTI	9.8 per 1,000 device-days	2006	[45]
Colombia	Multicenter adult ICU	CAUTI	4.3 per 1,000 device-days	2006	[50]
Croatia	Adult ICU	CAUTI	6.0 per 1,000 device-days	2006	[51]
Egypt	Pediatric ICU	CAUTI	25.5 per 1,000 device-days	2005	[52]
India	Multicenter adult ICU	CAUTI	5.7 per 1,000 device-days	2005	[53]
Mexico	Multicenter adult ICU	CAUTI	13.4 per 1,000 device-days	2006	[56]
Morocco	Adult medical ICU	CAUTI	12.5 per 1,000 device-days	2005	[57]
Peru	Multicenter adult ICU	CAUTI	6.2 per 1,000 device-days	2005	[58]
Philippines	Adult ICU	CAUTI	22.0 per 1,000 device-days	2006	[59]
Turkey	Multicenter adult ICU	CAUTI	11.1 per 1,000 device-days	2005	[66]
INICC	Multicenter adult ICU	CAUTI	8.9 per 1,000 device-days	2005	[155]

[a]IVD-BSI: Intravascular device-related bloodstream infection.
[b]VAP: Ventilator-associated pneumonia.
[c]International Nosocomial Infection Control Consortium.
[d]CAUTI: Catheter-associated urinary tract infection.

overall rate of VAP also was higher than the pooled NNIS rates, 24.1 vs. 5.1 per 1,000 ventilator-days, respectively, and the rate of CAUTI was 8.9 compared with 3.3 per 1,000 catheter-days [45,50,51,53,56–59,66,71].

There are a number of explanations for the higher rates of DAIs in developing country ICU patients [72,77,78]. Most developing countries do not have mandatory laws for HAI control programs and hospital accreditation is not mandatory. Hand hygiene is highly variable [79–81]. There are very limited funds and resources for IC [82–85], and nurse-to-patient staffing ratios are lower than in most industrialized countries. Use of outdated technology also is a factor (e.g., use of open rather than closed intravenous infusion and urinary collection systems [86]).

In developing countries, the perception is generally that HAI rates are low and that compliance with hand hygiene recommendations are high. However, frequently no formal outcome and process surveillance is conducted to validate the perception. Outcome surveillance of DAIs defines the magnitude of the problem, identifies the most high risk devices, and provides the framework for planning to reduce infection risk [3]. The second step is to implement targeted specific IC practices that have been shown to prevent HAI [87–91].

The authors have evaluated hospitals in which outcome and process surveillance has been the driving force to reduce HAI risk and related mortality. Targeted incidence of CVC-associated BSIs, CA-UTIs, and nosocomial pneumonia in many developing countries hospitals have been substantially reduced by the institution of outcome surveillance, process surveillance, and targeted performance feedback programs for hand hygiene, central venous catheter, ventilator, and urinary catheter care [92–106].

Process Surveillance

Process surveillance is the standardized collection of data regarding the IC practices actually used in the facility. This includes compliance with hand hygiene recommendations, vascular catheter care, urinary catheter care, measures to prevent VAP (such as position of the head and type of secretion suctioning), and measures to prevent SSI (e.g., presurgical shower, hair removal, antibiotic prophylaxis, etc.). Process surveillance usually is done by observation of actual practices, analysis of the data, and performance feedback to the healthcare personnel.

Hand hygiene is a fundamental aspect of IC; several studies reported a decline in HAI rates when compliance with hand hygiene is enhanced [107–112]. Despite universal acknowledgment of the pivotal role that hand hygiene and device care play in reducing HAI risk, hand hygiene compliance among healthcare workers in developing countries remains poor, with rates ranging from 9% to 75% [92,113–132] (Table 18-4).

A survey of 163 physicians reported that their compliance with hand hygiene recommendations was associated with awareness of being observed, and this is one of the key aspects of process surveillance [133]. Several interventions have been attempted to improve hand hygiene practices; among the most effective are those that emphasize targeted education, process surveillance, and frequent performance feedback [134–138]. Dubbert et al. found that while education alone improved compliance rates in a transient way, process surveillance and performance feedback resulted in sustained improvement in compliance [134].

In developing countries, implementation of education, process surveillance, and performance feedback considerably enhanced hand hygiene [92,114,116,126,139–142] [Table 18-5].

Numerous strategies have been attempted to enhance compliance with hand hygiene; some of them have resulted in improved short-term compliance [134,143,144], (but achievement of sustained improvement remains elusive [109]. In Argentina between April 1999 and October 2003, 15,531 patient contacts were observed in one hospital. The baseline rate of hand hygiene before contact with patients was 17%. With education, process surveillance, and performance feedback, hand hygiene before contact with the patients increased to 58% [114]. This program consisted of frequent focused education of healthcare workers, process surveillance, and performance feedback. Simultaneously, HAI rates were measured at baseline [71] and during the intervention to determine whether improved compliance would be associated with a reduction in HAIs. A 42% relative reduction in HAI rates was reported [92]. Lower adherence was found among physicians, similar to results reported in industrialized countries [133].

Process surveillance for vascular and urinary catheter care also has been effective in reducing associated HAIs in several previous studies conducted in developing countries, such as Argentina [92–94,139], Brazil [95,96], Colombia [97], India [98–100], Mexico [101,103], and Turkey [104–106] among others.

The International Nosocomial Infection Control Consortium (INICC) Program

INICC (www.INICC.org) is a nonprofit, open, multicenter, international, collaborative program modeled on the U.S. NNIS system. Formed in 1998, it is the first international research network and is responsible for much national and global progress. Founded in Argentina, it is a prospective, targeted, and outcome and process surveillance system designed to identify and reduce HAI rates and their consequences in the participating facilities. INICC employs a multiple-approach strategy combining the following interventions: outcome surveillance, process surveillance, performance feedback, targeted interventions guided by risk factor analysis, cost-effective interventions guided by cost analysis, tutorial for surveillance, training in IC guidelines application, secretarial and administrative support in entering data and developing charts, scientific

TABLE 18-4

BASELINE HAND HYGIENE COMPLIANCE BEFORE CONTACT WITH PATIENTS REPORTED BY HOSPITALS FROM COUNTRIES DEFINED AS LOW INCOME BY THE WORLD BANK

Country	Type of Study/Unit	Number of Observations	Hand Hygiene Compliance (%)	Year	Reference
Algeria	Multicenter hospitalwide		18.6	2006	[113]
Argentina	Multicenter adult ICU	15,531	17.0	2003	[114]
Argentina	Adult ICU	1,160	23.1	2005	[92]
Brazil	Multicenter adult ICU	3407	71.5	2004	[115]
China	Newborn ICU		40.0	2004	[116]
Eritrea (Africa)	Hospitalwide		30.0	2005	[117]
South Africa	Hospitalwide		65.2	2003	[118]
Colombia	Multicenter adult ICU	1,692	48.9	2004	[119]
Egypt	Multicenter hospitalwide		52.8	2006	[113]
India	Multicenter adult ICU	588	74.8	2005	[120]
Mexico	Multicenter adult ICU	6,861	35.8	2004	[121]
Mexico	Pediatric ICU	321	64.5	2004	[122]
Mexico	Newborn ICU	1,070	46.3	2005	[123]
Morocco	Adult ICU	139	64.0	2005	[124]
Morocco	Multicenter hospitalwide		16.9	2006	[113]
Peru	Multicenter adult ICU	1,329	63.1	2004	[125]
Russia	Newborn ICU	1,027	44.2	2003	[126]
Thailand	Hospitalwide		24.1	2003	[127]
Tunisia	Multicenter hospitalwide		32.3	2006	[113]
Turkey	Adult ICU		12.9	2002	[128]
Turkey	Multicenter adult ICU	4,657	28.8	2004	[129]
Turkey	Hospitalwide	1,400	31.9	2005	[130]
Turkey	Hematology unit	638	9.0	2005	[131]
INICC[a]	Multicenter adult ICU	62,626	50.9	2006	[132]

[a]International Nosocomial Infection Control Consortium.

data analysis and data interpretation to guide actions, sharing data at scientific meetings and in peer-reviewed journals, and cooperating with hospitals and organizations worldwide. Hospitals review the protocol with their research committees and agree to full participation by signing a commitment sheet and sending it to the INICC central office in Buenos Aires, which then provides analysis and reports monthly, answers questions, and augments the tutorial with personal instruction when needed.

Forms and software designed to record data and direct IC activity are used for both control patients without HAI and cases with HAI. These forms include name, medical record, age, gender, underlying diseases, and severity of illness score at the time of entrance to the ICU. On a daily basis, information regarding temperature, blood pressure, device-days, cultures taken, presence of clinical pneumonia, antibiotic use, and characteristics of any infection is collected both for cases and controls. Thus, it is

TABLE 18-5

RESULTS REPORTED BY PROGRAMS TO IMPROVE HAND HYGIENE COMPLIANCE IN HOSPITALS FROM COUNTRIES DEFINED AS LOW INCOME BY THE WORLD BANK

Country	Type of Study/Unit	Hand Hygiene Compliance Improvement (%)	Year	Reference
Argentina	Multicenter adult ICU	17.0 to 44.0	2003	[114]
Argentina	Adult ICU	23.1 to 64.5	2005	[92]
China	Newborn ICU	40.0 to 53.0	2004	[116]
Mexico	Multicenter adult ICU	35.8 to 75.8	2004	[140]
Mexico	Newborn ICU	46.3 to 67.7	2005	[141]
Russia	Newborn ICU	44.2 to 48.0	2003	[126]
Turkey	Multicenter adult ICU	11.9 to 43.9	2005	[142]

also possible to analyze cases and controls in a prospective cohort nested study [45,50,51,53,56–59,66,71].

At the same time, process surveillance and performance feedback are done for hand hygiene compliance, vascular and urinary catheter care, and mechanical ventilator care. Additional data collected include (1) placement of gauze on intravascular (IV) access insertion sites, marking the date on the IV administration set, condition of the gauze dressing (the presence or absence of moisture, blood, gross soilage, and the appearance of the insertion site), (2) position of the urinary catheter regarding the leg and position of urine bag regarding the bed, position of the bed head, cleanliness of tubes, aspiration technique, and (3) hand hygiene with alcohol hand rub or hand washing with water and antiseptic soap before patient contact. Data are entered into a standard form by local researchers who observed healthcare worker practices in the study units five days a week.

INICC has reported HAI and mortality results from several participating hospitals that applied both outcome and process surveillance (Table 18-6) [86,92–106,139].

Recently, INICC has joined with the International Federation of Infection Control (IFIC) to develop and test clinical definitions to facilitate surveillance in hospitals

that lack laboratory capabilities and thus prevent the hospitals from using the laboratory-based NNIS definitions.

ECONOMIC VALUATION: COSTS OF INFECTIONS, COSTS, AND BENEFITS OF IC

HAIs cost lives, reduce quality of life, and cause loss of productivity; occasionally, patients and/or their families are never whole again. Attributable costs include hospital stay (room and board), drugs and treatment, diagnostic tests, outbreak investigations, and surgical interventions; usually uncounted costs include time off work for patient and family, outpatient care, and societal loss of productivity. All of these costs cannot be adequately quantified, but some costs can be attached, mostly derived from sophisticated hospitals:

■ In the United Kingdom, Plowman reported an overall HAI rate of 7.8% based on 4,000 patients in a local hospital. These patients experienced a stay 11 days longer due to their HAI and costs 2.8 times higher than

TABLE 18-6
BEFORE AND AFTER STUDIES SHOWING HAI AND MORTALITY RATES REDUCTION BY APPLYING INICC STRATEGY

Country	Study Type	ICU	Reduction	RR[a]	CI[b] (95%)	p-Value	Ref
Argentina	Overall D-AI	A	41.0%; 47.56 to 27.9/1,000 bed-days	0.59	0.46–0.74	<0.0001	[92]
	IVD-BSI	A	75.0%; 45.9 to 11.1/1,000 catheter-days	0.25	0.17–0.36	<0.001	[93]
	IVD-BSI	A	64.0%; 6.5 to 2.4/1,000 catheter-days	0.36	0.14–0.94	0.02	[86]
	VAP[e]	A	31.0%; 51.3 to 35.5/1,000 ventilator-days	0.69	0.49–0.98	0.003	[139]
	CAUTI	A	42.0%; 21.3 to 12.4/1,000 catheter-days	0.58	0.39–0.86	0.006	[94]
Brazil	IVD-BSI	A	50.0%; 14.0 to 7.1/1,000 CVC-days	0.50	0.32–0.8	0.002	[95]
	IVD-BSI	A	54.0%; 7.1 to 3.2/1,000 CVC-days	0.46	0.23–0.91	0.02	[96]
Colombia	IVD-BSI	N	89.0%; 54.8 to 6.0/1,000 CVC-days	0.11	0.01–0.98	0.01	[97]
India	Overall D-AI	A	99.3%; 3.9 to 0.3/1,000 bed-days	0.07	0.02–0.34	0.000	[98]
	Overall D-AI	A	62.0%; 18.1 to 6.9/1,000 bed-days	0.38	0.19–0.78	0.006	[99]
	Mortality	A	78.0%; 1.9 to 0.4/1,000 bed-days	0.22	0.06–0.74	0.007	[100]
	IVD-BSI	A	54.0%; 22.6 to 10.3/1,000 bed-days	0.46	0.21–0.98	0.03	[99]
	VAP	A	50.6%; 29.1 to 14.4/1,000 ventilator-days	0.49	0.26–0.93	0.02	[100]
	CAUTI	A	88.8%; 4.5 to 0.5/1,000 catheter-days	0.11	0.01–0.86	0.01	[100]
Mexico	Overall D-AI	N	62.0%; 13.0% to 5.0%/1,000 bed-days	0.38	0.15–0.99	0.0	[103]
	Mortality	A	78.0%; 48.5% to 32.8%/1,000 bed-days	0.68	0.50–0.81	0.01	[101]
	Mortality	A	33.0%; 27.0% to 16.6%/1,000 bed-days	0.67	0.52–0.87	0.002	[102]
	IVD-BSI	A	58.0%; 46.3 to 19.5/1,000 CVC-days	0.42	0.27–0.66	0.0001	[101]
	IVD-BSI	A	82.0%; 17.0 to 3.0/1,000 CVC-days	0.18	0.10–0.32	0.000	[102]
	IVD-BSI	N	75.0%; 40.7 to 10.3/1,000 CVC-days	0.25	0.08–0.84	0.01	[103]
Turkey	Overall D-AI	A	39.0%; 30.0 to 18.3/1,000 bed-days	0.61	0.38–0.98	0.03	[104]
	IVD-BSI	A	82.0%; 10.0 to 1.8/1,000 CVC-days	0.18	0.05–0.6	0.001	[105]
	IVD-BSI	A	82.0%; 29.1 to 13.0/1,000 CVC-days	0.45	0.24–0.82	0.007	[106]

ICU: A, adult; N, neonatal; D-AI, device-associated infection; VAP, ventilator-associated pneumonia; CAUTI, catheter-associated urinary tract infection; IVD-BSI, intravenous device–associated bloodstream infection; CVC, central venous catheter.

uninfected, matched patients; 13% of infected patients died compared with 2% of uninfected patients [146].

- Stone reported results of a systematic audit linking costs of infections and IC interventions. Fifty-five IC studies published between 1990 and 2000 from North America, Europe, Australia, Asia, and South America were reviewed. The investigators found that length of stay decreased from 7.9 to 5.3 during the period but that HAI rates increased from 7.2 to 0.9 per 1,000 patient-days. The average cost for HAIs was $13,973US [146].
- Rosenthal reported HAI rates from ICUs in 10 developing countries to be 3 to 5 times higher than those reported by the NNIS system [45,50,51,53,56–59,66,71]
- Rosenthal also reported that in developing countries, VAP increased length of stay by 9 extra days and increased cost by $2,255 [147] and that CVC-BSIs increased length of stay by 12 extra days and increased cost by $4,888 in Argentina [148], and in Mexico, CVC-BSIs increased length of stay by 6 extra days and increased costs by $11,591 [149].

Who Pays for Infections?

Payer sources for hospitalization can be classified as follows:

- *Single payer systems, such as a government agency, in which all costs and savings accrue to a single budget.* The economic argument for establishing and funding an effective IC program is obvious.
- *Mixed payers such as a combination of government and insurance funding.* These still have a strong economic incentive for effective infection prevention even if there is a fee-for-service component.
- *Fee-for-service health care.* These facilities have little incentive to fund infection prevention, and cost-saving arguments are contrary to their interests. They may be persuaded to improve infection prevention by appealing to national pride, providing statistics from comparable countries, using adverse publicity, and threatening litigation.

Benefits of IC

Many studies have shown that effective infection prevention saves lives and money, but the data usually are from developed countries with single or mixed payer funding. In the United States, the CDC estimated in 2000 that the national cost for HAIs was $6 billion [150]. Haley reported that effective prevention programs in U.S. hospitals reduced HAI rates by 32%; HAIs rank in the top 10 causes of death in the United States. Effective programs conducted outcome surveillance, reported SSI rate data to surgeons, and had a trained physician directing the program and one infection control practitioner for every 250 beds [151]. HAIs are major contributors to complications of health care; one U.S. study reported that between 44,000 and 99,000 deaths

annually are attributable to HAIs. The study also reported that the NNIS system had a positive effect in reducing HAI rates among the participating hospitals [152].

The Keystone Project

Results from the Michigan Health and Hospital Association/Johns Hopkins Hospital Quality & Safety Research Group Keystone Project were announced in October 2005 for 120 hospital ICUs in the state of Michigan [153]. Participating hospitals enforced "best practices" derived from evidence-based studies. Using a predictive model and data collected from project participants, the study reported the total savings after 15 months of study and practice changes was follows:

- Patient lives saved: 1578
- Hospital-days saved: 81,020
- Healthcare dollars saved: $165,534,736

Hospitals participating in Keystone have reduced CVC-BSI infections by 50%. Sixty-eight of the participating ICUs reported no CVC-BSIs or VAPs for six months or more.

IC SOCIETIES: FORCE FOR CHANGE

During the 1950s, a pandemic of HAIs caused by a particularly virulent Staphylococcal 80/81 strain caught the attention of government agencies in the United States and England. Several national conferences were held in each country and, in the United States, led to recommendations from the CDC. The first formal IC program was in England, followed closely by two in the United States.

As the pandemic subsided in the early 1960s, major institutions in several countries began forming committees and appointing physicians, nurses, and laboratorians as IC coordinators. Because education and training in IC was not available as part of the undergraduate work in any of these fields, short workshops were developed, and the multidisciplinary participants began meeting together to share literature and information and to improve skills. By the late 1960s, many more hospitals were benefiting from IC programs and the need for training increased, resulting in 10–14-day workshops in several countries and languages, some of which continue now.

The first national, multidisciplinary IC societies were formed in the early 1970s and are responsible for much national and global progress: professionals are more likely to be effectively focused on the problem, education, research, and solutions than government agencies and are less likely to be distracted by political concerns. Just as the new IC professionals needed support, education, and a network of more experienced individuals, the new IC societies soon found that they also needed some of the same things. IC nurses from United States, United Kingdom, Sweden, Canada, and Denmark requested WHO support for an international IC meeting; WHO sponsored the meeting attended by 75 professionals from 25 countries in 1978, and the development of the International Federation of Infection Control (**www.theIFIC.org**) began soon after. IFIC members are the national IC societies of more than 55 countries [154]. The following are pertinent for the IFIC:

Vision: Every nation has a functioning IC organization.
Mission: The IFIC provides the essential tools, education materials, and communication that unite the existing IC societies and foster development of IC organizations where they are needed.

- IFIC fosters global development of IC societies and improvement in infection prevention practices by providing a communication network to promote education, training, and exchange of information among the member societies with particular emphasis on assisting those with limited resources.

Regional and international networks are an integral part of IFIC:

- Asia Pacific Society of Infection Control (APSIC).
- Eastern Mediterranean Regional Network for IC (EMR-NIC).
- Baltic Network for Infection Control and Containment of Antimicrobial Resistance (BALTICCARE).
- Southeastern Europe Infection Control (SEEIC).
- International Nosocomial Infection Control Consortium (INICC).

CONCLUSION

It is clear that HAIs are a huge and largely unrecognized threat to patient safety in the developing world, far greater than in the developed countries. Successful research in developing countries combined with intensive ongoing efforts to more consistently implement simple and inexpensive measures for prevention will lead to wider acceptance of IC practices in all hospitals of the developing countries.

REFERENCES

1. Nightingale F. *Notes on hospitals*. London: John W Parker, 1859.
2. Fauci AS. Infectious diseases: considerations for the 21st century. *Clin Infect Dis* 2001;32(5):675–685.
3. Hughes JM. Study on the efficacy of nosocomial infection control (SENIC Project): results and implications for the future. *Chemotherapy* 1988;34(6):553–561.
4. Jarvis WR. Selected aspects of the socioeconomic impact of nosocomial infections: morbidity, mortality, cost, and prevention. *Infect Control Hosp Epidemiol* 1996;17(8):552–527.
5. Diaz Molina C, Martinez de la Concha D, Salcedo Leal I, et al. Influence of nosocomial infection on mortality in an intensive care unit. *Gac Sanit* 1998;12(1):23–28.
6. Fagon JY, Chastre J, Vuagnat A, et al. Nosocomial pneumonia and mortality among patients in intensive care units. *JAMA* 1996;275(11):866–869.
7. Papazian L, Bregeon F, Thirion X, et al. Effect of ventilator-associated pneumonia on mortality and morbidity. *Am J Respir Crit Care Med* 1996;154(1):91–97.
8. Heyland DK, Cook DJ, Griffith L, et al. The attributable morbidity and mortality of ventilator-associated pneumonia in the critically ill patient: the Canadian Critical Trials Group. *Am J Respir Crit Care Med* 1999;159(4 Pt 1):1249–1256.
9. Digiovine B, Chenoweth C, Watts C, Higgins M. The attributable mortality and costs of primary nosocomial bloodstream infections in the intensive care unit. *Am J Respir Crit Care Med* 1999;160(3):976–981.
10. Laupland KB, Zygun DA, Doig CJ, et al. One-year mortality of bloodstream infection-associated sepsis and septic shock among patients presenting to a regional critical care system. *Intensive Care Med* 2005;31(2):213–219.
11. Blot S, De Bacquer D, Hoste E, et al. Influence of matching for exposure time on estimates of attributable mortality caused by nosocomial bacteremia in critically ill patients. *Infect Control Hosp Epidemiol* 2005;26(4):352–356.
12. Osmon S, Ward S, Fraser VJ, Kollef MH. Hospital mortality for patients with bacteremia due to Staphylococcus aureus or Pseudomonas aeruginosa. *Chest* 2004;125(2):607–616.
13. Tambyah PA, Knasinski V, Maki DG. The direct costs of nosocomial catheter associated urinary tract infection in the era of managed care. *Infect Control Hosp Epidemiol* 2002;23(1):27–31.
14. Emori TG, Culver DH, Horan TC, et al. National nosocomial infections surveillance system (NNIS): description of surveillance methods. *Am J Infect Control* 1991;19(1):19–35.
15. Horan TC, Emori TG. Definitions of key terms used in the NNIS System. *Am J Infect Control* 1997;25(2):112–116.
16. Garner JS, Jarvis WR, Emori TG, et al. CDC definitions for nosocomial infections, 1988. *Am J Infect Control* 1988;16(3):128–140.
17. Lynch P, Jackson M, Saint S. Research Priorities Project, year 2000: establishing a direction for infection control and hospital epidemiology. *Am J Infect Control* 2001;29(2):73–78.
18. Hauri AM, Armstrong GL, Hutin YJ. The global burden of disease attributable to contaminated injections given in health care settings. *Int J STD AIDS* 2004;15(1):7–16.
19. Zaidi AK, Huskins WC, Thaver D, et al. Hospital-acquired neonatal infections in developing countries. *Lancet* 2005;365(9465):1175–1188.
20. World Health Organisation. Removing obstacles to healthy development. 2006; (www.who.int/infectious-disease-report/index-rpt99.html) accessed February 28, 2006.
21. Lawn JE, Cousens S, Bhutta ZA, et al. Why are 4 million newborn babies dying each year? *Lancet* 2004;364(9432):399–401.
22. Pittet D, Donaldson L. Clean care is safer care: the first global challenge of the WHO World Alliance for Patient Safety. *Am J Infect Control* 2005;33(8):476–479.
23. www.who.int/en/, accessed April 29, 2006.
24. Diekema DJ, Pfaller MA, Schmitz FJ, et al. Survey of infections due to Staphylococcus species: frequency of occurrence and antimicrobial susceptibility of isolates collected in the United States, Canada, Latin America, Europe, and the Western Pacific region for the SENTRY Antimicrobial Surveillance Program, 1997–1999. *Clin Infect Dis* 2001;32 (suppl 2):S114–S132.
25. Gaynes R. The impact of antimicrobial use on the emergence of antimicrobial-resistant bacteria in hospitals. *Infect Dis Clin North Am* 1997;11(4):757–765.
26. Macdougall C, Polk RE. Antimicrobial stewardship programs in health care systems. *Clin Microbiol Rev* 2005;18(4):638–656.
27. Okeke IN, Lamikanra A, Edelman R. Socioeconomic and behavioral factors leading to acquired bacterial resistance to antibiotics in developing countries. *Emerg Infect Dis* 1999;5(1):18–27.
28. Gould IM. A review of the role of antibiotic policies in the control of antibiotic resistance. *J Antimicrob Chemother* 1999;43(4):459–465.
29. Borg MA, Scicluna E, de Kraker M, et al. Antibiotic Resistance in the South-Eastern Mediterranean—preliminary results from the ARMed Project: *Euro Surveill.* 2006;20:11–12.
30. Vandenesch F, Naimi T, Enright MC, et al. Community-acquired methicillin-resistant Staphylococcus aureus carrying Panton-Valentine leukocidin genes: worldwide emergence. *Emerg Infect Dis* 2003;9(8):978–984.
31. Gould IM. The clinical significance of methicillin-resistant Staphylococcus aureus. *J Hosp Infect* 2005;61(4):277–282.

32. Dumpis U, Balode A, Vigante D, et al. Prevalence of nosocomial infections in two Latvian hospitals. *Euro Surveill* 2003;8(3):73–78.

33. Valinteliene R, Jurkuvenas V, Jepsen OB. Prevalence of hospital-acquired infection in a Lithuanian hospital. *J Hosp Infect* 1996;34(4):321–329.

34. Brown S. Incidence of surgical site infection in Tbilisi, Georgia. 12th Annual Meeting of the Society for Healthcare Epidemiology of America, April 6–9, 2006, Salt Lake City, Utah.

35. Brown S, Kyrgyzstan. The incidence of surgical site infections in St. Petersburg, Russia. 11th Annual Meeting of the Society for Healthcare Epidemiology of America, April 1–3, 2001, Toronto, Canada.

36. Djumalieva GA, Kravtsov AA. Epidemiological estimation of prevalence of the surgical site infections and preventive action. *Central Asian Medical Journal* 2004;10(8):152–155.

37. National Nosocomial Infections Surveillance (NNIS) System Report. Data summary from January 1992 through June 2004. issued October 2004. *Am J Infect Control* 2004;32(8):470–485.

38. Richards MJ, Edwards JR, Culver DH, Gaynes RP. Nosocomial infections in coronary care units in the United States. National Nosocomial Infections Surveillance System. *Am J Cardio* 1998;82(6):789–793.

39. Barrett SP. Infection control in Britain. *J Hosp Infect* 2002;50(2):106–109.

40. Reed CS, Gorrie G, Spelman D. Hospital infection control in Australia. *J Hosp Infect* 2003;54(4):267–271.

41. Cook DJ, Walter SD, Cook RJ, et al. Incidence of and risk factors for ventilator-associated pneumonia in critically ill patients. *Ann Intern Med* 1998;129(6):433–440.

42. Gastmeier P, Hentschel J, de Veer I, et al. Device-associated nosocomial infection surveillance in neonatal intensive care using specified criteria for neonates. *J Hosp Infect* 1998;38(1):51–60.

43. Rosenthal VD, Guzman S, Orellano PW, Safdar N. Nosocomial infections in medical-surgical intensive care units in Argentina: attributable mortality and length of stay. *Am J Infect Control* 2003;31(5):291–295.

44. Pessoa-Silva CL, Richtmann R, Calil R, et al. Healthcare-associated infections among neonates in Brazil. *Infect Control Hosp Epidemiol* 2004;25(9):772–777.

45. Salomao R, Nouer S, Grinberg G, et al. Extra Length of stay of Nosocomial Infections at 5 Hospitals of Brazil. Findings of the International Nosocomial Infection Control Consortium (INICC). In: Proceedings and Abstracts of the 16th Annual Scientific Meeting of SHEA; 2006 March 18–21; Chicago, Illinois, USA; p. 91.

46. Nagata E, Brito AS, Matsuo T. Nosocomial infections in a neonatal intensive care unit: incidence and risk factors. *Am J Infect Control* 2002;30(1):26–31.

47. Febre N, de Medeiros ES, Wey SB, et al. Is the epidemiological surveillance system of nosocomial infections recommended by the American CDC applicable in a Chilean hospital? *Rev Med Chil* 2001;129(12):1379–1386.

48. Wang X, Zhou H, Wang X, et al. A study on nosocomial infection among inpatients in Beijing Hospital for elderly. *Zhonghua Liu Xing Bing Xue Za Zhi* 2001;22(3):212–214.

49. Efird MM, Rojas MA, Lozano JM, et al. Epidemiology of nosocomial infections in selected neonatal intensive care units in Colombia, South America. *J Perinatol* 2005.

50. Moreno CA, Rosenthal VD, Olarte N, et al. Device-associated infection rate and mortality in intensive care units of 9 Colombian hospitals: findings of the international nosocomial infection control consortium. *Infect Control Hosp Epidemiol* 2006;27(4):349–356.

51. Kalenic S, Mihaljevic L, Rosenthal VD, et al. Device associated infection rate, stay and mortality in Croatian critical patients: findings of International Nosocomial Infection Control Consortium, July 3–5, 2006, Spier Estate, Stellenbosch, South Africa.

52. El-Nawawy AA, El-Fattah MM, Metwally HA, et al. One year study of bacterial and fungal nosocomial infections among patients in pediatric intensive care unit (PICU) in Alexandria. *J Trop Pediatr* 2005.

53. Mehta Y., Chakravarthy M, Nair R, et al. Device-associated Nosocomial Infection Rates and Extra Length of Stay in Intensive Care Units of India. In: Proceedings and Abstracts of the 15th Annual Scientific Meeting of SHEA; 2005 April 9–12; Los Angeles, California, USA; p. 103.

54. Soto-Hernandez JL, Ramirez-Crescencio MA, Reyes-Ramirez G, et al. Nosocomial infections at a neurologic hospital, analysis of 10 years. *Gac Med Mex* 2002;138(5):397–404.

55. Ponce de Leon-Rosales SP, Molinar-Ramos F, Dominguez-Cherit G, et al. Prevalence of infections in intensive care units in Mexico: a multicenter study. *Crit Care Med* 2000;28(5):1316–1321.

56. Ramirez-Barba EJ, Rosenthal VD, Higuera F, et al. Device-associated nosocomial infection rates in intensive care units in four Mexican public hospitals. *Am J Infect Control* 2006;34(4):244–7.

57. Abouqal R, Madani N, Ali Zeggwagh A, Rosenthal VD. Extra Length of Stay and Device-Associated Nosocomial Infection Rates in Intensive Care Units in One Hospital of Morocco. In: Proceedings and Abstracts of the 45th Annual Scientific Meeting of ICAAC; 2005 December 16–19; Washington, DC, USA; p. 364.

58. Cuellar L, Fernández-Maldonado E, Castañeda-Sabogal A, et al. Extra Length of Stay and Device-Associated Nosocomial Infection Rates in Intensive Care Units in Three Hospitals of Peru. In: Proceedings and Abstracts of the 45th Annual Scientific Meeting of ICAAC; 2005 December 16–19; Washington, DC, USA; p. 364.

59. Ng J, Asetre-Luna I, Rosenthal VD, Yu C. Device-associated infection rate and length of stay in philippine critical patients: findings of International Nosocomial Infection Control Consortium. IFIC, July 3–5, 2006, Spier Estate, Stellenbosch, South Africa.

60. Al-Asmary SM, Al-Helali NS, Abdel-Fattah MM, et al. Nosocomial urinary tract infection: risk factors, rates and trends. *Saudi Med J* 2004;25(7):895–900.

61. Bilal NE, Gedebou M, Al-Ghamdi S. Endemic nosocomial infections and misuse of antibiotics in a maternity hospital in Saudi Arabia. *Apmis* 2002;110(2):140–147.

62. Al-Ghamdi S, Gedebou M, Bilal NE. Nosocomial infections and misuse of antibiotics in a provincial community hospital, Saudi Arabia. *J Hosp Infect* 2002;50(2):115–121.

63. Gosling R, Mbatia R, Savage A, et al. Prevalence of hospital-acquired infections in a tertiary referral hospital in northern Tanzania. *Ann Trop Med Parasitol* 2003;97(1):69–73.

64. Durmaz B, Durmaz R, Otlu B, Sonmez E. Nosocomial infections in a new medical center, Turkey. *Infect Control Hosp Epidemiol* 2000;21(8):534–536.

65. Yologlu S, Durmaz B, Bayindir Y. Nosocomial infections and risk factors in intensive care units. *New Microbiol* 2003;26(3):299–303.

66. Leblebicioglu H, Koksal I, Ulusoy S, et al. Prospective study on intensive care units of North of Turkey. Extra length of stay and device associated rates of nosocomial infections. In: Proceedings and Abstracts of Fifth Pan-American Congress of Infection Control and Hospital Epidemiology; 2004 October, 7–10; Lima, Peru. p. 15.

67. Esen S, Leblebicioglu H. Prevalence of nosocomial infections at intensive care units in Turkey: a multicentre 1-day point prevalence study. *Scand J Infect Dis* 2004;36(2):144–148.

68. Cevik MA, Yilmaz GR, Erdinc FS, Ucler S, Tulek NE. Relationship between nosocomial infection and mortality in a neurology intensive care unit in Turkey. *J Hosp Infect* 2005;59(4):324–330.

69. Taneja N, Emmanuel R, Chari PS, Sharma M. A prospective study of hospital-acquired infections in burn patients at a tertiary care referral centre in North India. *Burns* 2004;30(7):665–669.

70. Leblebicioglu H, Rosenthal VD, Arikan OA, et al. Device-associated hospital-acquired infection rates in Turkish intensive care units. Findings of the International Nosocomial Infection Control Consortium (INICC). *J Hosp Infect* 2007;65(3): 251–7.

71. Rosenthal VD, Guzman S, Crnich C. Device-associated nosocomial infection rates in intensive care units of Argentina. *Infect Control Hosp Epidemiol* 2004;25(3):251–255.

72. Martinez-Aguilar G, Anaya-Arriaga MC, Avila-Figueroa C. Incidence of nosocomial bacteremia and pneumonia in pediatric unit. *Salud Publica Mex* 2001;43(6):515–523.

73. Hosoglu S, Akalin S, Kidir V, Suner A, et al. Prospective surveillance study for risk factors of central venous catheter-related bloodstream infections. *Am J Infect Control* 2004;32(3):131–134.

74. Almuneef MA, Memish ZA, Balkhy HH, et al. Rate, risk factors and outcomes of catheter-related bloodstream infection in a paediatric intensive care unit in Saudi Arabia. *J Hosp Infect* 2006;62(2):207–213.

75. Li HY, He LX, Hu BJ, et al. A prospective cohort study of risk factors for ventilator-associated pneumonia in intensive care unit. *Zhonghua Nei Ke Za Zhi* 2004;43(5):325–328.

76. Almuneef M, Memish ZA, Balkhy HH, et al. Ventilator-associated pneumonia in a pediatric intensive care unit in Saudi Arabia: a 30-month prospective surveillance. *Infect Control Hosp Epidemiol* 2004;25(9):753–758.

77. Rezende EM, Couto BR, Starling CE, Modena CM. Prevalence of nosocomial infections in general hospitals in Belo Horizonte. *Infect Control Hosp Epidemiol* 1998;19(11):872–876.

78. Tinoco JC, Salvador-Moysen J, Perez-Prado MC, et al. Epidemiology of nosocomial infections in a second level hospital. *Salud Publica Mex* 1997;39(1):25–31.

79. Karabey S, Ay P, Derbentli S, et al. Handwashing frequencies in an intensive care unit. *J Hosp Infect* 2002;50(1):36–41.

80. Rosenthal VD, McCormick RD, Guzman S, et al. Effect of education and performance feedback on handwashing: the benefit of administrative support in Argentinean hospitals. *Am J Infect Control* 2003;31(2):85–92.

81. Higuera F, Rosenthal VD, Duarte P, Ruiz J, Franco G, Safdar N. The effect of process control on the incidence of central venous catheter-associated bloodstream infections and mortality in intensive care units in Mexico. *Crit Care Med* 2005;33(9):2022–7.

82. Merchant M, Karnad DR, Kanbur AA. Incidence of nosocomial pneumonia in a medical intensive care unit and general medical ward patients in a public hospital in Bombay, India. *J Hosp Infect* 1998;39(2):143–148.

83. Orrett FA, Brooks PJ, Richardson EG. Nosocomial infections in a rural regional hospital in a developing country: infection rates by site, service, cost, and infection control practices. *Infect Control Hosp Epidemiol* 1998;19(2):136–140.

84. Macias AE, Munoz JM, Bruckner DA, et al. Parenteral infusions bacterial contamination in a multi-institutional survey in Mexico: considerations for nosocomial mortality. *Am J Infect Control* 1999;27(3):285–290.

85. Chandra PN, Milind K. Lapses in measures recommended for preventing hospital-acquired infection. *J Hosp Infect* 2001;47(3):218–222.

86. Rosenthal VD, Maki DG. Prospective study of the impact of open and closed infusion systems on rates of central venous catheter-associated bacteremia. *Am J Infect Control* 2004;32(3):135–141.

87. Centers for Disease Control and Prevention. Guidelines for prevention of nosocomial pneumonia. *MMWR Recomm Rep* 1997;46(RR-1):1–79.

88. O'Grady NP, Alexander M, Dellinger EP, et al. Guidelines for the prevention of intravascular catheter-related infections. *Am J Infect Control* 2002;30(8):476–489.

89. Boyce JM, Pittet D. Guideline for hand hygiene in health-care settings: recommendations of the Healthcare Infection Control Practices Advisory Committee and the HICPAC/SHEA/APIC/IDSA Hand Hygiene Task Force. *MMWR Recomm Rep* 2002;51(RR-16):1–45.

90. Mangram AJ, Horan TC, Pearson ML, et al. Guideline for prevention of surgical site infection, 1999. *Am J Infect Control* 1999;27(2):97–132.

91. Garner JS. Guideline for isolation precautions in hospitals. *Infect Control Hosp Epidemiol* 1996;17(1):53–80.

92. Rosenthal VD, Guzman S, Safdar N. Reduction in nosocomial infection with improved hand hygiene in intensive care units of a tertiary care hospital in Argentina. *Am J Infect Control* 2005;33(7):392–397.

93. Rosenthal VD, Guzman S, Pezzotto SM, Crnich CJ. Effect of an infection control program using education and performance feedback on rates of intravascular device-associated bloodstream infections in intensive care units in Argentina. *Am J Infect Control* 2003;31(7):405–409.

94. Rosenthal VD, Guzman S, Safdar N. Effect of education and performance feedback on rates of catheter-associated urinary tract infection in intensive care units in Argentina. *Infect Control Hosp Epidemiol* 2004;25(1):47–50.

95. Salomao R, Blecher S, Maretti da Silva M, et al. Education and performance feedback effect on rates of central vascular catheter-associated bloodstream infections in adult intensive care units of one Brazilian hospital of Sao Paulo. June 19–23, 2005, Baltimore, Maryland.

96. Salomao R, Maretti Da Silva M, Vilins M, Da Silva E, Blecher S, Rosenthal VD. Prospective Study of the Impact of Switching from an Open IV Infusion System to a Closed System on Rates of Central Venous Catheter-Associated Bloodstream Infection in a Brazilian Hospital. In: Proceedings and Abstracts of the 45th Annual Scientific Meeting of ICAAC; 2005 December 16–19; Washington, DC, USA; p. 363.

97. Villamil-Gómez W, Ruiz-Vergara G. Pertuz AM, Rosenthal VD. Education and performance feedback effect on rates of central vascular catheter-associated bloodstream infections in newborn intensive care units in a private hospital in Colombia. In: Proceedings and Abstracts of the 32nd Annual Scientific Meeting of APIC; 2005 June 19–23; Baltimore, Maryland, USA; p. 82.

98. Chakravarthy M, Jawali V, Rosenthal VD, Venkatachalam N. Process and outcome surveillance plus education and feedback effect on device associated infections rates in Indian critical patients. July 3–5, 2006, Spier Estate, Stellenbosch, South Africa.

99. Mehta A, Rosenthal VD, Rodrigues C, et al. Process and outcome surveillance plus education and performance feedback effect on rates of device associated infections in adult intensive care units of one Indian hospital. VI Pan-American Infection Control and Hospital Epidemiology Meeting; September 11–15, 2006, Porto Alegre, Brazil.

100. Mehta Y, Rosenthal VD, Kapoor P, Pawar M, Tichan N. Effectiveness of Outcome and Process Surveillance for Reducing Ventilator-Associated Pneumonia and Mortality in a Hospital in India. Findings of the INICC. In: Proceedings and Abstract of 8th Annual Meeting of the IFIC; 2007 Oct 18–21; Budapest, Hungary.

101. Higuera F, Rosenthal VD, Duarte P, et al. The effect of process control on the incidence of central venous catheter-associated bloodstream infections and mortality in intensive care units in Mexico. *Crit Care Med* 2005;33(9):2022–2027.

102. Rangel-Frausto MS, Higuera F, Soto JM, Rosenthal VD. Cost effectiveness of switching from an open IV infusion system to a closed system on rates of central venous catheter-associated bloodstream infection in three Mexican hospitals. In: Proceedings and Abstracts of the 32nd Annual Scientific Meeting of APIC; 2005 June 19–23; Baltimore, Maryland, USA; p. 61.

103. Sobreyra Oropeza M, Herrera-Bravo M, Rosenthal VD. Nosocomial Infection Global Rates and Central Vascular Catheter—Associated Bloodstream Infections Rates Reduction in a Newborn Intensive Care Unit of One Mexican Public Hospital. In: Proceedings and Abstracts of the 15th Annual Scientific Meeting of SHEA; 2005 April 9–12, Los Angeles, California, USA; p. 123.

104. Koksal I, Aydin K, Rosenthal VD, Caylan R, Senel AC. Effectiveness of Outcome and Process Surveillance for Reducing Ventilator-Associated Pneumonia in a Hospital of Turkey. Findings of the INICC. In: Proceedings and Abstracts of the 34th Annual Scientific Meeting of APIC; 2007 June 24–28; San Jose, USA.

105. Ozgultekin A, Rosenthal VD, Turan G, Akgun N. Education and Performance Feedback Effect on Rates of Central Vascular Catheter—Associated Bloodstream Infections in Adult Intensive Care Units of One Turkish Hospital. In: Proceedings and Abstracts of the 33rd Annual Scientific Meeting of APIC; 2006 June 11–15; Tampa, Florida, USA; p. 24.

106. Ulger F, Esen S, Leblebicioglu H, Rosenthal VD. Process and outcome surveillance plus education and feedback effect on bloodstream infections in one Turkish intensive care unit. July 3–5, 2006, Spier Estate, Stellenbosch, South Africa.

107. Larson E. Skin hygiene and infection prevention: more of the same or different approaches? *Clin Infect Dis* 1999;29(5):1287–1294.

108. Doebbeling BN, Stanley GL, Sheetz CT, et al. Comparative efficacy of alternative hand-washing agents in reducing nosocomial infections in intensive care units. *N Engl J M* 1992;327(2):88–93.

109. Pittet D, Hugonnet S, Harbarth S, et al. Effectiveness of a hospital-wide programme to improve compliance with hand hygiene. *Lancet* 2000;356(9238):1307–1312.

110. Fendler EJ, Ali Y, Hammond BS, et al. The impact of alcohol hand sanitizer use on infection rates in an extended care facility. *Am J Infect Control* 2002;30(4):226–1233.

111. Zafar AB, Butler RC, Reese DJ, et al. Use of 0.3% triclosan (Bacti-Stat) to eradicate an outbreak of methicillin-resistant Staphylococcus aureus in a neonatal nursery. *Am J Infect Control* 1995;23(3):200–208.

112. Casewell M, Phillips I. Hands as route of transmission for Klebsiella species. *Br Med J* 1977;2(6098):1315–1317.

113. Amazian K, Abdelmoumene T, Sekkat S, et al. Multicentre study on hand hygiene facilities and practice in the Mediterranean area: results from the NosoMed Network. *J Hosp Infect* 2006;62(3):311–318.

114. Rosenthal VD, McCormick RD, Guzman S, et al. Effect of education and performance feedback on handwashing: the benefit of administrative support in Argentinean hospitals. *Am J Infect Control* 2003;31(2):85–92.

115. Salomao R, Maretti Da Silva M, Vilins M, et al. Multi-center prospective study to evaluate hand washing compliance in hospitals from Brazil: behaviour comparison between different stratums. Fifth Pan–American Congress of Infection Control and Hospital Epidemiology; October 7–10, 2004, Lima, Peru.

116. Lam BC, Lee J, Lau YL. Hand hygiene practices in a neonatal intensive care unit: a multimodal intervention and impact on nosocomial infection. *Pediatrics* 2004;114(5):e565–e571.

117. Samuel R, Almedom AM, Hagos G, et al. Promotion of handwashing as a measure of quality of care and prevention of hospital-acquired infections in Eritrea: the Keren study. *Afr Health Sci* 2005;5(1):4–13.

118. Jelly S, Tjale A. Hand decontamination practices in paediatric wards. *Curationis* 2003;26(4):72–76.

119. Álvarez Moreno C, Linares C, Agray M, et al. Multi-center prospective study to evaluate hand washing compliance in hospitals from Colombia: behaviour comparison between different stratums. Fifth Pan–American Congress of Infection Control and Hospital Epidemiology, October 7–10, 2004, Lima, Peru.

120. Mehta Y, Chakravarthy M, Nair R, Jawali V, Pawar M, Rosenthal VD. Prospective study to evaluate handwashing compliance in two Indian hospitals, in New Delhi and Bangalore. In: Proceedings and Abstracts of the 32nd Annual Scientific Meeting of APIC; 2005 June 19–23, Baltimore, Maryland, USA; p. 80.

121. Higuera F, Duarte P, Franco G, et al. Prospective Study to Evaluate Hand Washing Compliance In Public Hospitals From Mexico. Behaviour Comparison Between Different Stratums. In: Proceedings and Abstracts of Fifth Pan-American Congress Of Infection Control and Hospital Epidemiology; 2004 October, 7–10; Lima, Peru. p. 21.

122. Armas Ruíz A, Yberri I, Nuñez Espinoza E, et al. Prospective study to evaluate hand washing compliance in one pediatric intensive care unit of a Social Security hospital from mexico: behaviour comparison between different stratums. Fifth Pan-American Congress of Infection Control and Hospital Epidemiology, October 7–10, 2004, Lima, Peru.

123. Sobreyra-Oropeza M, Bravo MH, Rosenthal VD. Effect of education and performance feedback on handwashing in a public hospital in Mexico City. In: Proceedings and Abstracts of the 32nd Annual Scientific Meeting of APIC; 2005 June 19–23; Baltimore, Maryland, USA; p. 81.

124. Abouqal R, Zeggwagh A, Madani N, Rosenthal VD. Hand washing compliance in a hospital of Morocco. Difference between stratums. In: Proceedings and Abstracts of the 15th Annual Scientific Meeting of SHEA; 2005 April 9–12; Los Angeles, California, USA; p. 90.

125. Cuellar L, Rosales R, Castillo Bravo LI, et al. Multi-center national prospective study to evaluate hand washing compliance in hospitals from Peru: behaviour comparison between different stratums. Fifth Pan-American Congress of Infection Control and Hospital Epidemiology, October 7–10, 2004, Lima, Peru.

126. Brown SM, Lubimova AV, Khrustalyeva NM, et al. Use of an alcohol-based hand rub and quality improvement interventions to improve hand hygiene in a Russian neonatal intensive care unit. *Infect Control Hosp Epidemiol* 2003;24(3):172–179.

127. Paotong D, Trakarnchansiri J, Phongsanon K, et al. Compliance with handwashing in a university hospital in Thailand. *Am J Infect Control* 2003;31(2):128.

128. Karabey S, Ay P, Derbentli S, et al. Handwashing frequencies in an intensive care unit. *J Hosp Infect* 2002;50(1):36–41.

129. Cetinkaya Y, Yildirim G, Iskit A, et al. Multi-center national prospective study to evaluate hand washing compliance in hospitals from Turkey: behaviour comparison between different stratums. Fifth Pan-American Congress of Infection Control and Hospital Epidemiology, October 7–10, 2004, Lima, Peru.

130. Kuzu N, Ozer F, Aydemir S, et al. Compliance with hand hygiene and glove use in a university-affiliated hospital. *Infect Control Hosp Epidemiol* 2005;26(3):312–315.

131. Saba R, Inan D, Seyman D, et al. Hand hygiene compliance in a hematology unit. *Acta Haematol* 2005;113(3):190–193.

132. Rosenthal VD, Salomao R, Leblebicioglu H, Akan O, Sobreyra-Oropeza M. Hand Hygiene Compliance in Argentina, Brazil, Colombia, India, Mexico, Morocco, Peru and Turkey. Findings of the International Nosocomial Infection Control Consortium (INICC). In: Proceedings and Abstracts of the 33rd Annual Scientific Meeting of APIC; 2006 June 11–15; Tampa, Florida, USA; p. 31.

133. Pittet D, Mourouga P, Perneger TV. Compliance with handwashing in a teaching hospital: infection control program. *Ann Intern Med* 1999;130(2):126–130.

134. Dubbert PM, Dolce J, Richter W, et al. Increasing ICU staff handwashing: effects of education and group feedback. *Infect Control Hosp Epidemiol* 1990;11(4):191–193.

135. van de Mortel T, Bourke R, Fillipi L, et al. Maximising handwashing rates in the critical care unit through yearly performance feedback. *Aust Crit Care* 2000;13(3):91–95.

136. Tibballs J. Teaching hospital medical staff to handwash. *Med J Aust* 1996;164(7):395–398.

137. Aspock C, Koller W. A simple hand hygiene exercise. *Am J Infect Control* 1999;27(4):370–372.

138. Colombo C, Giger H, Grote J, et al. Impact of teaching interventions on nurse compliance with hand disinfection. *J Hosp Infect* 2002;51(1):69–72.

139. Rosenthal VD, Guzman S, Crnich C. Impact of an infection control program on rates of ventilator-associated pneumonia in intensive care units in 2 Argentinean hospitals. *Am J Infect Control* 2006;34(2):58–63.

140. Higuera F, Rangel-Frausto MS, Martinez Soto J, et al. National Multi-Center Study to Evaluate the Effect of Education and Performance Feedback on Hand Washing in the Intensive Care Units (ICUs) of Three Mexican Hospitals: Differences Between Gender, Health Care Workers and Type of Procedure. In: Proceedings and Abstracts of APIC meeting; 2004 June 7–10; Phoenix, Arizona, USA. p. 64.

141. Sobreyra Oropeza M, Herrera Bravo M, Rosenthal VD. Effect of education and performance feedback on handwashing in a Mexican public hospital of Mexico City. APIC meeting, June 19–23, 2005, Baltimore, Maryland.

142. Akan A, Özgultekin A, Rosenthal V. Effect of education and performance feedback on handwashing in two Turkish hospitals of Istanbul and Ankara. APIC meeting, June 19–23, 2005, Baltimore, Maryland.

143. Pittet D. Improving adherence to hand hygiene practice: a multidisciplinary approach. *Emerg Infect Dis* 2001;7(2):234–240.

144. Larson EL, Bryan JL, Adler LM, Blane C. A multifaceted approach to changing handwashing behavior. *Am J Infect Control* 1997;25(1):3–10.

145. Plowman R, Graves N, Griffin M, Roberts JA, Swan AV, Cookson BD, Taylor L. *Socioeconomic burden of hospital acquired infection.* London: PHLS, 1999.

146. Stone PW, Braccia D, Larson E. Systematic review of economic analyses of health care-associated infections. *Am J Infect Control* 2005;33(9):501–509.

147. Rosenthal VD, Guzman S, Migone O, Safdar N. The attributable cost and length of hospital stay because of nosocomial pneumonia in intensive care units in 3 hospitals in Argentina: a prospective, matched analysis. *Am J Infect Control* 2005;33(3):157–161.

148. Rosenthal VD, Guzman S, Migone O, Crnich CJ. The attributable cost, length of hospital stay, and mortality of central line-associated bloodstream infection in intensive care departments in Argentina: a prospective, matched analysis. *Am J Infect Control* 2003;31(8):475–480.

149. Higuera F, Rangel-Frausto MS, Rosenthal VD, et al. Attributable cost and length of stay for patients with central venous catheter-associated bloodstream infection in Mexico City intensive care units: a prospective, matched analysis. *Infect Control Hosp Epidemiol* 2007;28(1):31–5.

150. Centers for Disease Control and Prevention. *Hospital infections cost U.S. billions of dollars annually*. March 6, 2000.

151. Haley RW, Culver DH, White JW, et al. The efficacy of infection surveillance and control programs in preventing nosocomial infections in US hospitals. *Am J Epidemiol* 1985;121(2):182–205.

152. Kohn L, Corrigan J, Donaldson M. *To err is human:building a safer health system*. Washington, DC: Institute of Medicine, National Academy Press, 1999.

153. MHA Keystone Center for Patient Safety and Quality. Two-year project improves patient safety in Michigan Hospital ICUs. (www.MHAKeystoneCenter.org) Accessed October 13, 2005.

154. www.theific.org, [accessed March 6, 2006.]

155. Rosenthal VD, Maki DG, Salomao R, et al. Device-associated nosocomial infections in 55 intensive care units of 8 developing countries. *Ann Intern Med*, 2006;145(8):582–91.

Functional Areas of Concern

II

The Inanimate Environment*

William R. Jarvis

Concern about the infection hazard of environmental microorganisms arises because of our close interaction with the environment and its high content of microorganisms, including important human pathogens. Microbes are remarkably efficient at becoming dispersed to virtually all unprotected sites. Where there is moisture and organic material, proliferation to large numbers occurs. Even on dry, infertile surfaces, microbes survive in various relatively inactive states. Unfortunately, although it is easy to establish the presence of microorganisms in the environment, it is difficult to assess their role in causing human disease. Evaluating the evidence in this matter is the fundamental subject of this chapter.

The scope of this chapter is determined partly by logic and partly by tradition. The title itself is a misnomer: If the environment were inanimate, it would not require discussion. The major focus is on those normally nonsterile items that may serve as *fomites*, or vectors of infectious agents [1]. The word *fomite*, although in disfavor among some researchers, remains quite useful. A fomite is an inanimate object that may be contaminated with microorganisms and serve in their transmission. The origin of the term *fomites* is the Latin plural of *omes*, the genus of fungus that was used as tinder. The dried fungus is porous and, thus, was considered "capable of absorbing and retaining contagious effluvia." Consideration of this topic is extended to items that often are sterilized even though the need to do so is arguable (e.g., the internal surfaces of respirator and anesthesia breathing circuits, water in humidifier reservoirs [2],

endoscopes that are to be passed through nonsterile cavities, or reusable pressure transducer heads) [3]. The chapter does not discuss items that clearly must be sterile. Some inclusion distinctions are quite arbitrary. Pus while in a patient's wound or on the unwashed hands of a health-care worker (HCW) would not be considered part of the inanimate environment, but as soon as it is deposited on a surface, it would. Skin is not considered in this chapter, but airborne squamae are. Finally, elements traditionally considered environmental also are included, such as potted plants, cut flowers, insects, and problems associated with animal visitation in the hospital. This chapter also discusses the ultimate concern about the inanimate environment, ultraclean protective environments for immunosuppressed patients, disinfection and sterilization, and routine microbiologic monitoring of inanimate objects in the hospital.

The simplistic dichotomous view that we can apply to sterilization (i.e., an item is sterile or it is not) is not applicable to the factors under discussion. Instead, we must contend with the difficulty of determining the appropriate degree of contamination. In some instances, standards exist (e.g., dialysis water), but, for the most part, no standards have been set, and there is little rational basis for setting them. Setting such standards is made more difficult because microbiologic classification of environmental organisms is not as well developed as it is for organisms from clinical specimens.

There are paradoxes associated with microbiologic content of the environment. Some objects may be sterile as a by-product of manufacture. For instance, the protected outside surfaces of intravenous bottle stoppers usually are sterile, although manufacturers do not make the claim of sterility because it is burdensome to prove it to regulatory

---

*This chapter has been slightly revised from the previous edition version authored by Frank S. Rhame.

agencies. There are items that are not marketed as sterile but that usually are (and arguably should be). When contaminated, these items have been responsible for outbreaks including karaya ostomy bags or elastoplast, which have caused *Rhizopus* spp. [4,5] and *Clostridium perfringens* [6] skin infections; contaminated blood collection tubes have caused pseudobacteremias [7,8] and true bacteremias; and contaminated hand-care products have been implicated as a cause of infection [9,10]. Clinicians often perceive products that come in closed containers as sterile and use them as such even when they are not so marketed. Most would find surprising the frequency of contamination of oral medications (especially those of animal origin), ointments, nasal sprays, lotions, and mouthcare products [11].

The fomites discussed in this chapter include many entities for which no infection-causing potential has been established. Questions concerning the proper management of these items frequently confront infection control personnel. Even those skeptical of the infection-causing potential of environmental surfaces or ordinary objects used in patient care advocate processing and cleaning methods that may have a considerable financial impact. At times, procedures rest on aesthetic considerations. Carpets may not usually constitute an infection hazard, but fecal stains on them are unacceptable. Healthcare professionals may be convinced that microorganisms on the walls and floors play no role in causing human disease, but the lay public's perception is exactly the contrary. In an era of increasing attention to marketing and patient safety, visible dirt is undesirable. When standards have been set, formally or informally, they often have been based on the recognition of what reductions in microbial content can be consistently achieved with moderate resource use rather than on what levels prevent healthcare-associated infections (HAIs).

The fact that there are HAI outbreaks stemming from contaminated inanimate objects often is invoked as a basis for concern about endemic HAIs attributable to the inanimate environment. Publication bias brings forth the atypical, however. A single outbreak does not provide a basis for concern about environmental contamination.

ENVIRONMENTALLY ALTERED MICROORGANISMS

It seems paradoxical that environmental objects frequently can be contaminated by human pathogens but only rarely contribute to human infection. A potential explanation lies in the concept of environmentally damaged organisms. This concept has been rigorously demonstrated for *Streptococcus pyogenes* by Perry et al. and Rammelkamp et al. [12–14]. In a classic series of experiments, they studied streptococcal transmission in army barracks. Air, dust, or personal effects, such as blankets, were contaminated more often by streptococci when recruits had streptococcal illness or pharyngeal colonization. However, recruits who had

been issued freshly laundered, *Streptococcus*-free blankets acquired streptococcal infection or pharyngeal colonization just as often as barracks mates issued highly contaminated blankets [12]. The authors assessed the infectious potential of naturally contaminated barracks dust. Dust samples, dispersed in small enclosures, produced between 3,500 and 56,600 streptococci/m^3 air but did not result in pharyngeal colonization or infection in volunteers within the enclosures. Six volunteers had 17 direct inoculations of dust containing 1,800 to 42,000 streptococci onto the posterior pharynx. These resulted only in transient colonization lasting ≤30 minutes [12].

In contrast, fresh oropharyngeal secretions mixed with sterile dust and dried 4–8 hours produced streptococcal pharyngitis in two of eight volunteers after inoculation. Two of the remaining six volunteers developed pharyngitis on subsequent inoculation of smaller numbers of streptococci directly transferred on swabs of nasopharyngeal sections [14]. The designation of this phenomenon as *environmental damage* reflects a rather anthropocentric perspective. Streptococci presumably shift their metabolism to meet their needs. The physiologic basis of bacterial adaptation to desiccation has been explored [15] and involves substantial changes in internal constituents.

The loss of human pathogenicity associated with adaptation to the environment has been established for desiccated *S. pyogenes*. It seems plausible that other species have different adaptations to various environmental situations that also would reduce their pathogenicity for humans. For some organisms, however, it is reasonable to speculate that the required adaptations are less debilitating. "Water bacteria" in moist environments might be in metabolic states less different from their most pathogenic state. In contrast, *Legionella* spp. in their inanimate reservoir are hazardous, but person-to-person transmission does not take place. Viruses either are viable or not. *Clostridium difficile* as an environmental spore is more durable; if the spore is an infectious form for humans, environmental damage would not be relevant. These matters are, at present, largely unexplored.

EPISTEMOLOGY

With the foregoing generalities in mind, we confront the methodologic inadequacies that characterize most published studies asserting a causative role of inanimate objects in human disease. Evidence suggesting that a fomite has a role in causing disease due to a particular pathogen can be divided into seven categories. They are ordered here by the rigor with which they establish the point:

1. *The organism can survive after inoculation onto the fomite.* This is the weakest form of evidence, yet good journals allocate space to these studies, which sometimes gain widespread attention from the press. A case in point is the demonstration that herpes simplex

virus can survive when inoculated on hot-tub seats [16]. The finding was published despite the cogent words of the accompanying editorial [17], which pointed out the inconclusiveness of the observation.

2. *The pathogen can be cultured from in-use fomites.* A vast set of publications report the recovery of human pathogens from healthcare items. These demonstrations are a necessary but insufficient element in the assertion that a fomite causes infection. When the pathogen is present more frequently or in higher concentration in association with infected humans, this element is only marginally strengthened because the association is as likely to be due to the patient's infecting the environment as vice versa [18]. When the pathogen cannot be cultured, other markers may be used (e.g., hepatitis B surface antigen in the case of hepatitis B [19]). When it is suspected that environmental adaptation may lessen pathogenicity, it is desirable that the detection method simulate the natural infection (e.g., animal inoculation). Many recent studies have documented the ability to recover potential pathogens from computer keyboards, physician clothing, medical equipment, physician ties, and so on. The linkage to human disease as a result of such contamination is lacking.

3. *The pathogen can proliferate in the fomite.* Whether proliferation must be confirmed is largely a function of the size of the inoculum required to cause infection. For instance, this element is important for contaminated intravenous solutions: Most intravenous fluid contamination is at low concentrations, and humans ordinarily tolerate a few organisms given intravenously. For intravenous fluid contamination to be a hazard, the organisms must have the ability and time to proliferate. In general, contaminated objects do not cause infection in immunocompetent persons unless the contaminating organism can proliferate in the contaminated environment or the contamination is heavy and occurs shortly before exposure. However, immunocompromised persons may be more susceptible to becoming infected from such contaminated objects.

4. *Some fraction of acquisition cannot be accounted for by other recognized methods of transmission.* An example of this type of evidence is found in the last of a series of studies that began with the classic demonstration of the importance of hands and contact in nursery acquisition by newborns of *Staphylococcus aureus*. In the final study of the series, Mortimer et al. [20] went to great lengths to eliminate contact transmission in a nursery in which index babies were colonized by *S. aureus*. At least 9/158 contact-protected babies became colonized. This finding and the recovery of *S. aureus* on settle plates were interpreted as evidence that air was the vector of transmission. Another example was reported during a nursing-home outbreak of Norwalk agent diarrhea in which the authors suggested that airborne spread had occurred [21]. This element may

appear to be present simply because of the vicissitudes of biologic systems. It is inevitable that it will be difficult to account for all transmissions by any given mechanism. Implication of a fomite by exclusion of alternatives should be considered weak evidence unless a large fraction of transmissions cannot otherwise be explained.

5. *Retrospective case-control studies show an association between exposure to the fomite and infection.* The association must be verified by less frequent exposure in a comparison unaffected population. Such findings are strengthened when contamination can be confirmed microbiologically. The most common type of study reliably implicating a fomite in endemic or epidemic HAI is a case-control study of this type. The strengths and weakness of such studies are discussed in Chapters 7 and 8.

6. *Prospective observational studies may be possible when >1 similar type of "fomite" is in-use.* Such observations can be made without the need to randomize exposures.

7. *Prospective studies allocating exposure to the fomite to a subset of patients show an association between the exposure and infection.* Microbiologic confirmation of contamination assists in establishing a causal relationship. Ideally, the exposed group is selected randomly. There are two scenarios to consider: fomite A versus nothing when it is not important in patient care (e.g., potted plants) and fomite A versus fomite B when it is necessary in patient care (e.g., ≥2 different types of thermometers, endoscopes).

Only evidence from categories 5, 6, and 7 should be considered strong enough to securely implicate a fomite.

Strain analysis and molecular markers of clonality, so helpful in many areas of epidemiology [22], are less useful in this epistemology (Chapters 10 and 15). Strain differences can negate evidence in category 2. However, strain analysis usually does not substitute for evidence in categories 5, 6, or 7. For instance, most hospital outbreaks of vancomycin-resistant *enterococcus* (VRE) or *C. difficile* have been due to a particular strain. Strain homogeneity, compared with extra-hospital isolates, can establish that the "cases" among patients are nosocomial in origin. Finding the outbreak strain in the environment does not, however, establish its causal role. The transmissions could result from hand carriage or some other person-to-person contact and the infected patients could be contaminating the environment. Only when the direction is clear (there is no likely way for patients to contaminate a hot water tank with *Legionella* spp., for instance) can establishing strain identity between patient's and fomite isolates establish environmental causality. There is one last distinctive aspect of the application of strain identification techniques to environmentally caused outbreaks. A bona fide outbreak may arise from heterogeneous strains, because environmental isolates are generally heterogeneous. For instance, nosocomial *Aspergillus* spp. isolates in an outbreak due to a defect in air filtration will reflect the heterogeneity of environmental isolates [23].

AIR

There has probably been concern about air as a vehicle for transmission of infection for as long as there has been recognition of the transmissibility of disease. Surely, more data have been generated for this mode of transmission than for any other. Entire books have been devoted to the subject [24,25], suggesting that concise summarization is difficult. For much of human history, air was considered the primary carrier of contagion. The word "malaria" reflects the recognition that proximity to swamps increased the risk of illness (the ancients were correct, in a sense, since mosquitoes fly). However, the advent of scientific medicine caused the pendulum to swing too far in the opposite direction. By 1910, no illness was any longer thought to be airborne. Large droplets travel up to 1–2 m through the air but are not borne on it. In the context of infection transmission, airborne means "borne on the air" rather than "transported through the air." Large-droplet transmission is instead considered a type of contact spread [26] (Chapter 41). Only at the time of World War II did a more balanced view become established. Much of the subsequent work on air as a vector was done in the context of studies of biological warfare.

Although there are many concerns about air as a means of HAI pathogen transmission [27], the trend has been away from concern until very recently. Six articles dealing with airborne spread of HAI pathogens were presented at the initial International Conference on Nosocomial Infections in 1970, and Brachman estimated in 1970 [28] that between 10%–20% of endemic HAIs resulted from the airborne route. At the second International Conference on Nosocomial Infections in 1982, however, there was only one presentation about airborne organisms [29], and it dealt with the operating room. At the third and fourth International Conferences in 1990 and 2000, the topic was not discussed except for measles virus transmission.

Air may be sampled volumetrically or on settling plates (Chapter 10). Volumetric sampling produces quantitative data that are more readily conceptualized and seems more relevant to situations in which a pathogen is inhaled. It is the standard for rigorous studies. However, settling plates may be more appropriate to infections that result from settling organisms (e.g., wound infections), and such sampling can be performed without special equipment or expertise [30]. Unfortunately, there are few side-by-side surveys of air using volumetric and settling methods. In one study of air fungal content, 15-minute pairs compared volumetric sampling of 0.42 m^3 air with settling on a 100-mm plate (79 cm^2) [31]. A total of 127 sample pairs yielded total recoveries of 12,900 colony forming units (cfu) and 1,031 cfu, respectively, establishing one advantage for volumetric sampling. Furthermore, of the organisms captured by volumetric sampling, 9.2% were *Aspergillus* spp. while only 5.5% of the settling organisms were in that relatively buoyant genus, pointing out one of the complexities of interpreting settle plate results.

Assessment of the organism content of air is difficult because the concentration of certain organisms in the air is small compared with the volumes that can be conveniently assessed, producing considerable sampling error. Furthermore, there is tremendous variation in the microbial content of air, depending on location in the hospital, ventilation system, concurrent human activity, and proximity to sources of organisms. For a review of available air sampling methods, see Chapter 10 and Burge [32].

Few broad surveys of hospital air have complete microbial identification. In one set of studies, Greene et al. [33,34] found a mean organism count of 350–700 organisms/m^3. The highest counts were in laundry-handling areas followed closely by other storage and disposal areas. The lowest counts were in operating and delivery rooms. Approximately one-third of the organisms recovered were gram-positive cocci, another one-third were gram-positive bacilli, and the remainder were gram-negative bacilli or fungi. Gram-positive cocci constituted a higher proportion of the organisms in operating rooms, gram-positive bacilli (presumably mostly *Bacillus* spp.) made up a higher proportion of the organisms in the laundry and waste storage areas, and gram-negative bacilli were found in relatively high numbers in corridors.

More detailed consideration of air as a means of transmission is best made by considering the specific organism. There is convincing evidence for airborne transmission for only a small number of pathogens (e.g., varicella-zoster virus, influenza [including Avian Influenza], measles, or *Mycobacterium tuberculosi*). For others, airborne transmission has been reported in rare situations, but most transmission is by droplet or contact transmission (*e.g.*, Severe Acute Respiratory Syndrome Coronavirus (SARs-CoV), smallpox, *Brucella* spp., *Pseudomonas pseudomallei*, *Coxiella burnetii*, *Chlamydia psittaci*, *Francisella tularensis*, *Bacillus anthracis*, *Legionella* spp., *Yersinia pestis*, *Pneumocystis carinii*, *Aspergillus* spp., and other filamentous fungi). Additional organisms for example, mumps, rubella, *Mycobacterium avium* complex, *S. aureus* in very unusual circumstances, probably achieve airborne transmission. Some have argued that true airborne transmission (i.e., >3 feet) should be divided into intrinsic or opportunistic airborne-transmitted pathogens [27]. For most pathogens, humans (not the environment) are the major source of contagion. Control of airborne transmission in hospitals consists mainly of promptly identifying infectious patients and placing them in isolation rooms. Influenza control during community outbreaks is more complicated because of the high prevalence of infectious patients and personnel and because infectious persons may have subtle or no respiratory symptoms [35]. Preventing nosocomial influenza during community influenza outbreaks is one of the few solid rationales for human traffic control within hospitals.

Staphylococcus aureus

A solid theoretic basis exists for concern about the importance of airborne transmission of S. aureus (Chapter 40). Noble [36], probably the most avid student of this matter, summarizes information bearing on the origin of airborne S. aureus as follows. Humans liberate $\sim 3 \times 10^8$ squamae per day. Because the size distribution of airborne particles containing S. aureus (~ 4 to 25 μm in diameter] is nearly that of squamae and well above the diameter of naked, single S. aureus cells (~ 1 μm in diameter), it is presumed that most or all airborne S. aureus organisms are carried on these skin flakes. Because particles of this size become impacted on the nasal turbinates, a closed loop may exist: proliferation of S. aureus on the nasal mucosa, hand transfer of S. aureus to the skin, liberation on squamae, airborne transport of squamae, and impaction on the nasal mucosa. Hospital air contains ~ 0.7 S. aureus particles/m^3 [37].

Outbreaks of S. aureus (and S. pyogenes) surgical site infections (SSIs) have been solidly linked to airborne spread from dispersers in the operating room (Chapters 35, 40). In this context, surgical gowns make direct contact improbable and masks make droplet spread improbable. However, the importance of air as a medium for endemic S. aureus transmission in other settings is less clear. The strongest positive evidence is that of Mortimer et al. [20], who studied acquisition of staphylococcal colonization in newborn infants housed in a special nursery that also was used for the care of known colonized infants. Extraordinary measures were undertaken to eliminate contact transfer of S. aureus from the index babies to the study babies. Nevertheless, at least 9/158 newborns became colonized. The authors offered as evidence the following points that these acquisitions were airborne: (1) Contact transmission did not occur; (2) index strains of S. aureus were recovered on settling plates throughout the nursery; (3) the infants were ≥2 m apart, making large-droplet transmission unlikely; and (4) in the study, infants tended to be colonized in the nose first, whereas in previous studies infants acquiring S. aureus by physical transfer tended to be colonized at the umbilicus first.

Wenzel et al. [38] have critically analyzed nine additional articles published between 1966 and 1976 that purport to establish airborne transmission of S. aureus. None of these additional studies provides even strongly suggestive evidence of airborne spread. A bit of negative evidence with respect to endemic operating room acquisition of S. aureus came from the National Academy of Sciences–National Research Council study [39] of the influence of ultraviolet radiation on postoperative SSI (Chapter 33). In the study, high-intensity ultraviolet light in the operating room reduced airborne bacterial counts, as measured on settling plates, by 52% or 63%, depending on the ultraviolet intensity used. At neither intensity was there a similar reduction in postoperative SSI rates. More recently, Bischoff et al. have documented that those colonized with S. aureus are more likely to disseminate the pathogen when they have an upper respiratory viral infection, the so-called Cloud HCW [40].

Gram-Negative Bacilli

Volumetric sampling of ordinary hospital air with recovery of pathogenic Enterobacteriaceae and nonfermenters has been rare. Available studies tend to focus on specialized areas of the hospital (especially operating rooms), use settling-plate methods, assess outbreak situations, or provide incomplete microbiologic identification. Klebsiella or Pseudomonas spp. [41], and other gram-negative organisms can be recovered from hospital air, but the best correlation with acquisition by patients is via handborne rather than airborne organisms [42].

Clinicians have been particularly concerned about the spread of Pseudomonas aeruginosa and Burkholderia cepacia from or to hospitalized patients with cystic fibrosis. Molecular strain identification techniques establish that institutional person-to-person transmission occurs [43,44], but they do not identify the mechanism. P. aeruginosa has been recovered on settling plates near patients with cystic fibrosis [45]. Institution of isolation protocols has been associated with reduced transmission rates. However, the potential interactions between patients with cystic fibrosis are many, and air is not established as a path of transmission.

Two studies have described an association between airborne gram-negative bacilli and endemic HAI. The first and more convincing situation resulted from a very unusual circumstance. The newly constructed Hines Veterans Administration Hospital had a novel chute hydropulping waste disposal system that introduced malodorous bacteria-laden air throughout the hospital. Air sampling near the system demonstrated >5,600 cfu/m^3 of Pseudomonas organisms and Enterobacteriaceae (unfortunately, the relative amounts were unspecified) [46]. Concurrent continuous HAI surveillance found that the nosocomial BSI rate approximately doubled coincident with moving to the new hospital and fell to the baseline level after the chute hydropulping system was closed.

In a second study, carried out over a 5-year interval by Kelsen et al. [47], a significant positive correlation existed between the monthly rate of nosocomial respiratory tract infection in patients hospitalized in an intensive care unit and the average bacterial content of the air. During periods of heavy air contamination, the authors found an unusually high concentration of airborne gram-negative bacilli, ranging up to a P. aerugnosa content of 1,050 cfu/m^3 and a Klebsiella spp. content of 315 cfu/m^3. As the authors point out, the association may not imply that airborne gram-negative rods directly cause nosocomial respiratory tract disease; it is possible that airborne bacteria seeded nebulizers [48] or another intermediate reservoir. The association may have resulted from a third factor affecting both bacterial content of the air and the HAI rate. Finally, it is possible that the air may reflect patients' illnesses rather than the reverse.

Ultimately, the best evidence that endemic HAIs do not often result from airborne gram-negative bacilli probably arises from the repeated failure to recover such organisms in air cultures obtained during outbreak investigations. Although these situations may be atypical, as negative evidence they are convincing because this may be expected to be the situation most likely to produce positive air cultures. The widespread belief that gram-negative bacilli do not survive for prolonged periods when airborne, if true, may provide additional evidence. Here the experimental support is more tenuous than one might wish. Under certain conditions of humidity, temperature, and physiologic state, *Escherichia coli* can sustain up to 100% survival for half hours in microaerosols [49,50]. In general, *E. coli* survives better when aerosols are generated using broth cultures of organisms in relatively inactive states.

In summary, although there is insufficient evidence that airborne gram-negative bacilli constitute a source of endemic HAI to warrant changes in our current practices, situations that lead to high airborne concentrations of gram-negative bacilli should be avoided. Such situations include the use of aerosol-generating room humidifiers, which have been shown to cause considerable dissemination of *Pseudomonas* [51] or *Acinetobacter* spp. [52].

Legionella spp.

The original Legionnaires' outbreak included "Broad Street pneumonia" found among persons who remained outside the implicated hotel. These persons are presumed to establish airborne *Legionella pneumophilia* transmission, but they were not definitely proved to be due to *L. pneumophilia*. Subsequent outbreaks have been attributed to cooling tower contamination. Few of these studies have included long-term follow-up after cooling tower decontamination, nor have they demonstrated an association through strain identification. Although airborne transmission may take place, the emphasis for nosocomial legionellosis should be on control of contamination in the potable water supply.

Aspergillus spp.

Several lines of evidence strongly suggest that airborne *Aspergillus fumigatus* spores cause aspergillosis in immunosuppressed patients [53]:

1. *Aspergillus* spores are always present in unfiltered air, and the organism is highly adapted to airborne spread.

2. Most nosocomial aspergillosis appears first as pneumonia or nasopharyngeal infection. Even if there is an intermediate step of nasopharyngeal colonization, airborne spores would be the ultimate source.

3. Two hospitals have reported a decline in endemic nosocomial aspergillosis coincident with moving to new facilities with improved air filtration systems.

4. In virtually all reported nosocomial aspergillosis outbreaks, there has been an implicated airborne source of transmission stemming from a breakdown in the heating, ventilation, and air conditioning (HVAC) system; a breech of the building shell; or an in-hospital source of fungal spores.

5. Nosocomial aspergillosis arising in a patient cared for in a high-efficiency particulate air-(HEPA) filtered room has not been reported [54].

6. In one hospital, reductions in airborne *Aspergillus* spores coincided with a lowered rate of nosocomial aspergillosis in bone marrow transplant recipients.

It is likely that many other fungal organisms, such as *Mucor*, *Fusarium*, or *Pseudoallescheria* spp., also can in unusual situations be transmitted to patients through the air.

Occasionally, water reaches organic material within the hospital by penetration of the building shell, plumbing leakage, or condensation on chilled water lines or the inner surfaces of cold outside walls. Fungal growth may result within several days. Hospitals must act vigorously to stop the water leakage and promptly achieve drying. If growth of hazardous fungi has occurred, careful remediation is required.

Notwithstanding the occasional episode of in-hospital fungal growth, the majority of spores in hospital air are derived from outdoor air. Spores gain entrance into the hospital because of incomplete filtration—infiltrating around improperly seated filters, around window casings (especially when there is perpendicular wind), through entrances or via loading docks, and on the clothes of personnel and visitors. The better the filtration (i.e., the lower the spore counts), the more important the other sources of spores become. Spores may settle over time and be reaerosolized during manipulations of the HVAC systems while cleaning or during renovation that produces "mini-bursts" of spores. Explosive demolition produces very high *Aspergillus* spp. counts. Excavation can do so also, and renovation may [55] or may not [56].

Special efforts are required to protect bone marrow transplant (BMT) recipients (discussed later). Other patients are also highly susceptible to aspergillosis, including lymphoma and leukemia patients (especially those who are neutropenic for >7 days), solid organ transplant recipients, solid tumor chemotherapy patients, other recipients of cytotoxic therapy, patients with the acquired immunodeficiency syndrome, or steroid-treated patients. While special units for BMT patients are warranted, the potential for competition in room assignment and issues concerning where one draws the line for the remaining groups of patients make it desirable to achieve low spore counts throughout the hospital. In BMT units counts of <0.02 pathogenic *Aspergillus* spp./m^3 and, in the remainder of the hospital, counts of <0.05/m^3 can be achieved without undue burden.

Human Immunodeficiency Virus

There has been anxiety about airborne human immunodeficiency virus (HIV) transmission, especially in the operating room and the autopsy department (Chapter 42). This anxiety persists partly because of the potential for aerosol generation by mechanical saws [57] or other activities. Clearly, splatter of blood and tissue happens in these locations, and scrupulous attention should be paid to barriers for the surgeon or prosector. The available studies do not, unfortunately, distinguish adequately between those droplets and tissue fragments that travel <2 m in smooth arcs to the ground and aerosols (droplet nuclei) that remain airborne and threaten persons at a greater distance from the aerosol generation point. The hepatitis B precedent would suggest that only operating room or autopsy personnel in direct contact with blood are at risk. Special devices to protect against airborne HIV transmission are not warranted.

Laser Plumes

Surgical lasers generate visible smoke that could, in theory, contain viable airborne organisms [58]. Although pathogen transmission has not been verified, safety guidelines have been published [59].

WATER

Potable Water

Achievement of potability of water is a major public health activity, the discussion of which is beyond the scope of this book. Standard works may be consulted for details of water treatment and examination [60]. Verification of ordinary potability is of importance to infection control personnel only in hospitals with private water supplies where verification of water quality is a hospital's responsibility. It should be noted that U.S. federal drinking water regulations call for only one microbiologic assessment [61]: a coliform count (acceptable levels depend on sampling frequency but must average <1 per 100 ml). Even for community water, this sole criterion is probably inadequate, considering the variety of water sources, potential contaminants, and uses of water [62]. The European Community standards also include a limit on the total viable count [63]. Except for legionellosis (discussed later), there are few reports

of HAI arising from drinking water [64]; thus, further consideration of water in this chapter focuses on specialized uses in the hospital.

Potable water supply systems must be protected by vacuum breakers or other devices to keep water from being sucked back into the system during unusual events. To save expense, some building designers plan separate potable and nonpotable water systems. These systems must never be interconnected. Common sense requires that the potable water system be used for all hand washing, bathing of patients, cooking, washing of food and utensils for cooking and eating, food preparation or processing, and laundry. Given the few valid uses for nonpotable water in the hospital and the difficulty in forever preventing cross-connection, the value of designing hospitals with separate nonpotable water systems is questionable.

Dialysis Water

Detailed standards for hemodialysis water have been prepared by the Association for the Advancement of Medical Instrumentation (AAMI) and accepted by the American National Standards Institution [65]. The standard specifies that water used to prepare dialysate shall have a total microbial count of <200 per ml and the dialysate shall have <2,000 microbes per ml (Chapter 23). The rationale for the standard lies in studies carried out in the 1970s that indicated that pyrogenic reactions did not occur when dialysate had <2,000 organisms per ml [66,67]. Bacteria do not cross an intact dialysis membrane, but endotoxin may. The viable bacterial concentration is a rough measure of the endotoxin concentration. The rationale for the stricter (<200 organisms per ml) standard for water used to prepare dialysate is that organism multiplication may take place within the dialyzer. This is a more important problem for recirculating systems than for single-pass systems [68], a distinction not recognized in the AAMI standard. In recirculating systems, dialyzed materials can provide nutrition to contaminating bacteria. Many types of water treatment devices are available for use in preparing dialysate [69]. A more detailed discussion is available in a Food and Drug Administration (FDA) technical report [70].

Hydrotherapy Pools and Tanks

A number of features of hydrotherapy tanks have generated concern that they may transmit infection. Patients using them may have active infection, which may introduce hazardous bacteria and organic debris; patients may be incontinent of feces; warm temperature, water agitation, and a high number of successive patients per unit volume of water reduce available chlorine; the internal channels of agitators are difficult to disinfect; and highly contaminated water may be brought into close contact with potential portals of entry, such as pressure sores, Foley catheters, and percutaneous devices (see Chapter 45). One outbreak of

P. aeruginosa wound infections has been reliably linked to these tanks [71]. Because a wide variety of other human pathogens, such as coliforms, staphylococci, and fungi, have been isolated from immersion tanks [72], there is a broader potential of transmission.

Indeed, in a burn center where the infection potential of hydrotherapy tanks may be most severe, Mayhall et al. [73] have reported an *Enterobacter cloacae* BSI outbreak, which may have been associated with hydrotherapy transmission. To the extent that hydrotherapy tanks are similar to hot tubs and whirlpool spas, there is a more ominous possibility. Contamination of these water sources has resulted in *P. aeruginosa* folliculitis [74], urinary tract infections [75], and even pneumonia [76]. The danger from in-hospital hydrotherapy tanks is probably mitigated by higher standards of disinfection. In the outbreaks of community-acquired *P. aeruginosa* skin infections, even rudimentary standards of water maintenance were not in effect [74].

The Centers for Disease Control and Prevention (CDC) published recommendations for disinfection of hydrotherapy pools and tanks in 1974 [77]. For immersion tanks, the CDC recommended maintaining a free chlorine residual of 15 mg/L with a pH of 7.2 to 7.6, draining tanks between each patient's use, scrubbing out the tank with a germicidal detergent, and circulating chlorine solution through the agitator of the tank for ≥15 minutes at the end of each treatment day. For hydrotherapy pools, the CDC favored continuous filtration and the maintenance of free chlorine residuals of 0.4 to 0.6 mg/L. In the absence of continuous filtration, the CDC recommended potassium iodide and chloramine.

High-Purity Water

Distillation apparatus, reverse osmosis devices, and ion-exchange resin beds are all subject to contamination. Some hospital personnel erroneously assume this type of water is sterile. Distilled water, even if subsequently sterilized, may contain endotoxin. Febrile reactions caused by exposure to items rinsed in endotoxin-containing distilled water have occurred [78].

Water Bacteria

So-called water bacteria are organisms that proliferate in relatively pure water. The most adept species is *B. cepacia*. Carson et al. [79] reported on *B. cepacia* strains that could multiply to the levels of 10^7/ml and remain at these high levels for weeks in distilled water of very high resistivity. *P. aeruginosa* follows closely behind in this ability [80]. Furthermore, *P. aeruginosa* strains adapted to distilled water are relatively resistant to disinfectants [81]. *Acinetobacter calcoaceticus*, an emerging pathogen, seems particularly well adapted to highly aerated water sources. An enrichment technique for isolation

of *Acinetobacter* spp. from environmental samples using vigorous aeration has been described [82]. This feature of *Acinetobacter* spp. presumably accounts for its increased relative frequency of citation as a cause of humidifier or other respiratory device contamination [83,84]. Other water bacteria include *Flavobacterium meningosepticum* [85], other *Pseudomonas* species, *Acromobacter* species, *Aeromonas hydrophila*, *Flavimonas* [86], and certain nontuberculous mycobactria [87]. These last-named organisms are also relatively resistant to various disinfectants [88], including formaldehyde [89]. Among the water bacteria, *P. aeruginosa* and *Acinetobacter* [90] are unusual in that they also are common colonizers of healthy humans. Unprotected wet areas in a hospital should be considered contaminated with one or more water bacteria. These sources include tap water, drains and sinks, water baths, shower heads, flower water, ice machines, and water carafes.

Legionella spp.

Among the important HAI pathogens, *Legionellaceae* are the agents for which environmental sources are the most securely established. Person-to-person transmission of *L. pneumophila* is either very rare or nonexistent [91]. Nosocomial *L. pneumophila* pneumonia has been strongly associated with hot-water distribution systems and, perhaps, cooling towers (Chapter 31). *Legionella micdadei* appears to have a similar epidemiology [92]. Outbreaks of *Legionella dumofi* SSIs due to tap water contamination of fresh wounds appear to be a more atypical problem [93].

Muder et al. [94] have critically reviewed the mechanisms of transmission of *L. pneumophila*. Most of the initial outbreak reports, particularly outbreaks occurring in non-hospital settings, were associated with adjacent excavation or contaminated air-handling-system cooling towers. However, more recent hospital outbreaks have been securely linked to contamination of hot water systems. At the Wadsworth Veterans Administration Hospital in Los Angeles, where a large outbreak of nosocomial legionellosis took place over a period of several years, improvements in the air-handling system preceded efforts to eliminate *Legionella* spp. from the water system. Only the latter endeavor was followed by a reduction in the number of infections [95]. Many additional reports have attributed cessation of *Legionella* HAIs to reductions in the presence in hot-water systems of *L. pneumophila*. Unfortunately, with few exceptions [96], follow-up has been of more than one year's duration, and case ascertainment is unsure.

The way in which *L. pneumophila* contamination of hot water systems produces nosocomial pneumonia is not established. Presumably, inhalation of freshly aerosolized droplets predominates, although inhalation of particles (droplet nuclei) airborne from distant sources, aspiration of colonizing pharyngeal organisms, ingestion of drinking water, and contaminated respiratory therapy devices all remain possibilities [97]. An association of episodes with the use of contaminated shower heads has been found in some [98,99], but not the majority, of investigations.

L. pneumophila contamination of hot water distribution systems is variably present in hospitals; Vickers et al. [100] found it in 9/15 Pennsylvania hospitals. Systems more likely to be contaminated were older and tended to be in a vertical configuration, perhaps because of a greater tendency to have accumulated scale. Systems set at $>60°C$ were less likely to be contaminated. Given the exacting nutritional requirements of the *Legionellaceae*, it is not usual for this contamination to be widespread. A potential explanation is the promotion of *Legionella* spp. growth by other bacteria [101] or their ability to survive within amoebas [102]. In one investigation, shower heads contaminated with *L. pneumophila* were more likely to harbor amoebas [99]. These associations may ultimately permit indirect *Legionella* spp. decontamination.

The need to keep hospital hot water systems free of *Legionellaceae* and the role of routine culture confirmation of the presence of organisms are unresolved. Until recently, CDC personnel opposed culturing hospital water not associated with episodes of infection [103]. In 1995, an ambivalent stance was adopted [104]. Nosocomial *Legionella* spp. pneumonia often goes unrecognized unless the possibility is avidly investigated [97], making it difficult for any hospital to be complacent about its *Legionella* situation. There is at least one cited episode of a hospital with a contaminated potable water system and fairly secure evidence of the absence of nosocomial legionellosis [105], but such reports are rare. Yu [106] has advocated a 1-year quarterly cycle of hospital water cultures in hospitals where identification of nosocomial *Legionella* pneumonia patients is uncertain. The availability of commercial media for *Legionella* cultivation makes such surveillance relatively simple although some expertise is required for confirmation of recovered isolates. Vigorously swabbing scale from shower heads is more sensitive than culture of flushed water, but detailed protocols for routine culture programs are lacking. Shower head scale and water from the base of hot water storage tanks should be included in surveillance. Hospitals recovering *L. pneumophila* and, perhaps *L. micdadei*, should strengthen clinical case-ascertainment methods.

Hospitals with nosocomial *Legionella* spp. pneumonia episodes and contaminated hot water systems must strive to eliminate the latter. Superheating the water (to as high as 77°C [170°F]) provides an immediate solution but may cause scalding of patients or HCWs. Instituting long-term solutions is more difficult. Persistent colonization of hospital potable water systems by *L. pneumophila* arises, at least in part, because the organism can tolerate low levels of chlorine for relatively long periods of time [107]. Hyperchlorination damages some plumbing system components, and raising the pH aggravates scale formation [108]. Other possible ways to eliminate colonization include use of instantaneous steam water heaters, ultraviolet light, chloramines, and ozonation [101].

Eyewash Stations

Clinical laboratories have eyewash stations for emergency eye flushing. These often go unused for months. There have been reports that water in these stations becomes contaminated with *Acanthamoeba* and other amoebas [109] capable of causing chronic destructive keratitis. Although no such infections have been reported, a weekly flush reduces the contamination.

Walls, Floors, and Other Smooth Surfaces

Maki et al. [18] performed a landmark study assessing the relationship between organisms on environmental surfaces and HAI. During 1979, the University of Wisconsin Hospital moved to a new facility. There was no change in the HAI rate at any patient-care site or due to any pathogen associated with this change. Cultures of floors, walls, or other surfaces (including air, water, faucets, and sink drains) showed very similar organism profiles in the old facility and, after 6–12 months of occupancy, in the new facility. In contrast, corresponding cultures taken in the new facility before occupancy were relatively devoid of common HAI pathogens. The constancy of HAI rates provides strong evidence that the association between hospital environmental organism content and HAI arises because patients contaminate the environment, not vice versa. It is important to realize some limitations of the Maki study. The two pathogens for which environmental content is of primary importance (*Aspergillus* and *Legionella* spp.) were not assessed, and the environmental cultures were not processed for anaerobes (e.g., *C. difficile*) or viruses.

This study virtually rules out the environment as an important vector for the assessed organism-object combinations and severely undercuts the rationale for concern about other combinations in the absence of specific data to the contrary. In fact, one is forced to question seriously even such relatively modest recommendations as the use of antimicrobial detergents in hospital cleaning, terminal disinfection of isolation rooms, special cleaning of objects removed from isolation rooms, and wearing gowns and gloves when entering the room of patients in isolation when no contact with patients is anticipated (except for vancomycin-resistant enterococcus or *C. difficile*).

Respiratory Syncytial Virus

One pathogen clearly transmissible in the hospital by fomites is respiratory syncytial virus (RSV) (Chapter 41). Indirect evidence suggests that RSV transmission happens through contact; inoculation of RSV onto nasal or eye membranes causes infection quite efficiently [110]. Moreover, this virus survives for several hours on smooth surfaces [111]. Direct evidence of fomite transmission is now available [112]. Volunteers who entered a hospital room that had just been vacated by an RSV–infected patient became infected with RSV >50% after handling objects in the room and touching their eyes and nose as often as volunteers who cuddled RSV–infected babies. Volunteers sitting in the same room with an RSV–infected baby did not contract the illness. The relative importance of hand and fomite transmission is unknown, but it is of interest that RSV survives approximately 10 times better on smooth surfaces than on skin [111].

Clostridium difficile

Strain analysis techniques have unequivocally established that in-hospital transmission of C. difficile can take place (Chapter 33) [113]. Variation in hospital C. difficile transmission would provide a satisfactory explanation for the apparently wide variation in rates of C. difficile colitis in different hospitals. As with many HAI pathogens, increased environmental presence of C. difficile is associated with infected patients. In their excellent review, McFarland and Stamm [114] found five supportive studies. With regard to environmental concerns, what distinguishes C. difficile is its ability to form spores with the consequent prolonged survival of the organism in the environment and the plausibility that the spores retain full infectiousness. However, a controlled study of glove use suggested that most C. difficile transmissions arise from carriage by hands [115]. The same group has used restriction endonuclease strain analysis to establish that C. difficile acquisition does not geographically cluster within wards and is not more likely to be transmitted to a subsequent bed occupant [116]. No special environmental cleaning techniques for C. difficile contamination have been formally advocated, although the use of an agent such as bleach that is effective against spores is recommended. Emergence of a toxinotype III strain that is positive for binary toxin, an 18-base pair deletion in tcdC, and has increased resistance to fluoroquinolones is of concern.

Hepatitis B Virus

Concern about environmental hepatitis B virus (HBV) transmission arises from several lines of evidence. Clinical laboratories and hemodialysis units, areas frequently contaminated by blood, were foci of HBV transmission throughout the 1970s (Chapter 42). Many of the ward-acquired, and an even larger fraction of the laboratory-acquired, HBV episodes occurred without recognized percutaneous inoculation of blood. A decline in the incidence of hepatitis among HCWs began in the mid-1970s (before the introduction of HBV vaccine) when concern about blood contact became widespread [117]. Approximately 30%–40% of community-acquired episodes of HBV cannot be ascribed to sexual contact, needle sharing, or therapeutic blood component exposure [118]. Hepatitis B surface antigen (HBsAg) may be antigenically detected on surfaces in hospital areas likely to have been blood contaminated [19]. Surfaces not visibly contaminated with blood may also yield HBsAg. Even today, blood contamination can frequently be found on patient-care items [119]. In blood, HBV remains viable for ≤1 week after desiccation at room temperature [120], although inactivating it with disinfectant is not difficult [121]. Very high dilutions of HBV-containing blood can transmit hepatitis B.

These lines of evidence do not establish a role of the environment in HBV transmission. Coincident with efforts to eliminate or decontaminate environmental blood was the adoption of segregation of HBsAg-positive patients in dialysis and more widespread recognition of the hazard of needle sticks. Nevertheless, when contaminated objects have been in close proximity to a portal of entry, such as the finger platform of an automatic finger-stick device, HBV transmission by inanimate objects has been verified [122].

To clean blood spills, the CDC has recommended the use of any chemical germicide that is approved by the U.S. Environmental Protection Agency (EPA) as a "hospital disinfectant" and is tuberculocidal [123]. Because no contact time was specified, the recommendation is not that a tuberculocidal standard be met. Nevertheless, OHSA may arbitrarily enforce the germicide choice strictly. In areas where large blood spills are commonplace, such as around operating room tables, even this recommendation seems excessive. As long as such units have specialized cleaning protocols and good protective equipment, any hospital disinfectant should suffice. With large spills of cultured or concentrated agents in the laboratory, the contaminated area should be flooded with germicide before cleaning. Otherwise, the area should be cleaned and then decontaminated.

Viral Hemorrhagic Fever Agents

The Centers for Disease Control and Prevention (CDC) regards environmental surfaces to be a potential vector of viral hemorrhagic fever agent transmission. The 1980 recommendations [124] for the treatment of patients with Lassa fever and other acute viral hemorrhagic fevers included special isolation units with exhaust air filtration, use of a chemical toilet, disinfection of all items taken from the patient's room, and disinfection of the vacated room with gaseous formalin or paraldehyde. The CDC 1988 revision [125] restricted concern to patients with confirmed or suspected hemorrhagic fever due to the agents of Lassa, Marburg, Ebola or Crimean-Congo hemorrhagic fever. CDC statements in 1995 and 2005 [126] recommended the use of a negative pressure room with an anteroom and HEPA respirators for entering the room of patients with prominent cough, vomiting, diarrhea, or hemorrhage; minimizing laboratory testing; autoclaving, incinerating, or using bleach in washing linen; use of a chemical toilet or bleach disinfection of excretions and fluids before discarding them in the sewer; incineration or decontamination of solid medical waste; and processing clinical specimens in a class II biological safety cabinet following biosafety level 3 practices.

OTHER ENVIRONMENTAL FACTORS

Carpets

Carpeting a floor increases the microbiologic content per unit of floor surface by approximately four orders of magnitude [127]. Contaminating organisms include *S. aureus*, *E. coli*, and, more rarely, *Pseudomonas*. After removal of carpeting from hospital environments, the carpet content of *S. aureus* remains stable for more than a month and of other organisms for ≤6 months. In the best-controlled study, however, the total bacterial content of air was apparently unaffected by the presence or absence of carpet in the sampled area [128]. For areas with carpets, the air content also was not significantly influenced by vacuuming frequency (daily, every other day, or every third day) [128]. Unfortunately, these studies were carried out before the widespread adoption of large, self-propelled, high-pressure cleaner-extractors, which do create transient increases in air fungal content.

The infection hazard of carpets may be more important when patients have direct contact with carpeting (e.g., in pediatric areas) or when patients use wheelchairs. Wet machine cleaning has been associated with *Aspergillus flavus* proliferation. However, it has yet to be demonstrated that any HAI has arisen from a carpet. In recent years, manufacturers have marketed carpets with antimicrobial substances. As yet, these have not been rigorously assessed in independent studies.

Air-Fluidized Beds

Designed to prevent pressure sores by "flotation," air-fluidized beds have features posing a potential for infection transmission. Flotation is accomplished by driving air up through a 25-cm-deep layer of silicon-coated, soda lime glass microspheres 50–150 μm in diameter. The microspheres are held in the bed by a monofilament polyester filter sheet with openings of ~37 μm through which the microspheres cannot pass. Disinfection of the beds is accomplished by sieving out clumps of beads and organic debris and then operating the bed at high temperature and air flow to inactivate organisms by heat, abrasion [129], and desiccation.

Initial anxieties about the infection hazard from air-fluidized beds have largely dissipated. Beds spiked with *Staphylococcus epidermidis*, *P. aeruginosa*, or *Bacillus subtilis* did not cause airborne dissemination of these organisms, even shortly after inoculation [130]. The air over beds contaminated by use did not contain more organisms than control air over ordinary beds [131]. A single report of infection transmission, due to *Enterococci*, has appeared [132], suggesting that attention to proper decontamination of these beds is important. There remains the theoretic possibility that the air fluidization process renders airborne those organisms that usually remain harmlessly attached to surfaces (e.g., *M. tuberculosis*), and a study of the beds in the most heavily contaminated contexts has not been undertaken.

Soap

Given the emphasis on hand washing and hand hygiene, it is surprising that the problem of soap contamination is not better studied. Most soaps are not marketed as sterile. Recent outbreaks associated with either intrinsically or extrinsically contaminated soap reemphasize the potential danger of soaps as a cause of HAIs [133]. Other outbreaks have demonstrated the potential danger of intricately contaminated iodophors [10]. It is reasonable to postulate that it is advantageous to wash the hands with sterile soap (liquid or leaf) dispensed from forearm or leg-operated dispensers that are resistant to contamination. The use of contaminated hand lotion has been implicated in a *P. aeruginosa* outbreak [9].

Data confirming the expected contamination of in-use bar soap have been widely disseminated in the promotion of dispensed liquid soap [134]. However, data comparing the microbial burden on hands washed using a contaminated soap bar with that using uncontaminated nonmedicated soap are unavailable. At the least, it seems prudent to reduce the microbial content of soaps by using disposable liquid soap containers, thoroughly cleaning reusable liquid soap containers, or, if bar soap is used, purchasing small bars and providing soap racks that permit water drainage. The relative merits of these alternatives await additional study. In countries with limited resources, care should be taken not to use bar soap and, not to "top off" or refill liquid soap dispensers without disinfecting them between refilling to ensure that single-use paper towels are available for hand drying or to use waterless agents. The recent recommendations for use of waterless alcohol-based hand-hygiene agents enhance the availability of hand-hygiene facilities at the bedside, reduce the risk of soap contamination, and obviate the need for towels for drying (see Chapter 3).

Flowers

Flowers pose two theoretic infection hazards. Vase water inevitably contains large concentrations of potential HAI pathogens [135], and decaying organic matter in the dirt of potted plants provides a substrate for fungal growth. Although there are no convincing data establishing vase water as a seat of HAIs, many hospitals bar flowers in water and potted plants from the rooms of immunosuppressed or ICU patients. If vase water were to be disposed of gently and patients, personnel, and visitors washed their hands after touching the water, little danger should arise. Unfortunately, achieving uniform compliance with these precautions is improbable.

Animals

Sanctioned animal contact with hospital patients is of several types: blind or disabled patients or personnel may be accompanied by seeing eye or other service animals, pets may be brought to patients, animals may be used to entertain patients or provide pet therapy, and research animals may be housed in areas near patient-care units. Although Q fever is the only zoonosis shown to have been associated with epidemics in healthcare facilities, >100 organisms infect both humans and other animals [136]. Knowledge of transmission mechanisms of these organisms suggests several prudent measures.

Persons handling seeing eye or other dogs should be sure that the dogs are vaccinated against rabies, appear to be free of ectoparasites, and are healthy (in particular, ringworm should not be present). Arrangements should be made for walking the dogs and assuming responsibility for disposal of animal excreta. Pregnant ewes used in research centers have been the source of outbreaks of Q fever [137]. Hospitalized patients have not been affected in these outbreaks; however, airborne transmission to personnel having no direct contact with pregnant ewes has occurred. Although the hazard appears to be most severe at or near parturition [138], it seems prudent to bar all contact between patients and pregnant ewes and to ensure that pregnant ewes used for research are never, even during transportation, in areas from which airborne spread to patients can take place. More stringent recommendations for protection of personnel working with pregnant ewes have been published [139].

Certain animal contacts with children seem inadvisable in any circumstance. Reptiles cannot be reliably certified to be free of salmonellosis, wild carnivores (e.g., skunks, ferrets, raccoons) and bats pose an unacceptably high risk of rabies, and birds of virtually any species may transmit *C. psittaci*. Any contact with animal urine should be followed by hand hygiene and, if appropriate, more extensive disinfection procedures because of the possibility of leptospirosis. Contact with mouse or hamster urine also is hazardous to the immunocompromised patient because of the possibility of transmission of lymphocytic choriomeningitis virus. Household pets also can contaminate the hands of HCWs, who then can introduce the pathogen. This was illustrated by an outbreak of *Malassezia pachydermatis* in neonatal ICU patients [140].

Linen

Considering how heavily contaminated soiled linen is, it is remarkable how rarely it causes infection. Laundry workers, who have prolonged close contact with soiled linen, seem to be at risk only as a result of exposure to blood-contaminated sharp implements, hepatitis A [141], or other enteric pathogens [142], or unusually infectious organisms, such as *C. burnetii*. None of these dangers represents a meaningful hazard to patients. It seems prudent to handle soiled linen gently to reduce the dispersal of microorganisms in areas dedicated to the care of patients. Beyond that, there is little basis for employing special procedures. Given the improbability that soiled laundry reposing in a partially filled hamper adds organisms to the environment (much less causes HAI), it is difficult to understand the emphasis that hospital inspection agencies have previously placed on closing soiled-linen hampers.

Clean laundry, even after cold water processing, contains few pathogenic organisms. Sheets have a total aerobic colony-forming unit count of ~0.2 cfu/cm^3, and terry cloth items have ~2 cfu/cm^3. The profile of contaminating organisms (*Bacillus* spp, 58%; coagulase-negative staphylococci, 25%; *Corynebacterium* spp, 18%) after cleaning is markedly different from the prewash profile. Pathogenic species are rarely found in washed linen. The proper handling of clean linen during transportation and storage is probably the most important determinant of the microbial content at the time of use. Meyer et al. [143] studied newborn ICU laundry that had been washed at 75°C (167°F), dried at 96°C (205°F), and carefully handled. Rodac contact plates showed no organisms one-third of the time and >10 colonies per contact plate only 9% of the time. Linen near the top of the stack had a higher incidence of positivity and a higher number of colonies per plate than linen in the middle of the stack, suggesting that handling was the source of transfer of organisms.

Nosocomial *Bacillus cereus* infection has been attributed to clean linen [144,145]. The reported outbreak consisted of *B. cereus* umbilical colonization without clinical signs of infection in normal neonates and neonates in a special care unit. The source was considered to be contaminated clean diapers because the implicated *B. cereus* type was found in washed diapers and in the laundry machine. Because the implicated *B. cereus* type also was recovered from the hands of nursing staff, this attribution is unconvincing. Other reports of HAI due to clean linen—tinea pedis in a nursing home [146], staphylococcal disease in newborns [147], or urinary tract infection [148]—are likewise not persuasive.

The final revision of the American Hospital Association's *Infection Control in the Hospital* [149] recommended autoclaving linen for patients "particularly susceptible to infections," such as burn patients and in the nursery. The American Academy of Pediatrics [150] supported this recommendation until it softened its stance in 1983 [151]. No consensus body has such a recommendation at present. One line of argument against autoclaving linen arises after consideration of the panoply of techniques required to maintain sterility until the linen reaches the point of use. Applying these procedures to autoclaved linen would be burdensome and costly. Only one rationale for autoclaving laundry seems plausible. Laundry dried in unfiltered air becomes contaminated by *A. fumigatus*, and in specialized patient-care units with a very low fungal spore content and low air change rates, a few introduced spores can contribute a substantial portion of the ambient spores [152].

ULTRACLEAN PROTECTIVE ENVIRONMENTS

The ultimate expression of concern that environmental organisms pose an infection hazard is the ultraclean protective environment. When fully developed, these environments have HEPA air filtration with horizontal or vertical laminar airflow; sterile food or food with a low organism content; frequent disinfection of walls, floors, and other environmental surfaces; sterile linen and drinking water; toilet water disinfection; sterile booties, gowns, caps, and gloves for HCWs and visitors entering the room; and elaborate protective garb for patients leaving the room. Patients placed in such an environment are generally given oral nonabsorbable, topical, or systemic antimicrobials. This package of protective measures has been termed a *total protective environment, life island, protected environment,* or *barrier isolation.*

It has long been recognized that these special efforts can produce environmental surfaces and ambient air with markedly diminished organism content [153]. More important, a meta-analysis [154] of random allocation trials of various forms of ultraclean protective environments suggested that this package of techniques produces a statistically significant reduction in the incidence of infection. Of 10 trials [155–164], 5 showed a statistically significant reduction in overall, severe, or fatal infections. Of the remaining studies, three trials showed a trend to fewer infections in the protected patients, and one did not report infection rates. This infection prevention effect was generally noted after the second week, a finding in agreement with the view that there is a lag between becoming colonized with a HAI pathogen and subsequent infection.

However, the use of ultraprotective environments remains controversial for a number of reasons:

1. *Expense.* In new hospital construction, the capital cost of laminar airflow rooms is not great, especially when amortized over the life of a building. Modular units are commercially available. However, depending on what additional features are incorporated into the protective package, substantial ongoing expenses may be incurred.
2. *Deleterious effects.* During periods of severe illness, seeing only masked and gowned people, being served relatively unpalatable food, remaining confined to a small room, and consuming foul-tasting, diarrheagenic antibiotics aggravates the psychologic stress of having a potentially fatal condition. Premature withdrawal from protected environments, however, may predispose to gut colonization and subsequent disease caused by environmental pathogens.
3. *Difficulty in apportioning benefit among the various features of protected environments.* With few exceptions [162], the available studies deal with the impact of the total package versus conventional treatment of patients. If infections are prevented, it is difficult to factor out which component is responsible. It is even possible that the beneficial effect results from enhanced adherence to standard infection control procedures (e.g., vascular access cannula or Foley catheter management) rather than the protected environment per se.
4. *Doubts about study design.* Diagnosis of infection in very immunosuppressed patients with highly complicated profiles leads to problems. The physicians providing direct care of the patients and who are in the best position to make an assessment are also the least blinded with respect to the study group. All of these studies are described as using random allocation. However, the vicissitudes of room availability at the time of admission and the many factors involved in assigning patients to rooms make true randomization awkward. Only six of the studies provide detailed information about comparability of the groups of patients, and the studies conducted by the M. D. Anderson Hospital [155,160] have a troublesome design feature: The protected patients received more intensive chemotherapy. The investigators proceeded on the unproved but logical assumption that subsequent courses of induction could be more intensive in patients with no history of infection. The improved survival may have resulted from the more intensive therapy, which may not have been possible to administer to the control patients, who had been infected more often.
5. *Doubts about the larger significance of a real difference in infection rates.* In many of the studies, the lower infection rate provided only a brief postponement of death; longevity was most strongly influenced by the severity of the underlying illness. The reduction in infection, if real, may be most meaningful for patients treated with potentially curative therapies, such as children with acute lymphocytic leukemia or patients undergoing bone marrow transplantation.

Clearly, special efforts are warranted to lower the airborne fungal spore concentration in the rooms of highly immunosuppressed patients [165]. It is important to consider separately several features of air purification systems. Top-of-the-line bag filters probably remove nearly all fungal spores, but many hospitals prefer HEPA-filters because they add relatively little capital expense and meet standards more directly related to microbial filtration. The CDC has recommended HEPA filtration [104]. It may be desirable to place duct insulation outside the ducts [166].

Placing filters at the point of entrance of air into a patient's room permits safe local maintenance while the room is otherwise unoccupied and accommodates malfunction or maintenance of the central system. Sealing the room and placing it at positive pressure reduce infiltration of spores from the outside or adjacent hospital areas. Increasing the air change rate minimizes the potential exposure of a patient to infiltrating or introduced spores [152].

Air change rates of ≥10 per hour are desirable for BMT patients. Rates above 15–25 per hour are best accommodated by placing fans and filters next to the rooms because the caliber of ducts conveying air to and from central systems would have to be too large. Laminar airflow (a misnomer because objects in a room cause considerable turbulence) units are best thought of as ultrahigh air change rates. Air change rates of 100–400 per hour can be achieved. Attention to in-room air flow patterns [167] may lead to improvements in the safety of patients without requiring extra resources. Placing patients with infectious diseases or infected with the most infectious agents (e.g., *M. tuberculosis*) toward the exterior ward wall with windows in hospitals in countries with limited resources may reduce the risk of such agent transmission. Being cognizant of the air flow patterns in the room also may facilitate patient placement to minimize the risk of pathogen transmission.

Concerns are associated with other efforts to eliminate a patient's exposure to environmental organisms. Food with low organism content is unpalatable. Organisms on surfaces that do not come in contact with the patient probably are harmless. Elimination of environmental organisms can be very difficult. In one ultraprotective unit, there was a prolonged struggle to eliminate an unusual *Pseudomonas* spp. from toilet bowl water. Notably, although the organism was present for 20 months, no instance of HAI or colonization due to the organism was identified [168].

Except for fungal spore control, ultraprotective environments are not yet an established infection control measure. Even their advocates do not believe they truly are indicated *except for* patients undergoing BMT or intensive chemotherapy likely to produce >25 days of granulocytopenia [169]. What is critically needed is analysis of the relative benefit of the components of the protective package.

DISINFECTION AND STERILIZATION

This topic is addressed in Chapter 20.

Definitions

Sterilization means the complete elimination or rendering nonviable of all microorganisms, including all spores (Table 19-1). *Nonviable* is best taken to mean the irreversible loss of the ability to propagate indefinitely [170]. Ultraviolet light, although lethal, does not interrupt germination and temporary growth. Conversely, organisms seemingly killed by mercury can be resurrected by compounds that

displace mercury from sulfhydryl groups. Disinfection is divided into three levels [171]. *High-level disinfection* means the elimination of all viruses and vegetative microorganisms and most, but not necessarily all, bacterial or fungal spores. *Intermediate disinfection* means the elimination of all vegetative pathogenic bacteria, including *M. tuberculosis*, but not necessarily all viruses (nonenveloped or smaller viruses are more resistant to disinfection) or spores. Inactivation of *M. tuberculosis* is used in this definition not primarily because of concern about *M. tuberculosis* contamination. Mycobactericidal capacity is used because the organism is relatively resistant to disinfection compared with other vegetative bacteria, and a procedure to assess mycobactericidal activity has been established by the Association of Official Analytical Chemists (AOAC) [172], even its procedure has been challenged [173]. *Low-level disinfection*, roughly equivalent to *sanitization*, means the elimination of most pathogenic bacteria. *Cleaning* means the removal of all visible debris. All items should be scrupulously cleaned before disinfection because disinfecting methods may not penetrate debris. *Antisepsis* is the application of compounds to skin or mucous membranes to reduce microorganism content substantially.

Although the preceding definitions correspond best to practical use requirements, the Environmental Protection Agency (EPA), the main regulatory agency for disinfectants and sterilants until 1993, used a noncongruent classification of chemical germicides. *Sporicides* meet an AOAC standard for spore destruction [172]. They achieve sterilization or high-level disinfection depending on contact time. *Hospital disinfectants* inactivate *Salmonella choleraesuis*, *S. aureus*, and *P. aeruginosa* in highly specified AOAC tests [172]. *Disinfectants* and *sanitizers* meet other tests. The EPA registration categories made no reference to effectiveness against *M. tuberculosis*, the critical distinction between intermediate- and low-level disinfectants or to effectiveness in inactivating all viruses, the critical distinction between high- and intermediate-level disinfection. In the United States, the Food and Drug Administration (FDA) is now the regulatory agency for germicides that are sterilants or used for high-level disinfection. Its criteria for labeling are sufficiently stringent that few germicides have achieved sanction.

Kinetics of Microbial Killing

It is generally assumed, although not always supported by experimental evidence, that most microbial inactivation processes follow a "one-hit" killing curve. This presumption is equivalent to asserting that all the organisms in the population are equally susceptible to the process. These presumptions can be restated mathematically as follows. The number of microorganisms killed is proportional to the number present, and the proportion does not change as the population of remaining organisms decreases. When the logarithm of the concentration of organisms is displayed on the vertical scale and time on the horizontal scale, this

TABLE 19-1
MINIMUM STERILIZATION/DISINFECTION LEVEL REQUIREMENTS FOR VARIOUS ITEMS

Sterilization

Arthroscope
Cardiac catheter
Culdoscope
Cystoscope
Dental: forceps, scalpels, bone chisels, scalers, and other instruments; burrs, hand pieces, antiretraction valves, other intraoral devices attached to air or water lines, prophylaxis angles, ultrasonic scaler tips, air/water syringe tips, saliva ejectors, air evacuator tips prophylaxis cups and brushes
Dermabrasion wheel
Endoscopic biopsy forceps, cannulas, papillotomes, guide wires
Endoscope, rigid
Implantable device
Intravascular device
Needle
Peritoneoscope
Surgical instrument
Transducer head
Ureteroscope
Urinary catheter
Urological laser
Vaginal speculum (for use after rupture of membranes)

High-Level Disinfection

Bronchoscope
Cryoprobe
Dental: mirrors, amalgam condensers
Dialysis machine surfaces in contact with dialysate
Endoscope, flexible fiberoptic or video
Endotracheal tube
Laryngeal blades
Maschiadscope
Prostate ultrasound probe
Sinuscope
Tonometer tip

Intermediate-Level Disinfection

Anoscope
Bite blocks (between patients)
Breast pump surfaces in contact with milk
Breathing circuit
Dental: items to be handled in the laboratory, such as impressions, bite registrations, fixed and removable prosthesis, orthodontic appliances
Ear speculum and ear-examining instruments
EEG/EKG electrode
Electric razor head
Laryngeal mirror
Mouthpiece, anesthesia or pulmonary function testing
Nasal speculum
Thermometer (between patients)
Transesophageal electrode
Vaginal speculum (except during labor or after rupture of membranes)
Vaginal ultrasound probe
Ventilation bag connector

Low-Level Disinfection

Bathtub, infant
Bite blocks, radiation therapy (between uses by a single patient)
Hydrotherapy tanks
Infant furniture
Thermometers (between uses by a single patient)
Toy, infant

(continued)

TABLE 19-1
(CONTINUED)

Cleaning—between All Patients

Bathtubs, ceramic
Bedpans
Bed rails
Earphones
Blood pressure cuff
Electric razor body
Examination table
Cleaning—when visibly soiled
Food utensil
Nasal gas administration hood, dental
Shampoo tray

relationship results in the familiar straight-line killing curve. The slope of the killing curve is the measure of the rapidity of organism destruction. It often is expressed as the *decimal reduction time,* the time interval required to bring the concentration of organisms to 1/10 its previous concentration (i.e., 90% destruction). The difficulty in validating one-hit kinetics arises because of technical obstacles to experimentally ruling out the possibility that a very small fraction of the starting population of organisms is more resistant to killing. The potential difficulty in killing the last few (possibly more resistant) contaminating organisms is one basis for the overkill present in most sterility standards.

The preceding kinetics analysis establishes the importance of exposure time in accomplishing microbial destruction. A perfectly acceptable disinfection process will fail if not applied for sufficient time. If extremely high numbers of organisms must be inactivated with a very high probability that no survivors remain (e.g., manufacture of some vaccine), prolonged exposure times may be required. Furthermore, a given process may be sanitizing, disinfecting, or sterilizing, depending on the length of time it is applied.

Microbial Safety Index

The kinetics analysis also establishes that the operational assessment of sterility is a probabilistic assertion, not an all-or-nothing phenomenon [174]. This fact has led to the recommendation that the label *sterile* be supplemented by a microbial safety index (MSI) [175], defined as the absolute value of the logarithm of the probability that the item is contaminated.

For example, an item with an MSI of 3 would have a probability of 1 in 1,000 of containing a viable microorganism. As a practical matter, establishing that an item in a lot has an MSI >3 is extremely difficult by direct microbiologic assessment. With even the most rigorous culture technique, it is difficult to avoid introducing contamination at a level much less than 1 per 1,000 cultured items. Furthermore, the mathematics of sterility testing is unfavorable. For instance,

to establish with 95% confidence that a lot containing 10,000 items is contaminated at a rate of <1 per 1,000, almost 3,000 of the items must be cultured and found sterile.

Administrative Issues

The FDA requires that reusable medical devices be sold with specific instructions regarding reprocessing methods [171]. The use of alternate methods may invalidate a warranty or create a medicolegal dilemma. The latter problem arises if a product failure damages a patient. The manufacturer may try to shift liability to the hospital because the product was not used according to instructions. Manufacturers may thus escape the stringency of strict liability for product failure.

These same considerations apply to reprocessing disposable items. Through the early 1980s, relevant standard-setting organizations lined up fairly solidly against reprocessing disposable items. The CDC recommended in 1982 that "no disposable object designed for sterile, single use should be re-sterilized" [176]. This restriction was rescinded in 1985 [177]. Through 1984, the Joint Commission on Accreditation of Healthcare Organizations (JCAHO) flatly opposed any reprocessing. However, the 1995 JCAHO standards were less restrictive, merely requiring hospitals to have written policies that address reprocessing methods [178].

A 1977 FDA policy guide assigned full responsibility to the hospital when disposable medical devices were reused [179]. However, the FDA guide explicitly sanctioned the reuse of disposable items when the facility can establish that the item can be cleaned and sterilized adequately, that its "physical characteristics or quality are not adversely affected by their reprocessing," and, somewhat redundantly, that the product remains safe and effective for its intended use. None of these statements addresses the resterilization of an unused item. Occasionally, an item is removed from its package or its package has been damaged, but the item has not been used. Consistency requires that these items also be resterilized.

On August 14, 2000, the FDA released the document "Enforcement Priorities for Single-Use Devices Reprocessed by Third Parties and Hospitals" to provide guidance to third-party and hospitals reprocessors about their responsibilities as manufacturers engaged in reprocessing devices labeled for single use under the Federal Food, Drug, and Cosmetic Act (the FFDC Act), as amended by the Safe Medical Devices Act of 1990, the Medical Device Amendments of 1992, and the Food and Drug Modernization Act of 1997. Third-party and hospital reprocessors of single-use devices (SUDs) are subject to all regulatory requirements currently applicable to original equipment manufacturers, including premarket submission requirements (Section 513 and 515 of the FFDC Act; 21 *Code of Federal Regulations* Parts 807 and 814) (www.fda.gov/cdrh/ohip/guidance/1333.pdf).

A key question, begged by all the aforementioned bodies, is "How does one determine whether an item is disposable?" At present, the manufacturer makes the determination. An item is disposable if it comes in a package labeled with the words *disposable, single use only,* or the like. Some manufacturers have added such language to packages of products previously marketed with resterilization instructions. Indeed, manufacturers have little incentive, at least in the short term, to do otherwise. Labeling an item as disposable minimizes liability and maximizes sales volume.

The most compelling case for reuse of disposable items has been made for dialyzers [180–182] (see Chapter 23). First use of hollow-fiber dialyzers more often may be associated with mechanical failure and systemic reactions (fever, chest pain, transient fall in white blood cell count) due to chemicals leaching out of the membrane or increased complement activation by new dialysis membranes. Some first-use-type reactions continue to occur, however, with reused dialyzers [183]. Other items may be very expensive and capable of withstanding reprocessing methods. Because resterilization of an item costs a hospital between $10–$20, depending on the time required to clean and package it and the sterilization method used, the impetus to reuse exists only for expensive items. A detailed protocol for reuse of specific items has been successfully employed [184].

The JCAHO requires written hospital policies regarding decontamination and sterilization activities, the performance of sterilizing equipment, and the shelf life of all stored sterile items [178]. The CDC guidelines recommend weekly biologic monitoring of all sterilizers [177]. When an implantable device is sterilized, a biologic indicator should be used and found sterile before the device is implanted. A chemical indicator should be visible on the outside of all sterilized packages. Careful follow-up of unconverted indicators should be undertaken because investigation often turns up significant problems [185].

Choice of Sterilization or Disinfection Level

Support continues for Spaulding's classification scheme indicating the level of sterilization or disinfection required for various items [171,177,186]. *Critical* items enter tissue or the vascular space. *Semicritical* items come into contact with mucous membranes or nonintact skin. *Noncritical* items touch intact skin. Critical items are generally held to require sterilization, semicritical items to require high-level disinfection, and noncritical items to require intermediate- or low-level disinfection [171,176,187]. Virtually all germicides are effective against HIV [188].

High-level disinfection is, in fact, rather difficult to achieve. Most germicides require 20–45 minutes to attain tuberculobactericidal activity, exposure times well in excess of common usage [189]. Furthermore, if a device really has to be at a state of high-level disinfection at the time of subsequent use on another patient, it would have to be subject to sterile water rinsing, manipulation using sterile technique, air drying with filtered air, and protective wrapping. Such precautions are rarely part of hospital practice [189], nor are they called for in many specialty societies' published guidelines for the reprocessing of semicritical items [190]. This amounts to an acknowledgment that organisms carried over from the previous patient are the primary target of reprocessing techniques. This is a rational emphasis provided that the disinfected device is protected from "water bacteria" by complete drying and from gross recontamination or hand contact before subsequent usage.

The assertion that all semicritical items must be processed by high-level disinfection is difficult to justify. To make this claim is to suggest that items coming into contact with mucous membranes can be contaminated with no more than a few bacterial or fungal spores. High-level disinfection seems unwarranted for items that will touch normally contaminated mucous membranes, such as the mouth or the colon. The distinction made between mouthpieces, for which some authorities have recommended high-level disinfection [189], and silverware is difficult to understand. For items in contact with the gut, elimination of carryover enteric pathogens is the goal. Unfortunately, assessment of the ability to inactivate small nonenveloped viruses, which are the most resistant enteric pathogens, is not routinely available.

The evolution of the category of intermediate-level disinfection is intriguing. It was not included in the CDC guidelines published through 1983 [191]. The category was defined in the 1985 CDC revision [177], although there were no specific recommendations for how to achieve it nor distinctions made between items requiring low- vs. intermediate-level disinfection. In 1987, Rutala and Weber's table combined low- and intermediate-level disinfection [192]. In the 1990 Association for Practitioners in Infection Control (APIC) [193] guideline, the categories were separated and specific indications given for each. Both were described with *maximum* exposure times, suggesting that the briefest contact with the disinfectant suffices. Unfortunately, although the difficulty in achieving and maintaining high-level disinfection establishes the usefulness of a less-intensive disinfection level, there remains practically no rigorous study or body of evidence providing a foundation for the category of intermediate-level disinfection.

Special issues regarding certain devices should be recognized. Nebulizers produce, by design, particles that become deposited in the alveoli. Accordingly, nebulizer cups and solutions intended for nebulization must be sterile. Endoscopic retrograde cholangiopancreatography is potentially much more hazardous than all other forms of endoscopy as a result of the vulnerability of partially obstructed biliary tracts to infection and the severe nature of acute cholangitis. Contamination of the biliary tract can arise if the water channel in an endoscope used for the procedure holds contaminated water. When water is expelled from the catheter and then drawn back into the suction channel, organisms introduced into the suction channel can be picked up by the cannula before introduction above the ampulla of Vater.

Tonometers pose special difficulties. Numerous adenovirus outbreaks have resulted from inadequate disinfection procedures [194,195]. Adenoviruses, which are small and lipid free, are relatively difficult to disinfect. Furthermore, tonometer tips are expensive, harmed by many disinfectants, and used frequently. In addition, pneumotonometer tips have a cavity that can retain germicides with the potential for subsequent damage of a patient's cornea. The American Academy of Ophthalmology's recommendations for simple alcohol wiping do not achieve even intermediate-level disinfection [196]. Automated reprocessing machines also have produced disinfection failures [197]. Standards for evaluating these machines have been published [198].

Dental items are upgraded beyond the general scheme because of a consensus set of recommendations [199].

Many endoscopy systems, ultrasound probes, and other semicritical items are now marketed with disposable sheaths. In theory, the underlying item should need no reprocessing whatsoever after the sheath is discarded. Unfortunately, there is relatively little independent assessment of the integrity and durability of these sheaths. Clearly, if a defect in the sheath is detected after use or if the underlying item is visibly contaminated with a patient's secretions, the item should be reprocessed as if it had been used without a sheath. Otherwise, it is probably sufficient to reprocess the item using low-level disinfection.

Steam Sterilization

Steam sterilization is highly reliable and is the method of choice when the device can tolerate the procedure. Nevertheless, the subtleties to its use sometimes go unrecognized. Steam is more than an efficient conveyor of heat. The water molecules participate in the denaturation of proteins and the disruption of other complex molecules. Accordingly, it is essential that steam reach all the surfaces to be sterilized. In gravity displacement autoclaves, the introduced

steam, which is less dense than air, forces air down and out through the autoclave drain. Devices with depressions that are not placed on their side or that have curved lumens will not be completely exposed to steam. The American Association of Medical Instrumentation (AAMI) standard for 132°C (270°F) sterilization assumes that this problem can be overcome by extending the cycle to 10 minutes [69]. Unfortunately, if steam does not reach the surface, this is equivalent to dry heat, a process that is generally held to require 2 hours of exposure. The penetration of steam into wrapped packages, porous materials, or in overpacked chambers also is not secure in gravity displacement autoclaves. These problems are mitigated in vacuum displacement autoclaves, which are evacuated before the introduction of steam. Pulsed vacuum autoclaves are even more efficient because they go through several cycles of vacuum and steam replacement, thus more reliably eliminating air.

Flash autoclaving also has attendant problems. The term itself is used variably to refer to short-duration, high-temperature steam autoclaving; the autoclaving of devices without wrapping; gravity displacement autoclaving; or some combination of the foregoing procedures. There is doubtlessly a need for rapid sterilization of low-inventory instruments that inadvertently become contaminated during surgery or highly tailored implantable items for which it is difficult to maintain a complete sterile inventory. Recent evidence suggests that the widely accepted 3-minute standard for 132°C (270°F) autoclaving should be extended to 4 minutes [200]. Anxieties about the low margin of safety from the 3-minute autoclaving underlie the CDC's recommendation [176] that the 3-minute cycle is not sufficient for implantable objects. The CDC did not specify any minimum duration for implantable objects, although the AAMI suggests that 10 minutes will suffice [69].

The duration of sterilization cycles at standard sterilization temperatures (121°C [250°F]) for liquids also is somewhat arbitrary. In this situation, steam is conveying only heat; thus, by extension from the standard 30-minute cycle for solid objects, longer times should be required for large volumes of liquids. The fact that most standards recommend <30 minutes or, for volumes in excess of 1 L, only 45 minutes, probably reflects the low organism burden of most such materials before sterilization.

Selection and Use of Germicides

Many physical techniques and chemical agents are useful in various contexts for disinfection or sterilization [20]. A summary of methods appropriate for various uses has been updated periodically and was last published by the CDC in 1983 [176,191]. Unfortunately, the CDC was forced to refrain from tying recommendations closely to particular products. The substituted CDC environmental guideline published in 1985 and most recently in 2003 [176] discussed disinfectants and sterilants in a more general way. Revisions of the initial CDC summary have appeared [193,202]; they are presented in the Association for Professionals in Infection Control and Epidemiology's (APIC) "Guideline for Selection and Use of Disinfectants" written by Rutala [186]. Given the increase in type and composition of medical devices and the great variety of disinfection methods, this tabular approach is an oversimplification. The object categories overlap and are not comprehensive, and the descriptions of methods are largely references to manufacturers' recommendations for germicide concentrations, temperatures, and exposure times.

The APIC guideline [186] contains a superb discussion of the mechanisms of action, advantages and disadvantages, and tips on use of various disinfection methods. Besides the level of sterilization or disinfection, selection of a method necessitates considering its impact on the integrity of the device to be reprocessed, the possible effects on the warranty of the product and liability exposure, and occupational safety. Ethylene oxide, formaldehyde, or glutaraldehyde all pose potential risks to personnel. A proposed federal glutaraldehyde exposure standard, 0.2 parts per million (ppm) ceiling, will preclude glutaraldehyde use without evacuation hoods, personnel protection devices, or special enclosed reprocessors [203]. Whatever technique is selected, the manufacturer's instructions should be used to determine contact times and other use parameters. The disinfectant must be in contact with all relevant surfaces for the entire specified contact time.

It commonly is recommended that a particular product be purchased based on reference to standard guidelines, scientific literature, or manufacturers' recommendations. At a practical level, however, it is very difficult to use the first two. There is such a profusion of products that the standard recommendations [176,186] do not have enough specificity. Furthermore, manufacturers regularly modify their formulations and freely assert that flaws described in scientific publications [173,204] have been corrected. Thus, users are forced to rely on manufacturers' information. The only effectively regulated statement from manufacturers is that found on the label applied to the actual product.

The EPA has required that companies generate data underlying a claim that a product is a sporicide, hospital disinfectant (i.e., meets AOAC standards for disinfection of *S. aureus*, *P. aeruginosa*, and *S. choleraesuis*), or tuberculocide. The label has to specify the dilution, exposure time, and any other conditions required to achieve these disinfection. Reliance on the label is tricky for several reasons: the EPA or FDA can only irregularly independently verify manufacturers' claims [176,205,206], independent testing has revealed failures to meet standards [207], some disinfectant types may be inherently deficient [193], translating the EPA or FDA categories into the high-, intermediate-, and low-level disinfection system is somewhat arbitrary, and manufacturers do not always put all relevant information on the label. A manufacturer's written statement that a given product passes certain AOAC tests is important even if it is not independently verified.

Notwithstanding all of the difficulties attending reliance on the EPA registered product label and other written statements by manufacturers, most users must depend on them in product selection. At the University of Minnesota Hospital and Clinic, sterilization is considered achievable by any germicide that passes the AOAC test as a sporicide when it is used at the dilution, temperature, and exposure time required for sporicidal activity. In addition, steam, ethylene oxide, or dry heat are believed to produce sterilization. When a liquid germicide is used for sterilization, the item to be sterilized must be rinsed in sterile water, thoroughly dried, and enclosed in a sterile package.

High-level disinfection is considered possible using any germicide that passes AOAC tests as a sporicide and a tuberculocide when used at a dilution, temperature, and time required to produce tuberculocidal activity. After high-level disinfection, rinsing in tap water followed by thorough drying and low-touch handling is permitted. In addition, high-level disinfection is considered feasible with the use of sodium hypochlorite at 10,000 ppm for 5 minutes and 1,000 ppm for 20 minutes and pasteurization at 75°C (170°F) for 30 minutes or at 90°C (195°F) for 10 minutes [200]. Intermediate-level disinfection is believed to be effected by any germicide that passes AOAC tests as a hospital disinfectant and a tuberculocide when used at the concentration and temperature required to produce tuberculocidal activity with an exposure time of ≥10 minutes. Also accepted are sodium hypochlorite at 1,000 ppm or ethanol or isopropyl alcohol at 70% to 90% at an exposure time of 10 minutes. There is no actual evidence of effectiveness for the 10-minute exposure time. Finally, low-level disinfection is considered achievable through the use of any germicide that passes AOAC tests as a hospital disinfectant when used at the label concentration and temperature required to produce hospital disinfection—sodium hypochlorite at 100 ppm or ethanol or isopropyl alcohol at 70% to 90%. There is no specified minimum exposure time for low-level disinfection; merely wiping with the disinfectant is thought to be sufficient.

Creutzfeldt-Jakob Agent

The Creutzfeldt-Jakob agent and other prions are transmissible proteins in conformations that irreversibly autocatalyze conversion of the native proteins to the nonfunctional conformation. They are unusually resistant to inactivation. Transmission to humans has happened from stereotactic instruments, pituitary-derived growth hormone, corneal transplants, or dura mater grafts. Sporadic episodes in histopathology technicians have provoked anxiety about transmission to HCWs [209,210]. Critical or semicritical items previously in contact with brain tissue from Creutzfeldt-Jakob patients should be autoclaved for 1 hour at 132°C (270°F), immersed for 1 hour in 1 N sodium hydroxide, or both [211]. Although blood or spinal fluid has been found to transmit prions experimentally, there is no practical way to apply disinfecting methods to all the surfaces with which these body substances can come into contact. Given the frequency with which Creutzfeldt-Jakob disease remains undiagnosed, the potential for transmission by tissues other than brain, and the paucity of adequate disinfection methods, there is currently no practical way to accommodate fully the potential for transmission of this agent.

ENVIRONMENTAL SAMPLING

Routine Microbiologic Surveillance of Inanimate Objects

Environmental sampling accounted for a large fraction of HAI control efforts in the United States through 1970. As late as 1976, 74% of hospitals with ≥50 beds conducted routine environmental culturing [212] despite explicit statements by the CDC in 1970 [213] and the American Hospital Association in 1973 [214] recommending sharp circumscription of such routine culturing. These statements advocated abandonment of the practice of routinely culturing floors, walls, linens, and air but left open the possibility of conducting epidemiologically indicated cultures, spot-checking critical hospital equipment items (e.g., respiratory care equipment), undertaking routine microbial evaluation of hospital-prepared infant formula, and verifying sterilization procedures (176). Only the last procedure, however, was deemed necessary (see Chapter 20).

Possible grounds for routine culturing of inanimate objects include HAI prevention, education of HCWs, and responding to the guidelines put forth by a number of organizations or government agencies. To contribute to HAI prevention, the culture must at least have an interpretable result. When sterility is the goal, interpretation is possible. Culturing also may be of value, however, when the need for sterility is not established (e.g., infant formula, dialysis water). Perhaps the best operational definition of interpretability is that certain results lead to specific actions. An additional, less commonly articulated criterion is that the cultured object has a high enough probability of contamination with a severe enough consequence if contaminated to justify the culture. Routine culturing of purchased sterile supplies is not justified because of the very low chance of a positive culture.

The educational value of culturing inanimate objects is limited but may be a valid adjunct to other teaching efforts. Care must be taken to prevent such efforts from growing beyond the bounds of a specific educational objective. Responding to the guidelines of various organizations quickly becomes an arcane and ineffectual exercise. First, these organizations have considerably varied standings. One *must* comply with the rules of regulatory agencies, such as the FDA, the federal and state Occupational Health and Safety Administration, or the federal End Stage Renal Dialysis (ESRD) program. Any hospital with a training program must meet the standards of the JCAHO. However, compliance is less essential in recommendations from the many respected government (e.g., the CDC) or non-government (e.g., the AAMI, SHEA, or APIC) agencies/organizations.

A second problem in formulating a hospital's response to these various guidelines is that the statements themselves are sometimes frankly inconsistent. For instance, the CDC's Guideline for Prevention of Intravascular Device-Related Infections [215] made no mention of culturing hospital-compounded infusion solutions when the JCAHO seemed to require such culturing. A third problem, ambiguity, is illustrated by the JCAHO statement on monitoring parenteral medication. Through 1991 (but not thereafter), solutions "manufactured" in the hospital were supposed to "be examined on a sampling basis." We can only assume that the intent was to subject solutions to microbiologic examination.

A fourth problem is the lack of regular updating. Although some agencies, such as the JCAHO or AAMI, have instituted formal updating that includes specific rescission of previous statements, others have actually disbanded (e.g., the National Coordinating Committee on Large-Volume Parenterals (NCCLVP) sponsored by the USP and FDA [216]). A fifth complexity involves interlocking use of these dicta. The AAMI dialysis water–culturing protocol is explicitly intended to be flexible. However, the federal ESRD program requires exact compliance [217]. The American Society of Hospital Pharmacists has formally accepted the NCCLVP recommendations, giving them a longevity beyond that of their creator [216]. Despite these complexities, infection control personnel must consider the statements of these bodies in making decisions about culturing inanimate objects. If nothing else, these statements can assume substantial medicolegal importance.

A general problem that arises in considering culturing protocols for any product is determining when in the preparation-use sequence to perform the culture. It is logistically simpler to obtain the culture at the point of preparation, and the impetus to culture implements and objects used in the care of patients often comes from the quality control effort of the department preparing them. However, more relevant to patients' care is the status of the item at the time of its actual use. If cultures are positive at the end of the preparation-use sequence, efforts may be undertaken to determine the sources of contamination.

Some unusual biologic items probably should be routinely cultured. Organs, including corneas, bone, kidneys, livers, hearts, pancreases, and bone marrow for transplantation (especially if highly processed), may become contaminated in procurement, transportation, or storage. Positive cultures can have therapeutic implications in addition to suggesting the need for improvements in sterilization techniques. A biologic product that probably does not need routine culture is banked, expressed human milk intended for prompt ingestion by the donor's offspring.

It is administered orally and inevitably is frequently contaminated [218]. However, standards for donor selection, milk pasteurization, and microbiologic screening in other contexts have been published [219]. Consensus on two possible recommendations—routine culturing of hospital water for *Legionella* spp. and of air for fungi—may yet emerge. Routine culturing of air should be relevant only in hospitals with highly immunosuppressed patients.

Dialysis Water

The AAMI standard for culturing dialysis water (presented earlier) has been endorsed by the CDC [176] see also Chapter 23. Sampling should be conducted at least monthly. It is preferable to sample system water just before a disinfection cycle. Machine water should be taken from different machines to ensure that all defects are identified.

Hospital-Compounded Pharmacy Products

At present there is confusion regarding whether the production, mixing, or aliquoting of sterile materials by hospital pharmacies should be considered compounding or manufacturing. Preparations for individual patients clearly fall into the former category. Batches made in advance for many patients may be interpreted as being of the latter type. The implications are considerable. Compounding is governed by state boards of pharmacy and is subject to less stringent requirements. Manufacturing is regulated by the FDA and, thus, must comply with good manufacturing practice [220]. These standards, like JCAHO standards, are broadly phrased but are taken to require detailed compliance. With respect to sterility, these requirements call for culturing two items from batches of <20 items, 10% of lots of 20–200 items, and 20 units of larger lots [220]; detailed culturing procedures that include 14 days of observation for most items [220]; and quarantine of an entire batch until the sterility testing is completed [220]. These stipulations would be burdensome for hospital pharmacies.

Additional considerations apply to infusion solutions. A 1980 NCCLVP statement "endorses the concept of hospital pharmacies using sterility testing of IV admixtures as a method for monitoring the performances of pharmacy equipment and personnel" [216]. The rationale is worded to avoid the demand that sterility testing be completed before administering the solutions. The JCAHO eliminated an apparent requirement for culturing parenteral medications and solutions in 1992.

These recommendations may be challenged on several grounds. The bulk of infusion-caused infection arises from organisms ascending along the tissue-cannula interface rather than by fluid contamination (see Chapter 37). Much of the contamination of in-use infusion fluid probably arises during administration rather than compounding. Even the need for sterility of infusion fluid is arguable. Most in-use fluid contamination is present at very low concentrations, is due to relatively nonpathogenic strains, and has not been proved to be associated with illness. The least irrational program of infusion fluid culturing would focus on the in-use product, would use culture methods that do not yield positive cultures with very low levels of contamination, and would involve organism speciation to identify properly the few hazardous species capable of proliferating in the product.

Respiratory Therapy and Anesthesia Equipment

The current CDC Guideline for the Prevention of Healthcare-Associated Pneumonia [104] does not contain a recommendation for or against culturing respiratory therapy equipment. No recent organizational statement favors it. Advocates of routine culturing of breathing circuits must surmount two counterarguments: first, that there is no secure demonstration that small numbers of organisms on internal surfaces of breathing circuits cause disease and, second, that in-use breathing circuits frequently become contaminated with the patient's organisms, even if the circuits start out sterile [221]. Most reports of HAI caused by contamination of breathing circuits are not convincing. In others, it is not possible to be sure the contamination was of tubing rather than of a nebulizer or that the tubing was thoroughly dried after reprocessing [222]. Any program of routine culturing of these items should cope with the logistic problem of examining the most relevant specimens—those actually in use.

Laminar Airflow Hoods

Because HEPA filters do develop leaks, routine periodic evaluation is indicated. However, dioctyl phthalate testing is more reliable than using settling plates or other microbiologic assessments [223]. Through 1991, the JCAHO required microbiologic monitoring but in 1992 abridged the requirement to call for "a suitable area for manipulation of parenteral medications."

Formula

Through 1977, successive editions of *Standards and Recommendations for Hospital Care of Newborn Infants*, published by the American Academy of Pediatrics [150], recommended routine culturing of hospital-manufactured formula obtained from nursing units. Plate counts >25 cfu/ml were deemed to indicate that the technique was faulty and immediate corrective action required. The CDC supported this measure in 1982 [176]. The 1983 and 2002 American Academy of Pediatrics and American College of Obstetricians and Gynecologists publication, *Guidelines for Perinatal Care* [151], has superseded the former series, and it is silent with respect to culturing hospital-manufactured formula. Similarly, subsequent statements by the American Hospital Association [149] and the JCAHO contain no reference to this issue. Abandonment of this widely accepted practice—even by those skeptical of environmental culturing [224]—probably reflects a perception that most hospitals have switched to commercially prepared formulas. Although this is true of routine infant care, there is an increase in the development of hospital-prepared specialized enteral feedings, for which specific guidelines may need to be developed.

Clearly, it is necessary for infant formula and adult enteral supplements to be free of enteric pathogens and organisms capable of generating enterotoxins (e.g., *S. aureus*). It seems desirable that formula also be free of high concentrations of potent HAI pathogens. Neonatal *Klebsiella* bacteremia has followed oral ingestion of *Klebsiella*-contaminated breast milk [225]. *Enterobacter sakazakii* meningitis and death have resulted from imbibing contaminated powdered milk [226].

Freedom from *Aspergillus flavus* probably is desirable for all foodstuffs because of the potential of aflatoxin production. Nonetheless, previous recommendations do not call for organism identification, and it is unclear that even large numbers of organisms, excluding those mentioned previously, constitute any hazard.

Establishing protocols for culturing formula leads to many questions:

1. *Which of the many formulas hospitals now make must meet the standard?* The usual age cutoff for infants is 1 year, but it is likely that a contaminated enteral formula poses a greater hazard to an immunocompromised adult than to a relatively healthy 11-month-old baby.
2. *What culture methods should be used?* Because dry formula powder may contain high concentrations of

TABLE 19-2
AREAS OF FUTURE RESEARCH

Air

- Standardize the methodology and interpretation of microbiologic air sampling (e.g., determine action levels or minimum infectious dose for aspergillosis, and evaluate the significance of airborne bacteria and fungi in the surgical field and the impact on postoperative SSI).
- Develop new molecular typing methods to better define the epidemiology of healthcare-associated outbreaks of aspergillosis and to associate isolates recovered from both clinical and environmental sources.
- Develop new methods for the diagnosis of aspergillosis that can lead reliably to early recognition of infection.
- Assess the value of laminar flow technology for surgeries other than for joint replacement surgery.
- Determine whether particulate sampling can be routinely performed in lieu of microbiologic sampling for purposes such as determining air quality of clean environments (e.g., operating rooms, HSCT units).

Water

- Evaluate new methods of water treatment, both in the facility and at the water utility (e.g., ozone, chlorine dioxide, copper/silver/monochloramine) and perform cost-benefit analyses of treatment in preventing healthcare-associated legionellosis.
- Evaluate the role of biofilms in overall water quality and determine the impact of water treatments for the control of biofilm in distribution systems.
- Determine whether the use of ultrapure fluids in dialysis is feasible and warranted, and determine the action level for the final bath.
- Develop quality assurance protocols and validated methods for sampling filtered rinse water used with AERs, and determine acceptable microbiologic quality of AER rinse water.

Environmental Services

- Evaluate the innate resistance of microorganisms to the action of chemical germicides, and determine what, if any, linkage there may be between antibiotic resistance and resistance to disinfectants.

Laundry and Bedding

- Evaluate the microbial inactivation capabilities of new laundry detergents, bleach substitutes, other laundry additives, and new laundry technologies.

Animals in Healthcare Facilities

- Conduct surveillance to monitor incidence of infections among patients in facilities that use animal programs, and conduct investigations to determine new infection control strategies to prevent these infections.
- Evaluate the epidemiologic impact of performing procedures on animals (e.g., surgery or imaging) in human healthcare facilities.

Regulated Medical Waste

- Determine the efficiency of current medical waste treatment technologies to inactivate emerging pathogens that may be present in medical waste (e.g., SARS-co V).
- Explore options to enable healthcare facilities to reinstate the capacity to inactivate microbiological cultures and stocks on site.

(From [176])

spores, culture techniques that promote thermophilic organism growth frequently produce excessive counts from nonhazardous formulas.

3. *If counts exceed 25 cfu/ml, what actions should be taken?* Hospitals producing many small batches of highly individualized enteral formulas find it very burdensome to use sterile blenders and, when possible, sterile formula components. Blenders often are difficult to sanitize because of the crevices in the blade housing. Many specialized supplements rapidly lose nutritional value at 100°C (212°F), precluding postpreparation treatment.

The least arbitrary routine culturing program would focus on formula to be given to the most debilitated neonates or other patients, use culturing methods yielding only human pathogens—perhaps only enteric pathogens—and be considered only a marginal supplement to general sanitary measures.

Future Issues

The recent CDC environmental guideline identified a number of critical issues for future research. Answers to many of these and other questions could enhance our efforts in improving patient care and allocating resources to ensure that we appropriately address environmental issues that place our patients at increased risk of HAIs (Table 19-2).

REFERENCES

1. No author. *Oxford English dictionary.* Glasgow: Oxford University Press, 1971.
2. Cahill CK, Heath J. Sterile water used for humidification in low-flow oxygen therapy: Is it necessary? *Am J Infect Control* 1990;18:13.
3. Beck-Sague CM, Jarvis WR. Epidemic bloodstream infections associated with pressure transducers: A persistent problem. *Infect Control Hosp Epidemiol* 1989;10:54.
4. Mead JH, Lupton GP, Dillavon CL, Odom RB. Cutaneous *Rhizopus* infection: Occurrence as a postoperative complication associated with an elasticized adhesive dressing. *JAMA* 1979;242:272.
5. LeMaile-Williams M, Burwell LA, Salisbury D, et al. Outbreak of cutaneous *Rhizopus arrhizus* infection associated with karaya ostomy bags. *Clin Infect Dis* 2006;43:e83–88.
6. Pearson RD, Valenti WM, Steigbigel RT. *Clostridium perfringens* wound infection associated with elastic bandages. *JAMA* 1980;244:1128.
7. Hoffman PC, et al. False-positive blood cultures: Association with non-sterile blood collection tubes. *JAMA* 1976;236:2073.
8. Rogues AM, Sarlangue J, de Barbeyrac B, et al. *Agrobacterium radiobacter* as a cause of pseudobacteremia. *Infect Control Hosp Epidemiol* 1999;20:345–47.
9. Becks VE, Lorenzoni NM. *Pseudomonas aeruginosa* outbreak in a neonatal intensive care unit: A possible link to contaminated hand lotion. *Am J Infect Control* 1995;23:396.
10. Parrott PL, et al. *Pseudomonas aeruginosa* peritonitis associated with contaminated poloxamer-iodine solution. *Am J Infect Control* 1995;23:396–98.
11. Molina-Cabrillana J, Bolanos-Rivero M, Alvarez-Leon EE, et al. Intrinsically contaminated alcohol-free mouthwash implicated in a nosocomial outbreak of *Burkholderia cepacia* colonization and infection. *Infect Control Hosp Epidemiol* 2006;27:1281–82.
12. Perry WD et al. Transmission of group-A streptococci. I. The role of contaminated bedding. *Am J Hyg* 1957;66:85.
13. Perry WD, Siegel AC, Rammelkamp CH Jr. Transmission of group-A streptococci. II. The role of contaminated dust. *Am J Hyg* 1957;66:96.
14. Rammelkamp CH Jr, et al. Transmission of group-A streptococci. III. The effect of drying on the infectivity of the organism for man. *J Hyg* (London) 1958;56:280.
15. LeRudulier D, et al. Molecular biology of osmoregulation. *Science* 1984;224:1064.
16. Nerurkar LS, West F, Madden DL, Sever JL. Survival of herpes simplex virus in water specimens collected from hot tubs in spa facilities and on plastic surfaces. *JAMA* 1983;250:3081.
17. Douglas JM, Corey L. Fomites and herpes simplex viruses: A case for nonvenereal transmission? *JAMA* 1983;250:3093.
18. Maki DG, Alvarado CJ, Hassemer CA, Zilz MA. Relation of the inanimate hospital environment to endemic nosocomial infections. *N Engl J Med* 1982;307:1562.
19. Lauer JL, Van Drunen NA, Washburn JW, Balfour HH Jr. Transmission of hepatitis B virus in clinical laboratory areas. *J Infect Dis* 1979;140:512.
20. Mortimer EA Jr, Wolinsky E, Gonzaga AJ, Rammelkamp CH Jr. Role of airborne transmission in staphylococcal infections. *Br Med J* 1966;1:319.
21. Marx A, Shay DK, Noel JS, et al. An outbreak of acute gastroenteritis in a geriatric long-term-care facility: Combined application of epidemiological and molecular diagnostic methods. *Infect Control Hosp Epidemiol* 1999;20:306–11.
22. Maslow J, Mulligan ME. Epidemiologic typing systems. *Infect Control Hosp Epidemiol* 1996;17:595.
23. Rodriguez E, De Meeus T, Mallie M, et al. Multicentric epidemiological study of *Aspergillus fumigatus* isolates by multilocus enzyme electrophoresis. *J Clin Microbiol* 1996;34:2559.
24. Kundsin RB, ed. Airborne contagion. *Ann N Y Acad Sci* 1980;353:1.
25. Muilenberg ML, Burge HA. *Aerobiology.* Boca Raton: Lewis Publishers, 1996.
26. Eickhoff TC. Airborne disease: Including chemical and biological warfare. *Am J Epidemiol* 1996;144:S39.
27. Roy CJ, Milton DK. Airborne transmission of communicable infection—The elusive pathway. *N Engl J Med* 2004;350:1710–12.
28. Brachman PS. Nosocomial infection: Airborne or not? In: *Proceedings of the International Conference on Nosocomial Infections.* Chicago: American Hospital Association, 1970:189–92.
29. Lidwell OM. Airborne bacteria and surgical infection. *Am J Med* 1981;70:693.
30. Iwen PC, Davis JC, Reed EC, et al. Airborne fungal spore monitoring in a protective environment during hospital construction and correlation with an outbreak of invasive aspergillosis. *Infect Control Hosp Epidemiol* 1994;15:303.
31. Sayer WJ, Shean DB, Ghosseiri J. Estimation of airborne fungal flora by the Andersen sampler versus the gravity settling culture plate. I. Isolation frequency and number of colonies. *J Allergy* 1969;48:214.
32. Burge HA. *Bioaerosis.* Boca Raton: Lewis Publishers, 1995.
33. Greene VW, Vesley D, Bond RG, Michaelsen GS. Microbiological contamination of hospital air. I. Quantitative studies. *Appl Microbiol* 1962;10:561.
34. Greene VW, Vesley D, Bond RG, Michaelsen GS. Microbiological studies of hospital air. II. Qualitative studies. *Appl Microbiol* 1962;10:567.
35. Bean B, et al. Influenza B: Hospital activity during a community epidemic. *Diagn Microbiol Infect Dis* 1983;1:177.
36. Noble WC. Dispersal of microorganisms from skin. In: *Microbiology of human skin.* 2nd ed. London: Lloyd-Luke Ltd., 1981:79–85.
37. Shaffer JG, Key ID. A three-year study of carpeting in a general hospital. *Health Lab Sci* 1969;6:215.
38. Wenzel RP, Veazey JM Jr, Townsend TR. Role of the inanimate environment in hospital-acquired infections. In: Cundy KR, Ball W, eds. *Infection control in healthcare facilities: microbiological surveillance.* Baltimore: University Park Press, 1977:71–98.
39. Committee on Trauma, Division of Medical Sciences, National Academy of Sciences–National Research Council. Postoperative wound infections: The influence of ultraviolet irradiation of the

operating room and of various other factors. *Ann Surg* 1964;160 (suppl):1.

40. Bischoff WE, Wallis ML, Tucker BK, et al. "Gesundheit!" sneezing, common colds, allergies, and *Staphylococcus aureus* dispersion. *J Infect Dis* 2006;194:1119–26.

41. Dexter F. *Pseudomonas aeruginosa* in a regional burn center. *J Hyg* 1971;69:179.

42. Bauer TM, et al. An epidemiological study assessing the relative importance of airborne and direct contact transmission of microorganisms in a medical intensive care unit. *J Hosp Infect* 1990;15:301.

43. Cheng K, Smyth RL, Govan JRW, et al. Spread of β-lactam-resistant *Pseudomonas aeruginosa* in a cystic fibrosis clinic. *Lancet* 1996;348:639.

44. LiPuma JJ et al. Person-to-person transmission of *Pseudomonas cepacia* between patients with cystic fibrosis. *Lancet* 1990;336:1094.

45. Blessing-Moore J, Maybury B, Lewiston N, Yeager A. Mucosal droplet spread of *Pseudomonas aeruginosa* from cough of patients with cystic fibrosis. *Thorax* 1979;34:429.

46. Grieble HG, Bird TJ, Nidea HM, Miller CA. Chute-hydropulping waste disposal system: A reservoir of enteric bacilli and *Pseudomonas* in a modem hospital. *J Infect Dis* 1974;130:602.

47. Kelsen SG, McGuckin M. The role of airborne bacteria in the contamination of fine-particle nebulizers and the development of nosocomial pneumonia. *Ann N Y Acad Sci* 1980;353:218.

48. Kelsen SG, McGuckin M, Kelsen DP, Cherniak NS. Airborne contamination of fine-particle nebulizers. *JAMA* 1977;237:2311.

49. Dark FA, Callow DS. The effect of growth conditions on the survival of airborne *E. coli*. In: Hers JF, Winkler KC, eds. *Airborne transmission and airborne infection*. New York: Wiley, 1973:97–99.

50. Marthi B, Fieland VP, Walter M, Seidler RJ. Survival of bacteria during aerosolization. *Appl Environ Microbiol* 1990;56:3463.

51. Grieble HG, et al. Fine-particle humidifiers: Source of *Pseudomonas aeruginosa* infections in a respiratory-disease unit. *N Engl J Med* 1970;282:531.

52. Smith PW, Massanari RM. Room humidifiers as the source of *Acinetobacter* infections. *JAMA* 1977;237:795.

53. Rhame FS, Streifel AJ, Kersey JH Jr, McGlave PB. Extrinsic risk factors for pneumonia in the patient at risk. *Am J Med* 1984;76(5A):42.

54. Hahn T, Cummings KM, Michalek AM, et al. Efficacy of high-efficiency particulate air filtration in preventing aspergillosis in immunocompromised patients with hematologic malignancies. *Infect Control Hosp Epidemiol* 2002;23:525–31.

55. Kennedy HF, Michie JR, Richardson MD. Air sampling for *Aspergillus* spp. during building activity in a paediatric hospital ward. *J Hosp Infect* 1995;31:322.

56. Goodley JM, Clayton YM, Hay RJ. Environmental sampling for aspergilli during building construction on a hospital site. *J Hosp Infect* 1994;26:27.

57. Green FHY, Yoshida K. Characteristics of aerosols generated during autopsy procedures and their potential role as carriers of infectious agents. *Appl Occup Environ Hyg* 1990;5:853.

58. McKinley IB Jr, Ludlow MO. Hazards of laser smoke during endodontic therapy. *J Endodont* 1994;20:558.

59. Association of Operating Room Nurses. Proposed recommended practices: Laser safety in the practice setting. *AORN J* 1993;57:720.

60. American Public Health Association. *Standard methods for the examination of water and wastewater*. 17th ed. Washington, D.C.: American Public Health Association, 1989.

61. U.S. Environmental Protection Agency. National interim primary drinking water regulations. *Federal Register*, 1975;40:59566.

62. Geldreich EE. Current status of microbiological water quality criteria. *ASM News* 1981;47:23.

63. European Community Council directive no. 80/778/EEC of 15 July 1980 relating to the quality of water intended for human consumption. *Off J Eur Commun* 1980;L229:11.

64. Picard B, Goullet P. Seasonal prevalence of nosocomial *Aeromonas hydrophila* infection related to aeromonas in hospital water. *J Hosp Infect* 1987;10:152.

65. Association for the Advancement of Medical Instrumentation. *Hemodialysis systems*. ANSI/AAMI RD5:2003. Arlington, VA: Association for the Advancement of Medical Instrumentation.

66. Dawids SG, Vejlsgaard R. Bacteriological and clinical evaluation of different dialysate delivery systems. *Acta Med Scand* 1976;199:151.

67. Favero MS, et al. Gram-negative bacteria in hemodialysis systems. *Health Lab Sci* 1975;12:321.

68. Lauer JL, et al. The bacteriological quality of hemodialysis solution as related to several environmental factors. *Nephron* 1975;15:87.

69. Association for the Advancement of Medical Instrumentation. ANSI/AAMI RD52:2004: Dialysate for hemodialysis. Association for the Advancement of Medical Instrumentation, August 2004, American National Standards Institute, Inc.

70. Kesmaviam P, Luehmann D, Shapiro F, Comty C. *Investigation of the risks and hazards associated with hemodialysis systems*. Washington, DC: FDA Bureau of Medical Devices, 1980. (Technical report, contract no. 223–78–5046).

71. McGuckin MB, Thorpe RJ, Abrutyn E. An outbreak of *Pseudomonas aeruginosa* wound infections related to Hubbard tank treatments. *Arch Phys Med Rehabil* 1981;62:283.

72. Turner AG, Higgins MM, Craddock JG. Disinfection of immersion tanks (Hubbard) in a hospital burn unit. *Arch Environ Health* 1974;28:101.

73. Mayhall CG, Lamb VA, Gayle WE Jr, Haynes BW Jr. *Enterobacter cloacae* septicemia in a burn center: Epidemiology and control of an outbreak. *J Infect Dis* 1979;139:166.

74. Gustafson TL, Bank JD, Hutcheson RH Jr., Schaffner W. *Pseudomonas* folliculitis: An outbreak and review. *Rev Infect Dis* 1983;5:1.

75. Salmen P, Dwyer DM, Vorse H, Kruse W. Whirlpool-associated *Pseudomonas aeruginosa* urinary tract infections. *JAMA* 1983;260:2025.

76. Rose HD, et al. *Pseudomonas* pneumonia associated with use of a home whirlpool spa. *JAMA* 1983;250:2027.

77. Centers for Disease Control and Prevention. *Disinfection of hydrotherapy pools and tanks*. Atlanta: Hospital Infections Program, Center for Infectious Diseases, Centers for Disease Control and Prevention, 1974 [reprinted 1982].

78. Centers for Disease Control and Prevention. Endotoxic reactions associated with the reuse of cardiac catheters—Massachusetts. *MMWR* 1979;28:25.

79. Carson LA, Favero MS, Bond WW, Petersen NJ. Morphological, biochemical, and growth characteristics of *Pseudomonas cepacia* from distilled water. *Appl Microbiol* 1973;25:476.

80. Favero MS, Carson LA, Bond WW, Petersen NJ. *Pseudomonas aeroginosa*: Growth in distilled water from hospitals. *Science* 1971;173:836.

81. Carson LA, Favero MS, Bond WW, Petersen NJ. Factors affecting comparative resistance of naturally occurring and subcultured *Pseudomonas aeruginosa* to disinfectants. *Appl Microbiol* 1972;23:863.

82. Baumann P. Isolation of *Acinetobacter* from soil and water. *J Bacteriol* 1968;96:39.

83. Contant J, et al. Investigation of an outbreak of *Acinetobacter calcoaceticus* var. *anitratus* infections in an adult intensive care unit. *Am J Infect Control* 1990;18:288.

84. Gervich DH, Grout CS. An outbreak of nosocomial *Acinetobacter* infections from humidifiers. *Am J Infect Control* 1985;13:210.

85. Ratner H. *Flavobacterium meningosepticum*. *Infect Control Hosp Epidemiol* 1984;5:237.

86. Decker CF, Simon GL, Keiser JF. *Flavimonas oryzihabitans* (*Pseudomonas oryzihabitans*; CDC Group Ve-2) bacteremia in the immunocompromised host. *Arch Intern Med* 1991;151:603.

87. DuMoulin GC, Stottmeier KD. Waterborne mycobacteria: An increasing threat to health. *ASM News* 1986;52:525.

88. Carson LA, Petersen NJ, Favero MS, Aguero SM. Growth characteristics of atypical mycobacteria in water and their comparative resistance to disinfectants. *Appl Environ Microbiol* 1978;36:839.

89. Hays PS, McGiboney DL, Band JD, Feeley JC. Resistance of *Mycobacterium cheloneilike* organisms to formaldehyde. *Appl Environ Microbiol* 1982;43:722.

90. Bergogne-Baérezin E, Joly-Guillou ML, Vieu JF. Epidemiology of nosocomial infections due to *Acinetobacter calcoaceticus*. *J Hosp Infect* 1987;10:105.

91. Yu VL, Zuravleff JJ, Gavlik L, Magnussen MH. Lack of evidence for person-to-person transmission of Legionnaires' disease. *J Infect Dis* 1983;147:362.

92. Doebbeling BN, et al. Nosocomial *Legionella micdadei* pneumonia: 10 years experience and a case control study. *J Hosp Infect* 1989;13:289.

93. Lowry PW, et al. A cluster of *Legionella* sternal-wound infections due to postoperative topical exposure to contaminated tap water. *N Engl J Med* 1991;324:109.

94. Muder RR, Yu VL, Woo AH. Mode of transmission of *Legionella pneumophila*: A critical review. *Arch Intern Med* 1986;146:1607.

95. Shands KN, et al. Potable water as a source of Legionnaires' disease. *JAMA* 1985;253:1412.

96. Helms CM, et al. Legionnaires' disease associated with a hospital water system: A five-year progress report on continuous hyperchlorination. *JAMA* 1988;259:2423.

97. Muder RR, et al. Nosocomial Legionnaire's disease uncovered in a prospective study: Implications for underdiagnosis. *JAMA* 1983;249:3184.

98. Brady MT. Nosocomial Legionnaires' disease in a children's hospital. *J Pediatr* 1989;115:46.

99. Breiman RF, et al. Association of shower use with Legionnaires' disease. *JAMA* 1990;263:2924.

100. Vickers RM, et al. Determinants of *Legionella pneumophila* contamination of water distribution systems: 15-hospital prospective study. *Infect Control Hosp Epidemiol* 1987;8:357.

101. Kim BR, Anderson JE, Mueller SA, et al. Literature review—Efficacy of various disinfectants against *Legionella* in water systems. *Water Res.* 2002;36:4433–44.

102. Barbaree JM, et al. Isolation of protozoa from water associated with a legionellosis outbreak and demonstration of intracellular multiplication of *Legionella pneumophila*. *Appl Environ Microbiol* 1986;51:422.

103. Centers for Disease Control and Prevention. Should hospital water be checked for *Legionella*? *Hosp Infect Control* 1983;10:125.

104. Tablan OC, Anderson LJ, Besser R, et al. Healthcare Infection Control Practices Advisory Committee Guidelines for preventing health-care–associated pneumonia, 2003: Recommendations of CDC and the Healthcare Infection Control Practices Advisory Committee. *MMWR Recomm Rep* 2004;53(RR-3):1–36.

105. Plouffe JF, et al. Subtypes of *Legionella pneumophila* serogroup 1 associated with different attack rates. *Lancet* 1983;2:649.

106. Yu VL. Nosocomial legionellosis: Current epidemiological issues. In: Remington JS, Swartz MN, eds. *Current clinical topics in infectious diseases.* 7th ed. New York: McGraw-Hill, 1986:239–53.

107. Kuchta JM, et al. Susceptibility of *Legionella pneumophila* to chlorine in tap water. *Appl Environ Microbiol* 1983;46:1134.

108. States SJ, et al. Chlorine, pH, and control of *Legionella* in hospital plumbing systems. *JAMA* 1989;261:1882.

109. Bier JW, Sawyer TK. Amoebae isolated from laboratory eyewash stations. *Curr Microbiol* 1990;20:349.

110. Hall CB, Douglas RG Jr, Schnabel KC, Geiman JM. Infectivity of respiratory syncytial virus by various routes of inoculation. *Infect Immun* 1981;33:779.

111. Hall CB, Douglas RG Jr, Geiman JM. Possible transmission by fomites of respiratory syncytial virus. *J Infect Dis* 1980;141:98.

112. Hall CB, Douglas RG Jr. Modes of transmission of respiratory syncytial virus. *J Pediatr* 1981;99:100.

113. Wust J, Sullivan NM, Hardegger U, Wilkins TD. Investigation of an outbreak of antibiotic-associated colitis by various typing methods. *J Clin Microbiol* 1982;16:1096.

114. McFarland LV, Stamm WE. Review of *Clostridium difficile*–associated diseases. *Am J Infect Control* 1986;14:99.

115. Johnson S, et al. Prospective, controlled study of vinyl glove use to interrupt *Clostridium difficile* nosocomial transmission. *Am J Med* 1990;88:137.

116. Johnson S, et al. Nosocomial *Clostridium difficile* colonisation and disease. *Lancet* 1990;336:97.

117. Osterholm MT, Garayalde SM. Clinical viral hepatitis B among Minnesota hospital personnel. *JAMA* 1985;254:3207.

118. Alter MJ, et al. The changing epidemiology of hepatitis B in the United States: Need for alternative vaccination strategies. *JAMA* 1990;263:9.

119. Forester G, Joline C, Wormser GP. Blood contamination of tourniquets used in routine phlebotomy. *Am J Infect Control* 1990;18:386.

120. Bond WW, et al. Survival of hepatitis B virus after drying and storage for one week. *Lancet* 1981;1:550.

121. Bond WW, Favero MS, Petersen NJ, Ebert JW. Inactivation of hepatitis B virus by intermediate-to-high-level disinfectant chemicals. *J Clin Microbiol* 1983;18:535.

122. Douvin C, et al. An outbreak of hepatitis B in an endocrinology unit traced to a capillary-blood-sampling device. *N Engl J Med* 1990;322:57.

123. Centers for Disease Control and Prevention. Recommendations for prevention of HIV transmission in health-care settings. *MMWR* 1987;36(2S):1S.

124. Centers for Disease Control and Prevention. Recommendations for initial management of suspected or confirmed cases of Lassa fever. *MMWR* 1980;28(suppl):52.

125. Centers for Disease Control and Prevention. Management of patients with suspected viral hemorrhagic fever. *MMWR* 1988;37(S-3):1.

126. Centers for Disease Control and Prevention. Interim guidance for managing patients with suspected viral hemorrhagic fever in U.S. hospitals. *MMWR* 1995;44,475–79.

127. Anderson RL. Biological evaluation of carpeting. *Appl Microbiol* 1969,10.100.

128. Shaffer JG. Microbiology of hospital carpeting. *Health Lab Sci* 1966;3:73.

129. Winters WD. A new perspective of microbial survival and dissemination in a prospectively contaminated air-fluidized bed model. *Am J Infect Control* 1990;18:307.

130. Vesley D, Hankinson SE, Lauer JL. Microbial survival and dissemination associated with an air-fluidized therapy unit. *Am J Infect Control* 1986;14:35.

131. Bolyard EA, Townsend TR, Horan T. Airborne contamination associated with in-use air-fluidized beds: A descriptive study. *Am J Infect Control* 1987;15:75.

132. Freeman R, Gould FK, Ryan DW, et al. Nosocomial infection due to *Enterococci* attributed to a fluidized microsphere bed: The value of pyrolysis mass spectrometry. *J Hosp Infect* 1994;27:187.

133. Archibald LK, Corl A, Shah B, et al. *Serratia marcescens* outbreak associated with extrinsic contamination of 1% chlorxylenol soap. *Infect Control Hosp Epidemiol* 1997;18:704–9.

134. Heinze JE. Bar soap and liquid soap. *JAMA* 1984;251:3222.

135. Kates SG, McGinley KJ, Larson EL, Leyden JJ. Indigenous multiresistant bacteria from flowers in hospital and nonhospital environments. *Am J Infect Control* 1991;19:156.

136. Acha PN, Szyfres B. *Zoonoses and communicable diseases common to man and animals.* Washington, DC: Pan American Health Organization, 1980. (Scientific Publication No. 354.)

137. Hall CJ, et al. Laboratory outbreak of Q fever acquired from sheep. *Lancet* 1982;1:1004.

138. Abinanti FR, Welsh HH, Lennette EH, Brunetti O. Q fever studies. XVI. Some aspects of the experimental infection induced in sheep by the intratracheal route of inoculation. *Am J Hyg* 1953;57:170.

139. Bernard KW, Parham GL, Winkler WG, Melnick CG. Q fever control measures: Recommendations for research facilities using sheep. *Infect Control Hosp Epidemiol* 1982;3:461.

140. Chang HJ, Miller HL, Watkins N, et al. An epidemic of Malassezia pachydermatis in an intensive care nursery associated with colonization of health care workers' pet dogs. *N Engl J Med* 1998;338:706–11.

141. Centers for Disease Control and Prevention. Outbreak of viral hepatitis in the staff of a pediatric ward—California. *MMWR* 1977;26:77.

142. Standaert SM, Hutcheson RH, Schaffner W. Nosocomial transmission of *Salmonella* gastroenteritis to laundry workers in a nursing home. *Infect Control Hosp Epidemiol* 1994;15:22.

143. Meyer CL, et al. Should linen in newborn intensive care units be autoclaved? *Pediatrics* 1981;67:362.

144. Birch BR, et al. *Bacillus cereus* cross-infection in a maternity unit. *J Hosp Infect* 1981;2:349.

145. Public Health Laboratory Service. *Bacillus cereus* infections in hospitals. *Communicable Dis Rep* 1990;44:3.

146. English MP, Wethered RR, Duncan EHL. Studies in the epidemiology of tinea pedis. VIII. Fungal infection in a long-stay hospital. *Br Med J* 1967;3:136.

147. Gonzaga AJ, Mortimer EA Jr., Wolinsky E, Rammelkamp CH Jr. Transmission of staphylococci by fomites. *JAMA* 1964;189:711.

148. Kirby WMM, Corpron DO, Tanner DC. Urinary tract infections caused by antibiotic-resistant coliform bacilli. *JAMA* 1956;162:1.

149. American Hospital Association. *Infection control in the hospital.* 4th ed. Chicago: American Hospital Association, 1979.

150. American Academy of Pediatrics. *Standards and recommendations for hospital care of newborn infants.* 6th ed. Evanston, II: American Academy of Pediatrics, 1977.

151. American Academy of Pediatrics and American College of Obstetricians and Gynecologists. *Guidelines for perinatal care.* 5th ed. Evanston, II: American Academy of Pediatrics, 2002.

152. Rhame FS. Endemic nosocomial filamentous fungal disease: A proposed structure for conceptualizing and studying the environmental hazard. *Infect Control Hosp Epidemiol* 1986;7(suppl):124.

153. Solberg CO, et al. Laminar airflow protection in bone marrow transplantation. *Appl Microbiol* 1971;21:209.

154. Rhame FS. The inanimate environment. In: Bennett JV, Brachman PS, eds., *Hospital infections.* 3rd ed. Boston: Little, Brown, 1992:223–49.

155. Bodey GP, Rodriguez V, Cabanillas F, Freireich EJ. Protected environment–prophylactic antibiotic program for malignant lymphoma: Randomized trial during chemotherapy to induce remission. *Am J Med* 1979;66:74.

156. Buckner CD, et al. Protective environment for marrow transplant recipients: A prospective study. *Ann Intern Med* 1978;89:893.

157. Dietrich M, et al. Protective isolation and antimicrobial decontamination in patients with high susceptibility to infection: A prospective cooperative study of gnotobiotic care in acute leukemia patients. I. Clinical results. *Infection* 1977;5:107.

158. Klastersky J, Debusscher L, Weerts D, Daneau D. Use of oral antibiotics in protected environment units: Clinical effectiveness and role in the emergence of antibiotic-resistant strains. *Pathol Biol* (Paris) 1974;22:5.

159. Levine AS, et al. Protected environments and prophylactic antibiotics: A prospective controlled study of their utility in the therapy of acute leukemia. *N Engl J Med* 1973;288:477.

160. Rodriguez V, et al. Randomized trial of protected environment–prophylactic antibiotics in 145 adults with acute leukemia. *Medicine* 1978;57:253.

161. Schimpff SC, et al. Infection prevention in nonlymphocytic leukemia: Laminar air flow room reverse isolation with oral, nonabsorbable antibiotic prophylaxis. *Ann Intern Med* 1975;82:351.

162. Schimpff SC, et al. Comparison of basic infection prevention techniques with standard room reverse isolation or with reverse isolation plus added air filtration. *Leuk Res* 1978;2:231.

163. Storb R, et al. Graft-versus-host disease and survival in patients with aplastic anemia treated by marrow grafts from HLA-identical siblings: Beneficial effect of a protective environment. *N Engl J Med* 1983;308:302.

164. Yates JW, Holland JE A controlled study of isolation and endogenous microbial suppression in acute myelocytic leukemia patients. *Cancer* 1973;32:1490.

165. Rhame FS. Nosocomial aspergillosis: How much protection for which patients? *Infect Control Hosp Epidemiol* 1989;10:296.

166. Fox BC, et al. Heavy contamination of operating room air by *Penicillium* species: Identification of the source and attempts at decontamination. *Am J Infect Control* 1990;18:300.

167. Marshall JW, Vincent JH, Kuehn TH, Brosseau LM. Studies of ventilation efficiency in a protective isolation room by the use of a scale model. *Infect Control Hosp Epidemiol* 1996;17:5.

168. Newman KA, et al. Persistent isolation of an unusual *Pseudomonas* species from a phenolic disinfectant system. *Infect Control Hosp Epidemiol* 1984;5:219.

169. Pizzo PA. The value of protective isolation in preventing nosocomial infections in high risk patients. *Am J Med* 1981;70:631.

170. Davis BD. Growth and death of bacteria. In: Davis BD, Dulbecco R, Eisen HN, and Ginsberg HS, eds. *Microbiology.* 4th ed. Philadelphia: Lippincott, 1990:57–63.

171. Favero MS, Bond WW. Chemical disinfection of medical and surgical materials. In: Block SS, ed. *Sterilization and preservation.* 4th ed. Philadelphia: Lea & Febiger, 1991:617–41.

172. Helrich K, ed. *Official methods of analysis of the Association of Official Analytical Chemists.* 15th ed. Arlington, VA: Association of Official Analytical Chemists, 1990.

173. Cole EC, et al. Effect of methodology, dilution, and exposure time on the tuberculocidal activity of glutaraldehyde-based disinfectants. *Appl Environ Microbiol* 1990;56:1813.

174. Kelsen JC. The myth of surgical sterility. *Lancet* 1972;2:1301.

175. Campbell RW. Sterile is a sterile word. *Radiat Phys Chem* 1980;15:121.

176. Sehulster L, Chinn RY, CDC, and HICPAC. Guidelines for environmental infection control in health-care facilities. Recommendations of CDC and the Healthcare Infection Control Practices Advisory Committee (HICPAC). *MMWR Recomm Rep.* 2003;52(RR-10):1–42.

177. Boyce JM, Pittet D; Healthcare Infection Control Practices Advisory Committee. Society for Healthcare Epidemiology of America. Association for Professionals in Infection Control. Infectious Diseases Society of America. Hand Hygiene Task Force. Guideline for hand hygiene in health-care settings: Recommendations of the Healthcare Infection Control Practices Advisory Committee and the HICPAC/SHEA/APIC/IDSA Hand Hygiene Task Force. *Infect Control Hosp Epidemiol* 2002;23(12 Suppl):S3–40.

178. Joint Commission on Accreditation of Healthcare Organizations. *Accreditation manual for hospitals, 1996.* Oakbrook Terrace, II: Joint Commission on Accreditation of Healthcare Organizations, 1996.

179. Food and Drug Administration. Devices: Reuse of medical disposal devices. In: *Food and Drug Administration Compliance Policy Guide No. 7124.23.* Washington, DC: Executive Director of Field Operations, Division of Field Operations, 1977.

180. Alter MJ, et al. Reuse of hemodialyzers: Results of nationwide surveillance for adverse effects. *JAMA* 1988;260:2073.

181. Gordon SM, Tipple M, Bland LA, Jarvis WR. Pyrogenic reactions associated with the reuse of disposable hollow-fiber hemodialyzers. *JAMA* 1988;260:2077.

182. Pollak VE. Adverse effects and pyrogenic reactions during hemodialysis. *JAMA* 1988;260:2106.

183. Centers for Disease Control and Prevention. Update: Acute allergic reactions associated with reprocessed hemodialyzers—United States, 1989–1990. *MMWR* 1991;40:147.

184. Dunnigan A, et al. Success of re-use of cardiac electrode catheters. *Am J Cardiol* 1987;60:807.

185. Alvarado CJ, Stolz SM, Maki DG. Nosocomial *P. aeruginosa* infections from contaminated endoscopes. In: *ASM International Symposium on Chemical Germicides* [Abstract 39]. Madison: University of Wisconsin, 1990.

186. Rutala WA and the 1994, 1995, and 1996 APIC Guidelines Committee. APIC guideline for selection and use of disinfectants. *Am J Infect Control* 1996;24:313.

187. Rutala DR, Rutala WA, Weber DJ, Thomman CA. Infection risks associated with spirometry. *Infect Control Hosp Epidemiol* 1991;12:89.

188. Sattar SA, Springthorpe VS. Survival and disinfectant inactivation of the human immunodeficiency virus: A critical review. *Rev Infect Dis* 1991;13:430.

189. Rutala WA, Clontz EP, Weber DJ, Hoffmann KK. Disinfection practices for endoscopes and other semicritical items. *Infect Control Hosp Epidemiol* 1991;12:282.

190. Nelson DB, Jarvis WR, Rutala WA, et al. Multisociety guideline for reprocessing flexible gastrointestinal endoscopes. Society for Healthcare Epidemiology of America. *Infect Control Hosp Epidemiol* 2003;24:532–37.

191. Simmons BP. CDC guidelines for the prevention and control of nosocomial infections. *Am J Infect Control* 1983;11:97.

192. Rutala WA, Weber DJ. Environmental issues and nosocomial infections. In: Farber BF, ed. *Infection control in intensive care.* New York: Churchill Livingstone, 1987:131–71.

193. Rutala WA. APIC guideline for selection and use of disinfectants. *Am J Infect Control* 1990;18:99.

194. Montessori V, Scharf S, Holland S, et al. Epidemic keratoconjunctivitis outbreak at a tertiary referral eye care clinic. *Am J Infect Control* 1998;26:399–405.

195. Koo D, et al. Epidemic keratoconjunctivitis in a university medical center ophthalmology clinic; Need for re-evaluation of the design and disinfection of instruments. *Infect Control Hosp Epidemiol* 1989;10:547.

196. American Academy of Ophthalmology. *Updated recommendations for ophthalmic practice in relation to the human immunodeficiency virus.* San Francisco: American Academy of Ophthalmology, 1988.

197. Srinivasan A, Wolfenden LL, Song X, et al. An outbreak of *Pseudomonas aeruginosa* infections associated with flexible bronchoscopes. *N Engl J Med* 2003;348:221–27.

198. Rutala WA, Weber DJ. Reprocessing endoscopes: United States perspective. *J Hosp Infect* 2004;56 Suppl 2:S27–39.

199. Reichert M. Automatic washers/disinfectors for flexible endoscopes. *Infect Control Hosp Epidemiol* 1991;12:497.

200. Centers for Disease Control and Prevention. Guidelines for infection control in dental health-care settings—2003. *MMWR* 2003:52:RR–17.

201. Vesley D, Langholz AC, Rohlfing SR, Foltz WE. Fluorimetric detection of a *Bacillus stearothermophilus* spore-bound enzyme, alpha-D-glucosidase, for rapid indication of flash sterilization failure. *Appl Environ Microbiol* 1992;58:717–19.

202. Rutala WA. Disinfection, sterilization, and waste disposal. In: Wenzel RP, ed. *Prevention and control of nosocomial infections.* Baltimore: Williams & Wilkins, 1987:257–82.

203. Occupational Health and Safety Agency. Glutaraldehyde. *Federal Register,* 1989;54:2464.

204. Rutala WA, Cole EC. Ineffectiveness of hospital disinfectants against bacteria: A collaborative study. *Infect Control Hosp Epidemiol* 1987;8:501.

205. Groschell DHM. Caveat emptor: Do your disinfectants work? *Infect Control Hosp Epidemiol* 1983;4:144.

206. United States General Accounting Office. *Disinfectants: EPA lacks assurance they work* Gaithersburg, MD: GAO, 1990:64.

207. Rutala WA, Cole EC, Wannamaker NS, Weber DJ. Inactivation of *Mycobacterium tuberculosis* and *Mycobacterium bovis* by 14 hospital disinfectants. *Am J Med* 1991;91(suppl 3B):3B–267S.

208. Best M, Sattar SA, Springthorpe VS, Kennedy ME. Efficacies of selected disinfectant against *Mycobacterium tuberculosis.* *J Clin Microbiol* 1990;28:2234.

209. Miller DC. Creutzfeldt-Jakob disease in histopathology technicians. *N Engl J Med* 1988;318:853.

210. Sitwell L, et al. Creutzfeldt-Jakob disease in histopathology technicians. *N Engl J Med* 1988;318:854.

211. Weber DJ, Rutala WA. Managing the risk of nosocomial transmission of prion diseases. *Curr Opin Infect Dis* 2002;15:421–25.

212. Mallison GF, Haley RW. Microbiological sampling of the inanimate environment in U.S. hospitals, 1976–1977. *Am J Med* 1980;70:941.

213. Centers for Disease Control and Prevention. *Microbial environmental surveillance in the hospital* (National Nosocomial Infections Study report). Atlanta: Centers for Disease Control and Prevention, 1970.

214. American Hospital Association. Statement on microbiological sampling in the hospital. *Hospitals* 1974;48:125.

215. O'Grady NP, Alexander M, Dellinger EP, et al.; Healthcare Infection Control Practices Advisory Committee. Guidelines for the prevention of intravascular catheter-related infections. *Infect Control Hosp Epidemiol* 2002;23:759–69.

216. National Coordinating Committee on Large-Volume Parenterals. Recommended guidelines for quality assurance in hospital centralized intravenous admixture services. *Am J Hosp Pharm* 1980;37:645.

217. Department of Health and Human Services. Standards for the reuse of hemodialysis filters and other dialysis supplies. *Federal Register* 1987;52:36926.

218. Pejaver KR, Toonisi MA, Carg AK, Al-Hifzi I. Is expressed breast milk from home safe? A survey from a neonatal intensive-care unit. *Infect Control Hosp Epidemiol* 1996;17:356.

219. Arnold LDW, Tully MR, eds. Guidelines for the establishment and operation of donor human milk bank. Human Milk Banking Association of North America, 1993.

220. United States Pharmacopeial Convention, Inc. *The United States Pharmacopeia XXII The National Formulary XVII.* Rockville, MD: USP11989.

221. Craven DE, Goularte TA, Make BJ. Contaminated condensate in mechanical ventilation circuits: A risk factor for nosocomial pneumonia? *Am Rev Respir Dis* 1984;129:625.

222. Cefai C, Richards J, Gould FK, McPeake P. An outbreak of *Acinetobacter* respiratory tract infection from incomplete disinfection of ventilatory equipment. *J Hosp Infect* 1990;15:177.

223. National Sanitation Foundation. *Standard No. 49 for class II (laminar flow) biohazard cabinetry.* Ann Arbor: National Sanitation Foundation, 1976:B4.

224. McGowan JE Jr. Environmental factors in nosocomial infection: A selective focus. *Rev Infect Dis* 1981;3:760.

225. Donowitz LG, Marsik FJ, Fisher KA, Wenzel RP. Contaminated breast milk: A source of *Klebsiella* bacteremia in a newborn intensive care unit. *Rev Infect Dis* 1981;3:716.

226. Drudy D, Mullane NR, Quinn T, et al. *Enterobacter sakazakii:* An emerging pathogen in powdered infant formula. *Clin Infect Dis* 2006;42:996–1002.

Sterilization and Disinfection

20

William A. Rutala and David J. Weber

INTRODUCTION

In the United States in 1996, there were approximately 46,500,000 surgical procedures and an even larger number of invasive medical procedures [1]. For example, there are about 5 million gastrointestinal endoscopies per year [1]. Each of these procedures involves contact by a medical device or surgical instrument with a patient's sterile tissue or mucous membranes. A major risk of all such procedures is the introduction of pathogenic microbes that can lead to infection. For example, failure to properly disinfect or sterilize equipment has led to person-to-person transmission via contaminated devices (e.g., *M. tuberculosis*–contaminated bronchoscopes).

Achieving disinfection and sterilization through the use of disinfectants and sterilization practices is essential for ensuring that medical and surgical instruments do not transmit infectious pathogens to patients. Because it is not necessary to sterilize all patient-care items, healthcare policies must identify whether cleaning, disinfection, or sterilization is indicated based primarily on each item's intended use.

Multiple studies in many countries have documented lack of compliance with established guidelines for disinfection and sterilization [2,3]. Failure to comply with scientifically based guidelines has led to numerous outbreaks [3–7]. In this chapter, which is an updated version of other publications [8–12], a pragmatic approach to the judicious selection and proper use of disinfection and sterilization processes is presented.

DEFINITION OF TERMS

Sterilization describes a process that destroys or eliminates all forms of microbial life and is carried out in healthcare facilities by either physical or chemical methods. Steam under pressure, dry heat, ethylene oxide (ETO) gas, hydrogen peroxide gas plasma, and liquid chemicals are the principal sterilizing agents used in healthcare facilities. When chemicals are used for the purposes of destroying all forms of microbiological life, including bacterial spores, they may be called chemical sterilants. These same germicides used for shorter exposure periods also may be part of the disinfection process (i.e., high-level disinfection).

Disinfection describes a process that eliminates many or all pathogenic microorganisms on inanimate objects with the exception of bacterial spores. Disinfection usually is accomplished by the use of liquid chemicals or wet pasteurization in healthcare settings. The efficacy of disinfection is affected by a number of factors, each of which may nullify or limit the efficacy of the process. Some of the factors that affect both disinfection and sterilization efficacy are the prior cleaning of the object, the organic and inorganic load present, the type and level of microbial contamination, the concentration of and exposure time to the germicide, the design of the object (e.g., crevices, hinges, and narrow lumens), the presence of biofilms, the temperature and pH of the disinfection process, and, in some instances, the relative humidity of the sterilization process (e.g., ethylene oxide) [9,13].

By definition, then, disinfection differs from sterilization by its lack of sporicidal property, but this is an oversimplification. A few disinfectants will kill spores with prolonged exposure times (3–12 hours) and are called chemical sterilants. At similar concentrations but with shorter exposure periods (e.g., 20 minutes for 2% glutaraldehyde), these same disinfectants, called high-level disinfectants, will kill all microorganisms with the exception of large numbers of bacterial spores. Low-level disinfectants will kill most vegetative bacteria, some fungi, and some viruses in a practical period of time ($\leq$10 minutes), whereas intermediate-level disinfectants may be cidal for mycobacteria, vegetative bacteria, most viruses, and most fungi but do not necessarily kill bacterial spores. The germicides differ markedly among themselves primarily in their antimicrobial spectrum and rapidity of action. A number of products and processes can be used to disinfect or sterilize medical and surgical instruments based on the risk of infection involved in the use of the item (Table 20-1).

Terms with a suffix "cide" or "cidal" for killing action also are commonly used. For example, a germicide is an agent that can kill microorganisms, particularly pathogenic organisms ("germs"). The term germicide includes both antiseptics and disinfectants. Antiseptics are germicides applied to living tissue and skin while disinfectants are antimicrobials applied only to inanimate objects. In general, antiseptics are used only on the skin, not for surface disinfection, and disinfectants are not used for skin antisepsis because they may cause injury to skin and other tissues. Other words with the suffix "cide" (e.g., virucide, fungicide, bactericide, sporicide, and tuberculocide) can kill the type of microorganism identified by the prefix. For example, a bactericide is an agent that kills bacteria [8,11,14–18].

A RATIONAL APPROACH TO DISINFECTION AND STERILIZATION

More than 35 years ago, Earle H. Spaulding [15] devised a rational approach to disinfection and sterilization of patient-care items or equipment. This classification scheme is so clear and logical that it has been retained, refined, and successfully used by infection control professionals and others when planning methods for disinfection or sterilization [8,13,14,16,19,20]. Spaulding believed that the nature of disinfection could be understood more readily if instruments and items for patient care were divided into three categories based on the degree of risk of infection involved in the use of the items. The three categories he described were critical, semicritical, and noncritical. This terminology is employed by the CDC's "Guidelines for Environmental Infection Control in Healthcare Facilities" [21] and the CDC's "Guideline for Disinfection and Sterilization in Healthcare Facilities" [13].

Critical Items

Critical items are so called because of the high risk of infection if such an item is contaminated with any microorganism, including bacterial spores. Thus, it is critical that objects that enter sterile tissue or the vascular system be sterile because any microbial contamination could result in pathogen transmission. This category includes surgical instruments, cardiac and urinary catheters, implants, and ultrasound probes used in sterile body cavities. The items in this category should be purchased as sterile or be sterilized by steam sterilization if possible. If heat sensitive, the object may be treated with ethylene oxide (ETO) or hydrogen peroxide gas plasma or by liquid chemical sterilants if other methods are unsuitable. Tables 20-2 and 20-3 list several germicides categorized as chemical sterilants. These include $\geq$ 2.40% glutaraldehyde-based formulations, 1.12% glutaraldehyde with 1.93% phenol/phenate, 7.50% stabilized hydrogen peroxide, 7.35% hydrogen peroxide with 0.23% peracetic acid, 0.20% peracetic acid, and 1.00% hydrogen peroxide with 0.08% peracetic acid. With the exception of 0.20% peracetic acid (12 minutes at 50°–56°C), the indicated exposure times range from 3 to 12 hours [22]. Liquid chemical sterilants can be relied on to produce sterility only if cleaning, which eliminates organic and inorganic material, precedes treatment and if proper guidelines on concentration, contact time, temperature, and pH are met. Another limitation to sterilization of devices with liquid chemical sterilants is that the devices cannot be wrapped during processing in a liquid chemical sterilant; thus, it is impossible to maintain sterility following processing and during storage. Furthermore, devices may require rinsing following exposure to the liquid chemical sterilant with water that generally is not sterile. Therefore, due to the inherent limitations of using liquid chemical sterilants in a nonautomated reprocessor, their use should be restricted to reprocessing critical devices that are heat sensitive and incompatible with other sterilization methods.

Semicritical Items

Semicritical items are those that come in contact with mucous membranes or nonintact skin. Respiratory therapy and anesthesia equipment, some endoscopes, laryngoscope blades, esophageal manometry probes, vaginal and rectal probes, anorectal manometry catheters, and diaphragm fitting rings are included in this category. These medical devices should be free of all microorganisms (i.e., mycobacteria, fungi, viruses, bacteria), although small numbers of bacterial spores may be present. Intact mucous membranes, such as those of the lungs or the gastrointestinal tract, generally are resistant to infection by common bacterial spores but susceptible to other organisms such as bacteria, mycobacteria, and viruses.

TABLE 20-1
METHODS OF STERILIZATION AND DISINFECTION

	Sterilization		Disinfection		
	Critical Items (Will Enter Tissue or Vascular System or Blood Will Flow Through Them)		**High Level (Semicritical Items; [Except Dental] Will Come in Contact with Mucous Membrane or Nonintact Skin)**	**Intermediate-Level (Some Semicritical Items[a] and Noncritical Items)**	**Low-Level (Noncritical Items; Will Come in Contact with Intact Skin)**
Object	**Procedure**	**Exposure Time**	**Procedure (Exposure Time 12–30 min at ≥20°C)[b,c]**	**Procedure (Exposure Time ≥1 m)**	**Procedure (Exposure Time ≥1 m)**
Smooth, hard Surface[a,d]	A	MR	D	K	K
	B	MR	E	L[e]	L
	C	MR	F	M	M
	D	10 h at 20–25°C	H	N	N
	F	6 h	I[f]		O
	G	12 m at 50–56°C	J		
	H	3–8 h			
Rubber tubing and catheters[c,d]	A	MR	D		
	B	MR	E		
	C	MR	F		
	D	10 h at 20–25°C	H		
	F	6 h	I[f]		
	G	12 m at 50–56°C	J		
	H	3–8 h			
Polyethylene tubing and catheters[c,d,g]	A	MR	D		
	B	MR	E		
	C	MR	F		
	D	10 h at 20–25°C	H		
	F	6 h	I[f]		
	G	12 m at 50–56°C	J		
	H	3–8 h			
Lensed instruments[d]	A	MR	D		
	B	MR	E		
	C	MR	F		
	D	10 h at 20–25°C	H		
	F	6 h	J		
	G	12 m at 50–56°C			
	H	3–8 h			
Thermometers (oral and rectal)[h]				K[h]	
Hinged instruments[d]	A	MR	D		
	B	MR	E		
	C	MR	F		

Modified from Rutala (8,18,127) and Simmons (16). The selection and use of disinfectants in the healthcare field is dynamic, and products may become available that did not exist when this guideline was written. As newer disinfectants become available, persons or committees responsible for selecting disinfectants and sterilization processes should be guided by products cleared by the FDA and the EPA as well as information in the scientific literature.
A. Heat sterilization, including steam or hot air (see manufacturer's recommendations; steam sterilization processing time from 3–30 minutes).
B. Ethylene oxide gas (see manufacturer's recommendations, generally 1–6 hours processing time plus aeration time of 8–12 hours at 50–60°C).
C. Hydrogen peroxide gas plasma (see manufacturer's recommendations for internal diameter and length restrictions, processing time between 45–72 minutes).

TABLE 20-1
(CONTINUED)

	Sterilization		Disinfection		
	Critical Items (Will Enter Tissue or Vascular System or Blood Will Flow Through Them)		**High Level (Semicritical Items; [Except Dental] Will Come in Contact with Mucous Membrane or Nonintact Skin)**	**Intermediate-Level (Some Semicritical Items[a] and Noncritical Items)**	**Low-Level (Noncritical Items; Will Come in Contact with Intact Skin)**
Object	**Procedure**	**Exposure Time**	**Procedure (Exposure Time 12–30 min at $\geq 20°C)^{b,c}$**	**Procedure (Exposure Time $\geq$1 m)**	**Procedure (Exposure Time $\geq$1 m)**
	D	10 h at 20–25°C	H		
	F	6 h	I[f]		
	G	12 m at 50–56°C	J		
	H	3–8 h			

D. Glutaraldehyde-based formulations ($\geq$2% glutaraldehyde; caution should be exercised with all glutaraldehyde formulations when further in-use dilution is anticipated), glutaraldehyde (1.12%), and 1.93% phenol/phenate. One glutaraldehyde-based product has a high-level disinfection claim of 5 minutes at 35°C.
E. Ortho-phthalaldehyde (OPA) 0.55%.
F. Hydrogen peroxide 7.5% (will corrode copper, zinc, and brass).
G. Peracetic acid, concentration variable but 0.2% or greater is sporicidal. Peracetic acid immersion system operates at 50–56°C.
H. Hydrogen peroxide (7.35%) and 0.23% peracetic acid; hydrogen peroxide 1% and 0.08% peracetic acid (will corrode metal instruments).
I. Wet pasteurization at 70°C for 30 minutes with detergent cleaning.
J. Hypochlorite, single-use chlorine generated on-site by electrolyzing saline containing >650–675 active free chlorine (will corrode metal instruments).
K. Ethyl or isopropyl alcohol (70–90%).
L. Sodium hypochlorite (5.25–6.15% household bleach diluted 1:500 provides >100 ppm available chlorine).
M. Phenolic germicidal detergent solution (follow product label for use-dilution).
N. Iodophor germicidal detergent solution (follow product label for use-dilution).
O. Quaternary ammonium germicidal detergent solution (follow product label for use-dilution).
MR. Manufacturer's recommendations.
NA. Not applicable.
[a]Some items that may come in contact with nonintact skin for a brief period of time (e.g., hydrotherapy tanks) are usually considered noncritical surfaces and are disinfected with intermediate-level disinfectants (i.e., phenolic, iodophor, alcohol, chlorine).
[b]The longer the exposure to a disinfectant, the more likely it is that all microorganisms will be eliminated. Ten-minute exposure is not adequate to disinfect many objects, especially those that are difficult to clean because they have narrow channels or other areas that can harbor organic material and bacteria. Twenty-minute exposure at 20°C is the minimum time needed to reliably kill *M. tuberculosis* and nontuberculous mycobacteria with a 2% glutaraldehyde. With the exception of >2% glutaraldehydes, follow the FDA-cleared high-level disinfection claim. Some high-level disinfectants have a reduced exposure time (e.g., ortho-phthalaldehyde at 12 minutes at 20°C) because of their rapid activity against mycobacteria or reduced exposure time due to increased mycobactericidal activity at elevated temperature (e.g., 2.5% glutaraldehyde at 5 minutes at 35°C, 0.55% OPA at 5 min at 25°C in automated endoscope reprocessor).
[c]Tubing must be completely filled for high-level disinfection and liquid chemical sterilization; care must be taken to avoid entrapment of air bubbles during immersion.
[d]Material compatibility should be investigated when appropriate.
[e]A concentration of 1000 ppm available chlorine should be considered where cultures or concentrated preparations of microorganisms have spilled (5.25% to 6.15% household bleach diluted 1:50 provides >1000 ppm available chlorine). This solution may corrode some surfaces.
[f]Pasteurization (washer-disinfector) of respiratory therapy or anesthesia equipment is a recognized alternative to high-level disinfection. Some data challenge the efficacy of some pasteurization units.
[g]Thermostability should be investigated when appropriate.
[h]Do not mix rectal and oral thermometers at any stage of handling or processing.

Semicritical items minimally require high-level disinfection using chemical disinfectants. Glutaraldehyde, hydrogen peroxide, ortho-phthalaldehyde, peracetic acid with hydrogen peroxide, and chlorine are cleared by the Food and Drug Administration (FDA) [22] and are dependable high-level disinfectants provided the factors influencing germicidal procedures are met (Tables 20-2 and 20-3). The exposure time for most high-level disinfectants varies from 10–45 minutes at 20°–25°C. Outbreaks continue to occur when ineffective disinfectants, including iodophor, alcohol, and overdiluted glutaraldehyde [5], are used for "high-level disinfection." When a disinfectant is selected for use with certain patient-care items, the chemical compatibility after extended use with the items to be disinfected also must be considered. For example, compatibility testing by Olympus America of the 7.5% hydrogen peroxide found cosmetic and functional changes with the tested endoscopes (Olympus America, written communication, October 15, 1999). Similarly, Olympus does not endorse the use of the hydrogen peroxide with peracetic acid products due to cosmetic and functional damage (Olympus America, written communication, April 15, 1998 and September 13, 2000).

TABLE 20-2

COMPARISON OF THE CHARACTERISTICS OF SELECTED CHEMICALS USED AS HIGH-LEVEL DISINFECTANTS OR CHEMICAL STERILANTS

	HP (7.5%)	PA (0.2%)	Glut (≥2.0%)	OPA (0.55%)	HP/PA (7.35%/0.23%)
HLD claim	30 m @ 20°C	NA	20–90 m @ 20°–25°C	12 m @ 20°C, 5 m @ 25°C in AER	15 m @ 20°C
Sterilization claim	6 h @ 20°	12m @ 50°–56°C	10 h @ 20°–25°C	None	3 h @ 20°C
Activation	No	No	Yes (alkaline glut)	No	No
Reuse life[a]	21d	Single use	14–30 d	14d	14d
Shelf life stability[b]	2 y	6 mo	2 y	2 y	2 y
Disposal restrictions	None	None	Local[c]	Local[c]	None
Materials compatibility	Good	Good	Excellent	Excellent	No data
Monitor MEC[d]	Yes (6%)	No	Yes (1.5% or higher)	Yes (0.3% OPA)	No
Safety	Serious eye damage (safety glasses)	Serious eye and skin damage (conc soln)[e]	Respiratory	Eye irritant, stains skin	Eye damage
Processing	Manual or automated	Automated	Manual or automated	Manual or automated	Manual
Organic material resistance	Yes	Yes	Yes	Yes	Yes
OSHA exposure limit	1 ppm TWA	None	None[f]	None	HP-1 ppm TWA
Cost profile (per cycle)[g]	+ (manual), ++ (automated)	+++++ (automated)	+ (manual), ++ (automated)	++ (manual)	++ (manual)

Modified from Rutala, Weber (128).

Abbreviations: AER, automated endoscope reprocessor; HLD, high-level disinfectant; HP, hydrogen peroxide; PA, peracetic acid; Glut, glutaraldehyde; PA/HP, peracetic acid and hydrogen peroxide; OPA, ortho phthalaldehyde (FDA cleared as a high-level disinfectant, included for comparison to other chemical agents used for high-level disinfection); m, minutes; h, hours; NA, not applicable; TWA, time-weighted average for a conventional 8-hour workday.
[a]Number of days a product can be reused as determined by reuse protocol.
[b]Time a product can remain in storage (unused)
[c]No U.S. EPA regulations but some states and local authorities have additional restrictions.
[d]MEC = minimum effective concentration is the lowest concentration of active ingredients at which the product is still effective.
[e]Conc soln = concentrated solution.
[f]The ceiling limit recommended by the American Conference of Governmental Industrial Hygienists is 0.05 ppm.
[g]Per cycle cost profile considers cost of the processing solution and assumes maximum use life (e.g., 21 days for hydrogen peroxide, 14 days for glutaraldehyde), 5 reprocessing cycles per day, 1-gallon basin for manual processing, and 4-gallon tank for automated processing. + = least expensive; +++++ = most expensive.

Semicritical items that will have contact with the mucous membranes of the respiratory tract or gastrointestinal tract should be rinsed with sterile water, filtered water, or tap water followed by an alcohol rinse [13,23,24]. An alcohol rinse and forced-air drying markedly reduces the likelihood of contamination of the instrument (e.g., endoscope), most likely by removing the wet environment favorable for bacterial growth [24]. After rinsing, items should be dried and stored in a manner that protects them from damage or contamination. There is no recommendation to use sterile or filtered water rather than tap water for rinsing semicritical equipment that will have contact with the mucous membranes of the rectum (e.g., rectal probes, anoscope) or vagina (e.g., vaginal probes) [13].

Noncritical Items

Noncritical items are those that come in contact with intact skin but not mucous membranes. Intact skin acts as an effective barrier to most microorganisms; therefore, the sterility of items coming in contact with intact skin is "not critical." Examples of noncritical items are bedpans, blood pressure cuffs, crutches, bed rails, computers, linens, bedside tables, patient furniture, and floors. In contrast to critical and some semicritical items, most noncritical reusable items may be decontaminated where they are used and do not need to be transported to a central processing area. There is virtually no documented risk of transmitting infectious agents to patients via noncritical items [25] when they are used as noncritical items and do

TABLE 20-3

SUMMARY OF ADVANTAGES AND DISADVANTAGES OF CHEMICAL AGENTS USED AS CHEMICAL STERILANTS[a] OR AS HIGH-LEVEL DISINFECTANTS

Sterilization Method	Advantages	Disadvantages
Peracetic acid/hydrogen peroxide	■ No activation required ■ Odor or irritation not significant	■ Material compatibility concerns (lead, brass, copper, zinc) both cosmetic and functional ■ Limited clinical experience ■ Potential for eye and skin damage
Glutaraldehyde	■ Numerous use studies published ■ Relatively inexpensive ■ Excellent material compatibility	■ Respiratory irritation from glutaraldehyde vapor ■ Pungent and irritating odor ■ Relatively slow mycobactericidal activity ■ Coagulates blood and fixes tissue to surfaces ■ Allergic contact dermatitis
Hydrogen peroxide	■ No activation required ■ May enhance removal of organic matter and organisms ■ No disposal issues ■ No odor or irritation issues ■ Does not coagulate blood or fix tissues to surfaces ■ Inactivates *Cryptosporidium* ■ Use studies published	■ Material compatibility concerns (brass, zinc, copper, and nickel/silver plating) both cosmetic and functional ■ Serious eye damage with contact
Ortho-phthalaldehyde	■ Fast-acting, high-level disinfectant ■ No activation required ■ Odor not significant ■ Excellent materials compatibility claimed ■ Does not coagulate blood or fix tissues to surfaces claimed	■ Stains protein gray (e.g., skin, mucous membranes, clothing, and environmental surfaces) ■ More expensive than glutaraldehyde ■ Eye irritation with contact ■ Slow sporicidal activity ■ Exposure may result in hypersensitivity
Peracetic acid	■ Rapid sterilization cycle time (30–45 minutes) ■ Low temperature (50°–55°C) liquid immersion sterilization ■ Environmental friendly by-products (acetic acid, O_2, H_2O) ■ Fully automated ■ Single-use system eliminates need for concentration testing ■ Standardized cycle ■ May enhance removal of organic material and endotoxin ■ No adverse health effects to operators under normal operating conditions ■ Compatible with many materials and instruments ■ Does not coagulate blood or fix tissues to surfaces ■ Sterilant flows through scope facilitating salt, protein, and microbe removal ■ Rapidly sporicidal ■ Provides procedure standardization (constant dilution, perfusion of channel, temperatures, exposure)	■ Potential material incompatibility (e.g., aluminum anodized coating becomes dull) ■ Used for immersible instruments only ■ Biological indicator may not be suitable for routine monitoring ■ One scope or a small number of instruments can be processed in a cycle ■ More expensive (endoscope repairs, operating costs, purchase costs) than high-level disinfection ■ Serious eye and skin damage (concentrated solution) with contact ■ Point-of-use system, no sterile storage

Modified from (128).

[a]All products effective in presence of organic soil, relatively easy to use, and have a broad spectrum of antimicrobial activity (bacteria, fungi, viruses, bacterial spores, and mycobacteria). These characteristics are documented in the literature; contact the manufacturer of the instrument and sterilant for additional information. All products listed are FDA-cleared as chemical sterilants except OPA, which is an FDA-cleared, high-level disinfectant.

not contact non-intact skin and/or mucous membranes. However, these items (e.g., bedside tables, bed rails) could potentially contribute to secondary transmission by contaminating hands of healthcare workers or by contact with medical equipment that will subsequently come in contact with patients [26]. Table 20-1 lists several low-level disinfectants that may be used for noncritical items. The exposure time listed in the table is at least 1 minute.

AN OVERVIEW OF CLEANING, DISINFECTION, AND STERILIZATION

Cleaning

Cleaning is the removal of foreign material (e.g., soil and organic material) from objects, and it is normally accomplished using water with detergents or enzymatic products. Thorough cleaning is required before high-level disinfection and sterilization because inorganic and organic materials that remain on the surfaces of instruments interfere with the effectiveness of these processes. Also, if the soiled materials become dried or baked onto the instruments, the removal process becomes more difficult and the disinfection or sterilization process less effective or ineffective. Surgical instruments should be presoaked or rinsed to prevent drying of blood and to soften or remove blood from the instruments.

Cleaning is done manually when the use area does not have a mechanical unit (e.g., ultrasonic cleaner or washer disinfector) and for fragile or difficult-to-clean instruments. If cleaning is done manually, the two essential components are friction and fluidics. Using friction (e.g., rubbing/scrubbing the soiled area with a brush) is an old and dependable method. Fluidics (i.e., fluids under pressure) is used to remove soil and debris from internal channels after brushing and when the design does not allow the passage of a brush through a channel [27]. When using a washer-disinfector, care should be taken as to the method of loading instruments. Hinged instruments should be opened fully to allow adequate contact with the detergent solution. The stacking of instruments in washers should be avoided. Instruments should be disassembled as much as possible.

Disinfection

A great number of disinfectants are used alone or in combinations (e.g., hydrogen peroxide and peracetic acid) in the healthcare setting. These include alcohols, chlorine and chlorine compounds, formaldehyde, glutaraldehyde, ortho-phthalaldehyde, hydrogen peroxide, iodophors, peracetic acid, phenolics, and quaternary ammonium compounds. Commercial formulations based on these chemicals are considered unique products and must be registered with the Environmental Protection Agency

(EPA) or cleared by the FDA. In most instances, a given product is designed for a specific purpose and is to be used in a certain manner. Therefore, the label should be read carefully to ensure that the right product is selected for the intended use and applied in an appropriate manner.

Disinfectants are not interchangeable, so the user must have sufficient information to select an appropriate disinfectant for any item and use it in the most efficient way. An overview of germicides commonly used in healthcare can be found in other references [9,11,13]. It should be recognized that excessive costs may be attributed to incorrect concentrations and inappropriate disinfectants. Finally, occupational diseases among cleaning personnel have been associated with the use of several disinfectants such as formaldehyde, glutaraldehyde, chlorine, and others, and precautions (e.g., gloves, proper ventilation) should be used to minimize exposure [28–30].

Sterilization

Most medical and surgical devices used in healthcare facilities are made of materials that are heat stable and thus can be sterilized by heat, primarily steam sterilization. However, since 1950, there has been an increase in medical devices and instruments made of materials (e.g., plastics) that require low-temperature sterilization. Ethylene oxide gas has been used since the 1950s for heat- and moisture-sensitive medical devices. Within the past 20 years, a number of new, low-temperature sterilization systems (e.g., hydrogen peroxide gas plasma, peracetic acid immersion) have been developed and are being used to sterilize medical devices. Table 20-4 reviews sterilization technologies used in healthcare and makes recommendations for their optimum performance in the processing of medical devices [18,19,31–38].

Sterilization destroys all microorganisms on the surface of an item or in a fluid to prevent disease transmission associated with the use of that item. While the use of inadequately sterilized critical items represents a high risk of transmitting pathogens, documented transmission of pathogens associated with an inadequately sterilized critical item is exceedingly rare [39,40]. This is likely due to the wide margin of safety associated with the sterilization processes used in healthcare facilities. The concept of what constitutes "sterile" is measured as a probability of sterility for each item to be sterilized. This probability is commonly referred to as the sterility assurance level (SAL) of the product and is defined as the probability of a single viable microorganism occurring on a product after sterilization. SAL is normally expressed as 10^{-n}. For example, if the probability of a spore surviving were 1 in 1 million, the SAL would be 10^{-6} [41,42]. In short, an SAL is an estimate of lethality of the entire sterilization process and is a conservative calculation. Dual SALs (e.g., 10^{-3} SAL for blood culture tubes, drainage bags; 10^{-6} SAL for scalpels, implants) have been used in the United States for many

TABLE 20-4
SUMMARY OF ADVANTAGES AND DISADVANTAGES OF COMMONLY USED STERILIZATION TECHNOLOGIES

Sterilization Method	Advantages	Disadvantages
Steam	■ Nontoxic to patient, staff, environment ■ Cycle easy to control and monitor ■ Rapidly microbicidal ■ Least affected by organic/inorganic soils among sterilization processes listed ■ Rapid cycle time ■ Penetrates medical packing, device lumens	■ Deleterious for heat-sensitive instruments ■ Microsurgical instruments damaged by repeated exposure ■ May leave instruments wet, causing them to rust ■ Potential for burns (flash sterilization)
Hydrogen peroxide gas plasma	■ Safe for the environment ■ Leaves no toxic residuals ■ Cycle time is 28–75 minutes (varies with model type) and no aeration necessary ■ Used for heat- and moisture-sensitive items since process temperature <50°C ■ Simple to operate, install (208 V outlet), and monitor ■ Compatible with most medical devices ■ Requires only electrical outlet	■ Cellulose (paper), linens, and liquids cannot be processed ■ Sterilization chamber size from 1.8–9.5 ft³ total volume (varies with model type) ■ Endoscope or medical device restrictions based on lumen internal diameter and length (see manufacturer's recommendations) ■ Requires synthetic packaging (polypropylene wraps, polyolefin pouches) and special container tray ■ Hydrogen peroxide may be toxic at levels greater than 1 ppm TWA
100% ethylene oxide (ETO)	■ Penetrates packaging materials, device lumens ■ Single-dose cartridge and negative-pressure chamber minimizes the potential for gas leak and ETO exposure ■ Simple to operate and monitor ■ Compatible with most medical materials	■ Requires aeration time to remove ETO residue ■ Sterilization chamber size from 4 ft³ to 7.9 ft³ total volume (varies with model type) ■ ETO is toxic, a carcinogen, and flammable ■ ETO emission regulated by states but catalytic cell removes 99.9% of ETO and converts it to CO_2 and H_2O ■ ETO cartridges should be stored in flammable liquid storage cabinet ■ Lengthy cycle/aeration time
ETO Mixtures 8.6% ETO/91.4% HCFC 10.0% ETO/90.0% HCFC 8.5% ETO/91.5% CO_2	■ Penetrates medical packaging and many plastics ■ Compatible with most medical materials ■ Cycle easy to control and monitor	■ Some states require ETO emission reduction of 90–99.9% ■ CFC (inert gas that eliminates explosion hazard) banned in 1995 ■ Potential hazards to staff and patients ■ Lengthy cycle/aeration time ■ ETO is toxic, a carcinogen, and flammable
Peracetic acid	■ Rapid cycle time (30–45 minutes) Low temperature (50°–55°C) liquid immersion sterilization ■ Environmentally friendly by-products ■ Sterilant flows through endoscope which facilitates salt, protein, and microbe removal	■ Point-of-use system, no sterile storage ■ Biological indicator may not be suitable for routine monitoring ■ Used for immersible instruments only ■ Some material incompatibility (e.g., aluminum anodized coating becomes dull) ■ One scope or a small number of instruments processed in a cycle ■ Potential for serious eye and skin damage (concentrated solution) with contact ■ Must use connector between system and scope to ensure infusion of sterilant to all channels

Modified from (129).
Abbreviations: ETO, ethylene oxide; CFC, chlorofluorocarbon; HCFC, hydrochlorofluorocarbon.

years; the choice of a 10^{-6} SAL was strictly arbitrary and not associated with any adverse outcomes (e.g., patient infections) [41].

CURRENT ISSUES IN DISINFECTION AND STERILIZATION

Reprocessing of Endoscopes

Physicians use endoscopes to diagnose and treat numerous medical disorders. While endoscopes represent a valuable diagnostic and therapeutic tool in modern medicine and the incidence of infection associated with their use has been reported as very low (about 1 in 1.8 million procedures) [43], more healthcare-associated outbreaks have been linked to contaminated endoscopes than to any other medical device [3–5]. To prevent the spread of healthcare-associated infections (HAIs), all heat-sensitive endoscopes (e.g., gastrointestinal endoscopes, bronchoscopes, nasopharyngoscopes) must be properly cleaned and at a minimum subjected to high-level disinfection following each use. High-level disinfection can be expected to destroy all microorganisms; although when high numbers of bacterial spores are present, a few spores may survive.

Recommendations for the cleaning and disinfection of endoscopic equipment have been published and should be strictly followed [13,23]. Unfortunately, audits have shown that personnel do not adhere to guidelines on reprocessing [44–46] and outbreaks of infection continue to occur [47,48]. To ensure that reprocessing personnel are properly trained, there should be initial and annual competency testing for each individual who is involved in reprocessing endoscopic instruments [13,23,24,49].

In general, endoscope disinfection or sterilization with a liquid chemical sterilant or high-level disinfectant involves five steps after leak testing: (1) clean—mechanically clean internal and external surfaces, including brushing internal channels and flushing each internal channel with water and an enzymatic cleaner; (2) disinfect—immerse endoscope in high-level disinfectant (or chemical sterilant) and perfuse disinfectant (eliminates air pockets and ensures contact of the germicide with the internal channels) into all accessible channels such as the suction/biopsy channel and air/water channel and expose for a time recommended for the specific high-level disinfectant; (3) rinse—rinse the endoscope and all channels with sterile water, filtered water (commonly used with automated endoscope reprocessors), or tap water; (4) dry—rinse the insertion tube and inner channels with alcohol and dry with forced air after disinfection and before storage; and (5) store—store the endoscope in a way that prevents recontamination and promotes drying (e.g., hung vertically).

Unfortunately, there is poor compliance with the recommendations for reprocessing endoscopes. In addition,

there are rare instances when the scientific literature and recommendations from professional organizations regarding the use of disinfectants and sterilants may differ from the manufacturer's label claim. One example is the contact time used to achieve high-level disinfection with 2% glutaraldehyde. Based on FDA requirements (FDA regulates liquid sterilants and high-level disinfectants used on critical and semicritical medical devices), manufacturers test the efficacy of their germicide formulations under worst-case conditions (i.e., minimum recommended concentration of the active ingredient) and in the presence of organic soil (typically 5% serum). The soil is used to represent the organic loading to which the device is exposed during actual use and that would remain on the device in the absence of cleaning. These stringent test conditions are designed to provide a margin of safety by ensuring that the contact conditions for the germicide provide complete elimination of the test bacteria (e.g., 10^5 to 10^6 *M. tuberculosis* in organic soil and dried on a scope) if inoculated into the most difficult areas for the disinfectant to penetrate and in the absence of cleaning. However, the scientific data demonstrate that *M. tuberculosis* levels can be reduced by at least 8 $\log_{10}$ with cleaning (4 $\log_{10}$) followed by chemical disinfection for 20 minutes at 20°C (4 to 6 $\log_{10}$) [13,22,23,50]. Because of these data, professional organizations (at least 14 professional organizations worldwide) that have endorsed an endoscope reprocessing guideline recommend contact conditions of 20 minutes at 20°C (or less than 20 minutes outside the United States) with 2% glutaraldehyde to achieve high-level disinfection that differs from that of the manufacturer's label [23,51–54].

It is important to emphasize that the FDA tests do not include cleaning, a critical component of the disinfection process. Therefore, when cleaning has been included in the test methodology, 2% glutaraldehyde for 20 minutes has been demonstrated to be effective in eliminating all vegetative bacteria [13,50].

Disinfection of HBV-, HCV-, HIV-, or *M. tuberculosis*–Contaminated Devices

The CDC recommendation for high-level disinfection of HBV-, HCV-, HIV-, or *M. tuberculosis*–contaminated devices is appropriate because experiments have demonstrated the effectiveness of high-level disinfectants to inactivate these and other pathogens that may contaminate semicritical devices [55–79]. Nonetheless, some healthcare facilities have modified their disinfection procedures when endoscopes are used with a patient known or suspected to be infected with HBV, HIV, or *M. tuberculosis* [80,81]. This is inconsistent with the concept of Universal Precautions that presumes that all patients are potentially infected with bloodborne pathogens [65]. Several studies have highlighted the inability to distinguish HBV- or HIV-infected patients from noninfected patients on clinical grounds [82–84]. It also is likely that mycobacterial infection will not be clinically apparent in many patients. In most instances, hospitals that altered their disinfection procedure used ethylene oxide sterilization on the endoscopic instruments because they believed this practice reduced the risk of infection [80,81]. ETO is not routinely used for endoscope sterilization because of the lengthy processing time. Endoscopes and other semicritical devices should be managed the same way whether or not the patient is known to be infected with HBV, HCV, HIV, or *M. tuberculosis*.

An evaluation of a manual disinfection procedure to eliminate HCV from experimentally contaminated endoscopes provided some evidence that cleaning and 2% glutaraldehyde for 20 minutes should prevent transmission [77]. Using experimentally contaminated hysteroscopes, Sartor et al. detected HCV by polymerase chain reaction (PCR) in one (3%) of 34 samples following cleaning with a detergent, but no samples were positive following treatment with a 2% glutaraldehyde solution for 20 minutes [85]. Rey et al. demonstrated complete elimination of HCV (as detected by PCR) from endoscopes used on chronically infected patients following cleaning and disinfection for 3 to 5 minutes in glutaraldehyde [86]. Similarly, Chanzy et al. used PCR to demonstrate complete elimination of HCV following standard disinfection of experimentally contaminated endoscopes [77] while Ishino et al. found that endoscopes used on patients who were positive for HCV antibody had no detectable HCV RNA after high-level disinfection [87]. The inhibitory activity of a phenolic and a chlorine compound on HCV showed that the phenolic inhibited the binding and replication of HCV but the chlorine was ineffective, probably due to its low concentration and its neutralization in the presence of organic matter [88].

Occupational Safety and Health Administration Bloodborne Pathogen Standard

In December 1991, the Occupational Safety and Health Administration (OSHA) promulgated the standard "Occupational Exposure to Bloodborne Pathogens" to eliminate or minimize occupational exposure to bloodborne pathogens [89]. One component of this requirement is that all equipment and environmental and working surfaces be cleaned and decontaminated with an appropriate disinfectant after contact with blood or other potentially infectious materials. While the OSHA standard does not specify the type of disinfectant or procedure, the OSHA original compliance document [90] suggested that a germicide must be tuberculocidal to kill the HBV. To follow the OSHA compliance document, a tuberculocidal disinfectant (e.g., phenolic and chlorine) would be needed to clean a blood spill. However, in February 1997, OSHA amended its policy and stated that EPA-registered disinfectants that are labeled as effective against HIV and HBV would be considered

as appropriate disinfectants "provided such surfaces have not become contaminated with agent(s) or volumes of or concentrations of agent(s) for which higher level disinfection is recommended" [91]. When bloodborne pathogens other than HBV or HIV are of concern, OSHA continues to require the use of EPA-registered tuberculocidal disinfectants or hypochlorite solution (diluted 1:10 or 1:100 with water) [65,91]. Recent studies demonstrate that, in the presence of large blood spills, a 1:10 final dilution of EPA-registered hypochlorite solution initially should be used to inactivate bloodborne viruses [76,92] to minimize risk of disease to the healthcare worker from percutaneous injury during the clean-up process.

Inactivation of *Clostridium difficile*

The source of healthcare-associated acquisition of *C. difficile* in nonepidemic settings has not been determined. The environment and carriage on the hands of healthcare personnel have been considered as possible sources of colonization or infection [93,94]. Carpeted rooms occupied by a patient with *C. difficile* are more heavily contaminated with *C. difficile* than noncarpeted rooms [95]. Because *C. difficile* may display increased levels of spore production when exposed to non-chlorine-based cleaning agents and the spores are more resistant than vegetative cells to commonly used surface disinfectants [96], some investigators have recommended the use of dilute solutions of hypochlorite (1600 ppm available chlorine) for routine environmental disinfection of rooms of patients with *C. difficile*–associated diarrhea or colitis [97] to reduce the incidence of *C. difficile* diarrhea [98] or in units with high *C. difficile* rates [99]. Stool samples of patients with symptomatic *C. difficile* colitis must contain spores of the organism because ethanol treatment (active against vegetative bacteria but nor spore) of the stool is used for isolation of *C. difficile* in the laboratory to reduce the overgrowth by fecal flora [100,101]. Mayfield et al. showed a marked reduction in *C. difficile*–associated diarrhea rates in a bone-marrow transplant unit (from 8.6 to 3.3 episodes per 1,000 patient-days) during the period of bleach disinfection (1:10 dilution) of environmental surfaces compared to cleaning with a quaternary ammonium compound [99]. Because there are no EPA-registered products specifically approved for inactivating *C. difficile* spores, use of a diluted hypochlorite should be considered in units with high *C. difficile* rates. Thus, in units with high endemic *C. difficile* infection rates or in an outbreak setting, use dilute solutions of 5.25–6.15% sodium hypochlorite (e.g., 1:10 dilution of bleach) for routine environmental disinfection. Acidified bleach and regular bleach (5000 ppm chlorine) can inactivate 10^6 *C. difficile* spores in ≤10 minutes [102].

However, studies have shown that asymptomatic patients constitute an important reservoir within the healthcare facility and that person-to-person transmission is the principal means of transmission between patients. Thus, handwashing, barrier precautions, and meticulous environmental cleaning with an EPA-registered disinfectant (e.g., germicidal detergent) should be effective in preventing the spread of the organism in endemic situations [103].

Contaminated medical devices, such as colonoscopes and thermometers [104], have served as vehicles for the transmission of *C. difficile* spores. For this reason, investigators have studied commonly used disinfectants and exposure times to assess whether current practices may be placing patients at risk. Studies demonstrate that 2% glutaraldehyde [105–108] and peracetic acid [108,109] reliably kill *C. difficile* spores using exposure times of 5 to 20 minutes. Ortho-phthalaldehyde and $\geq 0.2\%$ peracetic acid (W. A. Rutala, written communication, April 2006) also can inactivate $\geq 10^4$ *C. difficile* spores in 10–12 minutes at 20°C [109].

Susceptibility of Antibiotic-Resistant Bacteria to Disinfectants

Several studies have found antibiotic-resistant hospital strains of common HAI pathogens (i.e., *Enterococcus*, *P. aeruginosa*, *Klebsiella pneumoniae*, *E. coli*, *S. aureus*, and *S. epidermidis*) to be equally susceptible to disinfectants as antibiotic-sensitive strains [110–113]. The susceptibility of glycopeptide-intermediate *S. aureus* was similar to vancomycin-susceptible, methicillin-resistant *S. aureus* [114]. Based on these data, routine disinfection and housekeeping protocols do not need to be altered because of antibiotic resistance provided the disinfection method is effective [115,116]. A study that evaluated the efficacy of selected cleaning methods (e.g., quaternary ammonium [QUAT]-sprayed cloth and QUAT-immersed cloth) for eliminating vancomycin-resistant enterococci (VRE) found that currently used disinfection processes are likely highly effective in eliminating VRE. However, surface disinfection must involve application to all potentially contaminated surfaces [115].

Inactivation of Creutzfeldt-Jakob Disease Agent

Creutzfeldt-Jakob Disease (CJD) is a degenerative neurologic disorder of humans with an incidence in the United States of approximately 1 case/million population/year [117]. CJD is thought to be caused by a proteinaceous infectious agent or prion. CJD is related to other human transmissible spongiform encephalopathies (TSEs) that include kuru (0 incidence, now eradicated), Gertsmann-Straussler-Sheinker syndrome (1/40 million), and fatal insomnia syndrome (FIS) (<1/40 million). The agents of CJD and other TSEs exhibit an unusual resistance to conventional chemical and physical decontamination methods. Because the CJD agent is not readily inactivated by conventional disinfection and sterilization procedures

and because of the invariably fatal outcome of CJD, the procedures for disinfection and sterilization of the CJD prion have been both conservative and controversial for many years.

The current recommendations consider inactivation data but also use epidemiological studies of prion transmission, infectivity of human tissues, and efficacy of removing proteins by cleaning. On the basis of scientific data, only critical (e.g., surgical instruments) and semicritical devices contaminated with high-risk tissue (i.e., brain, spinal cord, and eye tissue) from high-risk patients (e.g., known or suspected infection with CJD or other prion disease) require special prion reprocessing. For high-risk tissues, high-risk patients, and critical or semicritical medical devices, one of the following three methods should be used: (1) clean the device and sterilize using a combination of sodium hydroxide and autoclaving [118] (e.g., immerse in 1N NaOH for 1 hour; remove and rinse in water, and then transfer to an open pan and autoclave [121°C gravity displacement or 134°C porous or prevacuum sterilizer] for 1 hour); (2) autoclaving at 134°C for 18 minutes in a prevacuum sterilizer; or (3) 132°C for 1 hour in a gravity displacement sterilizer) [13,119]. The temperature should not exceed 134°C because the effectiveness of autoclaving may decline as the temperature is increased (e.g., 136°C, 138°C) [120]. Prion-contaminated medical devices that are impossible or difficult to clean should be discarded. Flash sterilization (i.e., steam sterilization of an unwrapped item at 132°C for 3 minutes) should not be used for reprocessing. To minimize environmental contamination, noncritical environmental surfaces should be covered with plastic-backed paper, and when contaminated with high-risk tissues, the paper should be properly discarded. Noncritical environmental surfaces (e.g., laboratory surfaces) contaminated with high-risk tissues should be cleaned and then spot decontaminated with a 1:10 dilution of hypochlorite solutions [119].

Emerging Pathogens, Antibiotic-Resistant Bacteria, and Bioterrorism Agents

Emerging pathogens are of growing concern to the general public and infection control professionals. Relevant pathogens include *Cryptosporidium parvum*, *Helicobacter pylori*, *E. coli* O157:H7, HIV, HCV, rotavirus, multidrug-resistant *M. tuberculosis*, human papilloma virus, norovirus, Severe Acute Respiratory Syndrome (SARS) coronavirus, avian influenza, and nontuberculosis mycobacteria (e.g., *M. chelonae*). Recent publications have highlighted the concern about the potential for biological terrorism [121]. The CDC has categorized several agents as "high priority" because they can be easily disseminated or transmitted person-to-person, cause high mortality, and are likely to cause public panic and social disruption [122]. These agents include *Bacillus anthracis* (anthrax), *Yersinia pestis* (plague), variola major (smallpox), *Francisella tularensis* (tularemia), filoviruses (Ebola hemorrhagic fever, Marburg hemorrhagic fever); and arenaviruses (Lassa [Lassa fever], Junin [Argentine hemorrhagic fever]), and related viruses [122].

With rare exceptions (e.g., human papilloma virus), the susceptibility of each of these pathogens to chemical disinfectants/sterilants has been studied and all of these pathogens (or surrogate microbes) such as feline-calicivirus for norovirus, vaccinia for variola [123], and *B. atrophaeus* (formerly *B. subtilis*) for *B. anthracis*, are susceptible to currently available chemical disinfectants/sterilants [124]. Standard sterilization and disinfection procedures for patient-care equipment (as recommended in this chapter) are adequate to sterilize or disinfect instruments or devices contaminated with blood or other body fluids from persons infected with bloodborne pathogens, emerging pathogens, and bioterrorism agents with the exception of prions (see previous comment). No changes in procedures for cleaning, disinfecting, or sterilizing need to be made for equipment [13].

In addition, there are no data to show that antibiotic-resistant bacteria (methicillin-resistant *Staphylococcus aureus* [MRSA], VRE, multidrug-resistant *M. tuberculosis*) are less sensitive to the liquid chemical germicides than antibiotic-sensitive bacteria at currently used germicide contact conditions and concentrations [110,125].

Advances in Disinfection and Sterilization Methods

In the past several years, new methods of disinfection and sterilization have been introduced in the healthcare setting. Ortho-phthalaldehyde (OPA) is a chemical sterilant that received FDA clearance in October 1999. It contains 0.55% 1,2-benzenedicarboxaldehyde. Studies have demonstrated excellent microbicidal activity in *in vitro* studies [13]. For example, Gregory et al. demonstrated that OPA has superior mycobactericidal activity (5-log_{10} reduction in 5 minutes) compared to glutaraldehyde [126]. The advantages, disadvantages, and characteristics of OPA are listed in Tables 20-2 and 20-3.

The FDA recently cleared a liquid high-level disinfectant (i.e., superoxidized water) that contains 650–675 ppm free chlorine, two chemical sterilants (i.e., 3.4% glutaraldehyde with 0.26% isopropanol, and 8.3% hydrogen peroxide with 7.0% peracetic acid) and a new sterilization system using ozone. Some of these processes may not be commercially available (e.g., 3.4% glutaraldehyde with 0.26% isopropanol, and 8.3% hydrogen peroxide with 7.0% peracetic acid), or there are only limited data in the scientific literature that assess the antimicrobial activity or material compatibility of these processes, so they have not yet been commonly integrated into clinical practice in the United States [13].

Several methods are used to sterilize patient-care items in healthcare, including steam sterilization, ethylene oxide, hydrogen peroxide gas plasma, and a peracetic acid immersion system. The advantages and disadvantages of these systems are listed in Table 20-4 [13].

New sterilization technology based on plasma was patented in 1987 and marketed in the United States in 1993. Gas plasmas have been referred to as the fourth state of matter (i.e., liquids, solids, gases, and gas plasmas). They are generated in an enclosed chamber under deep vacuum using radiofrequency or microwave energy to excite the gas molecules and produce charged particles, many of which are in the form of free radicals. This process has the ability to inactivate a broad spectrum of microorganisms, including resistant bacterial spores. Studies have been conducted against vegetative bacteria (including mycobacteria), yeasts, fungi, viruses, and bacterial spores [13]. The effectiveness of all sterilization processes can be altered by lumen length, lumen diameter, inorganic salts, and organic materials [13].

CONCLUSION

When properly used, disinfection and sterilization can ensure the safe use of invasive and non invasive medical devices. The method of disinfection and sterilization depends on the intended use of the medical device: Critical items (contact sterile tissue) must be sterilized before use; semi-critical items (contact mucous membranes or nonintact skin) must be high-level disinfected; and noncritical items (contact intact skin) should receive low-level disinfection. Cleaning should always precede high-level disinfection and sterilization. Current disinfection and sterilization guidelines must be strictly followed to prevent HAIs.

REFERENCES

1. Centers for Disease Control. *Ambulatory and inpatient procedures in the United States, 1996.* Atlanta, GA: November 1998.
2. McCarthy GM, Koval JJ, John MA, MacDonald JK. Infection control practices across Canada: do dentists follow the recommendations? *Journal/Canadian Dental Association. Journal de l Association Dentaire Canadienne* 1999;65(9):506–511.
3. Spach DH, Silverstein FE, Stamm WE. Transmission of infection by gastrointestinal endoscopy and bronchoscopy. *Annals of Internal Medicine* 1993;118(2):117–128.
4. Weber DJ, Rutala WA. Lessons from outbreaks associated with bronchoscopy. *Infect Control Hosp Epidemiol* 2001;22:403–408.
5. Weber DJ, Rutala WA, DiMarino AJ Jr. The prevention of infection following gastrointestinal endoscopy: the importance of prophylaxis and reprocessing. In: DiMarino AJ, Jr, Benjamin SB, eds. *Gastrointestinal diseases: an endoscopic approach.* 2nd ed. Thorofare, NJ: Slack, 2002:87–106.
6. Meyers H, Brown-Elliott BA, Moore D, et al. An outbreak of *Mycobacterium chelonae* infection following liposuction. *Clin Infect Dis* 2002;34:1500–1507.
7. Lowry PW, Jarvis WR, Oberle AD, et al. *Mycobacterium chelonae* causing otitis media in an ear-nose-and-throat practice. *N Engl J Med* 1988;319(15):978–982.
8. Rutala WA, 1994, 1995, and 1996 APIC Guidelines Committee. APIC guideline for selection and use of disinfectants. *American Journal of Infection Control* 1996;24(4):313–342.
9. Rutala WA, Weber DJ. Selection and use of disinfectants in healthcare. In: Mayhall CG, ed. *Hospital epidemiology and infection control.* 3rd ed. Philadelphia: Lippincott Williams & Wilkins, 2004:1473–1522.

10. Rutala WA, Weber DJ. Modern advances in disinfection, sterilization and medical waste management. In: Wenzel RP, ed. *Prevention and control of nosocomial infections*. 4th ed. Philadelphia: Lippincott Williams & Wilkins, 2003:542–574.

11. Rutala WA, Weber DJ. Disinfection, sterilization and control of hospital waste. In: Mandell GL, Bennett JE, Dolin R, eds. *Principles and practice of infections diseases*. Philadelphia: Elsevier Churchill Livingstone, 2005:3331–3347.

12. Rutala WA, Weber DJ. Disinfection and sterilization in health care facilities: What clinicians need to know. *Clin Infect Dis* 2004;39:702–709.

13. Rutala WA, Weber DJ, Healthcare Infection Control Practices Advisory Committee. Guideline for disinfection and sterilization in healthcare facilities: Recommendations of CDC. *MMWR* (In Press).

14. Favero MS, Bond WW. Chemical disinfection of medical and surgical materials. In: Block SS, ed. *Disinfection, sterilization, and preservation*. 5th ed. Philadelphia: Lippincott Williams & Wilkins, 2001:881–917.

15. Spaulding EH. Chemical disinfection of medical and surgical materials. In: Lawrence C, Block SS, eds. *Disinfection, sterilization, and preservation*. Philadelphia: Lea & Febiger, 1968:517–531.

16. Simmons BP. CDC guidelines for the prevention and control of nosocomial infections: guideline for hospital environmental control. *American Journal of Infection Control* 1983;11(3):97–120.

17. Block SS, ed. *Disinfection, sterilization, and preservation*. 5th ed. Philadelphia: Lippincott Williams & Wilkins, 2001.

18. Rutala WA. Disinfection, sterilization and waste disposal. In: Wenzel RP, ed. *Prevention and control of nosocomial infections*. 3rd ed. Baltimore: Williams and Wilkins, 1997:539–593.

19. Garner JS, Favero MS. CDC guideline for handwashing and hospital environmental control, 1985. *Infection Control* 1986;7(4):231–243.

20. Rutala WA. APIC guideline for selection and use of disinfectants. *American Journal of Infection Control* 1990;18(2):99–117.

21. Sehulster L, Chinn RYW, Healthcare Infection Control Practices Advisory Committee. Guidelines for environmental infection control in health-care facilities. *MMWR* 2003;52(RR-10):1–44.

22. Food and Drug Administration. FDA-cleared sterilants and high-level disinfectants with general claims for processing reusable medical and dental devices, May 13, 2005 (www.fda.gov/cdrh/ode/germlab.html).

23. Nelson DB, Jarvis WR, Rutala WA, et al. Multi-society guideline for reprocessing flexible gastrointestinal endoscopes. *Infect Control Hosp Epidemiol* 2003;24:532–537.

24. Gerding DN, Peterson LR, Vennes JA. Cleaning and disinfection of fiberoptic endoscopes: evaluation of glutaraldehyde exposure time and forced-air drying. *Gastroenterology* 1982;83(3):613–618.

25. Weber DJ, Rutala WA. Environmental issues and nosocomial infections. In: Wenzel RP, ed. *Prevention and control of nosocomial infections*. 3rd ed. Baltimore: Williams and Wilkins, 1997:491–514.

26. Weber DJ, Rutala WA. Role of environmental contamination in the transmission of vancomycin-resistant enterococci. *Infection Control & Hospital Epidemiology* 1997;18(5):306–309.

27. Reichert M. Preparation of supplies for terminal sterilization. In: Reichert M, Young JH, eds. *Sterilization technology for the health care facility*. Gaithersburg, MD: Aspen Publication, 1997:36–50.

28. Hansen KS. Occupational dermatoses in hospital cleaning women. *Contact Dermatitis* 1983;9(5):343–351.

29. Melli MC, Giorgini S, Sertoli A. Sensitization from contact with ethyl alcohol. *Contact Dermatitis* 1986;14(5):315.

30. Weber DJ, Rutala WA. Occupational risks associated with the use of selected disinfectants and sterilants. In: Rutala WA, ed. *Disinfection, sterilization, and antisepsis in healthcare*. Champlain, NY: Polyscience Publications, 1998:211–226.

31. Association for the Advancement of Medical Instrumentation. *Flash sterilization: steam sterilization of patient care items for immediate use*: report No. ANSI/AAMI ST37. Arlington, VA: AAMI, 1996.

32. Association for the Advancement of Medical Instrumentation. *Steam sterilization and sterility assurance in health care facilities*. Arlington, VA: ANSI/AAMI, 2002.

33. Association for the Advancement of Medical Instrumentation. Ethylene oxide sterilization in health care facilities: safety and effectiveness: report No. ANSI/AAMI ST41. Arlington, VA: AAMI, 1999.

34. Association of Peri-Operative Registered Nurses. Recommended practices for sterilization in the perioperative practice setting. *AORN Journal* 2006;83:700–722.

35. Association for Peri-Operative Registered Nurses. Recommended practices for cleaning and caring for surgical instruments and powered equipment. *AORN Journal* 2002;75:727–741.

36. Mangram AJ, Horan TC, Pearson ML, et al. Guideline for prevention of surgical site infection, 1999. Hospital Infection Control Practices Advisory Committee. *Infection Control & Hospital Epidemiology* 1999;20(4):250–278.

37. Education Design. *Best practices for the prevention of surgical site infection*. Denver Colorado: Education Design, 1998.

38. Association for the Advancement of Medical Instrumentation. *Comprehensive guide to steam sterilization and sterility assurance in health care facilities, AAMI ST79*. City: Publisher, 2006.

39. Singh J, Bhatia R, Gandhi JC, et al. Outbreak of viral hepatitis B in a rural community in India linked to inadequately sterilized needles and syringes. *Bulletin of the World Health Organization* Arlington, VA: Association for the Advancement of Medical Instrumentation, 1998;76(1):93–98.

40. Eickhoff TC. An outbreak of surgical wound infections due to Clostridium perfringens. *Surg Gynecol Obstet* 1962;114:102–108.

41. Favero MS. Sterility assurance: concepts for patient safety. In: Rutala WA, ed. *Disinfection, sterilization and antisepsis: principles and practices in healthcare facilities*. Washington, DC: Association for Professional in Infection Control and Epidemiology, 2001:110–119.

42. Oxborrow GS, Berube R. Sterility testing-validation of sterilization processes, and sporicide testing. In: Block SS, ed. *Disinfection, sterilization, and preservation*. 4th ed. Philadelphia: Lea & Febiger, 1991:1047–1057.

43. Schembre DB. Infectious complications associated with gastrointestinal endoscopy. *Gastrointestinal Endoscopy Clinics of North America* 2000;10(2):215–232.

44. Jackson FW, Ball MD. Correction of deficiencies in flexible fiberoptic sigmoidoscope cleaning and disinfection technique in family practice and internal medicine offices. *Archives of Family Medicine* 1997;6(6):578–582.

45. Orsi GB, Filocamo A, Di Stefano L, Tittobello A. Italian national survey of digestive endoscopy disinfection procedures. *Endoscopy* 1997;29(8):732–738.

46. Honeybourne D, Neumann CS. An audit of bronchoscopy practice in the United Kingdom: a survey of adherence to national guidelines. *Thorax* 1997;52(8):709–713.

47. Srinivasan A, Wolfenden LL, Song X, et al. An outbreak of *Pseudomonas aeruginosa* infections associated with flexible bronchoscopes. *N Engl J Med* 2003;348:221–227.

48. Cetse JC, Vanhems P. Outbreak of infection associated with bronchoscopes. *N Engl J Med* 2003;348:2039–2040.

49. Food and Drug Administration, Centers for Disease Control and Prevention. *FDA and CDC public health advisory: infections from endoscopes inadequately reprocessed by an automated endoscope reprocessing system*, Rockville, MD: FDA, 1999.

50. Rutala WA, Weber DJ. FDA labeling requirements for disinfection of endoscopes: a counterpoint. *Infection Control & Hospital Epidemiology* 1995;16(4):231–235.

51. Kruse A, Rey JF. Guidelines on cleaning and disinfection in GI endoscopy: update 1999. The European Society of Gastrointestinal Endoscopy. *Endoscopy* 2000;32(1):77–80.

52. British Society of Gastroenterology. Cleaning and disinfection of equipment for gastrointestinal endoscopy: report of a working party of the British Society of Gastroenterology Endoscope Committee. *Gut* 1998;42:585–593.

53. British Thoracic Society. British Thoracic Society guidelines on diagnostic flexible bronchoscopy. *Thorax* 2001;56(suppl 1): 1–21.

54. Rey JF, Kruse A. European Society of Gastrointestinal Endoscopy/European Society of Gastreointestinal Endoscopy Nurses and Associates technical note on cleaning and disinfection. *Endoscopy* 2003;35:869–877.

55. Sarin PS, Scheer DI, Kross RD. Inactivation of human T-cell lymphotropic retrovirus (HTLV-III) by LD. *N Engl J Med* 1985;313(22):1416.

56. Sarin PS, Scheer DI, Kross RD. Inactivation of human T-cell lymphotropic retrovirus. *Environ Microbiol* 1990;56:1423–1428.

57. Rutala WA, Cole EC, Wannamaker NS, Weber DJ. Inactivation of *Mycobacterium tuberculosis* and *Mycobacterium bovis* by 14 hospital disinfectants. *American Journal of Medicine* 1991;91(3B):267S–271S.

58. Ascenzi JM. Standardization of tuberculocidal testing of disinfectants. *Journal of Hospital Infection* 1991;18(suppl A):256–263.

59. Collins FM. Use of membrane filters for measurement of mycobactericidal activity of alkaline glutaraldehyde solution. *Applied & Environmental Microbiology* 1987;53(4):737–739.

60. Bond WW, Favero MS, Petersen NJ, Ebert JW. Inactivation of hepatitis B by intermediate-to-high-level disinfectant chemicals. *Journal of Clinical Microbiology* 1983;18(3):535–538.

61. Kobayashi H, Tsuzuki M. The effect of disinfectants and heat on hepatitis B virus. *Journal of Hospital Infection* 1984;5(suppl A):93–94.

62. Spire B, Barre-Sinoussi F, Montagnier L, Chermann JC. Inactivation of lymphadenopathy associated virus by chemical disinfectants. *Lancet* 1984;2(8408):899–901.

63. Martin LS, McDougal JS, Loskoski SL. Disinfection and inactivation of the human T lymphotropic virus type III/Lymphadenopathy-associated virus. *Journal of Infectious Diseases* 1985;152(2):400–403.

64. Resnick L, Veren K, Salahuddin SZ, et al. Stability and inactivation of HTLV-III/LAV under clinical and laboratory environments. *JAMA* 1986;255(14):1887–1891.

65. Centers for Disease Control. Recommendations for prevention of HIV transmission in healthcare settings. *MMWR* 1987;36:S3–S18.

66. Prince DL, Prince HN, Thraenhart O, et al. Methodological approaches to disinfection of human hepatitis B virus. *Journal of Clinical Microbiology* 1993;31(12):3296–3304.

67. Prince DL, Prince RN, Prince HN. Inactivation of human immunodeficiency virus type 1 and herpes simplex virus type 2 by commercial hospital disinfectants. *Chemical Times and Trends* 1990;13:13–16.

68. Sattar SA, Springthorpe VS. Survival and disinfectant inactivation of the human immunodeficiency virus: a critical review. *Reviews of Infectious Diseases* 1991;13(3):430–447.

69. Sattar SA, Springthorpe VS, Conway B, Xu Y. Inactivation of the human immunodeficiency virus: an update. *Rev Med Microbiol* 1994;5:139–150.

70. Kaplan JC, Crawford DC, Durno AG, Schooley RT. Inactivation of human immunodeficiency virus by Betadine. *Infection Control* 1987;8(10):412–414.

71. Hanson PJ, Gor D, Jeffries DJ, Collins JV. Chemical inactivation of HIV on surfaces. *Br Med J* 1989;298(6677):862–864.

72. Hanson PJ, Gor D, Jeffries DJ, Collins JV. Elimination of high titre HIV from fibreoptic endoscopes. *Gut* 1990;31(6):657–659.

73. Hanson PJ, Gor D, Clarke JR, et al. Recovery of the human immunodeficiency virus from fibreoptic bronchoscopes. *Thorax* 1991;46(6):410–412.

74. Hanson PJ, Jeffries DJ, Collins JV. Viral transmission and fibreoptic endoscopy. *Journal of Hospital Infection* 1991;18(suppl A):136–140.

75. Hanson PJ, Chadwick MV, Gaya H, Collins JV. A study of glutaraldehyde disinfection of fibreoptic bronchoscopes experimentally contaminated with *Mycobacterium tuberculosis*. *Journal of Hospital Infection* 1992;22(2):137–142.

76. Payan C, Cottin J, Lemarie C, Ramont C. Inactivation of hepatitis B virus in plasma by hospital in-use chemical disinfectants assessed by a modified HepG2 cell culture. *J Hosp Infect* 2001;47:282–287.

77. Chanzy B, Duc-Bin DL, Rousset B, et al. Effectiveness of a manual disinfection procedure in eliminating hepatitis C virus from experimentally contaminated endoscopes. *Gastrointestinal Endoscopy* 1999;50(2):147–151.

78. Druce JD, Russell JS, Birch CJ, et al. A decontamination and sterilization protocol employed during reuse of cardiac electrophysiology catheters inactivates human immunodeficiency virus. *Infect Control Hosp Epidemiol* 2003;24:184–190.

79. Payan C, Pivert A, Kampf G, et al. Assessment of new chemical disinfectants for HBV virucidal activity in a cell culture model. *J Hosp Infection* 2004;56 (suppl):S58–S63.

80. Rutala WA, Clontz EP, Weber DJ, Hoffmann KK. Disinfection practices for endoscopes and other semicritical items. *Infection Control & Hospital Epidemiology* 1991;12(5):282–288.

81. Reynolds CD, Rhinehart E, Dreyer P, Goldmann DA. Variability in reprocessing policies and procedures for flexible fiberoptic endoscopes in Massachusetts hospitals. *American Journal of Infection Control* 1992;20(6):283–290.

82. Handsfield HH, Cummings MJ, Swenson PD. Prevalence of antibody to human immunodeficiency virus and hepatitis B surface antigen in blood samples submitted to a hospital laboratory: implications for handling specimens. *JAMA* 1987;258(23):3395–3397.

83. Baker JL, Kelen GD, Sivertson KT, Quinn TC. Unsuspected human immunodeficiency virus in critically ill emergency patients. *JAMA* 1987;257(19):2609–2611.

84. Kelen GD, Fritz S, Qaqish B, et al. Unrecognized human immunodeficiency virus infection in emergency department patients. *N Engl J Med* 1988;318(25):1645–1650.

85. Sartor C, Charrel RN, de Lamballerie X, et al. Evaluation of a disinfection procedure for hysteroscopes contaminated by hepatitis C virus. *Infection Control & Hospital Epidemiology* 1999;20(6):434–436.

86. Rey JF, Halfon P, Feryn JM, et al. Risk of transmission of hepatitis C virus by digestive endoscopy. *Gastroenterologie Clinique et Biologique* 1995;19(4):346–349.

87. Ishino Y, Ido K, Sugano K. Contamination with hepatitis B virus DNA in gastrointestinal endoscope channels: risk of infection on reuse after on-site cleaning. *Endoscopy* 2005;37:548–551.

88. Agolini G, Russo A, Clementi M. Effect of phenolic and chlorine disinfectants on hepatitis C virus binding and infectivity. *American Journal of Infection Control* 1999;27(3):236–239.

89. Occupational Safety and Health Administration. Occupational exposure to bloodborne pathogens: final rule. *Federal Register* 1991;56:64003–64182.

90. Occupational Safety and Health Administration. OSHA instruction CPL 2-2.44C. Washington, DC: Office of Health Compliance Assistance, 1992.

91. Occupational Safety and Health Administration. OSHA Memorandum from Stephen Mallinger. EPA-registered disinfectants for HIV/HBV. Washington, DC: OSHA, 1997.

92. Weber DJ, Barbee SL, Sobsey MD, Rutala WA. The effect of blood on the antiviral activity of sodium hypochlorite, a phenolic, and a quaternary ammonium compound. *Infection Control & Hospital Epidemiology* 1999;20(12):821–827.

93. Kim KH, Fekety R, Batts DH, et al. Isolation of *Clostridium difficile* from the environment and contacts of patients with antibiotic-associated colitis. *J Infect Dis* 1981;143:42–50.

94. Bhalla A, Pultz NJ, Gries DM, et al. Acquisition of nosocomial pathogens on hands after contact with environmental surfaces near hospitalized patients. *Infect Control Hosp Epidemiol* 2004;25:164–167.

95. Skoutelis AT, Westenfelder GO, Beckerdite M, Phair JP. Hospital carpeting and epidemiology of *Clostridium difficile*. *American Journal of Infection Control* 1994;22(4):212–217.

96. Wilcox MH, Fawley WN. Hospital disinfectants and spore formation by *Clostridium difficile*. *Lancet* 2000;356(9238):1324.

97. Kaatz GW, Gitlin SD, Schaberg DR, et al. Acquisition of *Clostridium difficile* from the hospital environment. *American Journal of Epidemiology* 1988;127(6):1289–1294.

98. Wilcox MH, Fawley WN, Wigglesworth N, et al. Comparison of the effect of detergent versus hypochlorite cleaning on environmental contamination and incidence of *Clostridium difficile* infection. *J Hosp Infection* 2003;54:109–114.

99. Mayfield JL, Leet T, Miller J, Mundy LM. Environmental control to reduce transmission of *Clostridium difficile*. *Clinical Infectious Diseases* 2000;31(4):995–1000.

100. Marler LM, Siders JA, Wolters LC, et al. Comparison of five cultural procedures for isolation of *Clostridium difficile* from stools. *J Clin Microbiol* 1992;30:514–516.

101. Brazier JG. The diagnosis of *Clostridium difficile*-associated disease. *J Antimicrob Chemother* 1998;41(suppl):29–40.

102. Perez J, Springthorpe S, Sattar SA. Activity of selected oxidizing microbicides against spores of *Clostridium difficile*: Relevance to environmental control. *Am J Infect Control* 2005;33:320–325.

103. McFarland LV, Mulligan ME, Kwok RY, Stamm WE. Nosocomial acquisition of *Clostridium difficile* infection. *N Engl J Med* 1989;320(4):204–210.

104. Jernigan JA, Siegman-Igra Y, Guerrant RC, Farr BM. A randomized crossover study of disposable thermometers for prevention of *Clostridium difficile* and other nosocomial infections. *Infect Control Hosp Epidemiol* 1998;19:494–499.

105. Rutala WA, Gergen MF, Weber DJ. Inactivation of *Clostridium difficile* spores by disinfectants. *Infection Control & Hospital Epidemiology* 1993;14(1):36–39.

106. Hughes CE, Gebhard RL, Peterson LR, Gerding DN. Efficacy of routine fiberoptic endoscope cleaning and disinfection for killing *Clostridium difficile*. *Gastrointestinal Endoscopy* 1986;32(1):7–9.

107. Dyas A, Das BC. The activity of glutaraldehyde against *Clostridium difficile*. *Journal of Hospital Infection* 1985;6(1):41–45.

108. Wullt M, Odenholt I, Walder M. Activity of three disinfectants and acidified nitrite against *Clostridium difficile* spores. *Infect Control Hosp Epidemiol* 2003;24:765–768.

109. Block C. The effect of Perasafe and sodium dichloroisocyanurate (NaDCC) against spores of *Clostridium difficile* and *Bacillus atrophaeus* on stainless steel and polyvinyl chloride surfaces. *J Hosp Infection* 2004;57:144–148.

110. Rutala WA, Stiegel MM, Sarubbi FA, Weber DJ. Susceptibility of antibiotic-susceptible and antibiotic-resistant hospital bacteria to disinfectants. *Infection Control & Hospital Epidemiology* 1997;18(6):417–421.

111. Anderson RL, Carr JH, Bond WW, Favero MS. Susceptibility of vancomycin-resistant enterococci to environmental disinfectants. *Infection Control & Hospital Epidemiology* 1997;18(3):195–199.

112. Rutala WA, Barbee SL, Aguiar NC, et al. Antimicrobial activity of home disinfectants and natural products against potential human pathogens. *Infection Control & Hospital Epidemiology* 2000;21(1):33–38.

113. Sakagami Y, Kajimura K. Bactericidal activities of disinfectants against vancomycin-resistant enterococci. *J Hosp Infection* 2002;50:140–144.

114. Sehulster LM, Anderson RL. Susceptibility of glycopeptide-intermediate resistant *Staphylococcus aureus* (GISA) to surface disinfectants, hand washing chemicals, and a skin antiseptic. Abstract Y-3, 98th General Meeting of American Society for Microbiology, May 1998:547.

115. Rutala WA, Weber DJ, Gergen MF. Studies on the disinfection of VRE-contaminated surfaces. *Infection Control & Hospital Epidemiology* 2000;21(8):548.

116. Byers KE, Durbin LJ, Simonton BM, et al. Disinfection of hospital rooms contaminated with vancomycin-resistant *Enterococcus faecium*. *Infection Control & Hospital Epidemiology* 1998;19(4):261–264

117. Centers for Disease Control. Surveillance for Creutzfeldt-Jakob disease—United States. *MMWR* 1996;45:665–668.

118. World Health Organization. WHO infection control guidelines for transmissible spongiform encephalopathies, (www.who.int/csr/resources/publications/bse/whocdscsraph2003.pdf).

119. Rutala WA, Weber DJ. Creutzfeldt-Jakob disease: recommendations for disinfection and sterilization. *Clin Infect Dis* 2001;32:1348–1356.

120. Taylor DM. Inactivation of prions by physical and chemical means. *J Hosp Infection* 1999;43(suppl):S69–S76.

121. Henderson DA. The looming threat of bioterrorism. *Science* 1999;283:1279–1282.

122. Centers for Disease Control. Biological and chemical terrorism: strategic plan for preparedness and response. *MMWR* 2000;49 (no. RR-4):1–14.

123. Klein M, DeForest A. The inactivation of viruses by germicides. *Chem Specialists Manuf Assoc Proc* 1963;49:116–118.

124. Rutala WA, Weber DJ. Infection control: the role of disinfection and sterilization. *Journal of Hospital Infection* 1999;43(suppl):S43–S55.

125. Weber DJ, Rutala WA. Use of germicides in the home and health care setting: is there a relationship between germicide use and antimicrobial resistance. *Infect Control Hosp Epidemiol*. 2006;27:1107–19.

126. Gregory AW, Schaalje GB, Smart JD, Robison RA. The mycobactericidal efficacy of ortho-phthalaldehyde and the comparative resistances of *Mycobacterium bovis*, *Mycobacterium terrae*, and *Mycobacterium chelonae*. *Infection Control & Hospital Epidemiology* 1999;20(5):324–330.

127. Rutala WA. Selection and use of disinfectants in healthcare. In: Mayhall CG, ed. *Hospital Epidemiology and Infection Control.* 2nd ed. Philadelphia: Lippincott Williams & Wilkins, 1999:1161–1187.

128. Rutala WA, Weber DJ. Disinfection of endoscopes: review of new chemical sterilants used for high-level disinfection. *Infection Control & Hospital Epidemiology* 1999;20(1):69–76.

129. Rutala WA, Weber DJ. Clinical effectiveness of low-temperature sterilization technologies. *Infection Control & Hospital Epidemiology* 1998;19(10):798–804.

21

Foodborne Disease Prevention in Healthcare Facilities

Margarita E. Villarino and William R. Jarvis

Foodborne disease outbreaks may occur when food becomes contaminated with pathogenic organisms or toxins. When these contaminants are bacterial pathogens, food mishandling may permit proliferation of these organisms and subsequently cause illness when ingested by susceptible persons. Food service departments at hospitals and other healthcare facilities, such as nursing homes, must cope with problems associated with handling large amounts of raw food, serving many meals throughout the day, preparing and handling food for a variety of diets, and delays in serving. These challenges in food preparation and delivery in healthcare facilities are compounded by the necessity of serving many patients who are at high risk of contracting foodborne disease. Because of these problems, prevention of foodborne disease should be a high priority in healthcare facilities.

Foodborne disease outbreaks related to food service in healthcare facilities may affect patients [1–9], personnel [10,11], and visitors [12,13] and may involve food prepared in the facility itself [1,2,4] as well as food prepared elsewhere but served in the healthcare facility [14,15]. Generally, hospitalized persons are more likely than nonhospitalized persons to acquire disease when exposed to foodborne agents and to develop serious side effects associated with such diseases. This is most likely due to host factors (e.g., malignancy, achlorhydria, advanced age, diabetes mellitus, and acquired immunodeficiency syndrome [AIDS]) or iatrogenic factors (e.g., use of antibiotics, immunosuppressive agents, or antacids and gastric surgery). Small inocula of enteric pathogens that might be innocuous to most healthy people can cause disease and even death in highly susceptible patients.

Secondary transmission of foodborne pathogens also may come about when patients or healthcare facility personnel become infected and, in turn, expose other patients or personnel as a consequence of poor personal hygiene or improper patient care techniques. Epidemics resulting from person-to-person transmission occur most often in nurseries, pediatric wards, or nursing homes, where fecal-oral spread may be facilitated by difficulties in maintaining good hygiene [16]. Secondary transmission may involve persons within the healthcare facility (patients, personnel, and visitors) and others (such as family members) outside the hospital setting. Foodborne disease outbreaks affecting large numbers of hospital personnel have led to staffing problems and may hinder delivery of optimal care [11,12]. With assumptions made about the values of indirect costs, the cost of a hospital-based outbreak has been estimated to be as high as $400,000 [17].

The problems of food or dietetic services in healthcare facilities generally parallel those of large restaurants and catering firms but may be even more complex [18]. Healthcare facilities' food services typically operate 12–18 hours daily, 7 days per week. Similar to large restaurants, these institutions purchase and rapidly process quantities of food

TABLE 21-1

FOODS COMMONLY INVOLVED AND REPORTED CAUSE OF CONTAMINATION IN FOODBORNE OUTBREAKS OF BACTERIAL ETIOLOGY, UNITED STATES, 1975–1992

Cause	Numbers of Outbreaks	Typical Foods	Usual Reported Cause of Contamination			
			Improper Holding	Inadequate Cooling	Poor Hygiene	Contaminated Equipment
Salmonella	1,270	Poultry, eggs, beef, pork, ice cream	+	++	+	+
Staphylococcus aureus	355	Ham, poultry, pastries, beef	++	—	+	—
Clostridium botulinum	260	Vegetables, fish	+	++	—	—
Clostridium perfringens	206	Beef, poultry, Mexican food	++	+	—	—
Shigella	118	Salads	+	—	++	—
Bacillus cereus	77	Fried rice, Chinese food	++	+	—	—
Campylobacter jejuni	80	Milk	+	+	—	+
Vibrio parahaemolyticus	26	Shellfish	+	++	—	—

—, less frequent cause; +, frequent cause; ++, most frequent cause.
From Centers for Disease Control and Prevention, Foodborne Disease Surveillance.

that require large working surfaces, numerous utensils, and many working hands. They also must adhere to tight schedules, rapidly preparing and storing a large variety of foods. In addition, food services in such facilities have unique problems created by the need for a wide assortment of special diets, including enteral feedings. Meals and supplemental feedings must be provided from a central kitchen and sometimes from decentralized kitchens on wards. Finally, food often must be transported from a central preparation area throughout the institution. If food is not held at appropriate temperatures, delays between preparation and service present opportunities for proliferation of foodborne pathogens.

EPIDEMIOLOGIC ASPECTS OF FOODBORNE DISEASES

The epidemiology of foodborne disease outbreaks in the United Kingdom, Australia, and the United States has been reviewed extensively elsewhere [19–22]. In Scotland, during the 9-year period from 1978 to 1987, some 48 foodborne outbreaks were reported from hospitals, compared with 50 outbreaks during the previous 4 years (1973 to 1977) [19]. The decline in the overall incidence of food-poisoning outbreaks was attributed to an increased recognition by dietary departments of the principles of food temperature control. Reductions were seen in the number of outbreaks caused by *Clostridium perfringens* and *Staphylococcus* species while the number of outbreaks of salmonellosis rose. The average number of persons affected per outbreak of salmonellosis increased from 36 in 1973 to 81 in 1987. In contrast, in England and Wales during 1978 to 1987, a total of 248 outbreaks of salmonellosis was reported in hospitals compared with 522 outbreaks

reported during 1968 to 1977 [20]. This decline might have been a result of improved food-handling practices; environmental health officers in the United Kingdom have expanded the monitoring of hospital food service departments since 1977.

In the United States, from all foodborne outbreaks reported to the Centers for Disease Control and Prevention (CDC) during 1975 to 1992, the bacterial agents most frequently identified were *Salmonella, Staphylococcus aureus, C. botulinum,* and *C. perfringens* (Table 21-1). In healthcare facilities, *Salmonella* and *C. perfringens* are more significant than *C. botulinum* and *S. aureus.* Transmission of all four of these common foodborne bacterial pathogens was typically associated with certain food vehicles; likely sources of contamination varied for the different pathogens (Table 21-1). The number of reported foodborne outbreaks in known locations during 1975 to 1992 and the associated episodes and deaths in hospitals, nursing homes, and other known locations are shown in Table 21-2. Of these, hospitals and nursing homes accounted for 3.3% of the outbreaks, 4.8% of the episodes, and 28.9% of the deaths.

Only 123 foodborne disease outbreaks in hospitals were reported during this 17-year period. However, because foodborne disease outbreaks must be recognized, investigated, and reported to state health departments before being reported to the CDC, it is highly likely that foodborne outbreaks are underreported nationally. During 1975 to 1992, reported outbreaks in hospitals and nursing homes were significantly more likely to be caused by bacterial agents ($n = 143$) than by viruses, parasites, or chemicals ($n = 16$) (Table 21-3). Nonetheless, viral [13,23] and parasitic [24] foodborne outbreaks have been reported from healthcare facilities.

It is important to investigate foodborne disease outbreaks in hospitals, to define sources, modes of spread, and

TABLE 21-2

REPORTED FOODBORNE OUTBREAKS, CASES, AND DEATHS IN HOSPITALS, NURSING HOMES, AND OTHER KNOWN LOCATIONS, 1975–1992

	Hospitals		Nursing Homes		Other Known Locations	
	Total	Confirmed Cause	Total	Confirmed Cause	Total	Confirmed Cause
Number of outbreaks	123	67	168	92	8,631	3,225
Number of cases	6,638	3,941	6,783	3,665	268,009	135,035
Number of deaths	11	7	86	82	235	215
Deaths/1,000 cases	1.7	1.8	12.7	22.4	0.9	1.6

From Centers for Disease Control and Prevention, Foodborne Disease Surveillance.

methods for prevention and control of nosocomial foodborne disease. Of 233 hospital-based outbreaks of infection investigated by the CDC from 1956 to 1979, gastroenteritis was the most common cause; typical organisms were *Salmonella* spp. and enteropathogenic *Escherichia coli* [25]. In adult patients, contaminated food vehicles were frequently implicated in salmonellosis outbreaks. Outbreaks attributed to cross-infection, such as gastroenteritis in nurseries due to *E. coli* or *Salmonella*, were more difficult to recognize and control than were foodborne outbreaks. Most cross-infection outbreaks were recognized because the infecting pathogen was unusual or distinguished by a

unique antimicrobial resistance pattern. In England and Wales from 1978 to 1987, 71 of 235 (30%) reported outbreaks of salmonellosis in hospitals were attributed to cross-infection, compared with 57 (24%) outbreaks attributed to foodborne transmission [20]. However, foodborne outbreaks affected more persons (n = 1,862) than did those due to cross-infection (n = 558). Since 1979, CDC investigation of such outbreaks has been uncommon.

In the United States during 1975 to 1992, 336 reported deaths were associated with foodborne disease outbreaks with known place of preparation (Table 21-4). Eighty-six (26%) took place in nursing homes and 11 (3%)

TABLE 21-3

CONFIRMED CAUSES OF REPORTED FOODBORNE OUTBREAKS RELATED TO HOSPITALS, NURSING HOMES, AND OTHER KNOWN LOCATIONS, UNITED STATES, 1975–1992

	Hospitals		Nursing Homes		Other Known Locations	
	Number of Outbreaks	% of Total[a]	Number of Outbreaks	% of Total[a]	Number of Outbreaks	% of Total[a]
Bacterial						
Salmonella	35	52	61	66	1,157	36
Staphylococcus aureus	5	8	14	15	332	10
Clostridium perfringens	7	11	8	9	202	6
Shigella	3	5	1	1	112	4
Bacillus cereus	1	2	2	2	74	2
Campylobacter jejuni	1	2	3	3	74	2
Other bacteria	1	2	1	1	304	9
Subtotal	53	79	90	98	2,255	70
Viral	1	2	0	0	166	5
Parasitic	1	2	1	1	116	4
Chemical						
Scombroid	8	12	0	0	244	8
Ciguatera	0	0	0	0	211	7
Other	4	6	1	1	233	7
Subtotal	12	18	1	1	688	21
Total	67	100	92	100	3,225	100

[a]Percentages may sum to >100% because of rounding.
From Centers for Disease Control and Prevention, Foodborne Disease Surveillance.

TABLE 21-4

CAUSES OF DEATHS ASSOCIATED WITH FOODBORNE DISEASES OUTBREAKS IN HOSPITALS, NURSING HOMES, AND OTHER KNOWN LOCATIONS, UNITED STATES, 1975–1992

Cause	Total Deaths	Deaths in Hospital Outbreaks		Deaths in Nursing Home Outbreaks		Deaths in Other Known Locations	
		No.	% of Total	No.	% of Total	No.	% of Total
Salmonella	121	2	2	70	58	49	41
Clostridium perfringens	11	5	45	3	27	3	27
Staphylococcus aureus	4	0	0	2	50	2	50
Escherichia coil	4	0	0	4	100	0	0
Other known cause	168	0	0	3	2	165	98
Unknown cause	28	4	14	4	14	20	71
Total	336	11	3	86	24	239	71

From Centers for Disease Control and Prevention, Foodborne Disease Surveillance.

in hospitals. Of the 97 deaths in hospitals and nursing homes, 72 (74%) were due to *Salmonella*. In the United States, isolation rates of *Salmonella* serotype enteritidis have been increasing since 1976 [26]. From 1985 to 1991, 380 *S. enteritidis* outbreaks were reported to the CDC, involving 13,056 ill persons, 1,512 hospitalizations, and 50 deaths [27]. Of these outbreaks, 59 (16%) were in nursing homes or hospitals, accounting for 1,512 illnesses (12%) and 45 (90%) deaths. Of 167 outbreaks in which a food vehicle was identified, 137 (82%) implicated fresh eggs in the shell. During this same period, 60% (9/15) reported nursing home outbreaks with a known vehicle implicated dishes containing shell eggs. Four (8%) of the 49 *S. enteritidis* outbreaks reported from January to October 31, 1990, occurred in hospitals or nursing homes, compared with 26% (20/77) of such outbreaks in 1989 [28]. This decline in hospital- and nursing home-associated *S. enteritidis* outbreaks may reflect efforts to improve food safety in these settings (e.g., by using pasteurized eggs).

Surveillance data can help elucidate the relative importance of various factors that contribute to the occurrence of foodborne disease outbreaks. During 1975–1992, food-handling errors were noted in 212 reported foodborne outbreaks in hospitals or nursing homes. Holding food at improper temperatures was the most common such error. Other important errors included inadequate cooking, poor personal hygiene of food handlers, use of food from unsafe sources, and use of contaminated equipment. Training personnel in proper food-handling practices can eliminate these errors and prevent outbreaks.

Food served from a healthcare facility kitchen can be contaminated before, during, or after preparation. When purchased, raw poultry and red meat might already be contaminated with organisms (e.g., *Salmonella, C. perfringens, Campylobacter jejuni* or, more rarely, *E. coli* 0157:H7). In a 1988 survey of broiler chicken specimens from 195 poultry-processing plants, the prevalence of *Salmonella* spp.

contamination was 21% of 15,391 specimens [29]. *Campylobacter jejuni* typically is present in >50% of poultry carcasses at the point of sale [30]. Raw fish and shellfish can be contaminated with such pathogens as *Vibrio parahaemolyticus, C. perfringens,* and *V. vulnificus.* Shell eggs may be contaminated with *S. enteritidis,* either externally through fecal contamination or internally through transovarian transmission [31,32]. During processing, food also may become contaminated with organisms through contact with dirty hands, infected aerosols spread by coughing or sneezing, and contaminated equipment, such as meat slicers and working surfaces [33]. Finally, bacteria may grow while food is stored (e.g., when cooked foods are stored in direct contact with raw foods or when foods are held at inadequate temperatures). *Listeria monocytogenes* can survive and grow in food even with adequate refrigeration [34].

FOODS AND THE IMMUNOCOMPROMISED HOST

Patients in healthcare facilities are more susceptible to certain foodborne infections than the general population. The elderly, the immunosuppressed, and persons with chronic underlying diseases are generally at higher risk of infection and associated morbidity and mortality. In particular, outbreaks of foodborne disease in nursing homes can be associated with serious morbidity and mortality; therefore, efforts to provide the safest possible food to the elderly in nursing homes should be maximized.

Among persons in hospitals and nursing homes, increased susceptibility to foodborne infections may be caused by associated physiologic changes or therapy of underlying disease. Although the gastrointestinal tract is normally resistant to colonization, this resistance can be substantially diminished by antimicrobial therapy, mucositis from cancer treatments, decreased stomach acidity, impaired intestinal motility, and diminished mucosal, humoral, and cellular immunity. Even in numbers smaller than the usual infective dose, ingested microorganisms may cause systemic infection in these patients.

Because *E. coli*, *Klebsiella* spp., and *Pseudomonas aeruginosa* can contaminate fresh fruits, salads, and vegetables [35], these foods should not be served to neutropenic patients [36]. Another potential contaminant of fresh vegetables is *L. monocytogenes*, a gram-positive bacterium that particularly affects the elderly, pregnant women, and the severely immunosuppressed [34]. In one *L. monocytogenes* outbreak involving 20 patients from eight hospitals, raw vegetables served in hospital meals may have been contaminated; 10 (50%) of these patients were immunosuppressed [37]. Dairy products and any raw food of animal origin also may be contaminated with *Listeria*, *Salmonella*, or *E. coli* 0157:H7. Outbreaks of *E. coli* 0157:H7 and *Salmonella* in nursing homes have been particularly devastating. In two such *E. coli* 0157:H7 outbreaks, 15 deaths occurred [1,38]. In an outbreak of *S. enteritidis* in a nursing home, 25/104 affected patients died [39].

Human immunodeficiency virus (HIV)–infected persons are at increased risk of infection with bacterial foodborne pathogens (see Chapter 42). Among persons with AIDS, the reported incidence of laboratory-confirmed salmonellosis was 20 times that reported for persons without AIDS [40]. Compared with immunocompetent persons, those with AIDS and salmonellosis are more likely to have initial and recurrent bloodstream infections [41,42]. The reported incidence of campylobacteriosis among persons with AIDS in Los Angeles County between 1983 and 1987 was 39 times higher than the rate in the general population [43]. Similarly, the incidence of listeriosis among persons with HIV infection is estimated to be 60 times that of the general population; among persons with AIDS, the relative risk is more than 140 times greater [44]. Ingestion of contaminated foods is likely to be an important source of enteric infections in persons with AIDS. All immunocompetent persons should cook raw foods of animal origin thoroughly and avoid eating raw shellfish, raw milk, raw meat, and raw eggs [45–47]. Dietary departments in health facilities should follow these recommendations for all hospitalized patients, particularly those who are immunocompromised.

Enteral feeding solutions are used frequently to provide nutritional support to seriously ill patients with a functional digestive tract. These solutions often are prepared in food service departments. Enteral feedings contaminated by bacteria can cause severe healthcare-associated infections (HAIs) [48–50]; therefore, infection control practices for their preparation and administration should be reviewed and implemented [51]. A high incidence of microbial contamination of enteral nutrition, including powdered feeds requiring reconstitution, has been described [47,48, 50,52–56]. Contamination also can occur during assembly of a delivery system on the ward [57] or by bacteria colonizing the nasogastric tube or ascending from the patient's gut [58].

Factors contributing to the microbial contamination of enteral feeding solutions include the composition of the feeding solution, the lack of preservatives, the number of manipulations involved in the feeding process, the mode and duration of administration, and the timing of sampling [50]. *Enterobacter sakazakii* outbreaks in neonates have been traced to both extrinsically and intrinsically contaminated powdered infant formula [49,50,54]. Although contamination is most frequently the result of manipulation during preparation, adherence to appropriate food-handling practices is essential to minimize bacterial contamination during preparation and administration and bacterial growth during storage. Public health authorities' monitoring of recommended manufacturing procedures and of the regulations governing the bacterial content of powdered feeds has been suggested [50].

PREVENTION OF FOODBORNE TRANSMISSION IN HEALTHCARE FACILITIES

Requirements and recommendations concerning food services are provided to hospitals and other healthcare facilities from the Joint Commission on Accreditation of Healthcare Organizations (JCAHO) and the Association for Professionals in Infection Control and Epidemiology, Inc. (APIC) (Table 21-5). Responsibilities for the inspection and certification of food service facilities in healthcare organizations vary by state. Accreditation by JCAHO does not ensure regular food service inspection or food handler training. The infection control committee of each healthcare facility has an important responsibility in the prevention of foodborne disease. This committee is responsible for cooperating with the food services department in developing written policies and procedures and for reviewing these policies at least annually [59].

To prevent foodborne disease, both the JCAHO requirements and the APIC recommendations focus prevention efforts by hospitals and other healthcare institutions in two areas: food hygiene (i.e., food preparation, storage, and distribution) and health and hygiene of food service personnel. Both of these areas need to be reinforced by specific training of food service workers in the basic principles of food safety. New personnel should receive prompt training in good food-handling practices. Food service personnel from all work shifts should receive regular in-service training stressing the prevention of foodborne diseases and appropriate food-handling practices.

General approaches to limiting contamination and destroying or inhibiting the growth of potential foodborne pathogens have been reviewed elsewhere [60,61]. Healthcare facilities should consult a dietitian with special training in food service sanitation, sanitarian, or both about

TABLE 21-5

SUMMARY OF REQUIREMENTS AND RECOMMENDATIONS OF THE JOINT COMMISSION ON ACCREDITATION OF HEALTHCARE ORGANIZATIONS AND THE ASSOCIATION FOR PROFESSIONALS IN INFECTION CONTROL, INC. FOR FOOD (DIETETIC) SERVICES

JCAHO	APIC
Dietetic services shall meet the nutritional needs of patients through the following standards: 1. Organization to provide optimal nutritional care and quality of service 2. Appropriate training of personnel 3. Written policies and procedures 4. Safe, sanitary, and timely provision of food to meet nutritional requirements 5. Diet in accord with care provider's order and appropriate recording of dietetic information in patient's chart 6. Appropriate quality control mechanisms 7. Regular evaluation of quality and appropriateness in accordance with JCAHO quality assurance characteristics	Infection control activities of the food service department should include: 1. Development of purchasing specifications that meet standards of safety and sanitation for food, equipment, and cleaning supplies 2. Maintenance and cleaning of work areas, storage areas, and equipment in accordance with state and local health department standards 3. Development of written standards for safe food handling; cleaning and sanitizing of trays, utensils, and tableware; and disposing of dietary waste 4. Compliance with local health department regulations for storage, handling, and disposal of garbage 5. Educational programs for personnel in food preparation and personal hygiene

Data adapted from Joint Commission on Accreditation of Healthcare Organizations, *Accreditation manual for hospitals. 1991.* Chicago: Joint Commission on Accreditation of Healthcare Organizations, 1990; and Association for Practitioners in Infection Control, *APIC infection control and applied epidemiology: Principles and practice.* St. Louis: Mosby–Year Book, Inc., 1996.

formulating and monitoring food-handling operations and procedures. In addition, local or state health departments should be consulted about regulations and standards concerning food service personnel, food sanitation, and waste disposal.

Food Hygiene

Two factors are critical in preventing bacterial foodborne disease: holding food at appropriate temperatures (that is, either >60°C [140°F] or <5°C [41°F]) and avoiding cross-contamination of cooked food by raw food or by infected food-handling personnel [62]. In addition, pasteurized milk and pasteurized egg products should be used in place of raw milk and shell eggs. Food must be purchased from reliable sources; commercially filled unopened packages should be used when possible. Microbial contaminants on some raw foods may be kept from multiplying during processing by proper storage, thawing meat products in refrigerators (<5°C [41°F]), and adequate heat treatment. Because work surfaces, knives, slicers, pots, pans, and other kitchen equipment can convey bacteria from contaminated food to other foods, food contact surfaces of equipment and utensils must be cleaned and decontaminated between preparation of food items. Items such as slicers must be easy to disassemble to ensure proper cleaning.

Workers should be trained to operate and maintain equipment properly. Hand hygiene by food service personnel is an essential component of food hygiene. All workers must thoroughly wash their hands after handling raw poultry, meat, fish, fruits, and vegetables; after contact with unclean equipment and work surfaces, soiled clothing, washrags, and other items; and, most important, after using the bathroom. Spilled food should be cleaned up immediately. Equipment and the kitchen layout should be designed to promote rapid processing to minimize chances for cross-contamination; to avoid producing aerosols, sprays, or splashing during processing; and to facilitate cleaning and sanitizing operations [61]. Contamination by insects, rodents, sewage backflow, and drips must be prevented by screening, proper storage (including separating raw meat from processed foods), and adequate plumbing. Garbage from hospital kitchens and wards should be enclosed to protect it from insects and rodents and transported or disposed of in a sanitary manner, according to state and local regulations.

Cross-contamination can be minimized by adopting standard techniques for cleaning work surfaces and kitchen utensils and by ensuring that raw foods are processed in areas of the kitchen and on work surfaces that are not subsequently used for cooked foods. Separate cutting boards may not be required when the boards used are nonabsorbent and can be cleaned and sanitized adequately between uses for different food categories. Dishwashing- and utensil-washing equipment and techniques that sanitize service ware and prevent recontamination should be used to ensure sanitary provision of food. Disposable containers and utensils should be properly discarded after one use. Food hygiene procedures should be reviewed periodically and whenever physical changes in the kitchen are made or new equipment is put into use.

Foodborne disease outbreaks have resulted from poor planning and a lack of understanding of appropriate food-handling practices (e.g., not allowing enough time before cooking for poultry to thaw or assuming that thawing is complete). This problem can result in undercooking and can be compounded by keeping undercooked food in the oven after the heat has been shut off, providing ideal incubation conditions for bacteria that survived the initial cooking. Potentially harmful bacteria in foods must be destroyed by thorough cooking or reheating to the proper internal temperatures for the appropriate length of time. For example, meat and poultry should generally be cooked to heat all parts of the food to 68°C (155°F) for 15 seconds [62]. Internal meat temperatures should be measured by bayonet-type thermometers. Periodically, the internal temperature of foods in serving lines should be checked.

A common error resulting in foodborne disease outbreaks is storage of food at inappropriate temperatures; this error is most often identified in staphylococcal food poisoning outbreaks and in short- and long-incubation *Bacillus cereus*, *C. perfringens*, and *Salmonella* spp. outbreaks. In some outbreaks, even when refrigerator temperatures have been adequate, the center temperature of perishable foods was warm enough to permit bacteria to grow or toxin to be produced because the foods were in inadequate holding containers. When cooked foods are kept at room temperature (or are refrigerated in large quantities) for a period of 4 hours, certain pathogens remaining in the food may be able to multiply to sufficient levels or produce enough toxin to cause disease. Cooked foods have been kept too long at room temperature because of inadequate refrigerator space and failure to perceive the importance of refrigeration. In general, cooked food that requires refrigeration should be cooled from 60°C (140°F) to 21°C (70°F) within 2 hours and from 21°C (70°F) to ≤5°C (41°F) within 4 hours; storage temperature should not exceed 5°C (41°F). Food should be placed in shallow containers so that the food is no more than 4 inches deep.

Storage is a particular problem when food must be delivered from a central kitchen to peripheral areas of the healthcare facility or other buildings either by truck or on food carts. Procedures for transporting food must include a way to keep hot foods hot and cold foods cold. Thermometers used to measure holding temperatures should be standard equipment in such conveyances. Standby equipment should be on hand or alternative plans formulated to handle emergency conditions arising from equipment failure. Food delivered to a kitchen or ward should be properly stored to prevent growth of bacteria, and it should be distributed with minimum handling by ward personnel. In the event that ward personnel must handle food, they should be carefully supervised to ensure

that the same high standards required of kitchen personnel are maintained.

In the past, problems have arisen because of preferences for raw or undercooked foods. Substitution of pasteurized egg products for fresh eggs in nursing homes and hospitals is strongly recommended. Several outbreaks have been traced to blenders used for both raw eggs and to pureed foods. Requiring the use of separate blenders to scramble eggs and to puree cooked foods would reduce the risk of cross-contamination. Routine disassembly and sanitation of blenders after blending raw eggs also is important. Avoiding consumption of raw milk is important in preventing outbreaks caused by *Salmonella* spp. and *C. jejuni*.

Health and Hygiene of Food Service Personnel

Supervision of food service personnel requires attention to work habits, personal hygiene, and health. The hands of food service personnel may be colonized or infected with microorganisms, such as *S. aureus*, or may become contaminated by organisms from raw foods (*Salmonella* spp., *C. jejuni*, or *C. perfringens*) or human excreta (*Salmonella* spp., *Shigella* spp., Norovirus, or hepatitis A virus). These organisms may then contaminate food. Although thorough cooking of food just before consumption will eradicate the risk of many illnesses, staphylococcal food poisoning will not be eliminated because staphylococcal enterotoxins are heat stable.

Hand hygiene facilities should be conveniently located to permit use by employees in food preparation and utensil-washing areas and in or immediately adjacent to toilet facilities. Each hand hygiene facility should be provided a continuous supply of waterless agents, or hand-washing facilities should have clean water; a supply of hand-cleaning liquid, powder, or bar soap; and individual sanitary towels from a continuous towel system supplied with a clean towel or a heated-air hand-drying device. Common hand-drying towels are prohibited. If disposable towels are used, a waste receptacle should be located next to the hand-washing facility.

Various strategies have been used to monitor the health of food service personnel, including periodic stool examinations for certain pathogens. However, such measures may not be effective. One stool culture is not sufficient to detect the small number of organisms in the stool of an infected person who does not have diarrhea. For example, one rectal swab detected only 47% of chronic *Salmonella* serotype Derby carriers, and seven consecutive daily swabs were needed to detect 95% of known carriers [63]. Such extensive culturing is impractical and costly. Periodic stool cultures of food handlers may miss persons who excrete organisms intermittently or who become infected during the interval between cultures. In Jordan, a large outbreak of nosocomial salmonellosis caused by an asymptomatic infected food handler occurred despite the institution of routine quarterly stool cultures for kitchen employees [64].

In addition, cultures of nose and throat secretions and feces may reveal potential foodborne pathogens, such as *S. aureus*, but this carriage may be of no danger to others: most *S. aureus* carriers do not usually disseminate the organisms. Laboratory monitoring of food handlers actually could be counterproductive by instilling a false sense of security. Negative culture reports could be interpreted by the employee to indicate that he or she is not capable of contaminating food. From the management standpoint, laboratory monitoring of food handlers may convey the false impression that food safety is being enhanced. Thus, routine laboratory testing of food service personnel should not be performed [65].

The proper approach to managing the personal aspects of hygiene is to establish and pursue a policy of training food service managers and workers. The healthcare facility infection control committee should ensure a program comprising a comprehensive training course in the appropriate languages for all new employees at the onset of employment and in-service training at regular intervals for all food service personnel (see Chapter 4). As appropriate to the workers' level of responsibility, such courses should cover the basic principles of personal hygiene, emphasizing the need for good hand hygiene practices; the importance of informing supervisors of acute intestinal diseases, boils, and any skin infection, particularly on the fingers and hands; properly inspecting, handling, preparing, serving, and storing food; the proper cleaning and safe operation of equipment; general food service sanitation safety; the proper method of waste disposal; portion control; writing modified diets using the diet manual or handbook; diet instruction; and the recording of pertinent dietetic information in each patient's medical record [66]. In addition to training, a liberal medical leave policy will ensure that employees are not penalized financially when they report that they are ill.

SURVEILLANCE AND CONTROL

The responsibility for preventing, detecting, and investigating foodborne disease outbreaks rests with the healthcare facility infection control committee and the infection control professional (see Chapter 2). They can begin by carefully reviewing the results of recent hospital kitchen inspections by the local health department and the food safety training program currently in place for kitchen staff. In addition, they can ensure that, whenever possible, pasteurized eggs are used instead of shell eggs and verify that the risks of using a common blender to mix raw eggs and other foods are well understood by all employees. It is important that the infection control committee meet with the kitchen staff and communicate to them that food safety is of the highest priority.

Surveillance for illness among the kitchen staff may prevent some foodborne outbreaks and also may provide an early warning when such an outbreak occurs because they, too, eat the food. A monitoring procedure should be established to ensure that food service personnel are free from open skin lesions. Designated infection control staff should be informed of acute illnesses among food service workers that could potentially be transmitted by food. It is important to create an atmosphere that does not penalize food handlers for reporting illness. Any work restriction policy should encourage personnel to report their illnesses or exposures and not penalize them with loss of wages, benefits, or job status [67].

Appropriate culture specimens should be obtained and processed during such illnesses. In episodes of acute diarrhea, rectal swab or fecal specimens promptly inoculated onto appropriate laboratory media are recommended. Workers should not be permitted to return to their assigned jobs until their diarrhea has resolved and two stool cultures obtained ≥ 24 hours apart show negative results (see Chapter 33). If antimicrobial agents are used, follow-up cultures should be obtained after treatment has been completed. Personnel with boils, open sores, or cellulitis of the fingers, hands, and face should be excluded until they are adequately treated. The infection control professional's judgment should prevail in deciding when the worker can return to work.

Routine surveillance of patients and employees should detect any episodes of gastrointestinal disease related to the healthcare institution's food service. Temporal clustering of such episodes should alert the infection control personnel to the possibility of an outbreak. Promptly investigating and reporting outbreaks to the appropriate health authorities is essential to identifying and correcting food-handling error(s), preventing additional primary and secondary transmission of disease, and limiting outbreaks caused by commercially distributed foods.

REFERENCES

1. Carter AO, Borczyk AA, Carlson JAK, et al. A severe outbreak of *Escherichia coli* 0157:H7-associated hemorrhagic colitis in a nursing home. *N Engl J Med* 1987;317:1496–1500.
2. Lynch M, Painter J, Woodruff R, et al. Surveillance for foodborne-disease outbreaks—United States, 1998–2002. *MMWR Surveill Summ* 2006;55:1–42.
3. Giannella RA, Brasile L. A hospital foodborne outbreak of diarrhea caused by *Bacillus cereus*: clinical, epidemiologic, and microbiologic studies. *J Infect Dis* 1979;139:366–70.
4. Telzak EE, Budnick LD, Greenberg MSZ, et al. A nosocomial outbreak of *Salmonella enteritidis* infection due to the consumption of raw eggs. *N Engl J Med* 1990;323:394–97.
5. Thomas M, Noah ND. Hospital outbreak of *Clostridium perfringens* food poisoning. *Lancet* 1977;1:1046–48.
6. Yamagishi T, Sakamoto K, Sakurai S, et al. A nosocomial outbreak of food poisoning caused by enterotoxigenic *Clostridium perfringens*. *Microbiol Immunol* 1983;27:291–96.
7. Pavia AT, Nichols CR, Green DP, et al. Hemolytic-uremic syndrome during an outbreak of *Escherichia coli* 0157:H7 infections in institutions for the mentally retarded: Clinical and epidemiologic observations. *J Pediatr* 1990;116:544–51.

8. Standaert SM, Hutcheson RH, Schaffner W. Nosocomial transmission of *Salmonella* gastroenteritis to laundry workers in a nursing home. *Infect Control Hosp Epidemiol* 1994;15:22–26.

9. Holtby I, Stendon P. Food poisoning in two homes for the elderly. *Communicable Dis Rep* 1992;2:R125–26.

10. Khatib R, Naber M, Shellum N, et al. A common source outbreak of gastroenteritis in a teaching hospital. *Infect Control Hosp Epidemiol* 1994;15:534–35.

11. Centers for Disease Control and Prevention. Shigellosis in children's hospital—Pennsylvania. *MMWR* 1979;28:498–99.

12. Centers for Disease Control and Prevention. Hospital-associated outbreak of *Shigella dysenteriae* type 2—Maryland. *MMWR* 1983;32:250–52.

13. Meyers JD, Frederic JR, Tithen WS, Bryan JA. Foodborne hepatitis A in a general hospital: Epidemiologic study of an outbreak attributed to sandwiches. *JAMA* 1975;231:1049–53.

14. Centers for Disease Control and Prevention. Multistate outbreak of salmonellosis caused by precooked roast beef. *MMWR* 1981;30:391–92.

15. Spitalny KC, Okowitz EN, Vogt RL. Salmonellosis outbreaks at a Vermont hospital. *South Med J* 1984;77:168–72.

16. Linnemann CC Jr., Cannon CG, Stancek JL, et al. Prolonged hospital epidemic of salmonellosis: Use of trimethoprim-sulfamethoxazole for control. *Infect Control Hosp Epidemiol* 1985;6:221–25.

17. Yule BF, MacLeod AF, Sharp JCM, Forbes GI. Costing of a hospital-based outbreak of poultry-borne salmonellosis. *Epidemiol Infect* 1988;100:35–42.

18. No author. Food poisoning in hospitals [editorial]. *Lancet* 1980;1:576.

19. Collier PW, Sharp JC, MacLeod AF, et al. Food poisoning in hospitals in Scotland, 1978–1987. *Epidemiol Infect* 1988;101:661–67.

20. Joseph CA, Palmer SR. Outbreaks of *Salmonella* infection in hospitals in England and Wales, 1978–1987. *Br Med J* 1989;298:1161–64.

21. Dalton CB, Gregory J, Kirk MD, et al. Foodborne disease outbreaks in Australia, 1995 to 2000. *Commun Dis Intell* 2004;28:211–24.

22. Bean NH, Griffin PM, Goulding JS, Ivey CB. Foodborne disease outbreaks in the United States, 1973–1987. *J Food Protect* 1990;53:711–30.

23. Lopman BA, Reacher MH, Vipond IB, et al. Clinical manifestation of norovirus gastroenteritis in health care settings. *Clin Infect Dis* 2004;39:318–24. Epub 2004 Jul 9.

24. Levine WC, Smart JF, Archer DL, et al. Foodborne disease outbreaks in nursing homes, 1975 to 1987. *JAMA* 1991;266:2105–09.

25. Stamm WE, Weinstein RA, Dixon RE. Comparison of endemic and epidemic nosocomial infections. *Am J Med* 1981;70:393–97.

26. Tauxe RV. *Salmonella*: A postmodern pathogen. *J Food Protect* 1991;54:563–68.

27. Mishu B, Koehler J, Lee LA, et al. Outbreaks of *Salmonella enteritidis* infections in the United States, 1985–1991. *J Infect Dis* 1994;169:547–52.

28. CDC. Update: *Salmonella enteritidis* infections and shell eggs—United States, 1990. *MMWR* 1990;39:909–12.

29. Lee L, Threatt VL, Puhr ND, et al. Antimicrobial-resistant *Salmonella* spp. isolated from healthy broiler chickens after slaughter. *J Am Vet Med Assoc* 1993;202:752–55.

30. Tauxe RV. Epidemiology of *Campylobacter jejuni* infections in the United States and other industrialized nations. In: Nachamkin T, Blaser MJ, Tompkins LS, eds. Campylobacter jejuni: *Current status and future trends.* Washington, DC: American Society for Microbiology, 1992:9–19.

31. St. Louis ME, Morse DL, Potter ME, et al. The emergence of grade A eggs as a major source of *Salmonella enteritidis* infection. *JAMA* 1988;259:2103–07.

32. Gast RK, Beard CW. Production of *Salmonella enteritidis* contaminated eggs by experimentally infected hens. *Avian Dis* 1990;34:438–46.

33. Jordan MC, Powell KE, Corothers TE, Murray RJ. Salmonellosis among restaurant patrons: The incisive role of a meat slicer. *Am J Public Health* 1973;63:982–85.

34. Schucat A, Swaminathan B, Broome C. Epidemiology of human listeriosis. *Clin Microbiol Rev* 1991;4:169–83.

35. Shooter RA, Cooke EM, Faiers MC, et al. Isolation of *Escherichia coli, Pseudomonas aeruginosa,* and *Klebsiella* from food in hospitals, canteens, and schools. *Lancet* 1971;2:390–92.

36. Remington JS, Schimpff SC. Please don't eat the salads. *N Engl J Med* 1981;304:433–35.

37. Ho JL, Shands KN, Fredland G, et al. An outbreak of type 4b *Listeria monocytogenes* infection involving patients from eight Boston hospitals. *Arch Intern Med* 1986;146:520–24.

38. Ryan CA, Tauxe RV, Hosek GW, et al. *Escherichia coli* 0157:117 diarrhea in a nursing home: Clinical, epidemiological, and pathological findings. *J Infect Dis* 1986;154:631–38.

39. Centers for Disease Control and Prevention. Salmonellosis—Baltimore, Maryland. *MMWR* 1970;19:340.

40. Celum CL, Chaisson RE, Rutherford GW, et al. Incidence of salmonellosis in patients with AIDS. *J Infect Dis* 1987;156:998–1002.

41. Gruenewald R, Blum S, Chan J. Relationship between human immunodeficiency virus infection and salmonellosis in 20- to 59-year-old residents of New York City. *Clin Infect Dis* 1994;18:358–63.

42. Sperber SJ, Schleupner CJ. Salmonellosis during infections with human immunodeficiency virus. *Rev Infect Dis* 1987;9:925–34.

43. Sorvillo FJ, Lieb LE, Waterman SH. Incidence of campylobacteriosis among patients with AIDS in Los Angeles County. *J Acquir Immune Defic Syndr* 1991;4:598–602.

44. Jurado RL, Farley MM, Pereira E, et al. Increased risk of meningitis and bacteremia due to *Listeria monocytogenes* in patients with human immunodeficiency virus infection. *Clin Infect Dis* 1993;17:224–27.

45. Archer DL. Food counseling for persons infected with HIV: Strategy for defensive living. *Public Health Rep* 1989;104:196–98.

46. Griffin PM, Tauxe RV. Food counseling for patients with AIDS [Letter]. *J Infect Dis* 1988;158:668.

47. Angulo FK, Swerdlow DL. Bacterial enteric infections in persons infected with human immunodeficiency virus. *Clin Infect Dis* 1995;21 (suppl 1):S84–93.

48. Thum J, Crossley K, Gerdts A, et al. Enteral hyperalimentation as a source of nosocomial infection. *J Hosp Infect* 1990;15:203–17.

49. Mathus-Vliegen EM, Bredius MW, Binnekade JM. Analysis of sites of bacterial contamination in an enteral feeding system. *J Parenter Enteral Nutr* 2006;30:519–25.

50. Centers for Disease Control and Prevention (CDC). *Enterobacter sakazakii* infections associated with the use of powdered infant formula—Tennessee, 2001. *MMWR Morb Mortal Wkly Rep.* 2002;51:297–300

51. Levy J. Enteral nutrition: An increasingly recognized cause of nosocomial bloodstream infection. *Infect Control Hosp Epidemiol* 1989;10:395–97.

52. Anderson KR, Norris DJ, Godfrey LB, et al. Bacterial contamination of tube feeding formula. *J Parenter Enter Nutr* 1984;8:673–78.

53. Patchell CJ, Anderton A, MacDonald A, et al. Bacterial contamination of enteral feeds. *Arch Dis Child* 1994;70:327–30.

54. Simmons BP, Gelfand MS, Haas M, et al. Enterobacter sakazakii infections in neonates associated with intrinsic contamination of a powdered infant formula. *Infect Control Hosp Epidemiol* 1989;10:398–401.

55. Bowen AB, Braden CR. Invasive *Enterobacter sakazakii* disease in infants. *Emerg Infect Dis* 2006;12:1185–89.

56. U.S. Food and Drug Administration. *Bacterial contamination of enteral formula products.* Washington, DC: Public Health Service, Food and Drug Administration Bulletin, 1988.

57. Anderton A, Aidov KE. The effect of handling procedures on microbial contamination of enteral feeds. *J Hosp Infect* 1988;11:364–72.

58. de Leeuw I, Van Alsenoy L. Bacterial contamination of the feeding bag during catheter jejunostomy: Exogenous or endogenous origin? *J Parenter Enter Nutr* 1984;9:591–92.

59. Joint Commission on Accreditation of Healthcare Organizations. *Accreditation manual for hospitals, 1991.* Chicago: Joint Commission on Accreditation of Healthcare Organizations, 1990.

60. Bryan FL. Prevention of foodborne diseases in food-service establishments. *J Environ Health* 1979;41:198–206.

61. Bryan FL. Factors that contribute to outbreaks of foodborne disease. *J Food Protect* 1978;41:816–27.

62. U.S. Department of Health and Human Services. *Food code, 1993*. Washington, DC: Public Health Service, Food and Drug Administration, 1993.

63. McCall CE, Martin WT, Boring JR. Efficiency of cultures of rectal swabs and faecal specimens in detecting *Salmonella* carriers: Correlation with number of salmonellas excreted. *J Hyg* (London) 1966;64:261–69.

64. Khuri-Bulos NA, Khalaf MA, Shehabi A, Shami K. Foodhandler-associated *Salmonella* outbreak in a university hospital despite routine surveillance cultures of kitchen employees. *Infect Control Hosp Epidemiol* 1994;15:311–14.

65. World Health Organization. *Health surveillance and management procedures for foodhandling personnel*. Geneva, Switzerland: World Health Organization, 1989. (WHO Technical Report Series, no. 785.)

66. Association for Practitioners in Infection Control. *APIC infection control and applied epidemiology: Principles and practice*. St. Louis: Mosby-Year Book, 1996.

67. Bolyard EA, Tablan OC, Williams WW, et al. Guideline for infection control in healthcare personnel, 1998. Hospital Infection Control Practices Advisory Committee. *Infect Control Hosp Epidemiol* 1998;19:407–63.

Clinical Laboratory-Acquired Infections

22

Michael L. Wilson and L. Barth Reller

Clinical laboratories are an area of special concern in hospital infection control. Laboratory workers may be exposed to infectious agents during all steps of collection, transport, processing, and analysis of patients' specimens. The clinical microbiology staff in particular are at risk of occupational infection because the clinical specimens submitted for cultures are likely to contain infectious agents and the process of isolation and culture generates large numbers of pathogenic microorganisms.

The goals of this chapter are to provide an overview of the epidemiology of laboratory-acquired infections, to highlight those infections of special concern to laboratories, and to make specific recommendations for the prevention and control of laboratory-acquired infections. Not discussed in this chapter are the individual problems of clinical virology, research, anatomic pathology, commercial reference laboratories, or laboratories involved in the production or processing of large volumes of pathogenic microorganisms. The reader is referred to Collins' monograph for an extensive review of the subject of laboratory-acquired infections [1]. The roles of the clinical microbiology laboratory in infection surveillance, investigation of endemic and epidemic hospital infections, and the control of healthcare-associated infections are discussed in Chapters 6, 7, and 10, respectively.

INCIDENCE, CAUSATIVE AGENTS, AND COST

The true incidence of laboratory-acquired infections remains unknown. Early data were derived from surveys, personal communications, and literature reports, information that cannot be used to calculate incidence rates [2–5]. More recent data are derived from surveys, which again cannot be used to calculate true incidence rates. One survey [6] did report an annual incidence of three laboratory-acquired infections per 1,000 employees, and another [7] reported annual incidences of 1.4 and 3.5 per 1,000 employees among workers in hospital-based and public health laboratories, respectively. A recent survey from U.K. laboratories during 1994–1995 reported an incidence rate of 16.2 infections per 100,000 person-years, compared with a rate of 82.7 infections per 100,000 person-years during 1988–1989 [8]. Despite the limitations of the published data, it seems reasonable that the annual incidence of laboratory-acquired infections is between 1–5 infections per 1,000 employees. There is some evidence that the annual incidence is declining [2], particularly for hepatitis B virus (HBV) infections [9], owing to HBV immunization and adoption of standard precautions [10].

In years past, the most common laboratory-acquired infections were brucellosis, Q fever, typhoid fever, HBV, or tuberculosis [3,4]. More recent data show that the infections now most commonly acquired in clinical laboratories are HBV, shigellosis, or tuberculosis [6,11]. Other agents continue to pose a hazard to laboratory workers, however, as demonstrated by continuing reports of laboratory-acquired brucellosis [12–17], *Escherichia coli* 0157:H7 [18,19], salmonellosis [20–23], and meningococcemia [24–26].

The cost to healthcare systems for these infections is unknown. In one report [7], each laboratory-acquired infection resulted in an average of 1.2 lost work days for hospital-based laboratories and 1.3 lost work days for public health laboratories. The latter figure, however, does not include the 48 work days lost when one employee was hospitalized for a laboratory-acquired infection.

An accurate estimate of the cost to healthcare systems may not be possible without additional data or further studies, but it is clear that the cost to an infected individual can be high. It has been estimated that 200 to 300 healthcare workers (HCWs) die each year as a consequence of chronic HBV infection [27]. Because the risk to laboratorians of acquiring HBV equals or exceeds that of other HCWs [28,29], it seems reasonable that a substantial proportion of these deaths occur among laboratorians. There also are fatal laboratory-acquired infections caused by other pathogens [21,25]. Laboratory-acquired infection with human immunodeficiency virus (HIV), resulting in acquired immunodeficiency syndrome, has been reported in laboratory workers [30–32] who account for ~25% of reported occupational transmissions.

SOURCES OF INFECTIONS

Pike [2,3] and others [6,7,33,34] have attempted to determine which laboratory procedures, accidents, or other exposures to infectious agents are the source of laboratory-acquired infections (Table 22-1). These data indicate that the source of infection is unknown in ≤20% of episodes and that the infected individual is known only to have worked with the agents in the past in another 21% of episodes [3]. Thus, the exact source, procedure, or breach in technique can be identified in just over 50% of episodes. Among the recognized sources are accidents, which account for 18% of episodes. The types of accidents that lead to laboratory-acquired infections are listed in Table 22-2.

Laboratory accidents associated with exposure to infectious materials include creation of aerosols from spatters or spills; exposure of skin defects (cuts, abrasions, ulcers, dermatitis, etc.), conjunctivas, or mucosal surfaces; accidental aspiration or ingestions; and traumatic implantation [3]. Needle-stick injuries (NSI) and cuts with broken glass and other sharp objects account for up to 50% of accidents associated with laboratory-acquired infections [35,36]. The microbiological hazards associated

TABLE 22-1

SOURCES OF LABORATORY-ACQUIRED INFECTIONS IN THE UNITED STATES AND ABROAD

Proved or Probable Source	Number of Infections	Percentage of Total
Working with agent	827	21.1
Unknown and other	783	20.0
Known accident	703	17.9
Animal or arthropod	659	16.8
Aerosol	522	13.3
Patient's specimen	287	7.3
Human autopsy	75	1.9
Discarded glassware	46	1.2
Intentional infection	19	0.5
Total	3,921	100.00

Adapted from Pike RM. Laboratory-associated infections: summary and analysis of 3,921 cases. *Health Lab Sci* 1976;13:105–114.

with injuries from needle sticks and sharp objects have recently been reviewed [35,36], despite the fact that such behavior is proscribed in all laboratories [37–39].

Aerosol droplets vary in size, with larger droplets rapidly settling onto exposed surfaces. These droplets may carry infectious agents and can thus contaminate environmental surfaces. Smaller droplets remain suspended in the air for a longer period of time and, under the appropriate environmental conditions, can remain suspended indefinitely. Aerosols with droplets measuring <5 mm in diameter can be inhaled directly into alveoli; those measuring ~1 mm are the most likely to be retained within alveoli [40]. Many common laboratory procedures have been shown to produce aerosols in the size range [41–44]. Both *Mycobacterium tuberculosis* and nontuberculous mycobacteria may be transmitted by the aerosol route [45].

TABLE 22-2

KINDS OF LABORATORY ACCIDENT RESULTING IN INFECTION

Known Accident	Number of Infections	Percentage of Total
Spill or spatter	188	26.7
Needle stick	177	25.2
Broken glass injury	112	15.9
Bite or scratch	95	13.5
Mouth pipetting	92	13.1
Other	39	5.5
Total	703	99.9

Adapted from Pike RM. Laboratory-associated infections: summary and analysis of 3,921 cases. *Health Lab Sci* 1976;13:105–114.

Laboratory personnel have among the highest rates of NSI in HCWs [36,46]. Most NSI occur during disposal of used needles, assembly or disassembly of intravenous infusion sets, administration of parenteral injections or infusion therapy, drawing of blood, recapping of needles, or handling of waste that contains needles [36,46–48]. Recapping needles is particularly hazardous, causing 12%–30% of NSI [36,46]. It should be noted, however, that not recapping needles also may be hazardous [49]. The epidemiology of NSI among laboratory personnel has not been studied, but because activities such as intravenous infusion and handling infusion sets are not carried out in laboratories, recapping needles and handling waster are likely to be the most common causes of NSI among laboratory personnel. One-handed recapping before disposal of needles may reduce this risk.

INFECTIOUS AGENTS OF SPECIAL CONCERN IN CLINCAL LABORATORIES

The risk of acquiring infections in a clinical laboratory depends on several factors, the most important of which is the likelihood of exposure to an infectious agent [50]. The probability that such an exposure will result in infection depends on inoculum size, viability of the infectious agent, immune status of the exposed individual, and availability of effective postexposure prophylactic (PEP) therapy.

Human Immunodeficiency Virus (HIV)

Although the prevalence of HIV in laboratory specimens depends on the patient population served by that laboratory, a significant minority of clinical specimens will contain HIV in most healthcare settings. As a result, all clinical laboratory personnel can expect to eventually work with HIV-infected clinical specimens. Transmission of HIV during an occupational exposure occurs as a result of contact with contaminated material with nonintact skin or mucosal surfaces or as a result of traumatic implantation of infectious material. It is estimated that the risk of acquiring HIV infection from a NSI is ~0.3% to 0.5% [50–52]. The frequency of exposures among laboratory personnel has not been reported, but based on the epidemiology of HBV infection among laboratory personnel [29,51], it is likely that these personnel are among those HCWs most commonly exposed to HIV-contaminated specimens. The prevalence of HBV serological markers among clinical laboratory workers who handle blood or serum matches or exceeds that of other HCWs, including nurses and surgeons [53].

Although effective PEP protocols exist, prevention of HIV infection among HCWs depends primarily on prevention of exposure to the virus. Guidelines for preventing HIV exposure in the workplace have been published; they are based on the principle of standard precautions (see Chapter 42). These guidelines also are useful in preventing occupational exposure to other BBPs, particularly HBV. The guidelines are based on a common-sense approach to infection control, and there is evidence that occupational exposures to HIV in patient specimens have been reduced when standard precautions are used [10,54]. Even though the cost of implementing standard precautions is substantial (and may have been significantly underestimated heretofore [55,56]), standard precautions provide the most rational approach to minimizing the risk of acquiring BBPs [54].

Hepatitis B Virus

Despite the availability of safe and effective vaccines and of effective postexposure treatment regimens, HBV infection (see Chapters 4 and 42) remains a common HAI [7,14,28]. Surveys repeatedly have shown that laboratorians are among the most frequently infected HCWs [6,19,28,53], with seropositivity rates between 2–27 times that of the general population [53,56–60]. It is estimated that of the 300,000 new episodes of HBV infection in the United States each year, 1% to 6% (6,000 to 18,000) occur in HCWs [9, 61]. One report estimates that 12% of HBV-infected persons require hospitalization for HBV infections [9].

Because the incidence of HBV infection in a given population of patients may be high and is often underestimated and because compliance with barrier precautions often is inconsistent, the easiest way to prevent occupational HBV infection is by vaccination (see Chapters 4 and 42). The reported decrease in the incidence of laboratory-acquired HBV infection has been attributed to the introduction of HBV vaccine in 1982, since the decrease has occurred despite continued exposures [6,9,29,62,63]. Since 1992, the Occupational Safety and Health Administration has required that all employers have an exposure plan [65]. As part of this plan, employees are categorized as to the likelihood of occupational exposure to blood; those with such exposure are to be provided with HBV vaccination at no cost to the employee [64].

Employers should focus vaccination strategies on those employees most likely to be exposed because vaccinating employees with little or no risk of occupational exposure diverts resources from those employees who are at the highest risk [63]. Similarly, there is no compelling evidence to routinely perform postvaccination testing or provide booster doses; employers should not divert resources for either purpose [63]. Until all HCWs are willing to complete HBV vaccination, HBV is likely to remain a serious infection control issue in healthcare settings. Requiring HBV vaccination as a condition of employment may be the simplest way to ensure compliance.

Most laboratory-acquired HBV infections probably are not acquired via NSI or cuts with infected instruments but via clinically inapparent cutaneous or mucosal exposure to blood or blood products [28,58,60,65,66]. Therefore, rigid adherence to standard precautions should be followed by all laboratory personnel. Percutaneous exposure is not limited to those employees working directly with body fluids. One outbreak of laboratory-acquired HBV infections occurred among clerical employees whose only risk factor was exposure to HBV-contaminated computer requisitions [67]; in another study, the highest prevalence of seropositivity in a laboratory was among persons employed as glassware washers [68].

Hepatitis C Virus

Hepatitis C virus (HCV) (see Chapter 32) is transmitted via the same routes as HBV. Unlike HBV, HCV is not readily transmitted via NSI; estimates of the risk of transmission following NSI are in the range of 0%–10% [51,69–71]. Nonetheless, exposure is to be avoided because ≥50% of HCV-infected persons progress to chronic liver disease and cirrhosis or hepatocellular carcinoma or both will develop in many of them. As with HBV and HIV, HCV infection is highly prevalent in some populations of patients, such as injection drug users [72].

Mycobacterium Tuberculosis

Employees involved in the processing of clinical specimens or cultures from patients with tuberculosis (TB) (see Chapter 33) are at a much greater risk of acquiring TB than is the general population [11,73]. Once thought to be controlled in the United States, TB has reemerged as an important public health problem. Two issues are of particular importance to laboratory employees: the increasing incidence of TB and the development of strains that are resistant to several or all first-line chemotherapeutic agents. All healthcare facilities should have a comprehensive plan for the prevention, control, and treatment of TB [74].

Bacteria and Fungi

Bacterial infections of special concern to laboratory personnel are primarily those caused by highly virulent pathogens, such as *Brucella*, *N. meningitidis*, or *Francisella tularensis* [3,5,12–16,24–26] and the enteric pathogens *Shigella*, *Salmonella*, or *E. coli* O157:H7 [5,17–23,75]. Fungal pathogens of significance to laboratory employees include *Coccidioides immitis*, *Blastomyces*, *dermatitidis*, or *Histoplasma capsulatum* [76]. Recommendations for the safe processing of clinical specimens and cultures suspected of containing these agents are given later herein.

PREVENTION OF LABORATORY–ACQUIRED INFECTIONS

Each clinical laboratory must develop policies and procedures to prevent, document, and treat laboratory-acquired infections. The laboratory director, in conjunction with a designated laboratory safety officer, should take the lead role in developing and implementing these policies and should integrate them into the laboratory procedure manual [1,37–39,75,77]. All employees should receive the appropriate education and training necessary to perform their jobs safely. They should be aware of hazards associated with various infectious agents and exactly what should be done should an exposure take place. Immunization against HBV should be required for all laboratory workers. Initial and follow-up tuberculin skin testing or serologic testing for *M. tuberculosis* antibodies should be given according to current guidelines. Finally, a method for maintaining compliance with these policies and procedures must be implemented along with the appropriate documentation, counseling, and, if necessary, disciplinary action to ensure that employees work safely.

Biosafety Levels

The Centers for Disease Control and Prevention (CDC) and National Institute of Health have published a document defining four biosafety levels based on "the potential hazard of the agent and the laboratory function or activity" [37]. Laboratory design, equipment, and procedures necessary to achieve each biosafety level are detailed in that document. Most common pathogens may be handled under biosafety level 2 conditions. Cultures suspected of containing *Brucella*, *F. tularensis*, *M. tuberculosis*, *C. immitis*, *B. dermatitidis*, or *H. capsulatum* should be processed only under biosafety level 3 conditions. Biosafety level 4 conditions are not needed in general clinical microbiology laboratories.

Standard Precautions

Special policies and procedures are necessary for the safe handling and disposal of certain highly virulent pathogens. Rigorous adherence to standard precautions is sufficient to lessen or eliminate the risk of acquiring an infection from most patients' specimens processed in clinical laboratories. Implementation of standard precautions will be successful only if laboratory administrators and workers integrate standard precautions into routine laboratory operations and make every reasonable attempt to maintain and enforce such policies. Standard precautions have been shown to decrease the number of occupational exposures to blood and other body fluids among one group of HCWs [10,53]. The CDC recommendations for standard precautions for all HCWs and clinical laboratories are given in Tables 22-3 and 22-4, respectively.

Standard Microbiological Practices

When used in conjunction with standard precautions, the following practices should be effective in preventing

TABLE 22-3

STANDARD PRECAUTIONS FOR PREVENTION OF TRANSMISSION OF HIV, HBV, AND OTHER BLOODBORNE PATHOGENS IN HEALTHCARE SETTINGS

1. All healthcare workers should routinely use appropriate barrier precautions to prevent skin and mucous membrane exposure when contact with blood or other body fluids of any patient is anticipated. Gloves should be worn for touching blood and body fluids, mucous membranes, or non-intact skin of all patients; for handling items or surfaces soiled with blood or body fluids; and for performing venipuncture and other vascular access procedures. Gloves should be changed after contact with each patient. Masks and protective eyewear or face shields should be worn during procedures that are likely to generate droplets of blood or other body fluids to prevent exposure of mucous membranes of the mouth, nose, and eyes. Gowns or aprons should be worn during procedures that are likely to generate splashes of blood or other body fluids.
2. Hands and other skin surfaces should be washed immediately and thoroughly if contaminated with blood or other body fluids. Hands should be washed immediately after gloves are removed.
3. All healthcare workers should take precautions to prevent injuries caused by needles, scalpels, and other sharp instruments or devices during procedures; when cleaning used instruments; during disposal of used needles; and when handling sharp instruments after procedures. To prevent needle stick injuries, needles should not be recapped, purposely bent or broken by hand, removed from disposable syringes, or otherwise manipulated by hand. After they are used, disposable syringes and needles, scalpel blades, and other sharp items should be placed in puncture-resistant containers for disposal; the puncture-resistant containers should be located as close as practical to the use area. Large-bore reusable needles should be placed in a puncture-resistant container for transport of the reprocessing area.
4. Although saliva has not been implicated in HIV transmission, to minimize the need for emergency mouth-to-mouth resuscitation, mouthpieces, resuscitation bags, or other ventilation devices should be available for use in areas in which the need for resuscitation is predictable.
5. Healthcare workers who have exudative lesions or weeping dermatitis should refrain from all direct care of patients and from handling equipment used in the care of patients until the condition resolves.
6. Pregnant healthcare workers are not known to be at greater risk of contracting HIV infection than healthcare workers who are not pregnant; however, if a healthcare worker develops HIV infection during pregnancy, the infant is at risk of infection resulting from perinatal transmission. Because of this risk, pregnant healthcare workers should be especially familiar with and strictly adhere to precautions to minimize the risk of HIV transmission.

TABLE 22-4

STANDARD PRECAUTIONS FOR WORKERS IN DIAGNOSTIC PATHOLOGY LABORATORIES

1. All specimens of blood and body fluids should be put in a well-constructed container with a secure lid to prevent leaking during transport. Care should be taken when collecting each specimen to avoid contaminating the outside of the container and of the laboratory form accompanying the specimen.
2. All persons processing blood and body-fluid specimens (e.g., removing tops from vacuum tubes) should wear gloves. Masks and protective eyewear should be worn if mucous membrane contact with blood or body fluid is anticipated. Gloves should be changed and hands washed after completion of specimen processing.
3. For routine procedures, such as histologic and pathologic studies or microbiologic culturing, a biological safety cabinet is not necessary. However, biological safety cabinets (class I or II) should be used when conducting procedures that have a high potential for generating droplets, including activities such as blending, sonicating, and vigorous mixing.
4. Mechanical pipetting devices should be used for manipulating all liquids in the laboratory. Mouth pipetting must not be done.
5. Use of needles and syringes should be limited to situations in which there is no alternative, and the recommendations for preventing injuries with needles outlined under standard precautions in healthcare settings (Table 22-3) should be followed.
6. Laboratory work surfaces should be decontaminated with an appropriate chemical germicide after a spill of blood or other body fluids and when work activities are completed.
7. Contaminated materials used in laboratory tests should be decontaminated before reprocessing or be placed in bags and disposed of in accordance with institutional policies for disposal of infective waste.
8. Scientific equipment that has been contaminated with blood or other body fluids should be decontaminated and cleaned before being repaired in the laboratory or transported to the manufacturer.
9. All persons should wash their hands after completing laboratory activities and should remove protective clothing before leaving the laboratory.

most laboratory-acquired infections. These or equivalent procedures should be routine practice in all clinical laboratories [38,39,78–84].

Laboratory Access

Only trained personnel should be allowed in a laboratory under ordinary circumstances. Maintenance personnel, delivery persons, and other visitors with legitimate reason for being in the laboratory should either be escorted or be closely supervised to prevent unnecessary exposure to infectious agents. Laboratory trainees, house staff, and students also should be supervised closely. Children should not be allowed in laboratories.

Personnel Policies

All HCWs should have training commensurate with the level of expertise needed to safely perform all necessary procedures. Suggested topics for such training are given in Table 22-5 [39]. All HCWs should receive the necessary continuing education and training to ensure job safety. Employee job appraisals should document lapses in safety, techniques, or other behaviors that could result in occupational exposure to infectious agents. Persons exhibiting such behavior should be counseled and/or retrained.

Laboratory Facility

Laboratories should be designed to minimize traffic and unnecessary access to work areas. Laboratory furniture should be sturdy and easy to clean, and laboratories themselves should be uncluttered and easy to clean. Foot-, knee-, or elbow-operated hand-washing sinks or waterless agents for hand hygiene should be available and located near laboratory exits. The laboratory facility should be designed and constructed to meet criteria recommended for the appropriate biosafety level [37].

TABLE 22-5

A 10-STEP PROGRAM FOR TRAINING LABORATORY WORKERS IN BIOHAZARD SAFETY

1. Using standard precautions for handling blood and body fluids
2. Using aseptic technique and procedures
3. Following personal hygiene and wearing protective equipment
4. Establishing criteria for biosafety levels 1–4
5. Effectively using biological safety cabinets classes I–III
6. Safely using centrifuges and autoclaves
7. Decontaminating, disinfecting, and sterilizing
8. Handling, packaging, and disposing of biohazardous waste
9. Packaging, transporting, and shipping biohazardous waste
10. Reporting incidents and accidents

Hygiene for Workers

Eating, drinking, smoking, and applying cosmetics should be strictly prohibited within the laboratory [37]. All HCWs should wear and button full-length white laboratory coats while in the laboratory. HCWs and visitors should perform hand hygiene before leaving the laboratory. Food and other personal items should not be stored in refrigerators or freezers used to store clinical specimens or cultures. Refrigerators, freezers, and microwave ovens used to store or prepare food must be located outside the laboratory.

Clinical Specimens

Specimens must be labeled with the patient's full name, hospital identification number, and date drawn. Specimens received in damaged, leaking, or contaminated containers should not be processed; the person who collected the specimen should be notified and the specimens recollected.

Microbiological Techniques

Mouth pipetting should be strictly prohibited; mechanical pipetting devices should be used for all pipetting. All procedures should be performed in a way to minimize or prevent aerosols. Procedures that generate aerosols should be performed in a biological safety cabinet. Cylindrical electric burners are preferable to flame burners for sterilizing inoculating loops or needles and the tips of other small instruments. If flame burners are used, care should be taken to avoid spattering. This can be achieved by slowly drawing loops or needles through the flame with the loop entering the flame last. Cool inoculating loops and needles should be used when touching plates, colonies, or broth cultures. Work surfaces should be decontaminated at least once a day with an acceptable germicide. Work surfaces also should be decontaminated after spills (discussed later). Infectious wastes and patients' specimens should be disinfected before disposal (see later herein). Needles, blades, and other sharp items should be disposed of in rigid, tamper-resistant, puncture-proof, marked containers. Materials removed from the laboratory should be free of infectious hazard. Clinical specimens, cultures, or other potentially infectious materials should be packaged, labeled, and shipped according to federal regulations [39,85].

Safety Procedure Manual

Every laboratory should have an up-to-date safety manual that includes the following information:

1. A designated laboratory safety officer and explicit instructions on how to contact that individual in the event of an accident or exposure. This officer should lead the educational program for biohazard safety (Table 22-5).
2. Synopsis of safety components of good laboratory practice and hospital policies for infection control, including standard precautions.

3. A program for the prevention of transmission of *M. tuberculosis* to laboratory workers, developed in accordance with current recommendations.
4. Location of necessary emergency equipment and spill cleanup kits.
5. Detailed procedures for cleanup of spills.
6. Instructions for the effective use of biological safety cabinets.
7. Procedures for safe use of centrifuges and autoclaves.
8. Vaccination policies.
9. Procedures for PEP or treatment and counseling.

SAFETY IN HANDLING ACCIDENTS, USING EQUIPMENT, AND DISPOSING OF WASTES

Procedures for Spills and Accidents

Because of the potential for high concentration of microorganisms in patients' specimens and cultures in clinical laboratories, special procedures must be used to disinfect spills and other laboratory accidents [39,84]. The current CDC recommendation is to use "chemical germicides that are approved for use as 'hospital germicides' and are tuberculocidal when used at recommended dilutions" [50,63]. This recommendation applies to all types of spills or other laboratory accidents.

Written procedures should be in the laboratory safety manual. Employees should be trained to safely decontaminate and clean up spills involving those microorganisms cultured or studied in their laboratory. All necessary disinfectants and cleaning supplies must be readily available in the laboratory. Because spills may occur at any stage of transport, plating, processing, or storage of microbiological cultures, specific protocols should be available for spills occurring at each stage and for spills involving commonplace moderate-risk microorganisms and those of higher risk, such as *M. tuberculosis*.

The hazard associated with a spill depends on the nature of the spilled agent, the volume of material spilled, the concentration of the agent within the material, and where the spill takes place. Spills involving microorganisms such as *M. tuberculosis*, *F. tularensis*, *Brucella* spp, *C. immitis*, or *H. capsulatum* may pose a major hazard to laboratory workers. Spills of large volumes of moderate-risk microorganisms or those occurring in such a manner that aerosols might be generated also should be treated as a major hazard to laboratory workers.

Procedures Used for Routine Spills of Small Volumes of Moderate-Risk Microorganisms
1. The affected area should immediately be flooded with a suitable disinfectant and covered with paper towels.
2. Other workers should be warned to avoid the contaminated area.

3. Personnel should wear gloves and use an autoclavable dustpan and squeegee or forceps to pick up solid materials.
4. Any remaining fluids or other materials should be wiped up with paper towels.
5. Contaminated materials should be disposed of as infectious waste.
6. Unless the laboratory worker is injured or otherwise exposed during the spill or cleanup, no other specific action need be taken.

Procedures for Spills of Large Volumes of Moderate-Risk Agents or Highly Pathogenic Agents Outside a Biological Safety Cabinet
1. Employees should hold their breath, immediately evacuate the room, and close the door.
2. Employees should assist others as needed to protect them from potential exposure.
3. Other personnel should be warned to avoid the contaminated area. Personnel in adjacent areas should be warned of any potential hazard to their safety.
4. Contaminated clothing and protective equipment should be removed and discarded as biohazardous waste.
5. Employees should thoroughly wash exposed skin surfaces.
6. The laboratory safety officer and director should be immediately notified.
7. Biological safety cabinets should be left running to help decrease the concentration of aerosols in the contaminated room.
8. If the spill occurs in a room under negative pressure, >30 minutes should pass before personnel re-enter the affected room.
9. If the spill occurs in a room not under negative pressure, the cleanup should begin immediately.
10. Protective clothing, including a cap, mask, long-sleeved gown, shoe covers, and gloves, should be worn.
11. Because a disinfectant poured directly on the spills may generate aerosols, an appropriate disinfectant should be allowed to run into the spill from the sides.
12. The area should be covered with paper towels and allowed to stand for 20 minutes.
13. An autoclave dustpan and squeegee or forceps should be used to clean up pieces of broken glass and other sharp objects.
14. Remaining liquids should be wiped up with paper towels.
15. All materials, including protective clothing, should be discarded as biohazardous waste.

Procedures for Spills in Biological Safety Cabinets
1. Biological safety cabinets (BSCs) should be allowed to operate to minimize further risk to laboratory workers.

2. Cleanup should begin immediately.

3. Gloves, mask, and a gown should be worn during the cleanup.

4. Work surfaces and any catch pans or basins should be flooded with an adequate volume of disinfectant.

5. The flooded area should be allowed to stand for 20 minutes.

6. During this time, the BSC walls, work surfaces, and any equipment within the BSC should be cleaned with a germicidal disinfectant (e.g., phenolic or iodophor compounds). Flammable organic solvents, such as alcohols, should not be used because these compounds may reach dangerous concentrations within certain BSCs.

7. All contaminated materials and fluids should be disposed of as biohazardous waste.

8. Catch pans and basins should be cleaned per the manufacturer's recommendations.

9. High-efficiency particulate air (HEPA) filters and other components of the BSC should not be cleaned or disinfected by laboratory personnel. This is not necessary with most spills and should be done only by factory-trained and certified personnel. Major spills or those involving high-risk agents may necessitate formaldehyde decontamination of the BSC. Such decontamination should be performed only by qualified personnel.

LABORATORY EQUIPMENT

Laboratory safety and diagnostic equipment must be of the proper type and should be tested and maintained according to the manufacturer's recommendations. Equally important is its proper use by laboratory personnel. All personnel should be instructed on the proper use, care, and maintenance of laboratory equipment.

Biological Safety Cabinets

Biological safety cabinets are essential for the safe handling of infectious agents. Different BSCs are available; which one to use depends primarily upon the infectious agents to be handled [86]. Class I BSCs (Figure 22-1) have an open front into which room air flows. All of the exhaust air is discharged through HEPA filters to the outside environment. Although Class I BSCs protect the user from exposure to agents within the cabinet, they do not protect materials within the cabinet against contamination; Class I BSCs are unsuitable for use in clinical microbiology laboratories [39].

Class II BSCs (Figure 22-2) also have an open front into which room air flows. These BSCs differ from Class I BSCs in that a portion of the exhausted air passing through HEPA filters is recirculated into the cabinet. Then

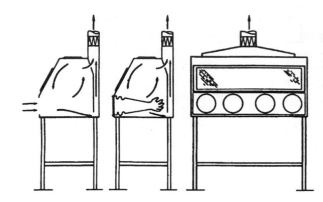

Figure 22-1 Design of class I biological safety cabinet

the filtered air is used to protect clinical specimens or cultures from contamination. Two basic types of Class II BSCs are available. Class II type A BSCs are the most commonly used in clinical laboratories and are sufficient for meeting biosafety level 2 or 3 criteria. Class II type B BSCs also may be used for this purpose but usually are more expensive to purchase and to operate [39,86]. Class III (Figure 22-3) BSCs provide the greatest protection to laboratory personnel, but their use usually is restricted to working with highly virulent pathogens in biosafety level 4 laboratories.

Laboratory workers must remember that BSCs are not chemical fume hoods. Toxic, noxious, or flammable chemicals must not be used in these hoods because the recirculation of exhaust air may allow these chemicals to reach dangerously high levels in the cabinet. BSCs should be installed, tested, and maintained only by qualified personnel. Regular testing and certification of BSCs is essential to ensure the safety of users. Laboratory personnel should be instructed in the proper use of BSCs and should be aware of their limitations in controlling aerosols. Personnel working in BSCs can adversely affect the ability of cabinets to contain infectious aerosols [82]. Users should consult the manufacturer on the potential effect of this and other factors (e.g., use of equipment within BSCs) before using a BSC. Finally, personnel should be aware that cabinet function depends on proper airflow patterns and that change in airflow patterns because of alterations in air supplies, temporary shutdowns for repairs, and so on, may adversely affect the functioning of BSCs.

Centrifuges

Centrifuges used to process clinical specimens or cultures should be equipped with sealable, autoclavable, breakage-resistant cups to prevent contamination of the centrifuge and the release of aerosols should centrifuge tubes break during processing. These cups must be removable from the centrifuge rotor so that they can be cleaned and autoclaved.

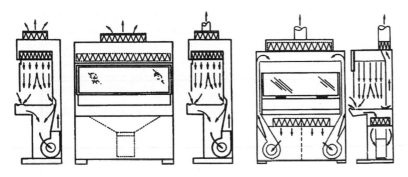

Figure 22-2 Design of class II biological safety cabinets types A and B

Autoclaves

An autoclave should be readily accessible to clinical laboratories. Routine maintenance, testing, and cleaning are essential. Autoclaves should be tested for their ability to kill standard bacterial spores [39]. It should be emphasized that autoclave tape indicates that an object has been autoclaved but not necessarily sterilized [83,84].

Laboratory and Protective Equipment

Other laboratory equipment should be of a type and design that allows for easy cleaning and disinfection. Safety equipment for the cleanup and disinfection of laboratory spills should be readily available. Proper gloves, gowns, masks, and shoe covers should be handy.

Both latex and vinyl disposable gloves have been shown to vary widely in their permeability [78,80]. It has been found that washing and reusing gloves is inadvisable and that the proportion of hands contaminated with test microorganisms after gloves are removed varies from 5% 50% [79]. Therefore, HCWs should wash their hands/perform hand hygiene after removing gloves. The issue of wearing two pairs of gloves ("double-gloving") is more contentious. Although it is logical to assume that two barriers offer more protection than one, concerns about loss of tactile sensation and dexterity have led to recommendations against double-gloving during routine laboratory procedures [80]. Wearing two pairs of gloves for autopsies and in other situations where large amounts of blood are present has been recommended [38].

Disposal of Infectious Materials

Materials contaminated with infectious agents must be disposed of properly to protect HCWs and the general public [39,83]. Safe disposal of infectious materials begins at the source where these materials are generated. The following procedures are recommended for the safe disposal of infectious materials and waste [39,83].

1. Adequate waste bins and containers for disposal of sharp objects must be readily available.
2. Waste bins should be lined with two autoclavable bags.
3. All containers should be clearly marked.
4. Laboratory and maintenance personnel should avoid physical contact with these materials; leaking containers should be treated as spills.
5. Infectious materials should be transported in or on carts that can be easily cleaned and disinfected.
6. Infectious materials should be autoclaved before disposal; double-bagging and overfilling should be avoided because these practices limit the effectiveness of autoclaving as a means of sterilization.
7. Regular monitoring of the adequacy of autoclave sterilization should be part of routine laboratory quality control procedures.

PREVENTION, POSTEXPOSURE TREATMENT, AND FOLLOW-UP

Vaccination

Laboratory workers may or may not have contact with patients, but they should still follow recommendations regarding vaccinations for all HCWs. All HCWs should be vaccinated against HBV. If possible, such vaccination should be given during the training years because the risk of occupational exposure to HBV appears to be greatest

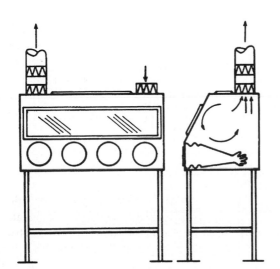

Figure 22-3 Design of class III biological safety cabinet

during that period. In addition, before employment, all HCWs should provide evidence of immunity to rubella. Persons lacking protective antibody to rubella virus should be vaccinated. Influenza, measles, mumps, and polio vaccines and tetanus-diphtheria toxoid immunization should comply with current guidelines from the Advisory Committee on Immunization Practices of the U.S. Public Health Service (see Chapter 4).

Postexposure Treatment and Prophylaxis

Specific treatment, prophylaxis, and counseling should be available for all HCWs after exposure to infectious agents. Of special importance to clinical laboratory workers are recommendations for prophylaxis or treatment of exposures to specimens taken from patients who are infected with HBV, HCV, or HIV. HCWs working in the mycobacteriology laboratories and those involved in the processing or disposal of materials likely to be contaminated with mycobacteria should receive pre-employment screening for *M. tuberculosis* and appropriate testing following a suspected exposure. The reader is referred to Chapter 4 for additional information.

Postexposure Investigation

Laboratory exposure of a HCW to a pathogen should prompt an immediate investigation into the reason(s) for the exposure. The investigation should include a review of relevant microbiologic practices, laboratory policies and procedures, and equipment and facilities. For example, when an HCW who works with mycobacteria has a tuberculin skin test conversion or develops active pulmonary TB, the BSC and air-handling systems should be checked, serviced, and balanced by qualified personnel. If the investigation does not provide a satisfactory explanation for the source of the exposure, it may be necessary to broaden the investigation. Using the same example, an HCW who works with mycobacteria but has other responsibilities outside the laboratory (e.g., phlebotomy) could conceivably have been exposed to a patient with active TB. If no source of exposure is found, the investigation should be expanded as appropriate to include potential sources of exposure outside the healthcare facility (e.g., family members).

CONCLUSIONS

Although the incidence of laboratory-acquired infections appears to be declining, infections still occur at a low rate and are associated with significant morbidity and mortality. Infections caused by HBV or HIV are of particular concern. Laboratory personnel should make every attempt to follow recommended guidelines, policies, and procedures designed to minimize the risk of working with infectious materials. Each laboratory must be designed and constructed to minimize accidents and facilitate cleanups. It must contain proper and well-maintained safety and diagnostic equipment. Most important, however, is the proper training and supervision of laboratory personnel and adherence to policies and procedures designed to provide a safe working environment. It is the obligation of laboratory directors and administrators to provide such an environment.

REFERENCES

1. Collins CH, Kennedy DA. *Laboratory-acquired infections.* 4th ed. London: Butterworth Heinemann, 1999.
2. Pike RM. Laboratory-associated infections: incidence, fatalities, causes, and prevention. *Annu Rev Microbiol* 1979;33:41–66.
3. Pike RM. Laboratory-associated infections: summary and analysis of 3,921 cases. *Health Lab Sci* 1976;13:105–114.
4. Sewell DL. Laboratory associated infections and biosafety. *Clin Microbiol Rev* 1995;8:389–405.
5. Harrington JM. Health and safety in medical laboratories. *Bull WHO* 1982;60:9–16.
6. Jacobson JT, Orlob RB, Clayton JL. Infections acquired in clinical laboratories in Utah. *J Clin Microbiol* 1985;21:486–489.
7. Vesley D, Hartmann HM. Laboratory-acquired infections and injuries in clinical laboratories: a 1986 survey. *Am J Public Health* 1988;78:1212–1215.
8. Walker D, Campbell D. A survey of infections in United Kingdom laboratories, 1994–1995. *J Clin Pathol* 1999;52:415–418.
9. Alter MH, Hadler SC, Margolis HS, et al. The changing epidemiology of hepatitis B in the United States: need for alternative vaccination strategies. *JAMA* 1990;263:1218–1222.
10. Fahey BJ, Koziol DE, Banks SM, et al. Frequency of nonparenteral occupational exposures to blood and body fluids before and after universal precautions training. *Am J Med* 1991;90:145–153.
11. Grist NR. Infections in British clinical laboratories 1980-1. *J Clin Pathol* 1983;36:121–126.
12. Yagupsky P, Peled N, Riesenberg K, Banai M. Exposure of hospital personnel to Brucella melitensis and occurrence of laboratory-acquired disease in an endemic area. *Scand J Infect Dis* 2000;32:31–35.
13. Noviello S, Gallo R, Kelly M, et al. Laboratory-acquired brucellosis. *Emerg Infect Dis* 2004;10:1848–1850.
14. Robichaud S, Libman M, Behr M, Rubin E. Prevention of laboratory-acquired brucellosis. *Clin Infect Dis* 2004;38: e119–e122.
15. Bouza E, Sanchez-Carrillo C, Haernangomez S, Gonzalez MJ; The Spanish Co-operative Group for the study of laboratory-acquired brucellosis. *J Hosp Infect* 2005;61:80–83.
16. Yagupsky P, Baron EJ. Laboratory exposures to brucellae and implications for bioterrorism. *Emerg Infect Dis* 2005;11:1180–1185.
17. Grist NR, Emslie JAN. Association of Clinical Pathologists surveys of infections in British clinical laboratories, 1970–1989. *J Clin Pathol* 1994;47:391–394.
18. Coia JE. Nosocomial and laboratory-acquired infection with *Escherichia coli* O157. *J Hosp Infect* 1998;40:107–113.
19. Spina N, Zansky S, Dumas N, Kondracki S. Four laboratory-associated cases of infection with *Escherichia coli* O157:H7. *J Clin Microbiol* 2005;43:2938–2939.
20. Blaser MJ, Hickman FW, Farmer JJ III, et al. *Salmonella typhi*: the laboratory as a reservoir of infection. *J Infect Dis* 1980;142:934–938.
21. Blaser MJ, Lofgren JO. Fatal salmonellosis originating in a clinical microbiology laboratory. *J Clin Microbiol* 1981;13:855–858.
22. Holmes MB, Johnson DL, Fiumara NJ, et al. Acquisition of typhoid fever from proficiency-testing specimens. *N Engl J Med* 1980;303:519–521.
23. Steckelberg JM, Terrell CL, Edson RS. Laboratory-acquired *Salmonella typhimurium* enteritis: association with erythema nodosum and reactive arthritis. *Am J Med* 1988;85:705–707.
24. Boutet R, Stuart JM, Kaczmarski EB, et al. Risk of laboratory-acquired meningococcal disease. *J Hosp Infect* 2001;49:282–284.
25. Centers for Disease Control and Prevention. Laboratory-acquired meningococcal disease—United States, 2000. *MMWR* 2002;51:141–144.

26. Sejvar JJ, Johnson D, Popovic T, et al. Assessing the risk of laboratory-acquired meningococcal disease. *J Clin Microbiol* 2005;43:4811–4814.
27. Williams WW, Preblud SR, Reichefderfer PS, et al. Vaccines of importance in the hospital setting: problems and development. *Infect Dis Clin North Am* 1989;3:701–722.
28. Leers W-D, Kouroupis GM. Prevalence of hepatitis B antibodies in hospital personnel. *Can Med Assoc J* 1975;113:844–847.
29. Pattison CP, Maynard JE, Berquist KR, et al. Epidemiology of hepatitis B in hospital personnel. *Am J Epidemiol* 1975;101:59–64.
30. Centers for Disease Control and Prevention. Guidelines for prevention of transmission of human immunodeficiency virus and hepatitis B virus to health-care and public-safety workers. *MMWR* 1989;38 (no. S-6):1–37.
31. Centers for Disease Control and Prevention. Surveillance for occupationally acquired HIV—United States, 1981–1992. *MMWR* 1992;41:823–825.
32. Marcus R, Centers for Disease Control Cooperative Needlestick Surveillance Group. Surveillance of healthcare workers exposed to blood from patients infected with human immunodeficiency virus. *N Engl J Med* 1988;319:1118–1122.
33. Evans MR, Henderson DK, Bennett JE. Potential for laboratory exposures to biohazardous agents found in blood. *Am J Public Health* 1990;80:423–427.
34. Miller CD, Songer JR, Sullivan JF. A twenty-five-year review of laboratory-acquired human infections at the National Animal Disease Center. *Am Ind Hyg Assoc J* 1987;48:271–275.
35. Collins CH, Kennedy DA. Microbiological hazards of occupational needlestick and "sharps" injuries. *J Appl Bacteriol* 1987,62:385–402.
36. McCormick RD, Maki DG. Epidemiology of needle-stick injuries in hospital personnel. *Am J Med* 1981;70:928–932.
37. Centers for Disease Control and Prevention, National Institutes of Health. *Biosafety in microbiological and biomedical laboratories.* 3rd ed. Atlanta: U.S. Department of Health and Human Services, Public Health Services, Centers for Disease Control; Bethesda: National Institutes of Health, 1993.
38. Clinical Laboratory Standards Institue. *Protection of laboratory workers from occupationally acquired infections; approved guideline.* 3rd ed. Villanova, PA.: CLSI, 2005.
39. U.S. National Research Council, Committee on Hazardous Biological Substances in the Laboratory. *Biosafety in the Laboratory: prudent practices for the handling and disposal of infectious materials.* Washington, DC: National Academy of Sciences, 1989.
40. Brown, JH, Cook KM, New FG, et al. Influence of particle size upon the retention of particulate matter in the human lung. *Am J Public Health* 1950;40:450–458.
41. Kenny MT, Sabel FL. Particle size distribution of *Serratia marcescens* aerosols created during common laboratory procedures and simulated laboratory accidents. *Appl Microbiol* 1968;16:1146–1155.
42. Stern EL, Johnson JW, Vesley D, et al. Aerosol production associated with clinical laboratory procedures. *Am J Clin Pathol* 1974;62:591–600.
43. Tomlinson AJH. Infected air-borne particles liberated on opening screwcapped bottles. *Br Med J* 1957;1:15–17.
44. Wedum AG. Laboratory safety in research with infectious aerosols. *Public Health Rep* 1964;79:619–633.
45. Loudon RG, Bumgarner R, Lacy J, et al. Aerial transmission of mycobacteria. *Am Rev Respir Dis* 1969;100:165–171.
46. Jagger J, Hunt EH, Brand Elnaggar J, et al. Rates of needle-stick injury caused by various devices in a university hospital. *N Engl J Med* 1988;319:284–288.
47. Weltman AC, Short LJ, Mendelson MH, et al. Disposal-related sharps injuries at a New York City teaching hospital. *Infect Control Hosp Epidemiol* 1995;16:268–274.
48. Anglim AM, Collmer JE, Loving TJ, et al. An outbreak of needlestick injuries in hospital employees due to needles piercing infectious waste containers. *Infect Control Hosp Epidemiol* 1995;16:570–576.
49. Jagger J, Hunt EH, Pearson RD. Recapping used needles: is it worse than the alternative? *J Infect Dis* 1990;162:784–785.
50. Henderson DK, Fahey BJ, Willy M, et al. Risk for occupational transmission of human immunodeficiency virus type 1 (HIV-1) associated with clinical exposures: a prospective evaluation. *Ann Intern Med* 1990;113:740–746.

51. Gerberding JL. Incidence and prevalence of human immunodeficiency virus, hepatitis B virus, hepatitis C virus, and cytomegalovirus among healthcare personnel at risk for blood exposure: final report from a longitudinal study. *J Infect Dis* 1994;170:1410–1417.
52. Mangione CM, Gerberding JL, Cummings SR. Occupational exposure to HIV: frequency and rates of underreporting of percutaneous and mucocutaneous exposures by medical housestaff. *Am J Med* 1991;90:85–90.
53. West DJ. The risk of hepatitis B infection among health professionals in the United States: a review. *Am J Med Sci* 1984;287:26–33.
54. Wong ES, Stotka JL, Chinchilli VM, et al. Are universal precautions effective in reducing the number of occupational exposures among healthcare workers? a prospective study of physicians on a medical service. *JAMA* 1991;265:1123–1128.
55. Bachner P. The epidemiology of fear: scientific, social, and political responses to the occupational risk of blood-borne infection. *Arch Pathol Lab Med* 1990;114:319–323.
56. Doebbeling BN, Wenzel RP. The direct costs of universal precautions in a teaching hospital. *JAMA* 1990;264:2083–2087.
57. Skinhøj P, Søeby M. Viral hepatitis in Danish healthcare personnel, 1974–8. *J Clin Pathol* 1981;34:408–411.
58. Hirschowitz BI, Dasher CA, Whitt FJ, et al. Hepatitis B antigen and antibody and test of liver function: a prospective study of 310 laboratory workers. *Am J Clin Pathol* 1980;73:63–68.
59. Levy BS, Harris JC, Smith JL, et al. Hepatitis B in ward and clinical laboratory employees of a general hospital. *Am J Epidemiol* 1977;106:330–335.
60. Osterholm M, Andrews JS. Viral hepatitis in hospital personnel in Minnesota: report of a statewide survey. *Minn Med* 1979;62:683–689.
61. Pantelick EL, Steere AC, Lewis HD, et al. Hepatitis B infection in hospital personnel during an eight-year period: policies for screening and pregnancy in high risk areas. *Am J Med* 1981;70:924–927.
62. Kane MA, Alter MJ, Hadler SC, et al. Hepatitis B infection in the United States: recent trends and future strategies for control. *Am J Med* 1989;87 (suppl 3A):11S–13S.
63. Lanphear BP, Linnemann CC, Cannon CG, et al. Decline of clinical hepatitis B in workers at a general hospital: relation to increasing vaccine-induced immunity. *Clin Infect Dis* 1993;16:10–14.
64. Agerton TB, Mahoney FJ, Polish LB, et al. Impact of the bloodborne pathogens standard on vaccination of healthcare workers with hepatitis B vaccine. *Infect Control Hosp Epidemiol* 1995;16:287–291.
65. U.S. Department of Labor, Occupational Safety and Health Administration. Occupational exposure to bloodborne pathogens: final rule. *Federal Register*, 1991;56:64175–64182.
66. Lauer JL, VanDrunen Na, Washburn, JW, et al. Transmission of hepatitis B virus in clinical laboratory areas. *J Infect Dis* 1979;140:513–516.
67. Pattison CP, Boyer KM, Maynard JE, et al. Epidemic hepatitis in a clinical laboratory: possible association with computer card handling. *JAMA* 1974;230:854–857.
68. Anderson RA, Woodfield DG. Hepatitis B virus infections in laboratory staff. *N Z Med J* 1982;95:69–71.
69. Kiyosawa K, Sodeyama T, Tanaka E, et al. Hepatitis C in hospital employees with needlestick injuries. *Ann Intern Med* 1991;115:367–369.
70. Puro V, Petrosillo N, Ippolito G, et al. Occupational hepatitis C virus infection in Italian healthcare workers. *Am J Public Health* 1995;85:1272–1275.
71. Suzuki K, Mizokami M, Lau JYN, et al. Confirmation of hepatitis C virus transmission through needlestick accidents by molecular evolutionary analysis. *J Infect Dis* 1994;170:1575–1578.
72. Kelen GD, Green GB, Purcell RH, et al. Hepatitis B and hepatitis C in emergency department patients. *N Engl J Med* 1992;326:1399–1404.
73. Reid DD. Incidence of tuberculosis among workers in medical laboratories. *Br Med J* 1957;2:10–14.
74. Centers for Disease Control and Prevention. Essential components of a tuberculosis prevention and control program: screening for tuberculosis and tuberculosis infection in high-risk populations:

recommendations of the Advisory Council for the Elimination of Tuberculosis. *MMWR* 1995;44(no. RR-11):1–34.

75. Harrington JM, Shannon HS. Survey of safety and healthcare in British medical laboratories. *Br Med J* 1977;1:626–628.

76. Standard PL, Kaufman L. Safety considerations in handling exoantigen extracts from pathogenic fungi. *J Clin Microbiol* 1982;15:663–667.

77. Centers for Disease Control and Prevention. Public health burden of vaccine-preventable diseases among adults: standards from adult immunization practice. *MMWR* 1990;39:725–729.

78. DeGroot-Kosolcharoen J, Jones JM. Permeability of latex and vinyl gloves to water and blood. *Am J Infect Control* 1989;17:196–201.

79. Doebbeling BN, Pfaller MA, Houston AK, et al. Removal of nosocomial pathogens from the contaminated glove: implications for glove reuse and handwashing. *Ann Intern Med* 1988;109:394–398.

80. Kotilainen HR, Brinker JP, Avato JL, et al. Latex and vinyl examination gloves: quality control procedures and implications for healthcare workers. *Arch Intern Med* 1989;149:2749–2753.

81. Kubica GP. Your tuberculosis laboratory: Are you really safe from infection? *Clin Microbiol Newslett* 1990;12:85–87.

82. Macher JM, First MW. Effects of airflow rates and operator activity on containment of bacterial aerosols in a class II safety cabinet. *Appl Environ Microbiol* 1984;48:481–485.

83. Reinhardt PA, Gordon JG. *Infectious and medical waste management.* Chelsea, MI: Lewis Publisher, 1991.

84. Vesley D, Lauer JL. Decontamination, sterilization, disinfection, and antisepsis. In: Fleming DO, Richardson JH, Tulis JJ, Vesley D, eds. *Laboratory safety: principles and practices.* 2nd ed. Washington, DC: American Society for Microbiology, 1995:219–237.

85. McVicar JW, Suen J. Packaging and shipping biological materials. In: Fleming DO, Richardson JH, Tulis JJ, Vesley D, eds. *Laboratory safety: principles and practices.* 2nd ed. Washington, DC: American Society of Microbiology, 1995:239–246.

86. Kruse RH, Puckett WH, Richardson JH. Biological safety cabinetry. *Clin Microbiol Rev* 1991;4:207–241.

Dialysis-Associated Complications and Their Control*

Matthew J. Arduino

INTRODUCTION

The number of patients who have end stage renal disease (ESRD) has increased dramatically in the past 40 years. ESRD patients are treated by three major forms of renal replacement therapy: hemodialysis applications (conventional dialysis, hemofiltration, or hemodiafiltration), peritoneal dialysis (continuous ambulatory peritoneal dialysis, intermittent peritoneal dialysis, or automated peritoneal dialysis), or kidney transplant. Data from the U.S. Renal Data System (USRDS) suggests that by 2003 there were approximately 453,000 patients with ESRD. In the United States, the predominant form of renal replacement therapy (for approximately 298,000) is maintenance hemodialysis. Only about 6–7% of all patients receiving dialysis therapies are treated by one form of peritoneal dialysis [1].

In 1967, approximately 1,000 patients were undergoing maintenance or chronic hemodialysis. In 1973, when full Medicare coverage was extended to ESRD patients, approximately 11,000 patients were undergoing dialysis in independent or hospital-based centers and in homes in the United States. At the end of 2002, approximately 264,000 patients were undergoing maintenance hemodialysis at 4,035 dialysis centers with 58,000 staff members throughout the United States [2]. The ESRD program is administered by the Center for Medicare and Medicaid Services (CMS) of the Department of Health and Human Services. It is the only Medicare entitlement that is based on the diagnosis of a medical condition.

The technology for performing dialysis as well as the potential for complications has changed significantly over the years. In the early 1960s, hemodialysis was used almost exclusively for the treatment of acute renal failure. Subsequently, the development of the arteriovenous shunt and certain other ancillary technologic advances in dialysis equipment expanded the use of hemodialysis to maintenance therapy for ESRD. In the 1970s, the primary mode for dialysis treatment was hemodialysis performed with various types of artificial kidney machines. Subsequently, the use of peritoneal dialysis, accomplished by automated machines or by intermittent cycling, increased. By the end of 2003, only 25,825 (approximately 8%) patients were being treated by peritoneal dialysis applications. Continuous ambulatory peritoneal dialysis (CAPD), automated peritoneal dialysis (APD), or intermittent peritoneal dialysis (IPD) modality is more popular among pediatric nephrology programs (approximately 40% of all pediatric dialysis patients) [1]. One must also recognize that patients may change modality due to vascular access failure, peritonitis, peritoneal transport issues, and so on.

*The findings and conclusions in this chapter are those of the author and do not necessarily represent the views of the Centers for Disease Control and Prevention/the Agency for Toxic Substances and Disease Registry.

All patients with chronic kidney disease, including dialysis patients, have a compromised immune system and other co-morbidities that place them at increased risk for infectious diseases. This chapter describes the major infectious diseases and several toxic complications due to chemical contamination that can be acquired in the dialysis center setting, the important epidemiologic and environmental microbiologic considerations, and infection control strategies.

The Centers for Disease Control and Prevention (CDC) compiled date from two sources. The first includes outbreak investigations in dialysis settings conducted by CDC and National Surveillance studies. During the past 33 years, the CDC investigated 36 outbreaks in the dialysis setting; 17 involved bacterial infections or pyrogenic reactions, 10 viral infections, 8 toxic chemical complications, and 1 allergic complication of dialysis. In addition, the CDC performed national surveys of Hepatitis B virus (HBV) incidence and prevalence in the early 1970s. These national surveys subsequently evolved into the National Surveillance of Dialysis-Associated Diseases in the United States performed by CDC in collaboration with CMS in 1976, 1980, 1982–1997, and 1999–2002 [2–15]. The data collected includes hemodialysis practices, infection control precautions, and the occurrence of certain hemodialysis-associated diseases.

BACTERIAL AND CHEMICAL CONTAMINANTS IN HEMODIALYSIS SYSTEMS

A typical hemodialysis system consists of a water supply, a system for mixing water and dialysis fluid concentrates, and a machine to pump the dialysis fluid through the artificial kidney (commonly referred to as the *hemodialyzer* or *dialyzer*). The dialyzer is connected to the patient's circulatory system and pumps blood through it to accomplish dialysis through a membrane to remove waste products from the patient's blood by both diffusion and convection.

Microbial Contamination of Water

Technical development and clinical use of hemodialysis delivery systems improved dramatically in the late 1960s and early 1970s. However, a number of microbiologic parameters were not accounted for in the design of many hemodialysis machines and their respective water supply systems. In many situations, certain types of gram-negative water bacteria can persist and actively multiply in aqueous environments associated with hemodialysis equipment. This can result in the production of massive levels of gram-negative bacteria, which can directly or indirectly cause septicemia or endotoxemia in patients [16–19].

A number of factors can influence microbial contamination of fluids associated with hemodialysis systems

(Table 23-1). The gram-negative water bacteria can be significant contaminants in hemodialysis systems (Table 23-2), and virtually all disinfection strategies for fluid water distribution lines and dialysis machines are targeted to this group of bacteria. Gram-negative water bacteria are capable of multiplying rapidly in all types of waters, even those containing relatively small amounts of organic matter, such as water treated by distillation, softening, deionization, or reverse osmosis. These organisms can attain levels ranging from 10^5 to 10^7 per milliliter of water and, under certain circumstances, can be a health hazard for patients undergoing dialysis; they constitute a direct threat of bacteremia, and they contain bacterial endotoxin (lipopolysaccharide) that can cause pyrogenic reactions [17–21]. It should be emphasized that virtually any gram-negative water bacterium that can grow in water systems represents a potential problem in a hemodialysis unit. These bacteria adhere to surfaces and can form biofilms (glycocalyxes) that can make them virtually impossible to eradicate [18,22–24]. In fact, control strategies are designed to reduce levels of microbial contamination in water and dialysis fluid to relatively low levels but not to completely eradicate them.

Gram-negative water bacteria can grow even more rapidly in treated water mixed with dialysate concentrate. This mixture results in dialysis fluid that is a balanced salt solution and growth medium that is almost as rich in nutrients as conventional nutrient broth [19,25,26]. Gram-negative water bacteria growing in distilled, deionized, or reverse osmosis treated water can reach levels of 10^5–10^7 organisms per milliliter, but these cell populations are not visibly turbid. On the other hand, these same bacteria growing in dialysis fluids can achieve levels of 10^8–10^9 organisms per milliliter and often are associated with noticeable turbidity [25].

Nontuberculous mycobacteria also can multiply in water (Table 23-2). Although they do not contain bacterial endotoxin, they are comparatively resistant to chemical germicides and, as will be discussed later, have been responsible for patient infections due to inadequately disinfected dialyzers that are reprocessed and inadequately disinfected peritoneal dialysis machines [27–30].

The strategy for controlling massive accumulations of gram-negative water bacteria or nontuberculous mycobacteria in dialysis systems primarily involves preventing their growth. This can be accomplished by proper disinfection of water treatment system and hemodialysis machines. Gram-negative water bacteria and their associated lipopolysaccharides (bacterial endotoxins) and nontuberculous mycobacteria ultimately come from the community water supply, and levels of these bacteria can be amplified depending on the water treatment systems, dialysate distribution systems, type of dialysis machine, and method of disinfection [17,27,28,31,32] (see Table 23-1). Each of these components is discussed separately in some detail.

TABLE 23-1
FACTORS INFLUENCING MICROBIAL CONTAMINATION IN HEMODIALYSIS SYSTEMS

Factors	Comments
Water supply	
Source of community water	
Groundwater	Contains endotoxin and bacteria
Surface water	Contains high levels of endotoxin and bacteria
Water treatment at dialysis center	
None	Not recommended
Filtration	
Prefilter	Uses particulate filter to protect equipment; does not remove microorganisms
Absolute filter (depth or membrane)	Removes bacteria but, unless changed frequently or disinfected, bacteria will accumulate and grow through filter; acts as significant reservoir of bacteria and endotoxin
Activated carbon filter	Removes organics and available chlorine or chloramine; significant reservoir of water bacteria and endotoxin
Water treatment devices	
Ion-exchange softener	Both softeners and de-ionizers are significant reservoirs of bacteria and do not remove endotoxin
Deionization	
Reverse osmosis	Removes bacteria and endotoxin but must be disinfected; operates at high water pressure
Ultraviolet light	Kills some bacteria, but there is no residual, and ultraviolet-resistant bacteria can develop
Ultrafilter	Removes bacteria and endotoxin; operates on normal line pressure; can be positioned distal to de-ionizer; must be disinfected
Water and dialysate distribution system	
Distribution pipes	
Size	Oversized diameter and length decrease fluid flow and increase bacteria reservoir for both treated water and centrally prepared dialysate
Construction	Can act as bacterial reservoirs because of rough joints, dead ends, and unused branches
Elevation	Outlet taps should be located at highest elevation to prevent loss of disinfectant
Storage tanks	Is undesirable because they act as reservoir of water bacteria; if present, must be designed properly, and routinely scrubbed and disinfected
Dialysis machines	
Single pass	Disinfectant should have contact with all parts of machine that are exposed to water or dialysis fluid
Recirculating single pass or overnight recirculating (batch)	Recirculating pumps and machine design allow for massive contamination levels if not properly disinfected. Chemical germicide treatment recommended

Water Supply

Dialysis centers use water from a public supply that may be derived from surface, ground, or blends of surface and ground waters. The source of the water may be important in terms of chemical, bacterial, and endotoxin content. Surface waters frequently contain endotoxin from gram-negative water bacteria and from certain types of blue-green algae (Cyanobacteria). Endotoxin levels are not substantially reduced by conventional municipal water treatment processes and can be high enough to cause pyrogenic reactions in patients undergoing dialysis [33].

Essentially all public water supplies are contaminated with water bacteria; consequently, a dialysis center's water treatment and distribution systems and dialysis machines are challenged repeatedly with continuous inoculation of these ubiquitous bacteria. Even adequately chlorinated water supplies commonly contain low levels of these microorganisms. Whereas chlorine and other disinfectants added to the city water may prevent high levels of contamination, the presence of these chemicals in dialysis fluids is undesirable because of adverse effects on patients undergoing dialysis [34–38]. Furthermore, the dialysis water treatment systems described in the following section

TABLE 23-2
TYPES OF WATER MICROORGANISMS THAT HAVE BEEN FOUND IN DIALYSIS SYSTEMS

Gram-Negative Water Bacteria
   Pseudomonas spp.
   Flavobacterium spp.
   Enterobacter cloacae
   Klebsiella pneumoniae
   Burkholderia cepacia complex
   Pseudomonas aeruginosa
   Ralstonia pickettii
   Serratia liquefaciens
   S. marcescens
   Stenotrophomonas maltophilia
Nontuberculous mycobacteria
   Mycobacterium chelonae
   M. abscessus
   M. mucogenicum
   M. fortuitum
   M. gordonae
   M. scrofulaceum
Fungi
   Candida parapsilosis
   C. albicans
   Phialemonium curvatum

effectively remove chlorine, allowing for the unrestricted growth of water microorganisms.

Water Treatment Systems

Water used to produce dialysis fluid must be treated to remove chemical contaminants. The Association for the Advancement of Medical Instrumentation (AAMI) has published guidelines for the chemical and bacteriologic quality of water used to prepare dialysis fluid [39,40]. Since 1997, most maintenance dialysis facilities (at least 97%) use water treatment that includes reverse osmosis either alone or in combination with deionization [13]. Water systems are divided into three types of components: pretreatment, treatment, and posttreatment. Some components may vary based on the area of the United States and local water quality. A variety of different water treatment system components is used, but most of them are associated with amplification of water bacteria (Table 23-1). The most common treatment component is ion exchange using water softeners (pretreatment) and deionizers (treatment or posttreatment polisher). However, neither of these components removes endotoxins or bacteria, and both provide sites of significant bacterial multiplication [41]. An effective means of treating water for dialysis is reverse osmosis. Reverse osmosis or deionization water treatment systems are used in 99% of U.S. dialysis centers [13]. Reverse osmosis possesses the singular advantage of being able to remove both bacterial endotoxins and bacteria from supply water. However, low numbers of gram-negative or nontuberculous mycobacteria water bacteria can either

penetrate this barrier, or by other means colonize the downstream portion of the reverse osmosis unit. Consequently, reverse osmosis systems must be disinfected routinely.

Various filters are marketed to control bacterial contamination in water and dialysis fluids. Most of these are inadequate, especially if they are not routinely disinfected or changed frequently. Particulate filters, commonly called *prefilters*, operate by depth filtration and do not remove bacteria or bacterial endotoxins. These filters can become colonized with gram-negative water bacteria, resulting in amplification of the levels of both bacteria and endotoxin in the filter effluent. Absolute filters, including the membrane types, temporarily remove bacteria from passing water. However, some of these filters tend to clog, and gram-negative water bacteria can "grow through" the filter matrix and colonize the downstream surface of the filters within a couple of days. Furthermore, absolute filters do not reduce levels of endotoxin in the effluent water. These types of filters should be changed regularly in accordance with the manufacturer's directions and disinfected in the same manner and at the same time as the dialysis system.

Activated carbon filters/tanks remove certain organic chemicals and available chlorine (free and combined chlorine) from water by adsorption, but the filters also significantly increase the level of water bacteria and do not remove bacterial endotoxins.

Germicidal ultraviolet irradiation (GUI) lamps are sometimes used to reduce bacterial contamination in water. These lamps should operate at a wavelength of 254 nm and provide a dose of radiant energy of 30 milliwatt-sec/cm^2. Several studies have demonstrated that a dose of 30 milliwatt-sec/cm^2 will kill more than 99.99% of a variety of bacteria, including Pseudomonas species, in a flow-through device [42,43]. However, certain gram-negative water bacteria appear to be more resistant to GUI than others, and using sublethal doses of GUI or exposing water for an insufficient contact time may lead to proliferation of these resistant bacteria in the water system [19,44]. This problem may be accentuated in recirculating dialysis systems in which repeated exposures to sublethal doses of GUI are used to ensure adequate disinfection. The multiplication of those microorganisms surviving initial exposure enhanced resistance to GUI. In addition, bacterial endotoxins are not affected by GUI.

As mentioned, an effective means of treating water for dialysis is the correct use of a reverse osmosis unit. This author recommends using a water treatment system that produces chemically adequate water without massive levels of microbial contamination. Such a system is well suited for hard water and involves the following procedure [45]: community-supplied water is passed through a pretreatment chain consisting of prefilters, softener, carbon adsorption media (filters or tanks), and a particulate filter and then is passed through the treatment components, a reverse osmosis unit, and finally a deionization unit. Through these phases, the water becomes progressively more pure chemically, but the level of bacterial contamination increases. To compensate, an ultrafilter can be included in the final step of the system to remove bacteria and bacterial endotoxins. The ultrafilter consists of similar types of membranes as in a reverse osmosis unit or a polysulfone membrane, but it can be operated at ordinary water line pressure. This entire system can be augmented with other source-water treatment devices, depending on the chemical quality of the water in question. If this system is adequately disinfected, the microbial content of water should be well within the recommended guidelines discussed Microbiologic Monitoring of Water and Dialysis Fluid.

Distribution Systems

Dialysis centers use one of two general systems for delivering dialysis fluids to individual dialysis machines. The first type treats the incoming supply water and distributes it to individual free-standing dialysis stations either in a direct feed system or an indirect feed system (recirculating system). At each station, the water is mixed with a dialysate concentrate according to automatic proportioning by the dialysis machine. A second type of system, usually found in large dialysis centers, involves the automatic mixing of treated water and dialysate concentrate at a central location followed by distribution of the warmed dialysis fluid through pipes to individual dialysis stations. In both designs, the distribution system consists of plastic pipes (usually polyvinyl chloride) and appurtenances.

These distribution systems can contribute to microbial contamination in two ways. First, they frequently use pipes that are larger in diameter and longer than necessary to handle the required fluid flow. This slows the fluid velocity and increases both the total fluid volume and the wetted surface area of the system. Gram-negative bacteria in fluids remaining in pipes may multiply rapidly and colonize the wetted surfaces of the pipes, producing bacterial populations and endotoxin quantities in proportion to the volume and surface area. Such colonization results in bacterial formation of protective biofilm, which is difficult to remove and protects the bacteria from disinfection [46].

Because pipes can constitute a source of water bacteria in a distribution system, routine disinfection should be performed at least weekly. To ensure that the disinfectant cannot drain from pipes by gravity before contact time is adequate, distribution systems should be designed with all outlet taps at equal elevation and at the highest point of the system. Furthermore, the system should be free of rough joints, dead-end pipes, and unused branches and taps. Fluid trapped in such stagnant areas can serve as reservoirs of bacteria capable of continuously inoculating the entire volume of the system [21].

Incorporation of a storage tank in a distribution system greatly increases the volume of fluid and surface area available to act as reservoirs for the multiplication of water bacteria. Storage tanks should not be used in dialysis systems unless they are properly designed, frequently drained, and adequately disinfected, including scrubbing the sides of the tank to remove bacterial biofilm. It is also recommended that an ultrafilter be used distal to the storage tank [47,48].

Hemolysis Machines

Currently in the United States, virtually all centers use single-pass hemodialysis machines. In the 1970s, most machines were of the recirculating or recirculating single-pass type. The nature of their design contributed to a relatively high level of gram negative bacterial contamination in dialysis fluid. Single-pass dialysis machines tend to respond to adequate cleaning and disinfection procedures and, in general, have lower levels of bacterial contamination in their dialysis fluid than do recirculating machines. Levels of contamination in single-pass machines depend primarily on the bacteriologic quality of the incoming water and on the method of machine disinfection [17–19].

A frequent error in disinfecting single-pass systems occurs when the disinfectant is introduced in the same manner and through the same port as the dialysate concentrate. By so doing, the pipes and tubing of the incoming water are not exposed to a disinfectant; thus, the environment is such that bacteria can readily colonize and proliferate, acting as a constant reservoir of contamination. To adequately disinfect a single-pass system, the disinfectant must reach all parts of the system's fluid pathways.

Dialyzers

The dialyzer (artificial kidney) usually does not contribute significantly to bacterial contamination of the dialysate. Most dialysis centers use hollow-fiber dialyzers [5,7,8], which tend not to amplify bacterial contamination in the dialysis systems. The percentage of centers that reported reuse of disposable dialyzers on the same patient increased from 18–82% during the period from 1976 to 1997 but declined slightly over the next 5 years to 63% in 2002 [2]. Improper reprocessing techniques have been associated with outbreaks of bacteremia and pyrogenic reactions in dialysis patients (Table 23-3).

Disinfection of Hemodialysis Systems

The objective of a dialysis system disinfection procedure is to primarily inactivate bacteria and fungi in the fluid pathways associated with the dialysis system and to prevent these organisms from growing to significant levels once the system is in operation. Routine disinfection of isolated components of a dialysis system frequently produces inadequate results in which the hazard to the

TABLE 23-3

OUTBREAKS ASSOCIATED WITH DIALYZER REUSE

Description	Cause(s) of Outbreak	Corrective Measure(s) Recommended	Reference
Mycobacterial infections in 27 patients	Inadequate concentration of dialyzer disinfectant	Increase formaldehyde concentration used to disinfect dialyzers to 4%	[27]
Mycobacterial infections in 5 high-flux dialysis patients; 2 deaths	Inadequate concentration of dialyzer disinfectant and inadequate disinfection of water treatment system	Use higher concentration of Peracetic acid for reprocessing dialyzers and follow manufacturers labeled recommendations; increase frequency of disinfecting the water treatment system	[29]
Bacteremia in 6 patients	Inadequate concentration of dialyzer disinfectant; water used to reprocess dialyzers did not meet AAMI standards	Use AAMI quality water; ensure proper germicide concentration in the dialyzer	[CDC unpublished data]
Bacteremia and pyrogenic reactions in 6 patients	Dialyzer disinfectant diluted to improper concentration	Use disinfectant at the manufacturers recommended dilution and verify concentration	[49]
Bacteremia and pyrogenic reactions in 6 patients	Inadequate mixing of dialyzer disinfectant	Thoroughly mix disinfectant and verify proper concentration	[50]
Bacteremia in 33 patients at 2 dialysis centers	Dialyzer disinfectant created holes in the dialyzer membrane	Change disinfectant (product was withdrawn from the marketplace by the manufacturer)	[51]
Bacteremia in 6 patients; all blood isolates had similar plasmid profiles	Dialyzers were contaminated during removal and cleaning of headers with gauze; staff was not routinely changing gloves; dialyzers not reprocessed for several hours after disassembly and cleaning	Do not use gauze or similar material to remove clots from header; change gloves frequently; process dialyzers after rinsing and cleaning	[52]
Pyrogenic reactions in 3 high-flux dialysis patients	Dialyzer reprocessed with 2 disinfectants; water for reuse did not meet AAMI standards	Do not disinfect dialyzers with multiple germicides; more frequent disinfection of water treatment system and conduct routine environmental monitoring of water for reuse	[53]
Pyrogenic reactions during high-flux dialysis	Dialyzers rinsed with city (tap) water containing high levels of endotoxin; water used to reprocess dialyzers did not meet AAMI standards	Do not rinse or reprocess dialyzers with tap water; use AAMI quality water for rinsing and preparing dialyzer disinfectant	[CDC unpublished data]
Pyrogenic reactions in 18 patients	Dialyzers rinsed with city (tap) water containing high levels of endotoxin; water used to reprocess dialyzers did not meet AAMI standards	Do not rinse or reprocess dialyzers with tap water; use AAMI quality water for rinsing and preparing dialyzer disinfectant	[54]
Pyrogenic reactions in 22 patients	Water for reuse did not meet AAMI standards; improper microbiological technique was used on samples collected for monthly monitoring	Use the recommended assay procedure for water analysis of water and dialysate; disinfect water distribution system	[55]
Bacteremia and Candidemia among patients in 7 dialysis units (Minnesota and California)	Dialyzers were not reprocessed in a timely manner; some dialyzer refrigerated for extended periods of time before reprocessing; company recently made changes to header cleaning protocol	Reprocess dialyzers as soon as possible; follow joint CDC and dialyzer reprocessing equipment and disinfectant manufacturer guidance for cleaning and disinfecting headers of dialyzer	[CDC unpublished data]

patient persists. Consequently, the total dialysis system (water treatment system, distribution system, and dialysis machine) needs to be considered when selecting and applying disinfection procedures.

Chlorine-based disinfectants (e.g., sodium hypochlorite solutions) are convenient and effective in most parts of the dialysis system when used at the manufacturer's recommended concentration. Also, the test for residual available chlorine to confirm adequate rinsing is simple and sensitive. However, because of the corrosive nature of chlorine, the disinfectant normally is rinsed from the system after a short (20–30 minute) exposure time. This practice commonly negates the disinfection procedure because the rinse water is not sterile and invariably contains waterborne microorganisms that immediately resume multiplication. If permitted to stand overnight, the water may contain significant microbial contamination levels. Therefore, chlorine disinfectants are most effective when applied just before the start-up of the dialysis system rather than at the end of the daily operation. In some large centers with multiple shifts, it may be reasonable to use sodium hypochlorite disinfection between shifts (this may not be necessary with some single-pass machines if the levels of bacterial contamination are below AAMI action limits [40]) and formaldehyde, peracetic acid, hydrogen peroxide, ozone, and hot water disinfection at the end of the day.

Aqueous formaldehyde, hydrogen peroxide, and peracetic acid solutions can produce good disinfection results. They are not as corrosive as hypochlorite solutions and can be allowed to remain in the dialysis system for long periods when it is not operational, thereby preventing the growth of bacteria in the system. Formaldehyde has good penetrating characteristics but is considered an environmental hazard and potential carcinogen and is associated with irritating qualities that are objectionable to staff members. Commercial tests (e.g., Formalert, Organon Teknika, Durham, NC) are available that are sensitive for testing for formaldehyde in water at concentrations as low as 1 part per million (ppm). (Use of trade name and commercial products is for identification purposes only and does not imply endorsement by the Centers for Disease Control and Prevention of the U.S. Public Health Service.) When used according to the manufacturers' recommendations, commercially available peracetic acid disinfectants for dialysis systems are not corrosive to machines and are good germicides [56].

Some dialysis systems use hot-water disinfection (pasteurization) to control microbial contamination. In this type of system, water heated to >80°C (176°F) is passed through all proportioning, distribution, and patient-monitoring devices before use. This system is excellent for controlling bacterial contamination [47,57]. Use of ozone also has been increasing as a means of sanitizing water treatment distribution loops and central bicarbonate delivery systems [47,57–59].

Monitoring Water and Dialysis Fluid

Bacteriologic assays of water and dialysis fluids should be performed at least once a month. Chemical analysis of water used for dialysis should be done before the system is designed and then at least seasonally (since feed water quality changes) to ensure that the water is of sufficient quality for hemodialysis applications [39,40]. The recommended levels of microbial contamination in water used to prepare dialysis fluid should not exceed 200 colony forming units per ml (CFU/ml) and contamination levels should not exceed 2000 CFU/ml in dialysis fluids [60,61]. These

TABLE 23-4

AAMI MICROBIAL QUALITY STANDARDS FOR DIALYSIS FLUIDS

Type of Fluid	Microbial Bioburden		Endotoxin	
	Maximum Contaminant Level	Action Level	Maximum Contaminant Level	Action Level
Water for all purposes	200 CFU/ml	50 CFU/ml	2 Eu/ml	1 Eu/ml
Conventional dialysate	200 CFU/ml	50 CFU/ml	2 Eu/ml	1 Eu/ml
Ultrapure dialysate	1 CFU/10 ml		0.03 Eu/ml	
Dialysate for infusion	1 CFU/1000 l[a]		0.03 Eu/ml	

[a]Compliance with a maximum bacterial level of 10^{-6} cfu/ml cannot be demonstrated by culturing but by processes developed by the machine manufacturers.

particular numbers are based on bacteriologic assays during epidemiologic investigations. However, an increasing body of evidence indicates that dialysate may be responsible in part for the chronic inflammatory state in dialysis patients [62–69]. In response to these studies, AAMI has published new recommendations, which begin to lower the maximum microbial contaminant levels in dialysis fluids. In these new recommendations, water and conventional dialysate have the same maximum contaminant levels (200 cfu/ml and 2 endotoxin units per ml (Eu/ml)). They also have included standards for ultrapure dialysate and dialysate for infusion (Table 23-4) [40].

The microbiological assay is quantitative rather than qualitative, and a standard technique for enumeration should be used; the standard recommended method is membrane filtration [40]. Water samples should be collected at a point that is as close as possible to where water enters the dialysate concentrate-proportioning unit. Samples should be collected at least monthly for established units and weekly for new units until an established pattern is determined. Repeat samples should be collected when microbial counts exceed the action level (Table 23-4) and after disinfection changes have been instituted. Dialysis fluid samples should be collected at the start or termination of dialysis close to the point where the dialysis fluid either enters or leaves the dialyzer. These types of samples also should be taken at least once monthly and after suspected pyrogenic reactions or changes in the water treatment system or disinfection protocols.

Samples should be assayed within 30 minutes or refrigerated (4°C) and assayed within 24 hours of collection. Total viable counts (standard plate counts) are the objective of the assays, and conventional laboratory procedures, such as membrane filtration technique or spread plate, can be used; calibrated loops should not be used because they sample a small volume and are inaccurate. Although standard methods such as agar, blood agar, and trypticase soy agar were considered equivalent in the earlier recommendations of the AAMI, research has since shown that many gram-negative bacterial flora of bicarbonate dialysis fluid require a small amount of NaCl for optimal growth. Consequently, trypticase soy agar currently is considered the culture medium of choice; other acceptable media include standard methods of agar and plate count agar (also known as TGYE). Colonies should be counted after 48 hours of incubation at 35°C–37°C (95°C–98.6°F) [40,60,61,70,71]. This method indicates water and dialysate fluid quality only and is not to be confused with total heterotrophic plate counts, which require much longer incubation times at 28°C. There has been discussion in the dialysis community that these methods infact under estimate the actual contamination of dialysis fluids [72,73].

In the event of an outbreak investigation, the assay may need to be qualitative and quantitative, and samples may have to be cultured using additional microbiological culture media and methods as is the case with nontuberculous mycobacteria and fungi (Table 23-2). In such instances, plates should be incubated for 5–14 days.

If centers reprocess dialyzers for reuse on the same patient, water used to rinse dialyzers and prepare dialyzer disinfectants also should be assayed at least monthly in the manner described previously. It is recommended that microbial or endotoxin contaminations not exceed 200 cfu/ml and 2 eu/ml (Table 23-4) [40,74].

Pyrogenic Reactions and Septicemia/Fungemia

Pyrogenic reactions and gram-negative sepsis are the most common complications associated with high levels of gram-negative bacterial contamination of dialysis fluid. Pyrogenic reactions can result from either the passage of bacterial endotoxin (lipopolysaccharide) in the dialysis fluid across the dialyzer membrane [75–79] or the transmembrane stimulation of cytokine production in the patient's blood by endotoxins in the dialysis fluid [80,81]. In other instances, endotoxins can enter the bloodstream directly with fluids that are contaminated with gram-negative bacteria [51,82]. Studies indicate that chronic hemodialysis patients have enhanced cytokine response compared to nonhemodialysis patients, which may account for the high rate of fatal sepsis in uremic patients [83].

The higher the level of bacteria and endotoxin in dialysis fluid, the higher the probability that bacteria or endotoxin will pass through the dialysis membrane or stimulate cytokine production. In an outbreak of febrile reactions among patients undergoing dialysis, the attack rates were directly proportional to the level of bacterial contamination in the dialysis fluid [19]. Prospective studies also demonstrated a lower pyrogenic reaction rate among patients when they underwent dialysis with dialysis fluid that had been filtered and from which most bacteria had been removed compared to patients who underwent dialysis with dialysis fluid that was highly contaminated (mean 19,000 cfu/ml) [84,85].

In 1997, 21% of U.S. hemodialysis centers reported at least one pyrogenic reaction in the absence of septicemia in patients undergoing dialysis [13]. This reported rate was fairly stable from 1989–1997 (range: 19–22%) [13]. An active surveillance system is essential for early detection and control of these complications. Clinical reactions should be defined as they occur because doing so may be the first clue that a problem exists. In addition, the dialysis system should be microbiologically monitored periodically by methods described previously.

Among 11 outbreaks of bacteremia and pyrogenic reactions not related to dialyzer reuse investigated by the CDC, inadequate disinfection of the water distribution or storage system was implicated in 4 of them (Table 23-5). The most recent outbreaks occurred at centers using dialysis machines having a port to dispose of dialyzer priming fluid (waste handling option) [89–91,95,96, CDC unpublished data, 2006]. One-way check valves in the waste-handling option had not been maintained, checked for competency, or disinfected as recommended, allowing backflow from the drain, contamination of the port, and backflow of fluid into the patients' blood lines.

Surveillance of Pyrogenic Reactions and Infections

Pyrogenic reactions in patients undergoing dialysis are associated with shaking chills, fever, and hypotension. Depending on the type of dialysis system and the level of initial contamination, the onset of an elevated temperature and chills can occur 1–5 hours after the initiation of dialysis and usually are associated with a decrease in systolic blood pressure of at least 30 millimeters of mercury (mm Hg). Other less frequent but characteristic symptoms may include headache, myalgia, nausea, and vomiting. We define a case of pyrogenic reaction as the onset of objective chills (visible rigors), fever (oral temperature ≥37.8°C [100°F]), or both in a patient who was afebrile (oral temperature ≤37.0°C [98.6°F]) and who had no signs or symptoms of infection before the dialysis treatment [33,54,82,85].

Differentiating gram-negative bacterial sepsis from a pyrogenic reaction can be difficult because the initial signs and symptoms of the two conditions are identical. The most reliable means of detecting sepsis is by culturing blood taken at the time of the reaction. However, because the results of these cultures take at least 18–24 hours to obtain and because therapy for sepsis should not be withheld for this length of time, other less reliable criteria must be used. Many pyrogenic reactions are not associated with bacteremia, and the preceding signs and symptoms generally abate within a few hours after dialysis has been

TABLE 23-5

CDC INVESTIGATED OUTBREAKS OF BACTEREMIA, FUNGEMIA, OR PYROGENIC REACTIONS UNRELATED TO HEMODIALYZER REUSE

Description	Cause(s) of Outbreak	Corrective Measure	Reference
Pyrogenic reactions in 49 patients	Untreated city (tap) water with high level of endotoxin	Install reverse osmosis system	[33]
Pyrogenic reactions in 45 patients	Inadequate disinfection of the fluid distribution system	Increase disinfection frequency and contact time for the disinfectant	[86]
Pyrogenic reactions in 14 patients; two bacteremias; one death	Reverse osmosis water storage tank contaminated with bacteria	Remove or properly disinfect and maintain storage tank	[18]
Pyrogenic reactions in 6 patients; 7 bacteremias	Inadequate disinfection of water distribution system and dialysis machines; improper microbial assay procedure	Use correct microbial assay procedure; disinfect water distribution system and dialysis machines according to manufacturer's recommendations	[87]
Bacteremia in 35 patients with central vein catheters (CVC)	CVCs used as primary access; median duration of infected catheters was 311 days; improper aseptic technique	Use CVCs only when necessary; use appropriate aseptic techniques when inserting and performing catheter care	[88]
Three pyrogenic reactions and 10 bacteremias in patients treated on machines with a port (WHO) for disposal of dialyzer priming fluid	Incompetent valve allowing backflow from the drain to the WHO and contamination of the blood lines; bacterial contamination of the WHO	Routine maintenance, disinfection, and determination of valve competency of the WHO	[89, 90]
Bacteremia in 10 patients treated on machines with a port for disposal of dialyzer prime	Incompetent valve allowing backflow from the drain to the WHO and contamination of the blood lines; bacterial contamination of the WHO	Routine maintenance, disinfection, and determination of valve competency of the WHO	[89, 91]
Outbreak of pyrogenic reactions and gram-negative bacteremia in 11 patients (four with bacteremia)	Water distribution system and machines not routinely disinfected according to manufacturer's recommendations; water and dialysate samples cultured using calibrated loops and blood agar plates	Disinfect machines according to manufacturer's instructions; include water distribution system in the weekly disinfection of the system; perform environmental monitoring of dialysis fluids using recommended methods	[92]
In a one-month period, 10 bacteremias and 6 pyrogenic reactions occurred in patients at a hemodialysis center	Preservative-free, single-use vials of epoetin alfa punctured multiple times, and residual epoetin alfa from multiple vials pooled and administered to patients	Follow manufacturer's recommendations for use of preservative free injectable medications	[93]
Phialemonium curvatum access infections in four hemodialysis patients; two died of systemic disease	Observations at the facility noted some irregularities in site prep for needle insertion; all affected patients had synthetic grafts; one environmental culture was positive of P. curvatum (condensate pan of HVAC) serving the dialysis facility	Review infection control practices; clean and disinfect the condensate HVAC system where water accumulates; perform surveillance on patients	[CDC unpublished data, 94]
Phialemonium curvatum blood stream infections in patients treated on the same hemodialysis machine	Patients dialyzed on a machine with a WHO port; P. curvatum isolated from treated water supplied to the station where the dialysis machine was located; water distribution system is disinfected once per year and cultures monitoring dialysis fluids were not performed on a routine basis	Eliminate dead legs in the distribution loop and disinfect the water distribution system on a regular schedule; follow manufacturer's instruction for disinfection and maintenance	[CDC unpublished data]

stopped. With gram-negative bacterial sepsis, fever and chills may persist, and hypotension is more refractory to therapy [33,82].

The early detection of pyrogenic reactions or gram-negative sepsis depends on a thorough understanding of the signs and symptoms of these entities by the dialysis staff and on the careful charting of the patient's symptoms and changes in blood pressure and temperature. The following diagnostic procedures are recommended for patients who meet the criteria of a pyrogenic reaction: a careful physical examination to rule out other causes of chills and fever (e.g., pneumonia, vascular access infection, urinary tract infection); blood cultures, other diagnostic tests (e.g., chest radiograph), and cultures as clinically indicated; collection of dialysis fluid from the dialyzer (downstream side) for quantitative and qualitative bacteriologic assays; and recording the incident in a log or other permanent record. Determining the cause of these episodes is important because they may be the first indication of a remediable problem.

Hemodialyzer Reuse

In the early 1960s, the most common dialyzer used in dialysis centers was the Kiil plate dialyzer, which was cleaned and disinfected after each patient use and supplied with a new set of cuprophane membranes. The dialyzer housing, however, was reused each time. With the development of disposable coil and hollow-fiber dialyzers, the use of the Kiil dialyzer was discontinued. Disposable dialyzers are medical devices that are supplied in a sterile state and were initially intended by the manufacturer for one-time use and since 1995 have required specific labeling that identified single use or multiple use [97]. In recent years, as a cost-saving effort, more centers are reusing dialyzers on the same patient after employing an appropriate disinfection procedure. Although it has caused some controversy, this is now standard practice in the dialysis community. From 1976–1983, the percentage of U.S. dialysis centers that reported reuse of disposable dialyzers increased from 18–52%. This upward trend in reuse continued until 1997 when 82% of centers reported that they reused disposable dialyzers on ≥1 patients [13]. In 1997, the average number of times a dialysis center reused dialyzers was 17 (range, 1–65). The mean number of times a dialyzer was reused was 38 (range, 1–179) [13]. Dialysis centers most likely to report reuse of dialyzers were those with larger patient populations (>40), those located in free-standing facilities, and those operated for profit compared with centers with smaller patient populations, those located in hospitals, and those not operated for profit [5,7,8,10,13]. However, within the last 6 years, one of the large U.S. dialysis provider organizations made a decision to discontinue reuse, which would account for the drop in reuse as of 2002 to 63% of facilities [2] and may eventually fall to the share of the dialysis market not represented by this provider.

CDC's surveillance project has not shown a correlation between HBV incidence or anti-Hepatitis C Virus (HCV) prevalence and dialyzer reuse. A study has shown a statistical association between the reuse of dialyzers disinfected with glutaraldehyde or peracetic acid/hydrogen peroxide and increased death rates at dialysis centers [98]. However, other factors may have contributed to what appears to be a causal relationship between reuse and a higher death rate, or the association may be due to unmeasured confounding factors [99–101].

In 1986, the U.S. Public Health Service (PHS) subsumed the AAMI's guidelines for reusing hemodialyzers [74] and recommended them as PHS guidance to the CMS, which, in turn, made them conditions for participation in Medicare/Medicaid. In effect, the AAMI guidelines, which became PHS guidance, resulted in CMS regulations. In general, if the procedures involved in reprocessing hemodialyzers are performed according to established and strict protocols, patients do not appear to have harmful effects. However, the practice of reusing disposable hemodialyzers should not be considered risk free. Outbreaks of patient infections and pyrogenic reactions associated with user error have occurred (Table 23-3). Many of these episodes were the result of inadequate reprocessing procedures, such as the use of incorrect concentrations of chemical germicides and failure to maintain standards for water quality [102]. In addition, in 1986, six dialysis centers reported outbreaks of pyrogenic reactions and septicemia that were associated with the use of a new germicide, the active ingredient of which was chlorine dioxide. That germicide, although efficacious for disinfecting dialyzers, appeared to degrade the integrity of cellulosic dialyzer membranes to such an extent that leaks in the membranes developed [103]. Centers that reported using this germicide employed manual reprocessing systems, and most of these centers reused their dialyzers >20 times.

In each of 3 successive years (1985–1988), reprocessing dialyzers in a manual reprocessing system was shown consistently to be significantly associated with a higher reported frequency of pyrogenic reactions, even with the use of other germicides, and was not necessarily related to the absolute number of reuses [4,104]. Some dialyzer membrane defects may go undetected when manual reprocessing systems are used because testing for dialyzer membrane integrity, as with an air-pressure leak test, generally is not performed with this type of system [105]. It is emphasized that adverse reactions associated with reuse of dialyzers are accentuated in dialysis centers that are having problems and that, for the most part, only a small number of centers are experiencing an increased risk with dialyzers that are reused >20 times or that include a manual reprocessing system. In 1993, only a modest and insignificant association between dialyzer reuse and reporting of pyrogenic reactions at U.S. hemodialysis centers occurred [10].

The procedures used in dialysis centers for reprocessing hemodialyzers usually cannot be classified as sterilization procedures but constitute high-level disinfection [70,105]. In 1983, most centers in the United States (94%) used 2% aqueous formaldehyde with a contact time of approximately 36 hours for high-level disinfection of disposable dialyzers [5]. Although this procedure may be satisfactory against the presumed microbiologic challenge of gram-negative water bacteria, it is inadequate for the highly germicide-resistant nontuberculous mycobacteria (Table 23-2).

CDC investigated an outbreak of infections caused by nontuberculous mycobacteria during which 27 infections occurred among 140 patients [27]. The source of the non-tuberculous mycobacteria appeared to be the water used in processing the dialyzers. It was evident that 2% formaldehyde did not effectively inactivate populations of these mycobacteria within 36 hours. It was subsequently shown that 4% formaldehyde with a minimum contact time of 24 hours can inactivate high numbers of nontuberculous mycobacteria; as a consequence, 4% formaldehyde is recommended as a minimum solution for disinfection of dialyzers [70,105,106].

A similar outbreak of systemic mycobacterial infections in five dialysis patients, resulting in two deaths, occurred when high-flux dialyzers were contaminated with mycobacteria during manual reprocessing and were then disinfected with a commercial dialyzer disinfectant prepared at a concentration that did not ensure complete inactivation of mycobacteria [29]. These two outbreaks emphasize the need to use dialyzer disinfectants at concentrations that are effective against the more chemically resistant microorganisms, such as mycobacteria.

Formaldehyde (a chemical solution obtained from chemical supply houses) for reprocessing dialyzers is now considered to be both environmentally hazardous and hazardous to use in the dialysis setting; it has recently been classified as a human carcinogen (cancer-causing substance) by the International Agency for Research on Cancer and as a probable human carcinogen by the U.S. Environmental Protection Agency. The use of formaldehyde in the dialysis setting has been decreasing due to limits on the allowable amounts in the wastewater stream and to reduce potential occupational and patient exposures. During 1983–2002, the centers using formaldehyde for reprocessing dialyzers decreased from 94% to 22% while the use of peracetic acid increased to 72% [2]. A number of chemical germicides specifically formulated for reprocessing hemodialyzers have been shown to be effective and are approved by the Food and Drug Administration (FDA).

Pyrogenic reactions in dialysis patients caused by reprocessing dialyzers with water that did not meet AAMI standards have been frequently associated with epidemics investigated by the CDC (Table 23-3). In most of these outbreaks, the water used to rinse dialyzers or to prepare dialyzer disinfectants exceeded allowable AAMI microbial or endotoxin standards because the water distribution system was not disinfected frequently, the disinfectant was improperly prepared, or routine microbiologic assays were improperly performed.

The California Department of Health Services conducted a series of investigations of outbreaks of bloodstream infections (BSIs) associated with dialyzer reuse in 2001 and 2002. It found that the BSI clusters caused by *Stenotrophomonas maltophilia, Burkholderia cepacia* complex, *Ralstonia pickettii,* or *Candida parapsilosis* were more likely to occur in dialysis facilities that refrigerated dialyzers before reprocessing them [107].

High-Flux Dialysis

High-flux dialysis is a very efficient hemodialysis treatment that uses dialyzer membranes with hydraulic permeabilities 5–10 times greater than those of conventional dialyzer membranes. By using highly permeable membranes in dialyzers that have larger membrane surface areas than conventional dialyzers and higher blood flow rates, dialysis treatment times can be reduced from 4–5 hours to 2–3 hours. Between 1988 and 1999, the U.S. hemodialysis centers reported using high-flux dialyzer membranes on at least some patients increased from 23% to approximately 58% [5,108]. Because high-flux membranes are so permeable, there is concern that bacteria or endotoxin in the dialysate may penetrate these membranes, causing infections or pyrogenic reactions in the patient. Another concern is that high-flux dialysis requires the use of bicarbonate dialysate, which, unlike the acetate-based dialysate used almost exclusively since the 1970s, is prepared from a concentrate that can support rapid bacterial growth. Acetate dialysate is prepared from a single concentrate with such a high salt molarity (4.8 M) that most bacteria cannot grow in it. Bicarbonate dialysate, in contrast, must be prepared from two concentrates, an acid concentrate with a pH of 2.8 that is not conducive to bacterial growth and a bicarbonate concentrate with a relatively neutral pH and a salt molarity of 1.2 molar (M). Because the bicarbonate concentration will support rapid bacterial growth [25,109], its use can increase bacterial and endotoxin concentrations in the dialysate and, theoretically, may contribute to an increase in pyrogenic reactions, especially when it is used during high-flux dialysis.

Some of this concern may be justified. In 1980s and 1990s, surveillance data showed a significant association between use of high-flux dialysis and reporting of pyrogenic reactions during dialysis [5–10]. However, a prospective study of pyrogenic reactions in patients receiving >27,000 conventional, high-efficiency, or high-flux dialysis treatments with a bicarbonate dialysate containing high concentrations of bacteria and endotoxin found no association between pyrogenic reactions and the type of dialysis treatment [84,85]. Although there seem to be conflicting data on the relationship between high-flux dialysis and pyrogenic reactions, centers providing high-flux dialysis should be especially mindful of ensuring that dialysate meets AAMI microbial standards (Table 23-4).

Other Infections

Vascular Access Site Infections

Hemodialysis procedures depend on direct and repeated access to large blood vessels that can provide rapid extracorporeal blood flow. Scribner developed a method for vascular access by surgically inserting plastic tubes, one into an artery and one into a vein. After treatment, the circulatory access would be kept open by connecting the two tubes outside the body using a small U-shaped device, which would shunt the blood from the tube in the artery back to the tube in the vein [110,111]. Although the external arteriovenous (AV) shunts were the foundation on which modern dialysis grew, their use in recent years has been limited to patients who require temporary access to treatment. The material used for these shunts can be biologic or synthetic. External shunts are primarily used for those in emergent need for continuous renal replacement therapy (CRRT) when catheters (central or femoral lines cannot be placed [112]). Three primary types of vascular access are used for hemodialysis therapy: native AV fistulas, AV grafts, and central hemodialysis catheters [113].

The AV fistula is believed to provide the best long-term access to circulation with the least number of complications. However, only 33% of all U.S. hemodialysis patients have AV fistulas; 42% have AV grafts, and 26% use a central line for dialysis. The use of central venous catheters (CVCs) for vascular access has doubled since 1995 while the use of AV grafts has declined from 65% to 42% of patients. AV fistula use has increased from 22% of patients in 1995 to 33% of patients in 2002 [2].

Access site infections are particularly important because they can cause disseminated bacteremia/fungemia or loss of the access. Local signs of vascular access infection include erythema, warmth, induration, swelling, tenderness, skin breakdown, loculated fluid, or purulent exudate [114–117]. Vascular access site infections may account for 15–20% of all access-related complications. In general, the length of time that a catheter is left in place and the duration of cannulation can be important factors predisposing to infection. In addition, the type of fistula, nature of the access site dressing, number of needle access events, movement of the site, and personal hygiene of the patient may play a role in the acquisition of infection. BSIs can occur, either by migration of bacteria down the outer surface of a hemodialysis catheter (tunnel) or by contamination of the lumen of the catheter during attachment or detachment during dialysis. Infections of the vascular access site can lead to sepsis, septic pulmonary emboli, endocarditis, or meningitis. No controlled prospective studies have been performed; thus, reported rates of access site infections among hemodialysis patients vary. Although the most frequent pathogens are *Staphylococcus aureus* or *S. epidermidis*, gram-negative bacteria also can be responsible for access site infections, especially if the site is in the patient's lower extremities. Transmission of these types of bacterial infections among patients or from staff members to patients in the hemodialysis center setting is primarily due to cross-contamination, which results in colonization and subsequent infection in a subset of these patients. Transmission can be controlled by good hand-hygiene and gloving techniques as well as good puncture techniques [118–124].

For many years, central (subclavian or jugular) catheters have been used for temporary venous access for hemodialysis. Recent technical improvements have made it feasible to use these catheters for permanent access, usually in patients for whom no other access is available [125]. However, CVCs have high rates of failure due to thrombosis and infection (Figure 23-1) [125]. In 1991, CDC investigated 35 BSIs among 68 patients receiving

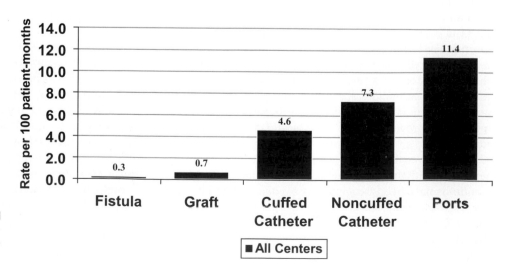

Figure 23-1 Rates of blood stream infection by access type—Dialysis Surveillance Network, 1999–2005.

hemodialysis through CVCs; one patient died and one developed endocarditis and required aortic valve replacement [126].

Infections Associated with Peritoneal Dialysis

As mentioned earlier, approximately 6–7% of U.S. ESRD patients were treated by peritoneal dialysis at the end of 2003 [1]. In peritoneal dialysis, the patient's peritoneal membrane is used to dialyze waste products from the patient's blood. In the mid-1970s, the development of automated peritoneal dialysis systems made intermittent peritoneal dialysis a viable alternative to hemodialysis for long-term management of ESRD patients. Currently, this approach has been replaced by chronic ambulatory peritoneal dialysis (CAPD), continuous-cycling peritoneal dialysis (CCPD), and chronic intermittent peritoneal dialysis (CIPD) in which presterilized dialysis fluid is either introduced by gravity or is cycled into a patient's peritoneal cavity. In CAPD, commercially available sterile dialysate in a plastic bag is self-administered by the patient who has a surgically implanted catheter. The exchanges are done every 4 hours, and the patient can be mobile between exchanges [127]. The most persistent problem in the management of patients treated by peritoneal dialysis is peritonitis [128,129].

In the past, automated peritoneal machines were used to create dialysate from tap water. To prevent the growth of pathogenic microorganisms that cause infection, automated peritoneal dialysis machines had to be cleaned and maintained properly. In theory, the incidence of peritonitis should be low because the machine functions as a closed system. However, the machines may themselves provide a reservoir for pathogens that cause peritonitis. Several outbreaks of bacterial peritonitis among patients receiving intermittent peritoneal dialysis have been reported, and the etiologic agents have included *Mycobacterium chelonei*–like organisms or *Pseudomonas cepacia* [30,131]. Both organisms can grow in water; investigation of these outbreaks revealed that machines were inadequately cleaned and disinfected and that the product water and dialysis fluid contained the microorganisms responsible for peritonitis [132]. In addition, one group of organisms, the nontuberculous mycobacteria such as *M. chelonae*, is significantly and extraordinarily resistant to the commonly used disinfectants [133]. Berkelman et al. recommended a set of guidelines that can ensure the production of sterile dialysis fluid and reduce the likelihood of outbreaks of peritonitis for dialysis centers using automated peritoneal dialysis machines [135]. The precise details and protocols differ for each machine type, and the reader is referred to the guidelines for a more complete discussion [134]. It should be noted that, for all practical purposes, the use of these automated peritoneal dialysis machines has been discontinued in the United States, and the preceding information is cited for completeness and for historical considerations.

With CAPD, CCPD, or CIPD, catheter-related infections and peritonitis remain the most common cause of morbidity among peritoneal dialysis patients, contribute significantly to the cost of this treatment, and are the primary reason for the abandonment of peritoneal dialysis. Incidence rates for peritonitis vary widely among centers and among modalities. In general, peritonitis has dramatically decreased from the inception of CAPD; rates >0.5 episodes per patient per year are still common [135–138]. The use of CCPD or CIPD in centers with experienced staff, patients, and patient caregivers has resulted in substantially reduced infection rates compared to CAPD. The weak link with peritoneal dialysis and the present catheter technology is the associated risk of tunnel or exit site infections. These infections occur at a rate of 0.7 episodes per patient per year [128,138–140].

Clinical symptoms of peritoneal infection usually appear 12–36 hours after bacterial contamination of the peritoneal cavity. Symptoms include nausea, vomiting, and abdominal pain. Later, vague abdominal tenderness may progress to severe, diffuse, or localized pain associated with fever, abdominal distention, and gastrointestinal dysfunction. The clinical diagnosis should be confirmed by bacteriologic analysis of the peritoneal fluid. Cloudy peritoneal fluid often is the first sign of infection.

The etiologic agents of peritonitis associated with conventional peritoneal dialysis usually are *S. epidermidis*, *S. aureus*, and other gram-positive bacteria, which collectively account for 55–80% of episodes; 17–30% of episodes are caused by gram-negative organisms such as *Enterobacteriaceae*, *Pseudomonas aeruginosa*, *Burkholderia cepacia*, and *Acinetobacter* species; in a few instances (10%), peritonitis is caused by fungi, yeast, mycobacteria, or anaerobic bacteria. Approximately 10% of episodes will be culture negative [128,141,142].

The primary strategy for controlling peritonitis is to prevent contamination of the dialysis fluid that enters the peritoneal cavity and to prevent tunnel and exit site infections. Prevention involves (1) aseptic manipulation of the sterile disposable plastic lines leading into the abdominal catheter that deliver the dialysis fluid into the peritoneal cavity, (2) a system for aseptic connection of the tubing containing the sterile dialysis fluid and the patient's catheter, and (3) appropriate access site care [143,144].

Noninfectious Complications

First-Use and Allergic Reactions

A variety of symptoms attributed to hypersensitivity reactions may occur during dialysis. Symptoms variously reported include increased or decreased blood pressure, dyspnea, cough, conjunctival injection, flushing, urticaria, headache, and pains in the chest, back, and limbs. Such symptoms are more common during the first use of a dialyzer and have been termed the "first-use syndrome" [145,146]. These reactions are more common with cuprophan dialyzers; some may be attributable to residual ethylene oxide in dialyzers [147–149]. During 1992–1993, such reactions were reported by 24–27% of dialysis centers and were most strongly associated with the use of cuprophan and regenerated cellulose membranes [10]. Reports of first-use syndrome have decreased from 43% of centers in 1984 to 23% of centers in 1997 [13].

In 1990, several outbreaks of anaphylactoid reactions associated with angiotensin-converting enzyme (ACE) inhibitors were reported. Reactions occurred within 10 minutes of initiating dialysis and included nausea, abdominal cramps, burning, flushing, swelling of the face or tongue, angioedema, shortness of breath, and hypotension. One outbreak was linked to the reuse of dialyzers [150], but other reports implicated polyacrylonitrile (PAN) dialyzers in the reactions [151–154]. In 1992, the FDA issued a safety alert regarding anaphylactoid reactions in patients on ACE inhibitors, especially those using PAN dialyzers [155].

Dialysis Dementia

Dialysis encephalopathy, or dialysis dementia, is a disorder that affects dialysis patients who, for a variety of reasons, are subjected to water that has a relatively high content of aluminum, such as community water supplies treated with alum. This complication was first described in 1972 by Alfrey et al. [156]. Schreeder et al. [157] first demonstrated the role of aluminum as a significant contributing factor in this disorder in an epidemiologic study. Case definitions of dialysis encephalopathy include three different groups of objective findings:

1. Speech impairment (stuttering, stammering, dysnomia, hypofluency, mutism).
2. Seizure disorder (generalized tonic-clonic, focal, or multifocal seizures).
3. Motor disturbance (myoclonic jerks, motor apraxia, immobility).

Schreeder et al. [157] showed that patients were at increased risk of dialysis dementia when the aluminum content of water used to prepare dialysate was high (>100 ng/L). The number of episodes of dialysis dementia reported to CDC has decreased from 0.4% in the years 1980 and 1983–1985 to 0.1% in 1990 ($N = 129$; case-fatality rate = 21%) [7]. Although it is not clear what was responsible for this decrease, we believe it may be related to increased awareness in the dialysis community of the requirement for good water treatment systems. In 1980, only 26% of U.S. hemodialysis centers reported that they employed a reverse osmosis system, either alone or with deionization in their water treatment systems. By 1988, 91% of the centers were using reverse osmosis alone or in combination with deionization as an integral part of their water treatment system [5]. Control of dialysis dementia revolves around adequate water treatment systems and invariably requires the use of reverse osmosis, either alone or with deionization.

It also is important to ensure that all components of the water treatment and dialysis fluid preparation and delivery systems be compatible with all fluid with which they are in contact in order to eliminate the possibility of leaching of harmful substances. In one outbreak, 58/85 (68%) dialysis patients at a dialysis center were diagnosed with acute or chronic aluminum intoxication that resulted in three deaths. Investigation revealed that the acidified portion (pH = 2.7) of the bicarbonate-based dialysate solution was passed through a pump with an aluminum housing, and aluminum was leached out of the pump and into the dialysate solution in concentrations exceeding 200 ppm and was present in the dialysis fluid [158].

Toxic Reactions

Chemicals in water or as residuals in dialysis fluid can affect dialysis patients. Certain chemicals in water may not be toxic when ingested by humans, but the hemodialysis patient may be exposed directly to 150 L of water per treatment. Two examples will illustrate this problem.

Occasionally, suppliers of community water change their water disinfection patterns by increasing chlorine dosages or by using monochloramine. These changes usually occur without the knowledge of the dialysis staff. Monochloramine (combined chlorine) in water used to prepare dialysis fluid must be removed or the patient will experience acute hemolysis. Patients will be exposed to this chemical if the correct water treatment system component (activated carbon) is not present or operating in the dialysis center. In one instance, a dialysis center changed from acetate to bicarbonate dialysate, adding an additional reverse osmosis unit and tanks for preparation and dilution of the dialysate. No changes were made to increase the capacity of the carbon filter, and within a few weeks, approximately 100 of the center's dialysis patients were exposed to chloramine-contaminated dialysate when the undersized carbon filters failed. A total of 41 patients required transfusion to treat hemolytic anemia caused by the chloramine exposure [34].

Another example of chemical intoxication occurred when a city water treatment plant accidentally fed excessive levels of fluoride into the community water supply, resulting in the death of one dialysis patient and acute illness in several other patients in a hemodialysis center receiving this community water supply. The center's water treatment system was not adequate to remove excessive fluoride from water [159].

In both of the preceding examples, a properly designed water treatment system consisting of adequate carbon filtration for the fluid flow and volume plus the use of reverse osmosis, deionization, and ultrafiltration would have prevented toxic reactions.

There also have been instances in which a disinfectant, such as formaldehyde, was not sufficiently removed from dialysis systems, and patients were exposed to the chemical.

TABLE 23-6

CDC-INVESTIGATED OUTBREAKS OF CHEMICAL INTOXICATIONS IN HEMODIALYSIS FACILITIES

Description	Cause(s) of Outbreak	Corrective Measure	Reference
Hemolytic anemia in 41 patients	Monochloramine in city water not removed completely by carbon filters	Size carbon adsorption media and place in series configuration (worker + polisher); monitor chloramines before each patient shift	[34]
Decreased hemoglobin in 3 pediatric patients	Disinfectant (30% hydrogen peroxide) not adequately rinsed from the water distribution system	Thoroughly rinse germicide from the system; use an appropriate test kit to confirm rinse out	[160]
Severe hypotension in 9 patients	Dialysate contaminated with sodium azide from new ultrafilters	Rinse system after modification or installation of new components; use equipment suitable for medical use	[161]
Aluminum intoxication in 27	Exhausted deionization tanks unable to remove aluminum from city water	Monitor deionization tanks daily; install reverse osmosis system	[162]
Formaldehyde intoxication in 5 patients, 1 death	Disinfectant not properly rinsed from the system	Eliminate stagnant flow areas; test for residual germicide	[163]
Aluminum intoxication in 27; 3 deaths	Aluminum pump was used to transfer acid concentrate to the treatment area	Use components that do not leach harmful substances into dialysis fluids.	[158]
Fluoride intoxication in 8; 1 death	Excess fluoride in city water; no water treatment by center	Install reverse osmosis system	[159]
Fluoride intoxication in 9 patients; 3 deaths	Exhausted deionization tanks discharge a bolus of fluoride	Deionization tanks should be monitored by resistivity meters with audible and visual alarms	[164, 165]
126 patients were exposed to microcystins in the dialysate; 47 patients died	Untreated water delivered to dialysis facility by tanker truck; by water system	Install appropriate water treatment equipment (granular activated carbon and reverse osmosis)	[166]
Sudden death in at least 50 patients in Spain, Croatia, Italy, Germany, Taiwan, Colombia and the United States	A perfluorohydrocarbon-based performance fluid used to detect in manufacturing the dialyzers was not adequately rinsed from all of the dialyzers	Improve quality control mechanisms at the manufacturing level before release of products; improve dialyzer priming at the facility level	[167, 168, CDC unpublished data, 2001]
16 patients exposed to volatile sulfur compounds, 2 deaths	Volatile sulfur-containing compounds (ie, methanethiol, carbon disulfide, dimethyldisulfide, and sulfur dioxide) were detected by gas chromatography and mass spectrometry in 8 of 12 water samples from the RO unit	Water treatment system including reverse osmosis system should be maintained; include distribution loop when disinfecting the reverse osmosis	[169]

This can be prevented by monitoring the system for complete rinsing using a chemical assay sensitive to the chemical.

A summary of toxic reactions in hemodialysis patients that have been investigated by the CDC is given in Table 23-6.

BLOOD BORNE VIRUSES: VIRAL HEPATITIS AND ACQUIRED IMMUNODEFICIENCY SYNDROME

Introduction

Shortly after the art and science of hemodialysis was institutionalized, it was recognized that both patients and staff members were at risk of acquiring viral hepatitis. The development and use of specific serologic testing identified HBV, and later HCV, as those most likely to be transmitted within the hemodialysis environment. Other blood borne pathogens that need to be considered as potentially transmissible in hemodialysis centers include hepatitis delta virus (HDV) and human immunodeficiency virus (HIV). The CDC has conducted 19 investigations involving the transmission of blood borne pathogens (Table 23-7). Hepatitis A virus (HAV), which is spread by the fecal-oral route and rarely by blood, has not been associated with hemodialysis.

Since HBV is the most efficiently transmitted blood borne virus in the dialysis setting, long-standing precautions developed for and shown to be effective in its control will be used, in part, as a model for the prevention of transmission of other blood borne infections. The primary rationale is that infection control practices that effectively control HBV transmission also would be effective

TABLE 23-7
TRANSMISSION OF BLOOD BORNE PATHOGENS IN HEMODIALYSIS FACILITIES

Description	Cause(s) of Outbreak	Corrective Measure	Reference
26 patients seroconverted to HBsAg positive over a 10-month period	Leakage of coil dialyzer membranes and use of a dialysis machine employing a recirculating bath	Separate HBsAg-positive patients and their equipment from other patients	[170]
19 Patients and 1 staff seroconverted to HBsAg positive during a 14-month period	No specific cause determined; false positive HBsAg results caused some susceptible patients to be dialyzed with HBsAg-positive patients	Laboratory confirmation of HBsAg-positive results; strict adherence to glove use and use of separate equipment	[171]
24 patients and 6 staff seroconvert to HBsAg positive during 10-month period	Staff not wearing gloves; surfaces not properly cleaned and disinfected; improper handling of needles/sharps resulting in many needlesticks	Separation of HBsAg-positive patients and equipment from other patients; proper precautions by staff (e.g. glove use; handling of needles/sharps)	[172]
13 patients and 1 staff seroconverted to HBsAg positive during a 1-month period	Extrinsic contamination of intravenous medication being prepared adjacent to area where blood work handled	Separate medication preparation area and blood processing for diagnostic tests	[173]
10 patients seroconverted from HBsAg positive in 1 month	Extrinsic contamination of a multidose intravenous medication vial shared by HBsAg-positive and negative patients	No sharing of supplies, equipment, and medications between patients	[174]
8 patients seroconverted to HBsAg positive during a 5-month period	Sporadic screening for HBsAg; HBsAg carriers not separated	Monthly screening of HBsAg-positive patients from other patients and have dedicated equipment and staff; vaccination of susceptible	[CDC unpublished data]
7 patients seroconverted to HBsAg positive during 3-month period	Same staff caring for HBsAg-positive and negative patients	Separation of HBsAg-positive patients from other patients; same staff should not care for HBsAg-positive and negative patients on the same shift	[175]
8 patients seroconverted to HBsAg positive during 1 month	Not consistently using pressure transducer protectors; same staff members cared for HBsAg-positive and negative patients on the same shift	Use pressure transducer protectors and replace after each use; same staff should not care for HBsAg-positive and negative patients on the same shift	[176]
14 patients seroconverted to HBsAg positive during a 6-week period	Failure to review results on admission and monthly HBsAg testing; inconsistent hand washing and use of gloves; adjacent clean and contaminated areas; <20% of patients vaccinated	Proper infection control precautions for dialysis units; routine review of serologic testing; hepatitis B vaccination of all susceptible patients	[177]
7 patients seroconvert to HBsAg positive during a 2-month period	Same staff member cared for both HBsAg-positive and negative patients on the same shift; common medication and supply carts were moved between patient stations, and medication vials were shared; no patients were vaccinated	Dedicate staff for HBsAg-positive patients; no sharing of medications or supplies between any patients; centralized medication and supply areas; hepatitis B vaccination of all susceptible patients	[177]
4 patients seroconverted to HBsAg positive during a 3-month period	Transmission appeared to occur during hospitalization at an acute facility	Vaccinated all susceptible patients against hepatitis B	[177]
11 patients seroconverted to HBsAg positive during a 3-month period	Staff, equipment, and supplies were shared between HBsAg-positive and negative patients; no patients vaccinated	Dedicate staff for HBsAg-positive patients; no sharing of medications or supplies between any patients; hepatitis B vaccination of all susceptible patients	[177]
2 patients seroconverted to HBsAg positive during a 4-month period	Same staff member cared for both HBsAg-positive and negative patients; no patients were vaccinated	Dedicate staff for HBsAg-positive patients; vaccinate all susceptible patients	[178]
36 patients with elevated liver enzymes consistent with non A, non-B hepatitis	Environmental contamination with blood	Monthly liver enzyme screening; proper precautions (i.e., gloves) by staff	[179]

TABLE 23-7
(CONTINUED)

Description	Cause(s) of Outbreak	Corrective Measure	Reference
35 patients with elevated liver enzymes consistent with non-A, non-B hepatitis during a 22-month period; 82% of probable cases were anti-HCV positive	Inconsistent use of infection control precautions, especially hand washing and glove use	Strict compliance to aseptic techniques and dialysis unit precautions	[180]
HCV infection developed in 7/41 (17.1%) patients; shift specific attack rates of 29% to 36%	Multidose vials left on top of machine and used by multiple patients; cleaning and disinfection of surfaces and equipment not routinely done; arterial lines for draining prime waste dropped into bucket that was not routinely cleaned or emptied between patients	Strict compliance with infection control precautions recommended for all patients; routine testing for HCV	[181]
HCV infection developed in 5/75 (6.7%) of patients	Sharing equipment and supplies between chronically infected and susceptible patients; gloves not routinely used; clean and contaminated areas not separated	Strict compliance with infection control precautions recommended for all patients	[182]
HCV infection developed in 3/23 (13%) of patients	Supply carts moved between stations and contained both clean supplies and blood-contaminated items; medications prepared in the same area used for disposal of used injection equipment	Strict compliance with infection control precautions recommended for all patients	[183]
13 patients found to be HIV positive; 9 seroconverted after the admission of a known HIV-positive patient	Access needles reprocessed by soaking in a common container with a low-level disinfectant, benzalkonium chloride; access needles reused on different patients	Do not reuse access needles	[184]
39 patients at 2 dialysis centers developed HIV infection	Sharing of syringes among patients was observed at both centers	Do not share syringes between patients; infection control guidelines for hemodialysis settings	[185]

for other blood borne viruses such as HCV and HIV because their efficiency of transmission is much less than that of HBV.

Viral Hepatitis

Hepatitis B Virus

Epidemiology

Hepatitis B Virus (HBV) is transmitted by percutaneous or per mucosal exposure to infectious blood or body fluids that contain blood. Hepatitis B surface antigen (HBsAg)-positive persons who also are positive for hepatitis B e antigen (HBeAg) have an extraordinary level of HBV circulating in their blood, approximately 10^8 virions per milliliter. With virus titers this high, body fluids containing serum or blood also may contain appreciable levels of HBV, and HBV can be present on environmental surfaces in the absence of any visible blood and still contain 10^2–10^3 infectious virions per milliliter [186]. Furthermore, HBV is relatively stable in the environment, and has been shown to remain viable for at least 7 days on environmental surfaces at room temperature [187]. Thus, wherever there is a good deal of blood exposure, the risk of HBV transmission can be high if proper control measures are not practiced. This is especially true in a hemodialysis center setting.

In the past, HBV infection could be acquired by patients in a dialysis unit by transfusion of infectious blood or blood products. This is very unlikely now since all blood is screened for HBsAg and antibody to hepatitis B core antigen (anti-HBc) and with the use of erythropoietin in dialysis patients. Dialysis patients, once infected, frequently become chronically infected but asymptomatic and are sources of HBV contamination of many environmental surfaces.

Given the extraordinarily high level of HBV in blood, the various modes of HBV transmission can be categorized based on efficiency as follows:

1. Direct percutaneous inoculation of HBV by needle from contaminated blood, serum, or plasma.
2. Percutaneous transfer of blood, serum, or plasma, such as may occur through cuts, scratches, abrasions, or other breaks in the skin.

3. Transfer of infected blood, serum, or plasma onto mucosal surfaces such as may occur through inadvertent introduction of these fluids into the mouth or eyes.
4. Introduction of other known infectious secretions, such as saliva and peritoneal fluid, onto mucosal surfaces.
5. Indirect transfer of HBV from blood, serum, or plasma by means of environmental surface contamination.

There is no epidemiologic or laboratory evidence of airborne HBV transmission [188,189], and no disease transmission occurs by the intestinal route. Splashes of infectious blood that enter the oral cavity may result in HBV infection because the virus enters the vascular system through the buccal cavity but not the intestinal tract.

V transmission can occur by a number of routes in the hemodialysis center setting. Staff members may become infected with HBV through accidental needle punctures or breaks in their skin or mucous membranes. These staff members have frequent and continuous contact with blood and blood-contaminated surfaces. Dialysis patients may acquire HBV infection in several ways, including (1) internally contaminated dialysis equipment (e.g., venous pressure gauges or venous pressure isolators or filters used to prevent reflux of blood into gauges) not routinely changed after each use, (2) injections (by contamination of the site of injection or the material being injected), or (3) breaks in the skin or mucous membranes that have contact with blood-contaminated objects. Patients who are dialyzed in centers that routinely reuse dialyzers are not at increased risk of HBV infection because of this practice [190].

There is no documentation that HBV has been transmitted from infected hemodialysis staff members to dialysis patients. Hypothetically, this route of transmission is possible but not likely because infectious blood and body fluids of dialysis personnel are not readily accessible to patients. However, dialysis staff members may physically carry HBV from infected patients to susceptible patients by means of contaminated hands, gloves, and other objects.

Environmental surfaces in the hemodialysis center can play a role in HBV transmission. It has been shown that HBsAg, which is considered a "footprint" of HBV, can be detected on environmental surfaces (especially those often touched) in dialysis center settings [186]. For example, HBsAg has been detected on clamps, scissors, dialysis machine control knobs, doorknobs, and other surfaces. If these surfaces or objects are not cleaned or disinfected frequently and are shared among patients using the same or neighboring machines, an almost unnoticeable infection transmission route is created. Although dialysis staff members may routinely change gloves after caring for each patient, a new pair of gloves can become contaminated when the staff member touches surfaces previously contaminated with blood from an HBsAg-positive patient. HBV can be transmitted from patient to patient when a staff member wearing the contaminated gloves searches for

the patient's best site of injection by applying finger pressure or by otherwise contaminating that site before injection. When donning a pair of new gloves, staff members should refrain from touching any environmental surfaces before performing the injection on the patient. Other environmental sources of contamination include shared items, such as multiple dose medication vials that can become contaminated with blood and serve as sources of patient-to-patient transmission.

This potential for the environmentally mediated mode of virus transmission rather than any phenomenon dealing with internal contamination of dialysis machines is the basis for the infection control strategies recommended for preventing HBV transmission in dialysis centers.

Surveillance data from the CDC show that, between 1972 and 1974, the incidence of HBsAg positivity among patients or staff increased by >100% to 6.2% and 5.2%, respectively [191,192]. In a separate survey of 15 hemodialysis centers during the same 2-year period, Szmuness et al. [193] showed that the point prevalence of a positive test for HBsAg was 16.8% among patients and 2.4% among staff. During this time, HBV infection in dialysis units had become highly endemic, and outbreaks were common because of the presence of chronically infected patients who were asymptomatic, the absence of sufficient disease and serologic surveillance systems to detect these chronic infections, and the lack of infection control measures to prevent transmission [170,172].

Subsequently, infection control strategies were developed to incorporated precautions for preventing exposures to blood and body fluids among both patients and staff with several extra precautions [194]. As will be discussed, these extra precautions included routinely testing all dialysis patients and staff members for HBsAg, dialyzing HBsAg-positive patients in separate areas or rooms in the dialysis center using dedicated dialysis machines and staff, rather than including HBsAg-positive patients in dialyzer reuse programs.

Continued nationwide surveillance by the CDC found that, by 1983, the incidence of HBV infection had declined to 0.5% among both patients and staff members [195]. Over the same period, the proportion of centers using separation practices increased from 75% to 86%, and the proportion of centers that screened patients monthly for HBsAg increased from 57% to 84%. In addition, the risk of acquiring HBV infection for patients was shown to be highest in those centers that provided dialysis to HBsAg-positive patients but did not separate these patients by room and machine. Other investigators also have shown that segregation of HBsAg-positive patients and their equipment reduces the incidence of HBV infection in hemodialysis units [196,197]. The success of separation practices in preventing HBV transmission can be linked to other control recommendations, including frequent serologic surveillance. Routine serologic surveillance facilitates the rapid identification of patients who become HBsAg-positive, which allows for the rapid implementation of isolation procedures before cross-infection can occur.

In 2002, the prevalence of HBsAg positivity among patients was 1.0%, a figure that has not changed substantially during the past decade. Similarly, the incidence of HBV infection in hemodialysis patients has not changed substantially during the past decade and in 2002 was 0.12% [2]. In 1994, an increasing number of centers reported to CDC episodes of HBV transmission among their patients. During a 5-month period in 1994 alone, five HBV outbreaks in chronic hemodialysis centers were investigated by CDC and/or state and local health authorities [177]. All were the result of failure to follow ≥1 recommended infection control practices for the prevention of HBV transmission in these settings including the failure to routinely screen patients for HBsAg or routinely review results of testing to detect infected patients; assignment of staff to the simultaneous care of infected and susceptible patients; and sharing supplies, particularly multidose medication vials, among patients. These same factors have typically been responsible for most other hemodialysis-associated HBV outbreaks reported in the past [170,172,175]. In addition, few patients in these centers had received HBV vaccine. Although HBV vaccine has been recommended for all hemodialysis patients since it became available in 1982, it has been shown to reduce the costs of serologic screening [198]. From 1983–2002, the percentage that had ever received at least three doses of HBV vaccine increased from 5.4% to 56% among patients and from 26.1% to 90% among staff [2]. As these outbreaks illustrate, the generally low incidence of HBV infection among hemodialysis patients does not preclude the need to maintain infection control measures that were specifically formulated to prevent the transmission of blood borne pathogens in these settings.

Screening and Diagnostic Tests

Several well-defined antigen-antibody systems are associated with HBV infection, including HBsAg and anti-HBs; hepatitis B core antigen (HBcAg) and anti-HBc; and HBeAg and antibody to HBeAg (anti-HBe). Serologic assays are commercially available for all of these except HBcAg because no free HBcAg circulates in blood. One or more of these serologic markers are present during different phases of HBV infection (Table 23-8) [199].

The presence of HBsAg indicates ongoing HBV infection and potential infectiousness. In newly infected persons, HBsAg is present in serum 30–60 days after exposure to HBV and persists for variable periods. Transient HBsAg positivity (lasting <18 days) can be detected in some patients during vaccination [200,201]. Anti-HBc develops in all HBV infections, appearing at onset of symptoms or liver test abnormalities in acute HBV infection, rising rapidly to high levels, and persisting for life. Acute or recently acquired infection can be distinguished by the presence of the immunoglobulin M (IgM) class of anti-HBc, which persists for approximately 6 months.

TABLE 23-8
INTERPRETATION OF SEROLOGIC TEST RESULTS FOR HEPATITIS B VIRUS INFECTION

Serological Markers

HBsAg[a]	Total Anti-HBc[b]	IgM[c] Anti-HBc	Anti-HBS[d]	Interpretation
—	—	—	—	Susceptible, never infected
+	—	—	—	Acute infection, early incubation[e]
+	+	+	—	Acute infection
—	+	+	—	Acute resolving infection
—	+	—	+	Past infection, recovered and immune
+	+	—	—	Chronic infection
—	+	—	—	False positive (i.e., susceptible), past infection, or "low-level" chronic infection
—	—	—	+	Immune if titer is >10 mIU/mL

[a]Hepatitis B surface antigen.
[b]Antibody to hepatitis B core antigen.
[c]Immunoglobulin M.
[d]Antibody to hepatitis B surface antigen.
[e]Transient HBsAg positivity (lasting <18 days) might be detected in some patients during vaccination.

In persons who recover from HBV infection, HBsAg is eliminated from the blood, usually in 2–3 months, and anti-HBs develop during convalescence. The presence of anti-HBs indicates immunity from HBV infection. After recovery from natural infection, most persons will be positive for both anti-HBs and anti-HBc whereas only anti-HBs develop in persons who are successfully HBV vaccinated. Persons who do not recover from HBV infection and become chronically infected remain positive for HBsAg (and anti-HBc), although a small proportion (0.3% per year) eventually clear HBsAg and might develop anti-HBs [202].

In some persons, the only HBV serologic marker detected is anti-HBc (i.e., isolated anti-HBc). Among most asymptomatic persons in the United States tested for HBV infection, an average of 2% (range: <0.1–6%) test positive for isolated anti-HBc [203]; among injecting-drug users, however, the rate is 24% [204]. In general, the frequency of isolated anti-HBc is directly related to the frequency of previous HBV infection in the population and can have several explanations. This pattern can occur after HBV infection among persons who have recovered but whose anti-HBs levels have waned or among persons who failed to develop anti-HBs. Persons in the latter category include those who circulate HBsAg at levels not detectable by current commercial assays. However, HBV DNA has been detected in <10% of persons with isolated anti-HBc, and these persons are unlikely to be infectious to others except under unusual circumstances involving direct percutaneous exposure to large quantities of blood (e.g., transfusion) [205]. In most persons with isolated anti-HBc, the result appears to be a false positive. Data from several studies have demonstrated that a primary anti-HBs response develops in most of these persons after a three-dose series of HBV vaccine [206,207]. No published data exist on response to HBV vaccination among hemodialysis patients with this serologic pattern.

A third antigen, HBeAg, can be detected in serum of persons with acute or chronic HBV infection. The presence of HBeAg correlates with viral replication and high levels of virus (i.e., high infectivity). Anti-HBe correlates with the loss of replicating virus and with lower levels of virus. However, all HBsAg-positive persons should be considered potentially infectious, regardless of their HBeAg or anti-HBe status.

Hepatitis C

Epidemiology

Data are limited on the current incidence or prevalence of HCV infection among maintenance hemodialysis patients. In 2002, 63% of dialysis centers tested patients for anti-HCV, and 11.5% reported having ≥1 patient who became anti-HCV positive in 2002 The incidence rate in 2002 was 0.34%; among centers that tested for anti-HCV, the prevalence of anti-HCV among patients was 7.8%, a decrease of 25.7% since 1995 [2]. In the facilities that tested, the reported incidence was 0.34%, and the prevalence was 7.8% (range among ESRD networks, 5.7% to 9.8%). Only 11.5% of dialysis facilities reported newly acquired HCV infection among their patients. Higher incidence rates have been reported from cohort studies of U.S. dialysis patients (<1–3%), Japan (<2%), or Europe (3–10%) [208–216]. Higher prevalence rates (10–76%) also have been reported in individual facilities [208,217–222].

HCV is most efficiently transmitted by direct percutaneous exposure to blood, and like HBV, the chronically infected person is central to the epidemiology of HCV transmission. Hemodialysis staff members have rates of anti-HCV comparable to those (1–2%) reported in other healthcare workers [223]. Risk factors associated with HCV infection among hemodialysis patients include blood transfusions from unscreened donors and years on dialysis [208,219,224,225]. The number of years on dialysis is the major risk factor that is independently associated with higher HCV infection rates. As the time patients spent on dialysis increased, their prevalence of HCV infection increased from an average of 12% for patients receiving dialysis <5 years to an average of 37% for patients receiving dialysis >5 years [208,219,226,227].

These studies and investigations of dialysis-associated HCV outbreaks indicate that HCV transmission most likely occurs because of inadequate infection control practices. During 1999 to 2000, CDC investigated three outbreaks of HCV infection among patients in chronic hemodialysis centers [CDC, unpublished data, 1999, 2000]. In two of the outbreaks, multiple HCV transmissions occurred during periods of 16–24 months (attack rates: 6.6–17.5%), and seroconversions were associated with receiving dialysis immediately after a chronically infected patient. Multiple opportunities for cross-contamination among patients were observed including (1) equipment and supplies that were not disinfected between patient use, (2) use of common medication carts to prepare and distribute medications at patient stations, (3) sharing of multidose vials, which were placed at patients' stations on the top of the hemodialysis machine, (4) contaminated priming buckets that were not routinely changed or cleaned and disinfected between patients; (5) machine surfaces that were not routinely cleaned and disinfected between patients; and (6) blood spills that were not cleaned up promptly. In the third outbreak, there were multiple infections clustered at one point in time (attack rate of 27%), suggesting a common exposure event. Multiple opportunities for cross-contamination from chronically infected patients also were observed in this unit. In particular, supply carts were moved from station to station and contained both clean supplies and blood-contaminated items, including small biohazard containers, sharps disposal boxes, and used Vacutainers containing patients' blood.

Other risk factors for acquiring HCV include injection drug use, exposure to an HCV-infected sexual partner or household contact, multiple sexual partners, and perinatal exposure [223,228]. The efficiency of transmission in settings involving sexual or household exposure to infected contacts is low, and the magnitude of risk and the circumstances under which these exposures result in transmission are not well defined.

Screening and Diagnostic Tests

FDA-licensed or approved anti-HCV screening tests used in the United States comprise three immunoassays; two enzyme immunoassays (EIA) and one enhanced chemiluminescence immunoassay (CIA) [229,230]. Although no true confirmatory test has been developed, supplemental tests for specificity are available. The FDA-licensed or approved supplemental tests include a serologic anti-HCV assay, the strip immunoblot assay (Chiron RIBA® HCV 3.0 SIA, Chiron Corp., Emeryville, California), and nucleic acid tests (NAT) for HCV RNA (including reverse transcriptase polymerase chain reaction [RT-PCR] amplification [231] and transcription mediated amplification [TMA]).

Anti-HCV testing includes initial screening with an EIA immunoassay. However, interpretation of the results of EIAs that screen for anti-HCV is limited by several factors: (1) these assays will not detect anti-HCV in approximately 10% of persons infected with HCV, (2) these assays do not distinguish between acute, chronic, or past infection,

(3) in the acute phase of hepatitis C, the interval between onset of illness and seroconversion may be prolonged, and (4) in populations with a low prevalence of infection, the rate of false positivity for anti-HCV is high. If the screening test is positive, supplemental testing with a test with high specificity should be performed to verify the results. Among hemodialysis patients, the proportion of false-positive screening test results averages approximately 15% [229]. For this reason, one should not rely exclusively on a positive anti-HCV screening test to determine whether a person has been infected with HCV.

Routine testing of hemodialysis patients for anti-HCV on admission and every 6 months thereafter has been recommended since 2001 [232]. For routine HCV testing of hemodialysis patients, the anti-HCV screening immunoassay is recommended, and if positive, supplemental anti HCV testing using RIBA (Table 23-9). RIBA is recommended rather than NAT because serologic assay can be performed on the same serum or plasma sample collected for the screening anti-HCV screening assay. In addition, in certain situations, the HCV RNA result can be negative in persons with active infection. As the titer of anti-HCV increases during acute infection, the titer of HCV RNA declines [233]. Thus, HCV RNA is not detectable in certain persons during the acute phase of their infection, but this finding can be transient and chronic infection can develop [234]. In addition, intermittent HCV positivity has been observed among patients with chronic HCV infection [235–237]. Therefore, the significance of a single negative HCV RNA result is unknown, and the need for further investigation or follow-up is determined by verifying anti-HCV status. Detection of HCV RNA also requires that serum or plasma sample be collected and handled in a manner suitable for NAT and that testing be performed in a laboratory with appropriate facilities established for NAT testing [229]. Although in rare instances, detection of HCV RNA might be the only evidence of HCV infection, a recent study conducted among almost 3,000 U.S. hemodialysis patients found that only 0.07% were HCV RNA positive but antibody negative [CDC, unpublished data].

Delta Hepatitis

Delta hepatitis is caused by the HDV, a relatively small defective virus that causes infection only in persons

TABLE 23-9

RECOMMENDATIONS FOR REPORTING RESULTS OF TESTING FOR ANTIBODY TO HEPATITIS C VIRUS (ANTI-HCV) BY TYPE OF REFLEX SUPPLEMENTAL TESTING PERFORMED

Anti-HCV Screening Test Result	Supplemental Test Result	Interpretation	Comments
Negative	Not applicable	Anti-HCV-negative	Not infected with HCV unless recent infection is suspected or other evidence exists to indicate HCV infection
Positive with high signal-to-cut-off ration	Not done	Anti-HCV-positive	Probably indicates past or present infection; supplemental serological testing not performed; samples with high signal-to-cut-off rations usually ($\geq$95%) confirm positive, but <5 of every 100 might represent false positives; more specific testing may be requested if indicated.
Positive	Recombinant immunoblot assay (RIBA®) positive	Anti-HCV positive	Indicates past or present HCV infection
Positive	RIBA negative	Anti-HCV negative	Not infected with HCV unless recent infection is suspected or other evidence exists to indicate HCV infection
Positive	RIBA indeterminate	Anti-HCV indeterminate	HCV antibody and infection status cannot be determined; another sample should be collected for repeat anti-HCV testing (>1 month) or for HCV RNA testing
Positive	Nucleic acid test (NAT) positive	Anti-HCV positive, HCV-RNA positive	Indicates active HCV infection
Positive	NAT negative RIBA positive	Anti-HCV positive, HCV-RNA negative	Presence of anti-HCV indicates past or present infection; single negative HCV-RNA result does not rule out active infection
Positive	NAT negative RIBA negative	Anti-HCV negative, HCV-RNA negative	Not infected with HCV
Positive	NAT negative RIBA indeterminate	Anti-HCV indeterminate, HCV-RNA negative	Screening test anti-HCV result probable false positive, which indicates no HCV infection

with active HBV infection. The prevalence of HDV infection is low in the United States with rates <1% among HBsAg-positive persons in the general population and >10% among HBsAg-positive persons with repeated percutaneous exposures (e.g., injecting drug users, persons with hemophilia) [238]. Areas of the world with high endemic rates of HDV infection include southern Italy, parts of Africa, and the Amazon basin.

Few data exist on the prevalence of HDV infection among chronic hemodialysis patients; a few studies have reported nonexistent to low prevalence among hemodialysis patients [239,240]. In endemic areas, prevalence rates may be relatively high among hemodialysis patients who are HBsAg-positive [241]. Only one transmission of HDV has been reported in the United States [242]. In this episode, transmission occurred from a patient who was chronically infected with HBV and HDV to an HBsAg-positive patient after a massive bleeding incident; both patients received dialysis at the same station.

HDV infection may occur as either co-infection with HBV or as a superinfection in a person with chronic HBV infection. Co-infections usually resolve, but superinfection frequently results in chronic HDV infection and severe disease. High mortality rates are associated with both types of infection. A serologic test that measures total antibody to HDV is commercially available.

Human Immunodeficiency Virus (HIV) Infection

During 1985–2002, the U.S. hemodialysis centers that reported providing chronic hemodialysis for patients with HIV infection increased from 11% to 39%, and the patients with known HIV infection increased from 0.3% to 1.5% [2]. Although the proportion of patients with HIV infection has remained fairly stable during the past decade, the number of infected patients has increased, as has the number of centers treating patients with HIV infection. HIV is transmitted by blood and other body fluids that contain blood. No patient-to-patient transmission of HIV has been reported in a U.S. hemodialysis center. However, there have been reports of transmission of HIV among patients in other countries. All of these outbreaks have been attributed to several breaks in infection control: (1) reusing access needles and inadequately disinfected equipment [184], (2) sharing of syringes among patients [185], and (3) sharing dialyzers among different patients [243]. HIV infection usually is diagnosed with assays that measure antibody to HIV, and a repeatedly positive EIA test should be confirmed by Western blot or other confirmatory test.

PREVENTING INFECTIONS AMONG CHRONIC HEMODIALYSIS PATIENTS

Preventing transmission among chronic hemodialysis patients of blood borne viruses and pathogenic bacteria from both recognized and unrecognized sources of infection requires implementation of a comprehensive infection control program. The components of such a program include infection control practices specifically designed for the hemodialysis setting, including routine serologic testing and immunization, surveillance, and training and education. CDC has published recommendations describing these components in detail [232].

The infection control practices recommended for hemodialysis units (Table 23-10) will reduce opportunities for patient-to-patient transmission of infectious agents, directly or indirectly via contaminated devices, equipment and supplies, environmental surfaces, and hands of personnel. These practices should be carried out routinely for all patients in the chronic hemodialysis setting because of the increased potential for blood contamination during hemodialysis and because many patients are colonized or infected with pathogenic bacteria.

Such practices include additional measures to prevent HBV transmission because of the high titer of HBV and its ability to survive on environmental surfaces (Table 23-10). The potential for environmentally mediated transmission of HBV rather than internal contamination of dialysis machines is the focus of infection control strategies for preventing HBV transmission in dialysis centers. For patients at increased risk for transmission of pathogenic bacteria, including antimicrobial-resistant strains, additional precautions also might be necessary in some circumstances. Furthermore, surveillance for infections and other adverse events is required to monitor the effectiveness of infection control practices, and training and education of both staff members and patients are critical to ensure that appropriate infection control behaviors and techniques are fully implemented.

In each chronic hemodialysis unit, policies and practices should be reviewed and updated to ensure that infection control practices recommended for hemodialysis units are implemented and rigorously followed. Intensive efforts must be made to educate new staff members and reeducate existing staff members regarding these practices. Readers should consult the CDC recommendations for details on these practices [232].

Routine Testing

All chronic hemodialysis patients should be routinely tested for HBV and HCV infection and the results promptly reviewed to ensure that patients are managed appropriately based on their testing results (Tables 23-10, 23-11). Test results (positive and negative) must be communicated to other units or hospitals when patients are transferred for care. Routine testing for HDV and HIV infection for purposes of infection control is not recommended.

Before admission to the hemodialysis unit, the HBV serologic status (i.e., HBsAg, total anti-HBc, and anti-HBs) of all patients should be known. Test results for patients

TABLE 23-10

RECOMMENDATIONS FOR PREVENTING INFECTIONS IN HEMODIALYSIS CENTERS

Infection control precautions for all patients

Wear disposable gloves when caring for the patient or touching the patient's equipment at the dialysis station; remove gloves and perform hand hygiene between each patient or station.

Items taken into the dialysis station should be disposed of, dedicated for use only on a single patient, or cleaned and disinfected before being taken to a common clean area or used on another patient.

When multiple-dose medication vials are used (including vials containing diluents), prepare individual patient doses in a clean (centralized) area away from dialysis stations and deliver separately to each patient. Do not carry multiple-dose medication vials from station to station.

Do not use common medication carts to deliver medications to patients. Do not carry medication vials, syringes, alcohol swabs, or supplies in pockets. If trays are used to deliver medications to individual patients, they must be cleaned between patients.

Clean areas should be clearly designated for the preparation, handling, and storage of medications and unused supplies and equipment. Clean areas should be clearly separated from contaminated areas where used supplies and equipment are handled. Do not handle and store medications or clean supplies in the same or an adjacent area where used equipment or blood samples are handled.

Use external venous and arterial pressure transducer protectors for each patient treatment to prevent blood contamination of the dialysis machines' pressure monitors. Change the external transducer protectors between each patient treatment, and do not reuse them. Internal transducer protectors do not need to be changed routinely between patients.

Clean and disinfect the dialysis station, all frequently touched surfaces. Discard all fluid and clean and disinfect all surfaces and containers associated with the prime waste (including chairs, beds, tables, machines, buckets attached to the machines) between patients.

For dialyzers and blood tubing that will be reprocessed, cap dialyzer ports and clamp tubing. Place all used dialyzers and tubing in leak proof containers for transport from station to reprocessing or disposal area.

Vaccinate all susceptible patients against hepatitis B; test for anti-HBs 1–2 months after last dose. If <10 mIU/ml consider patient susceptible, revaccinate with an additional three doses, and retest for anti-HBs. If ≥10 mIU/ml, consider patient immune, and retest annually. Give booster dose of vaccine if anti-HBs declines to <10 mIU/mL and continue to retest annually.

Additional precautions of HBsAg-positive patients

Dialyze HBsAg-positive patients in a separate room using separate machines, equipment, instruments, and supplies.

Staff members caring for HBsAg positive patients should not care for HBV-susceptible patients at the same time (e.g., during the same shift or during patient changeover).

TABLE 23-11

SCHEDULE FOR ROUTINE TESTING FOR HEPATITIS B VIRUS (HBV) AND HEPATITIS C VIRUS (HCV) INFECTIONS

Patient Status	On Admission	Monthly	Semiannual	Annual
All patients	HBsAg,[a] Anti-HBc[a] (total), Anti-HBs,[a] Anti-HCV, ALT[b]			
HBV susceptible, including nonresponders to vaccine		HBsAg		
Anti-HBs positive (≥10 milli-International Units/ml), anti-HBc negative				Anti-HBs
Anti-HBs and anti-HBc positive		No additional HBV testing needed		
Anti-HCV negative		ALT	Anti-HCV	

[a]Results of HBV testing should be known before the patient begins dialysis.

[b]HBsAg, hepatitis B surface antigen; anti-HBc, antibody to hepatitis B core antigen; anti-HBs, antibody to hepatitis B surface antigen; anti-HCV, antibody to hepatitis C virus; ALT, alanine aminotransferase.

transferred from another unit should be obtained before hand. If a patient's HBV serologic status is not known at the time of admission, testing should be completed within 7 days. The hemodialysis unit should ensure that the laboratory performing the testing for anti-HBs can detect a 10 milli-International Units per mL (mIU/mL) concentration to determine protective levels of antibody.

Routine HCV testing should include the use of both a screening immunoassay to test for anti-HCV and supplemental or confirmatory testing with an additional, more specific assay. Use of NAT for HCV RNA as the primary test for routine screening is not recommended because few HCV infections will be identified in anti-HCV negative patients. However, if ALT levels are persistently abnormal in anti-HCV negative patients in the absence of another etiology, testing for HCV RNA should be considered. Blood samples collected for NAT should not contain heparin, which interferes with the accurate performance of this assay.

HBV vaccination is an essential component of prevention in the hemodialysis setting. All susceptible patients and staff should receive HBV vaccine. Susceptible patients who have not yet received HBV vaccine, are in the process of being vaccinated, or have not adequately responded to vaccination should continue to be tested regularly for HBsAg. Detailed recommendations for vaccination and follow-up of hemodialysis patients have been published elsewhere [232].

Management of Infected Patients

HBV

HBsAg-positive patients should undergo dialysis in a separate room designated only for them. They should use separate machines, equipment, and supplies, and—most important—staff members should not care for both HBsAg-positive and susceptible patients at the same time or while the HBsAg-positive patient is in the treatment area. Dialyzers should not be reused on HBsAg-positive patients. Because HBV is efficiently transmitted through occupational exposure to blood, reprocessing dialyzers from HBsAg-positive patients might place HBV-susceptible staff members at increased risk for infection.

HBV chronically infected patients (i.e., those who are HBsAg positive, total anti-HBc positive, and IgM anti-HBc negative) are infectious to others and are at risk for chronic liver disease. These patients should be counseled regarding preventing transmission to others, and their household and sexual partners should receive HBV vaccine and should be evaluated (by consultation or referral, if appropriate) for the presence or development of chronic liver disease according to current medical practice guidelines. Persons with chronic liver disease should be vaccinated against HAV if susceptible.

HBV chronically infected patients do not require any routine follow-up testing for purposes of infection control. However, annual testing for HBsAg is reasonable to detect the small percentage of HBV-infected patients who might lose their HBsAg.

HCV

HCV-positive patients do not have to be isolated from other patients or dialyzed separately on dedicated machines. The purpose of routine testing is to monitor potential transmission within centers and ensure that appropriate practices are being properly and consistently used. Furthermore, HCV-positive patients can participate in dialyzer reuse programs. Unlike HBV, HCV is not transmitted efficiently through occupational exposures. Thus, reprocessing dialyzers from HCV-positive patients should not place staff members at increased risk for infection.

HCV-positive persons should be evaluated (by consultation or referral, if appropriate) for the presence or development of chronic liver disease according to current medical practice guidelines. They also should receive information concerning how they can prevent further harm to their liver and prevent transmitting HCV to others [244,245]. Persons with chronic liver disease should be vaccinated against HAV if susceptible.

HDV

Because HDV depends on an HBV-infected host for replication, prevention of HBV infection will prevent HDV infection in a person susceptible to it. Patients known to be infected with HDV should be isolated from all other dialysis patients, especially those who are HBsAg positive.

HIV

Infection control precautions recommended for all hemodialysis patients are sufficient to prevent HIV transmission between/among patients. HIV-infected patients do not have to be isolated from other patients or dialyzed separately on dedicated machines. In addition, they can participate in dialyzer reuse programs. Because HIV is not transmitted efficiently through occupational exposures, reprocessing dialyzers from HIV-positive patients should not place staff members at increased risk for infection.

Bacterial/Fungal Infections

Contact transmission can be prevented by hand hygiene [246], glove use, and disinfection of environmental surfaces. Infection control precautions recommended for all hemodialysis patients are adequate to prevent transmission for most patients infected/colonized with pathogenic bacteria, including antimicrobial-resistant strains. However, additional precautions should be considered for treatment of patients who might be at increased risk for transmitting pathogenic bacteria. Such patients include those with either an infected skin wound with drainage that is not contained by dressings (the drainage does not have to be culture positive for MRSA, VRE, or any specific pathogen) or fecal incontinence or diarrhea uncontrolled with personal hygiene measures. For these patients, consider using the following additional precautions: (1) staff members treating the patient should wear a separate gown over their usual clothing and remove the gown when finished caring for the patient and (2) dialyze the patient at a station with as few adjacent stations as possible (e.g., at the end or corner of the unit) [232].

Vancomycin is used commonly in dialysis patients in part because vancomycin can be conveniently administered to patients when they come in for hemodialysis treatments. Prudent antimicrobial use is an important component of preventing the spread of vancomycin resistance [247]. This CDC guideline states that vancomycin is not indicated for therapy (chosen for dosing convenience) of infections due to ß-lactam sensitive gram-positive microorganisms in patients with renal failure. Depending on the situation, alternative antimicrobials (e.g., cephalosporins) with dosing intervals >48 hours, which would allow postdialytic dosing, could be used. Recent studies suggest that cefazolin given three times a week in the dialysis unit provides adequate blood levels and could be used to treat many infections in hemodialysis patients [248,249].

Disinfection, Sterilization, and Environmental Hygiene

Good cleaning, disinfection, and sterilization procedures are important components of infection control in the hemodialysis center. The procedures do not differ from those recommended for other healthcare settings [250, 251], but the high potential for blood contamination makes the hemodialysis setting unique. Additionally, the need for routine aseptic access of the patient's vascular system makes the hemodialysis unit more similar to a surgical suite than to a standard hospital room. Medical items are categorized as critical (e.g., needles and catheters), which are introduced directly into the bloodstream or normally sterile areas of the body; semicritical (e.g., fiberoptic endoscopes), which come in contact with intact mucous membranes; and noncritical (e.g., blood pressure cuffs), which touch only intact skin [246,250].

Cleaning and housekeeping in the dialysis center have two goals: to remove soil and waste on a regular basis, thereby preventing the accumulation of potentially infectious material, and to maintain an environment that is conducive to good patient care. Crowding patients and overtaxing staff members may increase the likelihood of microbial transmission. Adequate cleaning may be difficult if there are multiple wires, tubes, and hoses in a small area. There should be enough space to move completely around each patient's dialysis station without interfering with the neighboring stations. When space is limited, the following can improve accessibility for cleaning: eliminating unneeded items; arranging required items in an orderly manner; and removing excess lengths of tubes, hoses, and wires from the floor. Because of the special requirements for cleaning in the dialysis center, staff should be specially trained in this task.

After each patient treatment, frequently touched environmental surfaces, including external surfaces of the dialysis machine, should be cleaned (with a good detergent) or disinfected (with a detergent germicide). It is the cleaning step that is important for interrupting the cross-contamination transmission routes. Antiseptics, such as formulations with povidone iodine, hexachlorophene, or chlorhexidine, should not be used because they are formulated for use on skin and are not designed for use on hard surfaces.

There is no evidence that medical waste is any more infectious than residential waste or has caused disease in the community [252]. Wastes from a hemodialysis center that are actually or potentially contaminated with blood should be considered infectious and handled accordingly. Eventually, these items of solid waste should be disposed of properly in an incinerator or sanitary landfill, depending on state or local laws.

Standard protocols for sterilization and disinfection are adequate for processing any items or devices contaminated with blood. Historically, there has been a tendency to use "overkill" strategies for instrument sterilization or disinfection and housekeeping protocols. This is not necessary. The floors in a dialysis center are routinely contaminated with blood, but the protocol for floor cleaning is the same as for floors in other healthcare settings. Usually, this involves the use of a good detergent germicide; the formulation can contain a low or intermediate level disinfectant.

Blood borne viruses, such as HBV and HIV, are inactivated by any standard sterilization systems such as standard steam autoclave cycles of 121°C (249.8°F) for 15 minutes, ethylene oxide gas [250], and low temperature hydrogen peroxide gas plasma [253]. Large blood spills should be cleaned to remove visible material, and then the area should receive low- to intermediate-level disinfection after the directions of the germicide manufacturer.

Blood and other specimens, such as peritoneal fluid, from all patients should be handled with care. Peritoneal fluid can contain high levels of HBV and should be handled in the same manner as the patient's blood. Consequently, if the center performs peritoneal dialysis, the same criteria for separating HBsAg-positive patients who are undergoing hemodialysis apply to those undergoing peritoneal dialysis.

HBV has not been grown in tissue cultures, and without a viral assay system, studies on the precise resistance of this virus to various chemical germicides and heat have not been performed. However, the resistance of HBV to both heat and chemical germicides may approach that of some other viruses and bacteria, but certainly not that of the bacterial endospore or the tubercle bacillus. Furthermore, studies have shown that HBV is not resistant to commonly used high level and intermediate level disinfectants [254,255].

Blood contamination of venous pressure monitors has been implicated in HBV transmission [176]. Therefore, if venous pressure transducer filters are used, they should not be reused.

In single-pass artificial kidney machines, the internal fluid pathways are not subject to contamination with blood. Although the fluid pathways that exhaust dialysis fluid from the dialyzer may become contaminated with blood in the event of a dialyzer leak, it is unlikely that this blood contamination will reach a subsequent patient. Therefore, disinfection and rinsing procedures should be designed to control contamination with bacterial rather than blood borne pathogens.

For dialysis machines that use a dialysate recirculating system (e.g., some ultrafiltration control machines and those that regenerate the dialysate), a blood leak in a dialyzer, especially a massive leak, can result in contamination of a number of surfaces that will contact the dialysis fluid of subsequent patients. However, the procedures that are normally practiced after each use of a recirculating machine—draining of the dialysis fluid, subsequent rinsing, and disinfection—will reduce the level of contamination below infectious levels. In addition, an intact dialyzer membrane will not allow passage of bacteria or viruses. Consequently, if a blood leak does occur with either type of dialysis machine, the standard disinfection procedure used for machines in the dialysis center to control bacterial contamination also will prevent transmission of blood borne pathogens.

REFERENCES

1. U.S. Renal Data System. USRDS 2005 Annual data report: Atlas of end-stage renal disease in the United States, National Institutes of Health, National Institute of Diabetes and Digestive and Kidney Diseases. Bethesda: 2005.
2. Finelli L, Miller JT, Tokars JI, et al. National surveillance of dialysis-associated diseases in the United States, 2002. *Seminars Dialysis* 2005;18:52–61.
3. Alter MJ, Favero MS, Petersen NJ, et al. National surveillance of dialysis-associated hepatitis and other diseases, 1976 and 1980. *Dialysis Transplant* 1983;12:860–61, 864–65, 868.
4. Alter MJ, Favero MS, Miller JK, et al. National surveillance of dialysis-associated diseases in the United States, 1987. *ASAIO Trans* 1989;35:820–31.
5. Alter MJ, Favero MS, Moyer LA, et al. National surveillance of dialysis-associated diseases in the United States, 1988. *ASAIO Trans* 1990;36:107–18.
6. Alter MJ, Favero MS, Moyer LA, Bland LA. National surveillance of dialysis-associated diseases in the United States, 1989. *ASAIO Trans* 1991;37:97–109.
7. Tokars JI, Alter MJ, Favero MS, et al. National surveillance of hemodialysis associated diseases in the United States, 1990. *ASAIO J* 1993;39:71–80.
8. Tokars JI, Alter MJ, Favero MS, et al. National surveillance of dialysis associated diseases in the United States, 1991. *ASAIO J* 1993;39:966–75.
9. Tokars JI, Alter MJ, Favero MS, et al. National surveillance of dialysis associated diseases in the United States, 1992. *ASAIO J* 1994;40:1020–31.
10. Tokars JI, Alter MJ, Favero MS, et al. National surveillance of dialysis associated diseases in the United States, 1993. *ASAIO J* 1996;42:219–29.
11. Tokars JI, Alter MJ, Miller E, et al. National surveillance of dialysis associated diseases in the United States, 1994. *ASAIO J* 1997;43:108–19.
12. Tokars JI, Miller ER, Alter MJ, Arduino MJ. National surveillance of dialysis associated diseases in the United States, 1995. *ASAIO J* 1998;44:98–107.
13. Tokars JI, Miller ER, Alter MJ, Arduino MJ. National surveillance of dialysis-associated diseases in the United States, 1997. *Seminars Dialysis* 2000;13:75–85.
14. Tokars JI, Frank M, Alter MJ, Arduino MJ. National surveillance of dialysis-associated diseases in the United States, 2000. *Seminars Dialysis* 2002;15:162–71.
15. Tokars JI, Finelli L, Alter MJ, Arduino MJ. National surveillance of dialysis-associated diseases in the United States, 2001. *Seminars Dialysis* 2004;17:310–19.
16. Favero MS, Carson LA, Bond WW, Petersen NJ. Pseudomonas aeruginosa: Growth in distilled water from hospitals. *Science* 1971;173:836–38.
17. Favero MS, Carson LA, Bond WW, Petersen NJ. Factors that influence microbial contamination of fluids associated with hemodialysis machines. *Appl Microbiol* 1974;28:822–30.
18. Favero MS, Petersen NJ, Boyer KM, et al. Microbial contamination of renal dialysis systems and associated health risks. *Trans Am Soc Artif Intern Organs* 1974;20A:175–83.
19. Favero MS, Petersen NJ, Carson LA, et al. Gram-negative water bacteria in hemodialysis systems. *Health Lab Sci* 1975;12:321–34.
20. Carson LA, Petersen NJ, Favero MS. Use of the Limulus amoebocyte lysate assay system for detection of bacterial endotoxin in fluids associated with hemodialysis procedures. In: Cohen E, ed. *Biomedical applications of the horseshoe crab (limulidae)*. New York: Alan R. Liss, 1979:453–64.
21. Petersen NJ, Boyer KM, Carson LA, Favero MS. Pyrogenic reactions from inadequate disinfection of a dialysis fluid distribution system. *Dialysis Transplant* 1978;7:52–57
22. Phillips G, Hudson S, Stewart WK. Persistence of microflora in biofilm within fluid pathways of contemporary haemodialysis monitors (Gambro AK-10). *J Hosp Infect* 1994;27:117–25.
23. Lonnemann G. When good water goes bad: How it happens, clinical consequences and possible solutions. *Blood Purif* 2004;22:124–29.
24. Hoenich NA, Ronco C, Levin R. The importance of water quality and haemodialysis fluid composition. *Blood Purif* 2006;24:11–18.
25. Arduino MJ, Bland LA, Favero MS. Microbiology of bicarbonate dialysate. *Nephrol News Issues* 1992;5:7–8
26. Bland LA, Favero MS. Microbial contamination control strategies for hemodialysis systems. *JCAHO Plant Technol Safety Series* 1989;3:30–36
27. Bolan G, Reingold AL, Carson LA, et al. Infections with Mycobacterium chelonei in patients receiving dialysis and using processed hemodialyzers. *J Infect Dis* 1985;52:1013–19.
28. Carson LA, Bland LA, Cusick LB, et al. Prevalence of nontuberculous mycobacteria in water supplies of hemodialysis centers. *Appl Environ Microbiol* 1988;54:3122–25.
29. Lowry PW, Beck-Sague CM, Bland LA, et al. Mycobacterium chelonae infection among patients receiving high-flux dialysis in a hemodialysis clinic in California. *J Infect Dis* 1990;161:85–90.
30. Band JD, Ward JI, Fraser DW, et al. Two outbreaks of peritonitis due to a Mycobacterium chelonei-like organism associated with intermittent chronic peritoneal dialysis. *J Infect Dis* 1982;145:9–17.
31. Poty F, Denis C, Baufine-Ducrocq H. Nosocomial Pseudomonas pickettii infection: Danger of the use of ion-exchange resins. *Presse Med* 1987;16:1185–87.
32. Carson LA, Bland LA, Cusick LB, et al. Factors affecting endotoxin levels in fluids associated with hemodialysis procedures. In: Novitsky TJ, Watson SW, eds. *Detection of bacterial endotoxins with the Limulus amoebocyte lysate test*. New York: Alan R. Liss, 1987:223–34.
33. Hindman SH, Favero MS, Carson LA, et al. Pyrogenic reactions during hemodialysis caused by extramural endotoxin. *Lancet* 1975;2:732–34.
34. Tipple MA, Shusterman N, Bland LA, et al. Illness in hemodialysis patients after exposure to chloramine contaminated dialysate. *ASAIO Trans* 1991;37:588–91.

35. Calderaro RV, Heller L. Outbreak of hemolytic reactions associated with chlorine and chloramine residuals in hemodialysis water. *Rev Saude Publica* 2001;35:481–86.

36. Arduino MJ. CDC investigations of noninfectious outbreaks of adverse events in hemodialysis facilities, 1979–1999. *Seminars Dialysis* 2000;13:86–91.

37. Fenves AZ, Gipson JS, Pancorvo C. Chloramine-induced methemoglobinemia in a hemodialysis patient. *Seminars Dialysis* 2000;13:327–29.

38. Villforth JC. FDA safety alert: Chloramine contamination of hemodialysis water supplies. *Am J Kidney Dis* 1988;11:447.

39. Association for the Advancement of Medical Instrumentation. *American national standard: Water treatment equipment for hemodialysis applications. ANSI/AAMI RD62-2001.* Arlington, VA: Association for the Advancement of Medical Instrumentation, 2001.

40. Association for the Advancement of Medical Instrumentation. *American national standard: Dialysate for hemodialysis. ANSI/AAMI RD52-2004.* Arlington, VA: Association for the Advancement of Medical Instrumentation, 2004.

41. Stamm JM, Engelhard WE, Parsons JE. Microbiological study of softener resins. *Appl Microbiol* 1969;18:376–86.

42. Martiny H, Wlodavezyz K, Harms G, Rueden H. The use of UV-irradiation for the disinfection of water. I. Communication: Microbiological investigations in drinking water. *Zb Bak Hyg B* 1988;185:350–67.

43. Martiny H, Brust H, Rueden H. The use of UV radiation for the disinfection of water. IV. Microbiological studies of the UV sensitivity of different aged cells of E. faecium, E. coli and P. aeruginosa. *Zbl Hyg Umweltmed* 1990;190:39–50.

44. Carson LA, and Petersen NJ. Photoreactivation of Pseudomonas cepacia after ultraviolet exposure: A potential source of contamination in ultraviolet-treated waters. *J Clin Microbiol* 1975;1:462–64.

45. Favero MS. Microbiological contaminants. In: *Proceedings of the Association for the Advancement of Medical Instrumentation Technology Assessment Conference: Issues in hemodialysis.* Arlington, VA: Association for the Advancement of Medical Instrumentation, 1981:30–33.

46. Anderson RL, Holland BW, Carr JK, et al. Effect of disinfectants on pseudomonads colonized on interior surface of PVC pipes. *Am J Public Health* 1990;80:17–21.

47. Arduino MJ. Microbiologic quality of water used for hemodialysis. *Contemp Dial Nephrol* 1996;17:17–19.

48. Arduino MJ, Favero MS. Microbiologic aspects of hemodialysis. In: *Water quality for hemodialysis.* Arlington, VA: Association for the Advancement of Medical Instrumentation, 1998:16–22.

49. Centers for Disease Control and Prevention. *Clusters of bacteremia and pyrogenic reactions in hemodialysis patients. Epidemic Investigation Report EPI 86-65, April 22, 1987.* Atlanta: CDC.

50. Beck-Sague CM, Jarvis WR, Bland LA, et al. Outbreak of gram-negative bacteremia and pyrogenic reactions in a hemodialysis center. *Am J Nephrol* 1990;10:397–403.

51. Murphy J, Parker T, Carson L, et al. Outbreaks of bacteremia in hemodialysis patients associated with alteration of dialyzer membranes following chemical disinfection. *ASAIO Trans* 1987;16:51.

52. Welbel SF, Schoendorf K, Bland LA, et al. An outbreak of gram-negative bloodstream infections in chronic hemodialysis patients. *Am J Nephrol* 1995;15:1–4.

53. Centers for Disease Control. *Pyrogenic reactions in patients undergoing high-flux hemodialysis, California. Epidemic Investigation Report EPI 86-80, June 1, 1987.* Atlanta: CDC, 1987.

54. Gordon S, Tipple M, Bland L, Jarvis W. Pyrogenic reactions associated with the reuse of disposable hollow fiber hemodialyzers. *JAMA* 1988;260:2077–81.

55. Rudnick JR, Arduino MJ, Bland LA, et al. Pyrogenic reactions associated with hemodialysis reuse. *Artif Organs* 1995;19:289–94.

56. Townsend TR, Siok-Bi W, Bartlett J. Disinfection of hemodialysis machines. *Dialysis Transplant* 1985;14:274, 78, 80, 82–83, 87.

57. Amato RL. Water treatment for hemodialysis—updated to include the latest AAMI standards for dialysate (RD52: 2004) continuing. *Nephrol Nurs J* 2005;32:151–67.

58. Smeets E, Kooman J, van der Sande F, et al. Prevention of biofilm formation in dialysis water treatment systems. *Kidney Int* 2003;2003;63:1574–76.

59. Amato RL, Curtis J. The practical application of ozone in dialysis. *Nephrol News Issues* 2002;16:27–30.

60. Favero MS, Petersen NJ. Microbiologic guidelines for hemodialysis systems. *Dialysis Transplant* 1977;6:34–36.

61. Association for the Advancement of Medical Instrumentation. *American national standard for hemodialysis systems. ANSI/AAMI RD5-1992.* Arlington, VA: Association for the Advancement of Medical Instrumentation, 1992.

62. Sitter T, Bergner A, Schiffl H. Dialysate related cytokine induction and response to recombinant human erythropoietin in haemodialysis patients. *Nephrol Dial Transplant* 2000;15:1207–11.

63. Vaslaki LR, Berta K, Major L, et al. On-line hemodiafiltration does not induce inflammatory response in end-stage renal disease patients: Results from a multicenter cross-over study. *Artif Organs* 2005;29:406–12.

64. Lacson E Jr., Levin NW. C-reactive protein and end-stage renal disease. *Seminars Dialysis* 2004;17:438–48.

65. Hsu PY, Lin CL, Yu CC, et al. Ultrapure dialysate improves iron utilization and erythropoietin response in chronic hemodialysis patients—a prospective cross-over study. *J Nephrol* 2004;17:693–700.

66. Kleophas W, Haastert B, Backus G, et al. Long-term experience with an ultrapure individual dialysis fluid with a batch type machine. *Nephrol Dial Transplant* 1998;13:3118–25.

67. Baz M, Durand C, Ragon A, et al. Using ultrapure water in hemodialysis delays carpal tunnel syndrome. *Int J Artif Organs* 1991;14:681–85.

68. Richardson D. Clinical factors influencing sensitivity and response to epoetin. *Nephrol Dial Transplant* 2002;17:53–59.

69. Schiffl H, Lang SM, Stratakis D, Fischer R. Effects of ultrapure dialysis fluid on nutritional status and inflammatory parameters. *Nephrol Dial Transplant* 2001;16:1863–69.

70. Favero MS, Bland LA. Microbiologic principles applied to reprocessing hemodialyzers. In: Deane N, Wineman RJ, Bemis JA, eds. *Guide to reprocessing of hemodialyzers.* Boston: Martinus Nijhoff, 1986:63–73.

71. Arduino MJ, Bland LA, Aguero SM, et al. Comparison of microbiologic assay methods for hemodialysis fluids. *J Clin Microbiol* 1991;29:592–94.

72. Klein E, Pass T, Harding GB, et al. Microbial and endotoxin contamination in water and dialysate in the central United States. *Artif Organs* 1990;14:85–94.

73. van der Linde K, Lim BT, Rondeel JM, et al. Improved bacteriological surveillance of haemodialysis fluids: A comparison between Tryptic soy agar and Reasoner's 2A media. *Nephrol Dial Transplant* 1999;14:2433–37.

74. Association for the Advancement of Medical Instrumentation. *American national standard: Reuse of hemodialyzers ANSI/AAMI RD47-2002/A1:2003.* Arlington, VA: Association for the Advancement of Medical Instrumentation, 2003.

75. Gazenfeldt-Gazit E, Elaihou HE. Endotoxin antibodies in patients on maintenance hemodialysis. *Israel J Med Sci* 1969;5:1032–36.

76. Lonnemann G, Behme TC, Lenzner B, et al. Permeability of dialyzer membranes to TNF-α inducing substances derived from water bacteria. *Kidney Int* 1992;42:61–68.

77. Laude-Sharpe M, Canoff M, Simard L, et al. Induction of IL-1 during hemodialysis: Trans-membrane passage of intact endotoxin (LPS). *Kidney Int* 1990;38:1089–94.

78. Kumano K, Yokota S, Nanbu M, Sakai T. Do cytokine-inducing substances penetrate through dialysis membranes and stimulate monocytes? *Kidney Int Suppl* 1993;41:S205–8.

79. Yamagami S, Adachi T, Sugimura T, et al. Detection of endotoxin antibody in long-term dialysis patients. *Int J Artif Organs* 1990;13:205–10.

80. Henderson LW, Koch KM, Dinarello CA, et al. Hemodialysis hypotension: The interleukin hypothesis. *Blood Purif* 1983;1:3–8.

81. Port FK, VanDerKerkhove KM, Kunkel SL, Kluger MJ. The role of dialysate in the stimulation of interleukin-1 production during clinical hemodialysis. *Am J Kidney Dis* 1987;10:118–22.

82. Kantor RJ, Carson LA, Graham DR, et al. Outbreak of pyrogenic reactions at a dialysis center: Association with infusion of heparinized saline solution. *Am J Med* 1983;74:449–56.

83. Powell AC, Bland LA, Oettinger CW, et al. Enhanced release of TNF-α, but not IL-1β, from uremic blood after endotoxin stimulation. *Lymphokine Cytokine Res* 1991;10:343–46.

84. Pegues DA, Oettinger CU, Bland LA, et al. A prospective study of pyrogenic reactions in hemodialysis patients using bicarbonate dialysis fluids filtered to remove bacteria and endotoxin. *J Am Soc Nephrol* 1992;3:1002–7.

85. Gordon SM, Oettinger CW, Bland LA, et al. Pyrogenic reactions in patients receiving conventional, high-efficiency or high-flux hemodialysis with bicarbonate dialysate containing high concentrations of bacteria and endotoxin. *J Am Soc Nephrol* 1992;2:1436–44.

86. Petersen NJ, Boyer KM, Carson LA, et al. Pyrogenic reactions from inadequate disinfection of a dialysis fluid distribution system. *Dialysis Transplant* 1978;7:52, 57–60.

87. Centers for Disease Control and Prevention. Pyrogenic reactions and gram-negative bacteremia in a hemodialysis center. *Epidemic investigation report EPI 91-37*. Atlanta: CDC, 1991.

88. Centers for Disease Control and Prevention. *Bacteremia in hemodialysis patients. Epidemic Investigation Report EPI 92-10*. Atlanta: CDC, 1992.

89. Centers for Disease Control and Prevention. *Outbreaks of gram negative bacterial bloodstream infections traced to probable contamination of hemodialysis machines*—Canada, 1995; United States, 1997; and Israel, 1997. *MMWR* 1998;47:55–59.

90. Jochimsen EM, Frenette C, Delorme M, et al. A cluster of bloodstream infections and pyrogenic reactions among hemodialysis patients traced to dialysis machine waste-handling option units. *Am J Nephrol* 1998;18:485–89.

91. Wang SA, Levine RB, Carson LA, et al. An outbreak of gram-negative bacteremia in hemodialysis patients traced to hemodialysis machine waste drain ports. *Infect Control Hosp Epidemiol* 1999;20:746–51.

92. Jackson BM, Beck-Sague CM, Bland LA, et al. Outbreak of pyrogenic reactions and gram-negative bacteremia in a hemodialysis center. *Am J Nephrol* 1994;14:85–89.

93. Grohskopf LA, Roth VR, Feikin DR, et al. Serratia liquefaciens bloodstream infections from contamination of epoetin alfa at a hemodialysis center. *N Engl J Med* 2001; 17;344:1491–97.

94. Proia LA, Hayden MK, Kammeyer PL, et al. Phialemonium: An emerging mold pathogen that caused 4 cases of hemodialysis-associated endovascular infection. *Clin Infect Dis* 2004;39:373–79.

95. Arnow PM, Garcia-Houchins S, Neagle MB, et al. An outbreak of bloodstream infections arising from hemodialysis equipment. *J Infect Dis* 1998;178:783–91.

96. Block C, Backenroth R, Gershon E, et al. Outbreak of bloodstream infections associated with dialysis machine waste ports in a hemodialysis facility. *Eur J Clin Microbiol Infect Dis* 1999;18:723–25.

97. Food and Drug Administration. *Guidance for hemodialyzer reuse*. Rockville: Food and Drug Administration, Center for Devices and Radiologic Health, 1995.

98. Held PJ, Wolfe RA, Gaylin DS, et al. Analysis of the association of dialyzer reuse practices and patient outcomes. *Am J Kidney Dis* 1994;23:692–708.

99. Collins AJ, Ma JZ, Constantini EG, Everson SE. Dialysis unit and patient characteristics associated with reuse practices and mortality: 1989–1993. *J Am Soc Nephrol* 1998;9:2108–17.

100. Collins AJ, Liu J, Ebben JP. Dialyzer reuse-associated mortality and hospitalization risk in incident Medicare haemodialysis patients, 1998–1999. *Nephrol Dial Transplant* 2004;19:1245–51.

101. Feldman HI, Bilker WB, Hackett MH, et al. Association of dialyzer reuse with hospitalization and survival rates among U.S. hemodialysis patients: Do comorbidities matter? *J Clin Epidemiol* 1999;52:209–17.

102. Roth VR, Jarvis WR. Outbreaks of infection and/or pyrogenic reactions in dialysis patients. *Seminars Dialysis* 2000;13:92–96.

103. Centers for Disease Control. Bacteremia associated with reuse of disposable hollow-fiber hemodialyzers. *MMWR* 1986;35:417–18.

104. Alter MJ, Favero MS, Miller JK, et al. Reuse of hemodialyzers. Results of nationwide surveillance for adverse effects. *JAMA* 1988;260:2073–76.

105. Bland L, Alter M, Favero M, et al. Hemodialyzer reuse: Practices in the United States and implications for infection control. *ASAIO Trans* 1985;31:556–59.

106. Favero MS. Distinguishing between high level disinfection, reprocessing, and sterilization. In: *Association for the Advancement of Medical Instrumentation, Reuse of disposables: Implications for quality health care and cost containment. Technical Assessment Report No. 6*. Arlington, VA: AAMI, 1983:19–20.

107. Rosenberg J. Primary blood stream infections associated with dialyzer reuse in California dialysis centers. *Proceedings of the 43rd Annual Meeting of the Infectious Diseases Society of America*. IDSA, Alexandria, VA, 2005.

108. Tokars JI, Miller ER, Alter MJ, Arduino MJ. *National surveillance of dialysis-associated diseases in the United States, 1999*. Atlanta: Centers for Disease Control and Prevention, 2001.

109. Bland LA, Ridgeway MR, Aguero SM, et al. Potential bacteriologic and endotoxin hazards associated with liquid bicarbonate concentration. *ASAIO Trans* 1987;33:542–45.

110. Quinton W, Dillard D, Scribner DH. Cannulation of blood vessels for prolonged hemodialysis. *Trans Soc Artif intern Organs* 1960;6:104–13.

111. Foran RF, Golding AL, Treiman RL, et al. Quinton-Scribner cannulas for hemodialysis. Review of four years' experience. *Calif Med* 1970;112:8–13.

112. Coronel F, Herrero JA, Mateos P, et al. Long-term experience with the Thomas shunt, the forgotten permanent vascular access for haemodialysis. *Nephrol Dial Transplant* 2001;16:1845–49.

113. Bell PRF, Veitch PS. Vascular access for hemodialysis. In: Jacobson HR, Striker GE, Klahr S, eds. *The principles and practice of nephrology*. Philadelphia: BC Decker, 1991:26–44.

114. Bonomo RA, Rice D, Whalen C, et al. Risk factors associated with permanent access-site infections in chronic hemodialysis patients. *Infect Control Hosp Epidemiol* 1997;18:757–61.

115. Kaplowitz LG, Comstock JA, Landwehr DM, et al. A prospective study of infections in hemodialysis patients: Patient hygiene and other risk factors for infection. *Infect Control Hosp Epidemiol* 1988;9:534–41.

116. Tokars JI, Miller ER, Stein G. New national surveillance system for hemodialysis-associated infections: Initial results. *Am J Infect Control* 2002;30:288–95.

117. Padberg FT Jr, Lee BC, Curl GR. Hemoaccess site infection. *Surg Gynecol Obstet* 1992;174:103–8.

118. Mehta S. Statistical summary of clinical results of vascular access procedures for hemodialysis. In: Jacobson HR, Striker GE, Klahr S, eds. *The priciples and practice of nephrology*. Philadelphia: BC Decker, 1991:145–57.

119. Whelchel JD. Central venous hemodialysis access catheters: A review of technical considerations and complications. In: Sommer BG, Henry ML, eds. *Vascular Access for Hemodialysis II*. Chicago: WL. Gore and Associates and Precept Press, 1991:123–38.

120. Goldstein MB. Prevention of sepsis from central vein dialysis catheters. *Seminars Dialysis* 1992;5:106–8.

121. Counts CS. Potential complications of the internal vascular access: Implications for nursing care. *Dialysis Transplant* 1993;22:75–79.

122. Dryden MS, Samson A, Ludlam HA, Wing AJ. Infective complications associated with the use of the Quinton Permacath for long-term central vascular access in hemodialysis. *J Hosp Infect* 1991;19:257–62.

123. Carlisle EJF, Blake P, McCarthy F, et al. Septicemia in long-term jugular hemodialysis catheters: Eradicating infection by changing the catheter over a guidewire. *Int J Artif Organs* 1991;14:150–53.

124. Saxena A, Panhotra BR. Haemodialysis catheter-related bloodstream infections: Current treatment options and strategies for prevention. *Swiss Med Wkly* 2005;135:127–38.

125. Klevens M, Tokars JI, Andrus MA. Electronic reporting of infections associated with hemodialysis. *Nephrol News Issues* 2005;19:37–38, 43.

126. Welbel SF, Williams D, Ray B, et al. Central venous catheter-associated bloodstream infections in a dialysis unit, Texas. In:

Abstracts of the 1993 Epidemic Intelligence Service Conference, Atlanta, April 19–23, 1993. Washington, DC: Department of Health and Human Services, 1993:59.

127. Gokal R, Khanna R, Krediet R Th, and Nolph KD. *Textbook of peritoneal dialysis.* 2nd ed. Dordrecht: Kluwer Academic Publishers, 2000.

128. Peterson P, Matzke G, Keane WF. Current concepts in the management of peritonitis in patients undergoing continuous ambulatory peritoneal dialysis. *Rev Infect Dis* 1987;9:604–12.

129. Walshe JJ, Morse GD. Infectious complications of peritoneal dialysis. In: Nissenson AR, Fine RN, Gentile DE, eds. *Clinical Dialysis* Norwalk,CT: Appleton, 1990:301–18.

130. Piraino B. Peritoneal dialysis infections recommendations. *Contrib Nephrol* 2006;150:181–86.

131. Berkelman RL, Godley J, Weber JA, et al. Pseudomonas cepacia peritonitis associated with contamination of automatic peritoneal dialysis machines. *Ann Intern Med* 1982;96:456–58.

132. Petersen NJ, Carson LA, Favero MS. Microbiological quality of water in an automatic peritoneal dialysis system. *Dialysis Transplant* 1977;6:38–40, 86.

133. Carson LA, Petersen NJ, Favero MS, Aguero SM. Growth characteristics of atypical mycobacteria in water and their comparative resistance to disinfection. *Appl Environ Microbiol* 1978;36:839–46.

134. Berkelman RL, Band JD, Petersen NJ. Recommendations for the care of automated peritoneal dialysis machines: Can the risk of peritonitis be reduced? *Infect Control* 1984;5:85–87.

135. Zelenitsky S, Barns L, Findlay I, et al. Analysis of microbiological trends in peritoneal dialysis-related peritonitis from 1991 to 1998. *Am J Kidney Dis* 2000;36:1009–13.

136. Oxton LL, Zimmerman SW, Roecker EB, Wakeen M. Risk factors for peritoneal dialysis-related infections. *Perit Dial Int* 1994;14:137–44.

137. Salusky IB, Holloway M. Selection of peritoneal dialysis for pediatric patients. *Perit Dial Int* 1994;17:S35–37.

138. Vas S, Oreopoulos DG. Infections in patients undergoing peritoneal dialysis. *Infect Dis Clin North Am* 2000;15:743–74.

139. Copley JB. Prevention of peritoneal dialysis catheter-related infections. *Am J Kidney Dis* 1987;10:401–7.

140. Thodis E, Passadakis P, Ossareh S, et al. Peritoneal catheter exit-site infections: Predisposing factors, prevention and treatment. *Int J Artif Organs* 2003;26:698–714.

141. Vas S. Microbiologic aspects of chronic ambulatory peritoneal dialysis. *Kidney Int* 1983;23:83–92.

142. Szeto CC, Chow VC, Chow KM, et al. Enterobacteriaceae peritonitis complicating peritoneal dialysis: A review of 210 consecutive cases. *Kidney Int* 2006;69:1245–52.

143. Pegues DA, Arduino MJ, Bland LA, Jarvis WR. Infectious complications in continuous ambulatory peritoneal dialysis. *Asepsis* 1989;11:6–12.

144. Piraino B, Bailie GR, Bernardini J, et al. Ad Hoc Advisory Committee. Peritoneal dialysis-related infections recommendations: 2005 update. *Perit Dial Int* 2005;25:107–31.

145. Hakim RM, Breillatt J, Lazarus JM, Port FK. Complement activation and hypersensitivity reactions to dialysis membranes. *N Engl J Med* 1984;311:878–82.

146. Villarroel F. First-use syndrome in patients treated with hollow-fiber dialyzers. *Blood Purif* 1987;5:112–4.

147. Ing TS, Ivanovich PT, Daugirdas JT. First-use syndrome and hypersensitivity during hemodialysis: Some pieces of the puzzle are falling into place. *Artif Organs* 1987;11:79–81.

148. Daugirdas JT, Potempa LD, Dinh N, et al. Plate, coil, and hollow-fiber cuprammonium cellulose dialyzers: Discrepancy between incidence of anaphylactic reactions and degree of complement activation. *Artif Organs* 1987;11:140–43.

149. Daugirdas JT, Ing TS. First-use reactions during hemodialysis: A definition of subtypes. *Kidney Int Suppl* 1988;24:S37–43.

150. Pegues DA, Beck-Sague CM, Woollen SW, et al. Anaphylactoid reactions associated with reuse of hollow-fiber hemodialyzers and ACE inhibitors. *Kidney Int* 1992;42:1232–37.

151. Teileans C, Madhoun P, Lenaers M, Schandene L. Anaphylactic reactions during hemodialysis on AN69 membranes in patients receiving ACE inhibitors. *Kidney Int* 1990;38:982–84.

152. Verresen L, Waer M, Vanrenterghem Y, Michielsen P. Angiotensin converting enzyme inhibitors and anaphylactoid reactions to high-flux membrane dialysis. *Lancet* 1990;336:1360–62.

153. van Es A, Henny FC, Lobatto S. Angiotensin-converting enzyme inhibitors and anaphylactic reactions to high-flux membrane dialysis. *Lancet* 1991;337:112–13.

154. Jadoul M, Struyven J, Stragier A, Van Ypersele De Strihou C. Angiotensin-converting enzyme inhibitors and anaphylactic reactions to high-flux membrane dialysis [Letter]. *Lancet* 1991;337:112.

155. Federal Drug Administration. Anaphylactoid reactions associated with ACE inhibitors and dialyzer membranes. *FDA Safety Alert,* March 6, 1992.

156. Alfrey AC, Mishell JM, Burks J, et al. Syndrome of dyspraxia and multifocal seizures associated with chronic hemodialysis. *Trans Am Soc Artif Intern Organs* 1972;18:257–61, 266–67.

157. Schreeder MT, Favero MS, Hughes JR, et al. Dialysis encephalopathy and aluminum exposure: an epidemiologic analysis. *J Chronic Dis* 1983;36:581–93.

158. Burwen DR, Olsen SM, Bland LA, et al. Epidemic aluminum intoxication in hemodialysis patients traced to use of an aluminum pump. *Kidney Int* 1995;48:469–74.

159. Centers for Disease Control and Prevention. Fluoride intoxication in a dialysis unit—Maryland. *MMWR* 1980;29:134–36.

160. Gordon SM, Bland LA, Alexander SR, et al. Hemolysis associated with hydrogen peroxide at a pediatric dialysis center. *Am J Nephrol* 1990;10:123–27.

161. Gordon SM, Drachman J, Bland LA, et al. Epidemic hypotension in a dialysis center caused by sodium azide. *Kidney Int* 1990;37:110–15.

162. Centers for Disease Control. *Dialysis dementia from aluminum. Epidemic Investigation Report EPI 81-39.* Atlanta: CDC, 1982.

163. Centers for Disease Control. *Formaldehyde intoxication associated with hemodialysis—California. Epidemic investigation report EPI 81-73.* Atlanta: CDC, 1984.

164. Arnow PM, Bland LA, Garcia-Houchins S, et al. An outbreak of fatal fluoride intoxication in a long-term hemodialysis unit. *Ann Intern Med* 1994;121:339–44.

165. Bland LA, Arnow PM, Arduino MJ, et al. Potential hazards of deionization systems used for water purification in hemodialysis. *Artif Organs* 1996;20:2–7.

166. Jochimsen EM, Carmichael WW, An JS, et al. Liver failure and death after exposure to microcystins at a hemodialysis center in Brazil. *N Engl J Med* 1998 26;338:873–78.

167. Food and Drug Administration. FDA investigating roles of Baxter's recalled dialyzers in dialysis patient deaths. *Medical Device Recalls* November 7, 2001.

168. No author. Caunaud B. performance liquid test as a cause for sudden deaths of dialysis patients: Perfluorohydrocarbon, a previously unrecognized hazard for dialysis patients. *Nephrol Dial Transplant* 2002;17:545–48.

169. Selenic D, Alvarado-Ramy F, Arduino M, et al. Epidemic parenteral exposure to volatile sulfur-containing compounds at a hemodialysis center. *Infect Control Hosp Epidemiol* 2004;25:256–61.

170. Snydman DR, Bryan JA, London WT, et al. Transmission of hepatitis B associated with hemodialysis: Role of malfunction (blood leaks) inside dialysis machines. *J Infect Dis* 1976;134:562–70.

171. Kantor RJ, Hadler SC, Schreeder MT, et al. Outbreak of hepatitis B in a dialysis unit, complicated by false positive HBsAg test results. *Dial Transplant* 1979;8:232–35.

172. Snydman DR, Bryan JA, Macon EJ, Gregg MB. Hemodialysis-associated hepatitis: Report of an epidemic with further evidence on mechanisms of transmission. *Am J Epidemiol* 1976;104:563–70.

173. Carl M, Francis DP, Maynard JE. A common source outbreak of hepatitis B in a hemodialysis unit. *Dialysis Transplant* 1983;12:222–29.

174. Alter MJ, Ahtone J, Maynard JE. Hepatitis B virus transmission associated with a multiple dose vial in a hemodialysis unit. *Am J Med* 1983;99:330–33.

175. Niu MT, Penberthy LT, Alter MJ, et al. Hemodialysis-associated hepatitis B: Report of an outbreak. *Dialysis Transplant* 1989;18:542–55.

176. Centers for Disease Control and Prevention. *Outbreak of hepatitis B in a dialysis center. Epidemic investigation report EPI 91-17.* Atlanta: CDC, 1993.

177. Centers for Disease Control and Prevention. Outbreaks of hepatitis B virus infection among hemodialysis patients—California, Nebraska, and Texas, 1994. *MMWR* 1996;45:285–89.

178. Hutin YJ, Goldstein ST, Varma JK, et al. *An outbreak of hospital acquired hepatitis B virus infection among patients receiving chronic hemodialysis. Infect Control Hosp Epidemiol* 1999;20:731–35.

179. Centers for Disease Control. *Non-A, Non-B hepatitis in a dialysis center, Nashville Tennessee. Epidemic investigation report EPI 78–96.* Phoenix: CDC, 1979.

180. Niu MT, Alter MJ, Kristensen C, et al. Outbreak of hemodialysis-associated non-A, non-B hepatitis and correlation with antibody to hepatitis C virus. *Am J Kidney Dis* 1992;19:345–52.

181. Centers for Disease Control and Prevention. *Possible ongoing transmission of hepatitis C virus in a hemodialysis unit. Epidemic investigation report EPI 99-38.* Atlanta: CDC, 1999.

182. Centers for Disease Control and Prevention. *Transmission of hepatitis C virus among hemodialysis patients. Epidemic investigation report EPI-2000.* Atlanta: CDC, 2000.

183. Centers for Disease Control and Prevention. *Transmission of hepatitis C virus in a hemodialysis unit. Epidemic investigation report EPI-2000-64.* Atlanta: CDC, 2000.

184. Velandia M, Fridkin SK, Cardenas V, et al. Transmission of HIV in dialysis centre. *Lancet* 1995;345:1417–22.

185. El Sayed NM, Gomatos PJ, Beck-Sague CM, et al. Epidemic transmission of human immunodeficiency virus in renal dialysis centers in Egypt. *J Infect Dis* 2000;181:91–97.

186. Favero MS, Maynard JE, Petersen NJ, et al. Hepatitis B antigen on environmental surfaces [Letter]. *Lancet* 1973;2:1455.

187. Bond WW, Favero MS, Petersen NJ, et al. Survival of hepatitis B virus after drying and storage for one week. *Lancet* 1981;1:550–51.

188. Petersen NJ. An assessment of the airborne route in hepatitis B transmission. *Ann NY Acad Sci* 1980;353:157–66.

189. Favero MS, Bolyard EA. Microbiologic considerations, disinfection and sterilization strategies and the potential for airborne transmission of bloodborne pathogens. *Surgical Clinics North America* 1995;75:1071–89.

190. Favero MS, Deane N, Leger RT, Sosin AE. Effect of multiple use of dialyzers on hepatitis B incidence in patients and staff. *JAMA* 1981;245:166–67.

191. Snydman DR, Bryan JA, Hanson B. Hemodialysis-associated hepatitis in the United States—1972. *J Infect Dis* 1975;132:109–13.

192. Snydman DR, Bregman D, Bryan JA. Hemodialysis-associated hepatitis in the United States, 1974. *J Infect Dis* 1977;135:687–91.

193. Szmuness W, Prince AM, Grady GF, et al. Hepatitis B infection. A point prevalence study in 15 US dialysis centers. *JAMA* 1974;227:901–6.

194. Centers for Disease Control and Prevention. Control measures for hepatitis B in dialysis centers. In: *Viral Hepatitis Investigation and Control Series.* Atlanta: CDC, 1977.

195. Alter MJ, Favero MS, Maynard JE. Impact of infection control strategies on the incidence of dialysis-associated hepatitis in the United States. *J Infect Dis* 1986;153:1149–51.

196. Marmion BP, Burrell CJ, Tonkin RW, Dickson J. Dialysis-associated hepatitis in Edinburgh: 1969–1978. *Rev Infect Dis* 1982;4:619–37.

197. Najem GR, Louria DB, Thind IS, Lavenhar MA, Gocke DJ, Basking SE, Miller AM, Frankel HJ, Notkin MG, Weiner B. Control of hepatitis B infection. The role of surveillance and an isolation hemodialysis center. *JAMA* 1981;245(2):153–57.

198. Alter MJ, Favero MS, Francis DP. Cost benefit of vaccination for hepatitis B in hemodialysis centers. *J Infect Dis* 1983;148:770–71.

199. Hoofnagle JH, Di Bisceglie AM. Serologic diagnosis of acute and chronic viral hepatitis. *Semin Liver Dis* 1991;11:73–83.

200. Kloster B, Kramer R, Eastlund T, et al. Hepatitis B surface antigenemia in blood donors following vaccination. *Transfusion* 1995;35:475–77.

201. Lunn ER, Hoggarth BJ, Cook WJ. Prolonged hepatitis B surface antigenemia after vaccination. *Pediatrics* 2000;105:E81.

202. McMahon BJ, Alberts SR, Wainwright RB, et al. Hepatitis B-related sequelae: Prospective study in 1400 hepatitis B

surface antigen—positive Alaska Native carriers. *Arch Intern Med* 1990;150:1051–54.

203. Hadler SC, Murphy B, Schable CA, et al. Epidemiological analysis of the significance of low-positive test results for antibody to hepatitis B surface and core antigens. *J Clin Microbiol* 1984;19:521–25.

204. Levine OS, Vlahov D, Koehler J, et al. Seroepidemiology of hepatitis B virus in a population of injecting drug users: Association with drug injection patterns. *Am J Epidemiol* 1995;142:331–41.

205. Silva AE, McMahon BJ, Parkinson AJ, et al. Hepatitis B virus DNA in persons with isolated antibody to hepatitis B core antigen who subsequently received hepatitis B vaccine. *Clin Infect Dis* 1998;26:895–97.

206. McMahon BJ, Parkinson AJ, Helminiak C, et al. Response to hepatitis B vaccine of persons positive for antibody to hepatitis B core antigen. *Gastroenterology* 1992;103:590–94.

207. Lai C-L, Lau JYN, Yeoh E-K, et al. Significance of isolated anti-HBc seropositivity by ELISA: Implications and the role of radioimmunoassay. *J Med Virol* 1992;36:180–83.

208. Niu MT, Coleman PJ, Alter MJ. Multicenter study of hepatitis C virus infection in chronic hemodialysis patients and hemodialysis center staff members. *Am J Kidney Dis* 1993;22:568–73.

209. Sypsa V, Psichogiou M, Katsoulidou A, et al. Incidence and patterns of hepatitis C virus seroconversion in a cohort of hemodialysis patients. *Am J Kidney Dis* 2005;45:334–43.

210. Fabrizi F, Martin P, Dixit V, et al. Acquisition of hepatitis C virus in hemodialysis patients: A prospective study by branched DNA signal amplification assay. *Am J Kidney Dis* 1998;31:647–54.

211. Petrosillo N, Gilli P, Serraino D, et al. Prevalence of infected patients and understaffing have a role in hepatitis C virus transmission in dialysis. *Am J Kidney Dis* 2001;37:1004–10.

212. dos Santos JP, Loureiro A, Cendoroglo Neto M, Pereira BJ. Impact of dialysis room and reuse strategies on the incidence of hepatitis C virus infection in haemodialysis units. *Nephrol Dial Transplant* 1996;11:2017–22.

213. Forns X, Fernandez-Llama P, Pons M, et al. Incidence and risk factors of hepatitis C virus infection in a haemodialysis unit. *Nephrol Dial Transplant* 1997;12:736–40.

214. Hmaied F, Ben Mamou M, Saune-Sandres K, et al. Hepatitis C virus infection among dialysis patients in Tunisia: Incidence and molecular evidence for nosocomial transmission. *J Med Virol* 2006;78:185–91.

215. Kobayashi M, Tanaka E, Oguchi H, et al. Prospective follow-up study of hepatitis C virus infection in patients undergoing maintenance haemodialysis: Comparison among haemodialysis units. *J Gastroenterol Hepatol* 1998;13:604–9.

216. McLaughlin KJ, Cameron SO, Good T, et al. Nosocomial transmission of hepatitis C virus within a British dialysis centre. *Nephrol Dial Transplant* 1997;12:304–9.

217. Silva LK, Silva MB, Rodart IF, et al. Prevalence of hepatitis C virus (HCV) infection and HCV genotypes of hemodialysis patients in Salvador, Northeastern Brazil. *Braz J Med Biol Res* 2006;39:595–602.

218. Chandra M, Khaja MN, Hussain MM, et al. Prevalence of hepatitis B and hepatitis C viral infections in Indian patients with chronic renal failure. *Intervirology* 2004;47:374–76.

219. Sivapalasingam S, Malak SF, Sullivan JF, et al. High prevalence of hepatitis C infection among patients receiving hemodialysis at an urban dialysis center. *Infect Control Hosp Epidemiol* 2002;23:319–24.

220. Carneiro MA, Martins RM, Teles SA, et al. Hepatitis C prevalence and risk factors in hemodialysis patients in Central Brazil: A survey by polymerase chain reaction and serological methods. *Mem Inst Oswaldo Cruz* 2001;96:765–69.

221. Covic A, Iancu L, Apetrei C, et al. Hepatitis virus infection in haemodialysis patients from Moldavia. *Nephrol Dial Transplant* 1999;14:40–45.

222. Fissell RB, Bragg-Gresham JL, Woods JD, et al. Patterns of hepatitis C prevalence and seroconversion in hemodialysis units from three continents: The DOPPS. *Kidney Int* 2004;65:2335–42.

223. Alter MJ. Epidemiology of hepatitis C in the west. *Sem Liv Dis* 1995;15:5–14.

224. Khokhar N, Alam AY, Naz F, et al. Risk factors for hepatitis C virus infection in patients on long-term hemodialysis. *J Coll Physicians Surg Pak* 2005;15:326–28.

225. Othman B, Monem F. Prevalence of antibodies to hepatitis C virus among hemodialysis patients in Damascus, Syria. *Infection* 2001;29:262–65.

226. Hardy NM, Sandroni S, Danielson S, Wilson WJ. Antibody to hepatitis C virus increases with time on hemodialysis. *Clin Nephrol* 1992;38:44–48.

227. Selgas R, Martinez-Zapico R, Bajo MA, et al. Prevalence of hepatitis C antibodies (HCV) in a dialysis population at one center. *Perit Dial Int* 1992;12:28–30.

228. Alter MJ. Prevention of spread of hepatitis C. *Hepatology* 2002;365(suppl 1):S93–98.

229. Dufour DR, Talastas M, Fernandez MD, Harris B. Chemiluminescence assay improves specificity of hepatitis C antibody detection. *Clin Chem* 2003;49:940–44.

230. Centers for Disease Control and Prevention. Guidelines for laboratory testing and result reporting of antibody to hepatitis c virus. *MMWR* 2003;52(RR-03):1–16.

231. Houghton M, Weiner A, Han J, et al. Molecular biology of the hepatitis C viruses: Implications for diagnosis, development and control of viral disease. *Hepatology* 1991;14:381–88.

232. Centers for Disease Control and Prevention. Recommendations for preventing transmission of infections among chronic hemodialysis patients. *MMWR* 2001;50(RR-5):1–43.

233. Busch MP, Kleinman SH, Jackson B, et al. Committee report. Nucleic acid amplification testing of blood donors for transfusion-transmitted infectious diseases: Report of the Interorganizational Task Force on Nucleic Acid Amplification Testing of Blood Donors. *Transfusion* 2000;40:143–59.

234. Williams IT, Gretch D, Fleenor M, et al. Hepatitis C virus RNA concentration and chronic hepatitis in a cohort of patients followed after developing acute hepatitis C. In: Margolis HS, Alter MJ, Liang TJ, et al., eds. *Viral hepatitis and liver disease.* Atlanta: International Press, 2002:341–44.

235. Alter MJ, Margolis HS, Krawczynski K, et al. The natural history of community-acquired hepatitis C in the United States. The Sentinel Counties Chronic non-A, non-B Hepatitis Study Team. *N Engl J Med* 1992;327:1899–905.

236. Thomas DL, Astemborski J, Rai RM, et al. The natural history of hepatitis C virus infection: Host, viral, and environmental factors. *JAMA* 2000;284:450–56.

237. Larghi A, Zuin M, Crosignani A, et al. Outcome of an outbreak of acute hepatitis C among healthy volunteers participating in pharmacokinetics studies. *Hepatology* 2002;36:993–1000.

238. Hadler SC, Fields HA. Hepatitis delta virus. In: Belshe RB, ed. *Textbook of human virology.* St Louis: Mosby Year Book, 1991:749–65.

239. Pol S, Dubois F, Mattlinger B, et al. Absence of hepatitis delta virus infection in chronic hemodialysis and kidney transplant patients in France. *Transplantation* 1992;54:1096–97.

240. Aghanashinikar PN, al-Dhahry SH, al-Marhuby HA, et al. Prevalence of hepatitis B, hepatitis delta, and human immunodeficiency virus infections in Omani patients with renal diseases. *Transplant Proc* 1992;24:1913–4.

241. Rezvan H, Forouzandeh B, Taroyan S, et al. A study on delta virus infection and its clinical impact in Iran. *Infection* 1990;18:26–28.

242. Lettau LA, Alfred HJ, Glew RH, et al. Nosocomial transmission of delta hepatitis. *Ann Intern Med* 1986;104:631–35.

243. Dyer E. Argentinian doctors accused of spreading AIDS. *BMJ* 1993;307:584.

244. Centers for disease Control. Recommendations for preventing transmission of hepatitis C virus (HCV infection and HCV-related chronic diseases. *MMWR* 1998;47(RR-19):1–39.

245. National Institutes of Health. *Chronic hepatitis C: Current disease management.* Washington, DC: National Institute of Diabetes, Digestive, and Kidney Diseases, 2000:1–21.

246. Boyce JM, Pittet D. Guideline for hand hygiene in healthcare-settings. Recommendations of the Healthcare Infection Control Practices Advisory Committee and the HICPAC/SHEA/APIC/IDSA Hand Hygiene Task Force. *Am J infect Control* 2002;30:S1–46.

247. Centers for Disease Control and Prevention. Recommendations for preventing the spread of vancomycin resistance. *MMWR* 1995;44 (RR-12):1–13.

248. Fogel MA, Nussbaum PB, Feintzeig ID, et al. Cefazolin in chronic hemodialysis patients: A safe, effective alternative to vancomycin. *Am J Kidney Dis* 1998;32:401–9.

249. Marx MA, Frye RF, Matzke GR, Golper TA. Cefazolin as empiric therapy in hemodialysis-related infections: Efficacy and blood concentrations. *Am J Kidney Dis* 1998;32:410–14.

250. Favero MS, Bond WW. Chemical disinfection of medical and surgical materials. In: Block SS, ed. *Disinfection, sterilization, and preservation.* 4th ed. Philadelphia: Lea & febiger, 1991:617–11.

251. Favero MS, Bolyard EA. Microbiologic considerations. Disinfection and sterilization strategies and the potential for airborne transmission of bloodborne pathogens. *Surg Clin North Am* 1995;75:1071–89.

252. Centers for Disease Control. Recommendations for prevention of HIV transmission in healthcare facilities. *MMWR* 1987;36:1S–18S.

253. Roberts C, Antonoplos P. Inactivation of human immunodeficiency virus type 1, hepatitis A virus, respiratory syncytial virus, vaccinia virus, herpes simplex virus type 1, and poliovirus type 2 by hydrogen peroxide gas plasma sterilization. *Am J Infect Control* 1998;26:94–101.

254. Bond WW, Favero MS, Petersen NJ, Ebert JW. Inactivation of hepatitis B virus by intermediate-to-high-level disinfectant chemicals. *J Clin Microbiol* 1983;18:535–38.

255. Sattar SA, Tetro J, Springthorpe VS, Giulivi A. Preventing the spread of hepatitis B and C viruses. Where are germicides relevant? *Am J Infect Control* 2001;29:187–97.

The Intensive Care Unit: Part A. HAI Epidemiology, Risk Factors, Surveillance, Engineering and Administrative Infection Control Practices, and Impact

Didier Pittet and Stephan J. Harbarth

The care of critically ill patients in specialized high-technology units is a primary component of modern medicine, although the efficacy and long-term benefit of critical care has been established for only a few conditions. Invasive diagnostic and therapeutic procedures are essential for the diagnosis and treatment of critically ill patients. However, life support systems often disrupt normal host defense mechanisms, affecting patients with already impaired immune response. Given the severity of the illnesses affecting patients in intensive care units (ICUs), it is not surprising that mortality rates can exceed 25%. In addition, more than one-third of the patients admitted to ICUs experience unexpected complications of medical care [1]. Healthcare-associated infection (HAI) is one of the most common medical complications affecting ICU patients. Although ICUs make up only 5–10% of

hospital beds, infections acquired in these units account for >20% of HAIs [2–4]. Fortunately, systematic studies of the determinants of HAIs, HAI surveillance, and adherence to protocols for preventing HAIs have been effective in reducing the risk for patients admitted to ICUs.

ICU-ACQUIRED HAIs

Pathogenesis

The dynamics of ICU-acquired HAIs are complex and depend on the contribution of the host's underlying conditions, the infectious agents, and the unique environment of the ICU. The following discussion considers the role of each component in the development of HAIs.

Host Defenses

The ability of patients in ICUs to ward off infections is seriously compromised. Natural host defense mechanisms may be impaired by underlying diseases or as a result of medical or surgical interventions. All patients admitted to an ICU will have at least one, often several, indwelling devices that break the normal skin barriers and establish direct access between the external environment and normally sterile body sites. Natural chemical barriers in the stomach are neutralized by administering H2-blockers or antacids that reduce acidity and allow growth of enteric flora. Physiologic mechanisms for evacuating and cleansing hollow organs are disrupted and circumvented by insertion of endotracheal tubes, nasogastric tubes, or urinary catheters.

Specific host defense mechanisms also may be impaired by the underlying diseases. Patients with malignant disorders may have abnormal immune responses as a result of their disease or from therapies that diminish the number of effective phagocyte cells and blunt the normal immune response. ICU patients who are at the extremes of age exhibit selected impairments in natural and specific defense mechanisms that increase the HAI risk [5,6].

Because of the precarious condition of ICU patients, normal food intake often is suspended, leading to under- or malnutrition [7]. Injured tissue, perfusion deficits, and infection cause fever and tachycardia through mechanisms mediated by hormones and cytokines, such as endotoxin. The physiologic response to these mediators is an increase in oxygen consumption stemming from an increase in metabolic demand. This response results in breakdown of muscle to meet the body's demand for energy. The lean body mass declines, resulting in deficits in substrates necessary for recovery [8].

Although its clinical significance in hospitals is not well established, malnutrition has been associated with increased complication rates and delayed wound healing [9,10]. Several studies suggest that poor nutritional status is a predisposing factor for HAIs [11–13]. Recent studies have confirmed that the use of enteral nutrition vs. total parenteral nutrition (TPN), early initiation of enteral nutrition, and use of enteral and parenteral glutamine and intensive insulin therapy are all associated with reduced infectious morbidity in critically ill patients [14–16]. For instance, early or glutamine-enriched enteral nutrition in critically ill patients has been reported to decrease HAIs and other complications [17,18]. Conversely, a meta-analysis including 26 studies that examined the relationship between TPN and mortality rates in critically ill patients showed that TPN had no effect on mortality and only lowered complication rates in malnourished patients [19]. In a meta-analysis of trials comparing enteral nutrition to TPN in ICU patients, Simpson et al. reported that TPN was associated with an increase in infectious complications (odds ratio [OR] = 1.47; 95% confidence intervals [CI] = 0.90 to 2.38) [20].

Important alterations in T- and B-cell function affecting host defense and resistance to infection are found in critically ill and traumatized patients [21]. Alterations in T-cell activation and cytokine production are frequently associated with trauma and hemorrhage. Injury and blood loss result in activation of CD8 T-cell populations capable of altering bacterial antigen-specific B-cell repertoires and suppressing the function of other T-cells.

Systemic hypoxia and hypovolemia also are significant contributors to the development of infection. However, significant changes in perioperative care have been suggested in recent years [22,23]. The maintenance or restoration of normal physiologic characteristics after surgery becomes the key to preventing complications [24].

Medical Devices

The results of the European Prevalence of Infection in Intensive Care (EPIC) study [25] highlighted the relative importance of medical devices as risk factors for HAIs compared with other factors. Factors were collected from >10,000 ICU patients, of whom 2,064 had ICU-acquired HAIs. Among the seven independent risk factors identified, four were associated with medical devices commonly used in ICUs: central venous catheters (CVC) (OR = 1.35, 95% CI = 1.60 to 1.57), pulmonary artery catheters (OR = 1.20, 95% CI = 1.01 to 1.43), urinary catheters (OR = 1.41, 95% CI = 1.19 to 1.69), and mechanical ventilation (OR = 1.75, 95% CI = 1.51 to 2.03). Other independent risk factors for ICU-acquired HAIs were stress ulcer prophylaxis (OR = 1.38, 95% CI = 1.20 to 1.60), the presence of trauma on admission (OR = 2.07, 95% CI = 1.75 to 2.44), and the length of ICU stay. The latter constituted the strongest predictor of HAIs and showed a linear increase in the odds for HAI with time spent in the ICU [25].

In a recently published study [26], McLaws and Berry analyzed the rate for CVC-associated bloodstream infection (BSI) in 1,375 patients who were monitored for 7,467 days of CVC use. They found significant differences in the BSI rate depending on the length of catheterization (Figure 24A-1). The probability of BSI with a CVC in place was 6% by day 15, 14% by day 25, 21% by day 30, and 53% by day 320. Thus, the risk of BSI is not homogenous and increases substantially after prolonged CVC-insertion (>2 wks).

Underlying Diseases

ICUs, by design, serve patients with severe illnesses that compromise host defense. Each patient must be assessed individually to determine how the underlying illness might interfere with host defense mechanisms. A simple assessment of the severity of underlying illness was developed by McCabe and Jackson [27], who stratified patients according to whether the underlying disease was fatal, ultimately fatal, or nonfatal. Subsequent studies by Britt et al. [28] demonstrated the utility of this simple assessment for estimating the risk of nosocomial BSI.

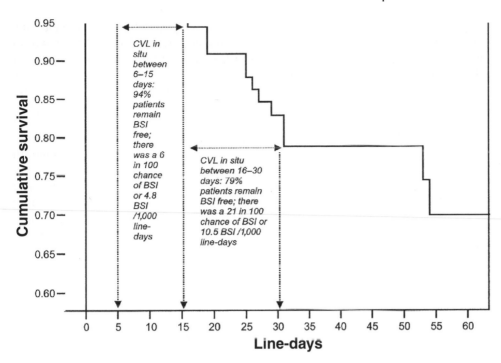

CVL in situ between 6–15 days: 94% patients remain BSI free; there was a 6 in 100 chance of BSI or 4.8 BSI /1,000 line-days

CVL in situ between 16–30 days: 79% patients remain BSI free; there was a 21 in 100 chance of BSI or 10.5 BSI /1,000 line-days

Figure 24A-1 Kaplan–Meier survival curve of a nonuniform hazard for the development of bloodstream infection (BSI) beginning with all patients (cumulative survival, 1.00) free of BSI. By day 5, 99% of the patients remained free of BSI. By day 16, 94% remained free of BSI. CVL-central venous catheter. (Adapted from McLaws ML, Berry G. Nonuniform risk of bloodstream infection with increasing central venous catheter-days. *Infect Control Hospital Epidemiol* 2005; 26:715–719 with permission.)

Numerous studies have found increasing rates of HAIs among patients with more severe illnesses [29].

Although McCabe's classification has been useful, it was not designed to assess ICU patients. Therefore, several severity-of-illness scoring systems have been proposed to estimate a patient's risk of death in ICUs objectively. Great progress has been observed in the last 10 years in the accuracy of statistical models to assess critically ill patients and predict survival [30,31]. Customized or modified versions of the most frequently used scoring systems (e.g., simplified acute physiology score [SAPS] III and Acute Physiology, Age, and Chronic Health Evaluation [APACHE] III) have been proposed to provide satisfactory estimates of the probability of death in ICU patients, which depends on the severity of illness, the number of acute organ failures, and the characteristics of underlying disease [32–35]. Nevertheless, limitations persist about the capacity of these scoring systems to integrate differences in overall quality of care [36]. Moreover, older versions of these scores, which were developed in the early 1990s, have shown a decline in predictive accuracy as the models age. Therefore, mortality tends to be overpredicted when older models are applied to more contemporary data, which, in turn, leads to biased benchmarking data of different ICUs [37]. Thus, care should be taken when using outdated severity scoring models to contemporary populations.

A group of critical care physicians developed, by consensus, the so-called "Sepsis-Related Organ Failure Assessment" (SOFA) score in December 1994, a severity scoring system that targets septic patients [38]. Because the score is not specific for sepsis, it was later called "Sequential Organ Failure Assessment." The SOFA score is composed of scores from six organ systems, graded from 0 to 4 according to the degree of dysfunction [39]. While primarily designed to describe morbidity, several analyses showed a relationship between the SOFA score and mortality [40,41]. These analyses indicated a good correlation of the score with survival and a good distribution of patients among the different score values.

Infectious Agents and Antimicrobial Resistance

In ICUs where antibiotics are used more frequently and in larger amounts than in almost any other hospital area, antimicrobial resistance ensures the survival of some HAI pathogens [42]. Moreover, the close proximity of patients facilitates transfer of resistant organisms from patient to patient [43,44]. It is noteworthy that trends in the pathogens responsible for HAIs in the ICU have shown an increase in infections due to multiply-resistant gram-positive bacteria (e.g., coagulase-negative staphylococci, *S. aureus*, *E. faecium*), gram-negative bacteria (GNB) (e.g., *Enterobacter* spp, *Acinetobacter baumannii*) and fungi such as *Candida* spp. [4,45,46]. The emergence of these pathogens is due, at least in part, to patterns of antibiotic use and selection pressure and to the development of antibiotic resistance among these isolates [47].

Recent data from the Center for Disease Control and Prevention's (CDC's) National Nosocomial Infections Surveillance (NNIS) system shows alarming trends in the nosocomial transmission rates of multiresistant organisms in the United States [48]. This voluntary surveillance system receives monthly reports of HAIs data from a nonrandom sample of >300 hospitals in 42 U.S. states. The microbiological data include antimicrobial susceptibility test results on all nonduplicate clinical isolates processed by the microbiology laboratories during each month stratified by patients' hospital location. The most recent NNIS report [48] shows that in 2003, 60% of all *Staphylococcus aureus* isolates in the participating U.S. ICUs were methicillin resistant, 29% of all enterococci were vancomycin resistant, and 89% of all coagulase-negative staphylococci were methicillin resistant. More than 30% of all *Pseudomonas aeruginosa* isolates from ICU patients were resistant to fluoroquinolones or ceftazidime. Of note, there has been a nearly 50% increase in nonsusceptible *Klebsiella pneumoniae* isolates to third-generation cephalosporins between 2002 and 2003. Likewise, methicillin-resistant *S. aureus* (MRSA) account for ≥30% of *S. aureus* isolates in most European ICUs and are a growing problem, especially in southern Europe, where rates of antibiotic resistance are alarmingly high with a prevalence of methicillin resistance among *S. aureus* isolates of ≥50% [49,50].

Organisms such as *Klebsiella* spp. and *Escherichia coli* are important sources of transferable antibiotic resistance, and multiresistant *Enterobacteriaceae* are now endemic in many countries and settings [45,51–54]. Numerous reports have demonstrated spread of antibiotic resistance from ICUs to other hospital units and vice versa [55–57]. D'Agata et al. [56,58] prospectively examined sporadic and endemic colonization with resistant GNB in a Boston ICU. The study showed that most resistant GNB were imported from outside but detected within the ICU by intensive microbiologic surveillance. Routine clinical cultures would have detected multiresistant GNB in only 5% (3/60) of patients. The most important risk factor for colonization with resistant GNB except for severity of illness and previous hospitalization was the duration of exposure to antibiotic prophylaxis with first-generation cephalosporins [56]. The authors concluded that inappropriate antibiotic use outside the ICU increases the chances of developing resistant GNB for patients admitted to the ICU.

Another HAI pathogen that is increasingly colonizing and infecting patients is *A. baumannii*. Patients with debilitating conditions are at especially high risk of acquiring pneumonia or bacteremia with this pathogen [59–62]. Observational studies may help to identify modifiable risk factors for *A. baumannii* HAI so that preventive measures can be implemented. The wide use of broad-spectrum antibiotics may be one of the most important risk factors for *A. baumannii* colonization and infection [63,64]. Villers et al. [65] illustrated the complex relation between the use of fluoroquinolones and the occurrence of *A. baumannii* infections in a French ICU. They showed that epidemic infections coexisted with endemic infections favored by the selection pressure of intravenous fluoroquinolones.

Different types of epidemiological studies have been used to quantify the association between antibiotic exposure and resistance in critically ill patients [66–70]. These studies included outbreak reports, laboratory-based surveys, randomized trials, and prospective or retrospective cohort studies based on analyses of individual patient data or aggregated data. The different methodological approaches are not mutually transposable, and the lack of uniformity makes the comparison of different studies difficult. For instance, aggregated data may be limited by "ecologic bias," which is the failure of group-level estimates to reflect the biological effect of antibiotic use at the individual-patient level. This bias is a result of the fact that, unlike individual-level studies, ecologic studies do not link individual outcome events to individual antibiotic exposure histories. Notwithstanding these difficulties, the majority of studies confirm that dramatic differences exist in the pattern of antimicrobial usage and antimicrobial resistance between different hospitals and ICUs. Use of antimicrobials may show important variations between institutions facing similar prevalences of highly resistant organisms, confirming that efforts to control resistance should focus on both antimicrobial use and infection control practices [71].

Sources of Colonization

Host colonization is a prerequisite for the development of infection. This process involves adherence of organisms to epithelial or mucosal cells, proliferation, and persistence at the site of attachment. Although the factors promoting the progression from colonization to infection are not well understood, almost 50% of ICU-acquired HAIs are preceded by host colonization with the same organism. Factors associated with microbial colonization are similar to those associated with development of infection. These risk factors include the duration of hospitalization and length of ICU stay, invasive devices, prolonged antibiotic therapy, and elimination of normal pharyngeal or bowel flora through the use of broad-spectrum antimicrobial agents [72]. Other factors promoting colonization of patients in ICUs include disruption of normal mechanical defense mechanisms (i.e., the bronchial mucociliary "escalator") by drugs or tracheal intubation, changes in protective antibacterial secretions (i.e., lysozyme, lactoferrin, saliva, and gastric acid) in response to stress and therapeutic agents, or disruption of "colonization resistance."

A vast literature exists regarding the development of colonization and subsequent infection [73]. A few important studies are summarized. The classic article [74] of Johanson et al., written in 1969, showed that severe illness predisposes to oropharyngeal GNB colonization. In 1974, Schimpff et al. [75] suggested that in critically ill patients, the origin of infection usually is the endogenous flora. Several studies have subsequently confirmed that patients are rapidly colonized by GNB after ICU admission and later develop infection with the same organisms [76–80].

In a recently published landmark study, Grundmann et al. [44] prospectively studied HAIs in patients admitted to five ICUs in Germany. During 28,498 patient days, 431 ICU-acquired HAIs and 141 episodes of nosocomial transmission were identified. A total of 278 HAIs were caused by the 10 species that were genotyped; only 41 (14.5%) could be associated with transmissions between patients. Thus, modern typing methods confirmed that the patients' endogenous flora is probably the most important source of HAI in the ICU setting.

The central role of gastric colonization in the pathogenesis of HAI and pneumonia has been called into question. Based on studying sequences of colonization in ICU patients, Bonten et al. [81] concluded that the stomach is unlikely to be an important source of pathogens leading to nosocomial pneumonia as diagnosed by bronchoalveolar lavage (BAL) or protected specimen brush (PSB). Furthermore, the initial site and route of colonization might not be the same for all organisms [81]. These results were confirmed in a large, observational cohort study conducted in two medical ICUs where specimens for culture were taken daily from nares, oropharynx, trachea, and stomach from the time of admission to the first signs of nosocomial pneumonia [82]. The stomach was an uncommon source of organisms that cause pneumonia in ventilated patients. Preventive regimens should thus be mainly directed against colonization of the oropharynx and trachea [83].

Epidemiology

Infection Sites and Types of ICU

In 1992, a total of 1,417 ICUs in 17 countries in Western Europe participated in a one-day point prevalence study [25]. The prevalence of ICU-acquired HAIs was 20.6% (2,064/10,038) and markedly varied from country to country, ranging from 9.7–31.6%. Trends toward higher ICU-acquired HAI prevalence paralleled trends toward higher mortality [84]. These differences are likely to reflect differences in ICU care practice between countries and underline the importance of controlling for case mix when interpreting and comparing HAI rates between hospitals or countries [85,86].

Not only at a national or international level, the frequency differs with which HAIs occur but also at different sites in the ICU and within a hospital. The annual NNIS report and data from the German ICU surveillance system Krankenhaus Infections Surveillance System illustrate these differences in the incidence of HAIs in different types of wards and ICUs [48,87]. First, urinary tract infections (UTIs) predominate in general wards, whereas the most common HAIs in ICUs are lower respiratory tract infections (LRTIs). Second, rates of HAI tend to be higher in surgical than medical ICUs, and rates in the adult ICUs are generally higher than in pediatric ICUs (except neonatal ICUs) [88]. Third, in adult ICUs, the lower respiratory tract (LRT) is the most common site of infection, whereas in pediatric ICUs, BSIs predominate (Table 24A-1). High rates of pulmonary infections relative to other HAI sites are unique to adult ICUs where patients are frequently admitted because of respiratory distress and require mechanical ventilation. Although primary BSIs and infections stemming from the

TABLE 24A-1

NOSOCOMIAL INFECTION RATES IN GERMAN INTENSIVE CARE UNITS; GERMAN KISS SURVEILLANCE SYSTEM, 1997 TO 2004, ACCORDING TO TYPE OF ICU AND INFECTION

Type of ICU	Urinary Tract Infection	Central Line-Associated Bloodstream Infection	Ventilator-Associated Pneumonia
	Rates Per 1,000 Device-Days		Rates Per 1,000 Days of Mechanical Ventilation
Inter-disciplinary	2.2	1.6	7.1
Surgery	3.6	2.0	9.5
Neurosurgery	4.5	1.4	10.8
Medical	2.9	2.2	6.9
Pediatric	2.4	4.0	1.9

www.nrz-hygiene.de.

presence of vascular cannulas are less common than LRTIs, the morbidity and mortality associated with these infections are particularly high [89,90].

In 2000, the CDC briefly reported a decrease in HAI rates in the ICUs of participating NNIS hospitals from 1990 to 1999 [91]. Device exposure–adjusted HAI rates decreased for three body sites (LRTIs, UTIs, and BSIs). The greatest decrease was observed for BSI rates, which decreased in medical ICUs by 44%, in coronary ICUs by 43%, in pediatric ICUs by 32%, and in surgical ICUs by 31%. However, because of a progressively shorter ICU length of stay over the last 20 years, the overall, hospitalwide rate of HAIs per 1,000 patient-days has actually increased by 36%, from 7.2 in 1975 to 9.8 in 1995 [92]. The variable use of different denominators also may have an important effect on trend analyses and may bias benchmarking [93].

When HAI rates have been compared over shorter increments of time (i.e., by month) wide variations have been noted. Observations in different ICUs suggested that the level of skilled nursing care relative to patient census may be an important determinant of this variation [94,95]. Indeed, there are a large number of studies showing that overcrowding, understaffing, or a misbalance between workload and resources are important determinants of HAIs and cross-transmission of organisms in ICUs [96–98]. Importantly, not only the number of staff but also the level of their training affects outcomes. The causal pathway between understaffing and HAI is complex, and factors might include lack of time to comply with infection control recommendations, job dissatisfaction, job-related burnout, absenteeism, and a high staff turnover [95].

In summary, rates of HAIs vary considerably within hospitals by type of ICU. Rates are generally lower in cardiac ICUs and higher in neonatal, surgical, trauma, and burn units, reflecting the higher risk of HAI of patients admitted to these latter types of units [48].

Impact of Infections Acquired in the ICU

HAIs in the ICU are harmful for the patients and expensive for society. Several studies suggest that nosocomial LRTIs and BSIs are associated with a two- to threefold increased risk of death in ICU patients [99,100]. Thus, in contrast to a widespread theory, a significant proportion of patients in the ICU dies due to HAIs.

Crude mortality rates in patients who acquire HAIs in the ICU are estimated to vary between 10% and 80%. The term attributable (or excess) mortality defines the mortality directly associated with the infection rather than the mortality attributable to underlying conditions. In ICU patients, underlying conditions other than HAI that may affect the outcome mainly include pre-existing comorbidities, severity of acute physiologic disturbance, and complications arising from these conditions [101].

Assessment of mortality attributable to HAIs in the ICU setting is difficult and not straightforward because HAIs and mortality attributable to other causes share common risk factors that may confound the cause-and-effect relationship. Thus, it is sometimes difficult to estimate whether the critically ill patient would have survived in the absence of HAI. The most often used approach to estimate the attributable mortality of HAIs in ICU patients is to conduct a matched cohort study. In this type of study design, cases are defined as patients in whom HAIs develop during their ICU stay. These case-patients are subsequently compared with noninfected controls. Case- and control-patients usually are matched for age, time of the year, underlying diseases, and additional variables that may contribute to excessive mortality rates of ICU stay independent of the HAI itself. In brief, the attributable mortality due to HAI defines the excess mortality due to the infection. As an example, Table 24A-2 summarizes estimates of excess mortality attributable to nosocomial pneumonia in ICU populations.

For the assessment of the economic burden associated with HAI in the ICU, matched cohort studies are not optimal. This study design has several limitations because of the time-varying nature of the exposure. One source of bias occurs when infected and uninfected patients are compared with regard to total hospital costs or total hospital length of stay [102]. For infected patients, only those costs incurred after the occurrence of the HAI are possibly secondary to infection. Before infection onset, patients are unexposed. The association between pre-infection outcome and HAI is entirely noncausal from the perspective of measuring the excess burden of infection. Therefore, combining pre-infection outcomes with

TABLE 24A-2
ATTRIBUTABLE MORTALITY OF VENTILATOR-ASSOCIATED PNEUMONIA: MATCHED COHORT STUDIES, 1993–2005

First Author, Year, Reference	Cases/ Controls	Mortality		
		Case	Control	Attributable
Fagon (1993) [242]	48/48	54.2	27.1	27.1
Papazian (1996) [243]	85/85	40.0	38.8	1.2
Baker (1996) [244]	29/58	24.0	24.0	0.0
Rello (1996) [245]	26/52	42.3	28.8	13.5
Heyland (1999) [246]	173/173	23.7	17.7	6.0
Bercault (2001) [247]	135/135	41.0	14.0	27.0
Rello (2002) [127]	816/2243	30.5	30.4	0.1
Hugonnet (2004) [126]	97/97	32.0	24.7	7.3
Rosenthal (2005) [248]	307/307	63.5	33.2	30.3

postinfection outcomes dramatically amplifies confounding [103].

Several recent studies have demonstrated the effect of this bias. Outcome analyses that did not account for the time before the occurrence of the HAI yielded different results than studies that did account for the time before the HAI. Schulgen et al. [104] tested different methods and showed that the use of unmatched or matched comparisons between non-infected and infected patients led to an overestimation of the excess length of stay due to nosocomial pneumonia compared to analyses based on a structural formulation of transitions between different states. In a recent study, Beyersmann et al. have confirmed the validity of this statistical approach [105]. They showed that HAI significantly reduced the discharge hazard (HR = 0.72; 95% CI = 0.63–0.82) (i.e., prolonged ICU stay). Prolongation of ICU length of stay due to HAI was estimated at 5.3 days ($\pm$1.6). Similarly, Asensio and Torres [106] found that regression models yielded lower estimates of the excess length of stay and cost due to HAI than a matched-pair comparison. Another approach to estimating cost and length of stay effects of adverse events is to apply survival models in which the adverse event is incorporated as a time-dependent variable. This strategy can be applied to costs and length of stay [103].

Even when the time-varying nature of the exposure is accounted for, it is still necessary to adequately adjust for traditional confounders, those factors that both increase the risk of HAI and affect the outcome of interest. For instance, Soufir et al. [107] investigated the excess risk of death due to catheter-related bloodstream infection (CR-BSI) in a cohort of critically ill patients. The crude case-fatality ratio was 50% and 21% in patients with and without CR-BSI, respectively. The statistical method of adjustment was based on Cox proportional hazards regression with inclusion of matching variables and prognostic factors for mortality. CR-BSI remained associated with mortality following adjustment for prognostic factors at ICU admission (HR = 2.0; P = 0.03). However, after controlling for severity scores calculated one week before CR-BSI, the increased mortality was no longer significant in the Cox model (HR = 1.4; P = 0.27).

In summary, HAIs in critically ill patients unquestionably have substantial impact on morbidity and mortality. However, the matched cohort study design may produce bias in the estimation of the effects of HAI on length of stay and costs. Cost effects or excess length of stay are likely to be overestimated if the interval to onset of HAI is not properly accounted for in the study design or analysis [103].

Causative Agents

Bacteria, fungi, and viruses have been reported as causative agents in HAIs, and many infections are polymicrobial. Data obtained from the NNIS System and the previously mentioned EPIC study (Table 24A-3) illustrate the trends in microbial etiology of HAIs responsible for disease in ICUs [25,108]. These data reflect a large geographic sample and are representative of ICUs in the industrialized world. Similar patterns of causative organisms have been noted in other studies [2,109–111]. For instance, recently reported data from the German KISS system identified the following as most commonly reported HAI pathogens [110]: S. aureus (16.5% of all HAIs), P. aeruginosa (14.2%), E. coli (13.9%), enterococci (13.4%), C. albicans (11.2%), Klebsiella spp. (9.1%), coagulase-negative staphylococci (9.1%), and Enterobacter spp. (7.4%). The recently published Sepsis Occurrence in Acutely ill Patients (SOAP) study [111] investigated a large cohort of septic patients in 198 ICUs in 24 European countries. Among the 279 patients with ICU-acquired HAIs, staphylococci, including MRSA, were most frequent (40%), followed by Pseudomonas spp. (21%), streptococci (19%), E. coli (17%), and C. albicans (16%). Patients with ICU-acquired HAIs had a higher incidence of mixed infections (23% vs. 16%) compared with those with non-ICU-acquired sepsis [111].

Table 24A-3 lists the most common HAI pathogens by infection site from U.S. or Western European ICUs. The leading pathogens causing nosocomial BSI and surgical site infections (SSIs) were staphylococci and enterococci. P. aeruginosa was the most common pathogen causing LRTI. Candida spp and E. coli were the most prevalent pathogens from UTIs. Overall, in contrast to the 1970s, major shifts in the etiology of HAIs occurred in the decades between 1980 and 2000 [29]. Gram-positive bacterial or fungal infections are becoming more common, and GNB such as Klebsiella spp. are becoming increasingly resistant to available antibiotics. Taken as a whole, the shifts are away from more easily treated pathogens

TABLE 24A-3

LEADING NOSOCOMIAL PATHOGENS BY SITE AND FREQUENCY

Sites	Pathogens	NNIS, ICU[a] (%)	EPIC, ICU[b] (%)
Blood	CNS	43%	34%
	S. aureus	14	22
	Enterococci	14	11
	Candida spp	NR	9
	E. coli	3	7
	Enterobacter spp	4	—
Surgical wound	S. aureus	23	27
	Enterococci	14	18
	CNS	16	14
	E. coli	7	13
	P. aeruginosa	9	22
	Enterobacter spp	9	8
Respiratory tract	P. aeruginosa	18	30
	S. aureus	28	32
	Enterobacter spp	10	7
	Acinetobacter spp	7	10
	K. pneumoniae	7	8
Urinary tract	E. coli	26	22
	Enterococci	17	15
	P. aeruginosa	16	19
	Candida spp	NR	21
	K. pneumoniae	10	—
	Enterobacter spp	7	—

CNS, coagulase-negative staphylococci. NR, not reported.
[a] [108]
[b] from Vincent JL, Bihari DJ, Suter PM, et al. The prevalence of nosocomial infection in intensive care units in Europe: results of the European Prevalence of Infection in Intensive Care (EPIC) study. JAMA 1995;274:639–644, and from Suter PM, personal communication (date unknown).

toward more resistant pathogens with fewer options for therapy [108].

Clusters of Infections in the ICU

Although <10% of hospitalized patients are treated in ICUs, many outbreaks of HAIs occur in these units, frequently related to breaks in technique or noncompliance with infection control guidelines. Other epidemics are associated with specific strains of bacteria, usually related to a contaminated inanimate or animate reservoir from which the organism may be transmitted to the patients [112].

A literature search in the Web-based repository **www.outbreak-database.com** for outbreaks occurring in ICUs identified more than 800 hits. Table 24A-4 summarizes important features of selected outbreaks [113–116]. Leading pathogens of outbreaks in the ICU setting were MRSA and GNB.

Although there were unique factors in each epidemic, several generalizations can be made. Epidemics associated with specific pathogens often were associated with bacteria that were relatively resistant to antibiotics, relatively

TABLE 24A-4
SELECTED OUTBREAKS IN DIFFERENT ICUs

Unit	Organism	Sites of Infection or Colonization	Transmission	Number of Patients	Duration	Reference
Medical ICU	Glycopeptide intermediate MRSA	Multiple sites	Cross-contamination	21	10 mo	[116]
Surgical ICU	Acinetobacter baumannii	Multiple sites	Respiratory equipment	10	4 mo	[115]
Surgical ICU	Arenavirus	Choriomeningitis	Transplanted organs from an infected donor	4	1 mo	[119]
Neonatal ICU	Pantoea spp	Sepsis	Contaminated parenteral nutrition	8	3 days	[249]
Pediatric ICU	Pneumocystis jirovecci	Pneumonia	Direct patient to patient	4	9 mo	[250]
Neonatal ICU	Pseudomonas aeruginosa	Bloodstream infection	Nurse with chronic otitis externa	5	7 mo	[114]
Neonatal ICU	MRSA	Multiple sites	Breast milk	3	1 mo	[113]
Mixed ICU	SARS	Pneumonia	Inhalation	51	3 mo	[251]
Mixed ICU	Serratia liquefaciens	Bloodstream infection	Pressure-monitoring equipment	16	3 mo	[252]
Neonatal ICU	Pseudomonas aeruginosa	Multiple sites	Artificial fingernails	46	15 mo	[253]
Neonatal ICU	Enterobacter cloacae	Multiple sites	Cross-contamination and multidose vials	8	2 mo	[96]
Neonatal ICU	Malassezia pachydermatis	Multiple sites	Health care workers' pet dogs	15	15 mo	[254]
Surgical ICU	Bacillus stearothermophilus	Sepsis	Contamination of plasma expanders	8	1 mo	[255]
Neonatal ICU	Hepatitis A	Hepatitis	Vertical transmission	10	1 mo	[256]
General ICU	Enterococcus faecium	Bacteremia	Electronic thermometer	9	3 mo	[257]

ICU, intensive care unit.

virulent when compared with normal endogenous and environmental flora, capable of withstanding variations in environmental conditions, and transmitted by hand from patient to patient [63]. Pathogens that exemplify these characteristics include *S. aureus* and *Serratia*, *Klebsiella*, and *Enterobacter* spp. Epidemics caused by unusual organisms, such as *Acinetobacter* spp, often were associated with contaminated equipment or with changes in the environment [117]. HAI outbreaks were more frequently reported from neonatal ICUs than from other types of ICUs [96]. It is important to remember that new equipment or a new procedure may introduce a new reservoir or mode of transmission into the ICU [118]. Finally, transplanted organs from infected donors also can serve as source of unusual HAIs in the critical care setting [119,120].

Clinical Aspects of Infections in the ICU

Critically ill patients are highly susceptible to HAIs. The importance of medical devices in catheter-associated UTIs, intravascular device–associated infections, and ventilator-associated pneumonia is discussed elsewhere. Only selected aspects of infections seen predominantly in ICU patients will be discussed in the following section.

Ventilator-Associated Pneumonia

Pneumonia is the most common ICU-acquired HAI, accounting for 25–50% of all HAIs in ICU patients [121]. In mechanically ventilated patients, pneumonia is associated with an excess mortality ranging between 0 and 30% (Table 24A-2) [104,122]. The attributable mortality varies according to underlying disease, type of pathogen, and adequacy of initial empiric antibiotic treatment [123–125]. For instance, in a matched cohort study conducted at Geneva University Hospitals, we analyzed 97 patients with ventilator-associated pneumonia (VAP) and observed an excess mortality rate of 7.3% (P = 0.26) [126]. Considering the studies shown in Table 24A-4 and the data generated by a recently published systematic review, critically ill patients who develop VAP appear to be 1.4–2.0 times as likely to die compared to patients without VAP [99]. In surviving patients, VAP causes substantial morbidity and extends hospital length of stay by at least 4 days.

Patients who have suffered severe trauma and those who have had major surgery are at particularly increased risk of subsequent LRTIs [127]. Exogenous infection is rare, but, on occasion, medication nebulizers, the endotracheal tube lumen, and other respiratory therapy equipment or

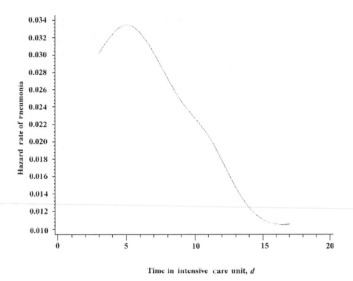

Figure 24A-2 Hazard rate for ventilator-associated pneumonia during the stay in the ICU. The hazard function presents the conditional probability of ventilator-associated pneumonia in the next day, given that a patient is event free. Estimation of the hazard function shows the event rate per day over the duration of ventilation. (Adapted from Cook et al. Incidence of and risk factors for ventillator-associated pneumonia in critically ill patients. *Ann Intern Med* 1998; 129:433–440 with permission.)

contaminated hospital water can serve as sources for the inoculation of organisms into the lung [115].

Although mechanical ventilation is not a necessary prerequisite for the development of ICU-acquired pneumonia, it substantially increases the LRTI risk. Cook et al. found that the daily risk of pneumonia was not linear: It was highest during the first week (3% per day) and decreased thereafter [128]. In the third week of mechanical ventilation, pneumonia developed in ~1% of patients with each additional day of mechanical ventilation (Figure 24A-2).

Cultures of the LRT are important in the diagnosis of ICU-acquired pneumonia [129]. Because the oropharynx of critically ill patients is frequently colonized with potentially pathogenic bacteria, care must be taken to avoid contaminating cultures of the lower airways. Retrieval of culture specimens by bronchoscope using either a PSB or BAL has been helpful for this purpose [130]. Although numerous studies have evaluated the performance of bronchoscopic and nonbronchoscopic procedures for the diagnosis of VAP, controversy persists about the optimal diagnostic strategy [131]. Fever, leukocytosis, and lung consolidation, hallmarks of pneumonia in otherwise healthy patients, can result from other pathogenic mechanisms in intubated patients (e.g., pulmonary edema, contusion, atelectasis, pleural effusion, or acute respiratory distress syndrome) [132]. Therefore, several authorities encourage the use of invasive techniques to diagnose VAP, including BAL, nonbronchoscopic ("blind") BAL, and "blind" PSB, to increase diagnostic accuracy and guide clinicians in their decision making [133]. Although diagnosis by invasive

methods requires a considerable commitment of resources, it can potentially reduce cost of care and may even lower mortality due to VAP [134,135]. Whatever method chosen, the interpretation of the sensitivity and specificity of any given sampling technique may be severely hampered by the distorting effect of previous antibiotic exposure on the yield of bacterial cultures [136].

Early Onset Pneumonia

Early onset VAP accounts for at least one-third of pneumonias in the ICU. This entity should be distinguished from late-onset episodes because of their different microbiologic spectrum, risk factors, and outcome. Because the pathogens causing aspiration pneumonia reflect the oropharyngeal microbial flora at time of aspiration, the pathogens that bring about early onset pneumonia are more likely to reflect normal oral flora or pathogens responsible for community-acquired pneumonia (*S. aureus, Streptococcus pneumoniae,* or *Hemophilus influenzae*). Nevertheless, antimicrobial-resistant pathogens also may be involved in early onset pneumonia, especially in settings with high prevalence of antibiotic overuse [137,138].

In a prospective cohort study of 747 critically ill patients, Bornstain et al. [139] reported that 80 patients (11%) experienced early onset pneumonia in their ICU. Aspiration of oropharyngeal flora was the presumed mode of inoculation. Male gender, impairment of reflexes that protect the airways, sucralfate use, or unplanned extubation were the most important risk factors. Use of certain antibiotics protected against early onset pneumonia. Other potentially modifiable risk factors for early onset and late-onset pneumonia have been summarized recently [140].

Nosocomial Sinusitis

Sinusitis frequently complicates nasotracheal or nasogastric intubation (2–25%) [141,142]. Mechanical obstruction of the maxillary sinuses usually initiates the process with subsequent spread to the ethmoid and sphenoid sinuses. Fever, leukocytosis, and purulent nasal discharge suggest the diagnosis, but their absence does not exclude it [143]. Conventional sinus radiographs and computed tomography scans are useful, but sinus aspirate allows confirmation of the diagnosis and identification of the causative agents [144]. In contrast to community-acquired sinusitis, GNB have predominated in this context. *Pseudomonas* spp., *Enterobacteriaceae,* and anaerobic bacteria have been the pathogens most commonly recovered [145,146]. In addition, *S. aureus* and *Candida* spp. also have been encountered, and polymicrobial infection has been documented in 40–100% of episodes. Nasotracheal intubation is associated with a significantly higher risk of infection than orotracheal intubation [147]. Complications include pansinusitis, orbital cellulitis, brain abscess, osteomyelitis, secondary BSI, and nosocomial pneumonia [142]. Treatment requires the removal of the device and adequate intravenous antibiotic therapy.

In summary, the existing studies establish that sinusitis joins pneumonia, catheter sepsis, SSIs, and UTIs as one of the "five horsemen" of clinically important HAIs in ICU patients. Therefore, a sinus computed tomography scan is a necessary component of the evaluation of intubated patients with fever or signs of sepsis from unknown origin [148]. Sinus aspiration is essential to confirm the diagnosis, direct antimicrobial therapy, and help drainage.

Other ICU-Specific Infectious Problems

Acalculous cholecystitis, also called postoperative cholecystitis, commonly complicates both abdominal and non-abdominal surgery in critically ill patients [149,150]. *P. aeruginosa*, *E. coli*, and *Enterobacter* spp. are the most commonly isolated pathogens. Severe complications can occur, including gangrene of the gallbladder, perforation, secondary peritonitis, intrahepatic abscesses, and ipsilateral empyema. Abdominal ultrasound has been found to be a reliable method of early detection of acalculous cholecystitis and for follow-up of possible complications. Diagnostic laparoscopy might be another accurate method to establish the early diagnosis. Treatment of acalculous cholecystitis requires surgery and appropriate antimicrobial therapy. Other important ICU–specific problems include *Pneumocystis jiroveci* pneumonia in patients with the acquired immunodeficiency syndrome, meningitis, and antibiotic-associated colitis, which are discussed in other chapters of this textbook.

The differentiation of the causes of fever in ICU patients is a daily challenge for physicians. Not all fevers result from infection; nosocomial fever often does not signal HAI and may augur a wide variety of other conditions. The most common causes of noninfectious fever are listed in Table 24A-5.

Control and Prevention of HAIs

Surveillance

Two types of measures are needed to control HAIs. Engineering controls are those controls that are incorporated

TABLE 24A-5
NONINFECTIOUS FEVER IN ICU PATIENTS

Atelectasis
Acute Respiratory Distress Syndrome
Central fever in head trauma patients
Chemical aspiration
Congestive heart failure
Deep venous thrombosis
Drug fever
Pancreatitis
Postoperative fever (during the first 72 hr after surgery)
Pulmonary embolism
Resorption of hematomas

into the structural design of the unit or equipment and over which there is limited human control. Administrative controls are guidelines that must be learned and executed by healthcare workers (HCWs). The latter are effective only if appropriate changes in behavior are incorporated into the routine activities of HCWs. For instance, we experienced a cluster of invasive pulmonary aspergillosis in nonimmunocompromised patients associated with room air filter replacement [151]. Such fatal infection could have been prevented by the establishment and application of guidelines for this procedure.

Engineering Controls

The contribution of the design of ICUs to the control of HAI is difficult to evaluate. However, it seems prudent to consider several issues when remodeling or designing new units [152]:

1. Adequate space around beds is important for placement of support and monitoring equipment, allowing staff access to both the patient and the equipment.
2. Individualized cubicles for each patient also may be important in reducing transmission of pathogens in the unit; the nurse-to-patient ratio should, however, not be affected by geographical distribution.
3. Alcohol-based hand rub dispensers should be located in convenient places within <2m from the point of care to facilitate hand hygiene by HCWs and to interrupt the most important mode of microbial transmission in the ICU [153].
4. Separate, designated sinks should be provided for cleaning equipment.
5. All ICUs should be equipped with one or more class A isolation rooms [154]. Class A isolation rooms include an anteroom for gowning and hand hygiene and should provide both positive or negative air pressure. Additional rooms for isolation precautions are necessary in units where patients are located in large open rooms [155].
6. Consideration also should be given to functional activities in the unit. Attention to traffic patterns and the location of clean and dirty utilities and janitors' closets may reduce opportunities for cross-contamination. Clean function and storage should be physically separated from dirty function and waste disposal. Housekeeping facilities and equipment should be designated for the specific unit and stored separately from clean and dirty utilities.

Administrative Controls for Medical Equipment

Medical technology is changing rapidly, and new diagnostic and therapeutic devices are constantly being introduced into ICUs. In many instances, the efficacy of the devices has not been adequately evaluated, and their effect on the HAI incidence is unknown. For example, vendors seeking to introduce new urinary catheters alleged to have antimicrobial activity should be challenged to provide data on the efficacy of their product [156].

Cleaning protocols for invasive devices should be provided by the industry and be reviewed by infection control professionals or hospital epidemiologists to ensure the adequacy of the recommendations. Sufficient numbers of frequently used instruments should be available to allow time for cleaning, disinfection, and sterilization, when recommended. An increase in the initial outlay for equipment may reduce costs and morbidity in the long term. The routine application of guidelines for the appropriate use of medical devices contributes significantly to the control of HAIs. Guidelines for the use and control of urinary tract catheters, intravascular devices, respiratory devices, and other products have been published by the CDC.

The Role of the Environment

For more than two decades, infection control has focused on patients rather than the patients' environment as the most important source of HAI pathogens. This attitude was based on studies that failed to find improvement in the HAI rates after the units were moved into new, "clean" structures [157,158]. However, there is a growing body of literature emphasizing that some HAI pathogens are ubiquitous in the environment of patient-care areas, waiting to be cross-transmitted on HCWs' hands [159]. Therefore, the widespread transmission of antibiotic-resistant pathogens that survive for considerable periods in the environment (VRE, MRSA, *A. baumannii*, *C. diffcile*) and recent advances in our knowledge of the transmission of HAI pathogens requires a change in hospital hygiene practices [160]. Appropriate cleaning and disinfection procedures are essential to decrease microbial burden in the close patient environment and minimize the likelihood of cross-infection of multiresistant pathogens in this high-risk area [161].

Oelberg et al. published a spectacular experimental study using non-infectious DNA markers designed from a cauliflower mosaic virus as surrogate markers to illustrate microbial transmission pathways [162]. These investigators demonstrated the rapid spread of the DNA markers via the hands of HCWs in a neonatal ICU. The most consistently positive sites within all pods were the blood-gas analyzers, computer mouse, telephone handles, medical charts, ventilator knobs, door handles, radiant warmer control buttons, patient monitors, and, of course, personnel hands [162]. These experimental findings were extended by Foca et al. [163], who conducted an epidemiological and molecular investigation of endemic *P. aeruginosa* transmission among infants in a neonatal ICU that was associated with widespread environmental contamination and carriage of the organisms on the hands of HCWs. A history of the use of artificial fingernails or nail wraps was an additional risk factor for colonization of the hands. Transmission of *P. aeruginosa* was stopped after re-emphasis of good hand-hygiene practices, the importance of reliable cleaning techniques of inanimate surfaces and equipment,

and the complete withdrawal of jewelry, cosmetic nail treatments, water baths, and unnecessary supplies kept by the patients' bedsides [163]. A recent investigation by Carling et al. corroborated the hypothesis that cleaning of the patients' close environment is suboptimal in most ICUs, which may play an important role as reservoir for transmitting HAI pathogens [164].

Administrative Controls for Healthcare Personnel
Staffing and Training

For the patient to benefit from technologic advances in medical care, HCWs must be well trained in state-of-the-art intensive care. Studies have documented that cooperation among critical care personnel can directly influence outcomes from intensive care, suggesting that the use of invasive technologies is important but not sufficient for optimal patient care [165,166]. Therefore, HCWs in ICUs should be involved in continuous postgraduate medical education to learn new technologies and the proper use of new medical devices and procedures [167]. They also need periodic updates on new disease entities peculiar to patients in ICUs, including psychologic problems and end-of-life issues associated with ICU hospitalization. Finally, the level of stress in ICUs exceeds that of most other areas of the hospital. As a result, rates of employee turnover are high. Loss of highly skilled healthcare workers requires extensive training of replacement workers, including in-depth training on infection control procedures. Changes in staff and unrecognized modifications in infection control procedures might contribute to HAI epidemics.

The extent and severity of illnesses afflicting ICU patients demand a high level of nursing care, and the high rate of HAIs mandate strict application of rigid barrier nursing techniques to control transmission. Breakdown in these techniques during periods of understaffing or overcrowding has been associated with HAI outbreaks [95]. A nurse-to-patient staffing ratio of 1:1 has been recommended to reduce lapses in techniques that lead to person-to-person transmission of pathogens within ICUs. A study from Geneva University Hospitals underlines the importance of an adequate nurse-to-patient ratio [96]. In this study, a low nurse-to-patient ratio was found to be an independent risk factor for transmission and acquisition of *Enterobacter cloacae* in neonates (Figure 24A-3). Thus, reductions in nursing staff below a critical level may cause an increase in HAIs in ICUs by making adequate patient care difficult [168].

It is important that HCWs in ICUs understand their responsibility in preventing transmission of infectious agents. This responsibility includes prevention of spread of pathogens from patient to patient and from the healthcare worker to the patient. Therefore, it is important that the hospital provide adequate staffing to cover medical absences and personal benefits that will not punish employees who are responsible enough to avoid working when ill.

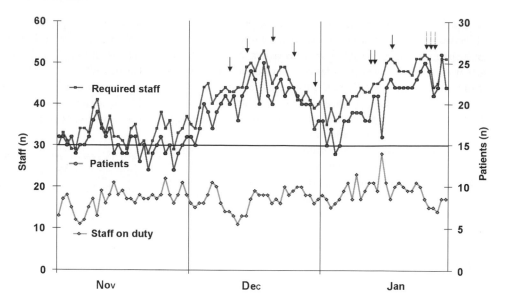

Figure 24A-3 Outbreak of *Enterobacter cloacae* at the neonatal ICU of Geneva University Hospitals, December 1996 to January 1997. Arrows indicate *Enterobacter cloacae* isolates. The horizontal line indicates the supposed maximum capacity (15 infants) of the unit.

Monitoring Quality of Care

The effectiveness of administrative controls will depend on compliance with established guidelines. Therefore, the performance and behavior of HCWs should be monitored [169]. Failure to comply with guidelines, whether on the part of physicians, nurses, or other support personnel, should be addressed promptly to prevent the establishment of bad habits that impose unnecessary risks on patients [170,171]. Monitoring the quality of medical care in ICUs is important, albeit controversial, given the complexity of the conditions of the patients and the procedures performed in these units [172].

Administrative Controls for Patients

Because of the risk of infection and other complications in ICUs, only patients who will benefit from high-intensity, high-risk care should be admitted to ICUs, and patients should be discharged from the ICU as soon as possible to lower the HAI risk. Unfortunately, there is little published information to assist the physician in making those important decisions. Surveillance for HAIs, monitoring HAI rates, and reporting results to personnel are important to ensure the quality of medical care in ICUs [173]. Properly conducted surveillance can identify behavioral, environmental, or treatment factors that, when corrected, will diminish endemic HAI rates in the unit [174]. Additional benefits of concurrent surveillance include early identification and intervention in epidemics [175].

Practical Aspects of Infection Control in the ICU

Methods for preventing HAIs are numerous. The principles are the same throughout the hospital, and many are discussed elsewhere in the text. Only selected measures

of prime importance in the ICU will be discussed in this section.

Patient Screening

Screening on ICU admission should be considered for control of highly transmissible HAI pathogens [176]. Patients colonized with multiresistant bacteria, such as MRSA or VRE, serve as a reservoir for spread within the healthcare environment, mainly through the hands of HCWs. Active surveillance by patient screening and intensive control measures attempt to decrease this reservoir with the ultimate goal of reducing infection rates [177]. Guidelines published by the CDC and Society for Healthcare Epidemiology of America (SHEA) are useful in this respect [178].

Nevertheless, the most efficient approach to control endemic MRSA in the ICU setting remains controversial [179–181]. Several authorities have suggested that screening on admission to ICUs and subsequent patient isolation may decrease the risk of cross-infection [182,183]. This may be particularly true when using a rapid screening test. We recently investigated the clinical usefulness of a rapid on-admission screening test for MRSA [184]. A substantial decrease in MRSA infections was seen in a medical ICU after increasing compliance with on-admission screening and implementing a strategy that linked the rapid test to pre-emptive isolation of MRSA patients. However, no effect on MRSA rates was observed in the surgical ICU, although a large number of unnecessary pre-emptive isolation-days could be saved by using the rapid MRSA test [184].

Despite the fact that culture-based MRSA screening techniques have proven inexpensive and sensitive if collected from several body sites, the time to report the results remains a major issue. Definitive identification and testing results are usually available only 48 to 96 hours after sample collection, a time delay that could allow MRSA cross-transmission if patients are not presumptively placed under contact precautions. This may be one of the reasons (besides low hand hygiene compliance) why the recently published study by Cepeda et al. did not show a significant effect of contact isolation for MRSA carriers identified by conventional methods [180].

Frequent transfers of patients through various units and levels of care increase the risk of transmission of resistant organisms throughout the hospital [54]. As mentioned earlier, colonized patients are important animate reservoirs of resistant organisms during interinstitutional or international transfers and probably account for the spread of multiresistant bacteria [61,185,186]. To control the spread of resistant organisms, it is important to document information regarding carriage of antibiotic-resistant microflora in the patient's medical record and to report it to receiving units and facilities. On-admission screening should be performed for any patient transferred from settings and institutions with endemic multiresistant pathogens

Patient Isolation

More than 50% of patients admitted to ICUs are colonized at the time of admission with the organism responsible for subsequent infections. Patients who are readmitted to the hospital may carry and transmit resistant organisms acquired during previous hospitalizations [187]. Not infrequently, unrecognized infection contributes to the decision for entry into the unit. The early diagnosis of potentially transmissible disease requires vigilance on the part of ICU physicians. Patients with suspected infections should be appropriately screened and segregated at the time of admission [188]. The level of isolation should account for each of the following factors: the site of infection, the mode of transmission, the amount of secretions or excretions, and the virulence and antimicrobial susceptibilities of the causative agent.

Discussion of specific isolation techniques are beyond the scope of this chapter. It should be recognized that as the duration of stay increases, the frequency of colonization with resistant microflora also grows. Patients become animate reservoirs that facilitate transmission to susceptible incoming patients [44]. It may be wise, therefore, to separate long-stay patients from the short-stay patients who make up the major portion of the population in the unit. This segregation may be accomplished by moving chronically ill patients to single rooms or relocating groups of patients to a physically separate part of the unit. A dedicated nursing staff for the long-term patients would provide an added barrier to transmission, but this is frequently impossible to implement. Adequate hand antisepsis certainly constitutes the most appropriate, least expensive, and highly effective measure, but lack of compliance is an issue [189,190].

Hand Hygiene

Routine hand hygiene before and between contact with patients is the most important feature of infection control.

Virtually all healthcare workers are aware of and agree with this concept [191]. It is dismaying, therefore, to see repeated reports of low levels of compliance with this simple and inexpensive technique. In ICUs, compliance usually does not exceed 40% and is frequently much lower [192]. Several reasons have been suggested to account for this low level of compliance, including lack of priority over other required procedures, insufficient time to accomplish hand hygiene, inconvenient placement of hand-hygiene tools, allergy or intolerance to the hand cleansing solutions, lack of leadership on the part of the senior medical staff, and lack of personal commitment to the routine of hand hygiene.

Grossly misleading impressions about the value of alcohol-based hand rubbing persisted widely during the 20th century [193]. Alcohol-based hand rubbing for HCWs has rarely been promoted systematically, and, consequently, sink-based handwashing with soap and water remained the predominant tool for reducing transient hand carriage of HAI pathogens in most ICUs. Only in the last five years has the strength of evidence in favor of alcohol-based hand rubbing become simply overwhelming so that infection-control experts around the world including the CDC and the World Health Organization (WHO) [153,192], have rewritten recommendations for hand hygiene in healthcare.

This breakthrough is due to the following important insights:

1. The time required for fully effective handwashing with soap and water is too long and, therefore, full compliance with handwashing recommendations is illusory, especially in ICUs [194].
2. If actively promoted, alcohol-based hand rubbing can improve compliance with hand-hygiene recommendations and can reduce HAI and transmission rates [195]. In high-demand settings, such as ICUs, an alcohol-based hand rub solution appears to be the only method that might allow reasonable compliance [190].
3. Various studies clearly demonstrate the improved antimicrobial efficacy of alcohol products relative to antiseptic soaps containing chlorhexidine or other antiseptics [196]. A few studies even raise doubts as to the efficacy of handwashing with soap and water in preventing the spread of multiresistant, gram-positive pathogens [197].
4. Alcohol-based hand rubbing with gels or liquid formulations containing emollients are less harmful to the skin than regular handwashing with soap and water [198,199].
5. Previous studies promoting handwashing with antimicrobial soap and water did not properly assess the independent value of alcohol-based hand rubbing [200].

Barrier Precautions

There is currently little evidence that the addition of gloves in the routine intensive care setting has any benefit over regular hand hygiene in controlling HAIs. Major arguments against the routine use of gloves in ICUs rely on the fact that HCWs frequently do not remove gloves when moving from patient to patient and forget to clean their hands after glove removal.

Whereas a number of studies have investigated the role of sophisticated forms of protective isolation in reducing high HAI rates in patients with profound granulocytopenia or full-thickness burns, only a few have evaluated whether simple protective isolation would be beneficial for ICU patients. Klein et al. [201] conducted a prospective, randomized trial in a pediatric ICU, assessing the benefit of simple barrier precautions (disposable gown and gloves) on both colonization and subsequent infection. Colonization with ICU-acquired bacterial strains occurred an average of 5 days later in isolated patients. The daily HAI rate for isolated patients was 2.2 times lower than among patients provided standard care.

Although previous studies have reported conflicting results concerning the value of protective isolation in ICU patients, gowns and gloves may be effective in dealing with selected high-risk patients [202]. The recent Severe Acute Respiratory Syndrome (SARS) epidemic has shown that hospitals with high compliance with barrier precautions had a lower impact and less viral transmission compared to institutions that lacked this response [203]. Further studies are necessary to determine the cost effectiveness of this approach in the general ICU population. To draw definitive conclusions, compliance with isolation precautions also should be evaluated. Only a few studies have analyzed compliance with isolation precautions, and most reported low compliance and insufficient knowledge of precautions for pathogens [204–206].

Controversies Specific to the ICU Setting

Selective Digestive Decontamination

Because many HAIs are believed to arise from endogenous flora in the oropharyngeal tract, innovations in prevention have focused on the control (decontamination) of potential pathogens with oral antimicrobial therapy. The aim of selective digestive decontamination (SDD) is to prevent overgrowth of pathogenic GNB and yeasts. It involves the use of topical oral and intestinal antibiotics, often with a systemic antibiotic added for the first few days of the regimen, with the goal being the elimination of potential pathogens from the gastrointestinal tract. With eradication of endogenous bacterial sources, infection may be avoided [207,208].

The role of SDD in preventing ICU-acquired HAI and mortality remains one of the most controversial issues in critical care medicine [209,210]. More than 30 randomized controlled trials that evaluated the efficacy of SDD in preventing VAP and reducing mortality have been published. Several meta-analyses of these studies showed a positive treatment effect, although the effect

appeared to be smaller when considering only high-quality studies [211,212]. The crucial concern associated with the use of SDD is the development and spread of antibiotic resistance; whether SDD contributes to or reduces antibiotic selection pressures by reducing the incidence of infection remains an open question. Nevertheless, some evidence supports the use of SDD as an effective strategy that may reduce morbidity and mortality in selected groups of critically ill patients hospitalized in those units where cross-transmission of multiresistant organisms (e.g., MRSA or *Acinetobacter* spp.) is not a predominant problem [213–216].

In spite of the data from many clinical trials and systematic reviews, it seems difficult to recommend that SDD be either abandoned or used routinely in the ICU setting. It may be premature to ignore the potential benefits of SDD because the results of most clinical trials have been encouraging in terms of reducing infection rates. Additional studies are clearly needed, especially about the overall mortality benefit of SDD [217]. It may be more practical to administer oropharyngeal decontamination without systematic antibiotic treatment; however, whether this approach has an impact on ICU-mortality remains to be shown [83,218–220]. Recently, a multicenter study investigated the potential preventive efficacy of an antimicrobial peptide (Iseganan) [221]. Although preliminary studies with this new agent were promising, the overall results of the clinical trial showed that the study drug was not effective in improving outcome in patients on prolonged mechanical ventilation.

Another potential role for SDD may be in the control of HAI outbreaks. Brun-Buisson et al. [222] reported that intestinal decontamination by oral nonabsorbable antibiotics was important in resolving an outbreak of multiresistant *Enterobacteriaceae* infections in a medical ICU. In units where routine infection control measures fail to control outbreaks, careful application of SDD, including the selection of appropriate oral antimicrobial agents and diligent monitoring for the emergence of new resistant strains, might be an important adjunct to conventional infection control procedures.

In summary, the use of SDD is more a question of philosophy and art rather than an exact science. We believe that SDD should be restricted to subgroups of patients at high risk of nosocomial pneumonia or to situations in which efficacy and cost effectiveness have been established. If used, surveillance for antimicrobial resistance must be done. Table 24A-6 summarizes situations and high-risk patients in which SDD may be beneficial.

Other Measures to Prevent VAP

Coma, prolonged mechanical ventilation through an endotracheal tube, repeated intubation, micro-aspiration events, and permanent supine position increase the risk of VAP [140]. A variety of strategies is recommended to prevent aspiration associated with enteral feeding:

TABLE 24A-6
POSSIBLE INDICATIONS FOR SELECTIVE DECONTAMINATION IN PATIENTS ADMITTED TO ICUs

- Prolonged neutropenia
- Multiple trauma
- Severe burns
- Outbreak of multiresistant gram-negative bacilli
- Esophageal resection
- Hepatic, renal, and pancreatic transplantation
- Prolonged ICU stay

---

discontinuation of enteral-tube feeding; removal of endotracheal devices as soon as possible; routine verification of the placement of the feeding tube and the patient's intestinal motility; and elevation of the head at an angle of 30°–45° [223,224]. The latter preventive measure has recently been questioned by a well-performed study by van Nieuwenhoven et al. [225] who showed that placing a patient into a semirecumbent position may be more difficult to achieve than previously thought. In that multicenter study, a 45° patient position did not appear to be achievable, and only a mean position of about 30° was achieved, which was not associated with a reduced VAP incidence [225].

Installation of effective drainage of subglottic secretions may reduce the risk for aspiration and VAP, as shown in several randomized trials [226,227]. Aspiration of subglottic secretions requires the use of specially designed endotracheal tubes containing a separate dorsal lumen that opens into the subglottic region. It is a promising new strategy for VAP prevention and should be considered in patients requiring prolonged mechanical ventilation. However, these specialized endotracheal tubes should be part of an organized VAP prevention strategy and should not be used in place of such efforts. In any case, the pressure of the endotracheal tube cuff should be adequate to prevent the leakage of colonized subglottic secretions into the lower airway.

Additional controversial issues surrounding VAP prevention, such as stress ulcer prophylaxis, postpyloric feeding, noninvasive positive-pressure ventilation, and ventilator circuit changes have been addressed in recently published reviews and position papers [140,223,224].

Preemptive Treatment of Fungal Infections

Candida spp infections in ICU patients have become increasingly important, particularly among surgical patients [4,228]. Infections mainly evolve from endogenous colonization facilitated by the use of broad-spectrum antibiotics [229,230]. It has been confirmed that sequential spread of candida spp. colonization from the abdominal cavity to other body sites takes place before candidemia

occurs [231]. In heavily colonized surgical ICU patients, *Candida* spp. colonization was patient specific and always preceded infection with a genotypically identical strain [232]. The intensity of *Candida* spp. colonization constitutes a strong predictor of subsequent infection [233]. In recognition of the high morbidity and mortality rates associated with those infections [100], an aggressive approach to suspected *Candida* spp. infections seems justified. Preemptive therapy in patients at high risk of infection has been tested in controlled clinical trials [234–236].

Multimodal Interventions Under Routine Working Conditions

It is unclear what proportion of ICU-associated HAIs is potentially preventable under routine working conditions. We recently performed a systematic review to describe multimodal intervention studies to provide a crude estimate of the proportion of potentially preventable HAIs [237]. The evaluation of 30 reports suggests that great potential exists to decrease HAI rates from a minimum reduction effect of 10% to a maximum effect of 70%, depending on the study design, baseline infection rates, and type of infection. The most important reduction effect was identified for CR-BSIs, whereas a smaller but still substantial potential for prevention seems to exist for other types of infections.

Although the optimal approach to reducing HAIs in critically ill patients is unclear, recent studies and quality improvement initiatives have shown that education-based programs with multiple interventions can substantially decrease infection rates in different ICUs and settings [238]. For instance, Berenholtz et al [239] have shown that multifaceted interventions that helped to ensure adherence with evidence-based guidelines nearly eliminated CR-BSIs in a surgical ICU in Baltimore. Education, process control, and feedback also were associated with significant reductions in rates of catheter-related infections in an ICU in Mexico [240]. Use of maximal barrier precautions during CVC insertion is a central part of these interventions and has been shown to be cost effective [241].

The "Bundle Approach": New Fashion or an Approach for Sustained HAI Prevention?

Approximately 50% of all U.S. hospitals have now joined the Institute for Healthcare Improvement (IHI) initiative, which is a nationwide quality improvement initiative to decrease HAIs and increase patient safety. As defined by IHI (**www.ihi.org**),

> care bundles, in general, are groupings of best practices with respect to a disease process that individually improve care, but when applied together result in substantially greater improvement. The science supporting the bundle components is sufficiently established to be considered standard of care.

Preliminary results posted on the IHI Web site indicate that this initiative has been successful in reducing infection and mortality rates in U.S. hospitals and ICUs.

CONCLUSIONS

Considerable progress has been made in providing intensive care and life support to patients who are acutely ill. Unfortunately, each new technologic advance is accompanied by potential risks for the patient, including HAIs. Clinical research is needed to address the benefits and risks associated with these new interventions. To achieve these objectives, collaboration is needed among critical care physicians, nursing staff, epidemiologists, and infection control professionals to design appropriate studies, interventions, and policies. Administrative and peer support is critical to the success of interventions to reduce HAI rates and improve patient safety. The challenge is to avoid undoing the benefits of intensive care by minimizing risk of complications.

REFERENCES

1. Buckley TA, Short TG, Rowbottom YM, Oh TE. Critical incident reporting in the intensive care unit. *Anaesthesia* 1997;52:403–409.
2. Legras A, Malvy D, Quinioux AI, et al. Nosocomial infections: prospective survey of incidence in five French intensive care units. *Intensive Care Med* 1998;24:1040–1046.
3. Laupland KB, Zygun DA, Davies HD, et al. Population-based assessment of intensive care unit-acquired bloodstream infections in adults: incidence, risk factors, and associated mortality rate. *Crit Care Med* 2002;30:2462–2467.
4. Wisplinghoff H, Bischoff T, Tallent SM, et al. Nosocomial bloodstream infections in U.S. hospitals: analysis of 24,179 cases from a prospective nationwide surveillance study. *Clin Infect Dis* 2004;39:309–317.
5. Gavazzi G, Krause KH. Ageing and infection. *Lancet Infect Dis* 2002;2:659–666.
6. Kaye KS, Schmit K, Pieper C, et al. The effect of increasing age on the risk of surgical site infection. *J Infect Dis* 2005;191:1056–1062.
7. De Jonghe B, Appere-De-Vechi C, Fournier M, et al. A prospective survey of nutritional support practices in intensive care unit patients: what is prescribed? What is delivered? *Crit Care Med* 2001;29:8–12.
8. Weissman C. Nutrition in the intensive care unit. *Crit Care* 1999;3:R67–R75.
9. Longo WE, Virgo KS, Johnson FE, et al. Risk factors for morbidity and mortality after colectomy for colon cancer. *Dis Colon Rectum* 2000;43:83–91.
10. Rapp-Kesek D, Stahle E, Karlsson TT. Body mass index and albumin in the preoperative evaluation of cardiac surgery patients. *Clin Nutr* 2004;23:1398–1404.
11. Delgado-Rodriguez M, Medina-Cuadros M, Gomez-Ortega A, et al. Cholesterol and serum albumin levels as predictors of cross infection, death, and length of hospital stay. *Arch Surg* 2002;137:805–812.
12. Rubinson L, Diette GB, Song X, et al. Low caloric intake is associated with nosocomial bloodstream infections in patients in the medical intensive care unit. *Crit Care Med* 2004;32:350–357.
13. Garrouste-Orgeas M, Troche G, Azoulay E, et al. Body mass index. An additional prognostic factor in ICU patients. *Intensive Care Med* 2004;30:437–443.
14. Heys SD, Schofield AC, Wahle KW. Immunonutrition in clinical practice: what is the current evidence? *Nutr Hosp* 2004;19:325–332.
15. Gramlich L, Kichian K, Pinilla J, et al. Does enteral nutrition compared to parenteral nutrition result in better outcomes in critically ill adult patients? a systematic review of the literature. *Nutrition* 2004;20:843–848.
16. Dhaliwal R, Heyland DK. Nutrition and infection in the intensive care unit: what does the evidence show? *Curr Opin Crit Care* 2005;11:461–467.
17. Houdijk AP, Rijnsburger ER, Jansen J, et al. Randomised trial of glutamine-enriched enteral nutrition on infectious morbidity in patients with multiple trauma. *Lancet* 1998;352:772–776.
18. Caparros T, Lopez J, Grau T. Early enteral nutrition in critically ill patients with a high-protein diet enriched with arginine, fiber, and antioxidants compared with a standard high-protein diet: the effect on nosocomial infections and outcome. *JPEN J Parenter Enteral Nutr* 2001;25:299–308.
19. Heyland DK, MacDonald S, Keefe L, Drover JW. Total parenteral nutrition in the critically ill patient: a meta-analysis. *JAMA* 1998;280:2013–2019.
20. Simpson F, Doig GS. Parenteral vs. enteral nutrition in the critically ill patient: a meta-analysis of trials using the intention to treat principle. *Intensive Care Med* 2005;31:12–23.
21. Abraham E. T- and B-cell function and their roles in resistance to infection. *New Horiz.* 1993;1:28–36.
22. Greif R, Akca O, Horn EP, et al. Supplemental perioperative oxygen to reduce the incidence of surgical-wound infection. *N Engl J Med* 2000;342:161–167.
23. Belda FJ, Aguilera L, Garcia de la Asuncion J, et al. Supplemental perioperative oxygen and the risk of surgical wound infection: a randomized controlled trial. *JAMA* 2005;294:2035–2042.
24. Heinzelmann M, Scott M, Lam T. Factors predisposing to bacterial invasion and infection. *Am J Surg* 2002;183:179–190.
25. Vincent JL, Bihari DJ, Suter PM, et al. The prevalence of nosocomial infection in intensive care units in Europe: results of the European Prevalence of Infection in Intensive Care (EPIC) study. *JAMA* 1995;274:639–644.
26. McLaws ML, Berry G. Nonuniform risk of bloodstream infection with increasing central venous catheter-days. *Infect Control Hosp Epidemiol* 2005;26:715–719.
27. McCabe WR, Jackson GG. Gram-negative bacteremia I. Etiology and ecology. *Arch Intern Med* 1962;110:847–855.
28. Britt MR, Schleupner CJ, Matsumiya S. Severity of underlying disease as a predictor of nosocomial infection. *JAMA* 1978;239:1047–1051.
29. Hugonnet S, Harbarth S, Ferriere K, et al. Bacteremic sepsis in intensive care: temporal trends in incidence, organ dysfunction, and prognosis. *Crit Care Med* 2003;31:390–394.
30. Timsit JF, Fosse JP, Troche G, et al. Accuracy of a composite score using daily SAPS II and LOD scores for predicting hospital mortality in ICU patients hospitalized for more than 72 h. *Intensive Care Med* 2001;27:1012–1021.
31. Leteurtre S, Martinot A, Duhamel A, et al. Validation of the paediatric logistic organ dysfunction (PELOD) score: prospective, observational, multicentre study. *Lancet* 2003;362:192–197.
32. Beck DH, Smith GB, Pappachan JV, Millar B. External validation of the SAPS II, APACHE II and APACHE III prognostic models in South England: a multicentre study. *Intensive Care Med* 2003;29:249–256.
33. Le Gall JR, Neumann A, Hemery F, et al. Mortality prediction using SAPS II: an update for French intensive care units. *Crit Care* 2005;9:R645–R652.
34. Metnitz PG, Moreno RP, Almeida E, et al. SAPS 3—from evaluation of the patient to evaluation of the intensive care unit, part 1. *Intensive Care Med* 2005;31:1336–1344.
35. Moreno RP, Metnitz PG, Almeida E, et al. SAPS 3—from evaluation of the patient to evaluation of the intensive care unit, part 2. *Intensive Care Med* 2005;31:1345–1355.
36. Metnitz PG, Lang T, Vesely H, et al. Ratios of observed to expected mortality are affected by differences in case mix and quality of care. *Intensive Care Med* 2000;26:1466–1472.
37. Kramer AA. Predictive mortality models are not like fine wine. *Crit Care* 2005;9:636–637.
38. Vincent JL, Moreno R, Takala J, et al. The SOFA (Sepsis-Related Organ Failure Assessment) score to describe organ dysfunction/failure. *Intensive Care Med* 1996;22:707–710.
39. Vincent JL, de Mendonca A, Cantraine F, et al. Use of the SOFA score to assess the incidence of organ dysfunction/failure in intensive care units: results of a multicenter, prospective study. *Crit Care Med* 1998;26:1793–1800.

40. Timsit JF, Fosse JP, Troche G, et al. Calibration and discrimination by daily Logistic Organ Dysfunction scoring comparatively with daily Sequential Organ Failure Assessment scoring for predicting hospital mortality in critically ill patients. *Crit Care Med* 2002;30:2003–2013.

41. Kajdacsy-Balla Amaral AC, Andrade FM, Moreno R, et al. Use of the sequential organ failure assessment score as a severity score. *Intensive Care Med* 2005;31:243–249.

42. Kollef MH, Fraser VJ. Antibiotic resistance in the intensive care unit. *Ann Intern Med* 2001;134:298–314.

43. Harbarth S. Nosocomial transmission of antibiotic-resistant microorganisms. *Curr Opin Infect Dis* 2001;14:437–442.

44. Grundmann H, Barwolff S, Tami A, et al. How many infections are caused by patient-to-patient transmission in intensive care units? *Crit Care Med* 2005;33:946–951.

45. Hanberger H, Garcia-Rodriguez JA, Gobernado M, et al. Antibiotic susceptibility among aerobic gram-negative bacilli in intensive care units in 5 European countries. *JAMA* 1999;281:67–71.

46. Fridkin SK, Steward CD, Edwards JR, et al. Surveillance of antimicrobial use and antimicrobial resistance in United States hospitals: project ICARE Project Intensive Care Antimicrobial Resistance Epidemiology (ICARE) hospitals. phase 2. *Clin Infect Dis* 1999;29:245–252.

47. Harbarth S, Albrich W, Goldmann DA, Huebner J. Control of multiply resistant cocci: do international comparisons help? *Lancet Infect Dis* 2001;1:251–261.

48. National Nosocomial Infections Surveillance (NNIS) System Report, data summary from January 1992 through June 2004, issued October 2004. *Am J Infect Control* 2004;32:470–485.

49. Tiemersma EW, Bronzwaer SL, Lyytikainen O, et al. Methicillin resistant *Staphylococcus aureus* in Europe, 1999–2002. *Emerg Infect Dis* 2004;10:1627–1634.

50. Orsi GB, Raponi M, Franchi C, et al. Surveillance and infection control in an intensive care unit. *Infect Control Hosp Epidemiol* 2005;26:321–325.

51. Wiener J, Quinn JP, Bradford PA, et al. Multiple antibiotic-resistant *Klebsiella* and *Escherichia coli* in nursing homes. *JAMA* 1999;281:517–523.

52. Hyle EP, Lipworth AD, Zaoutis TE, et al. Risk factors for increasing multidrug resistance among extended-spectrum beta lactamase-producing *Escherichia coli* and *Klebsiella* species. *Clin Infect Dis* 2005;40:1317–1324.

53. Zaoutis TE, Goyal M, Chu JH, et al. Risk factors for and outcomes of bloodstream infection caused by extended spectrum beta-lactamase-producing *Escherichia coli* and *Klebsiella* species in children. *Pediatrics* 2005;115:942–949.

54. Troche G, Joly LM, Guibert M, Zazzo JF. Detection and treatment of antibiotic-resistant bacterial carriage in a surgical intensive care unit: a 6-year prospective survey. *Infect Control Hosp Epidemiol* 2005;26:161–165.

55. Price DJ, Sleigh J. Control of infection due to *Klebsiella aerogenes* in a neurosurgical unit by withdrawal of all antibiotics. *Lancet* 1970;2:1213–1215.

56. D'Agata E, Venkataraman L, DeGirolami P, et al. Colonization with broad-spectrum cephalosporin-resistant gram-negative bacilli in intensive care units during a non-outbreak period: prevalence, risk factors, and rate of infection. *Crit Care Med* 1998;27:1090–1095.

57. Lucet JC, Decre D, Fichelle A, et al. Control of a prolonged outbreak of extended-spectrum beta-lactamase-producing enterobacteriaceae in a university hospital. *Clin Infect Dis* 1999;29:1411–1418.

58. D'Agata E, Venkataraman L, DeGirolami P, Samore M. Molecular epidemiology of acquisition of ceftazidime-resistant gram-negative bacilli in a nonoutbreak setting. *J Clin Microbiol* 1997;35:2602–2605.

59. Maniatis AN, Pournaras S, Orkopoulou S, et al. Multiresistant acinetobacter baumannii isolates in intensive care units in Greece. *Clin Microbiol Infect* 2003;9:547–553.

60. Villegas MV, Hartstein AI. Acinetobacter outbreaks, 1977–2000. *Infect Control Hosp Epidemiol* 2003;24:284–295.

61. Marais E, de Jong G, Ferraz V, et al. Interhospital transfer of pan-resistant Acinetobacter strains in Johannesburg, South Africa. *Am J Infect Control* 2004;32:278–281.

62. Van Looveren M, Goossens H. Antimicrobial resistance of Acinetobacter spp in Europe. *Clin Microbiol Infect* 2004;10:684–704.

63. Husni RN, Goldstein LS, Arroliga AC, et al. Risk factors for an outbreak of multi-drug-resistant Acinetobacter nosocomial pneumonia among intubated patients. *Chest* 1999;115:1378–1382.

64. Hsueh PR, Teng LJ, Chen CY, et al. Pandrug-resistant Acinetobacter baumannii causing nosocomial infections in a university hospital, Taiwan. *Emerg Infect Dis* 2002;8:827–832.

65. Villers D, Espaze E, Coste-Burel M, et al. Nosocomial Acinetobacter baumannii infections: microbiological and clinical epidemiology. *Ann Intern Med* 1998;129:182–189.

66. Fridkin SK, Edwards JR, Courval JM, et al. The effect of vancomycin and third-generation cephalosporins on prevalence of vancomycin-resistant enterococci in 126 U.S. adult intensive care units. *Ann Intern Med* 2001;135.175–183.

67. Harbarth S, Harris AD, Carmeli Y, Samore MH. Parallel analysis of individual and aggregated data on antibiotic exposure and resistance in gram-negative bacilli. *Clin Infect Dis* 2001;33:1462–1468.

68. Loeffler JM, Garbino J, Lew D, et al. Antibiotic consumption, bacterial resistance and their correlation in a Swiss university hospital and its adult intensive care units. *Scand J Infect Dis* 2003;35:843–850.

69. Neuhauser MM, Weinstein RA, Rydman R, et al. Antibiotic resistance among gram-negative bacilli in US intensive care units: implications for fluoroquinolone use. *JAMA* 2003;289:885–888.

70. Chastre J, Wolff M, Fagon JY, et al. Comparison of 8 vs 15 days of antibiotic therapy for ventilator-associated pneumonia in adults: a randomized trial. *JAMA* 2003;290:2588–2598.

71. Fridkin SK, Gaynes RP. Antimicrobial resistance in intensive care units. *Clin Chest Med* 1999;20:303–316.

72. Safdar N, Maki DG. The commonality of risk factors for nosocomial colonization and infection with antimicrobial-resistant *Staphylococcus aureus*, enterococcus, gram-negative bacilli, *Clostridium difficile*, and Candida. *Ann Intern Med* 2002;136:834–844.

73. Safdar N, Crnich CJ, Maki DG. The pathogenesis of ventilator-associated pneumonia: its relevance to developing effective strategies for prevention. *Respir Care* 2005;50:725–739.

74. Johanson WG, Pierce AK, Sanford J. Changing pharyngeal bacterial flora of hospitalized patients: emergence of gram-negative bacilli. *N Engl J Med* 1969;281:1137–1140.

75. Schimpff SC, Miller RM, Polkavetz S, Hornick R. Infection in the severely traumatized patient. *Ann Surg* 1974;179:352–357.

76. Atherton ST, White D. Stomach as source of bacteria colonising respiratory tract during artificial ventilation. *Lancet* 1978;2:968–969.

77. Garrouste-Orgeas M, Chevret S, Arlet G, et al. Oropharyngeal or gastric colonization and nosocomial pneumonia in adult intensive care unit patients: a prospective study based on genomic DNA analysis. *Am J Respir Crit Care Med* 1997;156:1647–1655.

78. Dent A, Toltzis P. Descriptive and molecular epidemiology of gram-negative bacilli infections in the neonatal intensive care unit. *Curr Opin Infect Dis* 2003;16:279–283.

79. Donskey CJ. The role of the intestinal tract as a reservoir and source for transmission of nosocomial pathogens. *Clin Infect Dis* 2004;39:219–226.

80. Blot S, Depuydt P, Vogelaers D, et al. Colonization status and appropriate antibiotic therapy for nosocomial bacteremia caused by antibiotic-resistant gram-negative bacteria in an intensive care unit. *Infect Control Hosp Epidemiol* 2005;26:575–579.

81. Bonten MJ, Gaillard CA, van Tiel FH, et al. The stomach is not a source for colonization of the upper respiratory tract and pneumonia in ICU patients. *Chest* 1994;105:878–884.

82. George DL, Falk PS, Wunderink RG, et al. Epidemiology of ventilator-acquired pneumonia based on protected bronchoscopic sampling. *Am J Respir Crit Care Med* 1998;158:1839–1847.

83. Bergmans DC, Bonten MJ, Gaillard CA, et al. Prevention of ventilator-associated pneumonia by oral decontamination: a prospective, randomized, double-blind, placebo-controlled study. *Am J Respir Crit Care Med* 2001;164:382–388.

84. Vincent JL. Nosocomial infections in adult intensive-care units. *Lancet* 2003;361:2068–2077.

85. Gastmeier P, Sohr D, Geffers C, et al. Are nosocomial infection rates in intensive care units useful benchmark parameters? *Infection* 2000;28:346–350.

86. Sax H, Pittet D. Interhospital differences in nosocomial infection rates: importance of case-mix adjustment. *Arch Intern Med* 2002;162:2437–2442.

87. Gastmeier P, Geffers C, Sohr D, et al. Surveillance of nosocomial infections in intensive care units: current data and interpretations. *Wien Klin Wochenschr* 2003;115:99–103.

88. Richards MJ, Edwards JR, Culver DH, Gaynes RP. Nosocomial infections in pediatric intensive care units in the United States. *Pediatrics* 1999;103:e39.

89. Pittet D, Tarara D, Wenzel RP. Nosocomial bloodstream infection in critically ill patients: excess length of stay, extra costs, and attributable mortality. *JAMA* 1994;271:1598–1601.

90. Digiovine B, Chenoweth C, Watts C, Higgins M. The attributable mortality and costs of primary nosocomial bloodstream infections in the intensive care unit. *Am J Respir Crit Care Med* 1999;160:976–981.

91. Center for Disease Control and Prevention. Monitoring hospital-acquired infections to promote patient safety—United States, 1990–1999. *MMWR Morb Mortal Wkly Rep* 2000;49:149–153.

92. Weinstein RA. Nosocomial infection update. *Emerg Infect Dis* 1998;4:416–420.

93. Eggimann P, Hugonnet S, Sax H, et al. Ventilator-associated pneumonia: caveats for benchmarking. *Intensive Care Med* 2003;29:2086–2089.

94. Tucker J. Patient volume, staffing, and workload in relation to risk-adjusted outcomes in a random stratified sample of UK neonatal intensive care units: a prospective evaluation. *Lancet* 2002;359:99–107.

95. Hugonnet S, Harbarth S, Sax H, et al. Nursing resources: a major determinant of nosocomial infection? *Curr Opin Infect Dis* 2004;17:329–333.

96. Harbarth S, Sudre P, Dharan S, et al. Outbreak of *Enterobacter cloacae* related to understaffing, overcrowding, and poor hygiene practices. *Infect Control Hosp Epidemiol* 1999;20:598–603.

97. Andersen BM, Lindemann R, Bergh K, et al. Spread of methicillin-resistant *Staphylococcus aureus* in a neonatal intensive unit associated with understaffing, overcrowding and mixing of patients. *J Hosp Infect* 2002;50:18–24.

98. Aiken LH, Clarke SP, Cheung RB, et al. Educational levels of hospital nurses and surgical patient mortality. *JAMA* 2003;290:1617–1623.

99. Safdar N, Dezfulian C, Collard HR, Saint S. Clinical and economic consequences of ventilator-associated pneumonia: a systematic review. *Crit Care Med* 2005;33:2184–2193.

100. Zaoutis TE, Argon J, Chu J, et al. The epidemiology and attributable outcomes of candidemia in adults and children hospitalized in the United States: a propensity analysis. *Clin Infect Dis* 2005;41:1232–1239.

101. Freeman J, Goldmann DA, McGowan JE. Methodologic issues in hospital epidemiology. IV. Risk ratios, confounding, effect modification, and the analysis of multiple variables. *Rev Infect Dis* 1988;10:1118–1141.

102. Whitehouse JD, Friedman ND, Kirkland KB, et al. The impact of surgical-site infections following orthopedic surgery at a community hospital and a university hospital: adverse quality of life, excess length of stay, and extra cost. *Infect Control Hosp Epidemiol* 2002;23:183–189.

103. Samore MH, Harbarth S. A methodologically focused review of the literature in hospital epidemiology and infection control. In: Mayhall CG, ed. *Hospital epidemiology and infection control.* 3rd ed. Philadelphia: Lippincott Williams & Wilkins, 2004:1645–1657.

104. Schulgen G, Kropec A, Kappstein I, et al. Estimation of extra hospital stay attributable to nosocomial infections: heterogeneity and timing of events. *J Clin Epidemiol* 2000;53:409–417.

105. Beyersmann J, Gastmeier P, Grundmann H, et al. Assessment of prolongation of intensive care unit stay due to nosocomial infections, using multistate models. *Infect Control Hosp Epidemiol* 2006; *Infect Control Hosp Epidemiol.* 2006;27:493–9.

106. Asensio A, Torres J. Quantifying excess length of postoperative stay attributable to infections: a comparison of methods. *J Clin Epidemiol* 1999;52:1249–1256.

107. Soufir L, Timsit JF, Mahe C, et al. Attributable morbidity and mortality of catheter-related septicemia in critically ill patients: a matched, risk-adjusted, cohort study. *Infect Control Hosp Epidemiol* 1999;20:396–401.

108. Gaynes R, Edwards JR. Overview of nosocomial infections caused by gram-negative bacilli. *Clin Infect Dis* 2005;41:848–854.

109. Alberti C, Brun-Buisson C, Burchardi H, et al. Epidemiology of sepsis and infection in ICU patients from an international multicentre cohort study. *Intensive Care Med* 2002;28:108–121.

110. Geffers C, Zuschneid I, Sohr D, et al. Microbiological isolates associated with nosocomial infections in intensive care units: data of 274 intensive care units participating in the German Nosocomial Infections Surveillance System (KISS). *Anasthesiol Intensivmed Notfallmed Schmerzther* 2004;39:15–19.

111. Vincent JL, Sakr Y, Sprung CL, et al. Sepsis in European intensive care units: results of the SOAP study. *Crit Care Med* 2006;34:344–353.

112. Harbarth S, Pittet D. Identification and management of infectious outbreaks in the critical care unit. *Curr Opin Crit Care* 1996;2:352–360.

113. Behari P, Englund J, Alcasid G, et al. Transmission of methicillin-resistant *Staphylococcus aureus* to preterm infants through breast milk. *Infect Control Hosp Epidemiol* 2004;25:778–780.

114. Zawacki A, O'Rourke E, Potter-Bynoe G, et al. An outbreak of *Pseudomonas aeruginosa* pneumonia and bloodstream infection associated with intermittent otitis externa in a healthcare worker. *Infect Control Hosp Epidemiol* 2004;25:1083–1089.

115. Pimentel JD, Low J, Styles K, et al. Control of an outbreak of multi-drug-resistant *Acinetobacter baumannii* in an intensive care unit and a surgical ward. *J Hosp Infect* 2005;59:249–253.

116. de Lassence A, Hidri N, Timsit JF, et al. Control and outcome of a large outbreak of colonization and infection with glycopeptide-intermediate *Staphylococcus aureus* in an intensive care unit. *Clin Infect Dis* 2006;42:170–178.

117. Zanetti G, Blanc DS, Federli I, et al. *Acinetobacter baumannii* epidemic in a burn unit: usefulness of improved culture medium to assess environmental contamination. In: IDSA, ed. *IDSA.* Boston: Infectious Disease Society of America. 2004:73.

118. Hamill RJ, Houston ED, Georghiou PR, et al. An outbreak of *Burkholderia* (formerly *Pseudomonas*) *cepacia* respiratory tract colonization and infection associated with nebulized albuterol therapy. *Ann Intern Med* 1995;122:762–766.

119. Lymphocytic choriomeningitis virus infection in organ transplant recipients—Massachusetts, Rhode Island, 2005. *MMWR Morb Mortal Wkly Rep* 2005;54:537–539.

120. Srinivasan A, Burton EC, Kuehnert MJ, et al. Transmission of rabies virus from an organ donor to four transplant recipients. *N Engl J Med* 2005;352:1103–1111.

121. Vincent JL. Ventilator-associated pneumonia. *J Hosp Infect* 2004;57:272–280.

122. Warren DK, Shukla SJ, Olsen MA, et al. Outcome and attributable cost of ventilator-associated pneumonia among intensive care unit patients in a suburban medical center. *Crit Care Med* 2003;31:1312–1317.

123. Moine P, Timsit JF, De Lassence A, et al. Mortality associated with late-onset pneumonia in the intensive care unit: results of a multi-center cohort study. *Intensive Care Med* 2002;28:154–163.

124. Garnacho J, Sole-Violan J, Sa-Borges M, et al. Clinical impact of pneumonia caused by *Acinetobacter baumannii* in intubated patients: a matched cohort study. *Crit Care Med* 2003;31:2478–2482.

125. Leroy O, Meybeck A, d'Escrivan T, et al. Impact of adequacy of initial antimicrobial therapy on the prognosis of patients with ventilator-associated pneumonia. *Intensive Care Med* 2003;29:2170–2173.

126. Hugonnet S, Eggimann P, Borst F, et al. Impact of ventilator-associated pneumonia on resource utilization and patient outcome. *Infect Control Hosp Epidemiol* 2004;25:1090–1096.

127. Rello J, Ollendorf DA, Oster G, et al. Epidemiology and outcomes of ventilator-associated pneumonia in a large U.S. database. *Chest* 2002;122:2115–2121.

128. Cook D, Walter S, Cook R, et al. Incidence of and risk factors for ventilator-associated pneumonia in critically ill patients. *Ann Intern Med* 1998;129:433–440.

129. Guidelines for the management of adults with hospital-acquired, ventilator-associated, and healthcare-associated pneumonia. *Am J Respir Crit Care Med* 2005;171:388–416.
130. Shorr AF, Sherner JH, Jackson WL, Kollef MH. Invasive approaches to the diagnosis of ventilator-associated pneumonia: a meta-analysis. *Crit Care Med* 2005;33:46–53.
131. Torres A, Ewig S. Diagnosing ventilator-associated pneumonia. *N Engl J Med* 2004;350:433–435.
132. Meduri GU, Mauldin GL, Wunderink RG, et al. Causes of fever and pulmonary densities in patients with clinical manifestations of ventilator-associated pneumonia. *Chest* 1994;106:221–235.
133. Chastre J, Fagon JY. Ventilator-associated pneumonia. *Am J Respir Crit Care Med* 2002;165:867–903.
134. Fagon JY, Chastre J, Wolff M, et al. Invasive and non-invasive strategies for management of suspected ventilator-associated pneumonia: a randomized trial. *Ann Intern Med* 2000;132:621–630.
135. Ost DE, Hall CS, Joseph G, et al. Decision analysis of antibiotic and diagnostic strategies in ventilator-associated pneumonia. *Am J Respir Crit Care Med* 2003;168:1060–1067.
136. Michaud S, Suzuki S, Harbarth S. Effect of design-related bias in studies of diagnostic tests for ventilator-associated pneumonia. *Am J Respir Crit Care Med* 2002;166:1320–1325.
137. Montravers P, Veber B, Auboyer C, et al. Diagnostic and therapeutic management of nosocomial pneumonia in surgical patients: results of the Eole study. *Crit Care Med* 2002;30:368–375.
138. Giantsou E, Liratzopoulos N, Efraimidou E, et al. Both early-onset and late-onset ventilator-associated pneumonia are caused mainly by potentially multiresistant bacteria. *Intensive Care Med* 2005;31:1488–1494.
139. Bornstain C, Azoulay E, De Lassence A, et al. Sedation, sucralfate, and antibiotic use are potential means for protection against early-onset ventilator-associated pneumonia. *Clin Infect Dis* 2004;38:1401–1408.
140. Bonten MJ, Kollef MH, Hall JB. Risk factors for ventilator-associated pneumonia: from epidemiology to patient management. *Clin Infect Dis* 2004;38:1141–1149.
141. Seiden AM. Sinusitis in the critical care patient. *New Horiz* 1993;1:261–270.
142. Stein M, Caplan ES. Nosocomial sinusitis: a unique subset of sinusitis. *Curr Opin Infect Dis* 2005;18:147–150.
143. Rouby JJ, Laurent P, Gosnach M, et al. Risk factors and clinical relevance of nosocomial maxillary sinusitis in the critically ill. *Am J Respir Crit Care Med* 1994;150:776–783.
144. Holzapfel L, Chastang C, Demingeon G, et al. A randomized study assessing the systematic search for maxillary sinusitis in nasotracheally mechanically ventilated patients. Influence of nosocomial maxillary sinusitis on the occurrence of ventilator-associated pneumonia. *Am J Respir Crit Care Med* 1999;159:695–701.
145. George DL, Falk PS, Umberto Meduri G, et al. Nosocomial sinusitis in patients in the medical intensive care unit: a prospective epidemiological study. *Clin Infect Dis* 1998;27:463–470.
146. Le Moal G, Lemerre D, Grollier G, et al. Nosocomial sinusitis with isolation of anaerobic bacteria in ICU patients. *Intensive Care Med* 1999;25:1066–1071.
147. Bach A, Boehrer H, Schmidt H, Geiss HK. Nosocomial sinusitis in ventilated patients. Nasotracheal versus orotracheal intubation. *Anaesthesia* 1992;47:335–339.
148. Heffner JE. Nosocomial sinusitis. Den of multiresistant thieves? *Am J Respir Crit Care Med* 1994;150:608–609.
149. Boland G, Lee MJ, Mueller PR. Acute cholecystitis in the intensive care unit. *New Horiz* 1993;1:246–260.
150. Laurila J, Syrjala H, Laurila PA, et al. Acute acalculous cholecystitis in critically ill patients. *Acta Anaesthesiol Scand* 2004;48:986–991.
151. Pittet D, Huguenin T, Dharan S, et al. Unusual cause of lethal pulmonary aspergillosis in patients with chronic obstructive pulmonary disease. *Am J Respir Crit Care Med* 1996;154:541–544.
152. Harvey MA. Critical-care-unit bedside design and furnishing: impact on nosocomial infections. *Infect Control Hosp Epidemiol* 1998;19:597–601.
153. WHO. Global Safety Challenge. (www.who.int/patientsafety/challenge/en/) accessed March 6, 2006.
154. Preston GA, Larson EL, Stamm W. The effect of private isolation rooms on patient care practices, colonization and infection in an intensive care unit. *Am J Med* 1981;70:641–645.
155. Ben-Abraham R, Keller N, Szold O, et al. Do isolation rooms reduce the rate of nosocomial infections in the pediatric intensive care unit? *J Crit Care* 2002;17:176–180.
156. Johnson JR, Kuskowski MA, Wilt TJ. Systematic review: antimicrobial urinary catheters to prevent catheter-associated urinary tract infection in hospitalized patients. *Ann Intern Med* 2006;144:116–126.
157. Maki DG, Alvarado CJ, Hassemer CA, Zilz MA. Relation of the inanimate hospital environment to endemic nosocomial infection. *N Engl J Med* 1982;307:1562–1566.
158. Huebner J, Frank U, Kappstein I, et al. Influence of architectural design on nosocomial infections in intensive care units—a prospective 2-year analysis. *Intensive Care Med* 1989;15:179–183.
159. Duckro AN, Blom DW, Lyle EA, et al. Transfer of vancomycin-resistant enterococci via health care worker hands. *Arch Intern Med* 2005;165:302–307.
160. Wendt C, Wiesenthal B, Dietz E, Ruden H. Survival of vancomycin-resistant and vancomycin-susceptible enterococci on dry surfaces. *J Clin Microbiol* 1998;36:3734–3736.
161. O'Connell NH, Humphreys H. Intensive care unit design and environmental factors in the acquisition of infection. *J Hosp Infect* 2000;45:255–262.
162. Oelberg DG, Joyner SE, Jiang X, et al. Detection of pathogen transmission in neonatal nurseries using DNA markers as surrogate indicators. *Pediatrics* 2000;105:311–315.
163. Foca M, Jakob K, Whittier S, et al. Endemic *Pseudomonas aeruginosa* infection in a neonatal intensive care unit. *N Engl J Med* 2000;343:695–700.
164. Carling PC, Briggs JL, Perkins J, Highlander D. Improved cleaning of patient rooms using a new targeting method. *Clin Infect Dis* 2006;42:385–388.
165. Pronovost PJ, Jenckes MW, Dorman T, et al. Organizational characteristics of intensive care units related to outcomes of abdominal aortic surgery. *JAMA* 1999;281:1310–1317.
166. Sherwood G, Thomas E, Bennett DS, Lewis P. A teamwork model to promote patient safety in critical care. *Crit Care Nurs Clin North Am* 2002;14:333–340.
167. Sherertz RJ, Ely EW, Westbrook DM, et al. Education of physicians-in-training can decrease the risk for vascular catheter infection. *Ann Intern Med* 2000;132:641–648.
168. Hugonnet S, Chevrolet JC, Pittet D. The effect of workload on infection risk in critically ill patients. *Crit Care Med* 2007;35:76–81.
169. Leape LL, Fromson JA. Problem doctors: is there a system-level solution? *Ann Intern Med* 2006;144:107–115.
170. Garland A. Improving the ICU, part 1. *Chest* 2005;127:2151–2164.
171. Garland A. Improving the ICU, part 2. *Chest* 2005;127:2165–2179.
172. Duke G, Santamaria J, Shann E, Stow P. Outcome-based clinical indicators for intensive care medicine. *Anaesth Intensive Care* 2005;33:303–310.
173. Zuschneid I, Schwab F, Geffers C, et al. Reducing central venous catheter-associated primary bloodstream infections in intensive care units is possible: data from the German nosocomial infection surveillance system. *Infect Control Hosp Epidemiol* 2003;24:501–505.
174. Eggimann P, Pittet D. Infection control in the ICU. *Chest* 2001;120:2059–2093.
175. Hugonnet S, Eggimann P, Sax H, et al. Intensive care unit-acquired infections: is postdischarge surveillance useful? *Crit Care Med* 2002;30:2636–2638.
176. Salgado CD, O'Grady N, Farr BM. Prevention and control of antimicrobial-resistant infections in intensive care patients. *Crit Care Med* 2005;33:2373–2382.
177. Harbarth S, Pittet D. MRSA—a European currency of infection control. *QJM* 1998;91:519–521.
178. Muto CA, Jernigan JA, Ostrowsky BE, et al. Guideline for preventing nosocomial transmission of multidrug-resistant strains of *Staphylococcus aureus* and *Enterococcus*. *Infect Control Hosp Epidemiol* 2003;24:362–386.

179. Marshall C, Wesselingh S, McDonald M, Spelman D. Control of endemic MRSA—what is the evidence? a personal view. *J Hosp Infect* 2004;56:253–268.

180. Cepeda JA, Whitehouse T, Cooper B, et al. Isolation of patients in single rooms or cohorts to reduce spread of MRSA in intensive-care units: prospective two-centre study. *Lancet* 2005;365:295–304.

181. Wernitz MH, Swidsinski S, Weist K, et al. Effectiveness of a hospital-wide selective screening programme for methicillin-resistant *Staphylococcus aureus* (MRSA) carriers at hospital admission to prevent hospital-acquired MRSA infections. *Clin Microbiol Infect* 2005;11:457–465.

182. Rubinovitch B, Pittet D. Screening for methicillin-resistant *Staphylococcus aureus* in the endemic hospital: what have we learned? *J Hosp Infect* 2001;47:9–18.

183. Lucet JC, Paoletti X, Lolom I, et al. Successful long-term program for controlling methicillin-resistant *Staphylococcus aureus* in intensive care units. *Intensive Care Med* 2005;31:1051–1057.

184. Harbarth S, Masuet-Aumatell C, Schrenzel J, et al. Evaluation of rapid screening and pre-emptive contact isolation for detecting and controlling methicillin-resistant *Staphylococcus aureus* in critical care: an interventional cohort study. *Crit Care* 2006;10:R25.

185. Harbarth S, Romand J, Frei R, et al. Inter- and intrahospital transmission of methicillin-resistant *Staphylococcus aureus*. *Schweiz Med Wochenschr* 1997;127:471–478.

186. Kassis-Chikhani N, Decre D, Gautier V, et al. First outbreak of multidrug-resistant *Klebsiella pneumoniae* carrying blaVIM-1 and blaSHV-5 in a French university hospital. *J Antimicrob Chemother* 2006;57:142–145.

187. Harbarth S, Sax H, Fankhauser-Rodriguez C, et al. Evaluating the probability of previously unknown carriage of MRSA at hospital admission. *Am J Med* 2006;119:275.e:15–23.

188. Bonten MJ, Slaughter S, Hayden MK, et al. External sources of vancomycin-resistant enterococci for intensive care units. *Crit Care Med* 1998;26:2001–2004.

189. Harbarth S, Pittet D, Grady L, et al. Interventional study to evaluate the impact of an alcohol-based hand gel in improving hand hygiene compliance. *Pediatr Infect Dis J* 2002;21:489–495.

190. Hugonnet S, Perneger TV, Pittet D. Alcohol-based handrub improves compliance with hand hygiene in intensive care units. *Arch Intern Med* 2002;162:1037–1043.

191. Pittet D, Simon A, Hugonnet S, et al. Hand hygiene among physicians: performance, beliefs, and perceptions. *Ann Intern Med* 2004;141:1–8.

192. Boyce JM, Pittet D. Guideline for hand hygiene in health-care settings: recommendations of the Healthcare Infection Control Practices Advisory Committee and the HIC-PAC/SHEA/APIC/IDSA Hand Hygiene Task Force. *Infect Control Hosp Epidemiol* 2002;23:S3–S40.

193. Harbarth S. Handwashing—the Semmelweis lesson misunderstood? *Clin Infect Dis* 2000;30:990–991.

194. Pittet D, Mourouga P, Perneger TV. Compliance with handwashing in a teaching hospital. *Ann Intern Med* 1999;130:126–130.

195. Pittet D, Hugonnet S, Harbarth S, et al. Effectiveness of a hospital-wide programme to improve compliance with hand hygiene. *Lancet* 2000;356:1307–1312.

196. Pittet D, Boyce JM. Hand hygiene and patient care: pursuing the Semmelweis legacy. *Lancet Infect Dis* 2001;1:9–20.

197. Goroncy-Bermes P, Schouten MA, Voss A. Effectiveness of a non-medicated handwash product, chlorhexidine, and an alcohol-based hand disinfectant against multiple-resistant Gram-positive microorganisms. *Infect Control Hosp Epidemiol* 2001;22:194–196.

198. Winnefeld M, Richard MA, Drancourt M, Grob JJ. Skin tolerance and effectiveness of two hand decontamination procedures in everyday hospital use. *Br J Dermatol* 2000;143:546–550.

199. Boyce JM, Kelliher S, Vallande N. Skin irritation and dryness associated with two hand-hygiene regimens: soap-and-water hand washing versus hand antisepsis with an alcoholic hand gel. *Infect Control Hosp Epidemiol* 2000;21:442–448.

200. Doebbeling BN, Stanley GL, Sheetz CT, et al. Comparative efficacy of alternative hand-washing agents in reducing nosocomial infections in intensive care units. *N Engl J Med* 1992;327:88–93.

201. Klein BS, Perloff WH, Maki D. Reduction of nosocomial infection during pediatric intensive care by protective isolation. *N Engl J Med* 1989;320:1714–1721.

202. Slota M, Green M, Farley A, et al. The role of gown and glove isolation and strict handwashing in the reduction of nosocomial infection in children with solid organ transplantation. *Crit Care Med* 2001;29:405–412.

203. Bell DM. Public health interventions and SARS spread, 2003. *Emerg Infect Dis* 2004;10:1900–1906.

204. Sax H, Perneger T, Hugonnet S, et al. Knowledge of standard and isolation precautions in a large teaching hospital. *Infect Control Hosp Epidemiol* 2005;26:298–304.

205. Askarian M, Shiraly R, McLaws ML. Knowledge, attitudes, and practices of contact precautions among Iranian nurses. *Am J Infect Control* 2005;33:486–488.

206. Pessoa-Silva CL, Posfay-Barbe K, Pfister R, et al. Attitudes and perceptions toward hand hygiene among healthcare workers caring for critically ill neonates. *Infect Control Hosp Epidemiol* 2005;26:305–311.

207. Bonten MJ, Kullberg BJ, van Dalen R, et al. Selective digestive decontamination in patients in intensive care. *J Antimicrob Chemother* 2000;46:351–362.

208. Krueger WA, Unertl KE. Selective decontamination of the digestive tract. *Curr Opin Crit Care* 2002;8:139–144.

209. Vincent JL. Selective digestive decontamination: for everyone, everywhere? *Lancet* 2003;362:1006–1007.

210. van Saene HK, Petros AJ, Ramsay G, Baxby D. All great truths are iconoclastic: selective decontamination of the digestive tract moves from heresy to level 1 truth. *Intensive Care Med* 2003;29:677–690.

211. Liberati A, D'Amico R, Pifferi S, et al. Antibiotics for preventing respiratory tract infections in adults receiving intensive care. *Cochrane Database Syst Rev* 2000(2):CD000022.

212. van Nieuwenhoven CA, Buskens E, van Tiel FH, Bonten MJ. Relationship between methodological trial quality and the effects of selective digestive decontamination on pneumonia and mortality in critically ill patients. *JAMA* 2001;286:335–340.

213. Krueger WA, Lenhart FP, Neeser G, et al. Influence of combined intravenous and topical antibiotic prophylaxis on the incidence of infections, organ dysfunctions, and mortality in critically ill surgical patients: a prospective, stratified, randomized, double-blind, placebo-controlled clinical trial. *Am J Respir Crit Care Med* 2002;166:1029–1037.

214. de Jonge E, Schultz MJ, Spanjaard L, et al. Effects of selective decontamination of digestive tract on mortality and acquisition of resistant bacteria in intensive care: a randomised controlled trial. *Lancet* 2003;362:1011–1016.

215. Acquarolo A, Urli T, Perone G, et al. Antibiotic prophylaxis of early onset pneumonia in critically ill comatose patients: a randomized study. *Intensive Care Med* 2005;31:510–516.

216. de La Cal MA, Cerda E, Garcia-Hierro P, et al. Survival benefit in critically ill burned patients receiving selective decontamination of the digestive tract: a randomized, placebo-controlled, double-blind trial. *Ann Surg* 2005;241:424–430.

217. Bonten MJ. Strategies for prevention of hospital-acquired pneumonia: oral and selective decontamination of the gastrointestinal tract. *Semin Respir Crit Care Med* 2002;23:481–488.

218. Pittet D, Eggimann P, Rubinovitch B. Prevention of ventilator-associated pneumonia by oral decontamination: just another SDD study? *Am J Respir Crit Care Med* 2001;164:338–339.

219. Fourrier F, Dubois D, Pronnier P, et al. Effect of gingival and dental plaque antiseptic decontamination on nosocomial infections acquired in the intensive care unit: a double-blind placebo-controlled multicenter study. *Crit Care Med* 2005;33:1728–1735.

220. Garcia R. A review of the possible role of oral and dental colonization on the occurrence of health care-associated pneumonia: underappreciated risk and a call for interventions. *Am J Infect Control* 2005;33:527–541.

221. Kollef M, Pittet D, Sanchez Garcia M, et al. A randomized double-blind trial of Iseganan in prevention of ventilator-associated pneumonia. *Am J Respir Crit Care Med* 2006;173:91–97.

222. Brun-Buisson C, Legrand P, Rauss A. Intestinal decontamination for control of nosocomial multiresistant gram-negative bacilli:

study of an outbreak in an intensive care unit. *Ann Intern Med* 1989;110:873–881.

223. Collard HR, Saint S, Matthay MA. Prevention of ventilator-associated pneumonia: an evidence-based systematic review. *Ann Intern Med* 2003;138:494–501.

224. Dodek P, Keenan S, Cook D, et al. Evidence-based clinical practice guideline for the prevention of ventilator-associated pneumonia. *Ann Intern Med* 2004;141:305–313.

225. Van Nieuwenhoven CA, Vandenbroucke-Grauls C, van Tiel FH, et al. Feasibility and effects of the semirecumbent position to prevent ventilator-associated pneumonia: a randomized study. *Crit Care Med* 2006;34:396–402.

226. Kollef MH, Skubas NJ, Sundt TM. A randomized clinical trial of continuous aspiration of subglottic secretions in cardiac surgery patients. *Chest* 1999;116:1339–1346.

227. Smulders K, van der Hoeven H, Weers-Pothoff I, Vandenbroucke-Grauls C. A randomized clinical trial of intermittent subglottic secretion drainage in patients receiving mechanical ventilation. *Chest* 2002;121:858–862.

228. Marchetti O, Bille J, Fluckiger U, et al. Epidemiology of candidemia in Swiss tertiary care hospitals: secular trends, 1991–2000. *Clin Infect Dis* 2004;38:311–320.

229. Eggimann P, Garbino J, Pittet D. Management of Candida species infections in critically ill patients. *Lancet Infect Dis* 2003;3:772–785.

230. Eggimann P, Garbino J, Pittet D. Epidemiology of Candida species infections in critically ill non-immunosuppressed patients. *Lancet Infect Dis* 2003;3:685–702.

231. Solomkin JS. Pathogenesis and management of Candida infection syndromes in non-neutropenic patients. *New Horiz* 1993;1:202–213.

232. Pittet D, Monod M, Filthuth I, et al. Contour-clamped homogeneous electric field gel electrophoresis as a powerful epidemiologic tool in yeast infections. *Am J Med* 1991;91:256S–263S.

233. Charles PE, Dalle F, Aube H, et al. Candida spp colonization significance in critically ill medical patients: a prospective study. *Intensive Care Med* 2005;31:393–400.

234. Pelz RK, Hendrix CW, Swoboda SM, et al. Double-blind placebo-controlled trial of fluconazole to prevent candidal infections in critically ill surgical patients. *Ann Surg* 2001;233:542–548.

235. Garbino J, Lew DP, Romand JA, et al. Prevention of severe Candida infections in nonneutropenic, high-risk, critically ill patients: a randomized, double-blind, placebo-controlled trial in patients treated by selective digestive decontamination. *Intensive Care Med* 2002;28:1708–1717.

236. Shorr AF, Chung K, Jackson WL, et al. Fluconazole prophylaxis in critically ill surgical patients: a meta-analysis. *Crit Care Med* 2005;33:1928–35.

237. Harbarth S, Sax H, Gastmeier P. The preventable proportion of nosocomial infections: an overview of published reports. *J Hosp Infect* 2003;54:258–266.

238. Larson E. State-of-the-science—2004: time for a "No Excuses/No Tolerance" (NET) strategy. *Am J Infect Control* 2005;33:548–557.

239. Berenholtz SM, Pronovost PJ, Lipsett PA, et al. Eliminating catheter-related bloodstream infections in the intensive care unit. *Crit Care Med* 2004;32:2014–2020.

240. Higuera F, Rosenthal VD, Duarte P, et al. The effect of process control on the incidence of central venous catheter-associated bloodstream infections and mortality in intensive care units in Mexico. *Crit Care Med* 2005;33:2022–2027.

241. Hu KK, Veenstra DL, Lipsky BA, Saint S. Use of maximal sterile barriers during central venous catheter insertion: clinical and economic outcomes. *Clin Infect Dis* 2004;39:1441–1445.

242. Fagon JY, Chastre J, Hance AJ, et al. Nosocomial pneumonia in ventilated patients: a cohort study evaluating attributable mortality and hospital stay. *Am J Med* 1993;94:281–288.

243. Papazian L, Bregeon F, Thirion X, et al. Effect of ventilator-associated pneumonia on mortality and morbidity. *Am J Respir Crit Care Med* 1996;154:91–97.

244. Baker AM, Meredith JW, Haponik EF. Pneumonia in intubated trauma patients: microbiology and outcomes. *Am J Respir Crit Care Med* 1996;153:343–349.

245. Rello J, Jubert P, Valles J, et al. Evaluation of outcome for intubated patients with pneumonia due to *Pseudomonas aeruginosa*. *Clin Infect Dis* 1996;23:973–978.

246. Heyland DK, Cook DJ, Griffith L, et al. The attributable morbidity and mortality of ventilator-associated pneumonia in the critically ill patient. *Am J Respir Crit Care Med* 1999;159:1249–1256.

247. Bercault N, Boulain T. Mortality rate attributable to ventilator-associated nosocomial pneumonia in an adult intensive care unit: a prospective case-control study. *Crit Care Med* 2001;29:2303–2309.

248. Rosenthal VD, Guzman S, Migone O, Safdar N. The attributable cost and length of hospital stay because of nosocomial pneumonia in intensive care units in 3 hospitals in Argentina: a prospective, matched analysis. *Am J Infect Control* 2005;33:157–161.

249. Habsah H, Zechaida M, Van Rostenberghe H, et al. An outbreak of *Pantoea spp* in a neonatal intensive care unit secondary to contaminated parenteral nutrition. *J Hosp Infect* 2005;61:213–218.

250. Hocker B, Wendt C, Nahimana A, et al. Molecular evidence of Pneumocystis transmission in pediatric transplant unit. *Emerg Infect Dis* 2005;11:330–332.

251. Ho AS, Sung JJ, Chan-Yeung M. An outbreak of severe acute respiratory syndrome among hospital workers in a community hospital in Hong Kong. *Ann Intern Med* 2003;139:564–567

252. Harnett SJ, Allen KD, Macmillan RR. Critical care unit outbreak of *Serratia liquefaciens* from contaminated pressure monitoring equipment. *J Hosp Infect* 2001;47:301–307.

253. Moolenaar RL, Crutcher JM, San Joaquin VH, et al. A prolonged outbreak of *Pseudomonas aeruginosa* in a neonatal intensive care unit: did staff fingernails play a role in disease transmission? *Infect Control Hosp Epidemiol* 2000;21:80–85.

254. Chang HJ, Miller HL, Watkins N, et al. An epidemic of *Malassezia pachydermatis* in an intensive care nursery associated with colonization of health care workers' pet dogs. *N Engl J Med* 1998;338:706–711.

255. Trilla A, Codina C, Salles M, et al. A cluster of fever and hypotension on a surgical ICU related to the contamination of plasma expanders by cell wall products of *Bacillus stearothermophilus*. *Infect Control Hosp Epidemiol* 1995;16:335–339.

256. Watson JC, Fleming DW, Borella AJ, et al. Vertical transmission of hepatitis A resulting in an outbreak in a neonatal intensive care unit. *J Infect Dis* 1993;167:567–571.

257. Livornese LL Jr., Dias S, Samel C, et al. Hospital-acquired infection with vancomycin-resistant *Enterococcus faecium* transmitted by electronic thermometers. *Ann Intern Med* 1992;117:112–116.

The Intensive Care Unit: Part B. Antibiotic Resistance and Prevention of CVC-BSIs, Catheter-Associated Urinary Tract Infections and C. *Difficile**

Nasia Safdar and Dennis G. Maki

INTRODUCTION

Intensive care units (ICUs) have revolutionized the care of critically ill patients with trauma, shock states, and other life-threatening conditions, leading to greatly improved outcomes [1,2]. However, nosocomial (ICU-acquired) infection remains a major challenge in the ICU patient; rates of infection in the ICU are 3–5 times higher than rates in other hospital wards [3,4]. Although patients in the ICU represent only 10% of all hospital admissions, they account for nearly 50% of all healthcare-associated infections (HAIs) in U.S. hospitals. Major advances in our understanding of the epidemiology and pathogenesis of ICU-acquired infections have occurred over the past two decades leading to the development of measures to greatly reduce or prevent HAIs.

Epidemiology

Currently, HAIs affect more than 2 million patients in U.S. hospitals annually and are associated with approximately 90,000 deaths each year [5].

Surveillance of HAIs, especially in high-risk hospital settings, such as the ICU, has become an integral feature of infection control and quality assurance in all U.S. hospitals. The Centers for Disease Control and Prevention (CDC) Study of the Efficacy of Nosocomial Infection Control

From the Section of Infectious Diseases, Department of Medicine, University of Wisconsin Medical School, and the Infection Control Department, University of Wisconsin Hospital and Clinics, University of Wisconsin-Madison, Madison, WI.

(SENIC) Project, showed that surveillance can help prevent HAIs [6].

The National Nosocomial Infections Surveillance (NNIS) system was established in the early 1970s to measure the impact of HAIs, better understand their associated risk factors, and develop effective strategies for their control [7]. NNIS, the only national system for tracking HAIs, includes approximately 350 hospitals. The NNIS system is currently being redesigned to cover new areas of patient safety monitoring and evaluation and will soon be called the National Healthcare Safety Network (NHSN). Surveillance of HAIs has been standardized by the NNIS System by providing simple unambiguous definitions, especially for device-associated infections [8]. Targeted surveillance and calculation of device-associated infection rates per 1000 device days allows benchmarking with similar hospitals and detection of unique institutional problems that need redress and a mechanism for assessing institutional trends and even HAI outbreaks.

Since the length of stay heavily impacts the HAI risk, infection rates should be expressed per 1000 patient-days. Device utilization affects device-associated infection rates, and the CDC recommends surveillance of device-associated infection and calculation of rates of device-associated infection per 1000 device days. Rates of HAI vary among the different types of ICUs and are highest in neonatal, surgical, and burn units followed by medical ICUs; Patients in coronary care units have a very low risk of infection (Table 24B-1) [9–11].

The epidemiology of ICU-acquired infection in developing countries has recently been characterized by a new large multinational surveillance system in developing countries in South and Central America, Asia, Africa, and the Middle East using NNIS definitions of HAI. In a recent report, overall rates of device-associated infection in 55 ICUs of the consortium were 22.5 infections per 1000 ICU-days; 41% of infections were ventilator-associated pneumonia (VAP), followed by CVC-related bloodstream infection (CVC-BSIs; 12.5 episodes per 1000 catheter-days) and catheter-associated urinary tract infections (CA-UTIs 8.9 episodes per 1000 catheter-days) [12]. These rates are two- to threefold higher than reported in North American ICUs and highlight the extraordinary vulnerability to HAIs in ICUs around the world.

Aerobic gram-negative bacilli, especially *Pseudomonas aeruginosa* account for 50% of ICU infections; gram-positive cocci (20%) and candida species (10%) make up the remainder [3,4]. Figures 24B-1–24B-4 show the microbiology of ICU infection overall and with VAP, CVC-BSIs, and CA-UTIs [4].

General Aspects of Infection Control

The U.S. Joint Commission on Accreditation of Healthcare Organizations (JCAHO) and similar regulatory agencies in many other countries mandate that every hospital have an active program for surveillance, prevention, and control of HAIs [13]. Surveillance is the cornerstone of an effective control program. In most institutions, surveillance focuses on infections caused by antibiotic-resistant bacteria and infections that greatly increase morbidity and mortality (e.g., surgical site infections [SSIs], BSIs and VAP).

Although it is unclear whether environmental contamination with resistant bacteria translates into greater infections in patients, the inanimate environment may be a reservoir of resistant HAI pathogens. Several studies have shown that methicillin-resistant *Staphylococcus aureus* (MRSA), vancomycin-resistant enterococcus (VRE), *Clostridium difficile*, and gram-negative bacteria can be recovered from a variety of hospital surfaces. Although the ICU environment cannot be made microbe free, certain architectural and environmental issues warrant attention. ICUs should be located in areas that limit traffic flow to essential ICU personnel. An adequate number of sinks and dispensers of waterless alcohol hand rub or antimicrobial soap must be available for all entering personnel who will have contact with the patient and the immediate

TABLE 24B-1

RATES OF DEVICE-ASSOCIATED INFECTIONS PER 1000 DEVICE-DAYS BY TYPE OF ICU IN NNIS HOSPITALS, JANUARY 2002–JUNE 2004

Infection	Type of ICU			
	Medical rate, mean (25%, 75%)	Medical-Surgical rate, mean (25%, 75%)	Surgical rate, mean (25%, 75%)	Coronary rate, mean (25%, 75%)
Catheter-associated urinary tract infection	5.1 (2.5, 7.1)	3.9 (2.1, 5.2)	4.4 (2.3, 6.5)	4.5 (2.6, 7.5)
Central line-associated bloodstream infection	5.0 (2.4, 6.4)	4.0 (2.6, 5.1)	4.6 (2.0, 5.9)	3.5 (1.5, 7.0)
Ventilator-associated pneumonia	4.9 (2.1, 6.2)	5.4 (2.6, 7.2)	9.3 (4.7, 12.2)	4.4 (1.9, 6.8)

(Adapted from [11])

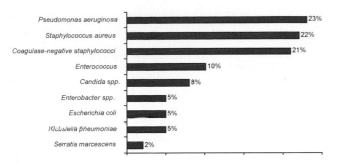

Figure 24B-1 Microbiology of infections in the ICU. (Adapted from [4])

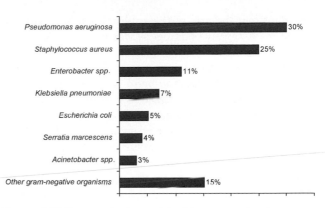

Figure 24B-3 Microbiology of healthcare-associated pneumonia in the ICU. (Adapted from [4])

environment. Separate areas and sinks should be used for cleaning, for storage, and for reprocessing contaminated equipment. All ICUs should have airborne infection isolation rooms for patients with tuberculosis or other airborne infections. For ICUs involved in the care of bone marrow transplant patients or hematologic malignancy, positive-pressure isolation rooms using high efficiency particulate air (HEPA) filtration should be available. All surfaces contiguous to the ICU patient should be wiped down with the general hospital disinfectant at least daily, and urine measuring devices, a frequent reservoir of gram-negative bacilli, should be rinsed with a disinfectant after each use. Each ICU patient should have a dedicated stethoscope and sphygmomanometer.

Hand Hygiene

Infected or colonized patients represent the main reservoir of HAIs in the ICU, and the major mechanism of spread of HAI pathogens in the ICU is by carriage on the hands, apparel, or equipment of healthcare workers (HCWs). This has been most clearly shown in outbreak settings and for gram-positive pathogens in studies predating the

advent of novel agents such as waterless alcohol based hand rubs for hand hygiene; the role played by HCWs in horizontal transmission of gram-negative bacilli in the ICU in the presence of waterless alcohol-containing hand rubs remains to be elucidated. In a recent well-conducted cohort study, Waters et al. sought to determine whether or not hand carriage of gram-negative bacilli by neonatal nurses was associated with endemic HAIs caused by gram-negative bacilli in neonates cared for by those nurses [14]. The investigators found that 192/2935 neonates enrolled acquired an infection caused by gram-negative bacilli; 70% of the isolates were available for molecular typing, and 9% (11/119) of strains causing infection were recovered from the hands of neonatal ICU nurses. An additional 33% (39/119) of strains were shared among infants providing indirect evidence of hand carriage by HCWs. In this study, sampling of nurses' hands was performed quarterly immediately after hand hygiene using waterless alcohol-containing hand rubs, and because carriage is typically transient, it is possible that more frequent culturing would have yielded a larger number of shared strains. It is

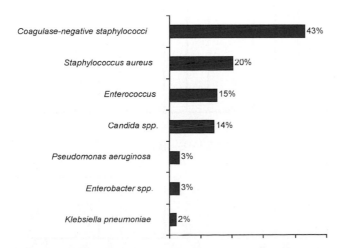

Figure 24B-2 Microbiology of bloodstream infections in the ICU. (Adapted from [4])

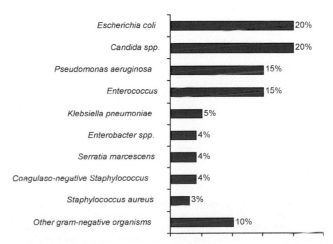

Figure 24B-4 Microbiology of catheter-associated urinary tract infections in the ICU. (Adapted from [4])

important that the role of the environment as a reservoir of HAI gram-negative pathogens was not assessed in this study.

Given the importance of hands as a major vehicle of horizontal transmission, hand hygiene remains the fundamental measure advocated to prevent HAIs [15–20]. Despite universal acknowledgement of hand washing as a cornerstone of HAI control programs, compliance rates >50% have been difficult to achieve, and hand-washing rates have ranged from 9% to 50% in HCW studies [21,22].

Recent investigations have strived to better understand the reasons for poor compliance in the face of the compelling evidence of the importance of hand washing for HAI prevention [21], identifying cutaneous irritation, inconvenient sink location, time constraints, high workload, and understaffing. Of concern, risk factors for noncompliance with hand hygiene include being a physician (rather than a nurse), working in an ICU, and, paradoxically, engaging in patient-care activities with a high risk of cross-transmission [21]. Interventions to redress these deficiencies have included targeted education; feedback; convenient location of sinks and hand-hygiene agents; use of alternative, less irritating hand-hygiene agents; and patient education [17]. Table 24B-2 summarizes strategies to enhance compliance with hand hygiene [23].

Hygienic hand care with antiseptics is clearly more effective than conventional hand washing with soap and water; the advantage is most pronounced when contamination is heavy [24,25]. Conventional handwashing with plain soap and water results in minimal reduction or even, paradoxically, an *increase* in bacterial counts compared to the baseline count before the hand washing

TABLE 24B-2
STRATEGIES TO IMPROVE HAND-HYGIENE COMPLIANCE

Healthcare worker education
Routine observation and feedback
Engineering controls
Easy, convenient availability of alcohol-based hand rub
Patient education
Reminders in workplace
Administrative sanctions or rewards
Improved skin care for healthcare workers
Active participation at individual and institutional level

(Adapted from [23]).

(Figure 24B-5) [18,26]. The increase is probably caused by promotion of bacterial release and dispersal through shedding of colonized skin squames [27,28]. In addition to superior antimicrobial activity, some antiseptics, such as chlorhexidine, bind to the stratum corneum, producing long-term anti-infective activity on the skin surface [29].

Antiseptics commercially available in the United States in a variety of formulations include chlorhexidine, iodophors, triclosan, Para-chloro-meta-xylenol, and alcohol based products [17]. A number of before–after studies using time-series analysis and HAIs as the primary outcome in ICUs [15,16,30–34] have shown that alcohol-containing waterless hand rubs were associated with significant HAI reductions. Three large, well-conducted, randomized trials assessing the efficacy of

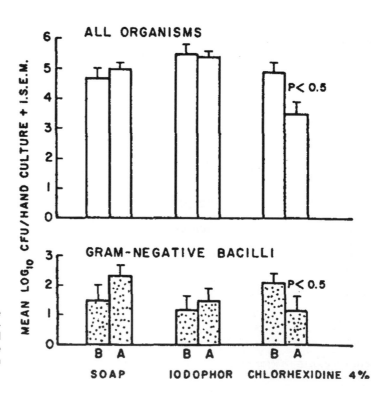

Figure 24B-5 Immediate bacterial removal with three hand-washing agents. Each agent was studied in 10 individuals with one week between tests. Cultures were obtained immediately before (B) and after (A) hand-washing with the agent. The bacterial count increased after hand washing with soap alone. (Adapted from [18].)

chlorhexidine-containing hand-hygiene products showed a 27–47% relative reduction in HAIs [30,33,34]. CDC recommendations for hand hygiene have recently been published [35], emphasizing hand antisepsis with an antiseptic containing-soap or detergent, or an alcohol-based hand rub: (1) before and after direct contact with patients or the environment and equipment in the immediate vicinity of the patient and (2) before performing invasive procedures, such as insertion of an intravascular device or urinary catheter. Alcohol-based, waterless hand rubs are now widely used in U.S. hospitals for hand hygiene because of their convenience and broadspectrum activity [17]. However, all have limited efficacy with gross soilage so that visibly soiled hands should always be washed with antiseptic soap and water [36].

The major factor limiting acceptance of alcohol products for hand antisepsis in the past was desiccation and irritation of skin. This is now obviated by incorporating emollients into alcohol-based hand rubs, which has enhanced HCW acceptance and may augment antibacterial activity by slowing the evaporation of alcohol [37]. A recent randomized clinical trial in 50 ICU HCWs compared a conventional 2% chlorhexidine gluconate wash with water to a waterless alcohol-based hand rub (61% ethanol with emollients) and showed that use of the waterless alcohol-based product produced significantly less skin

scaling and irritation [38]; unfortunately, degerming was not assessed.

The recent CDC guidelines have been endorsed by the American Medical Association [39] and the American Society for Microbiology [40], both of which have played an active role in emphasizing hand hygiene in all areas of health care. Institutional commitment is essential to improve compliance with recommended hand-hygiene practices. The CDC guideline recommends that institutions (1) monitor and record adherence to hand hygiene by ward or service, (2) provide feedback to HCWs about their performance, and (3) monitor the volume of alcohol hand rub used per 1000 patient-days. Table 24B-3 summarizes the recommendations for hand hygiene in the 2002 CDC Guideline [41].

Antimicrobial Resistance in the ICU

The global crisis in antimicrobial resistance has had a huge impact in the ICU where antibiotic pressure, critically ill patients, invasive devices, and procedures all contribute to increase nosocomial spread of multidrug-resistant pathogens (Figures 23b-6 and 23b-7) [42–44]. Stemming the tide of antimicrobial resistance mandates a multifaceted approach, encompassing antimicrobial stewardship, hand hygiene, and barrier precautions for HCWs in contact

TABLE 24B-3
HANDWASHING AND HAND ANTISEPSIS RECOMMENDATIONS FROM THE CDC/HICPAC GUIDELINE ON HAND HYGIENE.

	Strength of recommendation[a]
When hands are visibly dirty or contaminated with proteinaceous material or are visibly soiled with blood or other body fluids, wash hands with either a nonantimicrobial soap and water or an antimicrobial soap and water	IA
If hands are not visibly soiled, use an alcohol-based hand rub or wash hands with an antimicrobial soap and water for the following situations:	IB
Before direct contact with patients	
Before putting on sterile gloves when inserting a central vascular catheter	
Before inserting a urinary catheter, peripheral vascular catheter, or other invasive procedure not requiring surgery	
After contact with patient's intact skin	
After contact with body fluids, mucous membranes, and wound dressings if hands are not visibly soiled	
Moving from a contaminated body site to a clean body site during patient care	
After contact with inanimate objects in the immediate vicinity of the patient	
After removing gloves	
Before eating and after using a restroom, wash hands with a nonantimicrobial soap and water or with an antimicrobial soap and water	IB
Antimicrobial-impregnated wipes are not a substitute for using an alcohol-based hand rub or antimicrobial soap	IB
If exposure to bacillus anthracis, wash hands with nonantimicrobial soap and water or antimicrobial soap and water	II

(Adapted from [41]).
[a]Categorization of recommendations:
IA: strongly supported for implementation and strongly supported by well-designed experimental, clinical or, epidemiologic studies.
IB: strongly recommended for implementation and supported by certain clinical or epidemiologic studies and by strong theoretical rationale.
II: suggested for implementation and supported by suggestive clinical or epidemiologic studies or by strong theoretical rationale.

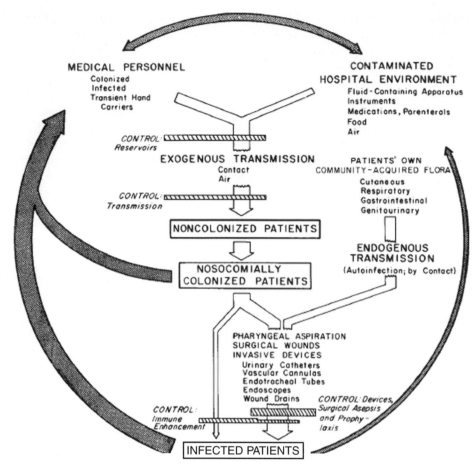

Figure 24B-6 The epidemiology of nosocomial infection. Transmission occurs mainly by contact spread to a much lesser extent by the airborne route. Aspiration, surgical wounds, exposure to invasive devices and antimicrobial use amplify transmission, colonization, and susceptibility to infection. (Adapted from [100] with permission.)

with high-risk patients. The CDC's Campaign to Prevent Antimicrobial Resistance aims to prevent antimicrobial resistance in healthcare settings [45]. The campaign centers on four main strategies: prevent infection, diagnose and treat infection, use antimicrobials wisely, and prevent transmission.

Control of Antimicrobial Resistance: Optimizing Antimicrobial Usage

Antimicrobial use drives antimicrobial resistance [46,47]. Studies have shown that inappropriate antimicrobial use is common in healthcare institutions [48,49]. Antimicrobial stewardship is essential to limit unnecessary antimicrobial use, optimize patient outcomes, and reduce the problem of antimicrobial resistance [50]. Various strategies have been proposed to improve antimicrobial use and limit emergence of resistance [43]. These include the use of protocols or guidelines, formulary restriction of key drugs, infectious disease consultation, computerized physician order entry, and increased use of diagnostics to confirm the presence of an infection (Table 24B-4).

Prevention of Nosocomial Spread of Resistant Organisms

Isolation of infected or colonized patients is widely regarded as the most important measure to prevent spread of

Figure 24B-7 Major antimicrobial resistant pathogens associated with nosocomial infections in ICUs in 1989, 1993, 1997 and 2002. (Adapted from National Nosocomial Infections Surveillance (NNIS) System Report, data summary from January 1992 to June 2002, issued August 2002 and [4].)

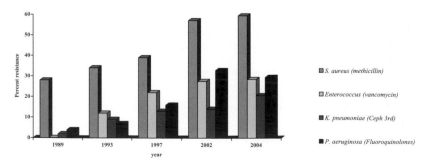

TABLE 24B-4

ANTIMICROBIAL USAGE STRATEGIES FOR REDUCING THE EMERGENCE OF ANTIMICROBIAL RESISTANCE IN THE INTENSIVE CARE UNIT

Recommendation	Strength of recommendation[a]
Limit unnecessary antibiotic administration	
Develop hospital-based guidelines for antibiotic use	II
Create an antibiotic use quality improvement team	II
Provide professional education and detailing on antibiotic use for physicians	II
Restrict hospital formulary	II
Use quantitative cultures for nosocomial pneumonia	I
Optimize antimicrobial effectiveness	
Avoid inadequate treatment by using automated guidelines	II
Use combination antimicrobial treatment	II
Consult with infectious diseases staff	II
Cycling antibiotics	II
Automatic stop orders for surgical prophylaxis	I
Avoid routine selective digestive decontamination	I
Computer–assisted provider order entry	II

(Adapted from [43]).
[a]Level I, supported by randomized controlled trials; Level II, supported by nonrandomized trials and observational studies.

resistant pathogens through the healthcare institution [51]. The most recent CDC guideline categorizes isolation precautions: (1) standard precautions and (2) transmission-based precautions [52]. Standard precautions specify the use of gloves for any anticipated contact with blood, any body fluid, secretions or excretions (except sweat), nonintact skin, and mucous membranes. Gowns are recommended if patient-care activities are likely to generate splashes of blood, body fluids, and secretions. Hand hygiene is expected after removing gloves and between patients. Standard precautions apply to *all* patients without regard to clinical diagnosis.

Transmission-based precautions include contact, droplet, and airborne precautions, each based on the mode of transmission of the infectious agent within the healthcare setting. Acknowledging that multidrug-resistant HAI pathogens, particularly MRSA or VRE, are spread primarily by direct (and indirect) contact with HCWs, the guideline specifies that patients known to be colonized or infected by resistant bacteria are to be placed in contact isolation, which requires a private room for the patient (or cohorting the patient in a semiprivate room with another patient who is also colonized or infected by the same organism). HCWs are expected to wear gloves on entry to the room and gowns if substantial contact with the patient or the environment is anticipated. Gloves and gowns should be removed and hands treated with a medicated hand-hygiene product while still in the isolation room. Noncritical patient-care items should be dedicated; if reused, they must be disinfected between patients.

Unfortunately, the existent paradigm for preventing spread of resistant organisms in the hospital—waiting until colonization or infection by MRSA, VRE or some other resistant organism is serendipitously identified by the clinical laboratory, following which the patient is placed in isolation, usually in a single room, requiring the use of gloves, with or without a gown, for all contacts with the patient—is failing dismally, viewing the inexorable growth in antimicrobial resistance [53].

A recent guideline from the Society for Healthcare Epidemiology of America [54] recommends that surveillance cultures to detect silent VRE or MRSA carriage be performed in roommates of VRE- or MRSA-colonized or infected patients and other high-risk patients at the discretion of infection control staff; patients found to be colonized must *also* be placed in contact isolation [54]. If these measures fail to contain spread, efforts should be intensified in the highest risk areas, such as the ICU. Cohorting of staff and screening of staff for carriage, if epidemiologic data point to a link, is recommended. Verification that environmental disinfection procedures are effective by environmental surveillance cultures before and after cleaning areas containing VRE- or MRSA-colonized or infected patients also is recommended.

We believe that a simpler strategy for preventing spread of all types of multidrug-resistant bacteria is the preemptive use of barrier isolation precautions (gowns and gloves) and dedicated patient-care items (e.g., stethoscopes and sphygmomanometers) for *all* high-risk patients from the time of admission to prevent HCWs from acquiring hand contamination by multidrug-resistant organisms when they have contact with patients with unrecognized colonization or infection and block transmission to other as yet uncolonized patients. Numerous studies have shown that the preemptive use of barrier precautions, also called "protective isolation," can effectively prevent the spread of multidrug-resistant organisms, such as MRSA or VRE, in an epidemic setting [55], and other studies have shown the effectiveness of protective isolation in high-risk populations, such as patients in an ICU, for prevention of endemic HAIs, including by multidrug-resistant organisms [56–59]. Three prospective randomized trials have been conducted to assess the efficacy of preemptive barrier precautions [56,57,60]; two showed benefit with a reduction in all HAIs in ICU patients (relative risk reduction, 52–81%) [56,57].

Specific Infections

Intravascular Device-Related Bloodstream Infections

The use of intravascular devices has become an essential component of delivering care to patients with cancer. Unfortunately, vascular access is associated with substantial and generally underappreciated potential for producing iatrogenic disease, particularly BSIs originating from infection of the percutaneous device used for vascular access. Nearly 40% of all nosocomial BSIs derive from vascular access in some form [61] and can be associated with excess mortality approaching 35% [62], increased length of hospitalization, and excess healthcare costs [63,64].

Individual types of intravascular devices (IVDs) pose different risks of infection. In a recent systematic review of 200 prospective studies, we showed that point incidence rates of IVD-related BSI were lowest with peripheral Intravenous (0.1%, 0.5 per 1000 IVD-days) or midline catheters (0.4%, 0.2 per 1000 catheter-days). Far higher rates were seen with short-term noncuffed and nonmedicated central venous catheters (CVCs) (4.4%, 2.7 per 1000 catheter-days). Arterial catheters used for hemodynamic monitoring (0.8%, 1.7 per 1000 catheter-days) and peripherally inserted central catheters (PICCs) used in hospitalized patients (2.4%, 2.1 per 1000 catheter-days) posed risks approaching those seen with short-term conventional CVCs used in the ICU. Surgically implanted long-term central venous devices—cuffed and tunneled catheters (22.5%, 1.6 per 1000 IVD-days) and central venous ports (3.6%, 0.1 per 1000 IVD-days)—appear to have high rates of infection when risk is expressed as BSIs per 100 IVDs but actually pose much lower risk when rates are expressed per 1000 IVD-days [65].

Figure 24B-3 summarizes the microbial profile of IVD-related BSIs (IVDR-BSIs) [4]. As might be expected from knowledge of the pathogenesis of these infections, skin microorganisms account for the largest proportion of IVDR-BSIs.

Recent evidence-based guidelines provide the best current information on the evaluation of the ICU patient with fever or other signs of sepsis [66]. Before any decision regarding initiation of antimicrobial therapy or removal of an IVD, the patient must be thoroughly examined to identify *all* plausible sites of infection, including ventilator-assisted pneumonia (VAP), CA-UTI, SSI, antibiotic-associated colitis, or line sepsis.

Despite the challenge of identifying the source of a patient's signs of sepsis [66], several clinical, epidemiologic, and microbiologic findings point strongly toward an IVD as the source of a septic episode. Patients with abrupt onset of signs and symptoms of sepsis without any other identifiable source should prompt suspicion of infection of an IVD. The presence of inflammation or purulence at the catheter insertion site is now uncommon in patients with IVDR-BSI [67]. However, if purulence is seen in combination with signs and symptoms of sepsis, it is highly likely the patient has IVDR-BSI and should prompt removal of the IVD. Finally, recovery of certain microorganisms in multiple blood cultures (e.g., Staphylococci, *Corynebacterium* or *Bacillus* species, or *Candida* or *Malassezia* spp.) strongly suggests infection of the IVD.

It is indefensible to start anti-infective drugs for suspected or presumed infection in the critically ill patient without first obtaining blood cultures from two separate sites, *at least one of which is drawn from a peripheral vein by percutaneous venipuncture*. In adults, if at least 30 milliliter (mL) of blood is cultured, 99% of detectable bacteremias should be identified [68–70]. Similar operating characteristics are achieved in the pediatric population using a weight-based graduated volume approach to blood cultures [71]. Standard blood cultures drawn through CVCs provide excellent sensitivity for diagnosis of BSI but are less specific than cultures obtained from a peripheral vein [72,73]. If the patient has a long-term multilumen catheter, a specimen should be obtained from each lumen of the catheter because studies have found a high rate of discordance (∼30%) between cultures obtained from different lumens of the same catheter [74].

Short-term IVDs should be removed from the outset in unstable patients with suspected IVDR-BSI (as follows); however, it often is undesirable or difficult to do this in patients with surgically implanted IVDs, such as Hickman and Broviac catheters. Only 15–45% of long-term IVDs that are removed for suspected infection are truly colonized or infected at the time of removal [75–77]. To avoid unnecessary removal of IVDs, methods have been developed to identify infection while allowing the device to stay in place: (1) paired quantitative blood cultures drawn from the IVD and percutaneously from a peripheral vein [78], (2) differential time to positivity (DTP) of paired standard blood cultures, one drawn from the IVD, the second from a peripheral vein [79], and (3) gram stain [80] or acridine orange staining of blood samples drawn through the IVD [81,82].

Quantitative blood cultures are labor intensive and cost almost twice as much as standard blood cultures. The DTP of paired blood cultures, one drawn through the IVD and the second concomitantly from a peripheral vein, has been shown to reliably identify IVDR-BSI of both short-term and long-term IVDs if the blood culture drawn from the IVD turns positive ≥ 2 hours before the culture drawn peripherally [83].

If a short-term vascular catheter is suspected of being infected because the patient has no obvious other source of infection to explain fever, there is inflammation at the insertion site, or cryptogenic staphylococcal sp. BSI or candidemia has been documented, blood cultures should be obtained and *the catheter should be removed and cultured*. Failure to remove an infected catheter puts the patient at risk of developing septic thrombophlebitis with peripheral IV catheters, septic thrombosis of a great central vein with CVCs [84], or even endocarditis. Continued access, if necessary, can be established with a new catheter inserted in a new site. Although small studies have found some utility of guidewire exchange in the management of CVCs suspected of being infected [85–88], we believe that, in the absence of randomized studies demonstrating its safety, guidewire exchange generally should not be performed if there is suspicion of IVDR-BSI, especially if there are signs of local infection such as purulence or erythema at the insertion site or signs of systemic sepsis without a source. In these instances, the old catheter should be removed and cultured and a new catheter should be inserted in a new site.

Prevention of IVDR-BSI

An updated guideline for the prevention of IVDR-BSIs was published in 2002 by the CDC's Healthcare Infection Control Practices Advisory Committee (HICPAC) (Table 24B-5) [89]

Ventilator-Associated Pneumonia

Mechanical ventilation is an essential feature of modern ICU care. Unfortunately, mechanical ventilation is associated with a substantial risk of VAP, the most common HAI in the ICU with an incidence ranging from 9–40% [90–92]; it is associated with prolonged hospitalization [93–95], increased healthcare costs [96], and a 15–45% attributable mortality [97–99].

Understanding the pathogenesis of VAP is essential to devising strategies for prevention of these infections [100]. Advances in our understanding of pathogenesis have led to the development of specific measures that can greatly reduce the risk of VAP [101–104].

In the mechanically ventilated patient, a number of factors conspire to compromise host defenses: critical illness, co-morbidities [105], and malnutrition impair the immune system [106], and, most important, endotracheal intubation thwarts the cough reflex [107], compromises mucociliary clearance [108], injures the tracheal epithelial surface [109], and provides a direct conduit for rapid access of bacteria from above into the lower respiratory tract [110,111]. It probably would be more accurate pathogenetically to rename VAP as "endotracheal intubation-related pneumonia." Invasive devices and procedures and antimicrobial therapy create a favorable milieu for antimicrobial-resistant HAI pathogens to colonize the aerodigestive tract [112]. This combination of impaired host defenses and continuous exposure of the lower respiratory tract to large numbers of potential pathogens through the endotracheal tube (Figure 24B-8) [113] put the mechanically ventilated patient at great jeopardy of developing VAP.

For microorganisms to cause VAP, they first must gain access to the normally sterile lower respiratory tract where they can adhere to the mucosa and produce sustained infection. Microorganisms gain access by one of four mechanisms: (1) aspiration of microbe-laden secretions, either from the oropharynx directly or, secondarily, by reflux from the stomach into the oropharynx and then into the lower respiratory tract [114–116], (2) direct extension of a contiguous infection, such as a pleural space infection, (3) inhalation of contaminated air or medical aerosols, and (4) hematogenous carriage of microorganisms to the lung from remote sites of local infection, such as CVC-BSI.

Outbreaks of VAP due to contamination of respiratory therapy equipment [117–125] and diagnostic equipment, such as bronchoscopes and endoscopes, have been well described [126–132]. For example, Takigawa et al. reported 16 episodes of hospital-acquired pneumonia due to *Burkholderia cepacia* caused by contamination of inhaled medication nebulizer reservoirs [125]. Likewise, Srinivasan et al. reported 28 episodes of pneumonia caused by *P. aeruginosa* linked epidemiologically to contaminated bronchoscopes with defective biopsy-port caps [132]. This outbreak occurred despite adherence to disinfection and sterilization guidelines [133].

Since the first reports of large outbreaks of severe acute respiratory syndrome (SARS) in 2003 in which more than 8,000 persons in China, Hong Kong, Singapore, Vietnam, Taiwan, and Canada ultimately became infected and 9.6% died [134], major advances have been made in our understanding of the epidemiology and mode of transmission of this new human Coronavirus [135]. SARS spreads almost exclusively through respiratory droplets from person to person, rarely by the airborne or contact route. The risk of SARS acquisition is far higher in the hospital than in the community, and nearly one-half of the early episodes involved HCWs or hospitalized patients infected secondarily upon admission [136]. Although SARS has been contained for now, if it returns, it will comprise an ongoing threat to patients and HCWs as a cause of nosocomial pneumonia. Outbreaks of other respiratory pathogens, such as *Legionella spp.*, influenza A or respiratory syncytial virus, are well described in nosocomial settings [65–71].

TABLE 24B-5

SUMMARY OF CDC/HICPAC GUIDELINE FOR PREVENTION OF INTRAVASCULAR DEVICE-RELATED BLOODSTREAM INFECTION

	Strength of recommendation[a]
General measures	
Educate all healthcare workers involved in intravascular device (IVD) care and maintenance	IA
Ensure adequate nursing staff levels in intensive care units (ICUs)	IB
Surveillance	
Monitor institutional IVD infection rates of IVD-related bloodstream infection (BSI)	IA
Express rates of CVC-related BSIs per 1000 CVC days	IB
At catheter insertion	
Aseptic technique:	
Hand hygiene before insertion or manipulation of any IVD	IA
Clean or sterile gloves during insertion and manipulation of noncentral IVDs	IC
Maximal barrier precautions during insertion of central venous catheters (CVCs): mask, cap, sterile gown, gloves and drapes	IA
Dedicated IVD team strongly recommended	IA
Chlorhexidine first choice for cutaneous antisepsis	IA
Subclavian vein rather than internal jugular vein catheter insertion	IA
Use of sutureless securement device	NR
Sterile gauze or a semipermeable polyurethane dressing to cover site	IA
No systemic or topical antibiotics at insertion	IA
Maintenance	
Remove IVD as soon as no longer required	IA
Monitor IVD site daily	IB
Change dressing of CVC insertion site at least weekly	II
Do not use topical antibiotic ointments	IA
Change needleless IV systems at least as frequently as the administration set; replace caps no more frequently than every 3 days or per manufacturers' recommendations	II
Complete lipid infusions within 12 hours	IB
Replace administration sets no more frequently than every 72 hours. When lipid-containing admixtures or blood products are given, sets should be replaced every 24 hours; with propofol every 6–12 hours	IA
Replace peripheral IVs every 72–96 hours	IB
Do not routinely replace CVCs or PICCs solely because of fever unless IVD infection is suspected, but replace catheter if there is purulence at the exit site, especially if the patient is hemodynamically unstable and IVD-related-BSI is suspected	IB
Technology	
Use antimicrobial-coated or antiseptic-impregnated CVC in adult patients if institutional rate of BSI is high despite consistent application of preventive measures and catheter likely to remain in place >5 days	IB
Use chlorhexidine-impregnated sponge dressing for patients with uncuffed CVCs or other catheters likely to remain in place for >5 days	NR
Use prophylactic antibiotic lock solution only in patients with long-term IVDs who have continued to experience IVD-related BSIs despite consistent application of infection control practices	II

(Adapted from [89]).

Note: BSI, bloodstream infection; CVC, central venous catheter; IVD, intravascular device; PICC, peripherally inserted central catheters.

[a]Taken from the CDC/HICPAC system of weighting recommendations based on scientific evidence.

IA: strongly supported for implementation and strongly supported by well-designed experimental, clinical, or epidemiologic studies.

IB: strongly recommended for implementation and supported by certain clinical or epidemiologic studies and by strong theoretical rationale.

IC: required for implementation as mandated by federal or state regulation or standard.

II: suggested for implementation and supported by suggestive clinical or epidemiologic studies or by strong theoretical rationale.

NR: no recommendation for or against at this time; unresolved issue involves practices for which insufficient evidence or no consensus exists about efficacy.

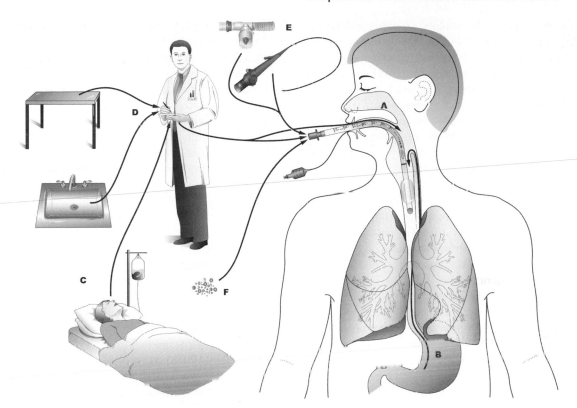

Figure 24B-8 Routes of colonization/infection in mechanically ventilated patients. Colonization of the aerodigestive tract may occur endogenously (A and B) or exogenously (C–F). Exogenous colonization may result in primary colonization of the oropharynx or may be the result of direct inoculation into the lower respiratory tract during manipulations of respiratory equipment (D), during using of respiratory devices (E), or from contaminated aerosols (C). (From [113].)

In the mid-1980s, tuberculosis (TB) rates in the United States rose after half a century of decline, and large nosocomial outbreaks with multidrug-resistant strains occurred. In one such outbreak investigated by the CDC, six episodes of TB occurred following exposure to a source-patient who had spent several weeks in the hospital before being placed in respiratory isolation [137]. Transmission of *Mycobacterium tuberculosis* through contaminated bronchoscopes and respiratory equipment also has been reported [138,139].

Although reported pseudo-outbreaks with nontuberculous mycobacteria far outnumber epidemics of true disease, HAI outbreaks caused by these ubiquitous environmental organisms are well described, most often in association with contaminated hospital water [140–142].

For most endemic VAPs, the most important mechanism of infection is aspiration of oropharyngeal organisms into the distal bronchi followed by bacterial proliferation and parenchymal invasion. Inflammation of the bronchiole wall involves the alveolar septi and airspaces leading to bronchopneumonia.

Pathogens causing VAP may be part of the host's endogenous flora at the time of hospitalization or may be acquired exogenously after admission to the healthcare facility from the hands, apparel, and equipment of HCWs, the hospital environment, and the use of invasive devices.

Although most VAP epidemics have stemmed from direct infection of the lower airway by exogenous organisms, such as gram-negative bacilli, Legionella spp., and aspergillus spp., epidemics can be more insidious with colonization of the upper airway and episodes of VAP occurring days or weeks later.

The normal flora of the oropharynx in the nonintubated patient without critical illness is composed predominantly of viridans streptococci, hemophilus spp., and anaerobes. Salivary flow and content (immunoglobulin, fibronectin) are the major factors maintaining the normal flora of the mouth (and dental plaque). Aerobic gram-negative bacilli rarely are recovered from the oral secretions of healthy patients [143,144]. During critical illness, especially in ICU patients, the oral flora shifts dramatically to colonization by aerobic gram-negative bacilli and *S. aureus* [145]. Bacterial adherence to the oro-tracheal mucosa of the mechanically ventilated patient is facilitated by reduced mucosal IgA and increased protease production, exposed and denuded mucous membranes, elevated airway pH, increased numbers of airway receptors for bacteria due to acute illness, and antimicrobial use.

A large number of studies show that colonization of the oropharynx by aerobic gram-negative and gram-positive pathogens, such as *S. aureus*, is a near-universal occurrence in critically ill patients receiving mechanical ventilation [114–116,146–149]. In a study of 80 ventilated patients, Torres et al. found that in 19 patients with secondary tracheal colonization, 46% of the microorganisms isolated in the trachea already had been isolated in the pharynx [114]. George et al. reported similar findings with 42% of the pathogens isolated in 26 patients with VAP previously recovered from the oropharynx [116]. In a more recent study performed in 48 trauma patients, Ewig et al. found that upon admission to the ICU, patients were colonized mainly with *S. aureus, H. influenzae,* or *Streptococcus pneumoniae.* However, follow-up cultures showed replacement of the normal oropharyngeal flora by enteric gram-negative bacilli and *P. aeruginosa.* Oropharyngeal colonization was a powerful independent predictor of subsequent tracheobronchial colonization ([Odds Ratio] OR 23.9, 95% [Confidence Interval] CI 3.8–153.3) [115].

Aspiration of oropharyngeal contents containing a large bacterial inoculum overwhelms host defenses already compromised by critical illness and the presence of an endotracheal tube, thus leading to the development of VAP.

Understanding this sequence of pathophysiologic events, it would seem logical that reducing concentrations of oral microorganisms should have a beneficial effect on VAP prevention. Five studies have evaluated the use of scheduled oral care with a chlorhexidine antiseptic solution for prevention of VAP [150–154]; chlorhexidine oral care reduced the incidence of oral microbial colonization *and* VAP. The use of chlorhexidine for oral antisepsis warrants further study and consideration for application in clinical practice.

The stomach has been posited to be an important reservoir of organisms that cause VAP [155]. In healthy persons, few bacteria entering the stomach survive in the presence of gastric acid. Conditions that reduce the gastric pH (e.g., achlorhydria, H2 antagonists, and enteral nutrition) predispose to bacterial proliferation in the stomach [156–159]. Several studies have shown a powerful relationship between a high gastric pH and massive overgrowth of gastric bacteria [156–159]. Gastric microorganisms reflux up the esophagus abetted by recumbent position and the ever-present naso- or oro-gastric tube and are aspirated into the trachea. Direct and indirect evidence exists to implicate the stomach as a potential reservoir of bacteria causing VAP [160–162]. Numerous studies have shown that gastric contents can be aspirated into the lower airways despite the presence of an endotracheal cuff [163,164]. However, recent literature suggests that the stomach, although a reservoir for enteric gram-negative bacteria, is not the primary site for colonization of pathogens and that the gastropulmonary route is not a major pathogenic route for development of VAP [146,165]. In a prospective, randomized, double-blind study in ICU patients, Bonten et al. compared antacids and sucralfate and measured intragastric acidity. Colonization by Enterobacteriaceae occurred in the stomach, trachea, and oropharynx; however, intragastric

acidity did not influence the incidence of VAP [166]. In another analysis of the same study, the same investigators showed that oropharyngeal colonization by Enterobacteriaceae was an important independent risk factor for VAP; in contrast, gastric colonization by Enterobacteriaceae was not found to increase the risk of VAP [167].

The diagnostic criteria and tests for VAP include clinical criteria, qualitative or quantitative endobronchial cultures, bronchoalveolar lavage (BAL) or culture of protected specimen brush samples obtained by bronchoscopic techniques, and specimens, including bronchial washings, mini-BAL, or protected specimen brush samples, obtained by blind non bronchoscopic procedures. Clinical criteria (e.g., fever, leukocytosis, purulent secretions, new or changing radiographic infiltrate) have high sensitivity but relatively low specificity. Clinical criteria are useful for initial screening for VAP and for selecting patients for invasive procedures that have sensitivities and specificities in the range of 80% [168]. The optimal methods for defining VAP in clinical practice and the impact of different diagnostic techniques on patient outcome are the subject of much debate [169].

NNIS data show that, based on clinical diagnosis, the most common pathogens isolated from pneumonia in patients in ICUs are *S. aureus, P. aeruginosa, Enterobacter* spp., and *Klebsiella pneumoniae,* with varying prevalences depending on the type of ICU [11] (Figure 24B-6). Early onset VAP, which manifests within the first 4 days of hospitalization, more often is caused by community-acquired pathogens, such as *S. pneumoniae* and *Haemophilus* spp.. When invasive techniques are used to diagnose VAP, the frequency of recovery of enteric gram-negative bacilli decreases from 50–70% of isolates to 35–45%. VAP is polymicrobial in as many as 20–40% of patients. A number of recent studies have shown that anaerobes do not play a major role in VAP [170].

Control Measures

A number of nonpharmacologic and pharmacologic preventive measures have been recommended for clinical use in ICUs (Table 24B-6) [171]. The use of nonabsorbable oral antibiotics to eradicate or reduce gastrointestinal carriage of pathogenic bacteria, a process widely termed *selective digestive decontamination (SDD),* has been extensively studied [172,173]. A short course of parenteral antimicrobials and a longer duration of topical antimicrobials have been used in most studies evaluating the efficacy of SDD for the prevention of VAP. More than 40 randomized controlled trials [174–176] and eight meta-analyses [177–181] have undertaken to determine the efficacy of SDD for reducing the incidence of VAP; most, but not all, have found a beneficial effect on VAP but an inconsistent effect on ICU mortality. Regardless of efficacy, a very real concern relates to the potential for antimicrobial resistance with long-term use of SDD [182,183]. Recent studies have justified this

TABLE 24B-6
MEASURES FOR PREVENTION OF VENTILATOR-ASSOCIATED PNEUMONIA

Recommendation	Strength of recommendation
General prophylaxis	
Effective infection control measures: staff education, compliance with alcohol-based hand disinfection, and isolation to reduce cross-infection with MDR pathogens should be used routinely	I
Surveillance of ICU infections to identify and quantify endemic and new MDR pathogens and prepare timely data for infection control and to guide appropriate antimicrobial therapy in patients with suspected HAP or other nosocomial infection, are recommended	II
Intubation and mechanical ventilation	
Intubation and ventilation should be avoided, if possible, because it increases the risk of VAP	I
Noninvasive ventilation should be used whenever possible in selected patients with respiratory failure	I
Orotracheal intubation and orogastric tubes preferred over nasotracheal intubation and nasogastric tubes to prevent nosocomial sinusitis and to reduce the risk of VAP	II
Continuous aspiration of subglottic secretions can reduce the risk of early-onset VAP and should be used, if available	I
Endotracheal tube cuff pressure should be maintained >20 cm H_2O to prevent leakage of bacterial pathogens around the cuff into the lower respiratory tract	II
Contaminated condensate should be carefully emptied from ventilator circuits and condensate should be prevented from entering either the endotracheal tube or inline medication nebulizers	II
Passive humidifiers or heat-moisture exchangers decrease ventilator circuit colonization but have not consistently reduced the incidence of VAP; thus, they cannot be regarded as a pneumonia prevention tool	I
Reduced duration of intubation and mechanical ventilation may prevent VAP and can be achieved by protocols to improve the use of sedation and to accelerate weaning	II
Maintaining adequate staffing levels in the ICU can reduce length of stay, improve infection control practices, and reduce duration of mechanical ventilation	II
Aspiration, body position, and enteral feeding	
Patients should be kept in the semirecumbent position	I
Enteral feeding is preferred over parenteral nutrition	I
Modulation of colonization: oral antiseptics and antibiotics	
Selective decontamination of the digestive tract is not recommended for routine use	II
Prior administration of systemic antibiotics has reduced the risk of nosocomial pneumonia in some patient groups, but if a history of prior administration is present at the time of onset of infection, there should be increased suspicion of infection with MDR pathogens	II
Prophylactic administration of systemic antibiotics for 24 hours at the time of emergent intubation has been demonstrated to prevent ICU-acquired HAP in patients with closed head injury, but routine use is not recommended until more data become available	I
Routine use of oral chlorhexidine is not recommended until more data become available	I
Use daily interruption or lightening of sedation to avoid constant heavy sedation and try to avoid paralytic agents	II
Stress bleeding prophylaxis, transfusion, and hyperglycemia	
If needed, stress bleeding prophylaxis with either H2 antagonists or sucralfate is acceptable	
Transfusion of red blood cell and other allogeneic blood products should follow a restricted transfusion trigger policy; leukocyte-depleted red blood cell transfusions can help to reduce HAP in selected patient populations	
Intensive insulin therapy is recommended to maintain glucose levels between 80 and 110 mg/dl in ICU patients	I

(Adapted from [171]).
Note: MDR, multidrug resistant; VAP, ventilator-associated pneumonia; HAP, hospital-acquired pneumonia.
[a]Level I, supported by randomized controlled trials; Level II, supported by nonrandomized trials and observational studies.

concern and further dampened enthusiasm for this approach. Moreover, most of the studies were not designed to assess the relative effect of the components of SDD (topical and systemic) on the prevention of VAP. Future studies need to more clearly evaluate antimicrobial resistance as a major endpoint, including the use of selective media for surveillance cultures to enhance recovery of nosocomial, antibiotic-resistant pathogens.

Use of sucralfate rather than H_2 blockers for stress ulcer prophylaxis, with a goal of maintaining gastric pH and thereby suppressing gastric colonization by potential VAP pathogens, initially appeared to be a promising preventive strategy but was not effective in a large, multi-center, randomized trial [143]. Preventive measures aimed at reducing the risk of aspiration, particularly by semirecumbent positioning of patients, have been among the more successful and less costly strategies. Measures aimed at improving host and lung defenses against aspirated pathogens are not yet ready for implementation.

Clostridium difficile-Associated Diarrhea

Clostridium difficile is the major infectious cause of nosocomial diarrhea and is associated with prolonged hospitalization and increased hospital costs [184]. The incidence of infection with this organism is increasing in hospitals worldwide due to the widespread use of broadspectrum antibiotics, with reported rates ranging from 1 to 10 episodes per 1000 discharges and 17 to 60 episodes per 100,000 bed-days [185].

Clostridium difficile infection encompasses a spectrum of conditions ranging from asymptomatic colonization to fulminant disease with toxic megacolon [186]. The usual presentation is acute watery diarrhea with lower abdominal pain and fever occurring during or shortly after beginning antimicrobial therapy. The antibiotics that most predispose to *C. difficile* infection are third- or fourth-generation cephalosporins, clindamycin, and penicillins [187]; however, virtually any antimicrobial may trigger *C. difficile* infection.

Diagnosis of *C. difficile*-associated diarrhea can be reliably made by detection of *C. difficile* toxins A and/or B by enzyme-linked immunoassay (ELISA) in a stool sample [188]. If this test is negative and *C. difficile* infection is strongly suspected, cytotoxin testing, widely regarded as the reference standard, should be performed. This test, while 94–100% sensitive and 99% specific, takes at least 48–72 hours before results are available. In severely ill patients, flexible sigmoidoscopy provides a rapid means of diagnosis because 90% of episodes of pseudo mebranous colitis involve the left side of the colon; the visualization of colonic pseudo membranes is essentially pathognomonic for *C. difficile* infection. Computerized tomography (CT) of the abdomen, while useful for identifying bowel wall thickness, does not differentiate between *C. difficile* and other causes of bowel wall thickening, such as ischemic colitis [189].

Clostridium difficile has become a major HAI pathogen widely prevalent in healthcare facilities, and control of nosocomial transmission is essential. A growing body of literature suggests that the inanimate environment may contribute to nosocomial transmission of *C. difficile*. Commonly used hospital disinfectants are not germicidal against *C. difficile* spores, which may persist for very prolonged periods on surfaces. A recent before–after study using sodium hypochlorite solution to disinfect a bone-marrow transplant ward found that rates of *C. difficile* infection decreased from 8.3 per 1000 patient-days to 3.4 per 1000 patient-days; when hypochlorite disinfection was discontinued, rates returned to baseline levels [190].

The Society for Healthcare Epidemiology of America has published a guideline for prevention and treatment of *C. difficile* infections (Table 24B-7) [191]. Patients with *C. difficile*-associated diarrhea should be placed in private rooms, and staff should wear gowns and gloves for all contacts with the patient. Hand hygiene with an antiseptic agent is essential. It is important to note that alcohol-based hand rubs do *not* have activity against the spore form of *C. difficile*. Equipment such as stethoscopes and sphygmomanometers should be dedicated to the patient, and consideration should be given to disinfecting the environment with sodium hypochlorite.

Catheter-Associated Urinary Tract Infection

Each year, urinary catheters are inserted in >5 million patients in acute-care hospitals and extended-care facilities [192]. CA-UTI is the most common HAI in hospitals and nursing homes, comprising >40% of all institutionally acquired infections [11]. Nosocomial bacteriuria or candiduria develops in up to 25% of patients requiring a urinary catheter for ≥7 days with a daily risk of 5% [192]. CAUTI is the second most common cause of nosocomial bloodstream infection [193]; some studies also have found increased mortality associated with it [194]. Although most CAUTIs are asymptomatic [195], rarely extend hospitalization, and add only $500 to $1,000 to the direct costs of acute-care hospitalization [196], asymptomatic infections commonly precipitate unnecessary antimicrobial therapy [197]. CAUTIs comprise perhaps the largest institutional reservoir of nosocomial antibiotic-resistant pathogens, the most important of which are multidrug-resistant Enterobacteriacae other than *Escherichia coli*, such as *Klebsiella*, *Enterobacter*, *Proteus*, or *Citrobacter*; *Pseudomonas aeruginosa*; enterococci and staphylococci; and *Candida* spp [198].

Excluding rare hematogenously derived pyelonephritis, caused almost exclusively by *S. aureus*, most microorganisms causing endemic CAUTI derive from the patient's own colonic or perineal flora or from the hands of HCWs during catheter insertion or manipulation of the collection system [199]. Organisms gain access in one of two ways. Extraluminal contamination may occur early by direct inoculation when the catheter is inserted or later by organisms ascending from the perineum by capillary action in the thin mucous film contiguous to the external catheter surface. Intraluminal contamination occurs by reflux of microorganisms gaining access to the catheter lumen from failure to maintain closed drainage or contamination of urine in the collection bag. Recent studies suggest that CAUTIs most frequently stem from microorganisms gaining access to the bladder extraluminally [200], but both routes are important.

Most infected urinary catheters are covered by a thick biofilm containing the infecting microorganisms embedded in a matrix of host proteins and microbial exoglycocalyx [201]. A biofilm forms intraluminally, extraluminally, or both ways, usually advancing in a retrograde fashion. The role of biofilms in the pathogenesis of CAUTI has

TABLE 24B-7

PREVENTION AND CONTROL OF *CLOSTRIDIUM DIFFICILE*-ASSOCIATED DIARRHEA (CDAD)

Recommendation	Strength of recommendation[a]
Surveillance and diagnosis	
Surveillance for CDAD should be performed in every institution	B-III
Appropriate and prompt diagnostic testing should be performed in patients with antibiotic-associated diarrhea	A-II
Diagnostic tests for *C. difficile* should be performed only on diarrheal (soft or unformed) stool specimens unless ileus is suspected	B-III
Testing of stool specimens from asymptomatic patients for *C. difficile* (including "test of cure" after treatment)	B-II
Prevention and control	
Implement policies to ensure prudent antimicrobial use	A-II
Surveillance of antimicrobial utilization in the facility should be conducted	B-III
Healthcare providers in the facility should be educated about the epidemiology of CDAD	B-III
Patients with CDAD and fecal incontinence should be in a private room. If possible, all patients with CDAD should be in private rooms	B-III
Meticulous hand hygiene with soap or an antiseptic agent is recommended after contact with patients, their body substances, or their potentially contaminated environment	B-III
Healthcare providers should wear gloves for contact with patients with CDAD	A-I
Use of disposable, single-use thermometers (rather than shared electronic thermometers) is recommended	A-II
Patient-care items, such as stethoscopes and sphygmomanometers, should be dedicated. If they must be shared, they should be disinfected between patients	B-III
Disinfection of the environment of a patient with CDAD should be done using sporocidal agents, such as a diluted sodium hypochlorite solution	B-II
Patients with CDAD may be removed from contact isolation when their diarrhea has resolved	B-III

(Adapted in part from the 2002 Society for Healthcare Epidemiology of America guidelines for the prevention of Clostridium difficile associated diarrhea, [191], and [207]).
Category:
A = good evidence to support a recommendation for use.
B = moderate evidence to support a recommendation for use.
Quality of evidence:
I = Evidence from ≥ properly randomized controlled trial.
II = evidence from ≥1 well-designed observational study, multiple time-series, or dramatic results of uncontrolled experiments.
III = expert opinion, descriptive studies.

not been established. However, anti-infective-impregnated or silver-hydrogel catheters, which inhibit adherence of microorganisms to the catheter surface, significantly reduce the risk of CAUTI [202], particularly infections caused by gram-positive organisms or yeasts, which are most likely to be acquired extraluminally from the periurethral flora. These data suggest that microbial adherence to the catheter surface is important in the pathogenesis of many, but not all, CAUTIs. Infections in which the biofilm does not play a pathogenetic role probably are caused by mass transport of intraluminal contaminants into the bladder by retrograde reflux of microbe-laden urine when a catheter or collection system is moved or manipulated.

Several catheter-care practices are universally recommended to prevent or at least delay the onset of CAUTI (Table 24B-8) [199,203]: avoid unnecessary catheterizations, consider a condom or suprapubic catheter, have a trained HCW insert the catheter aseptically, remove the catheter as soon as no longer needed, maintain closed drainage, ensure dependent drainage, minimize manipulations of the system, and separate catheterized patients.

Technologic innovations to prevent HAIs are likely to be most effective if they are based on a clear understanding of the pathogenesis and epidemiology of the infection. Novel technologies must be designed to block CAUTI by either the extraluminal or intraluminal routes or both. Impregnated catheters, which reduce adherence of microorganisms to the catheter surface, may confer the greatest benefit for preventing CAUTI. Two catheters impregnated with anti-infective solutions have been studied in randomized trials, one impregnated with the urinary antiseptic nitrofurazone [204] and the other with a new broad-spectrum antimicrobial combination of minocycline and rifampin [205]. Both catheters showed a significant reduction in bacterial CAUTIs; however, the studies were small, and selection of antimicrobial-resistant uropathogens was not satisfactorily resolved. Silver compounds also have been studied for coating urinary catheters. A meta-analysis of 8 randomized trials comparing silver oxide or silver alloy catheters with standard nonimpregnated catheters found that silver alloy but not silver oxide catheters were associated with a threefold reduced risk of CAUTI [206].

TABLE 24B-8

CENTERS FOR DISEASE CONTROL AND PREVENTION GUIDELINE FOR PREVENTION OF CATHETER-ASSOCIATED URINARY TRACT INFECTION

Recommendation	Strength of recommendation
Educate personnel in correct techniques of catheter insertion and care	I
Periodically reeducate personnel in catheter care	II
Catheterize only when necessary	I
Consider alternative techniques of urinary drainage before using an indwelling urethral catheter	III
Emphasize hand hygiene	I
Insert catheter using aseptic technique and sterile equipment	I
Use smallest bore catheter suitable	II
Secure catheter properly	I
Maintain closed sterile drainage	I
Replace the collecting system when sterile closed drainage has been violated	III
Avoid irrigation unless needed to prevent or relieve obstruction	II
Refrain from daily meatal care with povidone-iodine or soap and water	II
Obtain urine samples aseptically	I
Maintain unobstructed urine flow	I
Do not change catheters at arbitrary fixed intervals	II
Spatially separate infected and uninfected patients with indwelling catheters	III
Avoid routine bacteriologic monitoring	III
Medicated urinary catheters	NR

Adapted from [203].
Note: NR, no recommendation
[a]Level I, supported by randomized controlled trials
Level II, supported by nonrandomized trials and observational studies
III

Future Directions

It is clear that HAIs represent one of the most important causes of iatrogenic morbidity and mortality in patients who require prolonged life support in an ICU. Strategies to increase adherence to hand hygiene, to prevent patient colonization, and to prevention infection once colonization has occurred should be a major focus of ICU staff attention and a research priority. The importance of hand carriage of pathogens by HCWs, the role of airborne transmission in the ICU, and the relevance of contamination of the inanimate environment by mutidrug-resistant pathogens needs to be better delineated. More effective ways to enhance compliance with evidence-based guidelines for hand hygiene and to prevent VAP, IVDR-BSI, and CAUTI would have vast immediate benefits.

REFERENCES

1. Nathens AB, Rivara FP, MacKenzie EJ, et al. The impact of an intensivist-model ICU on trauma-related mortality. *Ann Surg* 2006;244:545–54.
2. Diringer MN, Edwards DF. Admission to a neurologic/neurosurgical intensive care unit is associated with reduced mortality rate after intracerebral hemorrhage. *Crit Care Med* 2001;29:635–40.
3. Vincent JL, Bihari DJ, Suter PM, et al. The prevalence of nosocomial infection in intensive care units in Europe. Results of the European Prevalence of Infection in Intensive Care (EPIC) Study. EPIC International Advisory Committee. *JAMA* 1995;274:639–44.
4. Richards M, Thursky K, Buising K. Epidemiology, prevalence, and sites of infections in intensive care units. *Semin Respir Crit Care Med* 2003;24:3–22.
5. Weinstein RA. Nosocomial infection update. *Emerg Infect Dis* 1998;4:416–20.
6. Haley RW, Culver DH, White JW, et al. The efficacy of infection surveillance and control programs in preventing nosocomial infections in US hospitals. *Am J Epidemiol* 1985;121:182–205.
7. Emori TG, Culver DH, Horan TC, et al. National nosocomial infections surveillance system (NNIS): Description of surveillance methods. *Am J Infect Control* 1991;19:19–35.
8. Garner JS, Jarvis WR, Emori TG, et al. CDC definitions for nosocomial infections, 1988. *Am J Infect Control* 1988;16:128–40.
9. Chandrasekar PH, Kruse JA, Mathews MF. Nosocomial infection among patients in different types of intensive care units at a city hospital. *Crit Care Med* 1986;14:508–10.
10. Brown RB, Hosmer D, Chen HC, et al. A comparison of infections in different ICUs within the same hospital. *Crit Care Med* 1985;13:472–76.
11. National Nosocomial Infections Surveillance (NNIS) System Report. Data summary from January 1992 through June 2004. *Am J Infect Control* 2004;32:470–85.
12. Rosenthal VD, Maki DG, Salomao R, et al. Device-associated nosocomial infections in 55 intensive care units of 8 developing countries. *Ann Intern Med* 2006;145:582–91.
13. Joint Commission on Accreditation of Healthcare Organizations. *Accreditation manual for hospitals.* Oak Brook, IL: JCAHO, 1989.
14. Waters V, Larson E, Wu F, et al. Molecular epidemiology of gram-negative bacilli from infected neonates and health care

workers' hands in neonatal intensive care units. *Clin Infect Dis* 2004;38:1682–87.

15. Simmons B, Bryant J, Neiman K, et al. The role of handwashing in prevention of endemic intensive care unit infections. *Infect Control Hosp Epidemiol* 1990;11:589–94.

16. Webster J, Faoagali JL, Cartwright D. Elimination of methicillin-resistant *Staphylococcus aureus* from a neonatal intensive care unit after hand washing with triclosan. *J Paediatrics & Child Health* 1994;30:59–64.

17. Pittet D, Boyce JM. Hand hygiene and patient care: Pursuing the Semmelweiss legacy. *Lancet Infectious Diseases* 2003;3:269–70.

18. Maki DG. The use of antiseptics for handwashing by medical personnel. *J Chemotherapy* 1989;1:3–11.

19. Jarvis WR. Handwashing—The Semmelweis lesson forgotten? *Lancet* 1994;344:1311–12.

20. Austin DJ, Bonten MJ, Weinstein RA, et al. Vancomycin-resistant enterococci in intensive-care hospital settings: Transmission dynamics, persistence, and the impact of infection control programs. *PNAS* 1999;96:6908–13.

21. Pittet D, Mourouga P, Perneger TV. Compliance with handwashing in a teaching hospital. Infection Control Program. *Ann Intern Med* 1999;130:126–30.

22. Larson E. A causal link between handwashing and risk of infection? Examination of the evidence. *Infect Control* 1988;9:28–36.

23. Pittet D. Improving adherence to hand hygiene practice: A multidisciplinary approach. *Emerg Infect Dis* 2001;7:234–40.

24. Eckert DG, Ehrenkranz NJ, Alfonso BC. Indications for alcohol or bland soap in removal of aerobic gram-negative skin bacteria. Assessment by a novel method. *Infect Control Hosp Epidemiol* 1989;10:306–11.

25. Ehrenkranz NJ, Alfonso BC. Failure of bland soap handwash to prevent hand transfer of patient bacteria to urethral catheters. *Infect Control Hosp Epidemiol* 1991;12:654–62.

26. Larson EL. Skin hygiene and infection prevention: More of the same or different approaches. *Clin Infect Dis* 1999;29:1287–94.

27. Meers PD, Yeo GA. Physiologic and microbiologic changes in skin related to frequent handwashing. *Infect Control* 1978;7:59–63.

28. Davies RR, Noble WC. Dispersal of bacteria on desquamated skin. *Lancet* 1962;2:1295–97.

29. Bruch M. Newer germicides: What they offer. In: Maibach H, Aly R, eds. *Skin microbiology: Relevance to clinical infection.* New York: Springer-Verlag, 1981:103–12.

30. Massanari RM, Hierholzer WJ. A crossover comparison of antiseptic soaps on nosocomial infection rates in intensive care units. *Am J Infect Control* 1984;12:247.

31. Brown SM, Lubimova AV, Khrustalyeva NM, et al. Use of an alcohol-based hand rub and quality improvement interventions to improve hand hygiene in a Russian neonatal intensive care unit. *Infect Control Hosp Epidemiol* 2003;24:172–79.

32. Lai KK, Fontecchio S, Melvin R. Impact of waterless handwashing foam on the incidence of vancomycin-resistant enterococci. Paper presented at 13th Annual Meeting of the Society for Healthcare Epidemiology of America 2001, Toronto, Canada.

33. Maki DG, Hecht J. Antiseptic containing hand-washing agents reduce nosocomial infections: A prospective study. Paper presented at Proceedings and Abstracts of the Twenty-Second Interscience Conference of Antimicrobial Agents and Chemotherapy, October 4–6, 1982, Miami.

34. Doebbeling BN, Stanley GL, Sheetz CT, et al. Comparative efficacy of alternative hand-washing agents in reducing nosocomial infections in intensive care units. *N Engl J Med* 1992;327:88–93.

35. Boyce JM, Pittet D. Guideline for hand hygiene in health-care settings. Recommendations of the Healthcare Infection Control Practices Advisory Committee and the HICPAC/ SHEA/APIC/IDSA Hand Hygiene Task Force. *MMWR Recomm Rep* 2002;51:RR-1-16.

36. Garner JS, Favero MS. CDC guidelines for the prevention and control of nosocomial infections. Guideline for handwashing and hospital environmental control, 1985. Supersedes guideline for hospital environmental control published in 1981. *Am J Infect Control* 1986;14:110–29.

37. Larson EL, Eke PI, Laughon BE. Efficacy of alcohol-based hand rinses under frequent-use conditions. *Antimicrob Agents Chemother* 1986;30:542–44.

38. Larson EL, Aiello AE, Bastyr J, et al. Assessment of two hand hygiene regimens for intensive care unit personnel. *Crit Care Med* 2001;29:944–51.

39. American Medical Association (www.ama-assn.org) accessed November 21, 2006.

40. American Society for Microbiology (www.asmusa.org) accessed November 21, 2006.

41. Boyce JM, Pittet D. Guideline for hand hygiene in health-care settings. Recommendations of the Healthcare Infection Control Practices Advisory Committee and the HICPAC/ SHEA/APIC/IDSA Hand Hygiene Task Force. Society for Health-care Epidemiology of America/Association for Professionals in Infection Control/Infectious Diseases Society of America. *MMWR Recomm Rep* 2002;51:1–45

42. Fridkin SK, Gaynes RP. Antimicrobial resistance in intensive care units. *Clin Chest Med* 1999;20:303–16.

43. Kollef MH, Fraser VJ. Antibiotic resistance in the intensive care unit. *Ann Intern Med* 2001;134:298–314.

44. National Nosocomial Infections Surveillance (NNIS) System Report. Data summary from January 1992 to June 2002. *Am J Infect Control* 2002;30:458–75.

45. Brinsley K, Srinivasan A, Sinkowitz-Cochran R, et al. Implementation of the Campaign to Prevent Antimicrobial Resistance in Healthcare Settings: 12 Steps to Prevent Antimicrobial Resistance Among Hospitalized Adults—Experiences from 3 institutions. *Am J Infect Control* 2005;33:53–54.

46. Mutnick AH, Rhomberg PR, Sader HS, Jones RN. Antimicrobial usage and resistance trend relationships from the MYSTIC Programme in North America (1999–2001). *J Antimicrob Chemother* 2004;53:290–96.

47. Neuhauser MM, Weinstein RA, Rydman R, et al. Antibiotic resistance among gram-negative bacilli in U.S. intensive care units: Implications for fluoroquinolone use. *JAMA* 2003;289:885–88.

48. Ena J, Dick RW, Jones RN, Wenzel RP. The epidemiology of intravenous vancomycin usage in a university hospital. A 10-year study. *JAMA* 1993;269:598–602.

49. Maki DG, Schuna AA. A study of antimicrobial misuse in a university hospital. *Am J Med Sci* 1978;275:271–82.

50. Fishman N. Antimicrobial stewardship. *Am J Med.* 2006;119: S53–61; discussion S62–70.

51. Boyce JM, Jackson MM, Pugliese G, et al. Methicillin-resistant Staphylococcus aureus (MRSA): A briefing for acute care hospitals and nursing facilities. The AHA Technical Panel on Infections Within Hospitals. *Infect Control Hosp Epidemiol* 1994;15:105–15.

52. Garner JS. Guideline for isolation precautions in hospitals. The Hospital Infection Control Practices Advisory Committee. *Infect Control Hosp Epidemiol* 1996;17:53–80.

53. Fridkin SK. Increasing prevalence of antimicrobial resistance in intensive care units. *Crit Care Med* 2001;29:N64–68.

54. Muto CA, Jernigan JA, Ostrowsky BE, et al. SHEA guideline for preventing nosocomial transmission of multidrug-resistant strains of *Staphylococcus aureus* and enterococcus. *Infect Control Hosp Epidemiol* 2003;24:362–86.

55. Maki DG, Zilz MA, McCormick R. The effectiveness of using preemptive barrier precautions routinely (protective isolation) in all high risk patients to prevent nosocomial infection with resistant organisms, especially MRSA, VRE and *C. difficile*. Paper presented at Thirty-Fourth Annual Meeting of the Infectious Disease Society of America, September 1996, New Orleans.

56. Klein BS, Perloff WH, Maki DG. Reduction of nosocomial infection during pediatric intensive care by protective isolation. *New Engl J Med* 1989;320:1714–21.

57. Slota M, Green M, Farley A, et al. The role of gown and glove isolation and strict handwashing in the reduction of nosocomial infection in children with solid organ transplantation. *Crit Care Med* 2001;29:405–12.

58. Safdar N, Marx J, Meyer N, Maki DG. The effectiveness of preemptive enhanced barrier precautions for controlling MRSA in a burn unit. *Am J Infect Control* 2006;34:476–83.

59. Montecalvo MA, Jarvis WR, Uman J, et al. Infection-control measures reduce transmission of vancomycin-resistant enterococci in an endemic setting. *Ann Intern Med* 1999;131:269–72.

60. Koss WG, Khalili TM, Lemus JF, et al. Nosocomial pneumonia is not prevented by protective contact isolation in the surgical intensive care unit. *Am Surg* 2001;67:

61. Crnich CJ, Maki DG. The role of intravascular devices in sepsis. *Current Infectious Disease Reports* 2001;3:497–506.

62. Pittet D, Tarara D, Wenzel R. Nosocomial bloodstream infection in critically ill patients. Excess length of stay, extra costs, and attributable mortality. *JAMA* 1994;271:1598–1601.

63. Digiovine B, Chenoweth C, Watts C, Higgins M. The attributable mortality and costs of primary nosocomial bloodstream infections in the intensive care unit. *Am J Resp Crit Care Med* 1999;160:976–81.

64. Rello J, Ochagavia A, Sabanes E, et al. Evaluation of outcome of intravenous catheter-related infections in critically ill patients. *Am J Resp Crit Care Med* 2000;162:1027–30.

65. Maki DG, Kluger DM, Crnich CJ. The risk of bloodstream infection in adults with different intravascular devices: A systematic review of 200 published prospective studies. *Mayo Clin Proc* 2006;81:1159–71.

66. O'Grady NP, Barie PS, Bartlett JG, et al. Practice guidelines for evaluating new fever in critically ill adult patients.Task Force of the Society of Critical Care Medicine and the Infectious Diseases Society of America. *Clin Infect Dis* 1998;26:1042–59.

67. Safdar N, Maki DG. Inflammation at the insertion site is not predictive of catheter-related bloodstream infection with short-term, noncuffed central venous catheters. *Crit Care Med* 2002;30:2632–35.

68. Weinstein MP, Murphy JR, Reller LB, Lichtenstein KA. The clinical significance of positive blood cultures: A comprehensive analysis of 500 episodes of bacteremia and fungemia in adults. II. Clinical observations, with special reference to factors influencing prognosis. *Rev Infect Dis* 1983;5:54–70.

69. Mermel LA, Maki DG. Detection of bacteremia in adults: Consequences of culturing an inadequate volume of blood. *Ann Intern Med* 1993;119:270–72.

70. Washington JAD, Ilstrup DM. Blood cultures: Issues and controversies. *Rev Infect Dis* 1986;8:792–802.

71. Gaur AH, Giannini MA, Flynn PM, et al. Optimizing blood culture practices in pediatric immunocompromised patients: Evaluation of media types and blood culture volume. *Ped Infect Dis J* 2003;22:545–52.

72. Norberg A, Christopher NC, Ramundo ML, et al. Contamination rates of blood cultures obtained by dedicated phlebotomy vs intravenous catheter. *JAMA* 2003;289:726–29.

73. Beutz M, Sherman G, Mayfield J, et al. Clinical utility of blood cultures drawn from central vein catheters and peripheral venipuncture in critically ill medical patients. *Chest* 2003;123:854–61.

74. Robinson JL. Sensitivity of a blood culture drawn through a single lumen of a multilumen, long-term, indwelling, central venous catheter in pediatric oncology patients. *J Ped Hematology Oncology* 2002;24:72–74.

75. Brun-Buisson C, Abrouk F, Legrand P, et al. Diagnosis of central venous catheter-related sepsis. Critical level of quantitative tip cultures. *Arch Intern Med* 1987;147:873–77.

76. Tacconelli E, Tumbarello M, Pittiruti M, et al. Central venous catheter-related sepsis in a cohort of 366 hospitalised patients. *Eur J Clin MicroInfect Dis* 1997;16:203–09.

77. Gowardman JR, Montgomery C, Thirlwell S, et al. Central venous catheter-related bloodstream infections: An analysis of incidence and risk factors in a cohort of 400 patients. *Intensive Care Med* 1998;24:1034–39.

78. Bouza E, Burillo A, Munoz P. Catheter-related infections: Diagnosis and intravascular treatment. *Clin Micro Infect* 2002;8:265–74.

79. Raad I, Hanna HA, Alakech B, et al. Differential time to positivity: A useful method for diagnosing catheter-related bloodstream infections. *Ann Intern Med* 2003;140:18–25.

80. Moonens F, el Alami S, Van Gossum A, et al. Usefulness of gram staining of blood collected from total parenteral nutrition catheter for rapid diagnosis of catheter-related sepsis. *J Clin Microbiol* 1994;32:1578–79.

81. Kite P, Dobbins BM, Wilcox MH, McMahon MJ. Rapid diagnosis of central-venous-catheter-related bloodstream infection without catheter removal. *Lancet* 1999;354:1504–7.

82. Bong JJ, Kite P, Ammori BJ, et al. The use of a rapid *in situ* test in the detection of central venous catheter-related bloodstream infection: A prospective study. *J Parenteral & Enteral Nutrition* 2003;27:146–50.

83. Raad I, Hanna HA, Alakech B, et al. Differential time to positivity: A useful method for diagnosing catheter-related bloodstream infections. *Ann Intern Med* 2004;140:18–25.

84. Verghese A, Widrich WC, Arbeit RD. Central venous septic thrombophlebitis—The role of medical therapy. *Medicine* 1985;64:394–400.

85. Duszak R, Jr., Haskal ZJ, Thomas-Hawkins C, et al. Replacement of failing tunneled hemodialysis catheters through pre-existing subcutaneous tunnels: A comparison of catheter function and infection rates for de novo placements and over-the-wire exchanges. *J Vascular & Interventional Radiology* 1998;9:321–27.

86. Robinson D, Suhocki P, Schwab SJ. Treatment of infected tunneled venous access hemodialysis catheters with guidewire exchange. *Kidney International* 1998;53:1792–94.

87. Beathard GA. Management of bacteremia associated with tunneled-cuffed hemodialysis catheters. *J Amer Soc Nephrol* 1999;10:1045–49.

88. Martinez E, Mensa J, Rovira M, et al. Central venous catheter exchange by guidewire for treatment of catheter-related bacteraemia in patients undergoing BMT or intensive chemotherapy. *Bone Marrow Transplantation* 1999;23:41–44.

89. O'Grady NP, Alexander M, Dellinger EP, et al. Guidelines for the prevention of intravascular catheter-related infections. Centers for Disease Control and Prevention. *MMWR Recomm Rep* 2002;51:1–29.

90. Ibrahim EH, Mehringer L, Prentice D, et al. Early versus late enteral feeding of mechanically ventilated patients: Results of a clinical trial. *J Parenter Enteral Nutr* 2002;26:174–81.

91. Kollef MH, Vlasnik J, Sharpless L, et al. Scheduled change of antibiotic classes: A strategy to decrease the incidence of ventilator-associated pneumonia. *Am J Respir Crit Care Med* 1997;156:1040–48.

92. Sirvent JM, Torres A, El-Ebiary M, et al. Protective effect of intravenously administered cefuroxime against nosocomial pneumonia in patients with structural coma. *Am J Respir Crit Care Med* 1997;155:1729–34.

93. Rello J, Ollendorf DA, Oster G, et al. Epidemiology and outcomes of ventilator-associated pneumonia in a large U.S. database. *Chest* 2002;122:2115–21.

94. Bercault N, Boulain T. Mortality rate attributable to ventilator-associated nosocomial pneumonia in an adult intensive care unit: A prospective case-control study. *Crit Care Med* 2001;29:2303–09.

95. Heyland DK, Cook DJ, Griffith L, et al. The attributable morbidity and mortality of ventilator-associated pneumonia in the critically ill patient. The Canadian Critical Trials Group. *Am J Respir Crit Care Med* 1999;159:1249–56.

96. Warren DK, Shukla SJ, Olsen MA, et al. Outcome and attributable cost of ventilator-associated pneumonia among intensive care unit patients in a suburban medical center. *Crit Care Med* 2003;31:1312–17.

97. Craig CP, Connelly S. Effect of intensive care unit nosocomial pneumonia on duration of stay and mortality. *Am J Infect Control* 1984;12:233–38.

98. Fagon JY, Chastre J, Hance AJ, et al. Nosocomial pneumonia in ventilated patients: A cohort study evaluating attributable mortality and hospital stay. *Am J Med* 1993;94:281–88.

99. Cunnion KM, Weber DJ, Broadhead WE, et al. Risk factors for nosocomial pneumonia: Comparing adult critical-care populations. *Am J Respir Crit Care Med* 1996;153:158–62.

100. Maki DG. Control of colonization and transmission of pathogenic bacteria in the hospital. *Ann Intern Med* 1978;89: 777–80.

101. Cassiere HA, Niederman MS. New etiopathogenic concepts of ventilator-associated pneumonia. *Semin Respir Infect* 1996;11: 13–23.

102. Collard HR, Saint S, Matthay MA. Prevention of ventilator-associated pneumonia: An evidence-based systematic review. *Ann Intern Med* 2003;138:494–501.

103. Kollef MH. Prevention of hospital-associated pneumonia and ventilator-associated pneumonia. *Crit Care Med* 2004;32:1396–1405.

104. Tablan OC, Anderson LJ, Besser R, et al. Guidelines for preventing health-care–associated pneumonia, 2003: Recommendations of

CDC and the Healthcare Infection Control Practices Advisory Committee. *MMWR Recomm Rep* 2004;53:1–36.

105. Johanson WG, Pierce AK, Sanford JP. Changing pharyngeal bacterial flora in hospitalized patients: Emergence of gram-negative bacilli. *New Engl J Med* 1969;281:1137–40.

106. Sigalet DL, Mackenzie SL, Hameed SM. Enteral nutrition and mucosal immunity: Implications for feeding strategies in surgery and trauma. *Can J Surg* 2004;47:109–116.

107. Gal TJ. How does tracheal intubation alter respiratory mechanics? *Probl Anesth* 1988;2:191–200.

108. Klainer AS, Turndorf H, Wu WH, et al. Surface alterations due to endotracheal intubation. *Am J Med* 1975;58:674–83.

109. Cooper JD, Grillo HC. Experimental production and prevention of injury due to cuffed tracheal tubes. *Surg Gynecol Obstet* 1969;129:1235–41.

110. Levine SA, Niederman MS. The impact of tracheal intubation on host defenses and risks for nosocomial pneumonia. *Clin Chest Med* 1991;12:523–43.

111. Bone DK, Davis JL, Zuidema GD, et al. Aspiration pneumonia: Prevention of aspiration in patients with tracheostomies. *Ann Thoracic Surgery* 1974;18:30–37.

112. Safdar N, Maki DG. The commonality of risk factors for nosocomial colonization and infection with antimicrobial-resistant *Staphylococcus aureus*, enterococcus, gram-negative bacilli, *Clostridium difficile* and Candida. *Ann Intern Med* 2002;136:834–44.

113. Crnich CJ, Safdar N, Maki DG. The role of the intensive care unit environment in the pathogenesis and prevention of ventilator-associated pneumonia. *Respir Care* 2005;50:813–36; discussion 836–18.

114. de Latorre FJ, Pont T, Ferrer A, et al. Pattern of tracheal colonization during mechanical ventilation. *Am J Respir Crit Care Med* 1995;152:1028–33.

115. Ewig S, Torres A, El-Ebiary M, et al. Bacterial colonization patterns in mechanically ventilated patients with traumatic and medical head injury. Incidence, risk factors, and association with ventilator-associated pneumonia. *Am J Respir Crit Care Med* 1999;159:188–98.

116. George DL, Falk PS, Wunderink RG, et al. Epidemiology of ventilator-acquired pneumonia based on protected bronchoscopic sampling. *Am J Respir Crit Care Med* 1998;158:1839–47.

117. Edmondson EB, Reinarz JA, Pierce AK, Sanford JP. Nebulization equipment. A potential source of infection in gram-negative pneumonias. *Am J Dis Child* 1966;111:357–60.

118. Mertz JJ, Scharer L, McClement JH. A hospital outbreak of Klebsiella pneumonia from inhalation therapy with contaminated aerosol solutions. *Am Rev Respir Dis* 1967;95:454–60.

119. Ringrose RE, McKown B, Felton FG, et al. A hospital outbreak of *Serratia marcescens* associated with ultrasonic nebulizers. *Ann Intern Med* 1968;69:719–29.

120. Grieble HG, Colton FR, Bird TJ, et al. Fine-particle humidifiers. Source of *Pseudomonas aeruginosa* infections in a respiratory-disease unit. *N Engl J Med* 1970;282:531–35.

121. Gorman GW, Yu VL, Brown A, et al. Isolation of Pittsburgh pneumonia agent from nebulizers used in respiratory therapy. *Ann Intern Med* 1980;93:572–73.

122. Cross AS, Roup B. Role of respiratory assistance devices in endemic nosocomial pneumonia. *Am J Med* 1981;70:681–85.

123. Hovig B. Lower respiratory tract infections associated with respiratory therapy and anaesthesia equipment. *J Hosp Infect* 1981;2:301–15.

124. Craven DE, Lichtenberg DA, Goularte TA, et al. Contaminated medication nebulizers in mechanical ventilator circuits. Source of bacterial aerosols. *Am J Med* 1984;77:834–38.

125. Takigawa K, Fujita J, Negayama K, et al. Nosocomial outbreak of *Pseudomonas cepacia* respiratory infection in immunocompromised patients associated with contaminated nebulizer devices. *Kansenshogaku Zasshi–J Japanese Assoc Infect Dis* 1993;67:1115–25.

126. Wheeler PW, Lancaster D, Kaiser AB. Bronchopulmonary cross-colonization and infection related to mycobacterial contamination of suction valves of bronchoscopes. *J Infect Dis* 1989;159:954–58.

127. Fraser VJ, Jones M, Murray PR, et al. Contamination of flexible fiberoptic bronchoscopes with *Mycobacterium chelonae* linked to an automated bronchoscope disinfection machine. *Am Rev Respir Dis* 1992;145:853–55.

128. Agerton T, Valway S, Gore B, et al. Transmission of a highly drug-resistant strain (strain W1) of *Mycobacterium tuberculosis*—Community outbreak and nosocomial transmission via a contaminated bronchoscope. *JAMA* 1997;278:1073–77.

129. Schelenz S, French G. An outbreak of multidrug-resistant *Pseudomonas aeruginosa* infection associated with contamination of bronchoscopes and an endoscope washer-disinfector. *J Hosp Infect* 2000;46:23–30.

130. Sorin M, Segal-Maurer S, Mariano N, et al. Nosocomial transmission of imipenem-resistant *Pseudomonas aeruginosa* following bronchoscopy associated with improper connection to the Steris System 1 processor. *Infect Control Hosp Epidemiol* 2001;22:409–13.

131. Weber DJ, Rutala WA. Lessons from outbreaks associated with bronchoscopy. *Infect Control Hosp Epidemiol* 2001;22:403–08.

132. Srinivasan A, Wolfenden LL, Song X, et al. An outbreak of *Pseudomonas aeruginosa* infections associated with flexible bronchoscopes. *N Engl J Med* 2003;348:221–27.

133. Walter VA, DiMarino AJ Jr. American Society for Gastrointestinal Endoscopy-Society of Gastroenterology Nurses and Associates Endoscope Reprocessing Guidelines. *Gastrointest Endosc Clin N Am* 2000;10:265–73.

134. World Health Organization. Summary of probable SARS cases with onset of illness from 1 November 2002 to 31 July 2003 (www.who.int/en) accessed November 21, 2006.

135. Peiris JSM, Yuen KY, Osterhaus ADME, Stohr K. The severe acute respiratory syndrome. *New Engl J Med* 2003;349:2431–41.

136. Lipsitch M, Cohen B, Cooper B, et al. Transmission dynamics and control of severe acute respiratory syndrome. *Science* 2003;300:1966–70.

137. No author. Tuberculosis outbreak in a community hospital—District of Columbia, 2002. *MMWR* 2004;19:214–16.

138. Michele TM, Cronin WA, Graham NM, et al. Transmission of *Mycobacterium tuberculosis* by a fiberoptic bronchoscope. Identification by DNA fingerprinting. *JAMA* 1997;278:1093–95.

139. Southwick KL, Hoffmann K, Ferree K, et al. Cluster of tuberculosis cases in North Carolina: Possible association with atomizer use. *Am J Infect Control* 2001;29:1–6.

140. Burns DN, Wallace RJ, Schultz ME, et al. Nosocomial outbreak of respiratory tract colonization with *Mycobacterium fortuitum*: Demonstration of the usefulness of pulsed field gel electrophoresis in epidemiological investigation. *Am Rev Respir Dis* 1991;144:1153–59.

141. Laussucq S, Baltch A, Smith RP, et al. Nosocomial *Mycobacterium fortuitum* colonization from a contaminated ice machine. *Am Rev Respir Dis* 1988;138:891–94.

142. Wallace RJ, Brown BA, Griffith DE. Nosocomial outbreaks/pseudo-outbreaks caused by nontuberculous mycobacteria. *Ann Rev Microbiol* 1998;52:453–90.

143. Estes RJ, Meduri GU. The pathogenesis of ventilator-associated pneumonia: I. Mechanisms of bacterial transcolonization and airway inoculation. *Inten Care Med* 1995;21:365–83.

144. Meduri GU, Estes RJ. The pathogenesis of ventilator-associated pneumonia: II. The lower respiratory tract. *Inten Care Med* 1995;21:452–61.

145. Scannapieco FA, Stewart EM, Mylotte JM. Colonization of dental plaque by respiratory pathogens in medical intensive care patients. *Crit Care Med* 1992;20:740–45.

146. Bonten MJ, Gaillard CA, van Tiel FH, et al. The stomach is not a source for colonization of the upper respiratory tract and pneumonia in ICU patients. *Chest* 1994;105:878–84.

147. Niederman MS, Mantovani R, Schoch P, et al. Patterns and routes of tracheobronchial colonization in mechanically ventilated patients. The role of nutritional status in colonization of the lower airway by Pseudomonas species. *Chest* 1989;95:155–61.

148. Cardenosa Cendrero JA, Sole-Violan J, Bordes Benitez A, et al. Role of different routes of tracheal colonization in the development of pneumonia in patients receiving mechanical ventilation. *Chest* 1999;116:462–70.

149. Niederman MS. Gram-negative colonization of the respiratory tract: Pathogenesis and clinical consequences. *Semin Respir Infect* 1990;5:173–84.

150. DeRiso AJ II, Ladowski JS, Dillon TA, et al. Chlorhexidine gluconate 0.12% oral rinse reduces the incidence of total nosocomial respiratory infection and nonprophylactic systemic antibiotic use in patients undergoing heart surgery. *Chest* 1996;109:1556–61.

151. Houston S, Hougland P, Anderson JJ, et al. Effectiveness of 0.12% chlorhexidine gluconate oral rinse in reducing prevalence of nosocomial pneumonia in patients undergoing heart surgery. *Am J Crit Care* 2002;11:567–70.

152. Fourrier F, Cau-Pottier E, Boutigny H, et al. Effects of dental plaque antiseptic decontamination on bacterial colonization and nosocomial infections in critically ill patients. *Inten Care Med* 2000;26:1239–47.

153. Fourrier F, Dubois D, Pronnier P, et al. Effect of gingival and dental plaque antiseptic decontamination on nosocomial infections acquired in the intensive care unit: A double-blind placebo-controlled multicenter study. *Crit Care Med* 2005;33:1728–35.

154. Koeman M, van der Ven AJ, Hak E, et al. Oral decontamination with chlorhexidine reduces incidence of ventilator-associated pneumonia. *Am J Respir Crit Care Med* 2006;173:1348–55.

155. Alcon A, Fabregas N, Torres A. Hospital-acquired pneumonia: Etiologic considerations. *Infect Dis Clin North Am* 2003;17:679–95.

156. du Moulin GC, Paterson DG, Hedley-Whyte J, Lisbon A. Aspiration of gastric bacteria in antacid-treated patients: A frequent cause of postoperative colonization of the airway. *Lancet* 1982;1:242–45.

157. Daschner F, Kappstein I, Engels I, et al. Stress ulcer prophylaxis and ventilation pneumonia: Prevention by antibacterial cytoprotective agents? *Infect Control Hosp Epidemiol* 1988;9:59–65.

158. Giannella RA, Broitman SA, Zamcheck N. Influence of gastric acidity on bacterial and parasitic enteric infections. A perspective. *Ann Intern Med* 1973;78:271–76.

159. Donowitz LG, Page MC, Mileur BL, Guenthner SH. Alteration of normal gastric flora in critical care patients receiving antacid and cimetidine therapy. *Infect Control* 1986;7:23–26.

160. Heyland D, Mandell LA. Gastric colonization by gram-negative bacilli and nosocomial pneumonia in the intensive care unit patient. Evidence for causation. *Chest* 1992;101:187–93.

161. Torres A, el-Ebiary M, Gonzalez J, et al. Gastric and pharyngeal flora in nosocomial pneumonia acquired during mechanical ventilation. *Am Rev Respir Dis* 1993;148:352–57.

162. Inglis TJ, Sherratt MJ, Sproat LJ, et al. Gastroduodenal dysfunction and bacterial colonization of the ventilated lung. *Lancet* 1993;341:911–13.

163. Torres A, Serra-Batlles J, Ros E, et al. Pulmonary aspiration of gastric contents in patients receiving mechanical ventilation: The effect of body position. *Ann Intern Med* 1992;116:540–43.

164. Ibanez J, Penafiel A, Marse P, et al. Incidence of gastroesophageal reflux and aspiration in mechanically ventilated patients using small-bore nasogastric tubes. *J Parenter Enteral Nutr* 2000;24:103–6.

165. Garrouste-Orgeas M, Chevret S, Arlet G, et al. Oropharyngeal or gastric colonization and nosocomial pneumonia in adult intensive care unit patients. A prospective study based on genomic DNA analysis. *Am J Respir Cri Care Med* 1997;156:1647–55.

166. Bonten MJ, Gaillard CA, van der Geest S, et al. The role of intragastric acidity and stress ulcur prophylaxis on colonization and infection in mechanically ventilated ICU patients. A stratified, randomized, double-blind study of sucralfate versus antacids. *Am J Respir Crit Care Med* 1995;152:1825–34.

167. Bonten MJ, Bergmans DC, Ambergen AW, et al. Risk factors for pneumonia, and colonization of respiratory tract and stomach in mechanically ventilated ICU patients. *Am J Respir Crit Care Med* 1996;154:1339–46.

168. Chastre J, Fagon JY. Ventilator-associated pneumonia. *Am J Respir Crit Care Med* 2002;165:867–903.

169. Chastre J, Fagon JY, Bornet-Lecso M, et al. Evaluation of bronchoscopic techniques for the diagnosis of nosocomial pneumonia. *Am J Respir Crit Care Med* 1995;152:231–40.

170. Marik PE, Careau P. The role of anaerobes in patients with ventilator-associated pneumonia and aspiration pneumonia: a prospective study. *Chest* 1999;115:178–83.

171. Guidelines for the management of adults with hospital-acquired, ventilator-associated, and healthcare-associated pneumonia. *Am J Respir Crit Care Med* 2005;171:388–416.

172. Krueger WA, Unertl KE. Selective decontamination of the digestive tract. *Curr Opin Crit Care* 2002;8:139–44.

173. de Jonge E, Schultz MJ, Spanjaard L, et al. Effects of selective decontamination of digestive tract on mortality and acquisition of resistant bacteria in intensive care: A randomised controlled trial. *Lancet* 2003;362:1011–16.

174. Sanchez Garcia M, Cambronero Galache JA, Lopez Diaz J, et al. Effectiveness and cost of selective decontamination of the digestive tract in critically ill intubated patients. A randomized, double-blind, placebo-controlled, multicenter trial. *Am J Respir Crit Care Med* 1998;158:908–16.

175. Winter R, Humphreys H, Pick A, et al. A controlled trial of selective decontamination of the digestive tract in intensive care and its effect on nosocomial infection. *J Antimicrob Chemother* 1992;30:73–87.

176. SanchezGarcia M, Cambronero Galache JA, Lopez Diaz J, et al. Effectiveness and cost of selective digestive decontamination of the digestive tract in critically ill intubated patients. A randomized, double-blind, placebo-controlled, multicenter trial. *Am J Respir Crit Care Med* 1998;158:908–16.

177. Meta-analysis of randomised controlled trials of selective decontamination of the digestive tract. Selective Decontamination of the Digestive Tract Trialists' Collaborative Group. *BMJ* 1993;307:525–32.

178. Safdar N, Said A, Lucey MR. The role of selective digestive decontamination for reducing infection in patients undergoing liver transplantation: A systematic review and meta-analysis. *Liver Transpl* 2004;10:817–27.

179. Nathens AB, Marshall JC. Selective decontamination of the digestive tract in surgical patients: A systematic review of the evidence. *Arch Surg* 1999;134:170–76.

180. Kollef MH. The role of selective digestive tract decontamination on mortality and respiratory tract infections. A meta-analysis. *Chest* 1994;105:1101–8.

181. Heyland DK, Cook DJ, Jaeschke R, et al. Selective decontamination of the digestive tract. An overview. *Chest* 1994;105:1221–29.

182. Bonten MJ, Grundmann H. Selective digestive decontamination and antibiotic resistance: A balancing act. *Crit Care Med* 2003;31:2239–40.

183. Ebner W, Kropec-Hubner A, Daschner FD. Bacterial resistance and overgrowth due to selective decontamination of the digestive tract. *Eur J Clin Microbiol Infect Dis* 2000;19:243–47.

184. Kyne L, Hamel MB, Polavaram R, Kelly CP. Health care costs and mortality associated with nosocomial diarrhea due to *Clostridium difficile*. *Clin Infect Dis* 2002;34:346–53.

185. Archibald LK, Banerjee SN, Jarvis WR. Secular trends in hospital-acquired *Clostridium difficile* disease in the United States, 1987–2001. *J Infect Dis* 2004;189:1585–89.

186. Bartlett JG. *Clostridium difficile* infection: Pathophysiology and diagnosis. *Semin Gastrointest Dis* 1997;8:12–21.

187. Bartlett JG. Antimicrobial agents implicated in *Clostridium difficile* toxin-associated diarrhea of colitis. *Johns Hopkins Med J* 1981;149:6–9.

188. Delmee M. Laboratory diagnosis of *Clostridium difficile* disease. *Clin Microbiol Infec* 2001;7:411–16.

189. Kawamoto S, Horton KM, Fishman EK. Pseudomembranous colitis: Spectrum of imaging findings with clinical and pathologic correlation. *Radiographics* 1999;19:887–97.

190. Mayfield JL, Leet T, Miller J, Mundy LM. Environmental control to reduce transmission of *Clostridium difficile*. *Clin Infect Dis* 2000;31:995–1000.

191. Simor AE, Bradley SF, Strausbaugh LJ, et al. *Clostridium difficile* in long-term-care facilities for the elderly. *Infect Control Hosp Epidemiol* 2002;23:696–703.

192. Warren JW. The catheter and urinary tract infection. *Med Clin North Am* 1991;75:481–93.

193. Bryan CS, Reynolds KL. Hospital-acquired bacteremic urinary tract infection: Epidemiology and outcome. *J Urol* 1984;132:494–98.

194. Platt R, Polk BF, Murdock B, Rosner B. Reduction of mortality associated with nosocomial urinary tract infection. *Lancet* 1983;1:893–97.

195. Tambyah PA, Maki DG. Catheter-associated urinary tract infection is rarely symptomatic: A prospective study of 1,497 catheterized patients. *Arch Intern Med* 2000;160:678–82.

196. Tambyah PA, Knasinski V, Maki DG. The direct costs of nosocomial catheter-associated urinary tract infection in the era of managed care. *Infect Control Hosp Epidemiol* 2002;23: 27–31.

197. Nicolle LE. Catheter-related urinary tract infection. *Drugs Aging* 2005;22:627–39.

198. Wazait HD, Patel HR, Veer V, et al. Catheter-associated urinary tract infections: Prevalence of uropathogens and pattern of antimicrobial resistance in a UK hospital (1996–2001). *BJU Int* 2003;91:806–9.

199. Maki DG, Tambyah PA. Engineering out the risk for infection with urinary catheters. *Emerg Infect Dis* 2001;7:342–47.

200. Tambyah PA, Halvorson KT, Maki DG. A prospective study of pathogenesis of catheter-associated urinary tract infections. *Mayo Clin Proc* 1999;74:131–36.

201. Saint S, Chenoweth CE. Biofilms and catheter-associated urinary tract infections. *Infect Dis Clin North Am* 2003;17:411–32.

202. Johnson JR, Kuskowski MA, Wilt TJ. Systematic review: Antimicrobial urinary catheters to prevent catheter-associated urinary tract infection in hospitalized patients. *Ann Intern Med* 2006;144:116–26.

203. Wong ES. Guideline for prevention of catheter-associated urinary tract infections. *Am J Infect Control* 1983;11:28–36.

204. Maki DG, Knasinski V, Halvorson KT, et al. A prospective, randomized, investigator-blinded trial of a novel nitrofurazone-impregnated urinary catheter. In: Proceedings and Abstracts of the Society for Healthcare Epidemiology in America Annual Meeting, April 5–7, 1998, Orlando, Florida.

205. Darouiche RO, Smith JA Jr., Hanna H, et al. Efficacy of antimicrobial-impregnated bladder catheters in reducing catheter-associated bacteriuria: A prospective, randomized, multicenter clinical trial. *Urology* 1999;54:976–81.

206. Saint S, Elmore JG, Sullivan SD, et al. The efficacy of silver alloy-coated urinary catheters in preventing urinary tract infection: A meta-analysis. *Am J Med* 1998;105:236–41.

207. Kish MA. Guide to development of practice guidelines. *Clin Infect Dis* 2001;32:851–54.

25

The Newborn Nursery and the Neonatal Intensive Care Unit

Jane D. Siegel

The newborn nursery includes healthy, full-term infants who weigh ≥2,000 grams (g) at birth in the normal newborn areas as well as high risk infants who weigh <2,000 g at birth and are term infants but have complex medical problems in the neonatal intensive care unit (NICU) or high-risk nursery (HRN) area. These infants have an increased risk of acquiring infection because all components of their host defense system are deficient compared with those of older infants or adults, and the severity of these deficiencies is increased as gestational age decreases [1]. Survival of prematurely born infants has improved in recent years as a result of more advanced high-risk obstetrical care and neonatal supportive care including the use of surfactant replacement for treatment of hyaline membrane disease, mechanical ventilation including conventional and high-frequency ventilation, extracorporeal membrane oxygenation (ECMO) and continuous hemofiltration to support cardiopulmonary and renal function, noninvasive ventilation (e.g., continuous positive airway pressure [CPAP]) and cardiac intervention techniques, improved surgical techniques, and screening and chemoprophylaxis for early onset group B streptococcal (GBS) diseases. Therefore, increasing numbers of infants of very low birth weight (VLBW) (500–1,000 g, ≥24 weeks gestation) are surviving but require prolonged length of NICU stay and are at increased risk for infection. The National Nosocomial Infections Surveillance (NNIS) system of the Center for Disease Control and Prevention (CDC) reported that the group of

VLBW infants (≤1,000 g) has the highest rates of central line including umbilical catheter-associated bloodstream infections (CLA-BSIs) (mean 9.1; range 1.6–16.1) CLA-BSIs per 1,000 central venous catheter (CVC)-days compared with all other intensive care units (ICUs) reporting in the NNIS system [2–5] (Table 25-1). The rates of infection caused by bacteria and *Candida* sp. vary considerably among NICUs in the United States [6,7] and Canada [8] even after adjustment for known risk factors that could be practice related. Identification of practices in the best performing units and of widespread implementation has been a successful strategy of the Vermont Oxford Collaborative to reduce infection and other complication rates associated with NICU care (**www.vtoxford.org/home.aspx**) [9–11]. Device-associated infection rates have decreased over time in NNIS HRNs as in other NNIS ICUs, most likely a reflection of the beneficial effect of consistent implementation of recommended practices, measurement of rates, and feedback to the primary caregivers.

In the absence of in utero infection, the neonate is first exposed to microorganisms during passage through the birth canal. Subsequently, the normal skin and mucous membrane microflora are derived from environmental sources. Healthy term infants usually have a short hospital stay of <72 hours and in the managed care era often barely 24 hours. Therefore, infections are acquired infrequently in the normal newborn nursery (<1% of all admissions) and could not become manifest until after discharge, making

TABLE 25-1

CENTRAL LINE (CL)–ASSOCIATED BLOODSTREAM INFECTION (BSI) (CLA-BSI) RATES[a] IN INTENSIVE CARE UNITS (ICUS)

ICU Type	Number of ICUs Reporting	Number of CLA-BSIs per 1,000 CL-DAYS Pooled Mean (Median, Range)	Median Device Utilization (DU) RATIO[b]
Trauma	22	7.4 (5.2, 1.9–11.9)	.60
Burn	14	7.0 (NA)	.56[c]
Pediatric	54	6.6 (5.2, 0.9–11.2)	.46
Medical	94	5.0 (3.9, 0.5–8.8)	.52
Respiratory	6	4.8 (NA)	.47
Surgical	99	4.6 (3.4, 0–8.7)	.63
Neurosurg	30	4.6 (3.1, 0–10.6)	.50
Coronary	60	3.5 (3.2, 1.0–9.0)	.36
Medical-Surgical			
Major teaching	100	4.0 (3.4, 1.7–7.6)	.56
All others	109	3.2 (3.1, 0.8–6.1)	.49
Cardiothoracic	48	2.7 (1.8, 0–4.9)	.83[c]
High-risk nursery[d]			
≤1,000 g	104	9.1 (8.5, 1.6–16.1)	.43
1001–1500 g	98	5.4 (4.0, 0–12.2)	.15
1501–2500 g	97	4.1 (3.2, 0–8.9)	.07
>2,500 g	94	3.5 (1.9, 0–7.4)	.11

(Adapted from [2])
[a](number of CLA − BSIs/number of central line-days) × 1,000
[b]Device utilization (DU) ratio = number of device days/number of patient-days
[c]Pooled mean rather than median used
[d]For the high-risk nursery, central line-days include umbilical line-days

surveillance particularly challenging. In contrast, VLBW infants could remain in the NICU for several weeks to months with continued exposure to many devices and invasive procedures, antibiotic-resistant hospital flora, and antimicrobial agents that further influence the composition of the microflora. Thus, meaningful analysis of healthcare-associated infection (HAI) rates in the newborn nursery must use consistent definitions and risk stratification to account for the heterogeneity of its population. The HRN is the focus of HAI surveillance and prevention because of the associated increase in morbidity and mortality.

DEFINITIONS

Time of Onset

Although the term *nosocomial* infection has been replaced by *healthcare-associated infection* in most populations studied by healthcare epidemiologists, *nosocomial* is an appropriate term for most NICU infections because neonates are generally not readmitted to nurseries after discharge. Occasionally, infants are transferred to other institutions for specialized surgical procedures and then return to the referring nursery for prolonged care, and HAI would be a more appropriate term for surgical site infections (SSIs) in such instances.

Various investigators define early onset disease as positive cultures of a normally sterile body fluid obtained within the first 3, 7, or 10 days of life. For the study of HAIs, the most appropriate time interval is 3 days. Infections that appear at <48 hours of age are considered to be maternally acquired. Approximately 15% of BSIs and pneumonias in the HRN are maternally acquired [4]. Outbreaks of early onset infections rarely are reported and have remained either unexplained [12] or have been associated with fetal scalp electrode placement during labor [13], contaminated resuscitation equipment in the delivery room [14,15], and contaminated materials used within the first few hours of life (e.g., hydrocolloid dressings manufactured in large sheets precut by healthcare workers [HCWs] and used to secure umbilical catheters or endotracheal tubes contaminated with *A. baumanni*) [16].

For the purposes of HAI tracking, positive cultures obtained >3 days of life are considered late onset disease. Because clinical manifestations of infection are often delayed and determining whether an infection was acquired from the mother or from transmission within the nursery is difficult, NNIS reports all infections except those that are transmitted transplacentally as HAIs [4]. Differentiation of early and late onset disease is most useful when designing prophylaxis regimens. It is recommended that bacterial infections other than urinary tract infection (UTI) occurring within the first month after discharge from the nursery be reported to the infant's nursery to facilitate prompt identification of an outbreak (e.g., skin infections associated with *Staphylococcus aureus* and streptococcus group A or B, omphalitis, and bacterial diarrhea, especially *Salmonella* species) [14,17–19].

Device-Related Infections

Standardized definitions developed and updated by CDC, are used to track rates of NICU infections associated with CVCs, including umbilical catheters and ventilator-associated pneumonia (VAP) [20]. Although the CDC definition of CLA-BSI includes culture negative, clinical sepsis in young infants, such infections are infrequently reported in NNIS, and it is likely that only laboratory-confirmed episodes will be reported to the National Healthcare Safety Network (NHSN), formerly NNIS. (www.cdc.gov/ncidod/hip/NNIS/members/pneumonia/Final/PneumoCriteriaV1.pdf)

Calculation of Device-Related Infection Rates in the High-Risk Nursery

Studies [3,21,22] have demonstrated the advantages of calculating device-associated HAI rates to control for duration of exposure to the primary risk factors. Device utilization (DU) ratios are useful for interhospital comparisons as long as each hospital has collected the data and the calculated ratios use the same definitions and methods. The DU ratio is the measure of an ICU's invasive practices that constitutes an extrinsic risk factor for HAI. The DU ratio also can serve as a marker for severity of illness or the patients' intrinsic susceptibility to infection. If the DU ratio is > the 90th percentile, a specific hospital is considered a high outlier and further investigation of that specific practice could be warranted. Device-associated infection rates and DU ratios are calculated as follows:

Central line-associated primary bloodstream infection (CLA-BSI) rate:

$$\frac{\text{Number of CLA-BSIs}}{\text{Number of central line days}} \times 1,000$$

Ventilator-associated pneumonia (VAP) rate:

$$\frac{\text{Number of VAPs}}{\text{Number of ventilator days}} \times 1,000$$

Device utilization (DU) ratio:

$$\frac{\text{Number of device days}}{\text{Number of patient days}}$$

Severity of Illness Scoring Systems

Measures of illness severity other than birth weight have been applied to the study of neonatal HAI risk since 1993 when several scoring systems were first described [23–27]. The Score for Neonatal Acute Physiology (SNAP) uses the worst recorded values of >24 routinely measured physiologic variables during the first 24 hours of stay. The SNAP-Perinatal Extension (SNAP-PE) adds scoring for birth weight, small for gestational age status, and low Apgar score (<7 at 5 minutes). Using multiple regression analysis, a study of coagulase-negative staphylococcal (CONS) BSIs demonstrated a 53.9% increase in a patient's risk of experiencing at least one nosocomial BSI episode associated with each 5-point increment in the admission day SNAP [24]. Further analysis of the association between admission-day therapies and BSI attack rates among these patients using the Neonatal Therapeutic Intervention Scoring System (NTISS) that bases severity of illness on 62 specific therapeutic interventions demonstrated a significant positive association of phototherapy and blood pressure support with colloid or vasopressor administration. One study that used SNAP and NTISS reported abnormal heart rate characteristics and worsening SNAP scores 24 hours before the clinical suspicion of sepsis [25]. A study of eradication of endemic methicillin-resistant *S. aureus* (MRSA) infections from the Parkland Health and Hospital System neonatal intensive care unit (NICU) [26] used the number of patient-care hours determined for each infant by the nursing staff according to a workload quantification method called the (GRASP) system [27] to calculate a time-and-intensity-of-care–adjusted HAI incidence density (see Chapters 6 and 8). Use of the sum of all infants' daily patient-care hours as the denominator effectively controlled for the difference in risk factors between the intensive care and intermediate care areas. Further validation is required before these scoring systems can be applied routinely.

A European scoring system, Clinical Risk Index for Babies (CRIB) also has been used but conflicting results concerning its accuracy in predicting outcome have been reported [28]. A model dependent on variables collected before admission to the NICU proposed by the National Institute of Child Health and Human Development (NICHD) neonatal research network has published performance worse than the CRIB and SNAP models. At this time, whether any of these scoring systems offer an advantage over birth weight, Apgar scores, and length of stay for risk stratification and predicting outcome is uncertain [5,23].

Distinguishing True Pathogens From Blood Culture Contaminants

Sepsis caused by pathogens that are common skin contaminants (e.g., CONS) can be associated with low colony counts [29–31] and relatively few symptoms. Analysis of sites from which isolates are recovered (e.g., peripheral, specific ports of CVCs and time to positivity) assists the clinician in distinguishing blood culture contaminants from true pathogens. Time to positivity is an indicator of the quantity of bacteria and is an easily implemented replacement for quantitative blood cultures. When there is a >2 hour difference in time to positivity for various sites, the site that turned positive first is more likely to be the source of the bacteremia or fungemia [32–34]. The following suggestions can optimize the clinician's accuracy in distinguishing true sepsis from contamination (see Chapter 9):

1. Obtain at least 0.5 to 2 milliliters (ml) of blood for culture from two separate sites (preferably one peripheral site in patients with an intravascular catheter) [29–34].
2. Isolates detected within 24–36 hours of submission are more likely to be true pathogens. If blood cultures from an asymptomatic neonate who is being evaluated at birth due to the presence of maternal risk factors remain negative at 36 hours, bacterial sepsis can be ruled out [34].
3. A clinical course or serial laboratory studies compatible with sepsis are documented (e.g., absolute total neutrophil [ATN], absolute total immature cell [ATI] counts and ratio of absolute total immature neutrophils to total neutrophils (I:T) $\geq$0.2 [35], and elevated C-reactive protein [36]). The likelihood of sepsis is <1% in the presence of 3 serial CBC and differential counts that remain normal over 36 hours.
4. The patient responds to antibiotics that are active against the isolate, usually vancomycin for CONS and MRSA. Clinical improvement and/or failure to recover the same pathogen from repeat blood cultures when an infant is being treated with an antimicrobial agent that is *not* active against the pathogen casts doubt on the validity of that isolate as a true pathogen.

RISK FACTORS FOR HAI

The intrinsic and extrinsic factors for HAI have been reviewed [37] and are summarized in Table 25-2.

Intrinsic Risk Factors

Birth weight and gestational age are the most important risk factors for the HAI development. The decreased function of the immune system in the most premature infants accounts for most of the increased intrinsic risk of infection [1]. There is minimal active transport of maternal IgG antibodies across the placenta until 32 weeks' gestation, neutrophils have defective chemotaxis or phagocytosis, and the classic and alternative complement pathways have decreased activity. Attempts to improve the neonate's immune function have included exchange transfusion [38], white blood cell transfusion [39], administration of intravenous immune globulin (IVIG) therapeutically [40] or prophylactically [41,42], and administration of recombinant human granulocyte colony-stimulating factor (G-CSF) [43]. Although these studies have been instructive, they have not demonstrated efficacy in adequately controlled trials, and no recommendations for routine use of these products have been made. In addition to providing enhanced opsonophagocytic activity, IVIG infusions are associated with a prompt release of neutrophils from the marrow

TABLE 25-2
RISK FACTORS FOR ACQUISITION OF NURSERY INFECTIONS

Intrinsic (host)
   Decreased function of the immune system
   Decreased protection from natural barriers (e.g., skin)
   Developing endogenous microflora
   Gestational age
   Severity of illness
   Underlying disease processes (e.g,. congenital organ system abnormalities, chronic lung disease, gastrointestinal tract pathology)
Extrinsic
   Use of devices
   Fetal scalp electrodes
   Umbilical, arterial, central venous catheters
   Mechanical ventilators
   Extracorporeal membrane oxygenation
   Ventriculoperitoneal shunts
   Fluids
   Total parenteral nutrition, intralipid
   Transfused blood products
   Respiratory care
   Breast milk
   Treatments
   Intravenous steroid therapy
   Use of H_2 blockers/proton pump inhibitors
Environment
   Acquisition of hospital flora
   Overcrowding, understaffing
   Contaminated equipment, fluids
   Traffic from other sections of hospital
   Radiology
   Laboratory
   Subspecialty consultants

neutrophil storage pool into the peripheral circulation and enhanced chemotaxis of neutrophils to the site of bacterial infection [40]. Antibody replacement could be more effective by using products containing high titers of antibody against the specific infecting agent, but such products are not yet available for routine use [44]. However, a significant protective effect has not been demonstrated in trials of two different preparations of intravenous *S. aureus* immune globulin [45,46].

Neonates are particularly vulnerable to colonization with virulent and/or antibiotic-resistant bacteria because their mucosal surfaces do not have the usual protective microflora of older infants and adults [47]. Immature, fragile skin of the VLBW neonate possibly does not serve as an adequate protective barrier against pathogens that colonize the skin and have the capacity to cause invasive disease [48].

Extrinsic Risk Factors

Many of the extrinsic HAI risk factors in the nursery are device- or environmentally related, as is observed in adult

ICUs. Extrinsic risk factors can be categorized as (1) medical devices and equipment, (2) medical treatments, (3) behavioral interventions, and (4) administrative and structural.

Medical Devices and Equipment

CVCs including peripherally inserted central catheters (PICC) are associated with increased risk of BSI caused by bacteria or fungi [4,5,49–52]. In fact, an increased risk of candidemia has been associated with each day of catheter use [52]. Various medical devices used for respiratory support (e.g., ventilators and noninvasive ventilatory devices including CPAP, ECMO, and Vapotherm 2000i™ [Vapotherm Inc, Stevensville, MD] oxygen delivery device) are associated with increased risk of infection [53,54]. The need by the neonate's with respiratory distress for increased humidification provides direct exposure of the respiratory mucosa to water that could be contaminated; therefore, the use of sterile water in such situations is recommended [55]. For example, contamination of the Vapotherm™ device with *Ralstonia* sp. during the manufacturing process that could not be eradicated with various disinfection procedures led to clinical infections and the withdrawal of this product from the market [56].

The use of umbilical catheters and the feeding of breast milk are unique to the nursery, and specific guidelines are required to care for the umbilicus and store breast milk for those infants who are too sick to suckle directly from the mother's breast. For example, breast milk from a mother who was infected with Group B Streptococcus (GBS) or *S. aureus* (MSSA or [MRSA]) has been implicated as the vehicle of transmission of these pathogens to infants and resulting severe sepsis [57–59]. Neonatal sepsis caused by *Klebsiella pneumoniae* has been associated with contaminated breast milk resulting from contamination of a component of a breast pump [60], and contamination of a milk bank pasteurizer was associated with an NICU outbreak of *Pseudomonas aeruginosa* infections [61]. Furthermore, viral agents that could be transmitted to infants in breast milk or in the blood contact associated with breast feeding from dry, cracked nipples include hepatitis B virus (HBV), human immunodeficiency virus (HIV), and human T-lymphotrophic virus type 1 (HTLV-1). Therefore, in countries where safe formula for bottle feeding is readily available, breast feeding is contraindicated for mothers known to be infected with HIV and HTLV-1. HBV vaccine given to neonates is protective against transmission by breast feeding. Although cytomegalovirus (CMV) is transmitted in breast milk, maternal antibody is protective against clinically significant disease. The CDC's strict guidelines developed for banking human milk obtained from unrelated donors include screening all donors for HIV, HTLV-1, and HBV surface antigen and pasteurization (62.5°C for 30 minutes) of all milk specimens. Bacterial counts of 10^4 colony-forming units (cfu)/ml or more of nonpathogenic organisms and

the presence of gram-negative bacteria (GNB), *S. aureus*, or α- or β-hemolytic streptococci preclude the use of milk the specimens come from [62]. Established guidelines for human breast milk banks (**www.hmbana.org**), personal hygiene, and handling and decontaminating the components of breast milk pumps [62] should be followed.

Medical Treatments

The use of steroids for treatment of chronic bronchopulmonary dysplasia has been associated with an increased risk of infection [63–65]. The finding of an increase in the incidence of disseminated *Candida* spp. infections associated with the unique practice of single-dose steroid administration in infants with prolonged hypotension shortly after birth further supports the role of steroids as an independent risk factor [64]. The risk–benefit ratio must be carefully considered before initiating a course of steroids in HRN infants. The use of H2 blocker/proton pump inhibitor therapy has been associated with an increased incidence of necrotizing enterocolitis [66], with sepsis associated with GNB in VLBW infants [50], and with candidemia [67]. An increased risk of invasive disease caused by extended-spectrum beta-lactamase (ESBL)-producing *Klebsiella* spp. [51] or *Candida* spp. [68] has been associated with the use of third-generation cephalosporins. Finally, topical petrolatum applied to the skin for improved moisturizing effect was associated with an increased risk of fungal infections [47].

Behavioral Interventions

There are theoretical concerns that infection risk can increase in association with the innovative practices of cobedding [69] and kangaroo care [70] used in the NICU to improve developmental outcomes as a result of increased opportunity for skin-to-skin exposure of multiple gestation infants to each other and to their mothers, respectively. However, the infection risk is actually reduced with kangaroo care. Although toys in NICU beds have been found to be contaminated with pathogenic bacteria [71], their role in transmission of infection has not been established.

Administrative and Structural Issues

Studies of outbreaks in the newborn nursery and NICUs were some of the first to demonstrate the relationship between rates of late onset infection and overcrowding and understaffing [26,72–76]. One study that evaluated staffing levels of registered nurses specifically found a significant reduction in the BSI risk when registered nurse staffing hours were increased in one NICU [76]. A movement toward constructing new NICUs with all single-patient rooms is emerging; its purpose is to improve the neurodevelopmental effects of lighting and sound, facilitating family-centered care, breast feeding, kangaroo care, and isolation precautions when needed, and thus reduce HAI rates [77,78]. Although data are not yet sufficient to support an evidence-based recommendation for single-patient rooms in NICUs, the most recent publication of recommended standards for NICU design and of experience suggests that this design will become more prevalent in the future. Finally, exposure to construction dust or to spores during transport could result in cutaneous or invasive aspergillosis in the neonate [79]; thus, dust containment and air filtration during construction, renovation, and any disruption of the integrity of the environment [80] are especially important for the NICU because the VLBW infant is at increased risk of developing disease after exposure.

Sites of Infection

The sites of HAIs in the HRN differ from those in adults [5]. Primary BSIs account for 30–50% of episodes in neonates, depending on birth weight, and SSIs and UTIs are rare. In contrast, >40% of HAIs in adults are UTIs, and 20% are SSIs (see UTI and SSI and ICU Chapters 24A, 24B, 30 and 35). Cutaneous sites are more likely to be involved in neonates. Clinical manifestations of MSSA and MRSA in otherwise healthy term neonates [81] or in those in the NICU [82] in the current era have been reviewed. Pustules, bullous impetigo, subcutaneous abscesses, scalded skin syndrome, and toxic shock syndrome associated with either MSSA or MRSA can be seen in outbreaks in term nurseries (often presenting after discharge) and NICUs. Omphalitis is rare (0.7%) in developed countries where deliveries are performed aseptically and cord care to prevent infection is performed routinely. However, occurence of omphalitis can involve serious complications including sepsis, superficial or deep abscesses, necrotizing fasciitis, peritonitis, and hepatic vein thrombosis [83]. Congenital mucocutaneous candidiasis in term infants generally is not associated with invasive disease whereas fungal dermatitis caused by *Candida albicans* is considered a manifestation of systemic disease when it occurs during the second week of life in extremely low birth weight (ELBW) infants after vaginal delivery, postnatal administration of steroids, or hyperglycemia [84]. Pulmonary infections result from exposure to respiratory viruses circulating in the community, and complications of respiratory support, gastroenteritis, and colitis can also occur following exposure to viruses and/or bacteria circulating in the community. Osteomyelitis/septic arthritis and conjunctivitis are other less common manifestations. Meningitis and brain abscess can also occur in neonates.

Necrotizing enterocolitis (NEC) is one of the most common gastrointestinal emergencies among neonates. In fact, >90% of episodes occur in infants who are born preterm, and the NEC risk is inversely related to birth weight and gestational age. Overall, there is about a 7% occurrence among VLBW infants with substantial variation over time and from center to center [85]. Factors that contribute to the development of NEC include developmental immaturity of the gastrointestinal tract function including circulatory regulation, hypoxic/ischemic injury, abnormal bacterial colonization, and early feeding of formula milk. The role of specific inflammatory cytokines in the pathogenesis of NEC is under investigation. Sporadic episodes and clusters can occur. Several different bacteria (e.g., *E. coli*, *Klebsiella pneumoniae*, *Enterobacter cloacae*, *Clostridium* sp.) and viruses (e.g., rotavirus, coronavirus, enterovirus) have been associated with NEC in some reports of clusters [86]. Outbreaks can be controlled by implementing infection control measures, including hand hygiene, contact precautions, cohorting of infants and staff, and restriction of HCWs with signs of gastrointestinal tract illness from duty until resolved [86].

Clinical manifestations include feeding intolerance; delayed gastric emptying; localized signs of abdominal distension, tenderness, cellulitis, peritonitis, occult, and grossly bloody stools; radiographic evidence of pneumatosis intestinalis or portal vein gas; and nonspecific systemic signs of sepsis with metabolic acidosis, thrombocytopenia, or disseminated intravascular coagulation (DIC). Mortality rates vary from 15–30%. When intestinal necrosis occurs, resecting is necessary, leaving the infant with short gut syndrome and totally parenteral nutrition dependent.

ETIOLOGY, CLINICAL MANIFESTATIONS, AND EPIDEMIOLOGY

Bacterial Outbreaks

Trends

Infections acquired in normal newborn nurseries are most frequently not invasive, usually involve the skin or mucous membranes, and result from HCW hand carriage, contaminated equipment, and medications. Impetigo (skin pustules), conjunctivitis [87], omphalitis, and soft tissue abscess are the most frequently observed clinical manifestations. *S. aureus* remains the most frequently isolated pathogen from such infants with MRSA causing infection more often than MSSA in communities with high prevalence of community-associated MRSA (CO-MRSA) infections [81]. Outbreaks of group A streptococcal [18,88] and of diarrhea caused by bacterial pathogens (e.g., *Salmonella* spp. or *Shigella* spp.) could occur in both term and preterm nurseries [17,89,90] but have been reported less frequently in recent years (see Chapters 34 and 41). CONS rarely cause early onset disease in otherwise healthy term neonates without any devices in place.

HCWs are rarely the *source* of outbreaks HAIs caused by bacteria and fungi, especially MRSA, but when they are, factors are usually present to increase the transmission of infectious agents to others (e.g., sinusitis, draining otitis externa, chronic otitis; respiratory tract infections, dermatitis, onychomycosis, and artificial nails) [91–97]. An HCW colonized with an epidemic strain of *S. aureus* rarely has been identified; when it has, the outbreak has been controlled by removing that individual from direct patient care [98]. Individual wearing artificial nail who have direct patient contact have been implicated in outbreaks of *Pseudomonas aeruginosa* [95,96] and ESBL-producing *Klebsiella pneumoniae* [97] in NICUs where molecular typing demonstrated that HCW and patient isolates were indistinguishable. These studies contributed substantially to the recommendation not to wear artificial nails or extenders when having direct contact with high-risk patients.

Unexplained shifts in the predominant etiology of bacterial infections in high-risk infants have been observed over time [99,100]. Invasive strains of *S. aureus* were predominant in the 1950s. For unexplained reasons, GNB, especially *Pseudomonas aeruginosa*, *Klebsiella* species, and *Escherichia coli* strains prevailed in the 1960s but were replaced by GBS in the 1970s. GBS remained the major pathogens of early onset disease throughout the 1980s and 1990s but manifested as late onset disease, most frequently meningitis, less commonly as osteomyelitis/septic arthritis, and rarely event [101] or horizontal transmission within the NICU. However, in the 1980s, MRSA and CONS emerged as prevailing HAI pathogens in the HRN. Although CONS continue to account for 40–50% of late onset infections in most NICUs in the 1990s, one NICU reported a shift to predominant GNB, especially ceftazidime-resistant *Enterobacter* sp., as the pathogen from 1996–2001 [102], and another reported an increase the number of commensals [100], similar to the experience of the National Institute of Child Health and Human Development Neonatal Research Network [6]. The following three pathogens associated with <15–20% of HRN infections are particularly problematic because of the difficulty in treatment: (1) enterococci, especially vancomycin-resistant enterococcus (VRE), (2) multidrug-resistant GNB, especially *Enterobacter* spp. and ESBL-producing *Klebsiella* spp, and (3) fungi, predominantly *Candida* spp., especially nonalbicans species.

Group B Streptococcus

From the late 1970s through the mid-1990s, GBS was the most frequently isolated pathogen from term infants with early onset disease, accounting for ~70% of episodes [6]. This pathogen was acquired from the mother in the peripartum period; in ~70% of infants <2,000 g at birth, GBS infections were acquired in utero with positive blood cultures obtained at birth. However, following the development and implementation of the evidence-based recommendations published collaboratively by CDC, American College of Obstetrics and Gynecology (ACOG), and the American Academy of Pediatrics (AAP) for the administration of chemoprophylaxis at the onset of labor to colonized women, those delivering prematurely, and those who have other risk factors that were published in 1996, there was a

65% reduction in the incidence of early onset GBS disease from 1993 to 1998 and a plateau in 1999–2001 [103]. The guidelines were updated to include a recommendation to screen all women at 35–37 weeks gestation based on a population-based study that demonstrated a greater reduction in disease associated with a screening-based strategy compared with a risk-based strategy [104]. This resulted in a further reduction in 2003–2004 to a rate of 0.34 per 1,000 live births reported by the CDC's active bacterial core (ABCS) surveillance network and a narrowing of the racial disparity in the rates of disease [105]. These data represent an 80% reduction from a rate in 1,000 live births of 1.7 in 1993 to 0.34 in 2004. A persistent reduction in early onset GBS disease has been reported also in the VLBW infants in the National Institute of Child Health and Human Development Neonatal Research Network [106] and by other groups who have been tracking rates of disease. Following publication of the GBS chemoprophylaxis guidelines, increased the rates of ampicillin resistant *E. coli* as a cause of early onset sepsis in VLBW infants have, but no association between intrapartum antibiotic exposure and overall or ampicillin-resistant *E. coli* sepsis has been found [106,107]. Continued population-based surveillance is needed.

Coagulase Negative Staphylococci

CONS account for nearly 50% of late onset HAIs in most recent reports [4–6,41,42,108]. Several reasons for the increased recognition of this organism as a neonatal pathogen follow:

1. Increased number and survival of the VLBW (<1,500 g at birth) infants.
2. Increased use of intravascular devices in the high risk neonate.
3. Increased likelihood of identifying a blood culture positive for CONS as a true bacteremia with the use of more consistent definitions and methods of obtaining blood cultures (e.g., two blood cultures, preferably one from a CVC and one from a peripheral site).

The epidemiology of neonatal CONS BSI has been studied extensively using pulsed-field gel electrophoresis (PFGE), ribotyping, DNA-DNA hybridization, and restriction endonuclease analysis in addition to the traditional methods of speciation, phage typing, and plasmid analysis. PFGE is the most reliable method for confirming identity of strains. Distinct clones of both *Staphylococcus haemolyticus* [109,110] and *Staphylococcus epidermidis* [111–113] can become endemic in HRNs and cause clusters of infections over periods of 6 months to as long as 10 years. At the same time, many completely unrelated strains can be isolated from infants within the same unit. Some HRNs possibly have no related strains identified during a specific period of time [114,115]. Eastick et al. [116] have reported relatively stable reservoirs of CONS in the feces, around the ear, and in the axillae and nares but small, unstable numbers on the skin of the forearm and leg. Thus, cross-contamination among sites on the same infant as well as horizontal spread among infants is an important mode of transmission. Infusion of parenteral fluids contaminated with CONS is a rare source of BSI in the HRN [117] (see Chapter 44).

The clinical manifestations of CONS-BSI are most often nonspecific, and this pathogen is rarely considered a cause of death [118]. The nonspecific signs of sepsis observed most frequently are fever, apnea and bradycardia, feeding intolerance, and lethargy. Temperature instability, thrombocytopenia, abdominal distention, and persistent BSI in the absence of a CVC have been associated with disease caused by CONS [119,120]. Specific delta toxin-producing strains have been found in pure culture in the stool or in the blood or peritoneal fluid of patients with a mild form of necrotizing enterocolitis [121, 122]. Focal infections associated with these pathogens include neck abscess, omphalitis, wound abscess, and mastitis [123]. Right-sided endocarditis caused by CONS must be considered in the presence of a CVC, persistent BSI (>48 hours), and thrombocytopenia during appropriate antimicrobial therapy for BSI [124]. Physical examination, could find no other abnormalities but an echocardiogram could demonstrate vegetations in the right atrium or on the tricuspid valve. Removal of the CVC is required for clearance of CONS if BSI persists >4 days [125].

Staphylococcus Aureus

After CONS, S. aureus was the second most frequently isolated pathogen from HRN infants in the 1986–1993 NNIS report [4] and in studies from the Neonatal Research Network [6]. In contrast, the point prevalence study of 29 NICUs performed in 1999 reported that enterococci were second after CONS, accounting for 15.5% of BSIs, and S. aureus accounted for only 3.4% of BSIs [5]. Since the late 1980s, S. aureus outbreaks in the HRN have been associated with both MSSA [73,98,126–129] and MRSA [26,130–134], and reports of outbreaks of MRSA have surpassed those of MSSA in recent years. Nurseries situated in large general hospitals that share services (laboratory, radiology) and HCWs (nurses, respiratory therapists, consulting physicians) are especially vulnerable to the acquisition of virulent strains from geographically distant foci of healthcare-associated MSSA or MRSA infection. A single or multiple virulent strains can be introduced into the nursery by a colonized infant, a visiting family member, and—rarely—an HCW [135–137]. However, the principal mode of transmission is horizontal via hands of HCWs who fail to follow recommendations for hand hygiene between patient contacts. PFGE is the most useful method to determine whether a single or multiple strains caused an outbreak [138]. High rates of colonization (30–70%) can become established before clinical disease is recognized. Environmental sources or chronic carriers have

rarely been implicated in nosocomial transmission in the NICU, but environmental contamination with S. aureus does occur and contributes to the overall burden of pathogens in high-risk units. *Unidentified* virulence factors and environmental conditions determine the persistence of the organism in the HRN. In Parkland Health and Hospital System's crowded HRN, MRSA persisted for a 3-year period from 1988 to 1991 [26]. Neither susceptible S. aureus and MRSA nursery outbreaks were controlled until conditions of overcrowding and understaffing were corrected [26,73]. Although MRSA is an important pathogen in NICUs, it is notable that in 2002, only 25% of S. aureus isolates from NICU patients in the NNIS system were resistant to methicillin compared with nearly 60% of S. aureus isolates from the NNIS ICU isolates overall [Fridkin, S, personal communication]. The prevalence of CO-MRSA strains that have antibiotic susceptibility and molecular profiles (staphylococcal chromosomal cassette [SCC] mec types IV or V) distinct from those of the traditional healthcare-associated MRSA strains [138] have increased in prevalence and transmission of those CO-MRSA strains have been reported within healthcare facilities [139–141]. Because CO-MRSA infections have been described in obstetrical patients [142] and 13/14 MRSA strains isolated from vaginal-rectal prenatal GBS screening cultures were CO-MRSA by SCCmec-typing [143], a likely source for neonatal infections is the colonized or infected mother. Trends in CO-MRSA strains as the etiology of HAIs are evolving.

Skin pustules, bullous impetigo, scalded skin syndrome [126–128], soft tissue abscesses, mastitis, conjunctivitis, pneumonia with or without empyema, osteomyelitis, septic arthritis, and SSIs are the most frequent manifestations of both MSSA and MRSA infections in neonates, and the case-fatality rate associated with invasive disease can be 15–30% [81,82]. BSIs with multiple foci of disease are characteristic of invasive S. aureus disease. Optimal diagnostic evaluation and treatment of neonates with only minor manifestations (e.g., pustules) of CO-MRSA are under investigation at the time of this publication.

Enterococcus

Enterococci have been recognized as important pathogens in the NICU since 1979 [144,145]. The incidence [4,5,100, 146] and number of reports of nursery outbreaks associated with susceptible *Streptococcus faecium* [147], *Streptococcus faecalis* [148], and, more recently, VRE [146,149–151] have increased substantially since the 1980s, but enterococci still account only for a relatively small proportion of neonatal infections. In regions of the United States where VRE have become problematic HAI pathogens, spread to the NICU has occurred [146]. Repetitive sequence polymerase chain reaction (rep-PCR) DNA fingerprinting is useful to distinguish outbreak strains from endemic strains and "background" nursery flora and to identify distinct clusters [150]. Invasion occurs most often from the infant's endogenous flora. In enterococcal outbreaks, however, environmental contamination, exposure to broadspectrum antimicrobials, horizontal transmission by HCW hands and, for VRE, repeated introduction by infants transferred to a regional NICU from a birth hospital with endemic VRE are important factors in the perpetuation of outbreaks.

Enterococci are associated only rarely with early onset sepsis. Most often, enterococci are isolated from the blood of low and VLBW infants with serious underlying conditions who have been in the NICU for >30–60 days. Prolonged use of CVCs, necrotizing enterocolitis, and bowel resection in addition to exposure to antibiotics are associated findings. Polymicrobial BSI is especially likely to occur in association with intra-abdominal disease, supporting the intestine as a point of invasion of enterococci. Clinical manifestations of enterococcal infections are nonspecific. The unusual episodes of meningitis [147] and endocarditis require prolonged (≥3 weeks and ≥6 weeks, respectively) treatment with combination therapy using a cell wall active agent combined with an aminoglycoside for cure. Successful treatment of endocarditis in a neonate with linezolid has been reported [152], but no experience with daptomycin in neonates has been published at this time. Linezolid should be restricted only when no other drugs are available to reduce the risk of emergence of resistance.

Gram-Negative Bacilli (GNB)

Infections caused by GNB are associated with the highest case-fatality rates: 40% (range, 24–62%) but approaching 90–100% in earlier studies. GNB infections in neonates have increased in many NICUs [6,100,102,106,153]. *E. coli* and *Klebsiella* or *Enterobacter* spp. are the most frequently isolated GNB in the absence of an outbreak [4–6,99,100,102,106]. ESBL-producing isolates of these species that have been reported by NICUs in recent years are especially problematic because of their resistance to the antimicrobial agents used routinely for empiric gram-negative coverage [51,94,97,154]. Of note, multispecies outbreaks of ESBLs can represent transfer of the same plasmid among species with person-to-person transmission [153]. Other GNB responsible for temporally related clusters in the NICU include *P. aeruginosa* [61,92,95,96], *Serratia* spp. [155–158], *Citrobacter diversus* [159–161], *Salmonella* spp. [17,162], *Acinetobacter* spp. [16], *Chryseobacterium* (*Flavobacterium*) *meningosepticum* [163], *Ralstonia pickettii* [56,164], and *Burkholderia cepacia* [164].

Molecular typing techniques (e.g., PFGE, ribotyping, polymerase chain reaction (PCR)-based methods) are valuable tools for defining the epidemiology of GNB infections in the NICU during both epidemic and nonepidemic periods [165,166] and should be used during outbreaks to determine whether horizontal transmission or selective antibiotic pressure is the predominant mechanism of spread

and to guide the development of effective interventions (see Chapter 16). Although nursery outbreaks of GNB infections have been associated with environmental contamination (e.g., antiseptic solutions [157], intravenous medications and solutions [157,158,164,167], human breast milk [58–60], sinks [158,163], respiratory therapy and resuscitation equipment [17,56], and bandages [16]), such contamination is implicated less frequently in well-developed countries with clean water supplies and well-defined protocols for sterilization of equipment and single use of disposable items (see Chapter 20). Some outbreaks of *Serratia marcescens* have been controlled by enforcing recommended general infection control measures, even when a source for the *Serratia* spp. cannot be determined or when isolates are unrelated by molecular typing [156]. In the absence of an environmental source, it is likely that a virulent epidemic strain is acquired from the infected mother or—rarely—from an colonized or infected HCW or emerges from the infant's endogenous flora and then is transmitted horizontally to HCW hands. Identical strains of *C. diversus* have been identified in maternal infant pairs [160] and in HCWs and infected neonates [161]. Prolonged rectal colonization in addition to hand colonization has been implicated in outbreaks of *C. diversus* meningitis that were not controlled until colonized HCWs were removed from the nursery [160,161]. In the absence of outbreaks, clones of resistant GNB have been shown to be acquired but cleared rapidly from the infants' flora after initial colonization. However, horizontal transmission of these organisms occurs and occasionally results in clinical disease [165]. Clones of multidrug-resistant *Enterobacter* spp. transmitted in the NICU also were found in geographically distinct areas of a children's hospital [166].

Clinical manifestations characteristic of GNB infections include necrotizing ophthalmitis, pneumonia, ecthyma gangrenosum, cardiovascular collapse, and meningitis. Although ecthymatous lesions are associated most frequently with *P. aeruginosa* invasive disease, they can be associated with other GNB pathogens or fungi. Biopsy and culture of such lesions are helpful in isolating the specific pathogen. *Salmonella* spp. have a proclivity for causing osteomyelitis and septic arthritis, and a meningitis that is especially difficult to cure even with prolonged courses of antibiotics that are highly active *in vitro* against the infecting strain. *C. diversus* meningitis is notable for occurring in clusters in NICUs and has an association with brain abscess in 77% of patients compared to 7% of patients with meningitis caused by other GNB [160]. *Flavobacterium meningosepticum*, an unusual GNB resistant to most antimicrobial agents used for empiric treatment of gram-negative meningitis in the newborn and is treated successfully by the combination of vancomycin and rifampin [168], is a less frequent cause of epidemic GNB meningitis [163].

The importance of antibiotic use in selecting multidrug-resistant strains of GNB in the NICU for aminoglycosides has been well documented [169,170] and for third-generation cephalosporins [51,171,172]. Monitoring for the development of resistance to the first-line aminoglycoside, usually gentamicin or tobramycin, is helpful to guide changes in antibiotic prescribing patterns. In the absence of multidrug-resistant strains, amikacin, third-generation cephalosporins, and meropenem are best reserved for rare individuals whose infection resistant routine treatment regimens. The combination of an aminoglycoside and third-generation cephalosporin is recommended to treat GNB meningitis even with organisms that are fully susceptible to aminoglycosides [62].

Bordetella Pertussis

Transmission of *B. pertussis* has been reported in normal newborn and intermediate care nurseries [173]. The source is usually an undiagnosed HCW [174] or visitor [175]; therefore, screening and administering the adult Tdap vaccine according to published recommendations [173] are especially important for family members likely to visit infants in the nurseries and for HCWs caring for such infants. Administration of adult Tdap vaccine to family members of infants in the NICU has been suggested as a method to improve vaccine uptake as demonstrated for influenza vaccine [176]. Healthcare facilities should provide the adult Tdap vaccine for HCWs.

Clostridium Difficile

Outbreaks of *Clostridium difficile*-associated colitis do not occur in the newborn nursery. In contrast to healthy adults who have an asymptomatic colonization rate of <5%, toxin-producing strains of *C. difficile* could be recovered from the stools of as many as 55% of asymptomatic neonates [177]. Disease usually does not occur because the immature intestinal mucosa of the neonate lacks receptors for the *C. difficile* toxin. This organism does not play a role in the pathogenesis of necrotizing enterocolitis, but an association with severe enterocolitis in infants with Hirschsprung's disease has been reported [178].

Fungal Infection

Of the subspecialty services in NNIS hospitals conducting hospitalwide surveillance, the HRN had one of the highest nosocomial fungal infection rates for the period 1986–1990: 7.6 per 1,000 discharges, after burn/trauma (16.1), cardiac surgery (11.2), and oncology (8.6) [179]. During this 5-year period, the fungal infection rate in the HRN increased from 4.7 to 9.6 per 1,000. In one study of candidemia in a pediatric population from 1988 to 1992, 25% of patients were premature infants [180]. In the 1986–1994 NNIS surveillance period, *Candida* spp. accounted for 7% of all BSIs in the HRN: it was fourth after CONS, GBS, and *S. aureus* [4]. The most recent data from 128 NICUs participating in the NNIS system showed

a 24% reduction in the number of infections per 1,000 patient-days among neonates <1,000 g from 3.5 during 1995–1999 to 2.68 ($p < .01$) during 2000–2004 with a stable rate in the larger neonates [181]. The decreases occurred among both *C. albicans* and *C. parapsilosis* BSI. There was no increase in species (e.g., *C. glabrata* or *C. krusei*) that would be expected to demonstrate resistance to fluconazole. NICU-specific rates of hospital-acquired candidemia for infants <1,000 g varied substantially: The median attack rate was 7.5%, but 25% of NICUs reported rates >13.5%; this is similar to the variation from 2.4–20.4% reported from the smaller National Institute of Child Health and Human Development Neonatal Network. However, data to identify practices in the NICUs with lower rates were insufficient.

The most consistent risk factors for candidemia in NICU infants reported in case-control studies using multivariate analyses are CVC use; previous bacterial BSIs; gastrointestinal pathology; abdominal surgery; gestational age <26 weeks; colonization, especially in multiple sites; and prolonged courses of broad-spectrum antibiotics (e.g., primarily third-generation cephalosporins) [67,68,182–186]. The importance of other risk factors, including infusion of hyperalimentation fluids, especially those containing lipid emulsions, delayed feedings, endotracheal intubation, administration of histamine-2 (H2) blocking agents, and corticosteroids as independent risk factors identified in some studies is not well established. In most instances, candidemia develops as a consequence of endogenous colonization rather than as a result of cross-contamination. Baley et al. [187] reported a 26.7% fungal colonization rate in infants weighing <1,500 g at birth who were followed prospectively. Two-thirds of these infants were colonized within the first week of life, probably reflecting maternal transmission during labor and delivery. Systemic disease developed in 7.7% of colonized infants. Although the National Epidemiology of Mycosis Survey (NEMIS) study group did not identify colonization as an independent risk factor in the six participating NICUs in 1993–1995, gastrointestinal (GI) tract colonization preceded candidemia in 43% of case-patients [67]. Once colonized, invasion arises most often from the GI tract. Early colonization is more likely to be associated with *Candida albicans*, whereas other species, such as *C. parapsilosis* and *C. tropicalis*, are more likely to be associated with late colonization that can result from horizontal transmission among infants or from HCWs.

C. parapsilosis is the most frequently reported cause of epidemic *Candida* spp. infections [188–190]. With the use of DNA fingerprinting, it has been possible to determine that several nursery outbreaks of invasive *Candida* spp. infections, including *C. albicans* [191–193], *C. tropicalis* [194], and *C. lusitaniae* [195] have been associated with cross-transmission from HCW hands [188,192–194], retrograde intravenous medication administration [191], and contamination of a multidose bottle of liquid glycerin used as a suppository [189]. The presence of onychomycosis in HCWs has been suggested as a possible source of nosocomial candidiasis spread by hand carriage [194]. Thus, it is likely that wide variation in rates of *Candida* BSIs is a marker for management choices and infection control practices [195].

Clinical manifestations of disseminated candidiasis usually are nonspecific. Neonates with a maternal history of vaginal moniliasis rarely contract congenital mucocutaneous candidiasis [84]. At birth, such infants have an intensely erythematous maculopapular eruption of the trunk and extremities that rapidly becomes vesicular and pustular and then resolves with extensive desquamation. Palms and soles are almost always affected. These infants who are otherwise asymptomatic do not have systemic involvement and respond well to topical antifungal therapy. In contrast, the development of a diffuse, erythematous, scaling, burnlike dermatitis in an infant <1,500 g birth weight is more likely to be a manifestation of invasive disease and requires systemic therapy [196].

Candida spp. are less frequently recovered from blood cultures of infants with invasive candidiasis than from infants with invasive bacterial disease. Candidemia is present most often in association with a CVC. In such patients, the CVC should be removed as soon as possible to facilitate clearance of the bloodstream. Persistently positive cultures of blood for *Candida* sp. is a risk factor for focal complications, and the risk increases with the increasing duration of positivity [197]. A minimum of two weeks of antifungal therapy is recommended when the CVC has been removed in the absence of other sites of focal infection to prevent the development of other foci. True candiduria can reflect disseminated disease or localized cystitis; thus, isolation of *Candida* sp. from the urine indicates the need to evaluate other sites of infection. Echocardiogram can best detect *Candida* spp. endocarditis associated with a CVC in an infant with a structurally normal heart. Large vegetations can be present in the absence of a murmur and signs of congestive heart failure [198]. At autopsy, fungal vegetations have been found in infants with endocarditis unsuspected before death. Osteomyelitis, septic arthritis, meningitis, and brain abscess are other foci of infection that can be present with relatively few specific physical signs. The most severe episodes of meningitis and endocarditis require prolonged treatment courses of amphotericin B, up to 40 to 50 milligrams per kilogram (mg/kg) total dose or at least 6 weeks of a liposomal amphotericin preparation, usually in combination with a second antifungal agent. At the time of publication, experience with the newer azoles (e.g., voriconazole) and echinocandins (e.g., caspofungin, micafungin) in neonates is not sufficient to determine whether these agents offer for treating any advantage serous invasive candidiasis. Medical therapy of VLBW infants with *Candida* spp. endocarditis with a combination of two antifungal agents has been successful and is often preferred due to the high risk of surgical excision of vegetations in

such infants. A review of the literature found little difference in survival between those neonates treated with antifungal therapy only (65%) compared with those who were treated with antifungal therapy and surgery (60%), $p = 1.0$ [199].

Other fungi associated with HAI in the NICU include *Aspergillus* spp. [199,200], *Malassezia* spp. [202,203], *Rhizopus* spp. [204], and *Trichosporon beigelii* [205]. *Aspergillus*, *Rhizopus*, and *Trichosporon* spp. are acquired from the environment via exposure to either construction dust or contaminated medical supplies. Infants with aspergillosis are notably not neutropenic but are premature and do not have normal chemotaxis and phagocytosis. Cutaneous aspergillosis can occur as the initial manifestation of disease or as one site of involvement in disseminated disease. Because of the risk of dissemination from primary cutaneous lesions and the difficulty in distinguishing primary from secondary lesions, aggressive systemic antifungal therapy is always indicated. Successful systemic voriconazole therapy of severe primary cutaneous aspergillosis that was refractory to amphotericin B in VLBW premature infants has been reported [201].

Both *Malassezia furfur* [202] and *Malassezia pachydermatis* [203] have been associated with BSI clusters in high-risk premature infants who have received intralipids through CVCs. *Malassezia* spp. isolates are most frequently isolated from blood obtained through a CVC and are rarely recovered from peripheral blood. *M. furfur* skin colonization rates of 25–84% have been reported for infants during prolonged NICU admissions, whereas >5% of infants hospitalized in a non-NICU setting or attending a well-baby clinic were colonized with this organism [202]. *Malessezia* spp. infections can manifest as a self-limiting condition, neonatal cephalic pustulosis on the face, scalp, or neck, and as a more severe clinical sepsis in neonates with CVCs. When temporally related episodes occur, these organisms most likely are carried from patient to patient on HCW hands. However, in one outbreak of *Malassezia* pachydermatis, transmission from pet dogs to HCWs and then to infants in the NICU was likely [203]. Because *M. furfur* requires an exogenous source of lipids to support its growth, the clinical microbiology laboratory inoculates the specimen on a solid agar plate that is then covered with a layer of sterile olive oil. The Isolator™ (Dupont Company, Wilmington, DE) blood culture system is the most convenient system available for isolating these organisms.

Viral Infections

Outbreaks of viral infections in the NICU have been recognized with increased frequency with the advent of improved techniques for viral isolation and identification of viral antigens using direct fluorescent antibody, enzyme-linked immuno assay (ELISA), and PCR technology (see Chapter 9). In nursery outbreaks of viral infections, the virus can be introduced by a staff member [206], and rates of infection of staff members could be high [207–211].

Because staff members have mild illness, they continue to work and to spread the pathogen by direct inoculation of their infected secretions. Respiratory syncytial virus (RSV) and rotavirus are the most frequently identified viral agents associated with nosocomial transmission [208,210] (see Chapters 32 and 34). Other respiratory viruses, notably influenza [211], parainfluenza [75], and adenoviruses [206] can be associated with clusters of respiratory infections having clinical manifestations similar to these of RSV. Manifestations of RSV infections in infants <3 weeks of age are atypical and more likely to include apnea, lethargy, and poor feeding in the absence of respiratory symptoms. Beyond 3 weeks of age, bronchiolitis and pneumonia are characteristic of RSV infections; apnea can precede the onset of respiratory symptoms. Infants with bronchopulmonary dysplasia requiring oxygen, congenital heart disease with pulmonary hypertension, and congenital immune deficiency syndromes are at the greatest risk for developing severe disease after infection with RSV. Substantial medical and economic impact of an RSV outbreak in an NICU has been quantified [212]. Several different types of adenovirus have been associated with nursery outbreaks [206,213]. The most common clinical manifestations are conjunctivitis and pneumonia. Direct inoculation by ophthalmologic instruments and transmission by the droplet route have been documented [213]; specific guidelines for retinopathy of prematurity (ROP) ophthalmologic examinations to prevent contact transmission include using gloves with change between patients, soaking instruments in 70% alcohol solution for 5–10 minutes, and changing alcohol solution twice daily have been issued [206]. Neonates can manifest multiorgan involvement with cardiovascular collapse and a bacterial sepsislike clinical syndrome with a case-fatality rate of 84%. Severity of illness can be determined by identifying the specific type of adenovirus causing the infections. The role of emerging respiratory viruses detected in infants and young children (e.g., human metapneumovirus, bocavirus) for neonates and potential for nursery outbreaks remains to be identified.

Nursery outbreaks of viruses with a gastrointestinal reservoir have been described, and those of coxsackie virus and echovirus infections have been reviewed [214]. In most outbreaks, the source patients acquired infection from their mothers and had severe disease. Case-fatality rates associated with hepatitis can be as high as 83%. Infants who acquire infection by nosocomial transmission have milder disease, with case-fatality rates of 12% or less. HCWs also can be vectors for spreading this group of viruses. The most common clinical manifestations of neonatal coxsackie virus and echovirus infections are hepatitis, meningoencephalitis, myocarditis, and pneumonia and are similar to the disease associated with neonatal herpes simplex encephalitis and disseminated infections. Specific diagnostic testing using sensitive and specific PCR assays is essential to distinguish these agents because no antiviral agents are available to treat coxsackie virus and echovirus infections.

Rotavirus and hepatitis A virus are transmitted by the fecal–oral route. Rotavirus transmission in the nursery is well documented; infection can be asymptomatic or associated with mild to moderate or severe diarrhea. Rotavirus-associated outbreaks of necrotizing enterocolitis have been reported [208]. HAI outbreaks of hepatitis A virus are extremely rare because of the relatively brief duration and low titer of viral shedding within the stool [215–217] (see Chapter 42). However, immunologically immature preterm infants can excrete hepatitis A viral antigen and RNA for as long as 4–5 months after the acute infection [216]. The source infants in reported outbreaks acquired hepatitis A virus either by vertical transmission from the mother before or during delivery [215] or by blood transfusion [216,217].

The following viruses are not transmitted horizontally in the nursery: human immunodeficiency virus (HIV), HBV, hepatitis C, and cytomegalovirus (CMV). Inadvertent exposure to expressed breast milk from a different mother who is infected with HIV has the theoretical risk of transmitting it. The source mother and the exposed infant should be tested for HIV under these circumstances [62]. Observing standard precautions and screening blood for transfusion and for CMV as well as using filtered blood or leukocyte-poor red blood cells have prevented transmission of infection (see Chapter 13). There is no significant increase in the excretion of CMV in infants in the nursery compared with patients in other areas of a pediatric hospital [218], nor is there a significant increase in the risk of acquisition of CMV infection among HCWs on pediatric or neonatal units compared with similar adults without hospital exposure [219,220]; thus, pregnant HCWs are not restricted from caring for infants known to excrete CMV [220]. Transmission of either herpes simplex [221,222] or varicella-zoster virus [223] in the nursery is extremely rare. Although transmission from oral lesions of nursery HCWs has been reported [222], the risk is so low that such individuals are no longer excluded from patient care as long as the lesion can be covered until dried [62]. In contrast, HCWs with herpetic whitlow are excluded from direct patient contact in the nursery. With widespread use of the varicella virus vaccine licensed in 1995, the number of susceptible or infected neonates, mothers, visitors, and HCWs has decreased substantially.

Tuberculosis

Congenital tuberculosis (TB) is extremely rare but can occur even when the mother is asymptomatic. Infants in the NICU who have TB are unlikely to transmit *Mycobacterium tuberculosis* to other infants and visitors but can transmit it to HCWs with unprotected close exposure [224]. However, *M. tuberculosis* has been transmitted to exposed neonates in the maternity unit, newborn nursery, and in recent years NICU and, to visitors and HCWs with active pulmonary TB in countries where TB is considered endemic [225] and in the United States [226–229]. The neonate is at great risk for developing a severe disseminated disease, including meningitis, once exposed to an individual with active TB. Thus, recognition of an exposure must be followed by a comprehensive evaluation and initiation of chemoprophylaxis when the exposure is significant. A decision analysis has been developed to assist neonatologists and infection control personnel in managing of *M. tuberculosis* exposures [229]. When a TB diagnosis is considered in a young infant, a liver biopsy that shows granulomas and acid fast bacilli is diagnostic.

HAI TREATMENT

Physicians treating specific HAI can consult their local nursery guidelines, the AAP *Redbook* [62], and Nelson's *Pocket Book of Pediatric Antimicrobial Therapy* [230] for specific recommendations concerning choice of agent, dosing regimen, and duration of therapy. Empiric therapy for early onset disease consists of ampicillin combined with an aminoglycoside. Ampicillin provides activity against GBS, enterococci, and *Listeria monocytogenes*. If *S. aureus* is suspected, methicillin, oxacillin, or—in areas with high prevalence of MRSA—vancomycin is recommended for gram-positive coverage. The choice of aminoglycoside is based on susceptibility patterns in the nursery, but amikacin usually is reserved because of its greater activity against some GNB resistant to gentamicin and tobramycin as well as its higher cost. In one study, empiric use of ampicillin and cefotaxime during the first three days of life was associated with an increased risk of death compared with ampicillin and gentamicin, but the mechanism is unknown [231].

When treating suspected late onset sepsis, the choice of antimicrobial agents varies substantially neonatologists [232]. Oxacillin can be used for gram-positive coverage safely in NICUs that do not have MRSA as a prevalent pathogen and in infants with CVCs who are minimally symptomatic. Blood cultures from two separate sites are helpful in distinguishing CONS that are skin contaminants from true pathogens. The advantage of not using vancomycin routinely is the reduced risk of emergence of VRE, vancomycin-resistant staphylococci, and GNB infections [232,233]. Third-generation cephalosporins are not recommended for routine empiric use because of the rapidity of emergence of resistance in an individual patient during therapy and in microflora of the unit [51,171,172,234] as well as the association with an increased risk of candidiasis in VLBW infants [66]. However, cefotaxime is added to the aminoglycoside if there is a strong suspicion of GNB meningitis. Once the identification and susceptibility of the GNB-causing meningitis is known, cefotaxime in combination with an aminoglycoside is continued for at least 10 days and a minimum of a 21-day course is completed. Cefatazidime, cefipime, piperacillin-tazobactam, and meropenem can be substituted for treatment of

susceptible strains of *Pseudomonas* and *Stenotrophomonas* spp. and other multidrug-resistant GNB. Ceftriaxone is not used in the neonate because of its displacement of bilirubin from albumin-binding sites [234] and its strong suppressive effect on the neonate's developing gastrointestinal flora [236]. Monitoring susceptibility patterns for GNB and antibiotic use is necessary to ensure that the currently recommended agents will be effective against the current pathogens (see Role of Microbiology in Chapter 15). With the exception of CONS-BSI, meningitis can be present in 10–20% of BSIs and in the absence of BSI or abnormalities of the cerebrospinal fluid (CSF) cell counts, glucose, and protein in 30–40% of infants with late onset sepsis. Therefore, a lumbar puncture for CSF culture and analysis is essential to diagnose meningitis [237,238]. Meningitic dosages of antimicrobial agents are recommended until meningitis has been ruled out.

Specific anaerobic coverage rarely is required in neonates. The most frequent indications are intra-abdominal sepsis, necrotizing enterocolitis, and intestinal perforation. Clindamycin, metronidazole, piperacillin-tazobactam, and meropenem provide activity against most anaerobes. Now that safer drugs for treating GNB infections are available, chloramphenicol is not recommended for neonates because of its toxicity and unpredictable pharmacokinetics, and trimethoprim-sulfamethoxazole is not used because of the rare idiosyncratic hepatotoxicity secondary to sulfa component.

Removing the catheter as soon as CLA BSIs associated with possible to clear the fungemia and prevent seeding other foci is essential for *Candida* sp. Traditionally, Amphotericin B and fluconazole have been the only treatment options for invasive fungal disease in the neonate. Although flucytosine was added to amphotericin B for enhanced activity in the most severe disease (e.g., endocarditis), its gastrointestinal toxicity prohibited its use for a prolonged course. While *C. albicans* had been nearly universally susceptible to fluconazole, the increasing frequency of infections caused by more resistant *Candida* spp. and the toxicity associated with amphotericin B have made antifungal treatment more difficult. Although most studies of fluconazole prophylaxis of high-risk neonates have not found emergence of resistance, one report described the emergence of fluconazole-resistant subclones of a single strain of *C. parapsilosis* that was a major cause of candidemia during a 12-year period when fluconazole prophylaxis was used [239]. Fortunately, The development of antifungal agents with less toxicity and greater activity against the more difficult to treat fungi has recently surged [240]. The new azole drug voriconazole now is preferred for the treatment of invasive aspergillosis. This drug has not been studied in neonates and there is theoretical concern about the effect on the developing retina because of the visual adverse events reported in adults and older children. The echinocandins represent a class of agents that interfere with fungal cell wall biosynthesis by inhibition of an enzyme present in fungi but absent in mammalian cells. These drugs are not substrates for the hepatic cytochrome p450 isoenzyme system or the intestinal glycopeptides, thereby reducing drug interactions. The echinocandins have excellent fungicidal activity against most *Candida* spp. and are fungistatic against *Aspergillus* sp. Caspofungin is the first in this class of agents to be studied. Although no large studies of the use of in neonates have been performed, two case-series [241,242] and individual case-reports indicate that it successfully treats refractory candidiasis in VLBW neonates and is well tolerated. Micafungin is another agent in this class that has undergone pharmacokinetic studies in neonates [243] and is now being used in larger neonatal studies.

Acyclovir is the preferred treatment for *Herpes simplex* and Varicella-Zoster viral infections. In a large, multicenter randomized controlled trial of ganciclovir therapy of infants with congenital CMV infection and central nervous system involvement, treatment prevented deterioration of hearing [244]. Studies to identify the patients who will experience the greatest benefit of treatment and to determine the optimal treatment regimen are ongoing. Treatment of RSV infections is primarily supportive. Recommendations for the use of aerosolized ribavirin therapy in RSV infections have been modified since the drug's licensure in 1986 because of the continuing questions concerning efficacy. Decisions concerning ribavirin use must be individualized and made with the knowledge of conflicting data concerning efficacy. Ribavirin can be considered for use in the infected, high-risk, low-birth-weight infant with chronic bronchopulmonary dysplasia, congenital heart disease, congenital immunodeficiency syndrome, and other serious underlying conditions such as neurologic and metabolic

disease and multiple congenital anomalies [62]. Ribavirin must be initiated early in the course of disease for optimum effectiveness. Some experts recommend the addition of the monoclonal antibody palivizumab to treat severe disease in high-risk patients based on anecdotal experience in adult bone marrow transplant patients [245]. No efficacy data in human infants have been published; therefore, further studies are needed.

HAI PREVENTION

Nursery Design and Staffing

The AAP and the ACOG collaborate to develop guidelines for all aspects of perinatal care, including infection control in the nursery [246]; they revise these guidelines at regular intervals; the next revision is scheduled for publication in 2007. Table 25-3 summarizes the recommended nurse/infant ratios based on the acuity of the medical condition and the amount and type of nursing care and support equipment needed. Nurse/infant ratios below those recommended have been associate with increased rates of bacterial invasive disease caused by MSSA [73], MRSA [26], *Enterobacter cloacae* [74], and other bacteria [72,76] and viral respiratory infections [75] in the nursery and NICU. Spatial requirements are defined in the 2006 Guidelines for Design and Construction of Health Care Facilities published by the American Institute of Architects (AIA) (www.aia.org/aah_gd_hospcons) and by the Consensus Committee on Recommended Standards for Newborn Intensive Care Unit Design [247] (Table 25-3). Single-patient rooms in the NICU can offer an infection control advantage,

---

TABLE 25-3

RECOMMENDED STAFFING RATIOS AND SPACE ACCORDING TO LEVEL OF CARE REQUIRED IN THE NEWBORN NURSERY (COMPILED FROM [246], [298], [247])

Care Provided	Registered Nurse-to-Infant Ratio	Floor Space (ft^2) Per Infant	Space Between Beds (ft)	Adjacent Aisle Width (ft)
Newborn admission and observation	1:4	40	NR	
Newborns requiring only *routine* care	1:6–8	30	3	a
Normal mother-newborn couplet care	1:3–4	NR	NR	NR
Newborns requiring *continuing* care	1:3–4	50	4	NR
Newborns requiring *intermediate* care	1:2–3	100–120	4	5
Newborns requiring *intensive* care	1:1–2	Multiple-bed rooms: 120–150	6	8
		Single-bed rooms: 150		8
Newborns requiring multisystem support[b]	1:1	b	b	b
Unstable newborns requiring complex critical care[b]	≥1:1	b	b	b

NR, No recommendation.
[a]No specific recommendation published; maximum 16 infant stations per nursery room
[b]Increased space requirements preferred, but no specific recommendations published

TABLE 25-4
DEFINITION OF EPIDEMIOLGICALLY IMPORTANT ORGANISMS

Any infectious agents transmitted in healthcare settings may, under defined conditions, become targeted for control because they are epidemiologically important. The strategies described in the Guidelines for Management of Multi-Drug Resistant Organisms (MDROs) in Healthcare Settings, 2006 may be applied to control epidemiologically important organisms other than MDROs. The presence of one or more of the following characteristics assist in recognition:

- *Propensity for transmission within healthcare facilities* based on published reports and the occurrence of temporal or geographic clusters of ≥2 patients (e.g., vancomycin-resistant enterococcus [VRE], methicillin-resistant *Staphyloccus aureus* [MRSA], methicillin-susceptible *S. aureus* [MSSA], *Clostridium difficile*, norovirus, respiratory syncytial virus [RSV], influenza, rotavirus, *Enterobacter* spp; *Serratia* spp., group A streptococcus). For susceptible bacteria known to be associated with asymptomatic colonization (e.g., MSSA), isolation from normally sterile body fluids in patients with significant clinical disease would be required for consideration as epidemiologically important.
  - Most experts agree that a single case of healthcare-associated invasive disease caused by certain pathogens (e.g., group A streptococcus postoperatively, in nurseries, in burn units; *Legionella* sp., *Aspergillus* sp.) is a trigger for investigation and the use of enhanced control measures because of the high risk of additional cases and the devastating outcomes associated with these infections.
- *Antimicrobial resistance implications*
  - Resistance to first-line therapies (e.g., MRSA, VISA, VRSA, VRE, ESBL-producing organisms).
  - Common and uncommon microorganisms with unusual patterns of resistance within a facility (e.g., the first isolate of *Burkholderia cepacia* complex or *Ralstonia* spp. in non-CF patients or a quinolone-resistant strain of *Pseudomonas aeruginosa* in a facility.
  - Difficulty in treating because of innate or acquired resistance to multiple classes of antimicrobial agents (e.g., *Stenotrophomonas maltophilia*, *Acinetobacter* spp.).
- *Association with serious clinical disease*, increased morbidity and mortality (e.g., MRSA and MSSA, group A streptococcus)
- *A newly discovered or reemerging pathogen*

(Adapted [250])

---

but more data are needed to support a universal recommendation.

Many experts recommend central high-efficiency particulate air (HEPA) filtration when constructing a new NICU due to the vulnerability of VLBW infants to infection caused by airborne spores and because surgical procedures (e.g., ECMO cannulation/decannulation, exploratory laparotomy in infants with necrotizing enterocolitis) are often performed in the NICU when high-risk infants are too unstable to withstand transport to the operating suite.

HAI Surveillance

An active surveillance program is an essential component of HAI prevention (see Chapter 5). In most hospitals, surveillance of positive clinical culture results is performed by infection control personnel who are responsible for several different units in the hospital. The CDC recommends the following: [1] prospective surveillance on a regular basis by trained infection control professionals using standardized definitions, [2] analysis of infection rates using established epidemiologic and statistical methods (e.g., calculating rates using appropriate denominators that reflect duration of exposure and using statistical process control charts for trending rates), [3] regularly using data in decision making, and [4] employing an effective and trained healthcare epidemiologist who develops infection control

strategies and policies and serves as a liaison with the medical community and the administration (2–22;248,249). For the NICU, birth-weight categories are used for risk stratification. A working definition of epidemiologically important organisms has been developed to assist the infection control team in recognizing pathogens that require further investigation and preventive measures; see Table 25-4 [250]. When infection control personnel identify temporally related clusters of clinical infections and/or epidemiologically important pathogens, especially those that are multidrug-resistant, they collaborate with the nursery staff to develop a prevention program (see Chapter 2). As soon as a cluster or outbreak is suspected, infection control personnel should notify the microbiology laboratory of the need for active surveillance cultures and to save isolates should molecular fingerprinting studies be indicated (see Chapter 6). Designating a nursery staff member who understands the psychology and operational logistics of the unit as the infection control liaison facilitates education and adherence to policies for hand hygiene, isolation precautions, cohorting of patients and staff, proper cleaning, disinfection and sterilization of medical equipment, and other aseptic practices [26,251,252]. Participation of nursery staff members in the design of prevention programs increases adherence and success. feedback of positive results is most important to the staff when they have succeeded in controlling an outbreak; guidelines to prevent a similar outbreak is essential.

Routinely culturing neonate body surfaces (i.e., skin, umbilicus, mucous membranes, tracheal aspirates, rectal swabs) is not recommended in nonoutbreak settings because they do not predict which infants are at risk for sepsis and are very costly [253,254]. In contrast, body surface cultures are helpful during an outbreak to identify infants who are colonized with the target pathogen in addition to infants who have positive clinical cultures for target pathogens (e.g., MRSA, VRE, and multidrug-resistant GNB). Newly admitted infants must be kept in cohorts separate from colonized and infected infants to limit horizontal transmission of the outbreak organism. In addition, it can be useful to take active MRSA and VRE surveillance cultures at regular intervals (e.g., 3, 6, or 12 months) in NICUs that have no clinical episodes of MRSA or VRE to detect the presence of target multidrug-resistant organisms (MDROs) establishing high colonization rates and clinical disease [130,250]. Regional collaboration for NICU surveillance and control of MRSA has proven particularly useful [130].

Isolation Precautions

The 2006 AAP *Redbook* [62] has incorporated the recommendations for standard and transmission-based precautions published by the CDC in 1996 [255] (revised for anticipated publication in 2007); the recommendations should be consulted for managing specific infections. Standard precautions remain the foundation in infection control to which other categories of precautions are added. Standard precautions have been expanded to include recommendations for respiratory hygiene/cough etiquette for individuals with symptoms of respiratory tract infection. However, such individuals should be restricted from entering the nursery. See the Tables 25-5 and 25-6, for the components of standard precautions and transmission-based precautions respectively. Table 25-7 summarizes the recommended precautions for the most frequently encountered neonatal infections that require contact, airborne, or droplet precautions in addition to standard precautions. In NICUs with single-patient rooms, personal protective equipment (PPE) needed for contact and droplet precautions should be donned upon entry into the room. In NICUs with multibed pods or bays, the space around the isolette of the infant who requires contact and/or droplet precautions is usually designated with tape on the floor and signs on the isolette. A separate room is not required for infants on contact or droplet precautions, but spatial separation from uninfected infants is preferred. Although enclosed isolettes provide a limited amount of barrier protection relative to open warmers or bassinets [129], they cannot be relied on to prevent pathogen spread to other infants by HCW hand carriage. Neonates usually are unable to generate large-particle droplets spontaneously, but endotracheal suctioning or administration of aerosol treatments can generate infectious droplets. According to standard precautions, masks are indicated if splatter of respiratory secretions is anticipated (e.g., endotracheal suctioning or intubation). At least one airborne infection isolation room (AIIR) with negative-pressure ventilation that meets standard requirements is recommended for every nursery/NICU to isolate neonates with perinatal exposure to maternal varicella and suspected or confirmed TB. Most other infections do not require special isolation rooms.

During outbreaks, the most effective method for preventing horizontal transmission is by cohorting infants who are colonized or infected with epidemiologically important pathogens away from newly admitted patients and ideally with dedicated personnel who do not care for newly admitted infants or infants who are not colonized or infected [26,130,256,257]. If transmission continues in the presence of strict cohorting, continual introduction of the epidemic organisms from a carrier or multiple different sources or from ineffective hand antisepsis is likely [159].

Hand Hygiene and Gloves

Performing hand hygiene between patient contacts is the single most important measure for preventing HAIs in the nursery [258](see Chapter 13). The scientific information documenting the role of transmission via the hands of HCWs, the efficacy for hand decontamination with either antimicrobial-containing soap or alcohol-based hand rubs, and the recommended use of gloves is summarized in the CDC/HICPAC Guideline for Hand Hygiene in Health-Care Settings [258]; an implementation guide has been developed through the collaboration of the Institute for Healthcare Improvement (IHI), CDC, Society of Healthcare Epidemiologists of America (SHEA), and the Professionals in Infection Control and Epidemiology (APIC) (www.IHI.org). The Guideline for Hand Hygiene summarizes nine studies, three of which were conducted in the NICU, newborn nursery, or general pediatrics units, that demonstrate a temporal relationship between the introduction of new hand-hygiene products and improved hand-hygiene practices and decreased MRSA infection rates when added to the other control measures that had been in place, including obtaining weekly active surveillance cultures and contact precautions. The important components of hand hygiene are consistency, duration of exposure, and antimicrobial content of the soap or waterless hand rub [258]. Alcohol-containing antiseptic hand gels and antimicrobial soap and water are preferred in nurseries and NICUs. A hands-free hand washing station should be provided in each single-patient room. Every infant bed in multi-bed rooms should be within 20 feet of a hand-washing station but should be no closer than 3 feet to other beds [247]. Having an alcohol gel dispenser mounted at each bedside provides the best opportunity for using hand hygiene consistently.

TABLE 25-5
RECOMMENDATIONS FOR APPLICATION OF STANDARD PRECAUTIONS FOR THE CARE OF ALL PATIENTS IN ALL HEALTHCARE SETTINGS

Component	Recommendations
Hand hygiene	After touching blood, body fluids, secretions, excretions, contaminated items; immediately after removing gloves; between patient contacts. Alcohol-containing antiseptic handrubs preferred *except* when hands are visibly soiled with blood and/or other proteinaceous materials or if exposure to spores (e.g., *C. difficile, B. antracis*) is likely to have occurred
Personal protective equipment (PPE)	
Gloves	For touching blood, body fluids, secretions, excretions, contaminated items, mucous membranes, nonintact skin
Gown	During anticipated procedures and patient-care activities with contact of clothing/exposed skin with blood/body fluids, secretions, and excretions
Mask, eye protection (goggles), face shield[a]	During procedures and patient-care activities likely to generate splashes or sprays of blood, body fluids, secretions, especially suctioning, endotracheal intubation to protect healthcare personnel
	Use of a mask by the individual inserting an epidural anesthesia needle or performing myelograms when prolonged exposure of the puncture site is likely to occur to project patient
Soiled patient-care equipment	Handle in a manner that prevents transfer of microorganisms to others and to the environment; wear gloves if visibly contaminated; perform hand hygiene
Environmental control	Develop procedures for routine care, cleaning, and disinfection of environmental surfaces, especially frequently touched surfaces in patient-care areas
Textiles and laundry	Handle in a manner that prevents transfer of microorganisms to others and to the environment
Injection practices (use of needles and other sharps)	Do not recap, bend, break, or hand-manipulate used needles; if recapping required, use a one-handed scoop technique only; use needle-free safety devices when available; place used sharps in puncture-resistant container. Use sterile, single-use, disposable needle and syringe for each injection given. Single dose medication vials preferred when medications are administered to >1 patient
Patient resuscitation	Use mouthpiece, resuscitation bag, other ventilation devices to prevent contact with mouth and oral secretions
Patient placement	Prioritize for single-patient room if patient is at increased risk of transmission, is likely to contaminate the environment, does not maintain appropriate hygiene, or is at increased risk of acquiring infection or developing adverse outcome following infection
Respiratory hygiene/cough etiquette (source containment of infectious respiratory secretions in symptomatic patients, beginning at initial point of encounter [e.g., triage and reception areas in emergency departments and physician offices])	Instruct symptomatic persons to cover mouth/nose when sneezing/coughing; use tissues, dispose of them in no-touch receptacle; observe hand hygiene after soiling hands with respiratory secretions; wear surgical mask if tolerated or maintain spatial separation, >3 feet if possible

A 2-minute scrub from hands to forearms with an antiseptic-containing soap is no longer recommended for nursery staff at the beginning of a work shift [258]. However, published recommendations in the AAP/ACOG Guidelines for Perinatal Care for the number of nursery scrub areas are to have (1) one scrub area at the entrance to each nursery with faucets operated by foot or knee controls and (2) one scrub sink for at least every 6–8 patient stations in the normal newborn nursery and for every 3–4 patient stations in the admission/observation, continuing care, intermediate care, and intensive care areas [246]. While some scrub sinks are required because surgical procedures are performed in the NICU, their number can likely be reduced. Hands should be washed thoroughly with an antimicrobial soap and water on entry into the nursery/NICU, and hand hygiene should be performed using either an antiseptic alcohol hand rub or antimicrobial soap and water between patient contacts. As part of good hand-hygiene practices, HCWs who have direct contact with high-risk patients should have well-groomed and short natural nails [258]. The evidence base to support the recommendations for HCWs with direct contact with patients in ICUs includes four studies performed in NICUs [94–97]. Novel strategies to improve adherence to recommendations for hand hygiene and monitoring adherence are needed in the nursery/NICU as in all other areas of healthcare facilities.

TABLE 25-6
TRANSMISSION-BASED PRECAUTIONS

In addition to standard precautions (SP), use transmission-based precautions for patients with highly transmissible or epidemiologically important pathogens for which additional precautions are needed

Component	Contact	Droplet	Airborne
Hand hygiene	Per SP Soap and water preferred over alcohol handrub for *C. difficile*, *Bacillus anthracis* spores	Per SP	Per SP
Gown	Yes, don upon room entry	Per SP	Per SP and if infectious, draining skin lesions present
Gloves	Yes, don upon room entry	Per SP	Per SP
Mask	Per SP	Yes, don upon room entry	N95 particulate respirator or higher
Goggles/face shield	Per SP	Per SP Always for SARS, avian influenza	Per SP Always for SARS, avian influenza
N95 or higher respirator	When aerosol-producing procedures performed for influenza, SARS, VHF	When aerosol-producing procedures performed for influenza, SARS, VHF	Yes, don upon entry
Room placement	Single-patient room preferred	Single-patient room preferred	Single-patient room
	Cohortlike infections if single-patient rooms unavailable	Cohortlike infections if single-patient rooms unavailable	Negative air pressure; 12 ACH/hr. for new construction, 6 ACH/hr. for existing rooms
Environmental measures	Increased frequency, especially in the presence of diarrhea	Routine	Routine
	Consider bleach solution for continued transmission of *C. difficile*, norovirus		
Transport	Mask patient if coughing	Mask patient	Mask patient
	Cover infectious skin, lesions		Cover infectious skin, lesions

Gloves must be worn when contact with blood or body fluids is anticipated or when handling anything on the transmission-based precautions list that has come in contact with an infant. Gloves are never washed between patients but must be changed between patient contacts. Hand hygiene is performed immediately upon glove removal.

Gowns, Caps, and Masks

The use of gowns on entrance into the nursery is a longstanding ritual that many nurseries are hesitant to relinquish. Studies of varying design conducted in the nursery and NICU confirm gown's lack of efficacy for preventing HAIs [259,260]. In alternate 2-month gowning and no-gowning cycles, Pelke et al. [260] demonstrated no significant differences in the rates of bacterial colonization, HAIs including RSV and necrotizing enterocolitis, and mortality. In addition, compliance with hand washing was not increased during the gowning cycles, nor was traffic into the unit changed. Thus, in a nonoutbreak setting, gowns are not required for staff or visitors upon entrance to the nursery but are indicated when there is soiling with blood or body fluids is anticipated, following contact precautions is necessary, clustered infections with epidemiologically important organisms that are considered to have been transmitted by the contact route are present, and parental concern exists for excessively soiled clothing. Some nurseries have continued to use gowns for handling newborn infants (e.g., cuddling, feeding).

Caps and masks are indicated when performing sterile procedures, including CVC placement. Masks also are used as part of standard precautions and droplet precautions to protect HCWs and an infant from an individual HCW with respiratory tract infection who is considered indispensable and cannot be removed from the nursery/NICU. Respirators of N95 or higher are indicated for HCWs having contact with a patient with suspected or confirmed TB.

Prevention of Transmission of Multidrug Resistant Organisms (MDROs)

Control of MDROs requires three groups of interventions: (1) prudent antimicrobial use to prevent emergence of resistance, (2) implementation of bundled practices to prevent device-related and SSIs (**www.ihi.org/IHI/Programs/Campaign**), and (3) infection control measures to prevent transmission within the NICU [250]. Based on the voluminous number of published studies of control of MDROs in NICUs and in other healthcare settings, it is clear that transmission of MDROs in healthcare settings can be controlled, but the single most effective strategy for all settings has not

TABLE 25-7

SUMMARY OF 1996 ISOLATION GUIDELINES FOR INFECTIONS ENCOUNTERED IN THE NURSERY

Infection	Type of precautions
Abscess	
Contained by dressing	Standard
Draining, not contained by dressing	Contact
Conjunctivitis (bacterial, chlamydia, gonococcal)	Standard
Cytomegalovirus	Standard
Enteroviruses (Coxsackievirus, echovirus)	Contact
Diarrhea (bacterial or viral)	Contact
Fungal (Candidiasis, aspergillosis, malassezia)	Standard
Hepatitis viruses	
Type A	Contact
All others	Standard
Herpes simplex (maternal exposure, disease)	Contact
Human immunodeficiency virus	Standard
Listeriosis	Standard
Measles	Airborne
Meningitis	
Neisseria meningitidis, Hemophilus influenzae, type B	Droplet × 24 hr
All others	Standard
Multidrug-resistant organisms (vancomycin-resistant enterococci, methicillin-resistant S. aureus, resistant gram-negative bacilli)	Contact
Necrotizing enterocolitis	Standard contact if cluster
Respiratory viruses	
Respiratory syncytial, parainfluenza	Contact
Adenovirus, influenza, rhinovirus	Droplet + contact
Rubella	Droplet
Streptococcal, Group A	Droplet × 24 hr Contact
Streptococcal, Group B	Standard
Syphilis	Standard
Toxoplasmosis	Standard
Tuberculosis	Airborne
Varicella	Airborne, contact

(Adapted from [255])

been established. Seven categories of measures are critical for preventing MDRO transmission [250]:

1. *Administrative measures* to ensure successful implementation of recommended practices including designating control of MDROs as an organizational patient safety priority, providing effective and timely communication of MDRO status of patients upon reentry or transfer to a facility, monitoring the implementation and adherence to precautions, providing feedback to HCWs, and supporting participation in regional coalitions.
2. *Education* of all HCWs, patients, families, and visitors.

3. *Judicious use of antimicrobials* including developing an active multidisciplinary antimicrobial management team. The influence of antimicrobial exposure on emergence of multidrug-resistant GNB has been demonstrated specifically in the NICU [51,169–172].
4. *Surveillance*, including tracking and trending MDRO rates and actively surveilling cultures in high-risk populations. Because HCWs rarely are the source of bacterial pathogens causing outbreaks, active surveillance cultures of HCWs are recommended only when epidemiologic evidence implicates them as a source of ongoing transmission.
5. *Infection control precautions*, including the use of hand hygiene, standard precautions and contact precautions with dedicated patient care equipment and cohorting patients infected with the same antibiotic-resistant pathogen(s) when single-patient rooms are not available.
6. *Environmental measures* (e.g., adherence to recommendations for cleaning and disinfecting potentially contaminated environmental surfaces and medical equipment). EPA-approved hospital-grade disinfectants are active against most pathogens, but disinfectants labeled as effective against specific pathogens could be required for *C. difficile* in the midst of an outbreak.
7. *MRSA decolonization* on a selective basis.

The most effective measure for MRSA and VRE control include a risk assessment, active surveillance testing for colonized patients, contact isolation for infected/colonized patients, and hand hand hygiene. Sole focus on MRSA or VRE may increase the possibility that multidrug-resistant GNB may emerge [261]. Expanding the program to include resistant GNB can be especially relevant for the NICU. The recommendations for implementing the baseline of these 7 measures in all healthcare facilities, especially in high-risk units within those facilities and defining target MDROs within a specific unit, assessing trends, and implementing a more intensified set of measures if rates of MDROs are not decreasing serve as a template for MDRO control in the NICU and include many studies of outbreak control in NICUs in the evidence base [250]. The NICU must participate in the overall facility strategies for MDRO control and interventions specific to its conditions.

Skin, Eye, and Cord Care

Initial cleansing of skin after birth is delayed until the neonate's temperature has stabilized. Warm water alone or warm water and a mild, nonmedicated soap are recommended when the skin is cleaned [246]. Hexachlorophene specifically is no longer recommended for routine daily bathing of neonates because of the neurotoxicity demonstrated previously when it is absorbed in large concentrations. However, chlorhexidine gluconate is poorly absorbed through intact skin and is therefore a suitable agent. When intramuscular injections are given in the delivery room as part of prophylaxis regimens (e.g., penicillin G to prevent early onset GBS disease or gonococcal ophthalmia, ceftriaxone to prevent gonococcal ophthalmia, and vitamin K to prevent hemorrhagic disease of the newborn), the injection site must first be cleansed well with alcohol. This prevents the introduction of microorganisms such as HIV, HBV, and herpes simplex virus in maternal blood and body fluids that could be contaminating the infant's skin.

A single application within 1 hour of delivery of topical tetracycline (1%) or erythromycin (0.5%) ophthalmic ointment is preferred to prevent gonococcal ophthalmia. The use of 1% silver nitrate drops is discouraged because of the associated chemical irritation. The eyes should not be irrigated after instillation of any of these agents. Single-use tubes or vials must be used to prevent cross-infection. A single dose of ceftriaxone, 125 mg (25 to 50 mg/kg for low-birth weight infants) intramuscularly or intravenously, is recommended for infants born to mothers with active gonorrhea at delivery [62].

The umbilical cord has been reported to become colonized with *S. aureus* in up to 70% of infants within 48 hours after birth and can potentially serve as a point of entrance for pathogens to cause invasive disease. High colonization rates in the nursery are associated with an increased rate of postdischarge infection for term infants and longer hospital stay for low-birth weight infants. Therefore, most nursery protocols include antiseptic treatment. Certainly, any nursery experiencing an increased rate of *S. aureus* infections uses topical antiseptics for cord care. In this era of increasing prevalence of CO-MRSA in many communities, cord care to prevent MRSA colonization could be even more important. The role of antimicrobial applications to the umbilical cord to prevent bacterial colonization and infection has been reviewed [262,263]. These reviews conclude that there is evidence that applying antiseptic to the cord reduces bacterial colonization, but there is insufficient evidence to determine whether any agent is preferred. The delay in time to cord separation >7 days in infants treated with topical antiseptics is not significant clinically and should not deter the use of antibacterial products. Use of dry cord care and isopropyl alcohol has been associated with higher colonization rates than of the following antiseptic agents: (1) triple dye, a combination of brilliant green (2.29 mg/mL), proflavine hemisulfate (1.14 mg/mL), and gentian violet (2.29 mg/mL), (2) bacitracin ointment, (3) chlorhexidine, and (4) silver sulfadiazine cream (1% Silvadene™). However, consistently greater efficacy has not been demonstrated for any one agent [262,263]. Iodine-containing agents are not recommended because of the possibility of transcutaneous absorption and suppression of neonatal thyroid function. Short-term use of mupiricin (Bactroban™) ointment to control an outbreak associated with susceptible *S. aureus* or MRSA may be considered, but mupiricin is not recommended routinely because of the emergence of resistant strains after its frequent or prolonged use [264]. If a nursery discontinues antimicrobial care of the umbilicus in favor of dry cord care, it is important to conduct postdischarge surveillance to ensure the absence of adverse effects.

Traditionally, triple dye has not been used in the NICU because of theoretical concern about increasing systemic absorption and rendering the umbilical stump unsuitable for vessel catheterization. However, adverse effects have been observed since a routine single application of triple dye to the umbilical stump was extended to infants in the intermediate care area of Parkland Health and Hospital System in 1988 and then to the NICU area in 1991. In the NICU, the application of triple dye after umbilical vessel catheterization in the first 12 hours after birth was instrumental in controlling a prolonged MRSA outbreak [26].

Intravascular Catheters and Respiratory Therapy Equipment

Few controlled investigations of care practices of intravascular catheter or respiratory therapy equipment specifically in the newborn nursery have been conducted. Consequently, nurseries usually follow guidelines for the care of catheters and respiratory equipment based on studies in older children and adults [55,265] (see Chapters 31 and 37). PICC and surgically placed tunneled CVCs are used in the NICU, which have no significant differences in the complication rate [266]. Application of the bundled practices for preventing CLA-BSIs in children (www.chca.com/news/camapign.html) have been applied to neonates and have reduced rates of CLA-BSI significantly. The bundled practices include (1) assessing daily the need for the catheter and goals for removal, (2) using chlorhexidine to prepare the insertion site and for maintenance, (3) using maximal sterile barrier precautions for catheter insertion, (4) consistently using recommended hand hygiene, and (5) observing insertion and maintenance practices. Femoral lines must be protected against contamination from urine and stool. Although chlorhexidine has not been approved for use in infants <2 months of age, ample experience indicates that it can be used safely in neonates. Minimizing catheter manipulation and paying specific attention to aseptic technique when catheters are manipulated (e.g., hub, exit site, blood sampling) are important for preventing CLA-BSIs [267]. Practices for which some but not enough data suggest efficacy in support of recommendations for routine use include chlorhexidine sponge dressings (Biopatch)™ [268] and vancomycin-heparin lock solution [269]. The chlorhexidine sponge dressing should not be used in neonates <1,000 g or <7 days old or of gestational age <26 weeks because of reports of exudative-type local reactions and pressure necrosis occurring under the patch in these very premature infants [265,268]. Unique to the nursery is the use of umbilical arterial and venous catheters for which many care issues remain unresolved. The rates of colonization and associated BSIs are similar for umbilical arterial and venous catheters. The umbilical insertion site must be cleansed with an appropriate antiseptic before catheter insertion. Tincture of iodine is not used because of the potential effect on the neonatal thyroid [246]. Umbilical arterial catheters should not be left in place >5 days. Removing umbilical venous catheters after 14 days is recommended, but a recent randomized trial reported no increased adverse events associated with umbilical venous catheters in neonates with birth weights <1,251 g for up to 28 days compared with removal of the umbilical venous catheter after 7–10 days and its replacement with a PICC [270].

Mouth-suctioning devices, such as the De Lee suction trap, are no longer used because of the risk of exposure to potentially infectious aspirated material that could enter the HCW's mouth. When a mechanical suction apparatus is used, the negative pressure should be no more than 100 millimeters of mercury when the suction tubing is occluded [246]. The optimal bundled practices for preventing ventilator-associated pneumonia in the NICU and PICU have not been determined, but the options for modifying the adult bundles and experiences in two institutions have been reviewed [271]. Only sterile water should be used for any device that provides humidification to the neonate, and all equipment must be cleaned and disinfected according to manufacturers' recommendations [55]. Isolation of pathogens such as *Burkholderia cepacia* and *Ralstonia* sp. from respiratory secretions should alert NICU personnel to the possibility of contaminated equipment [56,272].

Each nursery should develop protocols for care of the specific intravascular catheters and respiratory therapy equipment that are used in the specific unit. These protocols should be consistent with the current AAP or CDC guidelines.

Immunoprophylaxis

As described, the administration of both standard IVIG preparations [40–42] and high titer staphylococcal immunoglobulin products [44–46] either to treat or prevent neonatal sepsis has not been efficacious, even when serum IgG levels are maintained >400 millimeters per deciliter The largest multicenter, controlled trial, which enrolled 2,416 infants, reported lot-to-lot variation in antibody profile despite the use of thousands of donors for processing each batch of IVIG [42]. In contrast, palivizumab, a humanized mouse monoclonal antibody that neutralizes RSV and prevents viral binding to cells is recommended for monthly intramuscular injection during the RSV season for high-risk children to prevent severe disease and RSV-related hospitalizations [273]. High risk groups include (1) infants and children <2 years old with chronic lung disease who have required medical therapy for chronic lung disease within 6 months before the anticipated start of the RSV season,

(2) infants born at ≤32 weeks gestation even if they do not have chronic lung disease, (3) infants born at 32–35 weeks gestation with ≥2 risk factors for RSV-associated hospitalization, and (4) children ≤24 months of age with hemodynamically significant cyanotic and acyanotic congenital heart disease. Although efficacy and safety have been demonstrated, cost effectiveness has not; therefore, targeting only those for whom efficacy has been shown is important [274]. A large multicenter trial of Numax™, a novel recombinant humanized IgG1 monoclonal antibody derived from palivizumab, has been completed, but results a not yet have been published. It is possible that this product could has improved efficacy.

A single dose of palivizumab is recommended for high-risk neonates at the time of discharge during the RSV season. However, because very premature infants do not sustain protective serum concentrations until after the second dose, it has been suggested that such infants should receive a dose at 1 month before discharge from the NICU in addition to the dose at discharge [275]. The use of palivizumab to control an RSV outbreak has not been studied. However, there is one report of the successful use of palivizumab administration to all infants in an NICU during an RSV outbreak that was not controlled by standard infection control measures [276]. It is important to note that RSV transmission can be well controlled [210] by following contact precautions, screening visitors and cohorting infants.

Varicella-zoster immune globulin (VZIG™ [Massachusetts Public Health Bilogics Laboratory, Boston, MS], VariZIG™ [Cangene Corp., Winneped, Canada]) is indicated for susceptible high-risk individuals exposed to varicella [277]. After an exposure in the NICU, VZIG or VariZIG 125 units are administered to premature infants of >28 weeks' gestation whose mothers have no prior history of varicella or varicella immunization and to all premature infants <28 weeks' gestation or ≤1,000 g birth weight regardless of maternal history due to lack of placental transfer of antibody in earlier stages of pregnancy [62,277]. Most premature infants of ≥28 weeks' gestation whose mothers are immune have acquired sufficient maternal antibody to protect them from severe disease and complications. However, chronologic age >2 months and seven or more transfusions of packed red cells can be associated with increased rates of seronegativity in infants whose mothers are immune [278]. Neither VZIG or VariZIG is recommended for healthy, term infants postnatally exposed even if their mothers have a negative history of varicella. Before administrating VZIG or VariZIG in a nursery exposure, obtaining serum from the infants to confirm susceptibility is helpful. If antibody determinations are available within 72 hours of the exposure, VZIG or VariZIG administration can be delayed until results are available. If antibody is present, the infant does not require isolation during the 10–28 days after exposure. VZIG is not indicated if an infant has received an infusion of IVIG for other indications within the previous 3 weeks.

It is prudent to provide influenza vaccine to the visiting family members to protect them and the infants in the NICU [62,211]. The NICU also provides an excellent opportunity to counsel adolescent and adult family members about the importance of receiving Tdap to protect their own infants and others in the NICU and to provide it to them [176].

Chemoprophylaxis

Maternal screening and chemoprophylaxis have dramatically reduced the risk of early onset GBS disease [105]. However, the use of antimicrobial agents for HAI prevention in the NICU is strongly discouraged because of the risk of the emergence of resistant microorganisms that will require more broad-spectrum and potentially more toxic antimicrobial agents for treatment (see Chapters 14 and 15). Two groups of investigators have reported the efficacy of low-dose vancomycin, 25 µg/mL of total parenteral nutrition fluid, to decrease catheter colonization and BSI caused by CONS. In two different, prospective, randomized, controlled trials of 70 and 150 VLBW infants, CONS-BSI was decreased in infants weighing <1,500 g from 34% to 1.4%, respectively, and in infants weighing <1,000 g from 26–2.8%, respectively [279,280]. Despite the beneficial effect, neither set of investigators and an accompanying editorial recommends the routine use of this regimen because of the risk of the emergence of vancomycin-resistant organisms [281]. Continued exposure of the normal flora to low concentrations of vancomycin creates especially favorable conditions for resistance to occur. In addition, morbidity and mortality associated with CONS infection is not severe enough to justify the risks. In another randomized study of 148 infants weighing <1,500 g with percutaneous CVCs, the use of amoxicillin 100 mg/kg/day intravenously in three divided doses had a negligible effect on the incidence of septicemia because the rate in the control group was so low, 2.7% [282]. In conclusion, strict adherence to the recommended bundled practices for CVC insertion and maintenance remains the preferred method of prevention of CLA-BSIs.

Far more controversial is the role of fluconazole for prophylaxis of invasive candidiasis in the high-risk VLBW infant. Many studies of fluconazole prophylaxis have been published [283–288], and the results and cautions to neonatologists are best summarized in editorials by Long and Stevens [195] and by Fanaroff [284]. Published studies of fluconazole prophylaxis have demonstrated wide center-to-center variation in rates of invasive candidiasis before initiating prophylaxis, have targeted VLBW infants <1,500 g and ELBW infants <1,000 grams and/or gestational age <30 or 32 weeks, and have administered fluconazole (1) daily for the first 30 days of life (2) daily during periods of administration of antibiotics for >3 days [288], (3) every third day for 2 weeks followed by every other day for 2 weeks and then daily for 2 weeks [284,285], (4) twice

weekly for 6 weeks [284], or (5) every third day for 1 week followed by daily for 3 weeks [286,287]. All studies have been single-center studies, and most have been prepost intervention studies. Two small prospective, randomized placebo-controlled studies were published in 2001 [289, 290]; the more recent prospective randomized, double-blind clinical trial compared two different dosing schedules but did not have a control group [284]. The conclusion from these studies is that fluconazole prophylaxis does prevent *Candida* spp. BSIs and reduce *Candida*-related mortality in ELBW infants. Unfortunately, the recent publication from the NNIS HRNs that demonstrated a decreased incidence in *Candida* spp. BSIs in ELBW infants in 2000–2004 compared with 1995–1999 could not determine whether the reduced rate was associated with the use of fluconazole [7]. The concern is that there is evidence of the emergence of nonalbicans *Candida* strains that are resistant to fluconazole, there has been no multicenter trial, and *Candida* spp. BSIs are markers of management choices and infection control practices. Evidence-based practices relating to management of CVCs and prudent use of antimicrobials are more likely to be long-term safe and effective measures than the use of an antifungal agent for prophylaxis. Hence, caution is urged until more is known.

Visitation of Siblings and Others

Because the acquisition of a seemingly innocuous viral infection in high-risk neonates can result in unnecessary evaluation and empirical therapy for septicemia and serious life-threatening disease, special visitation policies are required in nurseries and NICUs. All visitors with signs or symptoms of respiratory or gastrointestinal tract infection should be restricted from visiting any patients in healthcare facilities. During the influenza season, it is preferred that all visitors have received influenza vaccine. Increased restrictions could be needed in the midst of a community outbreak (e.g., severe acute respiratory syndrome, influenza). For infants requiring contact precautions, the use of PPE by visitors is determined by the nature of the interaction with the patient and the likelihood that the visitor will frequent common areas in the nursery/NICU area or interact with other infants' family members. Although the neonatology staff encourage visits by siblings in the NICU, the medical risk must not outweigh the psychosocial benefit. Studies demonstrate that parents favorably regard sibling visitation [291] and that bacterial colonization [292,293] or subsequent infection [294] does not increase in the neonate who has been visited by siblings, but these studies are limited by small numbers. Strict guidelines for sibling visitation should be established and enforced to maximize visitation opportunities and minimize risks of transmission of infectious agents. The following visitation recommendations can guide policy development:

1. Sibling visitation should be encouraged in the well-child nursery and NICU.

2. Before visitation, a trained staff member or nurse should interview parents concerning the current health status of siblings. Siblings who are visiting should have received all vaccines recommended for their age. Children with fever or symptoms of an acute illness, such as upper respiratory tract infection, gastroenteritis, and dermatitis, should not be allowed to visit. Siblings who have been exposed to a known infectious disease and are still within the incubation period should not be allowed to visit. After the interview, the staff member or nurse should place a written consent for sibling visitation in the permanent patient record and provide a name tag for the sibling indicating that he or she has been approved for visitation for that day.

3. Asymptomatic siblings who recently have been exposed to Varicella virus but have been immunized can be assumed to be immune.

4. The visiting sibling should visit only his or her sibling and should not be allowed in playrooms with groups of patients.

5. Visitation should be limited to periods of time that ensure adequate screening, observation, and monitoring of visitors by medical and nursing staffs.

6. Children should observe hand hygiene before and after contact with the patient.

7. During the entire visit, sibling activity should be supervised by parents or a responsible adult.

Occupational and Employee Health

All HCWs in the all nursery areas must be immune to vaccine-preventable diseases. All nursery staff should be screened by history and, when indicated, serology for susceptibility to rubella, rubeola, varicella, and HBV (see Chapter 3). Appropriate immunizations must be provided for those who are seronegative. Annual influenza immunizations also should be administered to staff members, including pregnant women, in October and November of each year according to the CDC recommendations [295]. The cold-adapted, live-attenuated influenza vaccine (FLU-MIST™) can be administered safely to HCWs in the nursery without contraindications; because the amount of attenuated virus shed is below the infectious dose, the vaccine virus is unable to replicate at the higher temperatures of the lower respiratory tract, and no adverse effects have been reported in contacts of recipients of this vaccine [296]. This vaccine also offers the advantage of improved protection against drifted strains not contained in the vaccine as compared with the killed vaccine. The newest vaccine recommended for administration to HCWs in contact with young infants is the adult pertussis vaccine (Tdap) that should be administered as a single dose if ≥2 years have elapsed since the most recent Tetanus-diptheria vaccine (Td) [173]. Shorter intervals may be used in the midst of an outbreak. Guidelines for removing HCWs with highly contagious conditions from direct patient contact in the nursery should be consulted for specific recommendations [246,297]. Decisions concerning the removal of personnel with respiratory, gastrointestinal, or mucocutaneous infections must be made on an individual basis. Removal of all individuals with mild illnesses could be impractical in an overcrowded, understaffed nursery. Therefore, specific instructions concerning precautions to prevent transmission of infection to patients must be given. Individuals with pertussis, active TB, varicella, exudative skin lesions, or weeping dermatitis must be removed from direct patient contact until they are no longer infectious. HCWs with herpes labialis ("cold sores") are no longer excluded from the nursery because the transmission risk is so low. Such individuals are instructed to cover the lesions, not to touch the area surrounding the lesions, carefully observe hand-washing procedures, and not to kiss or cuddle neonates under their care. The role of topical penciclovir or oral acyclovir is not established but decreases the quantity and duration of viral shedding in treated individuals. HCWs with herpetic whitlow must be restricted from contact with neonates until the lesions are completely crusted. HCWs who are known to be carriers of hepatitis B surface antigen or infected with HIV are managed and counseled individually (see Healthcare worker and HIV Chapters 42 and 43). For those with HIV, continued patient contact is determined by the stage of disease and the absence of potentially transmissible infections and is governed by state law. Percutaneous and mucocutaneous exposures to blood-borne pathogens are managed according to standard protocols (see Chapter 44).

In the nursery, there has been much concern about the exposure of pregnant HCWs to neonates with congenital infections, especially CMV [220]. Frequently, the most anxiety is generated over infections that pose the least risk. Several epidemiologic studies in hospitals and day care centers have established that the nursery staff do not have an increased risk of acquiring CMV from their patients and that exposure to toddlers in day-care centers is associated with a significantly higher risk of seroconversion [218–220]. Therefore, pregnant women are not restricted from caring for infants who are identified as infected with CMV. All female HCWs in the childbearing age group must be taught to adhere strictly to standard precautions, especially hand hygiene and the use of gloves when contact with urine, saliva or blood is likely and that prepregnancy immunization against HBV, rubella, rubeola, and varicella is the most efficacious method of protecting themselves and their unborn children. Table 25-8 summarizes the relevant facts concerning infections that create the greatest concern among pregnant women in direct contact with young infants and as well as additional information [220]. We have found that pregnant HCWs are reassured greatly by reviewing this information with them.

The only restriction that is applied to pregnant HCWs is to avoid exposure to ribavirin. Although there are no data support the theoretic risks of teratogenicity in humans,

TABLE 25-8

THE PREGNANT HEALTH CARE WORKER: GUIDE TO MANAGEMENT OF OCCUPATIONAL EXPOSURE TO SELECTED INFECTIOUS AGENTS

Agent	In-Hospital Source	Potential Effect on the Fetus	Rate of Perinatal Transmission	Maternal Screening	Prevention
Bioweapons agents, Category A Smallpox (vaccinia)	Respiratory secretions, contents of pustule-vessicular lesions	Fetal vaccinia, premature delivery, spontaneous abortion, perinatal death		History of successful vaccination within previous 5 years	Preevent vaccination contraindicated during pregnancy;[b] vaccine and VIG (vaccinia-immune globulin) after exposure; preexposure vaccine only if smallpox present in the community and exposure to patients with smallpox likely
Cytomegalovirus (CMV)	Urine, blood, semen, vaginal secretion, immunosuppression, transplant, dialysis, day care	Classic cytomegalic inclusion disease (5–10%)[a] Hearing loss (10–15%)	Primary infection (25–50%) Recurrent infants 52% Symptomatic (5–15%)	Routine screening not recommended; antibody incompletely protective	Airborne plus contact precautions. Efficacy of CMV Immune globulin not established No vaccine available Standard precautions
Hepatitis A (HAV)	Feces (most common), blood (rare)	No fetal transmission described; transmission can occur at delivery if woman still in the infectious phase and cause hepatitis	None	Routine screening not recommended	Killed viral vaccine safely used in pregnancy; contact precautions during acute phase
Hepatitis B (HBV)	Blood, bodily fluids, vaginal secretions, semen	Hepatitis, early onset hepatocellular carcinoma	HbeAg HbsAg 10% HbeAg HbsAg 90%	Routine HBsAg testing advised	HBV vaccine during pregnancy if indications exist Neonate: HBIG plus vaccine at birth Standard precautions
Hepatitis C (HCV)	Blood, sexual	Hepatitis	5% (0–25%)	Routine screening not recommended	No vaccine or immune globulin available; post exposure treatment with antiviral agents investigational Standard precautions
Herpes simplex virus (HSV)	Vesicular fluid, oropharyngeal and vaginal secretions	Sepsis, encephalitis, meningitis, mucocutaneous lesions, congenital malformation (rare)	Primary genital 33–50% Recurrent genital 1–2%	Antibody testing minimally useful Genital inspection for lesions if in labor	Chemoprophylaxis at 36 weeks decreases shedding Standard precautions Contact precautions for patients with skin lesions
Human immunodeficiency virus (HIV)	Blood, bodily fluids, vaginal secretions, semen	No congenital syndrome. If fetus infected, AIDS in 2–4 yrs.	Depends on HIV viral titer and use of antiretroviral agents during pregnancy, labor, and postnatally in the infant If titer <1,000 virus; rate, 2% If titer ≥10,000; rate up to 25%	Routine maternal screening advised; if exposed, test every 3 months	Anti-retro-viral chemoprophylaxis available for exposures, postnatal chemoprophylaxis for HIV + mothers and their infants Standard precautions
Influenza	Sneezing, coughing, respiratory tract secretions	No congenital syndrome: influenza in mother could cause hypoxia in fetus	Rare	None	TIV for all pregnant women during influenza season to decrease risk of hospitalizations for cardio pulmonary complications in mother No risk if exposed to individuals who received live attenuated influenza vaccine (LAIV) Droplet precautions Add contact precautions for young infants

(From [240])

[a]Congenital syndrome: Varying combinations of jaundice, hepatosplenomegaly, microcephaly, thrombocytopenia, anemia, retinopathy, skin and bone lesions

[b]Live virus vaccine given before or after pregnancy.

VDRL, Venereal Disease research laboratory test; RPR, rapid plasma reagin test; FTA-ABS, Fluorescent Treponema Antigen-Antibody test.

hospitals should follow the manufacturer's recommendation to restrict exposure [62].

REFERENCES

1. Lewis DB, Wilson CB. Developmental immunology and role of host defenses in fetal and neonatal susceptibility to infection. In: Remington JS, Klein JO, Baker C, Wilson CB, eds. *Infectious diseases of the fetus and newborn infant.* 6th edition. Philadelphia: WB Saunders, 2005:87–210.
2. National Nosocomial Infections Surveillance (NNIS). NNIS System Report, data summary from January 1992 through June 2004, issued October 2004. *Am J Infect Control* 2004;32:470–85.
3. Gaynes RP, Martone WJ, Culver DH, et al. Comparison of rates of nosocomial infections in neonatal intensive care units in the United States. *Am J Med* 1991;91(suppl 3B):192S–96S.
4. Gaynes RP, Edwards JR, Jarvis WR, et al. Nosocomial infections among neonates in high-risk nurseries in the United States. *Pediatrics* 1996;98:357–61.
5. Sohn AH, Garrett DO, Sinkowitz-Cochran RL, et al. Prevalence of nosocomial infections in neonatal intensive care unit patients: Results from the first national point-prevalence survey. *J Pediatr* 2001;139(6):821–27.
6. Stoll BJ, Hansen N. Infections in VLBW infants: Studies from the NICHD neonatal research network. *Semin Perinatol* 2003;27:293–301.
7. Fridkin SK, Kaufman D, Edwards JR, et al. Changing incidence of Candida bloodstream infections among NICU patients in the United States:1995–2004. *Pediatrics* 2006;117:1680–87.
8. Aziz K., McMillan DD, Andrews W, et al. Variation in rates of nosocomial infection among Canadian neonatal intensive care units may be practice-related. *BMC Pediatrics* 2005;5:22.
9. Kilbride HW, Powers R, Wirstschafter DD, et al. Evaluation and development of potentially better practices to prevent neonatal nosocomial bacteremia. *Pediatrics* 2003;111:e504–18.
10. Kilbride HW, Wirstschafter DD, Powers R, Sheehan MB. Implementation of evidence-based potentially better practices decrease nosocomial infections. *Pediatrics* 2003;111:e519–33.
11. Horbar JD, Plsek PE, Schriefer JA, and Leahy K. Evidence-based quality improvement in neonatal and perinatal medicine: The neonatal intensive care quality improvement collaborative experience. *Pediatrics* 2006;118(suppl 2):S57–64.
12. Adams WG, Kinney JS, Schuchat A, et al. Outbreak of early onset group B streptococcal sepsis. *Pediatr Infect Dis J* 1993;12:675–70.
13. Ledger WJ. Complications associated with invasive monitoring. *Semin Perinatol* 1978;2:187–94.
14. Rubenstein AD, Fowler RN. Salmonellosis of the newborn with transmission by delivery room resuscitators. *Am J Public Health* 1955;45:1109–14.
15. Fierer J, Taylor PM, Gerzon HM. *Pseudomonas aeruginosa* epidemic traced to delivery-room resuscitators. *N Engl J Med* 1967;276:991–96.
16. Melamed R, Greenberg D, Porat N, et al. Successful control of an *Acinetobacter baumanni* outbreak in a neonatal intensive care unit. *J Hosp Infect* 2003;53:31–38.
17. Khan MA, Abdur-Rab M, Israr N, et al. Transmission of *Salmonella worthington* by oropharyngeal suction in hospital neonatal unit. *Pediatr Infect Dis J* 1991;10:668–72.
18. Isenberg HD, Tucci V, Lipsitz P, Facklam RR. Clinical laboratory and epidemiological investigations of a *Streptococcus pyogenes* cluster epidemic in a newborn nursery. *J Clin Microbiol* 1984;19:366–70.
19. Couto RC, Pedrosa TM, Tupinambas U, Rezende NA. The effect of post-discharge surveillance and control strategies on the course of a *Staphylococcus aureus* outbreak in a newborn nursery. *Braz J Infect Dis* 2000;4:296–300.
20. Garner JS, Jarvis WR, Emori TG, et al. CDC definitions for nosocomial infections 1988. *Am J Infect Control* 1988;16:128–40.
21. Pottinger JM, Herwaldt LA, Perl TM. Basics of surveillance—An overview. *Infect Control Hosp Epidemiol* 1997;18(7):513–27.
22. Haley RW. The scientific basis for using surveillance and risk factor data to reduce nosocomial infection rates. *J Hosp Infect* 1995;30(suppl):3–14.
23. Pollack MM, Koch MA, Bartel DA, et al. A comparison of neonatal mortality risk prediction models in very low birth weight infants. *Pediatrics* 2000;105:1051–57.
24. Gray JE, Richardson DK, McCormick MC, et al. Coagulase-negative staphylococcal bacteremia among very low birthweight infants: Relation to admission illness severity, resource use, and outcome. *Pediatrics* 1995;95:225–30.
25. Griffin MP and Moorman R. Toward the early diagnosis of neonatal sepsis and sepsis-like illness using novel heart rate analysis. *Pediatrics* 2001;107:97–104.
26. Haley RW, Cushion NB, Tenover FC, et al. Eradication of endemic methicillin-resistant *Staphylococcus aureus* infections from a neonatal intensive care unit. *J Infect Dis* 1995;171:614–24.
27. Trofino J. JCAHO nursing standards, nursing care hours and LOS per DRG: Part I. *Nurse Manager* 1986;17:19–24.
28. van der Zwet WC, Kaiser AM, van Elburg RM, et al. Nosocomial infections in a Dutch neonatal intensive care unit: Surveillance study with definitions for infection specifically adapted for neonates. *J Hosp Infect* 2005;61:300–11.
29. St. Geme JW III, Bell LM, Baumgart S, et al. Distinguishing sepsis from blood culture contamination in young infants with blood cultures growing coagulase-negative staphylococci. *Pediatrics* 1990;86:157–62.
30. Schelonka RL, Chai MK, Yoder BA, et al. Volume of blood required to detect common neonatal pathogens. *J Pediatr* 1996;129:275–78.
31. Jawaheer G, Neal TJ, Shaw NJ. Blood culture volume and detection of coagulase negative staphylococcal septicaemia in neonates. *Arch Dis Child* 1997;76:F57–58
32. Struthers S, Underhill H, Albersheim S, et al. A comparison of two versus one blood culture in the diagnosis and treatment of coagulase negative staphylococcus in the neonatal intensive care unit. *J Perinatol* 2002;22:547–49.
33. Garcia-Prats JA, Cooper TR, Schneider VF, et al. Rapid detection of microorganisms in blood cultures of newborn infants utilizing an automated blood culture system. *Pediatrics* 2000;105:523–27.
34. Kumar Y, Quinibi M, Neal TJ, Yoxall CW. Time to positivity of neonatal blood cultures. *Arch Dis Child Fetal Neonatal Ed* 2001;85:F182–86.
35. Engle WD, Rosenfeld CR, Mouzinho A, et al. Circulating neutrophils in septic preterm neonates: Comparison of two reference ranges. *Pediatrics* 1997;99:e10–16.
36. Madan A, Adams MM, Philip AGS. Frequency and timing of symptoms in infants screened for sepsis: Effectiveness of a sepsis screening pathway. *Clinical Pediatrics* 2003;42:11–18.
37. Jarvis WR, Robles B. Nosocomial infections in pediatric patients. *Adv Pediatr Infect Dis* 1996;12:243–59.
38. Vain NE, Mazglumian JR, Swarner W, et al. Role of exchange transfusion in treatment of severe septicemia. *Pediatrics* 1980;66:693–97.
39. Cairo MS, Worcester CC, Rucker RW, et al. Randomized trial of granulocyte transfusions versus intravenous immune globulin therapy for neonatal neutropenia and sepsis. *J Pediatr* 1992;120:281–85.
40. Christensen RD, Brown MS, Hall DC, et al. Effect on neutrophil kinetics and serum opsonic capacity of intravenous administration of immune globulin to neonates with clinical signs of early-onset sepsis. *J Pediatr* 1991;118:606–14.
41. Baker CJ, Melish ME, Hall RT, et al. Intravenous immune globulin for the prevention of nosocomial infection in low-birth-weight neonates. *N Engl J Med* 1992;327:213–19.
42. Fanaroff AA, Korones SB, Wright LL, et al. A controlled trial of intravenous immune globulin to reduce nosocomial infections in very-low-birth-weight infants. *N Engl J Med* 1994;330:1107–13.
43. Gillan ER, Christensen RD, Suen Y, et al. A randomized, placebo-controlled trial of recombinant human granulocyte colony-stimulating factor administration in newborn infants with presumed sepsis: Significant induction of peripheral and bone marrow neutrophilia. *Blood* 1994;84:1427–33.
44. Weisman LE, Cruess DF, Fisher GW. Standard versus hyperimmune intravenous immunoglobulin in preventing or treating neonatal bacterial infections. *Clin Perinatol* 1993;20:211–24.
45. Bloom B, Schelonka R, Kueser T, et al. Multicenter study to assess safety and efficacy of INH-A21, a donor-selected human

staphylococcal immunoglobulin for prevention of nosocomial infections in very low birth weight infants. *PIDJ* 2005;10:858–66.

46. Benjamin DK, Schelonka R, White R, et al. A blinded, randomized, multicenter study of an intravenous *Staphylococcus aureus* immune globulin. *J Perinatol* 2006;26:290–95.

47. Goldmann DA. Bacterial colonization and infection in the neonate. *Am J Med* 1981;70:417–22.

48. Edwards WH, Conner JM, Soll RF. The effect of prophylactic ointment therapy on nosocomial sepsis rates and skin integrity in infants with birth weights of 501 to 1000 g. *Pediatrics* 2004;113:1195–1203.

49. Brady MT. Health care-associated infections in the neonatal intensive care unit. *Am J Infect Control* 2005;33:268–75.

50. Graham PL, Begg MD, Larson E, et al. Risk factors for late onset gram-negative sepsis in low birth weight infants hospitalized in the neonatal intensive care unit. *PIDJ* 2006;25:113.

51. Pessoa-Silva CL, Meurer Moreira B, Camara Almeida V, et al. Extended-spectrum beta-lactamase-producing Klebsiella pneumoniae in a neonatal intensive care unit: Risk factors for infection and colonization. *J Hosp Infect* 2003;53:198–206.

52. Feja KN, Wu F, Roberts K, et al. Risk factors for candidemia in critically ill infants: A matched case-control study. *J Pediatr* 2005;147:156–61.

53. Apisarnthanarak A, Holzmann-Pazgal G, Hamvas A, et al. Ventilator-associated pneumonia in extremely preterm neonates in a neonatal intensive care unit: Characteristics, risk factors, and outcomes. *Pediatrics* 2003;112:1283–89.

54. Coffin SE, Bell LM, Manning M, Polin R. Nosocomial infections in neonates receiving extracorporeal membrane oxygenation. *ICHE* 1997;18(2):93–96.

55. CDC. Guidelines for preventing health-care-associated pneumonia, 2003: Recommendations of CDC and the Healthcare Infection Control Practices Advisory Committee (HICPAC). *MMWR* 2004;53(RR-3).

56. Jhung M, Sunenshine R, Noble-Wang J, et al. *Ralstonia* contamination of neonatal oxygen delivery device—United States, 2005. Presented at the 16th annual meeting of the Society for Healthcare Epidemiology of America (SHEA), March 19, 2006, Chicago, Illinois [abstract 21].

57. Bingen E, Denamur E, Lambert-Zechovsky N, et al. Analysis of DNA restriction fragment length polymorphism extends the evidence for breast milk transmission in *Streptococcus agalactiae* late-onset neonatal infection. *J Infect Dis* 1992;165:569–73.

58. El-Mohandes AE, Schatz V, Keiser JF, et al. Bacterial contaminants of collected and frozen human milk used in an intensive care nursery. *Am J Infect Control* 1993;21:226–30.

59. Gastelum DT, Dassey D, Mascola L, Yasuda LM. Transmission of community-associated methicillin-resistant Staphylococcus aureus from breast milk in the neonatal intensive care unit. *PIDJ* 2005;24:1122.

60. Donowitz LG, Marsik FJ, Fisher KA, Wenzel RP. Contaminated breast milk: A source of Klebsiella bacteremia in a newborn intensive care unit. *Rev Infect Dis* 1981;3(4):716–20.

61. Gras-Le Guen C, Lepelletier D, Debillon T, et al. Contamination of a milk bank pasteuriser causing a Pseudomonas aeruginosa outbreak in a neonatal intensive care unit. *Pediatrics* 2006;118:874–81.

62. Committee on Infectious Diseases, American Academy of Pediatrics. 2006 *Redbook: Report of the Committee on Infectious Diseases.* Elk Grove Village, IL: American Academy of Pediatrics, 2006.

63. Stoll BJ, Gordon T, Korones SB, et al. Late-onset sepsis in very low birth weight neonates: A report from the National Institute of Child Health and Human Development Neonatal Research Network. *J Pediatr* 1996;129:63–71.

64. Botas CM, Kurlat I, Young SM, et al. Disseminated candidal infections and intravenous hydrocortisone in preterm infants. *Pediatrics* 1995;95:883–87.

65. Kaempf JW, Campbell B, Sklar RS, et al. Implementing potentially better practices to improve neonatal outcomes after reducing postnatal dexamethasone use in infants born between 501 and 1250 grams. *Pediatrics* 2003;111:e534–41.

66. Guillet R, Stoll BJ, Cotten CM, et al. Association of H2-blocker therapy and higher incidence of necrotizing enterocolitis in very low birth weight infants. *Pediatrics* 2006;117:e137–42.

67. Saiman L, Ludington E, Pfaller M, et al. Risk factors for candidemia in Neonatal Intensive Care Unit patients. The National Epidemiology of Mycosis Survey study group. *PIDJ* 2000;19:319.

68. Cotton CM, McDonald S, Stoll B, et al. The association of third-generation cephalosporin use and invasive candidiasis in extremely low birth-weight infants. *Pediatrics* 2006;118:717–22.

69. Nyqvist KH, Lutes LM. Co-bedding twins: A developmentally supportive care strategy. *J Obstet Gynecol Neonatal Nurs* 1998;27(4):450–56.

70. Conde-Agudelo A, Diaz-Rossello JL, Belizan JM. Kangaroo mother care to reduce morbidity and mortality in low birth-weight infants. *Cochrane Database Syst Rev* 2003(2):CD002771.

71. Davies MW, Mehr S, Garland ST, Morley CJ. Bacterial colonization of toys in neonatal intensive care cots. *Pediatrics* 2000;106(2):e18.

72. Goldmann DA, Durbin WA Jr, Freeman J. Nosocomial infections in a neonatal intensive care unit. *J Infect Dis* 1981; 144(5):449–59.

73. Haley RW, Bregman DA. The role of understaffing and overcrowding in recurrent outbreaks of staphylococcal infection in a neonatal special-care unit. *J Infect Dis* 1982;145(6):875–85.

74. Harbarth S, Sudre P, Dharan S, et al. Outbreak of *Enterobacter cloacae* related to understaffing, overcrowding, and poor hygiene practices. *Infect Control Hosp Epidemiol* 1999;20(9):598–604.

75. Moisiuk SE, Robson D, Klass L, et al. Outbreak of parainfluenza virus type 3 in an intermediate care neonatal nursery. *Pediatr Infect Dis J* 1998;17(1):49–53.

76. Cimiotti JP, Haas J, Saiman L, Larson EL. Impact of staffing on bloodstream infections in the neonatal intensive care unit. *Arch Pediatr Adolesc Med* 2006;160:832–36.

77. White RD. Recommended standards for newborn ICU design. *J Perinatology* 2006;26:S2–18.

78. Harris DD, Shepley MM, Whie RD, et al. The impact of single family room design on patients and caregivers: Executive summary. *J Perinatol* 2006;26:S38–48.

79. Andresen J, Nygaard EA, Stordal K. Primary cutaneous aspergillosis (PCA)—A case report. *Acta Paediatr* 2005;94(6):761–62.

80. CDC. Guidelines for Environmental Infection Control in Health-Care Facilities. Recommendations of CDC and the Healthcare Infection Control Practices Advisory Committee (HICPAC). *MMWR* 2003;52(RR-10):1–42.

81. Fortunov RM, Hulten KG, Hammerman WA, et al. Community-acquired *Staphylococcus aureus* infections in term and near-term previously healthy neonates.

82. Healy CM, Palazzi DL, Edwards MS, et al. Features of invasive staphylococcal disease in neonates. *Pediatrics* 2004;114(4): 953–61.

83. Fraser N, Davies BW, Cusack J. Neonatal omphalitis: A review of its serious complications. *Acta Paediatr* 2006;95:519–22.

84. Rowen JL. Mucocutaneous candidiasis. *Semin perinatol* 2003;27: 406–13.

85. Lin PW and Stoll BJ. Necrotising enterocolitis. *Lancet* 2006;368: 1271–83.

86. Boccia D, Stolfi I, Lana S, Moro ML. Nosocomial necrotizing enterocolitis outbreaks: Epidemiology and control measures. *Eur J Pediatr* 2001;160:385–91.

87. Mooney BR, Green JA, Epstein BJ, et al. Non-gonococcal ophthalmitis associated with erythromycin ointment prophylaxis of gonococcal ophthalmia neonatorium. *Infect Control* 1984;5:138–40.

88. Campbell JR, Arango CA, Garcia-Prats JA, et al. An outbreak of M serotype 1 group A streptococcus in a neonatal intensive care unit. *J Pediatr* 1996;129:396–402.

89. Schroeder SA, Aserkoff B, Brachman PS. Epidemic salmonellosis in hospitals and institutions: A five-year review. *N Engl J Med* 1968;279:674–78.

90. Salzman TC, Scher CD, Moss R. Shigellae with transferable drug resistance: Outbreak in a nursery for premature infants. *J Pediatr* 1967;71:21–26.

91. Vonberg R, Stamm-Balderjahn S, Hansen S, et al. How often do asymptomatic healthcare workers cause methicillin-resistant *Staphylococcus aureus* outbreaks? A systematic evaluation. *Infect Control Hosp Epidemiol* 2006;27:1123–27.

92. Zawacki A, O'Rourke E, Potter-Bynoe G, et al. An outbreak of *Pseudomonas aeruginosa* pneumonia and bloodstream infection associated with intermittent otitis externa in a healthcare worker. *Infect Control Hosp Epidemiol* 2004;25(12):1083–89.

93. Bertin ML, Vinski J, Schmitt S, et al. Outbreak of methicillin resistant *Staphylococcus aureus* colonization and infection in a neonatal intensive care unit linked to a healthcare worker with chronic otitis. *ICHE* 2006;27:581–85.

94. Boszczowski I, Nicoletti C, Puccini DM, et al. Outbreak of extended spectrum beta-lactamase-producing Klebsiella pneumoniae infection in a neonatal intensive care unit related to onychomycosis in a health care worker. *Pediatr Infect Dis J* 2005;24(7):648–50.

95. Foca M, Jakob K, Whittier S, et al. Endemic Pseudomonas aeruginosa infection in a neonatal intensive care unit. *N Engl J Med* 2000;343(10):695–700.

96. Moolenaar RL, Crutcher JM, San Joaquin VH, et al. A prolonged outbreak of Pseudomonas aeruginosa in a neonatal intensive care unit: Did staff fingernails play a role in disease transmission? *Infect Control Hosp Epidemiol* 2000;21(2):80–85.

97. Gupta A, Della-Latta P, Todd B, et al. Outbreak of extended-spectrum beta-lactamase-producing Klebsiella pneumoniae in a neonatal intensive care unit linked to artificial nails. *Infect Control Hosp Epidemiol* 2004;25(3):210–15.

98. Nakashima AK, Allen JR, Martone WJ, et al. Epidemic bullous impetigo in a nursery due to a nasal carrier of *Staphylococcus aureus*: Role of epidemiology and control measures. *Infect Control* 1984;5:326–31.

99. Gladstone IM, Ehrenkranz RA, Edberg SC, et al. A ten-year review of neonatal sepsis and comparison with the previous fifty-year experience. *Pediatr Infect Dis J* 1990;9:819–25.

100. Bizzarro MJ, Raskind C, Baltimore RS, Gallagher PG. Seventy-five years of neonatal sepsis at Yale: 1928–2003. *Pediatrics* 2005;116:595–602.

101. Steere AC, Aber RC, Warford LR, et al. Possible nosocomial transmission of group B streptococci in a newborn nursery. *J Pediatr* 1975;87:784–87.

102. Nambiar S, Singh N. Change in epidemiology of health care-associated infections in a neonatal intensive care unit. *Pediatr Infect Dis J* 2002;21(9):839–42.

103. Schrag SJ, Zywicki S, Farley MM, et al. Group B streptococcal disease in the era of intrapartum antibiotic prophylaxis. *N Engl J Med* 2000;342:15.

104. CDC. Prevention of perinatal group B streptococcal disease: Revised guidelines from CDC. *MMWR* 2002;51(RR-11).

105. CDC. Early-Onset and Late-Onset Neonatal Group B Streptococcal Disease—United States, 1996—2004. *MMWR* 2005;54:1205–8.

106. Stoll BJ, Hansen NI, Higgins RD, et al. Very low birth weight preterm infants with early onset neonatal sepsis. The predominance of gram-negative infections continues in the National Institute of Child Health and Human Development Neonatal Research Network, 2002–2003. *PIDJ* 2005;24:635.

107. Schrag SJ, Stoll BJ. Early-onset sepsis in the era of widespread intrapartum chemoprophylaxis. *PIDJ* 2006;25:939–40.

108. Beck-Sague CM, Azimi P, Fonseca SN, et al. Bloodstream infections in neonatal intensive care unit patients: Results of a multicenter study. *Pediatr Infect Dis J* 1994;13:1110–16.

109. Low DE, Schmidt BK, Kirpalani IIM, et al. An endemic strain of *Staphylococcus haemolyticus* colonizing and causing bacteremia in neonatal intensive care unit patients. *Pediatrics* 1992;89:696–700.

110. Neumeister B, Kastner S, Conrad S, et al. Characterization of coagulase-negative staphylococci causing nosocomial infections in preterm infants. *Eur J Clin Microbiol Infect Dis* 1995;14:856–63.

111. Huebner J, Pier GB, Maslow JN, et al. Endemic nosocomial transmission of *Staphylococcus epidermidis* bacteremia isolates in a neonatal intensive care unit over 10 years. *J Infect Dis* 1994;169:526–31.

112. Lyytikainen O, Saxen H, Rylanen R, et al. Persistence of a multiresistant clone of *Staphylococcus epidermidis* in a neonatal intensive-care unit for a four-year period. *Clin Infect Dis* 1995;20:24–29.

113. Raimundo O, Heussler H, Bruhn JB, et al. Molecular epidemiology of coagulase-negative staphylococcal bacteremia in a newborn intensive care unit. *J Hosp Infect* 2002;51:33–42.

114. Kacia MA, Horgan MJ, Preston KE, et al. Relatedness of coagulase-negative staphylococci causing bacteremia in low-birthweight infants. *Infect Control Hosp Epidemiol* 1994;15:658–62.

115. Nesin M, Projan SJ, Kreisiverth B, et al. Molecular epidemiology of *Staphylococcus epidermidis* blood isolates from neonatal intensive care unit patients. *J Hosp Infect* 1995;31:111–21.

116. Eastick K, Leening JP, Bennet D, et al. Reservoirs of coagulase negative staphylococci in preterm infants. *Arch Dis Child* 1996;74:F99–104.

117. Fleer A, Senders RC, Visser MR, et al. Septicemia due to coagulase-negative staphylococci in a neonatal intensive care unit: Clinical and bacteriological features and contaminated parenteral fluids as a source of sepsis. *Pediatric Infectious Disease* 1983;2:428–31.

118. Hall SL. Coagulase-negative staphylococcal infections in neonates. *Pediatr Infect Dis J* 1991;10:57–67.

119. Patrick CC, Kaplan SR, Baker CJ, et al. Persistent bacteremia due to coagulase-negative staphylococci in low birth weight neonates. *Pediatrics* 1989;84:977–85.

120. Khasu M, Oslovich H, Henry D, et al. Persistent bacteremia and severe thrombocytopenia caused by coaguase negative staphylococcus in a neonatal intensive care unit. *Pediatrics* 2006;117:340–48.

121. Gruskay J, Abbasi S, Anday E, et al. *Staphylococcus epidermidis*-associated enterocolitis. *J Pediatr* 1986;109:520–23.

122. Scheifele DW, Bjornson GL. Delta toxin activity in coagulase-negative staphylococci from the bowels of neonates. *J Clin Microbiol* 1988;26:279–82.

123. Noel GJ, Edelson PJ. *Staphylococcus epidermidis* bacteremia in neonates: further observations and the recurrence of focal infection. *Pediatrics* 1984;74:832–37.

124. Noel GJ, O'Loughlin JE, Edelson PJ. Neonatal *Staphylococcus epidermidis* right-sided endocarditis: Description of five catheterized infants. *Pediatrics* 1988;82:234–39.

125. Karlowicz MG, Furigay PJ, Croitoru DP, Buescher S. Central venous catheter removal versus *in situ* treatment in neonates with coagulase-negative staphylococcal bacteremia. *PIDJ* 2002;21:22–27.

126. Dancer SJ, Simmons NA, Poston SM, et al. Outbreak of staphylococcal scalded skin syndrome among neonates. *J Infect* 1988;16:87–103.

127. Dave J, Reith S, Nash JQ, et al. A double outbreak of exfoliative toxin-producing strains of *Staphylococcus aureus* in a maternity unit. *Epidemiol Infect* 1994;112:103–14.

128. Mackenzie A, Johnson W, Heyes B, et al. A prolonged outbreak of exfoliative toxin A-producing *Staphylococcus aureus* in a newborn nursery. *Diagn Microbiol Infect Dis* 1995;21:69–75.

129. Graham PL, Morel A, Zhou J, et al. Epidemiology of methicillin susceptible *Staphylococcus aureus* in the neonatal intensive care unit. *Infect Control Hosp Epidemiol* 2002;23:677–82.

130. Gerber SI, Jones, RC, Scott MV, et al. Management of outbreaks of methicillin resistant *Staphylococcus aureus* infection in the neonatal intensive care unit: A consensus statement. *Infect Control Hosp Epidemiol* 2006;27:139–45.

131. Jernigan JA, Titus MG, Groschel DH, et al. Effectiveness of contact isolation during a hospital outbreak of methicillin-resistant Staphylococcus aureus. *Am J Epidemiol* 1996;143(5):496–504.

132. Mitsuda T, Arai K, Fujita S, et al. Epidemiological analysis of strains of methicillin-resistant Staphylococcus aureus (MRSA) infection in the nursery: Prognosis of MRSA carrier infants. *J Hosp Infect* 1995;31:123–34.

133. Noel GJ, Kreiswirth BN, Edelson PJ, et al. Multiple methicillin-resistant *Staphylococcus aureus* strains as a cause for a single outbreak of severe disease in hospitalized neonates. *Pediatr Infect Dis J* 1992;11:184–88.

134. Davies EA, Emmerson AM, Hogg GM, et al. An outbreak of infection with a methicillin resistant *Staphylococcus aureus* in a special care baby unit: Value of topical mupiricin and of traditional methods of infection control. *J Hosp Infect* 1987;10:120–28.

135. Hollis RJ, Barr JL, Doebbeling BN, et al. Familial carriage of methicillin-resistant *Staphylococcus aureus* and subsequent infection in a premature neonate. *J Infect Dis* 1995;21:328–32.

136. Al-Tawfiq JA. Father-to-infant transmission of community acquired methicillin resistant *Staphylococcus aureus* in a neonatal intensive care unit. *Infect Control Hosp Epidemiol* 2006;27:636–67.

137. Morel A, Wu F, Della-Latta P, et al. Nosocomial transmission of methicillin resistant *Staphylococcus aureus* from a mother to her preterm quadruplet infants. *Am J Infect Control* 2002;30:170–73.

138. McDougal LK, Steward CD, Killgore GE, et al. Pulsed-field gel electrophoresis typing of oxacillin resistant *Staphylococcus aureus* isolates from the United States: Establishing a national database. *J Clin Microbiol* 2003;41:5113–20.

139. Saiman L, O'Keefe M, Graham PL, et al. Hospital transmission of community-acquired methicillin-resistant Staphylococcus aureus among postpartum women. *Clin Infect Dis* 2003;37(10):1313–19.

140. Eckhardt C, Halvosa JS, Ray SM, Blumberg HM. Transmission of methicillin-resistant Staphylococcus aureus in the neonatal intensive care unit from a patient with community-acquired disease. *Infect Control Hosp Epidemiol* 2003;24(6):460–61.

141. Healy CM, Hulten KG, Palazzi DL, et al. Emergence of new strains of methicillin-resistant Staphylococcus aureus in a neonatal intensive care unit. *Clin Infect Dis* 2004;39(10):1460–66.

142. Laibl VR, Sheffield JS, Roberts S, et al. Clinical presentation of community-acquired methicillin resistant *Staphylococcus aureus* in pregnancy. *Obstet Gynecol* 2005;105:461–65.

143. Chen KT, Huard RC, Della-Latta P, Saiman L. Prevalence of methicillin sensitive and methicillin resistant *Staphylococcus aureus* in pregnant women. *Obstet Gynecol* 2006;108:482–87.

144. Buchino JJ, Ciamberella E, Light I. Systemic group D streptococcal infection in newborn infants. *Am J Dis Child* 1979;133:270–73.

145. Bavikatte K, Schreiner RL, Lemons JA, et al. Group D streptococcal septicemia in the neonate. *American Journal of Diseases of Children* 1979;133:493–96.

146. McNeeley DF, Saint-Louis F, Noel GE. Neonatal enterococcal bacteremia: An increasingly frequent event with potentially untreatable pathogens. *Pediatr Infect Dis J* 1996;15:800–5.

147. Coudron PE, Mayhall CG, Facklam RR, et al. *Streptococcus faecium* outbreak in a neonatal intensive care unit. *J Clin Microbiol* 1984;20:1044–48.

148. Luginbuhl LM, Rotbart HA, Facklan RR, et al. Neonatal enterococcal sepsis: Case–control study and description of an outbreak. *Pediatr Infect Dis J* 1987;6:1022–30.

149. Rupp ME, Marion N, Fey PD, et al. Outbreak of vancomycin resistant *Enterococcus faecium* in a neonatal intensive care unit. *ICHE* 2001;22:301–3.

150. Singh N, Leger M, Campbell J, et al. Control of vancomycin resistant enterococci in the neonatal intensive care unit. *ICHE* 2005;26:646–49.

151. Golan Y, Doron S, Sullivan B, Snydman DR. Transmission of vancomycin resistant enterococcus in a neonatal intensive care unit. *PIDJ* 2005;24:566–67.

152. Ang JY, Lua JL, Turner DR, Asmar BI. Vancomycin-resistant *Enterococcus faecium* endocarditis in a premature infant successfully treated with linezolid. *PIDJ* 2003;22:1101–3.

153. Hervas JA, Ballesteros F, Alomar A, et al. Increase of *Enterobacter* in neonatal sepsis: A twenty-two-year study. *PIDJ* 2001;20:134–40.

154. Linkin DR, Fishman NO, Patel J, et al. Risk factors for extended-spectrum beta-lactamase-producing enterobacteriaceae in a neonatal intensive care unit. *ICHE* 2004;25:781–83.

155. Campbell JR, Zaccaria E, Mason EO Jr, Baker CJ. Epidemiological analysis defining concurrent outbreaks of Serratia marcescens and methicillin-resistant Staphylococcus aureus in a neonatal intensive-care unit. *Infect Control Hosp Epidemiol* 1998;19(12):924–28.

156. David MD, Weller TMA, Lambert P, Fraise AP. An outbreak of *Serratia marcescens* on the neonatal unit: A tale of two clones. *J Hosp Infect* 2006;63:27–33.

157. McNaughton M, Mazinke N, Thomas E. Newborn conjunctivitis associated with triclosan 0.5% antiseptic intrinsically contaminated with *Serratia marcescens*. *Canadian Infect Control* 1995;10:7–8.

158. Fleisch F, Zimmerman-Baer U, Zbinden R, et al. Three consecutive outbreaks of *Serratia marcescens* in a neonatal intensive care unit. *Clin Infect Dis* 2002;34:767–73.

159. Goering RV, Ehrenkranz J, Sanders CC, et al. Long term epidemiological analysis of *Citrobacter diversus* in a neonatal intensive care unit. *Pediatr Infect Dis J* 1992;11:99–104.

160. Kline MW. *Citrobacter* meningitis and brain abscess in infancy: Epidemiology, pathogenesis, and treatment. *J Pediatr* 1988;113:430–34.

161. Lin FC, Devor WF, Morrison C, et al. Outbreak of neonatal *Citrobacter diversus* meningitis in a suburban hospital. *Pediatr Infect Dis J* 1987;6:50–55.

162. Schroeder SA, Aserkoff B, Brachman PS. Epidemic salmonellosis in hospitals and institutions: A five-year review. *N Engl J Med* 1968;279:674–78.

163. Hoque SN, Graham J, Kaufmann ME, Tabaqchali S. *Chryseobacterium (Flavobacterium) meningosepticum* outbreak associated with colonization of water taps in a neonatal intensive care unit. *J Hosp Infect* 2001;47:188–92.

164. Kimura AC, Calvet H, Higa JI, et al. Outbreak of *Ralstonia pickettii* bacteremia in a Neonatal Intensive Care Unit. *PIDJ* 2005;24:1099–1103.

165. Dent A, Toltzis P. Descriptive and molecular epidemiology of gram negative bacilli infections in the neonatal intensive care unit. *Current Opinion in Infect Dis* 2003;16:279–83.

166. de Man P, van der Veeke E, Leemreijze M, et al. *Enterobacter* sp. in a pediatric hospital: Horizontal transfer or selection of individual patients? *J Infect Dis* 2001;184:211–14.

167. Matsaniotis NS, Syriopoulou VP, Theodoridou MC, et al. *Enterobacter* sepsis in infants and children due to contaminated intravenous fluids. *Infect Control* 1984;5:471–77.

168. Di Pentima MC, Mason EO Jr, Kaplan SL. *In vitro* antibiotic synergy against *Flavobacterium meningosepticum*: Implications for therapeutic options. *Clin Infect Dis* 1998;26(5):1169–76.

169. Howard JB, McCracken GH Jr. Reappraisal of kanamycin usage in neonates. *J Pediatr* 1975;86(6):949–56.

170. van der Zwet WC, Parlevliet GA, Savelkoul PH, et al. Nosocomial outbreak of gentamicin-resistant *Klebsiella pneumoniae* in a neonatal intensive care unit controlled by a change in antibiotic policy. *J Hosp Infect* 1999;42(4):295–302.

171. Bryan CS, John JF Jr, Pai MS, Austin TL. Gentamicin vs cefotaxime for therapy of neonatal sepsis. Relationship to drug resistance. *Am J Dis Child* 1985;139(11):1086–89.

172. Acolet D, Ahmet Z, Houang E, et al. *Enterobacter cloacae* in a neonatal intensive care unit: Account of an outbreak and its relationship to use of third generation cephalosporins. *J Hosp Infect* 1994;28(4):273–86.

173. CDC. Preventing Tetanus, diphtheria, and pertussis among adults: Use of tetanus toxoid, reduced diphtheria toxoid and acellular pertussis vaccine: recommendations of the Advisory Committee on Immunization Practices (ACIP) and Recommendation of ACIP, supported by the Healthcare Infection Control Practices Advisory Committee (HICPAC), for use of Tdap among health-care personnel. *MMWR* 2006;55:(RR-17).

174. Bryant KA, Humbaugh K, Brothers K, et al. Measures to control an outbreak of pertussis in a neonatal intermediate care nursery after exposure to a healthcare worker. *ICHE* 2006;27:541–45.

175. Bamberger E, Starets-Haham O, Greenberg D, et al. Adult pertussis is hazardous for the newborn. *ICHE* 2006;27:623–25.

176. Shah S, Caprio M, Mally P, Hendricks-Munoz K. Rationale for the administration of acellular pertussis vaccine to parents of infants in the neonatal intensive care unit. *J Perinatol* 2007;27:1–3.

177. Donta ST, Myers MG. Clostridium difficile toxin in asymptomatic neonates. *J Pediatr* 1982;100(3):431–34.

178. Parsons SJ, Fenton E, Dargaville P. Clostridium difficile associated severe enterocolitis A feature of Hirschsprung's disease in a neonate presenting late. *J Paediatr Child Health* 2005;41:689–90.

179. Beck-Sague CM, Jarvis WR. National Nosocomial Infections Surveillance System: Secular trends in the epidemiology of nosocomial fungal infections in the United States, 1980–1990. *J Infect Dis* 1993;167:1247–51.

180. Stamos JK, Rowley AH. Candidemia in a pediatric population. *Clin Infect Dis* 1995;20:571–75.

181. Fridkin SK, Kaufman D, Edwards JR, et al. Changing incidence of *Candida* bloodstream infections among NICU patients in the United States: 1995–2004. *Pediatrics* 2006;117:1680–87.

182. Baley JE, Kliegman RM, Fanaroff AA. *Pediatrics* 1984;73:144–52.

183. Weese-Mayer DE, Fondriest DW, Brouillette RT, et al. Risk factors associated with candidemia in the neonatal intensive care unit: A case-control study. *Pediatr Infect Dis J* 1987;6:190–96.

184. Shetty SS, Harrison LH, Hajjeh RA, et al. Determining risk factors for candidemia among newborn infants from population-based surveillance: Baltimore, Maryland, 1998–2000. *PIDJ* 2005;24:601–4.

185. Feja KN, Wu F, Roberts K, et al. Risk factors for candidemia in critically ill infants: A matched case-control study. *J Pediatrics* 2005;147:156–61.

186. Manzoni P, Farina D, Leonessa M, et al. Risk factors for progression to invasive fungal infection in preterm neonates with fungal colonization. *Pediatrics* 2006;118:2359–64.

187. Baley JE, Kliegman RM, Boxerbaum B, et al. Fungal colonization in the very low birthweight infant. *Pediatrics* 1986;78:225–32.

188. Saxen H, Virtanen M, Carlson P, et al. Neonatal *Candida parapsilosis* outbreak with a high case fatality rate. *Pediatr Infect Dis J* 1995;14:776–81.

189. Welbel SF, McNeil MM, Kuykendall RJ, et al. *Candida parapsilosis* bloodstream infections in neonatal intensive care unit patients: Epidemiologic and laboratory confirmation of a common source outbreak. *Pediatr Infect Dis J* 1996;15:998–1002.

190. Lupetti A, Tavanti A, Davini P, et al. Horizontal transmission of *Candida parapsilosis* candidemia in a neonatal intensive care unit. *J Clin Microbiol* 2002;40:2363–69.

191. Sheretz RJ, Gledhill KS, Hampton KD, et al. Outbreak of *Candida* bloodstream infections associated with retrograde medication administration in a neonatal intensive care unit. *J Pediatr* 1992;120:455–61.

192. Betremieux P, Chevrier S, Quindos G, et al. Use of DNA fingerprinting and biotyping methods to study a *Candida albicans* outbreak in a neonatal intensive care unit. *Pediatr Infect Dis J* 1994;13:899–05.

193. Marco F, Lockhart SR, Pfaller MA, et al. Elucidating the origins of nosocomial infections with *Candida albicans* by DNA fingerprinting with the complex probe Ca3. *J Clin Microbiol* 1999;37:2817–28.

194. Finkelstein R, Reinhertz G, Hashman N, et al. Outbreak of *Candida tropicalis* fungemia in a neonatal intensive care unit. *Infect Control Hosp Epidemiol* 1993;14:587–90.

195. Long SS, Stevenson DK. Reducing *Candida* infections during neonatal intensive care: Management choices, infection control, and fluconazole prophylaxis. *J Pediatrics* 2005;147:135–40.

196. Baley JE, Silverman RA. Systemic candidiasis: Cutaneous manifestations in low birth weight infants. *Pediatrics* 1988;82:211–15.

197. Chapman RL, Faix RG. Persistently positive cultures and outcome in invasive neonatal candidiasis. *PIDJ* 2000;19:822–27.

198. Mayayo E, Moralejo J, Camps J, et al. Fungal endocarditis in premature infants. Case report and review. *Clin Infect Dis* 1996;22:366–68.

199. Levy I, Shalit I, Birk E, et al. *Candida* endocarditis in neonates: Report of five cases and review of the literature. *Mycoses* 2006;49:43–48.

200. Papouli E, Roilides E, Bibashi E, et al. Primary cutaneous aspergillosis in neonates: Case report and review. *Clin Infect Dis* 1996;22:1102–04.

201. Frankenbusch K, Eifinger F, Kribs A, et al. Severe primary cutaneous aspergillosis refractory to amphotericin B and the successful treatment with systemic voriconazole in two premature infants with extremely low birth weight. *J Perinatol* 2006;26:511–14.

202. Stuart SM, Lane AT. *Candida* and *Malassezia* as nursery pathogens. *Semin Dermatol* 1992;11:19–23.

203. Chang HJ, Miller HL, Watkins N, et al. An epidemic of *Malassezia pachydermatis* in an intensive care nursery associated with colonization of healthcare workers' pet dogs. *NEJM* 1998;338:706–11.

204. Mitchell SJ, Gray J, Morgan MEI, et al. Nosocomial infection with *Rhizopus microsporus* in preterm infants: Association with wooden tongue depressors. *Lancet* 1996;348:441–43.

205. Fisher DJ, Christy C, Spafford P, et al. Neonatal *Trichosporon beigelii* infection: Report of a cluster of cases in a neonatal intensive care unit. *Pediatr Infect Dis J* 1993;12:149–55.

206. Faden H, Wynn RJ, Campagna L, Ryan RM. Outbreak of adenovirus type 30 in a neonatal intensive care unit. *J Pediatrics* 2005;146:523–27.

207. Agah R, Cherry JD, Garakian AJ, et al. Respiratory syncytial virus (RSV) infection rate in personnel caring for children with RSV infections. *American Journal of Diseases of Children* 1987;141:695–97.

208. Rotbart HA, Levin MJ, Yolken RH, et al. An outbreak of rotavirus-associated neonatal necrotizing enterocolitis. *J Pediatr* 1983;103:454–59.

209. Finn A, Anday E, Talbot GH. An epidemic of adenovirus 7a infection in a neonatal nursery: Course morbidity and management. *Infect Control Hosp Epidemiol* 1988;9:398–404.

210. Hall CB. Nosocomial respiratory syncytial virus infections: The "Cold War" has not ended. *Clin Infect Dis* 2000;31(2):590–96.

211. Maltezou HC, Drancourt M. Nosocomial influenza in children. *J Hosp Infect* 2003;55(2):83–91.

212. Halasa NB, Williams V, Wilson GJ, et al. Medical and economic impact of a respiratory syncytial virus outbreak in a neonatal intensive care unit. *PIDJ* 2005;24:1040–44.

213. Piedra PA. Adenovirus in the neonatal intensive care unit: Formidable, forgotten foe. *J Pediatrics* 2005;146:447–48.

214. Modlin JF. Perinatal echovirus infection: Insights from a literature review of 61 cases of serious infection and 16 outbreaks in nurseries. *Rev Infect Dis* 1986;8:918–26.

215. Watson JC, Fleming DW, Borella AJ, et al. Vertical transmission of hepatitis A resulting in an outbreak in a neonatal intensive care unit. *J Infect Dis* 1993;167:567–71.

216. Rosenblum LS, Villarino ME, Nainan OV, et al. Hepatitis A outbreak in a neonatal intensive care unit: Risk factors for transmission and evidence of prolonged viral excretion among preterm infants. *J Infect Dis* 1991;164:476–82.

217. Azimi PH, Roberto RR, Guralnik J, et al. Transfusion-acquired hepatitis A in a premature infant with secondary nosocomial spread in an intensive care nursery. *Am J Dis Children* 1986;140:23–27.

218. Brady MT, Demmler GJ, Reis S. Factors associated with cytomegalovirus excretion in hospitalized children. *Am J Infect Control* 1988;16:41–45.

219. Balcarek KB, Bagley R, Cloud GA, et al. Cytomegalovirus infection among employees of a children's hospital: No evidence for increased risk associated with patient care. *JAMA* 1990;263:840–44.

220. Siegel J, Gall SA. The pregnant healthcare worker. In: Carrico R et al. eds. *APIC text of infection control and epidemiology*. 2nd ed. Washington DC 2005:1–13.

221. Hammerberg O, Watts J, Chernesky M, et al. An outbreak of herpes simplex virus type 1 in an intensive care nursery. *Ped Infect Dis* 1983;2:290–94.

222. Light IJ. Postnatal acquisition of herpes simplex virus by the newborn infant: A review of the literature. *Pediatrics* 1979;63:480–82.

223. Friedman CA, Temple DM, Robbins KK, et al. Outbreak and control of varicella in a neonatal intensive care unit. *Pediatr Infect Dis J* 1994;13:152–54.

224. Mouchet F, Hansen V, Van Herreweghe I, et al. Tuberculosis in healthcare workers caring for a congenitally infected infant. *ICHE* 2004;25:1062–66.

225. Heyns L, Gie RP, Goussard P, et al. Nosocomial transmission of *Mycobacterium tuberculosis* in kangaroo mother care units: A risk in tuberculosis-endemic areas. *Acta Paediatrica* 2006;95:535–39.

226. Nicholas NB, Gayer M, Frieden TR, Fujiwara PI. A continuing outbreak of multi-drug resistant tuberculosis, with transmission in a hospital nursery. *Clin Infect Dis* 1998;26:303–7.

227. Sen M, Gregson D, Lewis J. Neonatal exposure to active pulmonary tuberculosis in a health care professional. *CMAJ* 2005;172:1453–56.

228. CDC. *Mycobacterium tuberculosis* transmission in a newborn nursery and maternity ward—New York City, 2003. *MMWR* 2005;54:1280–83.

229. Berkowitz FE, Severens JL, Blumberg HM. Exposure to tuberculosis among newborns in a nursery: Decision analysis for initiation of prophylaxis. *ICHE* 2006;27:604–11.

230. Bradley JS, Nelson JD. *2006–2007 Nelson's Pocket Book of Pediatric Antimicrobial Therapy*. 16th ed. Buenos Aires, Argentina: Association for Health Research and Development, 2006.

231. Clark RH, Bloom BT, Spitzer AR, Gerstmann DR. Empiric use of ampicillin and cefotaxime, compared with ampicillin and gentamicin, for neonates at risk for sepsis is associated with an increased risk of neonatal death. *Pediatrics* 2006;117:67–74.

232. Rubin LG, Sanchez PJ, Siegel JD, et al. Evaluation and treatment of neonates with suspected late onset sepsis: A survey of neonatologists' practices. *Pediatrics* 2002;110(4):e42.

233. Van Houten MA, Uiterwaal C, Heesen G, et al. Does the empiric use of vancomycin in pediatrics increase the risk for gram-negative bacteremia? *PIDJ* 2001;20:171–77.

234. Heusser, MF, Patterson JE, Kuritza AP, et al. Emergence of resistance to multiple beta-lactams in *Enterobacter cloacae* during treatment for neonatal meningitis with cefotaxime. *Pediatr Infect Dis J* 1990;9:509–12.

235. Fink S, Karp W, Robertson A. Ceftriaxone effect on bilirubin-albumin binding. *Pediatrics* 1987;80:873–75.

236. McCracken GH, Siegel JD, Threlkeld N, et al. Pharmacokinetics of ceftriaxone in newborn infants. *Antimicrob Agents Chemother* 1983;23:341–43.

237. Stoll BJ, Hansen N, Fanaroff AA, et al. To tap or not to tap: High likelihood of meningitis without sepsis among very low birth weight infants. *Pediatrics* 2004;113:1181–86.

238. Garges HP, Moody A, Cotton CM, et al. Neonatal meningitis: What is the correlation among cerebrospinal fluid cultures, blood cultures, and cerebrospinal fluid parameters? *Pediatrics* 2006;117:1094–1100.

239. Sarvikivi E, Lyytikainen O, Soll DR, et al. Emergence of fluconazole resistance in a *Candida parapsilosis* strain that caused infections in a neonatal intensive care unit. *J Clin Microbiol* 2005;43:2729–35.

240. Steinbach WJ, Benjamin DK. New antifungal agents under development in children and neonates. *Curr Opin Infect Dis* 2005;18:484–89.

241. Odio CM, Araya R, Pinto LE, et al. Caspofungin therapy of neonates with invasive candidiasis. *PIDJ* 2004;23:1093–97.

242. Natarajan G, Lulic-Botica M, Rongkavilit C, et al. Experience with caspofungin in the treatment of persistent fungemia in neonates. *J Perinatol* 2005;25:770–77.

243. Heresi GP, Gerstmann DR, Reed MD, et al. The pharmacokinetics and safety of micafungin, a novel echinocandin, in premature infants. *PIDJ* 2006;25:1110–15.

244. Kimberlin DW, Lin CY, Sanchez PJ, et al. Effect of ganciclovir therapy on hearing in symptomatic congenital cytomegalovirus disease involving the central nervous system: A randomized, controlled trial. *J Pediatr* 2003;143:16–25.

245. Jafri HS. Treatment of respiratory syncytial virus: Antiviral therapies. *PIDJ* 2003;22(suppl):S89–93.

246. American Academy of Pediatrics Committee on Fetus and Newborn, American College of Obstetrics and Gynecology Committee on Obstetrics. *Guidelines for perinatal care*. 5th ed. Elk Grove Village, IL: American Academy of Pediatrics 2002;24:331–53.

247. White RD. Recommended standards for newborn ICU design. *J Perinatol* 2006;26(suppl):S2–S18.

248. Gaynes R, Richards C, Edwards J, et al. Feeding back surveillance data to prevent hospital-acquired infections. *Emerg Infect Dis* 2001;7(2):295–98.

249. Benneyan JC, Lloyd RC, Plsek PE. Statistical process control as a tool for research and healthcare improvement. *Qual Saf Health Care* 2003;12(6):458–64.

250. Management of multi-drug resistant organisms (MDROs) in Healthcare Settings, 2006 (www.cdc.gov/ncidod/dhqp/pdf/ar/mdroGuideline2006.pdf) posted 19 October 2006.

251. Dawson SJ. The role of the infection control link nurse. *J Hosp Infect* 2003;54(4):251–57.

252. Wright J, Stover BH, Wilkerson S, Bratcher D. Expanding the infection control team: Development of the infection control liaison position for the neonatal intensive care unit. *Am J Infect Control* 2002;30(3):174–78.

253. Lee PYC, Holliman RE, Davis EG. Surveillance cultures on neonatal intensive care units. *J Hosp Infect* 1995;29:233–37.

254. Evans ME, Schaffner W, Federspiel CF, et al. Sensitivity, specificity, and predictive value of body surface cultures in a neonatal intensive care unit. *JAMA* 1988;259:248–52.

255. Garner JS. The Hospital Infection Control Practices Advisory Committee: Guideline for isolation precautions in hospitals. *Infect Control Hosp Epidemiol* 1996;17:54–80.

256. Jernigan JA, Titus MG, Groschel DHM, et al. Effectiveness of contact isolation during a hospital outbreak of methicillin-resistant *Staphylococcus aureus*. *Am J Epidemiol* 1996;143:496–504.

257. Coovadia YM, Johnson AP, Bhana RH, et al. Multiresistant *Klebsiella pneumoniae* in a neonatal nursery: The importance of maintenance of infection control policies and procedures in the prevention of outbreaks. *J Hosp Infect* 1992;22:197–205.

258. CDC. Guideline for hand hygiene in health-care settings: Recommendations of the Healthcare Infection Control Practices Advisory Committee and the HICPAC/SHEA/APIC/IDSA Hand Hygiene Task Force. *MMWR* 2002;51(16)(RR-16):1–44.

259. Cloney DL, Donowitz LG. Overgrown use for infection control in nurseries and neonatal intensive care units. *Am J Dis Children* 1986;140:680–83.

260. Pelke S, Ching D, Easa D, et al. Gowning does not affect colonization of infection rates in a neonatal intensive care unit. *Arch Pediatr Adolesc Med* 1994;148:1016–20.

261. Strausbaugh LJ, Siegel JD, Weinstein RA. Preventing transmission of multidrug-resistant bacteria in health care settings: A tale of 2 guidelines. *Clin Infect Dis* 2006;42(6):828–35.

262. Mullany LC., Darmstadt GL, Tielsch JM. Role of antimicrobial applications to the umbilical cord in neonates to prevent bacterial colonization and infection: A review of the evidence. *PIDJ* 2003;22:996–1002.

263. Zupan J, Garner P, Omari AAA. Topical umbilical cord care at birth. *Cochrane Database of Systematic Reviews* 2004;3:CD001057.

264. Cookson BD. The emergence of mupiricin resistance: A challenge to infection control and antibiotic prescribing practice. *J Antimicrobials Chemother* 1998;41:11–18.

265. CDC. Guidelines for the prevention of intravascular catheter-related infections. *MMWR* 2002;51(10)(RR-10):1–26.

266. Foo R, Fujii A, Harris J, et al. Complications in tunneled CVL versus PICC lines in very low birthweight infants. *J Perinatol* 2001;21:525–30.

267. Mahieu LM, DeDooy JJ, Lenaerts AE, et al. Catheter manipulations and the risk of catheter-associated bloodstream infection in neonatal intensive care unit patients. *J Hops Infect* 2001;48:20–26.

268. Garland JS, Alex, CP, Mueller CD, et al. A randomized trial comparing povidone-iodine to a chlorhexidine gluconate-impregnated dressing for prevention of central venous catheter infections in neonates. *Pediatrics* 2001;107:1431–36.

269. Garland JS, Alex CP, Hendrickson KJ, et al. A vancomycin-heparin lock solution for prevention of nosocomial bloodstream infection in critically ill neonates with peripherally inserted central venous catheters: A prospective, randomized trial. *Pediatrics* 2005;116:e198–205.

270. Butler-O'Hara M, Buzzard CJ, Reubens L, et al. A randomized trial comparing long-term and short-term use of umbilical venous catheters in premature infants with birth weights of less than 1251 grmas. *Pediatrics* 2006;118:e25–35.

271. Curley M, Schwalenstocker E, Deshpande JK, et al. Tailoring the Institute for Health Care Improvement 100,000 lives campaign to pediatric settings: The example of ventilator-associated pneumonia. *Pediatr Clinics NA* 2006;53:1231–51.

272. Loukil C, Saizou C, Doit C, et al. Epidemiologic investigation of *Burkholderia cepacia* acquisition in two pediatric intensive care units. *ICHE* 2003;24:707–10.

273. Committee on Infectious Diseases and Committee on Fetus and Newborn. Revised indications for the use of palivizumab and respiratory syncytial virus immune globulin intravenous for the prevention of respiratory syncytial virus infections. *Pediatrics* 2003;112:1442–46.

274. Stevens TP, Hall CB. Controversies in palivizumab use. *PIDJ* 2004;25:1151–52.

275. Wu S-Y, Bonaparte J, Pyati S. Palivizumab use in very premature infants in the neonatal intensive care unit. *Pediatrics* 2004;114:e554–56.

276. Abadesso C, Almeida HI, Virella D, et al. Use of palivizumab to control an outbreak of syncytial respiratory virus in a neonatal intensive care unit. *J Hosp Infect* 2004;58:38–41.

277. CDC. A new product (VariZIG™) for postexposure prophylaxis of varicella available under an investigational new drug application expanded access protocol. *MMWR* 2006;55:209–10.

278. Lipton SV, Brunel PA. Management of varicella exposure in a neonatal intensive care unit. *JAMA* 1989;261:1782–84.

279. Spafford PS, Sinkin RA, Cox C, et al. Prevention of central venous catheter-related coagulase-negative staphylococcal sepsis in neonates. *J Pediatr* 1994;125:259–63.

280. Kacia MA, Horgan MJ, Ochoa L, et al. Prevention of gram-positive sepsis in neonates weighing less than 1500 grams. *J Pediatr* 1994;125:253–58.

281. Barefield ES, Philips JB. Vancomycin prophylaxis for coagulase-negative staphylococcal bacteremia. *J Pediatr* 1994;125:230–32.

282. Harms K, Herting E, Iron M, et al. Randomized, controlled trial of amoxicillin prophylaxis for prevention of catheter-related infections in newborn infants with central venous silicone elastomer catheters. *J Pediatr* 1995;127:615–19.

283. Fanaroff AA. Fluconazole for the prevention of fungal infections: Get ready, get set, caution. *Pediatrics* 2006;117:214–15.

284. Kaufman D, Boyle R, Hazen KC, et al. Twice weekly fluconazole prophylaxis for prevention of invasive *Candida* infection in high-risk infants of <1000 grams birth weight. *J Pediatr* 2005; 147:172–79.

285. Healy CM, Baker CJ, Zaccaria E, et al. Impact of fluconazole on incidence and outcome of invasive candidiasis in a neonatal intensive care unit. *J Pediatr* 2005;147:166–71.

286. Kerrini G, Perugi S, Dani C, et al. Fluconazole prophylaxis prevents invasive fungal infection in high-risk, very low birth weight infants. *J Pediatr* 2005;147:162–65.

287. Manzoni P, Arisio R, Mostert M, et al. Prophylactic fluconazole is effective in preventing fungal colonization and fungal systemic infections in preterm neonates: A single-center, 6 year, retrospective cohort study. *Pediatrics* 2006;117:e22–32.

288. Uko S, Soghier LM, Vega M, et al. Targeted short-term fluconazole prophylaxis among very low birth weight and extremely low birth weight infants. *Pediatrics* 2006;117:1243–52.

289. Kicklighter SD, Springer SC, Cox T, et al. Fluconazole for prophylaxis against candidal rectal colonization in the very low birth weight infant. *Pediatrics* 2001;107:293–98.

290. Kaufman D, Boyle R, Hazen KC, et al. Twice weekly fluconazole prophylaxis against fungal colonization and infection in preterm infants. *NEJM* 2001;345:1660–66.

291. Renaud MT. Parental response to family centered maternity care and the implementation of sibling visit. *Mil Med* 1981;146:850–52.

292. Wranesh BL. The effect of sibling visitation on bacterial colonization rate in neonates. *JOGN Nurse* 1982;11:211–13.

293. Umphenour JH. Bacterial colonization in neonates with sibling visitation. *JOGN Nurse* 1980;9:73–75.

294. Schwab F. Sibling visiting in a neonatal intensive care unit. *Pediatrics* 1983;71:835–38.

295. CDC. Influenza vaccination of healthcare personnel: Recommendations of the Healthcare Infection Control Advisory Committee (HICPAC) and the Advisory Committee on Immunization Practices (ACIP). *MMWR* 2005;55(RR-2).

296. Talbot T, Crocker DD, Peters J, et al. Duration of viral shedding after trivalent intranasal live attenuated influenza vaccination in adults. *ICHE* 2005;26:494.

297. Bolyard EA, Tablan OC, Williams WW, et al. Guideline for infection control in healthcare personnel, 1998. Hospital Infection Control Practices Advisory Committee. *Infect Control Hosp Epidemiol* 1998;19(6):407–63.

298. American Institute of Architects. 2006 Guidelines for design and construction of health care facilities (www.aia.org/aah_gd_hospcons).

The Operating Room

26

Joan Blanchard and Nancy Chobin

The perioperative setting has changed in healthcare facilities as regulatory requirements and agency recommendations continue to increase and the effect of healthcare personnel shortages is felt. The perioperative environment still is considered high risk for both the patient and the surgical team [1]. More than 90,000 patient deaths annually result from adverse events [2]. The second most common cause of healthcare-associated infection (HAI) is surgical site infection (SSI). Morbidity, mortality, and increased healthcare costs related to SSIs are of considerable concern [3]. The costs of an SSI can be significant; an SSI caused by methicillin-resistant *Staphylococcus* aureus (MRSA) can be as much as $92,363 or more [4]. Approximately 27 million people have surgery annually; about 500,000 of these patients will acquire an HAI [5]. It is estimated that 40% to 60% of SSIs are preventable [3].

Regulatory and recommending agencies are working closely with each other to change those statistics. These agencies and associations are represented by the American College of Surgeons (ACS), American Society of Anesthesia (ASA), Association of periOperative Registered Nurses (AORN), Association for Professionals in Infection Control and Epidemiology (APIC), Society for Healthcare Epidemiology (SHEA), Centers for Medicare and Medicaid (CMS), Joint Commission (JC), Centers for Disease Control and Prevention (CDC), and American Hospital Association (AHA), to name a few.

The JC works with the Sentinel Event Advisory Group to review pertinent literature and reports and identifies patient safety goals and requirements. In addition, the JC has created separate National Patient Safety Goals (NPSGs) for both inpatient and ambulatory healthcare facilities. The NPSGs were created to improve patient safety and may change each year [6].

The safety goal that applies to infection control is NPSG [7] to reduce the risk of healthcare-associated infections.

This goal outlines measures to reduce the transmission of pathogens from staff members to patients and complies with the CDC hand hygiene guidelines. In addition to HAIs, it addresses any infection that may result in the unanticipated death of a patient or any patient infection that may result in a loss of function or may become permanent. These infections must be reported as a sentinel event. A root cause analysis should be performed to establish what systems processes were in place that led to the occurrence [7].

The JC tracks sentinel events; however, due to poor reporting by healthcare facilities, the actual statistics concerning these events are unknown. The actual number of SSIs that cause sustained loss of function may be higher than currently accepted. All of these issues identify the increased hazards to patients and staff members in the operating room [8].

OPERATING ROOM (OR) HAI SURVEILLANCE

Exposure to blood, body fluid, and pathogens is common in the operating room (OR). The risk of transmitting a pathogen to an otherwise healthy patient exists as does the possibility of adding to the morbidity and mortality of already ill patients. As a result, classification systems have been developed to alert staff members to a patient's risk for an adverse event.

SSI RISK STRATIFICATION

The CDC's National Nosocomial Infections Surveillance (NNIS) system developed and uses an SSI risk index ranging from zero to three points. The patient's risk index points are assigned based on the surgical wound classification, ASA classification system, and length of the surgical procedure [9].

SURGICAL WOUND CLASSIFICATION

Wound classification should be made at the time of the operative procedure by the surgeon performing the procedure and documented by the circulating registered nurse as follows:

- Clean wounds are uninfected surgical wounds with no inflammation noted and that do not enter the respiratory, alimentary, genital, or urinary tract.
- Clean-contaminated wounds are operative wounds in which the respiratory, alimentary, genital, or urinary tract is entered under normal conditions and without unusual contamination.
- Contaminated wounds include open, new, or accidental wounds resulting from operations with major breaks in sterile technique or gross spillage from gastrointestinal tract and incisions in which acute, non-purulent inflammation is encountered.
- Dirty or infected wounds include old traumatic wounds with retained tissue that is not viable, tissue that has clinical infection, or perforated viscera [10,11].

ASA CLASSIFICATION SYSTEM

The ASA uses a point system to rate or classify the patient's health or condition before surgery. The patient assessment is done by the anesthesia care provider (Table 26-1) [12].

LENGTH OF SURGICAL PROCEDURE

Classifying a patient based on the length of a procedure is done after the procedure. Risk increases as the time of the procedure increases. If the total time for a surgical procedure extends beyond T hours (when T is the 75th percentile of the total time for procedures of that type), then the higher number of points equals the greater SSI risk [9].

The CDC defines SSIs that occur within 30 days of surgical procedures without an implant to be considered HAIs. In procedures with an implant placed, infections within one year of surgery are considered HAIs if the implant remains in place [13].

The CDC's NNIS has developed standardized surveillance definitions of SSIs (Figure 26-1). Consistently using recognized definitions of SSIs provides perioperative personnel with important data to change practice patterns and protect patients from acquiring HAIs [13].

TABLE 26-1
AMERICAN SOCIETY OF ANESTHESIA PHYSICAL STATUS CLASSIFICATION

Status	Definition of Patient Condition
P1	Healthy patient
P2	Patient with a mild systemic disease
P3	Patient with a severe systemic disease that limits activity but is not incapacitating
P4	Life-threatening, severe systemic disease
P5	Moribund patient who is not expected to live longer than 24 hours without the procedure
P6	Patient declared brain dead; organs being removed for donor purposes

With permission of the American Society of Anesthesia.

MICROORGANISMS IDENTIFIED IN THE PERIOPERATIVE SETTING

According to the CDC's NNIS, pathogens causing SSIs include the following:

- *Bacteroides fragilis.*
- *Candida albicans.*
- Coagulase-negative staphylococci.
- Enterobacter species.
- Enterococcus species.
- *Escherichia coli.*
- Group D streptococci (i.e., non-enterococci), other streptococcus species, and other gram-positive aerobes.
- *Klebsiella pneumoniae.*
- *Proteus mirabilis.*
- *Pseudomonas aeruginosa.*
- *Staphylococcus aureus* [13].

Many of the pathogens causing SSIs are from endogenous sources that may come from the patient's own skin, mucous membranes, or hollow viscera. Exogenous sources also can cause SSIs. These include surgical team members, equipment, instruments, or contaminated supplies on the sterile field used during the surgical procedure [14]. Preoperative colonization of the patient's nares with *Staphylococcus aureus* also can increase the risk of contracting an SSI [13].

Patient populations at greatest risk for developing an SSI include those who

- Are immunocompromised.
- Are malnourished.
- Are obese.
- Are older.
- Have a prolonged hospital stay.
- Have had blood transfusions of certain blood products.

Criteria for Defining a Surgical Site Infection (SSI)[1]

Superficial incisional SSI

Infection occurs within 30 days after the surgery *and* infection involves only skin or subcutaneous tissue of the incision *and* at least *one* of the following occurs.

- Purulent drainage, with or without laboratory confirmation, from the superficial incision.
- Organisms are isolated from an aseptically obtained culture of fluid or tissue from the superficial incision.
- At least one of the following signs or symptoms of infection is present: pain or tenderness, localized swelling, redness, or heat, and superficial incision is deliberately opened by the surgeon, unless the incision is culture-negative.
- A superficial incisional SSI is diagnosed by the surgeon or attending physician.

Do not report the following conditions as SSI:

- stitch abscess (ie, minimal inflammation and discharge confined to the points of suture penetration);
- infection of an episiotomy or newborn circumcision site;* or
- infected burn wound;* or
- incisional SSI that extends into the fascial and muscle layers (see deep incisional SSI).

Deep incisional SSI

Infection occurs within 30 days after the surgery if no implant** is left in place or within one year if implant is in place and the infection appears to be related to the surgery *and* infection involves deep soft tissues (eg, fascial and muscle layers) of the incision *and* at least *one* of the following occurs.

- Purulent drainage from the deep incision is present but not from the organ/space component of the surgical site.
- A deep incision spontaneously dehisces or is deliberately opened by a surgeon when the patient has at least one of the following signs or symptoms: fever (>38° C/100.4° F), localized pain, or tenderness, unless the site is culture-negative.
- An abscess or other evidence of infection involving the deep incision is found on direct examination, during reoperation, or by histopathologic or radiologic examination.

- A deep incisional SSI is diagnosed by a surgeon or attending physician.

Report the following as deep incisional SSIs:

- infection that involves both superficial and deep incision sites or
- an organ/space SSI that drains through the incision.

Organ/space SSI

Infection occurs within 30 days after the surgery if no implant** is left in place or within one year if implant is in place and the infection appears to be related to the surgery *and* infection involves any part of the anatomy (eg, organs, spaces) other than the incision that was opened or manipulated during surgery *and* at least *one* of the following occurs.

- Purulent drainage is present from a drain that is placed through a stab wound into the organ/space.#
- Organisms are isolated from an aseptically obtained culture of fluid or tissue in the organ/space.
- An abscess or other evidence of infection involving the organ/space is found on direct examination, during reoperation, or by histopathologic or radiologic examination.
- An organ/space SSI is diagnosed by a surgeon or attending physician.

* Specific criteria are used for identifying infected episiotomy and circumcision sites and burn wounds.
** The National Nosocomial Infection Surveillance System[2] defines an implant as a nonhuman derived implantable foreign body (eg, prosthetic heart valve, nonhuman vascular graft, mechanical heart, hip prosthesis) that is permanently placed in a patient during surgery.
 # If the area around a stab wound becomes infected, it is not an SSI. It is considered a skin or soft tissue infection, depending on its depth.

NOTES

1. *A J Mangram et al, "Guideline for prevention of surgical site infection, 1999,"* American Journal of Infection Control *27 (April 1999) 97-132.*
2. *National Nosocomial Infections Surveillance System, Centers for Disease Control and Prevention,* http://www.cdc.gov/ncidod/hip/SURVEILL/NNIS.HTM *(accessed 17 August 2004).*

Figure 26-1   Criteria for defining a surgical infection.

- Have diabetes and experience increased glucose levels (i.e., more than 200 mg/dL) in the immediate postoperative period.
- Smoke.

Knowing which patients are most at risk for developing SSIs and understanding the possible sources of pathogen transmission may help surgical team members protect patients and prevent SSIs. Using antibiotic prophylaxis appropriately, maintaining patients' temperatures, controlling patients' glucose levels, using clippers to remove hair, and adhering to the principles of asepsis are all proactive measures for preventing SSIs [15].

MODES OF PERIOPERATIVE PATHOGEN TRANSMISSION

HAIs originating in the perioperative suite, in general, result from a break in aseptic technique. It is impossible to exclude all microorganisms from the OR environment. For the safety of both patients and personnel, therefore, every effort should be made to minimize patient exposure to these microorganisms [16]. Perioperative personnel must be scrupulous in their aseptic technique and ensure that their practice is based on valid evidence-based research and supported by their professional organization. They must be familiar with their standards of practice and be aware of any breaks in technique. Every attempt must be made to provide quality care to patients and prevent the occurrence of adverse events.

Concerns have been raised that some common perioperative practices may result in patient HAIs. The following demonstrates how devastating poor aseptic practice habits can be to patients. The anesthesia care provider practice of administering medications to multiple patients from the same syringe, for example, is of concern. Even if the needle on the syringe has been changed, repeated use of the same syringe is never advisable [17]. A Hepatitis C outbreak in 52 patients at one hospital occurred as a result of the reuse of needles and syringes in October 2002 [18]. The anesthesia care provider was injecting medication into the intravenous (IV) tubing of multiple patients using the same syringe and needle. This practice was investigated and the risk of transmitting infection from patient to patient was studied. The blood contamination rate in IV tubing was 3.3% at the injection site and 0.3% farther away from the injection site. Having a one-way valve made no difference. It has also been found that even if the needle had been changed but the syringe had not, this did not reduce HAI rates [19]. A survey of 2,530 anesthesiologists in 1995 found that 39% reported reusing syringes from patient to patient. Another 1995 study found that 20% of anesthesiologists reused syringes from patient to patient, and 34% often did not disinfect the stopper on multidose vials [20].

The ASA recommendations for infection control for the practice of anesthesiology support the practice of using aseptic technique, using multiuse vials appropriately, and not reusing syringes and needles [21]. Preventing contamination of medications requires safe handling of parenteral medications to prevent HAIs in patients undergoing anesthesia or sedation. Many factors can influence contamination of medications that are likely to support the growth of organisms. Preservative-free medication ampules, vials, and prefilled syringes for single-patient, single-dose use should be checked for the presence of preservative agents. Single-use ampules and vials should be discarded after the content has been drawn up. Prefilled syringes should be discarded after they are used because a single dose ampule, vial, or prefilled syringe contains medication intended for

single use only and generally does not contain the bacteriostatic or preservative agents found in multidose vials. Additionally, the CDC Guidelines recommend that medications be drawn up as close to administration time as possible. These medications may become contaminated with bacteria or other microorganisms from nonsterile glass fragments, airborne contaminants, or failure to use aseptic technique. Postoperative fever, infection, sepsis, or other life-threatening illnesses and death have been reported after extrinsic contamination of propofol [22].

Syringes and needles are single-use sterile items as well. Medication from a syringe must not be administered to multiple patients even if the needle is changed. Connecting or entering a patient's IV infusion line contaminates these items. All used needles and syringes should be discarded immediately into a sharps container. Using single-use needles and syringes prevents a siphoning effect that aspirates the needle contents into the syringe when the needle is removed. A needle with viral or bacterial contamination will contaminate the syringe even if the needle is flushed before removing it from the syringe.

Blood-borne pathogens may contaminate the syringe when used with IV, intramuscular, or subcutaneous administration of medication. If backflow occurs during blood sample aspiration or from a transfusion, this also could lead to contamination. Reuse of syringes and needles puts patients at risk for cross-contamination and increases HCWs' risks if a needle-stick injury occurs [21].

Multidose vials may have suspected or visible contamination, and if so, should be discarded. For example, HAI outbreaks, including hepatitis B, have been traced to extrinsically contaminated multidose vials. Breaks in aseptic technique can introduce microbial contamination into the vial via the needle, syringe, or rubber stopper. Viral particles may survive in some multidose vials for at least one day. Outdated multidose vials should be discarded [21].

MEANS OF MONITORING PERIOPERATIVE SSIS

The CMS has been engaged since 2002 in active efforts to decrease SSIs by initiating two projects, the Surgical Infection Prevention (SIP) project and the national Surgical Care Improvement (SCIP) project [23]. The SCIP project is a national quality partnership of organizations that have made efforts to improve surgical patient care using evidence-based practice recommendations. The SCIP project followed the SIP.

The mission of this collaborative effort is to create systems that decrease SSI rates, which hospitals can do by implementing a systemwide model of care [24]. One goal within the CMS SIP project is to decrease morbidity and mortality associated with postoperative SSIs in the Medicare patient population by promoting the appropriate selection and timing of the administration of prophylactic antibiotics. A panel of multidisciplinary experts developed three performance measures for national surveillance and quality improvement:

- Receipt of prophylactic antibiotics within one hour before making the surgical incision.
- Receipt of prophylactic antibiotics consistent with current CMS recommendations.
- Discontinuation of prophylactic antibiotics within 24 hours after surgery.

The outcome indicators are to

- Double the number of surgical procedures between SSI occurrences.
- Reduce preventable SSIs by 90%.
- Achieve 100% compliance with appropriate selection and timing of prophylactic antibiotic administration [23].

The Quality Improvement Organization (QIO), formerly known as the Peer Review Organization in each state, will work with hospitals to improve these SSI prevention practice indicators. The QIOs assist healthcare facilities in providing high quality care by educating, analyzing data, providing quality improvement tools and techniques, and facilitating hospital compliance with the guidelines to enhance patient care and safety.

Hospitals may select other practices, such as maintaining patients' normothermia, glucose control, and oxygenation; hair removal with clippers; and other SSI prevention procedures. The procedures to be tracked are those commonly performed on Medicare patients: coronary artery bypass grafting; other open chest surgery; vascular surgery, including aneurysm repair; thromboendarterectomy and vein bypass procedures; hip and knee joint arthroplasty, excluding revision surgery; general abdominal colorectal surgery; and abdominal and vaginal hysterectomy [24].

This project uses evidence-based research. Hospitals must become involved and play a significant part in contributing to the prevention of SSIs. For more information regarding the SIP Project, visit **www.medqic.org/sip**.

The national SCIP project is derived from data accumulated in the SIP Project; it is a national quality partnership of organizations that have made efforts to improve surgical patient care using evidence-based practice recommendations [25]. The SCIP process and outcome measures for SSI prevention include these:

- SCIP INF 1—Prophylactic antibiotics are administered within one hour before the surgical incision.
- SCIP INF 2—Prophylactic antibiotic selection is appropriate for surgical patients.
- SCIP INF 3—Prophylactic antibiotics are discontinued within 24 hours after surgery end time and except for cardiac patients, when it is 48 hours after surgery end time.
- SCIP INF 4—Cardiac surgery patients experience controlled 6 AM postoperative serum glucose.

- SCIP INF 5—Postoperative wound infection has been diagnosed during index hospitalization (outcome measurement).
- SCIP INF 6—Surgery patients undergo appropriate hair removal.
- SCIP INF 7—Colorectal surgery patients experience normothermia in the immediate postoperative period.

SCIP also includes additional measures for cardiac, venous thromboembolism, and respiratory conditions. These make up the Interpretive Guideline Update [26]. For more information, visit the SCIP Questions & answers for hospital quality improvement at **www.medqic.org/scip/pdf/Q&A%20QIs%2007-05.pdf**.

The following are some examples of improvements made by healthcare partners involved in SCIP:

- After having used the national Surgical Quality Care Improvement Program, the Veterans Health Administration experienced a 27% drop in mortality in its surgical procedures [27].
- Facilities using the CDC's NNIS system experienced a 44% decrease in device-associated and SSI rates [27].
- A recent collaborative of the QIO's reduced SSIs by 27% at 56 facilities in the United States [28].

For more information, visit the Medicare Quality Improvement Community at **http://www.qnetquest.org/quest/index.do?mode=96&image=http://www.medqic.org/dcs/mq/images/medqic_banner_quest.gif**

PREVENTION OF NOSOCOMIAL SSIS

Perioperative personnel can do the following things to prevent or reduce SSIs in patients under their care.

Hand Hygiene and the Surgical Scrub

Hands can be a major source of transient flora (i.e., major vectors of cross contamination) [29]. Hand hygiene should be performed before and after patient contact, after removing gloves, before and after eating, before and after using the restroom, and any time that there is a possibility that hands have come in contact with blood or body fluids.

Hand rubs containing ≥60% alcohol have been recommended for use by the CDC in healthcare facilities. Access to scrub facilities or hand rubs must be convenient for staff member compliance. The National Fire Protection Association has added an amendment that now allows alcohol hand rubs in egress corridors. On March 25, 2006, the CMS filed an interim final rule approving the use of alcohol hand rubs in corridors. Local or state fire codes should be checked for requirements on alcohol hand rubs in healthcare facilities [30]. Placing these hand rubs in corridors should add to the ease of use for personnel and thus help to decrease the risk of pathogen transmission via the hands of HCWs.

The intent of hand antisepsis is to decrease any soil and transient pathogens that are on hands, nails, and forearms;

decrease resident pathogens; and reduce return growth of pathogens. The result of using an antiseptic should be a decrease in pathogens on intact skin. An antiseptic should be nonirritating, antimicrobial, broad spectrum, fast acting, and have a long-acting effect.

When using brushless hand scrubs, hands should be washed with soap and water first if they are visibly soiled. Hand scrub can be applied after washing. Data show that there may be better compliance when U.S. Food and Drug Administration (FDA)–compliant alcohol-based hand rubs are available rather than the traditional scrubs with brushes. Continued scrubbing with brushes can cause skin damage and encourage growing counts of gram-negative bacteria and *Candida* [29].

Jewelry (e.g., rings, watches, bracelets) should be removed before washing or scrubbing hands. The Chicago Antimicrobial Resistance Project (CARP) studied the use of three randomly chosen hand hygiene products. Hands were cultured before and after hand hygiene. The study revealed there was a 10-fold increase in skin organisms on nurses who were wearing rings. The pathogens that were isolated were *S. aureus*, gram-negative bacilli, and *Candida* species. If more than one ring is worn, there is increased risk of contamination [31–33].

Nail care is an important part of hand hygiene. Most of the microorganisms on the hands are in the subungual area on the hands. Use of a nail cleaner to remove the collected debris is important, especially under nails that are long. Long nails are a hazard that can cause injury to patients when moving or positioning them and can cause tears in gloves. Wearing artificial nails in the perioperative area has been associated with SSI outbreaks and may increase the risk of SSIs. Moisture can remain between the natural and the artificial nail, providing a good medium for microorganisms to grow. Gram-negative microorganisms (i.e., *Serratia marcescens*) have been cultured under these nails; fungal infections also can occur [13,34].

Preoperative Patient Skin Preparation

An assessment of hair at the surgical site should be done before hair removal. The amount of hair, area of the incision, and type of procedure should be determined. If hair must be removed, it should be performed by a person skilled in hair removal, outside the OR, and in a way that preserves the patient's privacy and comfort. Hair clippers provide less irritation and are easier to use to achieve effective hair removal. Razors should not be used. Clippers provide the least irritating and easiest way to achieve hair removal. Depilatories may cause skin reactions [13,35]. Testing for possible allergic reaction to the depilatory should be done before applying it. Manufacturer's guidelines should be followed.

Several antiseptic skin preparation products for surgical preps are available, but no comparative studies have been done to provide sufficient evidence that one product should

be used over another. In choosing an antiseptic, refer to current research as well as the CDC, APIC, and FDA guidelines [35]. In preparing the patient's skin, keep the following recommendations in mind.

- Prepare areas of higher microbial counts (e.g., the umbilicus, open wounds) last.
- Allow the antiseptic to remain on the skin for 1–2 minutes or until it dries naturally (without wiping or drying) to enable the agent to provide antisepsis
- Cover an open contaminated area, such as a colostomy, with an antiseptic soaked sponge while performing the prep. Leave the prepping of this open site for last.
- Use normal saline to prepare the area when prepping burn patients.
- Keep alcohol, alcohol-based products, and chlorohexidine gluconate away from the patient's mucous membranes.
- Be gentle with skin preparation of patients with diabetes, skin ulcerations, or delicate skin (e.g., premature infants, the elderly).
- Allow enough time for vapors from flammable antiseptic agents, such as alcohol or alcohol-based antiseptics, to completely dissipate to reduce the possibility of fire.
- Do not allow any pooling of the antiseptic under the patient, in the linens, on the grounding pad, and so on to prevent chemical burns or a fire [35].

Surgical Attire

Surgical attire consists of freshly laundered scrub clothes, a head cover or hood, and shoes that are clean, have no visible debris on them, and provide foot protection. Masks are worn wherever sterile supplies or scrubbed persons are present. Scrub clothes should be made of low-linting material that helps contain bacterial shedding. Warm-up jackets (i.e., long-sleeved jackets) that button or snap should be worn by nonscrubbed staff members. Jackets made of fleece are not appropriate because they are flammable and attract lint [13,34]. Surgical attire should be changed every day or when items become soiled, contaminated, or wet. Scrub clothing that is contaminated with blood/body fluids must remain at the healthcare facility to be laundered there or at a healthcare facility–approved laundry. This decreases the possibility of transmitting pathogens from the healthcare facility to HCWs' homes or to the public. Reusable scrub clothing should be placed in an assigned hamper for laundering after use [34]. AORN does not recommend home laundering.

Head Cover

Head covers or hoods should be made of low-linting material and should be changed daily. A head cover or hood helps to contain hair and decreases the possibility of hair or dandruff falling on surgical attire, on the sterile field, or in to a surgical wound. Bald or shaved heads must be covered to prevent epidermal shedding. Hair can serve as a filter and collect bacteria if left uncovered. Single-use head coverings should be disposed of at the end of the shift. Reusable head coverings should be placed in the appropriate hamper for laundering after use [32,34].

Masks

Masks that cover both the wearer's nose and mouth should be worn. Ties need to be secured to prevent venting. The purpose of the mask is to contain droplets or microorganisms from escaping [34]. According to the Occupational Safety and Health Administration (OSHA) Final Rule, masks are required and must be worn whenever splashes, spray or spatter, droplets of blood, or body fluids that may be potentially infectious and could contaminate the eyes, nose, or mouth can be anticipated [36]. Opinions may differ regarding the effectiveness of masks [37,38].

When removing masks, HCWs should remove them carefully to prevent possible pathogens from contaminating their hands. Masks should not be allowed to hang down around the neck or be placed in a pocket for later use. They should be discarded after use by handling only the ties or elastic [13,32,39].

With airborne diseases (e.g., *Mycobacterium tuberculosis*), OSHA requires that respiratory protection be certified by the National Institute for Occupational Safety and Health and the CDC. This level of particulate filter respirator (i.e., N-, R-, or P-95, 99, or 100) includes respirators that are disposable or powered air-purifying respirators (PAPRs). Particulate filter respirators (N-, R-, or P-95, 99, or 100) must be fitted to the wearer's face [40].

Gowns

Gowns should be made of protective material that is liquid resistant to prevent exposure to blood/body fluids that may be infectious [41]. The surgical team members wear sterile gowns to assist in maintaining a sterile field. Gowns may be reusable or disposable and must meet the standards set by the American Society for Testing and Materials (ASTM) [13].

Gloves

Glove selection should be based on the tasks to be performed. Sterile gloves are selected when performing sterile procedures, and nonsterile gloves are used for nonsterile procedures. Gloves help reduce gross contamination of the hands and need to be changed between patient procedures or contacts to prevent microorganism transmission. Hand hygiene should be performed after gloves are removed [34]. Gloves should be changed as soon as holes or tears are apparent. Double gloving (i.e, wearing two pairs of gloves) decreases the possibility of a bloodborne pathogen exposure [13].

Eyewear

HCWs should wear eyewear that forms a protective barrier over the eyes to prevent splashes, splatters, or sprays from contaminating the eyes when there is any possibility of this occurring. When the eyewear becomes contaminated, HCWs should discard or decontaminate them [34].

Shoe Covers

Wearing fluid-resistant shoe covers to prevent splashes or spills from contaminating the shoes is considered part of the Personal Protective Equipment (PPE) requirement when procedures involve irrigation or profuse loss of body fluids (e.g., orthopedic trauma, cases). Shoe covers assists in keeping the HCWs' feet dry [42]. There is no evidence that shoe covers reduce the incidence of SSIs. If shoe covers develop tears, holes, or become wet, they should be removed and replaced. Before leaving the perioperative area, HCWs should discard shoe covers [34].

Environmental Cleaning

Patients having an invasive procedure should be ensured a clean environment. Cleaning the OR should be done on a regular schedule to decrease dust, soil, and the microbial load that occurs in this setting. ORs should be cleaned at the beginning of the day and between each surgical patient. Terminal cleaning should be done at the end of the day. An Environmental Protection Agency (EPA)–registered hospital disinfectant should be used for cleaning. Manufacturer's guidelines should be followed. Alcohol should not be used for surface cleaning [43].

Blood/body fluid spills should be cleaned with an EPA–registered germicide with specific claims for the elimination of HIV and Hepatitis B. If needed, an intermediate germicide that is tuberculocidal can be used. Spills of blood/body fluid should be removed as soon as possible. If there is a possibility of splatter, additional PPE should be worn by the HCW. Persons cleaning the OR should wear protective gloves [44].

Sodium hypochlorite (i.e., bleach) may be used for blood/body fluid spill cleanup. It should be a fresh solution of sodium hypochlorite in a 1:10 dilution (i.e., 1 part sodium hypochlorite to 10 parts water). When mixed, the solution should be dated and discarded after 24 hours [44]. HCWs should read the label contents on the sodium hypochlorite container to ensure that the product is not diluted and is the percentage needed [45].

Areas of the floor that are noticeably soiled need to be cleaned with a new or laundered mop head in an EPA–registered, hospital-grade germicide. A mop head that has been used should not be dipped in the clean germicide solution again. If the mop head is redipped into the clean solution, the solution must be discarded. Mopping the floor helps eliminate dust, debris, and soil. Following a surgical procedure, only a 3- to 4-ft perimeter surrounding the surgical field needs to be mopped. It is important to move the OR bed to ensure that the floor is not soiled and has nothing left under it. There is no scientific evidence to support cleaning the entire floor for SSI reduction.

Terminal cleaning should be done once during every 24-hour period whether or not the OR has been used. This practice helps reduce resident microbial flora. Terminal cleaning includes the surgical lights and external tracks, ceiling-mounted equipment, all furniture and equipment (to include telephones and light switches), hallways and floors, handles on cabinets and push plates, ventilation faceplates, horizontal surfaces, substerile areas, scrub and utility areas, and scrub sinks. Soap dispensers that require refills are not recommended. Refilled soap dispensers can act as reservoirs for microorganisms [43].

Medical Waste

Contaminated items should be segregated into noninfectious and infectious waste. Waste that is contaminated with blood and/or tissue that would release blood/body fluids if compressed must be handled separately from other waste. Items that are infectious or could release blood should be placed in leak-proof, closable containers or bags that are color coded and tagged for easy identification as hazardous waste. Containers or bags are transported to a biohazardous waste area [43].

Medical waste is segregated into the following categories; laboratory and microbiology waste; bulk blood, blood products, and specimens containing blood and body fluids; pathology wastes (i.e., anatomical specimens); and sharps. Sharps should be disposed of in an impervious, puncture-proof container as near the patient care area as possible [44]. The perioperative area has one of the highest percutaneous injury rates of all practice areas, but perioperative staff are the least likely to report bloodborne pathogen exposures. Studies show that from 7% to 15% of all thoracic, trauma, burn, emergency orthopedic, major vascular, intra-abdominal, or gynecologic surgeries have sharps injuries incurred by the surgical team. Using the OSHA 300 Log or a Needlestick Injury Log will assist employees in determining the trends in injuries. This log also identifies the devices that are most often involved in exposures [46]. Personnel assigned to handle waste should be trained in the use of PPE and use it as needed. HCWs should use the same method for disposing of isolation waste as they would use with hazardous waste from the perioperative suite [44].

OPERATING ROOM DESIGN AND ENVIRONMENT

The OR design and its environment are very important in reducing SSI risk. A central core should be used for storing sterile equipment and supplies.

Heating, Ventilation, and Air Conditioning (HVAC)

The OR ventilation system should control the amount of particulates in the perioperative environment. Air is delivered from ceiling vents that should be located high on the walls of the room. The outlet exhaust vents should be located near the floor. These vents should be across from the inlet vents. The direction of incoming air should be downward with little flow of air toward the floor and exhaust outlets. The air pressure should be positive in the OR compared to the adjacent areas. This helps to decrease the amount of air moving into the OR from the adjacent areas [32]. There should be at least three outside air exchanges per hour in the total air exchange. This assists the exhaust requirements for the HVAC system. Portable air conditioners, humidifiers, or dehumidifiers should not be used in the perioperative area. These products may move air and microbes around, thereby increasing the possibility of an SSI [47].

Humidity levels should be controlled to decrease static electricity (i.e., a lower level of humidity increases the possibility of static electricity) and decrease the possibility of microbial growth (i.e., a higher level of humidity may increase microbial growth) [32]. Ideal ranges of temperature, levels of humidity, and number of air exchanges for perioperative areas are listed in Table 26-2.

Traffic Patterns in the Perioperative Suite

The number of HCWs present affects the level of microbes in the perioperative area; therefore, traffic should be

TABLE 26-2
TEMPERATURE/HUMIDITY/AIR EXCHANGES

Location	Operating Room
Temperature	68–73
Humidity	30–60%
Exchange per hour	15
Recirculation by room unit (fans)	No
Pressure relation to adjacent area	Positive
Exchange outdoor air per hour	3
Location	Anesthesia gas storage
Temperature	Not designated
Humidity	30–60%
Exchange per hour	8
Recircrulation by room unit fans	No
Pressure relation to adjacent area	Negative
Exchange outdoor air per hour	Not designated
Location	Recovery room
Temperature	70–75
Humidity	30–60%
Exchange per hour	6
Recirculation by room unit (fans)	No
Pressure relation to adjacent area	Not designated
Exchange outdoor air per hour	2

From American Institute of Architects Committee on Architecture for Health with assistance from the U.S. Department of Health and Human Services. *Guidelines for construction and equipment of hospital and medical facilities*, Washington DC: AIA Press, 2001, used with permission.

minimized [13]. The surgical suite has three delineated traffic sections: unrestricted, semirestricted, and restricted.

> **Unrestricted:** This area includes a control location where staff monitor the entrance of patients, personnel, and materials. Street clothes may be worn in this area. Traffic is not severely restricted, but only authorized individuals should be in this area.
>
> **Semirestricted:** This part of the perioperative suite includes the areas that support the surgical suite. Storage for clean and sterile supplies, work areas for storage and processing of instruments, and hallways lead to the restricted area of the surgical suite. Only authorized personnel and patients are permitted here. Scrub attire is worn in this area including long-sleeved jackets that are buttoned or snapped closed during use. A surgical cap or hood should completely cover the head and facial hair of all personnel.
>
> **Restricted:** This area includes the operating and procedure rooms, the clean core, and scrub sink areas. Full surgical attire including masks is required. Non-scrubbed personnel should wear long-sleeved jackets that are buttoned or snapped closed during use. In rooms with open sterile supplies, masks are required [48].

Movement into and out of the ORs should be kept to a minimum. Bacterial shedding increases with activity, and there may be more airborne contamination as a result of increased traffic. Talking and the number of people present during a surgical procedure should be limited [13].

Doors to individual ORs should remain closed except during the transporting of patients and the movement of staff, supplies, or equipment. This helps to maintain the appropriate number of air exchanges and levels of humidity.

Laminar Flow

The CDC suggests that healthcare facilities "consider performing orthopedic implant procedures in ORs supplied with ultra clean air" [13]. Laminar flow is listed as a category II recommendation, which means it is "suggested for implementation and supported by suggestive clinical or epidemiological studies or theoretical rationale" [13]. A study with 40 patients undergoing total hip replacement (THR) in an ultraclean and in a standard room was conducted. The objective was to use a molecular biological technique called polymerase chain reaction (PCR) to establish wound contamination rates after a THR in an ultra-clean and standard OR. The study covered a three-year period. Following skin incision, specimens of pericapsular tissue were obtained from each patient's posterior joint capsule. Surgeons obtained additional specimens at the end of the procedure and before closure. Gram stains and cultures were done immediately on one specimen. The other specimens were frozen for later PCR analysis.

The results indicated that the ultra-clean rooms had no impact on the contamination rate at the start or end of the procedure. None of the specimens ($n = 20$) at the start of the procedure in the standard room was positive by culture; two were positive by PCR. At the end of the procedure, none of the specimens was positive by culture; six were positive by PCR. The findings in the standard OR specimens showed a higher contamination rate at the end of the procedure than at the start of the procedure. There were no specimens ($n = 20$) at the start of the procedures positive by culture done in the standard OR; three were positive by PCR. Two of the specimens taken at the end of the procedure were positive by culture, and nine were positive by PCR. Eight infections were detected by PCR in the cases done in the ultra-clean OR; no infections were detected by culture. The contamination rate for the standard and ultra-clean ORs were the same. The clinical implication is that greater effort should be taken in both types of ORs to control traffic and keep doors closed, especially at the end of the case [49,50].

Ultraviolet Light (UVL)

The premise for using UVL for low-level disinfection is that it kills select vegetative bacteria, fungi, and lipoprotein viruses on contact. It may, however, actually sustain life for other organisms. The usefulness of UVL is very restricted because the UV rays must to be in direct and close contact with the organisms. Some healthcare facilities have ORs with UVL installed; however, the UVL cannot be used when the OR is occupied. Care should be taken to wear protective clothing and goggles if entering a room when UVL is activated because it can cause skin burns, and conjunctivitis [51]. The CDC does not recommend the use of UVL as a method of decreasing SSIs (Category IB) [13].

Scrub Sinks

A scrub sink should be located next to each OR, or one sink can serve two ORs. There should be no scrub sinks in the central core to prevent splashes and aerosolization that could occur in an area where sterile supplies are kept [32].

Floors

Floors should be seamless, have a hard surface, be easy to clean, and have cove fittings from the floor to the wall. All of these measures prevent microbes from accumulating [32].

STERILIZATION OF INSTRUMENTS AND DEVICES

Proper cleaning of instruments is critical for the sterilization process to be successful. Prior to transporting instruments to the decontamination area, an enzymatic solution, spray, or gel may be used on instruments that are difficult to clean. Instruments that can be should be opened/taken apart for thorough cleaning and removal of bioburden. If blood is allowed to remain on the instruments, corrosion and pitting may occur. A washer/sterilizer, ultrasonic cleaner, washer/decontaminator, or manual cleaning may be used for cleaning and decontaminating instruments. Personnel performing decontamination should wear PPE when working with contaminated instruments [52].

Prior to cleaning and decontamination, the following information needs to be determined:

1. Are written instructions for cleaning, positioning, and sterilization cycles available from the instrument(s) manufacturer? Without this information, the device may not be properly cleaned, positioned, and/or sterilized.
2. Are the OR staff able to replicate the recommended cleaning protocols? For example, does the OR have an ultrasonic cleaner if this process is recommended by the device manufacturer? Does the OR have the recommended cleaning agents/implements?

Flash sterilization (steam sterilization using the unwrapped method) can be performed using a gravity or prevacuum steam sterilizer. This type of sterilizer is routinely available in the surgical suite to provide quick sterilization of devices when there is insufficient time to perform the preferred wrapped instrument methods. Operating room personnel should complete competencies in the operation of flash sterilization equipment prior to using this method.

To operate the sterilizer in the flash cycle, the following needs to be determined:

1. Has proper cleaning been done prior to flash sterilization? If the device has not been thoroughly and properly cleaned, steam may not make contact with all surfaces of the device.
2. Did the instrument manufacturer provide flash sterilization instructions? Many manufacturers no longer recommend flash sterilization. Without this information, the facility bears the responsibility for the safety and efficacy of the device.

The use of flash sterilization containers may prevent contamination of the contents after completion of the flash cycle when transporting the container to the area needed. Flash sterilization containers present concerns including the requirement for special sterilization cycles, special biological testing, and various types of maintenance for the valves in the flash container.

Documentation of items processed in each flash cycle is recommended to track devices back to the patient. Flash sterilization of implants is not recommended. If an implant must be flash sterilized, the implant manufacturer's written instructions for cycle time and temperature must be followed. A biological test should be included in the cycle and the results documented.

Flash sterilization began as a means to quickly sterilize a single, one-of-a-kind device that was dropped or contaminated. Unfortunately, some facilities are using flash sterilization to compensate for inadequate instrument inventories, poor scheduling, and a lack of coordination/communication with vendors for loaner specialty instruments [53].

SURGICAL INSTRUMENT TRACKING

Tracking surgical instrument use and finding their location have become very important. Missing instrument(s) require personnel time to find them, can be costly, and most importantly, may compromise patient safety [54]. Instrument sets can be identified by bar coding and can be scanned before and after they are decontaminated. Another system involves radio frequency identification (RFID) technology that uses a small tag that stores a code with information that the Sterile Processing Department (SPD) determines [55]. SPDs may also develop their own system. A digital camera may be used to photograph instruments. These photographs may be downloaded to a software system and be customized for the individual setting. Video demonstrations can then created if a multimedia feature is available [56].

The advantage of using a surgical instrument tracking system is that it allows the data collected every time the instrument(s) is moved to be recorded and the location noted. The software systems can generate reports and documentation on patient safety and protect healthcare facilities against litigation. If the SPD had a sterilization cycle in which sterilization parameters were not met, SPD is able to identify the location of the instrument(s) by utilizing a computerized tracking system. If a patient develops a postoperative infection, reports may also be used to track whether the instrument(s) were sterilized appropriately. A tracking system is only as good as the data that are entered. It is crucial to have well-trained personnel who understand the tracking process [54].

SCHEDULING PERIOPERATIVE PROCEDURES

Surgical procedures may be scheduled in the OR at any time with the exception of patients who have a latex allergy. If possible, it would be best to schedule a patient with a latex allergy as the first procedure of the day. Theoretically, as the day progresses, latex may be aerosolized from the supplies and gloves used. As the first procedure of the day, this risk is reduced as the air exchanges through the night filter out the latex [43].

DISASTER MANAGEMENT IN THE PERIOPERATIVE AREA

Perioperative personnel need to be prepared to respond to disasters. Since the terrorist attacks of September 11, 2001, in the United States, healthcare facilities have expanded their disaster preparation to include not only natural but also human made disasters. State and federal governments now mandate that all healthcare facilities have emergency response plans. The JC has stressed the importance of a plan that is scalable, sustainable, and community integrated. Healthcare facilities accredited by JC must conduct two tests of their emergency management plan in hospitals and one in ambulatory care facilities. This can be an actual emergency or a drill [57].

CONCLUSION

SSIs continue to increase as the number of at-risk patients requiring surgical interventions increases. Patients representative of this rise in at-risk population include the elderly, premature infants, and patients who are obese, immunocompromised, diabetic, or smoke. The length of hospital stay is decreasing, and an increasing number of invasive procedures are being performed in outpatient settings which include hospital outpatient, free-standing surgery centers, and office-based surgeries. The perioperative environment continues to be a hazardous one for patients and staff. HCWs who follow OSHA, CDC, AORN, APIC, ASA, and JC regulations/guidelines/recommendations can reduce the risk of pathogen transmission or injury to themselves and their patients, thus increasing the culture of safety in the perioperative environment.

REFERENCES

1. Position statement on workplace safety. *Standards, Recommended Practices, and Guidelines.* Denver: AORN, 2006:385–386.
2. Burke JP. Infection control—a problem for patient safety. *N Engl J Med*; 2003;348:651–655.
3. Bratzler D. Other resource from SIP to SCIP. Surgical infection prevention and surgical care improvement national iniative to improve care for Medicare Patients. (www.medqic.org/dcs/ContentServer?cid=1107196774282&pagename=Medqic%2FOtherResource%2FOtherResourcesTemplate&c=OtherResource) accessed July 14, 2006.
4. Engenmann JJ, Carmeli Y, Cosgrove SE, et al. Adverse clinical and economic outcomes attributable to methicillin resistance among patients with *Staphyloccocus aureus* surgical site infection. *Clin Infec Dis* 2003;36:592–598.
5. Barnard BM. Fighting surgical site infections. *Infection Control Today* 2002:28–32.
6. Joint Commission on Accreditation of Healthcare Organizations. 2006 ambulatory care and office-based surgery National Patient Safety Goals. (http://www.jointcommission.org/PatientSafety/NationalPatientSafetyGoals/07_amb_obs_npsgs.htm) accessed July 11, 2006.
7. Joint Commission on Accreditation of Healthcare Organizations. *Comprehensive accreditation manual for hospitals: the official handbook.* Oakbrook, IL: JC, 2006:10–11.
8. 2006 National Patient Safety Goals. Joint Commission on Accreditation of Healthcare Organizations (www.legacyhealth.org/body.cfm?id=1140) accessed July 11, 2006.
9. Jannelle J, Howard R, Fry D. Surgical site infections. *APIC text of infection control and epidemiology.* 2nd ed. Chicago: APIC, 2005;23:1–10.
10. Garner JS. CDC guideline for prevention of surgical wound infection. 1985: Supercedes guideline for prevention of surgical wound infection, 1982, Revised. *Inf Control* 1986;3:193–200.
11. Simmons BP. Guideline for prevention of surgical wound infection. *Infection Control* 1982;3; 185–186.
12. Association American Society of Anesthesia. *Providers manual for anesthesia departments.* Park Ridge, IL: ASA, 1997:1–5.
13. Mangram AJ, Hovan TC, Pearson ML, et al. Guidelines for prevention of surgical site infection, 1999. *Am J Infect Control* 1999;27:97–132.
14. Tomaselli N. Prevention and treatment of surgical site infections. *Infection Control Resource* 2004;5:1–8.
15. Improving surgical care: preventing surgical complications: Surgical Care Improvement Project (www.medqic.org/scip/scip_impsurgcare.html) accessed July 11, 2006.
16. Fortunato NH. *Berry & Kohn's operating room technique.* 9th ed. St Louis: Mosby, 2000:221.
17. Koepke JW, et al. Viral contamination of intradermal skin tests syringes. *Annals of Allergy* 1985;55:776.
18. Greene E. Hepatitis C outbreak: more than 52 infected by reused needles and syringes. *American Society of Anesthesiologists ASA Newsletter* 2002;66:1–5
19. Trepanier CA, et al. Risk of cross-infection related to multiple use of disposable syringes. *Can J Anesth* 1990;37:156–159.
20. Rosenberg AD, et al. Accidental needlesticks: do anesthesiologists practice proper infection control precautions? *Am J Anesthesiol* 1995;22:125–132.
21. American Society of Anesthesiologists Task Force on Infection Control. *Recommendations for infection control for the practice of anesthesiology.* 2nd ed. Park Ridge, IL: ASA, 1999.
22. Revised statement on patients and HCWs with bloodborne diseases *Standards, recommended practices, and guidelines.* Denver: AORN, Inc, 2003.152.
23. Surgical infection prevention description. *Medicare quality improvement community* (www.medqic.org/content/nationalpriorities/topics/projectdes.jsp;jsessionid=3A2E3BB025DFA404DFDFC0F0F38B8B9D?g11n.enc=ISO-8859-1&topicID=461).
24. Strategy for redesign processes: sponsor collaborative to promote improvement. Centers for Medicare and Medicaid MEDQIC (www.medqic.org/dcs/ContentServer?cid=1116947499240&pagename=Medqic%2FContent%2FParentShellTemplate&parentName=StrategyForChange&c=MQParents).
25. SCIP: project information (www.medqic.org/scip/) accessed July 11, 2006.
26. Hospital CMS measures: SCIP process and outcome measures (http://www.medqic.org/dcs/ContentServer?cid=1136495755695&pagename=Medqic%2FOtherResource%2FOtherResourcesTemplate&c=OtherResource).
27. Surgical Care Improvement Project. Improving surgical care: preventing surgical complications (http://www.medqic.org/dcs/ContentServer?cid=1136495755695&pagename=Medqic%2FOtherResource%2FOtherResourcesTemplate&c=OtherResource) accessed July 12, 2006.
28. Dellinger EP, Hausmann SA, et al. Hospitals collaborate to decrease surgical site infections. (Excerpta) *Am J Surg* 2005;190:9–15.
29. Recommended practices for surgical hand antisepsis. *Standards, recommended practices, and guidelines.* Denver: AORN, 2006:537–545.
30. Centers for Disease Control and Prevention. CMS interim final rule regarding placement of alcohol-based hand-rub dispensers. *Hand hygiene in healthcare settings* (www.cdc.gov/handhygiene/firesafety/cmsRuling.htm) accessed July 12, 2006.
31. Phillips M. Attire, surgical scrub, gowning, and gloving. *Berry & Kohn's operating room technique.* 10th ed. St. Louis: Mosby, 2004:272.

32. Fogg DM. Infection prevention and control. In: Rothrock JC, ed. *Alexander's care of the patient in surgery.* 12th ed. St Louis: Mosby, 2003:97–158.

33. Trick WE, Vernon MO, et al. Impact of ring wearing on hand contamination and comparison of hand hygiene agents in a hospital. *Clin Infect Dis* 2003;36:1383–1390.

34. Recommended practice: surgical attire. In: *Standards, recommended, practices, and Guidelines.* Denver: AORN, 2006:451–457.

35. Recommended practice for skin preparation of patients. *Standards, recommended practices, and guidelines.* Denver: AORN, 2006: 603–605.

36. Occupational exposure to bloodborne pathogens; final rule (29 CFR Part 1910.1030). *Federal Register* 1991; 56:64004–64182; amended January 18, 2001.

37. Belkin BN. Surgical face masks in the operating theater: are they still necessary? *JHI* 2002;50:233–235.

38. Tunevall TG. Postoperative wound infections and surgical face masks: a controlled study. *World J Surg* 1991;15:383–387.

39. Emsley L. Why wear surgical face masks? *Nurs Times* 2000;96: 38–39.

40. Jensen PA, Lambert LA, et al. Guideline for preventing the transmission of Mycobacterium tuberculosis in health-care settings, 2005. *MMWR* 2005;54(RR-17):171–119.

41. Recommended practices for selection of gowns and drapes. In: *Standards, recommended practices, and guidelines.* Denver: AORN, 2006:531–535.

42. U.S. Department of Labor, Occupational Safety & Health Administration. Regulations (standards—29 CFR) bloodborne pathogens 1910.1030 2006:1–33 (www.osha.gov/pls/oshaweb/searchresults .category?p_text=Bloodborne%20Pathogen%20-1910.1030&p_ title=&p_status=CURRENT) accessed July 12, 2006.

43. Recommended practices for environmental cleaning in the surgical suite. *Standards, recommended practices, and guidelines.* Denver: AORN, 2006:517–523.

44. Schulster L, Chinn RY. Guidelines for environmental infection control in health-care facilities. *MMWR* 2003;52(RR-10):1–44.

45. Use of chlorine compounds as disinfectants, SafetyNet #68. Safety net. UC Davis Environmental Health and Safety. 2-1493. Available at: http://ehs.ucdavis.edu/ftpd/sftynet/sn_68.pdf.

46. ECRI. *Operating room risk management newsletter.* December 2004: 1–6.

47. American Institute of Architects Committee on Architecture for Health with assistance from the U.S. Department of Health and Human Services. *Guidelines for construction and equipment of hospital and medical facilities.* Washington, DC: AIA Press, 2001: 70–80.

48. Recommended practices for traffic patterns in the perioperative practice setting. *Standards, recommended practices, and guidelines.* Denver: AORN, 2006:659–662.

49. Allen G. Evidence for practice: contamination in standard versus ultra-clean ORs. *AORN Journal* 2005;81:890–892.

50. Clark MT, et al. Contamination of primary hip replacements in standard and ultra-clean operating theaters detected by polymerase chain reaction. *Acta Orthop Scand* 2004;75:544–548.

51. Phillips NH. Decontamination and disinfection. *Berry & Kohn's operating room technique.* 9th ed. St Louis: Mosby, 2000:293.

52. Recommended practices for cleaning and caring for surgical instruments and powered equipment. *Standards, recommended practices, and guidelines.* Denver: AORN, 2006:555–563.

53. Recommended practices for sterilization in the perioperative practice setting. *Standards, recommended practices, and guidelines.* Denver: AORN, 2006:629–641.

54. Neil R. Keeping track. *Mater Manag Health Care* 2004;13(11): 18–21.

55. Akridge, J. Operating room keeping track of surgical Instruments. *Healthcare Purchasing News* 2004;28(3):29–32.

56. Bersch, C. Operating room instrument tracking—a science of its own. *Healthcare Purchasing News* 2003;27(3):20–21.

57. Comments by Dennis O'Leary. "Homeland defense: blueprints for emergency management responses. Washington DC: Joint Commission on Accreditation of Healthcare Organizations Conference, October 23–25, 2002.

Ambulatory Care Settings

27

Candace Friedman and Kathleen H. Petersen

BACKGROUND

Healthcare is increasingly provided in ambulatory care settings. These settings include a wide variety of primary and specialty offices and clinics, urgent care centers, dental offices, and physical medicine and rehabilitation centers. Treatments once provided only in a hospital are now offered in outpatient settings, including infusion therapy, dialysis, and endoscopy. In addition, many surgical procedures formerly performed only on inpatients are now routine practice in ambulatory surgery centers.

Ambulatory care settings present unique challenges for infection prevention and control. High volume, complexity of care, increasingly vulnerable patients, and brief visits influence the development and recognition of healthcare-associated infections (HAI).

Medical procedures performed in the ambulatory setting may put patients at risk of infections. Use of intravascular devices may lead to infections such as catheter site infection, bloodstream infection, septic thrombophlebitis, or endocarditis. Other invasive procedures, including surgical procedures, endoscopies, bronchoscopies, and cystoscopies, pose a risk of infection due to the disruption of normal host barriers. In addition, there have been reports of outbreaks due to inadequate sterilization or disinfection of equipment, absent or inappropriate use of barriers, inappropriate work restrictions for ill health care workers, and poor hand hygiene. However, despite increasingly complex ambulatory care, overall risks of HAI continue to remain low [1].

There also is the risk of exposure to communicable diseases in ambulatory settings. The potential for infection transmission, including the spread of measles and tuberculosis, to patients and staff in ambulatory care has long been recognized [1]. Additionally, there are concerns about transmission of antibiotic resistant bacteria and the threat of biodisaster-related infections in these settings.

GENERAL PREVENTION

Several basic infection prevention [1–3] and control principles and practices to reduce the risk of infection are essential regardless of setting. These include hand hygiene, standard precautions, cleaning, disinfection, and sterilization of medical devices, management of infectious patients, and occupational health.

Hand Hygiene

Hands [4] must be cleaned as in any other healthcare setting. Plain or antimicrobial soap and an alcohol-based hand sanitizer should be readily available. Sinks must be conveniently located. Alcohol hand sanitizer containers should be placed in waiting areas, patient rooms, and support areas. For invasive procedures a surgical hand scrub is required. Staff should be offered a choice of antimicrobial scrub products. (See Chapter 3.)

An issue in ambulatory settings is how best to monitor appropriate hand hygiene. Observations are limited for areas where care is provided behind a door. Settings where observations are possible include surgery centers, infusion; dialysis, endoscopy, and physical medicine; and rehabilitation areas. A surrogate for observation can be an evaluation of the quantity of hand hygiene products used before and after any intervention designed to increase hand hygiene. The rate of use is then equal to the amount of product divided by the number of visits for a certain time period.

Standard Precautions

Use Standard Precautions for all patients. This includes the use of appropriate personal protective equipment (e.g., gloves, gowns, and face protection) as needed. The type of exposure expected will determine the specific barrier to use. Barriers should be readily available in examination and treatment rooms. Gloves must be worn for drawing blood, handling contaminated items, performing invasive procedures, and using certain chemicals. In addition, safety devices, especially intravenous catheters and blood drawing needles, must be accessible. Training regarding specific practices involved in standard precautions must be provided to staff.

Infectious Patients

Some method of isolation and barrier precautions must be used in any setting. Contact, droplet or airborne precautions may be implemented depending on the patient population and complexity of patient care [5].

A respiratory hygiene campaign should be routinely used instructing visitors, patients, and staff to "cover their cough." Signs providing instructions should be prominently displayed, and tissues, hand sanitizer, and masks made readily available.

There should be a method to identify potentially infectious patients. Early identification can assist with the use of appropriate isolation/precautions. A screening tool may be useful for assessing diseases such as tuberculosis, chickenpox, measles, and pertussis. Screening can be performed on the telephone. Patients meeting screening criteria should be provided a mask if appropriate and separated from others as much as possible—not remaining in waiting areas. Patients with rash or fever should be seen at times when there are the fewest patients.

Cleaning/Disinfection/Sterilization

Cleaning the environment [6,7] and equipment is important in any setting. Room furniture, floors, countertops, examination tables, and other equipment should be cleaned routinely using a low-level disinfectant. Disposable, single-use items must not be reprocessed unless Food and Drug Administration (FDA) requirements are met [8]. Any reusable instrument or equipment that enters sterile tissue or cavities must be sterilized before use. High-level disinfection may be used for items that contact mucous membranes or non-intact skin. (See Chapter 20.)

Written procedures should note how each instrument or piece of equipment will be processed. Outlining the barriers staff need to use, how to clean the item, the

TABLE 27-1
DEVELOPING PROCEDURES FOR DISINFECTION/STERILIZATION OF EQUIPMENT

- Meet with clinic managers, nurse, or medical assistant educators
- Develop procedures: use same procedures throughout institution
- Develop training and competency
- Implement procedures
- Perform site surveys to assess practice: process surveillance
- Evaluate assessment
- Implement changes
- Document and share with relevant staff

proper disinfection or sterilization method, and storage parameters makes the procedure a useful educational tool (see Table 27-1).

Steam autoclaves often are available in ambulatory care settings. Peel pouches may be used to package small items. There also may be items (e.g., vaginal specula) that can be steam sterilized unwrapped in place of high-level disinfection. Preventive maintenance is critical to ensure a safe, functional sterilizer.

Staff members must be educated on the practices required for safe and effective processing of items and how to properly use chemicals and sterilizers.

Storage

Store all clean or sterile items in a manner to prevent contamination. Sterile supplies should be kept in closed drawers or cupboards if not in a designated clean supply room. All supplies should be stored in a first-in, first-out manner to ensure the use of the oldest items first.

Occupational Health

Occupational health programs are important in ambulatory care settings. There should be a comprehensive vaccination program for employees including hepatitis B vaccine and influenza vaccine. A tuberculosis screening program also is important. There should be a system of follow-up for any body substance or chemical exposure. In addition, a program for prevention must include use of safety devices when applicable to prevent needlestick injuries. (See Chapter 4.)

SETTINGS, RISKS AND PREVENTION

Each of the following sections summarizes the application of infection prevention and control principles in various ambulatory care settings. Prevention of infections due to infusion therapy and dialysis is covered elsewhere. (See Chapters 23 and 37.)

Primary and Specialty Care Medical Offices and Clinics

Services in these areas range from non-invasive health maintenance examinations to procedures such as endoscopies, biopsies, and minor surgeries. Overall risk of infection in this setting is very low. Potential risks to staff include sharps injuries and exposure to communicable infections. Risks to patients include exposure to infectious agents in the waiting room and other common areas and ineffective reprocessing of medical devices. The role of computer keyboards, stethoscopes, and other environmental sources in the spread of communicable diseases is generally low in the medical office and clinic setting [1].

Reportable diseases diagnosed by the medical office or clinic must be reported to the local health department. Primary care can also play a major role in promoting community health (e.g., providing immunizations and teaching patients about hand hygiene, appropriate use of antibiotics, and prevention of sexually transmitted diseases).

Specific measures to prevent infections include the following:

- Triaging patients with possible airborne illness (e.g., chicken pox) to enter an alternate door when available and avoid time in the waiting room.
- Practicing aseptic technique for minor procedures including proper patient skin antisepsis, and no preset up of sterile trays.
- Cleaning surfaces (e.g., examination tables, examination lights, and blood pressure cuffs) on a regular basis.
- Disinfecting and sterilizing instruments safely, effectively, and reliably after each patient use and consistent with policies and procedures of the organization. Staff with expertise in infection prevention and control should assist in the evaluation of reprocessing practices before placing new equipment or devices into use. This is especially important in specialty clinics, such as ophthalmology, infertility, and urology, where technology is advancing rapidly and new devices are often introduced.
- Immunizing patients: appropriate vaccine storage, preparation, and record keeping.
- Cleaning toys after contamination (e.g., "mouthing") and on a regular basis [9].

Dental Offices

Dental and oral surgical procedures are among the most frequently performed procedures. Procedures vary from routine teeth cleaning to dental implants to temporomandibular joint surgery.

Risks of infection due to dental procedures include contaminated instruments and equipment (e.g., ultrasonic scaling, high-speed hand pieces, and waterlines). In addition, there is a risk of postsurgical infection after procedures due to microbes in the oral cavity (e.g., tooth extraction and dental implants). Dental healthcare workers may be exposed to infection due to contact with blood and oral/respiratory secretions, especially aerosols, and contaminated equipment and surfaces.

Specific measures to prevent infections include the following [1,10–12]:

- Performing a surgical scrub for oral surgical procedures.
- Using safety dental syringes/injectors and work practices to prevent body substance exposures.
- Decreasing aerosols generated during treatments through the use of rubber dams, high-velocity air evacuation, and proper patient positioning.
- Using water that meets Environmental Protection Agency standards for drinking.
- Sterilizing instruments that penetrate soft tissue, including reusable prophylaxis angles, high-speed dental hand pieces, and low-speed hand-piece components used intraorally.
- High-level disinfecting of instruments that contact oral tissues or heat-sensitive instruments.
- Cleaning hand pieces thoroughly both internally and externally. They must be run to discharge water and air after each patient.
- Flushing ultrasonic scalers and air/water syringes for 20–30 seconds after each patient.
- Cleaning the following areas with disinfectant cleaner after each patient: countertops, chair switches, light handles, dental unit surfaces, aspirator tube, edge of spittoon, and ultrasonic scaler hand piece.

Emergency Department

Services provided in an emergency or urgent care department (ED) [1,13–17] focus on the care of critically ill or injured individuals who are having various procedures performed. Some of these patients come to the ED with communicable diseases. In addition, individuals seeking treatment after a biological or chemical attack will be advised to go to an ED.

Risk of infection to patients arises primarily from invasive procedures performed (e.g., bloodstream infections related to intravascular catheter placement). Waiting and other common areas pose a risk of exposure to communicable diseases for patients, visitors, and staff. Staff are also at risk from aerosols and blood and body fluid exposure. ED staff are at a greater risk of exposure to bloodborne pathogens than other healthcare workers due to their frequent contact with blood.

Specific measures to prevent infections include the following:

- Using aseptic practices as in any healthcare setting for intravascular devices, ventilators, urinary catheterization, and any other procedure.

For suspected tuberculosis, chickenpox, measles, rubella, or other airborne infections and unidentified rashes:

The nurse will triage the patient on a phone call and will discuss with the physician or assigned clinician whether or not the patient must be seen, whether the visit can be rescheduled, or whether the case can be handled over the telephone.

If the patient will be seen:

1. Advise patient to come to an alternate door, not the main entrance, when available.

2. Determine immune status of staff. Recommend that only staff members who are immune care for patient. All nonimmune staff who must care for the patient must wear masks (assuming this is an airborne-spread disease).

3. At the time of entry to the facility, have the patient wear a mask (surgical or isolation).

4. Place the patient in an examination room immediately to avoid time in the waiting room.

5. Keep the examination room door closed.

6. When the patient leaves, clean surfaces contaminated with blood or body fluids as for any patient, using standard precautions.

Patients with suspected active, pulmonary TB (or other airborne-spread disease) must be handled according to airborne precautions. Patient is to be moved to a facility with negative pressure isolation rooms, such as _____ Hospital, as soon as possible or sent home with appropriate instructions.

If possible exposure occurs, contact _____ or _____
                                   (Infection Control)   (Employee Health)

Figure 27-1 Sample triage policy for infection prevention in ambulatory care.

■ Assessing patients for signs and symptoms of communicable diseases. A triage screening tool can be used to identify potentially contagious patients (see Figure 27-1). Mask identified patients promptly and separate them from others.

■ Having a system of isolation/precautions for management of potentially infectious patients.

■ Having an emergency response plan that includes biological threats.

Outpatient Surgery

Outpatient surgery is performed in traditional hospital settings or in stand-alone surgery centers that may or may not be affiliated with larger medical institutions. Surgical procedures commonly performed on outpatients include removal of cataracts, muscle/tendon procedures, reduction of fractures, laparoscopic cholecystectomies, tubal ligation, hernia repairs, knee arthroscopies, and many types of plastic and oral surgery.

The risk of surgical site infection (SSI) varies according to procedure; however, it is reported to be <1% overall and certainly less than for inpatient surgery [18]. Outpatient procedures are generally shorter and not as invasive or complicated as those performed in hospitals. Prevention of postsurgical infections is covered in Chapter 35; however, there are special standards for office-based surgery outlined by the Joint Commission [19]. Surgical team members are also at risk for infection due to the potential for blood and body fluid contamination and injuries from sharp items.

The strategy for surveillance of surgical site infections differs slightly from inpatient surveillance; however, it is necessary to evaluate infection trends, develop rates for new or more complex surgeries, and monitor changes in rates following interventions. Surveillance should include the following:

- Determining procedures to follow: Perform a risk assessment for high-volume, high-risk, problem-prone, and historically problematic procedures. Perform a medical literature search for articles on the procedures that will be followed to determine a benchmark. Once enough data have been collected, an internal baseline rate can be determined.
- Developing case findings of effective data sources, such as medical records, letters to surgeons, and contact with the medical offices where patients receive postsurgery care.
- Performing data analysis and follow-up: Determine who will collect the data, develop reports, receive reports, and the frequency of reports; outline who will be responsible for follow-up of recommendations or changes in practice.
- Reassessing rates after changes in practice.

DIAGNOSTIC AND TREATMENT

Endoscopy

Endoscopy procedures are among the most common of outpatient procedures. Infection risk related to endoscopy has been demonstrated to be very low [20]. Cross-infection has been traced to a failure to practice recommended cleaning and disinfection procedures of the endoscopes or ancillary equipment. These include *Mycobacterium tuberculosis* related to bronchoscopy, Hepatitis C related to colonoscopy, *Pseudomonas aeruginosa* related to endoscopic retrograde cholangiopancreatography, and Staphylococcal infections related to arthroscopy [1]. Patients also may develop infections from endogenous flora as the endoscopes are passed through the gastrointestinal, urinary, or respiratory tracts [21]. In addition, there have been reports of mucous membrane damage (i.e., colitis) linked to inadequate rinsing of disinfectant, specifically glutaraldehyde from sigmoidoscope channels [1]. Endoscopy staff members are at risk of exposure to body fluids during procedures and to chemicals during disinfecting procedures.

Endoscopes are inherently heat-sensitive, complex, and fragile instruments. This makes management of these devices critical. However, adhering to specific infection prevention and control activities reduces the risk of infection to a minimal level:

- Ensuring that all staff responsible for using and reprocessing the endoscopes are trained and competent.
- Reprocessing endoscopes consistently after each patient use. Most endoscopes are high-level disinfected. (See Chapter 20.)
- Following detailed procedures provided by each endoscope manufacturer and by professional organizations [20,21].

- In addition, because of the potential for tuberculosis related to bronchoscopies, performing these procedures using guidelines from the Centers for Disease Control and Prevention (CDC) [22].

Radiology

Radiology departments provide a number of services, including diagnostic radiography, computed tomography, fluoroscopy, ultrasound, and interventional procedures. Risks of infection are primarily related to intravascular catheter use, equipment (e.g., ultrasound probes and fluids, contrast medium). Because patients suspected of having tuberculosis or other communicable respiratory illness often are evaluated with diagnostic radiography, there is a risk of transmission to both patients and staff. Staff members also are at risk of bloodborne pathogen exposure due to their contact with blood during invasive procedures.

Specific measures to prevent infections include the following [1,23–27]:

- Using safety devices, especially intravenous catheters and needle holders/pads, and passing instruments safely.
- Using aseptic practices for intravascular devices and other procedures.
- Avoiding hair removal unless it interferes with the procedure. Clip the site, if necessary.
- Using appropriate techniques during invasive procedures, e.g., insertion of tunneled catheters, surgical scrub, and use of a sterile field system. Nonporous drapes must cover the area surrounding the wound; cover the patient and any hardware on the table that might come in contact with a long catheter/wire [28]. Operators should wear cap, mask, gown, and gloves [29]. Circulators should wear a scrub suit.
- High-level disinfecting endocavitary and vaginal ultrasound probes after each use, even when probe covers are used [27]. Reuse catheters in angiography only per FDA regulations [8].
- Implementing a protocol on how to manage patients suspected of having an airborne communicable disease, e.g., use of a mask on the patient when an identified patient is seen for chest radiography.

Cardiology: Cardiac Catheterization and Electrophysiology

Increasingly complex diagnostic and interventional procedures are performed on outpatients in the cardiac catheterization laboratory [28,30], including placement of pacemakers, stents and other implantable devices, angioplasty, and cardiac catheterizations.

Infections are rare after invasive cardiovascular procedures and usually are associated with the procedural site or the device. However, risks for infection have been linked to contaminated instruments and solutions or breaks in technique. When infection occurs, it is presumed that bacteria are introduced at the time of vascular puncture or incision. Infectious complications include bloodstream infection, endarteritis, pacemaker and defibrillator infections, coronary stent, and puncture site infections. Patients with implants also may develop late-onset infections. Skin microorganisms usually cause these infections. Endotoxin reactions after catheterization have also been reported. Risks for staff are mainly through exposure to blood from sharps injuries or splashing of blood.

Specific measures to prevent infections include the following:

- Preparing the patient: Follow standard vascular access and surgery site preparation. Do not remove hair unless it will interfere with the operation.
- Performing standard surgical hand antisepsis and avoid artificial nails, as described in Chapters 3 and 35.
- Using aseptic technique, as described in Chapter 3.
- Preparing staff [28]:
  - The cardiologist should wear mask, eye protection, cap, sterile gloves, and sterile gown.
  - Staff assisting within the sterile field should wear scrub suit, cap, mask, and gloves, adding eye protection if there is a splash potential during the specific procedure.
  - Circulators should wear scrub suits.
- Inserting intravascular catheters and maintenance: follow CDC guidelines on prevention of catheter-related infections [31].
- Controlling intravenous solutions (e.g., dyes, flush solutions). Ensure sterility; cold infusates need to be cooled without contact with tap water that might contaminate the infusate and then be inadvertently injected into vessels.
- Processing equipment: Most supplies used in the unit are disposable. However, single-use device (SUD) catheters can be reprocessed for reuse, following stringent requirements of the FDA. Most electrophysiology units use third-party reprocessors for these devices [8].
- Ensuring sterility of implants: any implant removed for infection must be reported to the FDA. Work with the institution's risk management department on appropriate protocols.
- Controlling the environment: Air handling is similar to that in operating rooms. This includes ensuring that the room is set at positive pressure with a minimum of 15 air exchanges per hour; make sure construction/renovation plans follow health department specifications [32].
- Cleaning procedure rooms after each case [32,33].
- Using safety devices and disposing of sharp instruments and needles safely.
- Using prophylactic antibiotics per recommendations [28].
- Developing written policies and procedures for infection prevention and control.

Surveillance for bloodstream infections (BSI) and SSIs is difficult unless patients return to the clinic affiliated with the cardiac area. However, there should be a system in place for follow-up of patients. Because reported rates of infection are low, any evidence of an outbreak or cluster should be carefully evaluated.

Physical Medicine and Rehabilitation

Rehabilitation services provide a multidisciplinary team approach to treat patients with often complex medical and physical conditions. Rehabilitation specialties include physical, occupational, and speech and language therapy; orthotics and prosthetics; recreational, art, and music therapy; and rehabilitation engineering. Programs often target special needs, such as sports or spinal injuries, traumatic brain injuries, or strokes.

Although services are wide ranging, few involve invasive procedures, and infections related to these services are rarely reported. Some exceptions include electromyography (EMG), wound irrigation [34], and hydrotherapy for patients with open wounds [1]. Speech therapists or others working with the mouth or items that contact oral secretions, such as during swallowing studies, may be exposed to respiratory infections of the patient. Rehabilitation patients at increased risk of infection include cystic fibrosis (CF) patients who may develop and/or spread *Pseudomonas* spp. or *Burkholderia* spp. to other CF patients, arthritis patients on high-dose steroids, patients with large wounds coming for irrigation or hydrotherapy, diabetic patients being fitted for orthotics or prosthetics, and spinal cord injury or other rehabilitation patients with indwelling urinary catheters.

Specific measures to prevent infections include the following:

- Practicing standard precautions: Evaluate the need for barriers during treatment of patients who may be incontinent, have open wounds, or have increased respiratory secretions.
- Applying precautions consistently for all patients who may have antibiotic-resistant microorganisms (e.g., treating CF patients colonized with *Burkholderia* spp. at the end of the day and/or individually when no other CF patients are being treated). Clean all equipment after each of these patients.
- Restricting children receiving speech and language therapy who have upper respiratory infections.
- Cleaning mats, walkers, canes, wheelchairs, weights, transfer devices, occupational and speech therapy tools, toys, and other equipment after use or place barriers between patients and equipment. Evaluate whether equipment touches skin, mucous membrane or sterile tissue. Establish a frequency of cleaning and which disinfectants will be used [35]. (See Chapter 20.)
- Using aseptic technique during wound care and dressing changes. Follow local health department regulations for medical/regulated/biohazardous waste for dressing disposal. When irrigation of large wounds is performed

(e.g., pulsatile lavage), follow specific recommendations to prevent aerosolization, including the use of barriers such as gloves, impervious gowns, and face protection [34].

- Draining and disinfecting hydrotherapy tank and agitator jets after each patient.
- Following state laws for treating (e.g., chlorinating) and testing the pool or whirlpool water in aquatic therapy. Develop consistent policies for restriction of patients due to open wounds or fecal incontinence.
- Disposing of electromyography needles and other sharp items carefully.

HOME CARE

Services provided in a home setting consist of skilled nursing care, respiratory therapy, infusion therapy, wound care, dialysis, nutrition therapy, physical and occupational therapy, and hospice care. Home healthcare is a growing segment of the healthcare delivery system. Many patients cared for at home are immunocompromised, are of advanced age, and/or have a chronic illness. In addition, they may have various types of devices, including intravascular and urinary catheters, and use equipment that require management (e.g., ventilators). Risks for infection are generally associated with these devices, for example, bloodstream infections due to intravascular devices (See Chapters 31, 37). Staff may be at risk during contact with patients who have communicable diseases.

Much of the care provided in the home is by someone other than a healthcare worker (e.g., family members). These individuals also play an important role in infection prevention. Education of caregivers in hand hygiene, aseptic practices, care of devices, use of barriers, disinfection practices, and other aspects of care are extremely important. Caregivers should also be informed of appropriate signs and symptoms of infection.

Surveillance for infections is a challenge for home care agencies due to the difficulty of obtaining information. Data should be collected for high-risk infections in the populations served; these may include urinary tract infections, BSI, pneumonia, and skin/soft tissue infections. Definitions on surveillance criteria have been published for home care [36].

Home care agencies should monitor for BSI and tunnel or exit site infections in their patients who receive home infusion. If patients are on ventilators, they should be monitored for the development of pneumonia. Clinical home care staff will need to help collect data by identifying patients with clinical signs and symptoms of infection. They can then report the information to a central individual responsible for infection prevention and control. That person will then apply the definitions and make recommendations for changes in practice when appropriate.

Specific measures to prevent infections include the following [37–41]:

- Using standard precautions with attention to hand hygiene. Alcohol-based hand sanitizers, soap, and clean paper or cloth towels should be brought to the home by the healthcare worker.
- Immunizing patients as necessary.
- Transporting clean and sterile supplies in a manner to prevent contamination (e.g., in a travel bag).
- Setting up a clean work surface.
- Using safety devices and carefully discarding sharp items; take a container to the home if necessary.
- Disinfecting urinary drainage bags per safe protocols.
- Handling fluids (e.g., sterile water) in a manner to prevent contamination. Use small bottles, carefully handle caps, and store properly.
- Providing enteral feedings safely: refrigerate, thoroughly clean blender parts, measuring utensils, and other reusable items after use. Allow to thoroughly dry. Hang for only recommended time limits. Use clean technique to prepare and administer enteral feedings.
- Following intravascular device guidelines and ensuring proper handling and storage of medications [31].
- Providing sterile solutions prepared for intravenous infusion.
- Developing procedures on frequency of ventilator tubing changes, tracheostomy care, use of gloves when suctioning and disinfecting suction catheters, canisters, and tracheostomy cannula. Suctioning is usually performed using clean rather than sterile technique.
- Developing procedures that outline maintenance requirements for respiratory care equipment. Room humidifiers should be dried between uses.
- Outlining aseptic practices related to urinary catheterization. Clean technique is appropriate (see Chapter 30)
- Using clean technique during wound care.
- Teaching caregivers methods to prevent pressure ulcers.
- Developing a system to manage equipment taken to/from the patient's home (e.g., clean items always placed in a clear bag and used items placed into a colored plastic bag). Separate clean and dirty areas and items.

INFECTION PREVENTION AND CONTROL PROGRAM

The infection prevention and control (IPC) program design must take into account factors that will influence its activities. These include the population served, demographics of the institution, clinical focus, volume of activity, and number of staff.

Infection Control Professional

Responsibility for IPC programs in ambulatory care settings may be designated to a staff member or an infection control professional (ICP) with specialized training. It should be clear who has the designated responsibility.

Specific activities include surveillance, data management, cluster investigations, quality improvement activities, patient and staff education, policy and procedure updates, product evaluation, and exposure investigations. A staff member may be assigned many of these responsibilities. However, if necessary, the services of a trained ICP should be obtained as a consultant.

Whoever is assigned responsibility for IPC must include both clinical and support teams in the program to ensure success. Specific information on designing an IPC program is outlined in Chapter 5.

Specific IPC Activities in Ambulatory Care [1,42–47]

Data Management

One of the major functions of an IPC program is data management. Chapter 6 discusses surveillance; therefore, this section focuses on issues pertinent in ambulatory care settings.

A surveillance plan should be developed. It should outline what types of infection will be monitored (outcome surveillance) [48–50] or what practices will be routinely evaluated (process surveillance) [51,52]. In addition, the plan should note the methods used to disseminate data to appropriate staff.

Healthcare-associated SSIs postambulatory care surgery or BSI after infusion therapy or dialysis are appropriate outcome measures for settings to perform these procedures. There are no specific definitions for HAIs in ambulatory settings. The general definition used for an HAI is the development of an infection not present or incubating at the time of the visit or intervention. Any definition must include a temporal association with the visit or care provided. For example, a BSI occurring within 48 hours of a visit to an infusion center may be considered an HAI.

Any surveillance measuring outcomes must consider how to obtain information. Patients in these settings may not return to the same provider for follow-up if an infection occurs. Systems to identify these patients may include coordination with hospitals, provider offices, and home care services. Methods to obtain information may consist of phone calls to patients or providers, patient mail-back questionnaires, or provider surveys; laboratory and radiology reports; risk management database; and communication with staff.

Surveillance of processes may be used to review the care and maintenance of instruments and equipment and practices at a site. This system focuses on observations using a survey tool to collect information. Table 27-2 is an example of questions that can be used on a survey tool. Process surveillance methods are used to measure compliance with policies and procedures; data can then be used to improve outcomes. Reports of findings should

TABLE 27-2 **EXAMPLE OF AN AMBULATORY CARE SURVEY TOOL**		
Safe, Effective High-Level Disinfectant	**Yes**	**No**
Are containers		
Completely covered?		
Labeled with chemical name and safety or environmental hazard?		
Checked each day of use for effectiveness?		
Results recorded?		
Labeled with expiration date?		
Are devices thoroughly cleaned before soaking in disinfectant?		
Are devices completely immersed in disinfectant?		
Are items soaked at least 20 minutes?		
Are devices rinsed thoroughly after soaking?		
Are competencies in place for staff?		

be sent to staff who can facilitate changes and monitor practices.

Patients and staff also are at risk of infection due to exposure to communicable diseases. If this is a potential risk in a setting, it should be part of the surveillance plan.

Reportable Diseases

Certain communicable diseases are reportable to state and local health departments. It is important to provide this information as appropriate to ensure communication with health departments and laboratories.

Construction/Renovation

All construction/renovation projects must have infection control input [53]. Specific concerns include the management of the project, especially minimizing dust generation, and review to ensure that basic infection prevention measures are included (e.g., sinks and proper air flow).

Biodisaster/Emerging Diseases

Patients with diseases suspected of being related to bioterrorism may be identified in ambulatory care sites. Each area should have a biological disaster plan that may be included in a general disaster plan. A method for early recognition of the illness is a key component of any plan [54,55].

REFERENCES

1. Friedman C, Petersen KH, ed. *Infection control in ambulatory care*. Sudbury, MA: Jones and Bartlett Publishers, 2004.
2. Herwaldt LA, Smith SD, Carter CD. Infection control in the outpatient setting. *Infect Control Hosp Epidemiol*. 1998; 19:41–74.
3. Jennings JA, Friedman C, Wideman JM. Ambulatory care. In: *APIC text of infection control and epidemiology*. 2nd ed. Washington, DC: Association for Professionals in Infection Control and Epidemiology, Inc. 2005.

4. Centers for Disease Control and Prevention. Guideline for hand hygiene in health-care settings: recommendations of the Healthcare Infection Control Practices Advisory Committee and the HICPAC/SHEA/APIC/IDSA Hand Hygiene Task Force. *MMWR* 2002; 51(No. RR-16).

5. Garner JS, Hospital Infection Control Practices Advisory Committee. Guideline for isolation precautions in hospitals. *Am J Infect Control* 1996; 24:24–52.

6. Rutala WA. APIC guidelines for selection and use of disinfectants. *Am J Infect Control* 1996; 24:3113–3342.

7. Rutala WA, Weber DJ. Cleaning, disinfection, and sterilization in healthcare facilities. In *APIC text of infection control and epidemiology*. 2nd ed. Washington, DC: Association for Professionals in Infection Control and Epidemiology, Inc. 2005.

8. Reuse of single use devices. U.S. Food and Drug Administration. (www.fda.gov/cdrh/reprocessing) accessed May 17, 2007.

9. Committee on Infectious Diseases. In: *2003 red book*. Elk Grove Village, IL: American Academy of Pediatrics, 2003.

10. Molinari JA, Harte JA. Dental services. In: *APIC text of infection control and epidemiology*. 2nd ed. Washington, DC: Association for Professionals in Infection Control and Epidemiology, Inc. 2005.

11. Kohn WG, Collins AS, Cleveland JL, et al. Centers for Disease Control and Prevention guidelines for infection control in dental health-care settings—2003. *MMWR* 2003; 52(RR-17):1–61.

12. Harrel SK, Molinari J. Aerosols and splatter in dentistry: a brief review of the literature and infection control implications. *JADA* 2004; 135:429–437, 505–508.

13. Talan DA. Infectious disease issues in the emergency department. *Clin Infect Dis* 1996; 23:1–14.

14. Kelen GD, Hansen KN, Green GB, et al. Determinants of emergency department procedure- and condition-specific universal (barrier) precaution requirements for optimal provider protection. *Ann Emerg Med* 1995; 25:743–750.

15. Schoolfield MB, Peters SJ. Infectious disease screening and isolation for pediatric patients in an emergency department. *J Emerg Nurs* 1995; 21:33–36.

16. Bloodborne infections in emergency medicine. American College of Emergency Physicians, 2004. (www.acep.org/webportal/PracticeResources/PolicyStatements/pubhlth/BloodborneInfectionsEM.htm) accessed April 24, 2006.

17. Keim M, Kaufmann AF. Principles for emergency response to bioterrorism. *Ann Emerg Med* 1999; 34:177–182.

18. Hirsemann S, Sohn D, Gastmeier K, Gastmeier P. Risk factors for surgical site infections in a free-standing outpatient setting. *Am J Infect Control* 2005; 33:6–10.

19. Joint Commission's Ambulatory Care Accreditation Program 2006. (www.jointcommission.org/AccreditationPrograms/Office-BasedSurgery/) accessed April 30, 2006.

20. American Society of Gastrointestinal Endoscopy. Multi-society guideline for reprocessing flexible gastrointestinal endoscopes 2006. (http://www.apic.org/AM/TemplateRedirect.cfm?template=/CM/ContentDisplay.cfm&ContentID=6381) accessed May 17, 2007.

21. Stricof RL. Endoscopy. In: *APIC text of infection control and epidemiology*. 2nd ed. Washington, DC: Association for Professionals in Infection Control and Epidemiology, Inc., 2005.

22. Guidelines for preventing the transmission of *Mycobacterium tuberculosis* in health-care settings, 2005. *MMWR* 2005; 54:1–141.

23. Hansen ME, Bakal CW, Dixon GD, et al. Guidelines regarding HIV and other bloodborne pathogens in vascular/interventional radiology. *J Vasc Interv Radiol* 2003; 14:375S–384S.

24. English JF, Malone JL, Waters CL, et al. Selection and use of disinfectants for transvaginal ultrasound probes. *Am J Infect Control* 1999; 27:191, abstract.

25. Nihill DM, Otten JE, Lynch P. Imaging services and radiation oncology. In: *APIC text of infection control and epidemiology*. 2nd ed. Washington, DC: Association for Professionals in Infection Control and Epidemiology, Inc., 2005.

26. Ustunsoz B. Hospital infections in radiology clinics. *Diagn Interv Radiol* 2005; 11(1):5–9.

27. Guidelines for cleaning and preparing endocavitary ultrasound transducers between patients (www.aium.org/publications/statements/_statementSelected.asp?statement=27) accessed April 24, 2006.

28. Chambers CE, Eisenhauer MD, McNichol LB, et al. Infection control guidelines for the cardiac catheterization laboratory. *Cathet Cardiovasc Interv* 2006; 67:78–86.

29. Miller DL, O'Grady NP. Guidelines for the prevention of intravascular catheter-related infections: recommendations relevant to interventional radiology. *J Vasc Interv Radiol* 2003; 14:133–136.

30. Aureden KL. Cardiac catheterization and electrophysiology. In: *APIC text of infection control and epidemiology*. 2nd ed. Washington, DC: Association for Professionals in Infection Control and Epidemiology, Inc., 2005.

31. Centers for Disease Control and Prevention. Guidelines for the prevention of intravascular catheter-related infections. *MMWR* 2002; 51(No. RR-10):1–29.

32. Sehulster L, Chinn RY. CDC; HICPAC guidelines for environmental infection control in health-care facilities: recommendations of CDC and the Hospital Infection Control Practices Advisory Committee. *MMWR Recomm Rep* 2003; 52(RR-10):1–42.

33. Mangram AJ, Horan TC, Pearson ML, et al. Guideline for the prevention of surgical site infection, 1999. *Infect Control Hosp Epidemiol* 1999; 20:247–280.

34. Maragakis LL, Cosgrove SE, Song X, et al. An outbreak of multidrug-resistant *Acinetobacter baumannii* associated with pulsatile lavage wound treatment. *JAMA* 2004; 292:3006–3011.

35. Felix K. Rehabilitation. In: *APIC text of infection control and epidemiology*. 2nd ed. Washington, DC: Association for Professionals in Infection Control and Epidemiology, Inc., 2005.

36. Embry FC, Chinnes LF. Draft definitions for surveillance of infections in home health care. *Am J Infect Control* 2000; 28:449–453.

37. Rhinehart E. Infection control in home care. *Emerg Infect Dis* 2001; 7:208–211.

38. Rhinehart E, McGoldrick M. Infection control in home care and hospice. 2nd ed. Sudbury, MA: Jones and Bartlett Publishers, 2006.

39. Morrison J. Health Canada, nosocomial and occupational infections section. Development of a resource model for infection prevention and control programs in acute, long term, and home care settings: Conference proceedings of the Infection Prevention and Control Alliance. *Am J Infect Control* 2004; 32:2–6.

40. Embry FC. Home care. In: *APIC text of infection control and epidemiology*, 2nd ed. Washington, DC: Association for Professionals in Infection Control and Epidemiology, Inc., 2005.

41. Smith PW, Roccaforte JS. Epidemiology and prevention of infections in home healthcare. In: Mayhall CG, ed. *Hospital epidemiology and infection control*. 3rd ed. Philadelphia: Lippincott Williams & Wilkins, 2004.

42. Friedman C, Barnette M, Buck AS, et al. Requirements for infrastructure and essential activities of infection control and epidemiology in out-of-hospital settings: a consensus panel report. *Am J Infect Control* 1999; 27:418–430.

43. Hurt N. The role of the infection control nurse in quality management in the ambulatory care setting. *J Healthcare Quality* 1993; 15:43–44.

44. Haim L. Recommendations for optimizing an infection control practitioner's effectiveness in an ambulatory care setting. *J Healthcare Quality* 1994; 16:31–34.

45. Jarvis WR. Infection control and changing health care delivery systems. *Emerg Infect Dis* 2001; 7:170–173.

46. Horan-Murphy E, Barnard B, Chenoweth C, et al. APIC/CHICA-Canada infection control and epidemiology: professional and practice standards. *Am J Infect Control* 1999; 27:47–51.

47. Friedman C. Infection control and prevention programs. In: *APIC text of infection control and epidemiology*. 2nd ed. Washington, DC: Association for Professionals in Infection Control and Epidemiology, Inc., 2005.

48. Arias KM. Surveillance. In: *APIC text of infection control and epidemiology*. 2nd ed. Washington, DC: Association for Professionals in Infection Control and Epidemiology, Inc., 2005.

49. Lee TB, Baker OG, Lee JT, et al. Recommended practices for surveillance. *Am J Infect Control* 1998; 26:277–288.

50. Manian FA. Surveillance of surgical site infections in alternative settings: exploring the current options. *Am J Infect Control* 1997; 25:102–105.

51. Infection control practitioner audit form for patient/resident service units. *Can J Infect Control* 2002; 17:23–26.

52. Baker OG. Process surveillance: an epidemiologic challenge for all health care organizations. *Am J Infect Control* 1997; 25:96–101.

53. Bartley J. Construction and renovation. In: *APIC text of infection control and epidemiology*. 2nd ed. Washington, DC: Association for Professionals in Infection Control and Epidemiology, Inc., 2005.

54. Rebmann T. Disaster management. In: *APIC text of infection control and epidemiology*. 2nd ed. Washington, DC: Association for Professionals in Infection Control and Epidemiology, Inc., 2005.

55. Rebmann T. Bioterrorism. In: *APIC text of infection control and epidemiology*. 2nd ed. Washington, DC: Association for Professionals in Infection Control and Epidemiology, Inc., 2005.

Infections in Long-Term Care Facilities

28

Chesley L. Richards, Jr. and Donna Lewis

INTRODUCTION

Long-term care has been defined as "an array of health, personal care, and social services provided over a sustained period of time to persons with chronic conditions and with functional limitations" [1]. These services can be provided in the home, in community settings, or in institutions. In contrast to acute care facilities, long-term care facilities (LCTFs) typically are residential. Consequently, staffing and policies are oriented toward maintaining independence, maximizing resident and family satisfaction, and promoting socialization. The traditional LTCF resident is a cognitively or functionally impaired elderly adult. However, recent trends have seen increases in the proportion of LTCF residents who receive postacute care services (e.g., rehabilitation following a surgical operation or acute illness) or skilled nursing services (e.g., intravenous antimicrobials, parenteral or enteral nutrition, or aggressive wound care). This chapter will review LTCF characteristics, selected infections in LTCF residents and facilities, and infection control issues in LTCF.

CHARACTERISTICS OF LTCF RESIDENTS, STAFF, AND CLINICIANS

LTCF Characteristics

In the United States, >40% of adults will reside in an LTCF at some point during their life [2,3]. Of 1.6 million LTCF residents in 1999 in the United States, most were female (72%), age ≥75 (78%), widowed (57%), and residing in nursing homes in the Midwest and South (63%) [4]. Before LTCF admission, most residents came from a hospital (46%) or private residence (30%). LTCF residents are highly dependent on staff for activities of daily living (ADLs). Of 5 ADLs (bathing, dressing, eating, transferring, or toileting), most residents (74%) require assistance with ≥3 ADLs (Figure 28-1). The most common ADL requiring assistance is bathing (94%).

LTCF staffing is lower than staffing in acute care hospitals. Nationally, LTCFs have one-third the number of full- or part-time employees (1.9 million vs. 5.3 million) as acute care hospitals, even though there are more LTCFs than acute care hospitals (16,000 vs. 5,800) and >50% more LTCF beds (1.6 million vs. 987,000) [5]. Nursing staff includes registered nurses (RN) (7.6 full-time employees [FTEs] per 100 beds), licensed practical nurses (LPN) (10.6 FTEs per 100 beds), or nurse's aides (32.9 FTEs per 100 beds) [4]. These FTE distributions represent the *entire staff*, not just staffing per shift. Consequently, these data emphasize that nurse's aides provide the bulk of direct resident care in most LTCFs. Especially during evening/night shifts or on weekends, a typical 100-bed LTCF may have only one or two RNs or LPNs on duty. Improving the ratio of nursing staff to residents and expanding the presence of RNs has been proposed as important steps toward improving the quality of care in nursing homes [1].

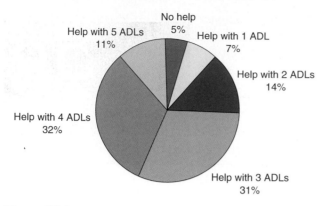

Figure 28-1 Percent distribution of residents with dependencies in activities of daily living and number of dependences: United States, 1999. *Vital Health Stat* 2002; 13 (152).

Direct medical care rarely is provided by physicians in the LTCF setting. The majority of physicians (77%) do not spend time caring for nursing home residents [6]. For physicians who provide nursing home care, the median effort is 2 hours per week, or approximately 4% of the physicians' overall practice. Very few physicians (3%) spend >5 hours per week providing medical care in nursing homes. Consequently, nonphysician clinicians provide much of the direct medical care in LTCFs. In a national survey of LTCFs, 63% reported having nurse practitioners with a median of two nurse practitioners per facility [7]. On-site nonphysician clinicians can reduce hospitalizations of LTCF residents and overall costs [8,9].

In addition to practicing clinicians, each nursing home is required to have a medical director who is responsible for providing "oversight and participate in drug utilization review and quality assurance programs and to work with attending physicians on appropriate drug therapies and medical care issues" [1]. Most medical directors are either internists or family physicians and on average spend 10–20 hours per month performing medical director responsibilities, which include infection control and resident safety. At a national level, the American Medical Director's Association (AMDA) is the primary professional organization for medical directors and provides training and certification for medical directors [10].

LTCFs often have consultant pharmacists on staff or available by contract who evaluate medication prescribing in the facility and provide consultation regarding drug therapy issues. In most LTCFs, consultant pharmacists perform mandatory medication reviews and provide feedback to the LTCF administrator and medical director. Consultant pharmacists may offer an important on-site perspective and expertise in improving the management of a wide range of medications, including antimicrobials, and should be seen as a potential resource for clinicians and medical directors regarding antimicrobial management [11]. During disease outbreaks in LTCFs, consultant pharmacists also may provide valuable resident and family counseling regarding medication side effects or support regarding the distribution of prophylactic antimicrobials (i.e., oseltamivir) [12].

RISK FACTORS FOR INFECTIONS IN LTCFS

Resident Level

Resident-level risk factors for infection include immunologic senescence, malnutrition, chronic diseases, medications (e.g., immunosuppressants, central nervous system agents that diminish cough reflex), cognitive deficits that may complicate resident compliance with basic sanitary practices (e.g., hand hygiene), and functional impairments (e.g., fecal and urinary incontinence, immobility, diminished cough reflex) [13–16] (Table 28-1). Medical interventions also may increase risk for infection. Indeed, with the growth of subacute or postacute care, many LTCFs now have residents receiving medical interventions or therapy (e.g., central venous catheters, hemodialysis, parenteral antimicrobial or nutrition therapy, or mechanical ventilation) equivalent in complexity to interventions performed in many acute care hospitals.

Facility Level

As residences, LTCFs typically promote activities and policies that foster socialization of residents through group

---

TABLE 28-1

INDIVIDUAL-LEVEL RISK FACTORS FOR INFECTION IN LTCF RESIDENTS

■ Immunologic senescence
■ Lack of vaccination
  ● Influenza, pneumococcal
■ Malnutrition
■ Chronic diseases
  ● Cancer
  ● Diabetes mellitus
  ● Emphysema, chronic bronchitis
  ● Congestive heart failure
  ● Peripheral vascular disease
■ Medications
  ● Immunosuppressants
  ● Central nervous system agents that diminish cough reflex
■ Cognitive deficits that may complicate resident compliance with basic sanitary practices (e.g., hand hygiene)
■ Functional impairments
  ● Fecal and urinary incontinence
  ● Immobility
  ● Diminished cough reflex
■ Medical interventions
  ● Central venous catheters, hemodialysis
  ● Urinary catheters, gastrostomy catheters
  ● Parenteral antimicrobial or nutrition therapy
  ● Mechanical ventilation

activities, both in and outside the nursing home. While these activities are important for promoting good physical and mental health for residents, they also may increase risk for exposure to and transmission of communicable infectious diseases [13–16]. While vital to restoring or maintaining physical and mental function, occupational and physical therapy activities may increase risk for person-to-person transmission or exposure to contaminated environmental surfaces (e.g., physical or occupational therapy equipment). In LTCFs, group bathing facilities or whirlpool therapy units may be potential sources of infection with waterborne pathogens. Finally, group dining is encouraged for nursing home residents. A common dining area may be used for all nursing home residents or for residents of a specific ward, hall, or wing in a large facility. Group dining may be an avenue for person-to-person transmission of infectious pathogens and for foodborne disease outbreaks [13–16]. Low rates of healthcare worker (HCW) immunization in LTCFs have been associated with outbreaks caused by vaccine-preventable respiratory pathogens (e.g., influenza, S. pneumoniae) [16–19]. Finally, specific institutional characteristics have been associated with disease outbreaks. In a study of outbreaks among New York LTCFs, institutional risk factors for respiratory or gastrointestinal infection outbreaks included larger homes (risk ratio 1.71 per 100 bed increase), nursing homes with a single nursing unit, or with multiple units but shared staff [20]. Risk for outbreaks was lower in LTCFs with paid employee sick leave.

ANTIMICROBIAL RESISTANT PATHOGEN INFECTIONS IN LTCFS

The introduction or emergence of antimicrobial resident bacteria in LTCFs has resulted in both regional outbreaks of antimicrobial-resistant pathogen (ARP) infections and increasing prevalence of ARPs [21,22]. In addition to the individual and institutional risk factors for infection discussed previously, colonization with ARPs (e.g., methicillin resistant *Staphylococcus aureus* (MRSA); vancomycin-resistant *enterococcus* (VRE), multidrug-resistant *E. coli*, *Acinetobacter*, *Enterobacter*, or *Pseudomonas aeruginosa*) increases the likelihood of both epidemics and high rates of endemic disease with ARPs in LTCFs [23]. Risk factors for the development of infection with multidrug-resistant pathogens include exposure to antimicrobials, lack of hand-washing sinks, and lower levels of registered nurse staffing [24].

SELECTED INFECTIONS

Evaluation of Fever and Infection in LTCF Residents

Recommendations outlining the minimum evaluation for infection in nursing home residents have been published

[25]. For residents with suspected infection, the guideline recommends that nurse's aides measure vital signs (e.g., temperature, blood pressure, pulse, respiratory rate, presence of pain), identify residents with fever or suspected infection, and relay this information to licensed nursing staff. Next, the licensed nursing staff (e.g., LPN or RN) should perform an initial clinical assessment on residents with fever or suspected infection, and significant findings should be relayed to clinicians [25]. LTCFs should have training and procedures in place to ensure that residents with suspected infection are quickly identified by nursing staff and appropriate information relayed to clinicians.

Only limited diagnostic testing for febrile or potentially infected residents is available in most LTCFs. Laboratory testing usually is sent to a hospital or reference laboratory. The delay between obtaining specimens and actual laboratory processing and in getting reports back to clinicians in LTCFs may be substantial. This delay may lead to poor decisions regarding empiric or continued antimicrobial use. Medical directors should work with nursing home administrators, directors of nursing, and laboratory providers to both improve specimen collection and reporting of results. When possible, laboratory providers should provide a facility-specific antibiotic susceptibility testing profile (i.e., antibiogram) either for the individual facility or for a network of LTCFs. Using acute care facility antibiograms may be misleading, and the availability of a LTCF specific antibiogram may improve the initial selection of empiric antimicrobial therapy. Clinicians should re-evaluate residents on antimicrobial therapy at 48 to 72 hours with the goal of tailoring antimicrobial therapy to the clinical course, identified pathogens, and antimicrobial susceptibility profile. Residents who require diagnostic studies not available in the LTCF or who are unstable should be transferred to acute care hospitals for further evaluation and therapy unless they have advanced directives (e.g., "living wills") for no hospitalization. Residents with presumed infections account for one-quarter of all hospital transfers from LTCFs [26].

The minimum recommended evaluation varies depending on the type of suspected infection [25]. First, LTCF residents may present atypically when developing infections. For example, altered mental status or a decline in oral intake without fever may be the initial presentation for pneumonia or urinary tract infection in some residents. In addition, residents with cognitive or speech impairment may not be able to communicate symptoms related to infection and may instead develop agitation or combativeness.

All residents with a presumed infection should have a complete blood count (CBC) performed. The presence of leukocytosis (white blood count [WBC] count $\geq 14,000$ cells/mm^3), even in the absence of a left shift, warrants further careful assessment for infection. Urinalysis and urine cultures are often overused in LTCFs and should be reserved for residents with symptoms of urinary tract infection without indwelling urinary catheters. In residents with chronic indwelling urinary catheters, urinalysis and urine cultures should be obtained only for symptoms or signs referable to the urinary tract or for presumed sepsis. For residents with suspected pneumonia, especially with tachypnea (respiratory rate > 25 breaths per minute), the minimum evaluation should include a chest radiograph and determination of oxygen saturation using pulse oximetry.

In addition to recommended tests, some laboratory tests may not be appropriate in LTCF residents. For example, properly collected sputum gram stain and culture can be very helpful in diagnosis and treatment of pneumonia. However, sputum studies should be obtained only if purulent sputum is available and if the sample can be transported to the clinical laboratory ≤2 hours of collection [25]. In most LTCFs, this will not be possible. In many LTCFs, blood cultures probably should not be obtained because of the high likelihood of contamination, low yield, and the recognition that residents with presumed sepsis or bacteremia probably should be transferred to acute care facilities for evaluation and management [25]. If blood cultures are obtained, LTCF medical directors should ensure that staff members (e.g., nurses) collecting the blood samples have been properly trained. Working with the hospital or commercial laboratory to monitor for probable contaminants in blood culture results (e.g., coagulase-negative *Staphylococcus*) may provide early clues when collection techniques are suboptimal. Similarly, surface cultures from infected wounds are not recommended because of the high likelihood of contamination and the low yield from these cultures.

Urinary Tract Infections (UTIs)

UTIs account for 25–30% of all bacterial infections in LTFC residents [4,7] and are among the most common bacterial infections in LTCF residents. Normally, the urinary bladder is sterile; however, in frail older adults, the bladder often becomes colonized with bacteria, typically from the gastrointestinal tract [27]. Determining whether bacteriuria represents colonization or true infection is both difficult and controversial. Accurate clinical diagnosis of symptomatic UTI in frail elderly LTCF residents may be difficult. In the institutionalized elderly, only 4–8% of residents with fever and bacteriuria have clinical findings consistent with UTI [28]. In residents with an indwelling urinary catheter, about 25% of individuals with fever and bacteriuria had UTI [28]. In cognitively impaired frail elderly people, eliciting symptoms or signs specific to the urinary tract (e.g., dysuria, frequency, flank pain) can be extraordinary difficult. Using more nonspecific symptoms (e.g., changes in mental status, decreased oral intake) can be misleading. In cognitively impaired elderly persons, new urinary incontinence should be considered as a potentially useful symptom or sign to indicate UTI, although further studies are needed to better define its sensitivity and specificity for predicting UTI.

Urinalysis (UA) in healthy, young adults is very useful in detecting UTIs. However, the presence of pyuria, either by direct microscopy (e.g., ≥5 WBCs on high powered field) or dipstick (e.g., positive leukocyte esterase) is less helpful in frail elderly. For example, in 214 chronically incontinent asymptomatic nursing home residents, 45% had pyuria, and 43% had bacteriuria. Of those who had pyuria, 59% had bacteriuria [29]. In a study of newly catheterized hospitalized patients of all ages (mean age = 60 years), the positive predictive value of pyuria was 32% [30]. Use of pyuria or bacteriuria as indicators of UTI in frail elderly patients without clinical symptoms is not recommended.

In LTCFs, chronic urinary catheters are used to manage patients who have neurogenic bladders or obstruction to urinary drainage. The presence of a urinary catheter increases risk for UTI dramatically. Consequently, primary prevention strategies in LTCF have focused on improved incontinence management and removal of catheters. Unfortunately, physicians may not always be aware that residents have urinary catheters, even when these catheters are considered inappropriate [31]. An alternative for residents who truly have a long-term indication for a urinary catheter, use of an antimicrobial- or silver-impregnated catheter may be beneficial [32]. Compared to standard urinary catheters, trials of antimicrobial- (e.g., nitrofurazone, minocycline-rifampin) and silver-impregnated catheters have demonstrated substantial reductions (30 to 70%) in bacteriuria and UTIs [33]. A recent decision analysis suggests that despite a higher catheter cost, use of silver impregnated catheters would probably be cost saving at a population level in addition to preventing UTIs [34].

Respiratory Tract Infections

Respiratory tract infection outbreaks in LTCFs are relatively common. In five Canadian LTCFs, 16 outbreaks over 3 years involving 480/1,313 residents were reported [35]. The outbreaks occurred year round, and the most common symptoms among residents during these outbreaks were cough (83%), fever (40%), and coryza (45%). A minority of residents developed pneumonia (15%). The most common pathogens were influenza, parainfluenza, or respiratory syncytial viruses; *Legionella* spp; or *Chlamydia pneumoniae*. Approximately 12% of residents were transferred to hospitals, and 8% died.

Influenza

The most important cause of respiratory tract disease outbreaks in LTCFs is influenza. Outbreaks of influenza A or B usually occur from early October to April but may sometimes extend into summer [36]. Of the 20,000 deaths from influenza each year, 90% occur in persons ≥65 years. Primary risk factors are lack of influenza vaccination among residents and HCWs. Ventilation and architectural issues also may play a role. In a report of an outbreak of influenza A affecting 68 residents, the LTCF had four separate buildings, one of which was newly constructed [37]. Interestingly, the attack rate in the new building was significantly lower than in the other buildings. Key differences in the new building included (1) a ventilation system that did not recirculate air, (2) more public space per resident, and (3) no office space in the building serving the entire facility. Even widespread use of immunization, the cornerstone of influenza prevention, may be insufficient to prevent some LTCF outbreaks. Especially in older residents, influenza vaccine effectiveness may be diminished, increasing the risk for influenza outbreaks. These failures may be secondary to poor immunologic response to the vaccine in this elderly population. In a LTCF with high rates (>85%) of resident influenza vaccination, outbreaks involving 172 residents were reported despite a match between the vaccine strain and outbreak strain [38]. Although influenza vaccination may not completely prevent clinical disease, clinical presentation often is ameliorated, especially if the match between influenza strains circulating in the LTCF and the vaccine strain is good.

Other Respiratory Viruses

In addition to influenza, infections with parainfluenza virus, respiratory syncytial virus, adenoviruses, and rhinoviruses can cause respiratory tract disease in LTCF residents. Parainfluenza virus type 3 was associated with an outbreak of respiratory disease on a 50 bed nursing unit of a large Wisconsin LTCF. The attack rate was 50% and resulted in 16% mortality within 9 days of symptom onset [39]. In contrast, a study of 30-day mortality suggested that non-influenza viruses have lower mortality than influenza viruses with mortality ranging from 6.1% (influenza B) and 5.4% (influenza A) to virtually nil for (RSV) and rhinoviruses [10]. The key observations from reports on respiratory tract outbreaks are that early identification of the infectious agents, institution of appropriate treatment or prophylaxis, and aggressive use of infection control precautions, especially isolation of residents and improved HCW compliance with hand hygiene recommendations, are critical to minimize serious morbidity and deaths.

Streptococcus Pneumoniae

Although not a common cause of outbreaks in LTCFs, *Streptococcus pneumoniae* is the most common pathogen identified in endemic respiratory tract disease in LTCF residents, is an important cause of invasive disease, and is increasingly resistant to antimicrobials. The incidence of invasive *S. pneumoniae* in LTCF residents is 4 times higher than in community living elderly individuals [41]. In a review of 26 *S. pneumoniae* outbreaks since 1990, the majority occurred in elderly patients in LTCFs or hospitals [42]. The most common serotypes identified in these outbreaks

were 23F, 14, and 4, all of which are included in current formulations of the pneumococcal vaccine. Outbreaks of *S. pneumoniae* pneumonia and bacteremia in Oklahoma, Massachusetts, and Maryland LTCFs were associated with low pneumococcal vaccination rates [43]. An LTCF outbreak of *S. pneumoniae* pneumonia in Massachusetts was associated with a 20% case-fatality rate. Antecedent infection with human parainfluenza virus was associated with increased risk of *S. pneumoniae* infection [44].

Legionnaire's Disease

Legionnaire's disease, caused by *Legionella pneumophilia*, remains an important consideration during respiratory tract disease outbreaks. Outbreaks in both LTCFs and hospitals generally are associated with contaminated water systems. *L. pneumophilia* may persist in healthcare facility water systems despite the use of a variety of interventions [45]. To identify these outbreaks earlier, LTCF clinicians and staff should maintain a high index of suspicion for Legionnaires's disease and obtain the proper laboratory support for microbiologic testing to identify *L. pneumophila*.

Nursing Home–Acquired Pneumonia

Pneumonia probably is the most serious common infection in LTCFs with regard to morbidity and mortality [46]. Independent risk factors for LTCF-acquired pneumonia include poor functional status, chronic lung disease, difficulty swallowing, presence of a tracheostomy, increasing age, and male gender. Aspiration of oropharyngeal contents is the usual mechanism, especially in frail, cognitively impaired or neurologically compromised residents. Diagnosis should include chest radiography and assessment of oxygenation (e.g., pulse oximetry) at a minimum but etiologic diagnosis often is lacking. Prevention interventions such as improving oral hygiene, swallowing evaluations, and dietary interventions (e.g., thickening of liquids) have had limited evaluation and success. Elevation of the head of the bed in a resident with high risk for aspiration may be beneficial but also may increase risk for other adverse events (e.g., falls). Influenza and pneumococcal vaccination are recommended to reduce risk for pneumonia.

Gastrointestinal Infections

Diarrhea in LTCF residents is common and may be due to both infectious and noninfectious causes. Diarrheal or gastrointestinal outbreaks in LTCFs are potentially explosive, have high attack rates once established, and can result in severe dehydration and death. Outbreaks can affect both residents and staff, causing severe disruption in the LTCF. The usual modes of transmission are through person-to-person transmission or, less commonly, foodborne transmission. The most common outbreaks are due to norovirus or rotavirus. Outbreaks due to bacterial pathogens are less commonly reported.

A few case reports illustrate key aspects of diarrheal or gastroenteritis outbreaks in LTCFs. In a 250-bed LTCF in Tennessee, 14% of residents developed gastroenteritis due to *Salmonella hadar* [47]. Among the 244 HCWs, the attack rate was 27% in laundry workers while only 3% in nursing staff and 4% in kitchen staff. Although the index case was probably a member of the kitchen staff, the high attack rate among the laundry staff was probably secondary to inconsistent use of gloves and lack of protective clothing while handling of increased volumes of soiled linen during the outbreak. In an Australian LTCF, 25 residents developed gastroenteritis caused by *Clostridium perfringens* due to contamination of pureed food [48]. Apparently, after the food was liquified, it was not reheated and subsequently became contaminated. Consequently, the authors recommended that pureed food be reheated to 70°C to inactivate potential contaminating pathogens before consumption. In Virginia LTCFs during one year, caliciviruses were responsible for eight different reported outbreaks [49]. In a Maryland LTCF with 121 residents, 51% of residents and 47% of the staff developed gastroenteritis due to a calicivirus over a four-month period [50]. The index case in the outbreak was a nurse who continued to work for two additional days after becoming ill. The outbreak illustrates the need to exclude ill employees in a timely fashion by providing sick leave and not expecting staff to take annual or vacation leave for illnesses. In a norovirus outbreak in an LTCF, the majority (57%) of residents developed acute gastroenteritis following exposure to an ill LTCF resident, the index case [51]. In the residents, prominent symptoms included vomiting (90%), diarrhea (70%), and fever (12%). Four residents required hospitalization, and three died. Many HCWs (35%) also developed gastroenteritis. Based on molecular typing, the outbreak appeared to occur among debilitated residents and their nurses, implying that the outbreak was propagated through LTCF staff rather than ambulatory residents. Cohorting of ill patients and strict adherence to infection control practices, such as hand hygiene, glove use, and barrier precautions, stopped the outbreak.

Skin Infections

Skin infections in LTCF residents usually are caused by fungi or bacteria, easily treated, and self-limited. However, LTCF residents have several risk factors that may promote both more serious infections and skin infection outbreaks. These risk factors include poor nutritional status, presence of surgical wounds or pressure ulcers, skin maceration or wetness due to contact with feces or urine, and the use of common bathing facilities. Examples of LTCF skin infection outbreaks due to bacteria include *S. pyogenes*–associated cellulitis, *Pseudomonas aeruginosa*

associated with a contaminated whirlpool bath, and group A *streptococcus* or ARPs causing infections of pressure ulcers. In addition to bacterial skin infections, scabies is an important parasitic skin infection that not infrequently causes outbreaks in LTCFs. Transmission of scabies may occur by contact with mite-contaminated inanimate objects (e.g., bed linens) or direct person-to-person contact. Outbreaks of scabies in three Norwegian LTCF lasted for five months and involved 27 patients or HCWs [52]. Initial treatments with permethrin were not successful; however, benzyl benzoate was effective. Ultimately, >600 residents and staff were treated. A key observation from these outbreaks was the need for simultaneous treatment of residents and staff and disinfection of bedding, clothing, and the environment. As with other outbreaks, early identification is optimal for management of scabies outbreaks and occasionally may require dermatological consultation or skin biopsy for diagnosis.

Infections with ARPs

Both endemic and epidemic infections in LTCFs occur due to ARPs [15]. Important ARPs include MRSA; VRE, or multidrug-resistant gram-negative rods such as *E. coli*, *Acinetobacter*, *Enterobacter*, or *Pseudomonas aeruginosa* [23,53]. Widespread colonization of residents in LTCFs with ARPs provides a potential reservoir for subsequent transmission and outbreaks. In Chicago, a citywide outbreak of multidrug-resistant *Klebsiella pneumoniae* and *Escherichia coli* demonstrated that LTCFs were important ARP reservoirs [54]. Furthermore, in a single Chicago skilled nursing facility, 43% of residents were colonized with ≥1 ARP [55]. Recent studies have demonstrated success in reducing VRE colonization or infection and may offer important intervention strategies for the future [56,57]. These studies have documented the importance of resident active surveillance cultures, isolation, HCW hand hygiene, and decreased inappropriate antimicrobial use.

In addition to cross-transmission, widespread antimicrobial use is a potential risk factor for the development of antimicrobial resistance within LTCFs. In Maryland, 54% of LTCF residents received ≥1 course of antimicrobial therapy [58]. In four New York LTCFs, the percentage of patient-days during which antimicrobials were given ranged from 2.7% to 6.8% [59]. In a Veterans Affairs LTCF, the majority (54%) of patient febrile episodes resulted in the initiation of antimicrobial therapy, with upper respiratory tract illnesses, bronchitis/pneumonia, or UTIs accounting for the majority of indications [60]. Following diagnostic evaluation, 39% of patients continued to receive antimicrobials despite negative laboratory and radiographic studies for bacterial infections. In general, previous studies have found substantial inappropriate use of antimicrobials in LTCF residents, ranging from 25–75% [61]. In addition to increasing the risk of ARP colonization or infection, inappropriate antimicrobial use adds to patient care costs and may place the patient at risk for adverse medication reactions [59,61].

INFECTION CONTROL IN LTCFS

Developing and implementing infection prevention and control programs in LTCFs is especially challenging. A comprehensive approach should include preventing infections through vaccinations, improving the diagnostic approach to infections and antimicrobial use and implementing effective infection control strategies [62].

Infection Control Program

Several reviews, guidelines, and position statements for infection control in LTCFs have been published previously [61,63,64]. In addition, guidelines from the Centers for Disease Control and Prevention for many aspects of infection control are available through the Internet (www.cdc.gov/ncidod/dhqp). The key components of a well-organized infection control program in LTCFs include (1) a well-trained infection control professional (ICP) to head the program, (2) an infection control committee, (3) a written and widely disseminated infection control plan, and (4) sufficient administrative support to undertake core infection control functions.

The two most important aspects of an LTCF infection control program are that the ICP is trained in infection control and that the LTCF administrator provides support and resources for the program. In a survey of LTCFs in the northeastern United States, most ICPs were registered nurses (90%) who performed infection control duties on a part-time basis (median = 8 hours per week) [65]. However, only half (52%) had formal training in infection control, and most had additional clinical or administrative nursing duties. These sobering statistics point out the difficulty faced in obtaining significant resources for LTCF infection control. However, the second component of the program, an infection control committee, can be instrumental in assisting the ICP in developing the infection control program. In smaller LTCFs, the committee may consist of the ICP, nursing director, medical director, and administrator. In larger LTCFs, the infection control committee also might include consultant pharmacists, an infectious disease expert, representatives from physical therapy or rehabilitation, and environmental services. In addition, the formation of teams including both geriatric clinicians, ICPs, and nursing staff may be especially beneficial in outbreak management [66]. To address resource limitations, LTCFs can seek to develop alliances with acute care hospitals, other LTCFs in the region, or have a corporate infection control program in a multifacility corporate chain. In some LTCFs, the infection control committee or its functions may be part of the facility's overall quality management or improvement committee.

In this setting, it is important to maintain a distinct focus, expertise, and resource commitment on infection control.

Immunization

Currently, LTCF residents should have yearly influenza vaccination and pneumococcal vaccination at least once after age 65, and LTCF HCWs should strongly consider receiving annual influenza vaccination [36,67,68]. Overall vaccination rates among LTCF residents for influenza vaccine (64%) and pneumococcal vaccine (28%) are suboptimal, and many LTCFs have inadequate policies addressing routine vaccination [69]. Preventing influenza and pneumococcal infections through an active immunization program is important not only for preventing these infections but also for limiting empiric antimicrobial use and avoiding post-influenza secondary bacterial infection. The components of a well-organized immunization program include a written facility policy and plan on immunization, an implementation manual, training for staff members including physicians on the immunization plan, collecting and recording baseline vaccination rates for current residents, and then initiation of vaccination of both current residents and new arrivals [69]. To monitor for outbreaks and institute timely control measures, LTCF infection control personnel should include active surveillance for acute febrile respiratory tract illnesses as part of the overall infection control plan. Furthermore, LTCF personnel should develop the surveillance system in conjunction with local and state health departments to enhance communication and ensure compliance with public health requirements [69]. Recently, implementation of standing orders for influenza and pneumococcal vaccination in LTCFs has been proposed as an effective intervention to increase vaccination rates [70].

Antimicrobial Prescribing

Decreasing inappropriate antimicrobial use in LTCFs should be an important component of an effective infection control program. Categories of inappropriate use include continued antimicrobial exposure despite no clinical evidence of infection, antimicrobial therapy with agents to which organisms from appropriate clinical cultures were not susceptible, and use of antimicrobials in residents with known allergies to the agent or with significant drug-drug interactions. Inappropriate use of an antimicrobial agent adds to patient care costs, may place the patient at risk for adverse medication reactions, and increases the risk of infections with ARPs.

In an effort to improve antimicrobial prescribing, minimum criteria for the initiation of antimicrobial therapy in LTCF residents have been proposed [71] (Table 28-2). These recommendations were not meant as strict management guidelines for clinically complex residents, and the residents' overall status must be considered by the clinician. The recommendations are useful in attempting to provide

TABLE 28-2
MINIMUM CRITERIA FOR THE INITIATION OF ANTIMICROBIAL THERAPY IN NURSING HOME RESIDENTS

Skin and Soft Tissue Infections

New **OR** increasing purulent drainage at the wound, skin, or soft tissue site

- **OR** two of the following:
  - Fever*
  - Redness
  - Warmth
  - Tenderness
  - New or increasing swelling at the affected site

Lower Respiratory Infections

- For residents with fever >38.9 C
  and at least one of the following
  - >25 breaths per minute
  - productive cough
- Fever >37.9 but <38.9
  - Cough and at least one of the following
    - Pulse >100
    - Delirium
    - Rigors
    - Respiratory rate >25
- Afebrile with COPD and age >65
  - New or increased cough with purulent sputum production
- Afebrile without COPD
  - New cough with purulent sputum
  - >25 breaths per minute or delirium

Urinary Tract Infection

- No indwelling catheter
  - Acute dysuria alone or fever
  - And at least one of the following: new or worsening urgency, frequency, suprapubic pain, gross hematuria, costovertebral angle tenderness, urinary incontinence
- With chronic indwelling catheter
  - And at least one of the following: Fever*, new costovertebral angle tenderness, rigors, new onset delirium

Fever with Unknown Focus of Infection

- Fever* and new onset of delirium or rigors

*Fever defined as >37.9 (100.0) or 1.5 C increase over baseline. Source: Loeb M, Bentley DW, Bradley S, et al. Development of minimum criteria for the initiation of antibiotics in residents of long-term care facilities: results of a consensus conference. *Infect Cont Hosp Epidemiol* 2001;22:120–124.

a rationale and guide for empiric antimicrobial therapy in otherwise stable residents. The guideline was based on expert opinion and remains to be tested in clinical trials. An important action that would potentially make a significant impact on antimicrobial prescribing in nursing homes is re-evaluation of residents with suspected infection after 48–72 hours of initial empiric antimicrobial therapy. For those residents in whom the clinical course (e.g., afebrile, no change in baseline functional status) and diagnostic study results (e.g., normal WBC count, negative culture results) do not suggest infection, clinicians should consider discontinuing antimicrobial therapy.

Hand Hygiene

Improved adherence to hand hygiene (i.e., hand washing or use of alcohol-based hand rubs) has been shown to terminate outbreaks in healthcare facilities, to reduce transmission of pathogens (e.g., MRSA), and to reduce overall infection rates. CDC has published guidelines to promote improved hand hygiene in healthcare settings including LTCFs [72]. In addition to traditional hand washing with soap and water, CDC recommends use of alcohol-based handrubs by HCWs for patient care because they address some of the obstacles that HCWs face in maintaining hand hygiene. When HCWs' hands are visibly soiled, they should wash with soap and water. The use of gloves does not eliminate the need for hand hygiene. Likewise, the use of hand hygiene does not eliminate the need for gloves. Gloves reduce hand contamination by 70–80%, prevent cross-contamination, and protect patients and HCWs from infection. Handrubs should be used before and after each patient contact, just as gloves should be changed before and after each patient contact. Alcohol-based handrubs should be applied to the palm of one hand and hands rubbed together, covering all surfaces of hands and fingers, until hands are dry. Alcohol-based hand rubs significantly reduce the number of microorganisms on skin, are fast acting, save time, and cause less skin irritation than soap and water.

When evaluating hand hygiene products for potential use in healthcare facilities, administrators or product selection committees should consider the relative efficacy of antiseptic agents against various pathogens and the acceptability of hand hygiene products by personnel. Characteristics of a product that can affect acceptance and therefore usage include its smell, consistency, color, and effect of dryness on hands. CDC recommends that healthcare facilities develop and implement a system for measuring improvements in adherence to these hand hygiene recommendations. Some of the suggested performance indicators include periodic monitoring of hand hygiene adherence and providing feedback to personnel regarding their performance, monitoring the volume of alcohol-based handrub used/1,000 patient-days, monitoring adherence to policies dealing with wearing artificial nails, and focused assessment of the adequacy of HCW hand hygiene when outbreaks of infection occur.

Infection Control Precautions

Infection control precautions are recommended, effective, and widely used in hospitalized patients who are colonized or infected with selected ARPs [73]. However, national guidelines for the use of infection control precautions in LTCF residents are used variably. Although use of active surveillance cultures and contact precautions in colonized

LTCF residents has been shown to reduce infections for some ARPs (e.g., VRE), widespread use of contact precautions has not occurred and would be challenging to implement in many LTCFs [56]. While also not widely used to date, universal glove use for contact with LTCF residents also may be effective [74]. However, simply having LTCF staff comply with standard precautions is likely to have an enormous impact in reducing ARP transmission. Often with bed-bound residents, HCWs are the usual vectors for transmission of pathogens. Because good hand hygiene is vital to reduce cross-transmission, LTCFs should consider the use of newly developed waterless alcohol-based hand hygiene agents to promote hand hygiene. Decisions about isolation of LTCF residents colonized or infected with ARPs must be considered on an individual resident and facility basis and must incorporate both an assessment of risk for cross-transmission and the impact on the resident's social and psychological health [61–64]. In addition to national guidelines, many state or local health departments have developed guidelines regarding the use of contact precautions or isolation of residents in LTCFs in that state or local jurisdiction. The LTCF medical director should be knowledgeable about these guidelines when making decisions regarding use of infection control precautions or isolating residents.

CONCLUSIONS

Infections in LTCF residents are an important public health concern, can result in serious illnesses and death in LTCF residents, and can be disruptive to LTCF staff. The major risk factors include the chronically ill population, the potential for cross-transmission during group activities and resident-HCW interactions, and the widespread empiric use of antimicrobial therapy. LTCFs can attempt to prevent or control ARP infections by ensuring that residents receive appropriate immunizations, supporting appropriate clinician evaluation for suspected infection, promoting good hand hygiene and appropriate empiric antimicrobial prescribing, and ensuring that the LTCF has a well-staffed and organized infection control program. Over the next several decades, the population of elderly LTCF residents will dramatically increase; resources for infection control programs in LTCF will be an important investment in improving the quality of care in this increasingly important healthcare setting. Likewise, the development of new knowledge regarding the epidemiology, prevention, and outcomes of infections in the LTCF residents is needed to make scientifically sound decisions regarding the use of limited infection control resources in LTCFs [75].

REFERENCES

1. Wunderlich GS, Kohler P, eds. *Improving the quality of long-term care.* Washington DC: National Academy Press, 2001; 1–20, 199–201.
2. Kemper P, Murtaugh CM. Lifetime use of nursing home care. *N Engl J Med* 1991;324:595–600.
3. Murtaugh CM, Kemper P, Spillman BC, Carlson BL. The amount, distribution, and timing of lifetime nursing home use. *Med Care* 1997;35:204–218.
4. Jones A. The national nursing home survey: 1999 summary. *Vital Health Stat* 2002; 13(152).
5. Eberhardt MS, Ingram DD, Makuc DM, et al. *Urban and rural chartbook: health,* United States 2001. Hyattsville, MD: National Center for Health Statistics, 2001.
6. Katz PR, Karuza J, Kolassa J, Hutson A. Medical practice with nursing home residents: results from the national physician professional activities census. *J Am Geriatr Soc* 1997;45:911–917.
7. Rosenfeld P, Kobayahsi M, Barber P, Mezey M. Utilization of nurse practitioners in long-term care: findings and implications of a national survey. *J Am Med Dir Assoc* 2004;51:9–15.
8. Ackermann RJ, Kemle KA. The effect of a physician assistant on the hospitalization of nursing home residents. *J Am Geriatr Soc* 1998;46:610–614.
9. Kane RL, Keckhafer G, Flood S, et al. The effect of evercare on hospital use. *J Am Geriatr Soc* 2003;51:1427–1434.
10. American Medical Directors Association (www.amda.com).
11. Harjivan C, Lyles A. Improved medication use in long-term care: building on the consultant pharmacist's drug regimen review. *Am J Managed Care* 2002;8:318–326.
12. Bowles SK, Kennie N, Ruston L, et al. Influenza outbreak in a long-term-care facility: considerations for pharmacy. *Am J Health-System Pharm* 1999;56:2303–2307.
13. Ouslander JG, Osterweil D, Morley J. *Medical care in the nursing home.* New York: McGraw-Hill, 1997.
14. Ouslander JG, Schnelle JF. Nursing home care. In Hazzard WR, Blass JP, Ettinger WH, et al. eds. *Principles of geriatric medicine and gerontology.* New York: McGraw-Hill, 1999.
15. Nicolle LE, Strausbaugh LJ, Garibaldi RA. Infections and antibiotic resistance in nursing homes. *Clin Micro Rev* 1996;9:1–17.
16. Nuorti JP, Butler JC, Crutcher JM, et al. An outbreak of multidrug resistant pneumococcal pneumonia and bacteremia among unvaccinated nursing home residents. *N Engl J Med* 1998;338:1861–1868.
17. Potter J, Stott DJ, Roberts MA, et al. Influenza vaccination of health care workers in long-term care hospitals reduces the mortality of elderly patients. *J Infect Dis* 1997;175:1–6.
18. Nichol KL, Grimm MB, Peterson DC. Immunizations in long-term care facilities: policies and practice. *J Am Geriatr Soc* 1996;44:349–355.
19. Carman WF, Elder AG, Wallace LA, et al. Effects of influenza vaccination of health-care workers on mortality of elderly people in long-term care: a randomized controlled trial. *Lancet* 2000;355:93–97.
20. Li J, Birkhead GS, Strogatz DS, Coles FB. Impact of institution size, staffing patterns, and infection control practices on communicable disease outbreaks in New York state nursing homes. *Am J Epidemiol* 1996;143:1042–1049.
21. Bonomo RA. Multiple antibiotic-resistant bacteria in long-term care facilities: an emerging problem in the practice of infectious disease. *Clin Infect Dis* 2000;31:1414–1422.
22. Wiener J, Quinn JP, Bradford PA, et al. Multiple antibiotic-resistant Klebsiella and *Escherichia coli* in nursing homes. *JAMA* 1999;281:517–523.
23. Strausbaugh LJ, Crossley KB, Nurse BA, Thrupp LD. Antimicrobial resistance in long-term-care facilities: antimicrobial use in long-term care facilities. *Infect Control Hosp Epidemiol* 1996;17:129–140.
24. Loeb MB, Craven S, McGeer AJ, et al. Risk factors for resistance to antimicrobial agents among nursing home residents. *Am J Epidemiol* 2003;157:40–47.
25. Bentley DW, Bradley S, High K, et al. Practice guidelines for evaluation of fever and infection in long-term care facilities. *Clin Infect Dis* 2000;31:640–653.
26. Irvine PW, Van Buren N, Crossley K. Causes for hospitalization of nursing home residents: The role of infection. *J Am Geriatr Soc* 1984;32:103–107.
27. Nicolle L. Urinary tract infection in long-term-care facility residents. *Clin Infect Dis* 2000;31:757–761.
28. Orr PH, Nicolle L, Duckworth H, et al. Febrile urinary tract infection in the institutionalized elderly. *Am J Med* 1996;100:71–77.

29. Ouslander JG, Schapira M, Schnelle JF, Fingold S. Pyuria among chronically incontinent but otherwise asymptomatic nursing home residents. *J Am Geriatr Soc* 1996;44:420–423.

30. Tambyah PA, Maki DG. The relationship between pyuria and infection in patients with indwelling urinary catheters. *Arch Intern Med* 2000;160:673–677.

31. Saint S, Wiese J, Amory JK, et al. Are physicians aware of which of their patients have indwelling urinary catheters? *Am J Med* 2000;109:476–480.

32. Maki D, Tambyah PA. Engineering out the risk of infection with urinary catheters. *Emerg Infect Dis* 2001;7:342–347.

33. Saint S, Elmore JG, Sullivan SD, et al. The efficacy of silver alloy-coated urinary catheters in preventing urinary tract infection: a meta-analysis. *Am J Med* 1998;105:236–241.

34. Saint S, Veenstra DL, Sullivan SD, et al. The potential clinical and economic benefits of silver alloy urinary catheters in preventing urinary tract infection. *Arch Intern Med* 2000;160:2670–2675.

35. Loeb M, McGeer A, McArthur M, et al. Surveillance for outbreaks of respiratory tract infections in nursing homes. *Can Med Assoc J* 2000;162:1133–1137.

36. Smith NM, Bresee JS, Shay DK, et al. Prevention and control of influenza: recommendations of the Advisory Committee on Immunization Practices. *Morb Mort Weekly Rep* 2006:55; 1–41.

37. Drinka PJ, Krause P, Schilling M, et al. Report of an outbreak: nursing home architecture and influenza-A attack rates. *J Am Geriatr Soc* 1996;44:910–913.

38. Ohmit SE, Arden NH, Monto AS. Effectiveness of inactivated influenza vaccine among nursing home residents during an influenza type A (H3N2) epidemic. *J Am Geriatr Soc* 1999;47:165–171.

39. Faulks JT, Drinka PJ, Shult P. A serious outbreak of parainfluenza type 3 on a nursing unit. *J Am Geriatr Soc* 2000;48:1216–1218.

40. Drinka PJ, Gravenstein S, Langer E, et al. Mortality following isolation of various respiratory viruses in nursing home residents. *Infect Cont Hosp Epidemiol* 1999;20:812–815.

41. Kupronis B, Richards C, Whitney C, and the ABC Surveillance Network. Invasive pneumococcal disease in older adults residing in long-term care facilities and in the community. *J Am Geriatr Soc* 2003;51:1520–1525.

42. Gleich S, Morad Y, Echague R, et al. *Streptococcus pneumoniae* Serotype 4 outbreak in a home for the aged: report and review of recent outbreaks. *Infect Cont Hosp Epidemiol* 2000;21:711–717.

43. Nuorti JP, Butler JC, Crutcher JM, et al. An outbreak of multidrug resistant pneumococcal pneumonia and bacteremia among unvaccinated nursing home residents. *N Engl J Med* 1998;338:1861–1868.

44. Fiore AE, Iverson C, Messmer T, et al. Outbreak of pneumonia in a long-term care facility: antecedent human parainfluenza virus 1 may predispose to bacterial pneumonia. *J Am Ger Soc* 1998;46:1112–1117.

45. Fiore AE, Nuorti JP, Levine OS, et al. Epidemic Legionnaires' disease two decades later: old sources, new diagnostic methods. *Clin Infect Diseases* 1998;26:426–433.

46. Mylotte JM. Nursing home-acquired pneumonia. *Clin Infect Dis* 2002;35:1205–1211.

47. Standaert SM, Hutcheson RH, Schaffner W. Nosocomial transmission of salmonella gastroenteritis to laundry workers. *Infect Cont Hosp Epidemiol* 1994;15:22–26.

48. Tallis G, Ng S, Ferreira C, et al. A nursing home outbreak of *Clostridium perfringens* associated with pureed food. *Aust New Zeal J Pub Health* 1999;23:421–423.

49. Jiang X, Turf E, Hu J, et al. Outbreaks of gastroenteritis in elderly nursing homes and retirement facilities associated with human caliciviruses. *J Med Virol* 1996;50:335–341.

50. Rodriguez EM, Parrott C, Rolka H, et al. An outbreak of viral gastroenteritis in a nursing home: importance of excluding ill employees. *Infect Cont Hosp Epidemiol* 1996;17:587–592.

51. Marx A, Shay DK, Noel JS, et al. An outbreak of acute gastroenteritis in a geriatric long-term care facility: combined application of epidemiological and molecular diagnostic methods. *Infect Cont Hosp Epidemiol* 1999;20:306–311.

52. Andersen BM, Haugen H, Rasch M, et al. Outbreak of scabies in Norwegian nursing homes and home care patients: control and prevention. *J Hosp Infect* 2000;45:160–164.

53. Trick WE, Kuehnert MJ, Quirk SB, et al. Regional dissemination of vancoymcin-resistant enterococci resulting from interfacility transfer of colonized patients. *J Infect Dis* 1999;180:391–396.

54. Wiener J, Quinn JP, Bradford PA, et al.. Multiple antibiotic-resistant Klebsiella and *Escherichia coli* in nursing homes. *JAMA* 1999;281:517–523.

55. Trick WE, Weinstein RA, DeMarais PL, et al. Colonization of skilled-care facility residents with antimicrobial-resistant pathogens. *J Am Geriatr Soc* 2001;49:270–276.

56. Ostrowsky BE, Trick WE, Sohn AH, et al. Control of vancomycin-resistant enterococcus in health care facilities in a region. *N Engl J Med* 2001;344:1427–1433.

57. Silverblatt FJ, Tibert C, Mikolich D, et al. Preventing the spread of vancomycin-resistant enterococci in a long-term care facility. *J Am Geriatr Soc* 2000;48:1211–1215.

58. Warren JW, Palumbo FB, Fitterman L, Speedie SM. Incidence and characteristics of antibiotic use in aged nursing home patients. *J Am Geriatr Soc* 1991;39:963–972.

59. Mylotte JM. Antimicrobial prescribing in long-term care facilities. *Infect Control Hosp Epidemiol* 1999;27:10–19.

60. Weinberg AD, Pals JK, Gurwitz JH. Are antibiotics over-utilized for treatment of early stage fevers in long-term care patients. *J Subacute Care* 1996:7–10.

61. Nicolle LE, Bentley D, Garibaldi R, et al. Antimicrobial use in long-term care facilities. *Infect Control Hosp Epidemiol* 2000;21:537–545.

62. Richards CL. Preventing antimicrobial-resistant bacterial infections among older adults in long term care facilities. *J Am Med Dir Assoc* 2005;6:144–151.

63. Friedman C, Barnette M, Buck AS, et al. Requirements for infrastructure and essential activities of infection control and epidemiology in out-of-hospital settings: a consensus panel report. *Am J Infect Control* 1999;27:695–705.

64. Nicolle LE. Infection control in long-term care facilities. *Clin Infect Dis* 2000;31:752–756.

65. Goldrick BA. Infection control programs in skilled nursing long-term care facilities: an assessment, 1995. *Am J Infect Control* 1999; 27:4–9.

66. Ahibrecht H, Shearen C, Degelau J, Guay DRP. Team approach to infection prevention and control in the nursing home setting. *Am J Infect Control* 1999;27:64–70.

67. Centers for Disease Control and Prevention. Prevention of pneumococcal disease: recommendations of the Advisory Committee on Immunization Practices (ACIP). *MMWR* 1997;46(RR-8):7–10.

68. Pearson M, Bridges C, Harper S. Influenza vaccination of healthcare personnel. *MMWR* 2006:55; 1–16.

69. Sneller VP, Izurieta H, Bridges C. Prevention and control of vaccine-preventable diseases in long-term care facilities. *J Am Med Dir Assoc* 2000;1:S1–S37.

70. Centers for Disease Control and Prevention. Use of standing orders programs to increase adult vaccination rates. *MMWR* 2000;49:15–26.

71. Loeb M, Bentley DW, Bradley S, et al. Development of minimum criteria for the initiation of antibiotics in residents of long-term care facilities: results of a consensus conference. *Infect Cont Hosp Epidemiol* 2001;22:120–124.

72. Boyce JM, Pittet D, and the Healthcare Infection Control Practices Advisory Committee. Guideline for hand hygiene in health-care settings: recommendations of the Healthcare Infection Control Practices Advisory Committee and the HIC-PAC/SHEA/APIC/IDSA Hand Hygiene Task Force. *MMWR* 2002;51(RR-16):1–45.

73. Muto CA, Jernigan JA, Ostrowsky BE, et al. SHEA guideline for preventing nosocomial transmission of multidrug-resistant strains of *Staphylococcus aureus* and *enterococcus*. *Infect Cont Hosp Epidemiol* 2003; 24:362–386.

74. Trick WE, Weinstein RA, DeMarais PL, et al. Comparison of routine glove use and contact-isolation precautions to prevent transmission of multidrug-resistant bacteria in a long-term care facility. *J Am Ger Soc* 2004;52:2003–2009.

75. Richards C. Infections in residents of long-term care facilities: an agenda for research: report of an expert panel. *J Am Geriatr Soc* 2002;50:570–576.

Endemic and Epidemic Hospital Infections

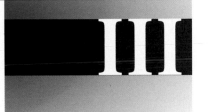

Incidence and Nature of Endemic and Epidemic Healthcare-Associated Infections

29

Lennox K. Archibald and William R. Jarvis

In the current era of managed care, U.S. healthcare systems are evolving from the traditional acute care hospital inpatient setting to a new integrated, extended care model that includes acute care hospitals, outpatient clinics, ambulatory center, long-term care facilities (LTCFs), and the home. As expected, healthcare-associated infections (HAIs) and antimicrobial resistance may occur at any of these levels of care. Except for the acute care hospitals, however, the relative importance of each of these settings for the acquisition of HAIs remains largely uncharacterized or unknown. The term nosocomial infection has traditionally defined infections acquired in the hospital inpatient setting [1]. Although the term has now been extrapolated to encompass infections acquired in other healthcare settings outside the acute care hospital, there is a paucity of published surveillance data regarding the occurrence of HAIs in LTCFs or the home. This chapter describes (1) the incidence and prevalence rates of common HAI pathogens in the United States, (2) secular trends in the occurrence of some sentinel HAIs, (3) the nature of HAI outbreaks in various healthcare settings, and (4) the implications for patient outcome and healthcare workers (HCWs).

Each year, approximately 35 million people are hospitalized in the United States, accounting for 168 million inpatient-days [2]. HAIs affect approximately 2 million (5.6%) of these patients and contribute to at least 90,000 deaths annually [3]. Almost 85% of these HAIs is associated with bacterial pathogens, and 33% is thought to be preventable just by maintaining infection surveillance and control programs without even taking individual preventive practices into consideration (e.g., catheter or wound care) [4]. The problem of HAIs is compounded by the emergence of antimicrobial resistant pathogens. Antimicrobial resistance contributes substantially to the higher death rates and escalating healthcare costs that currently are attributable to HAIs in the United States. A myriad of published data from single center studies has characterized the HAI pathogens and their susceptibility profiles to commonly available antimicrobials. The financial burden associated with HAIs includes the immediate costs of treating an unexpected infection, the added costs of antimicrobial resistance (e.g., inpatient care requirements, protracted duration of admissions, costly alternative antimicrobials, or toxicity to alternative antimicrobials) and the potential costs, such as lost productivity and untreatable infections.

ENDEMIC HAIS

Infection Rates

Because of their documented impact on prevention, surveillance and control of HAIs have become priorities within the various healthcare settings. A key objective of managed care is to improve the quality of medical care provided while controlling costs. To achieve this objective, key components of the managed care business model included substantial down sizing of general hospitals and monitoring quality of care and the occurrence, effects, and outcomes of HAIs through the estimation of infection rates using approaches that are strikingly similar to the principles of W. E. Deming for quality improvement in manufacturing [5]. However, to use HAI rates as a basis for measuring quality of care, rates must be valid to begin with and meaningful for comparison, either from one hospital to another or within a hospital over time [6]. Published reports have addressed the importance of adjusting for risk factors (e.g., device use, severity of illness) when comparing mortality rates among hospitals [7,8]. Similar approaches for HAI rates also are necessary [9].

A rate is an expression of the probability of occurrence of an event during a certain time interval. The numerator of an infection rate is always the number of infections of a particular type that have occurred within a particular group of patients over a particular period of time. The group of patients chosen and the choice of the denominator used in calculating the infection rates are what separate comparative rates from those that are not. The concept of a comparable rate is one that controls for variations in the distribution of a major risk factor associated with the event so that the rate could be meaningfully compared internally within the hospital or to an external standard or benchmark. Such risk factors could either be intrinsic or extrinsic: The former includes diseases (congenital or acquired), underlying conditions such as immunosuppression, age and gender, and severity of illness; extrinsic risk factors include various forms of therapy, exposure to antimicrobials, various treatments and procedures (including surgical), exposure to devices such as intravascular catheters, mechanical ventilators, urinary catheters, chest tubes or ventriculostomy catheters, receipt of solid organs or allograft tissues, duration of hospitalization, or exposure to HCWs. HAI surveillance enables healthcare facilities to objectively analyze and follow the trends of their own HAI over time.

The estimation of HAI rates in the United States began with surveillance studies of the prevalence and incidence of infections in individual hospitals [10–12]. The first systematic effort to estimate the magnitude of the problem on a wider scale was made by the Centers for Disease Control (now the Centers for Disease Control and Prevention [CDC]) in a collaborative study of eight community hospitals known as the Comprehensive Hospital Infections Project (CHIP) [10]. Performed in the late 1960s and early 1970s, this study involved intensive surveillance efforts to detect both nosocomial and community-acquired infections. At that time, data from these surveillance efforts suggested that approximately 5% of patients in community hospitals acquired ≥1 HAI, an estimate that was subsequently widely held to be the national HAI rate.

In 1970, CDC extended its HAI surveillance activities to a group of 80 volunteer hospitals of diverse sizes and types to help create a national HAI database, improve surveillance methods in acute care hospitals, guide the prevention efforts of infection control professionals (ICPs), and establish national risk-adjusted benchmarks for HAI rates [13–15]. This group of hospitals became the foundation of the National Nosocomial Infections Surveillance (NNIS) system, for many years the only source of national data on the epidemiology of HAIs, the pathogens that cause these infections and their respective antimicrobial susceptibility profiles [16]. Participation in the NNIS system is voluntary and is limited to U.S. acute care hospitals ≥100 beds. LTCFs, such as rehabilitation, mental health, or nursing homes, are not included in the NNIS system, which evolved over the years to a format in which participating hospitals collect and report to CDC their HAI data on medical and surgical intensive care unit (ICU) patients using standardized protocols, called surveillance components: adult and pediatric ICU, high-risk nursery, and surgical inpatient [15]. All HAIs in these groups of patients are collected using uniform definitions for HAIs and infection sites [1]. The identities of all NNIS hospitals remain confidential under section 308(d) of the U.S. Public Health Service Act.

In January 1999, the NNIS hospitalwide component was discontinued and a new component that included antimicrobial use data was incorporated. Reasons for eliminating the collection of hospitalwide data included the inordinate amount of time and resources required to collect these data, inaccurate case-finding in this setting, and the fact that hospitalwide rates are not amenable to risk adjustment and therefore not meaningful for national comparison [16]. During 2004, the NNIS system was combined with two other national healthcare surveillance systems into a single internet-based system—the National Healthcare Safety Network (NHSN) [17]. CDC has not yet released results of NHSN data analyses. Since the establishment of NHSN, approximately 243 hospitals regularly report ICU HAI data to CDC.

Various analyses of the NNIS data have yielded rough estimates of overall HAI rates that mirrored the 5% ascertained in the community hospitals that participated in CHIP. During 1974–1983, CDC carried out the Study on the Efficacy of Nosocomial Infection Control (SENIC) project [4]. One of the objectives of the SENIC project was to derive a more precise estimate of the nationwide HAI rate from a statistical sample of U.S. hospitals [18].

With 338 randomly selected general medical and surgical hospitals with ≥50 beds taking part and examination of more than one-third million patient medical records, two key findings of the SENIC project were first, that hospitals with the lowest HAI rates had both strong surveillance or prevention and control programs and second, different categories of HAIs required specific control programs whose effectiveness were not necessarily transferable when applied arbitrarily for control of any class of HAI. On the basis of direct estimates made in the 338 participating hospitals, it was estimated that ≥2.1 million HAIs occurred among the 37.7 million admissions to the 6,449 acute care U.S. hospitals in a 12-month period from 1975 to 1976 [19]. This gave rise to a nationwide overall rate of 5.7 HAIs per 100 admissions (i.e., ~4.5% of hospitalized patients experienced ~1 HAI).

CDC investigators recognized early on that overall HAI rates, such as those cited, were crude rates (i.e., imprecise, meaningless, and not valid unless they were risk adjusted). A crude overall HAI rate is the total number of HAIs at all sites (e.g., urinary tract infections [UTIs], pneumonias, surgical site infections [SSIs], bloodstream infections [BSIs], and others) divided by a measure of the population at risk (e.g., the number of admissions, discharges, or patient-days). Using a crude HAI rate to characterize a hospital's HAI problem has been seriously questioned or rejected [20,21]. Many investigators and organizations, including the Task Force on Infection Control for the Joint Commission on Accreditation of Healthcare Organizations (JCAHO), have rejected this rate as a valid indicator of quality of care [22]. The reasons were stated by Dr. Robert Haley himself, the task force chair and a principal investigator in the SENIC project: "A hospital's crude overall nosocomial infection rate was considered to be too time-consuming to collect because of the need to do continuous, comprehensive surveillance, unlikely to be accurate, and thus misleading to interpret, and unusable for interhospital comparison because of the lack of a suitable risk index of infection of all types" [23]. Before HAI rates are used for interhospital or intrahospital comparison or as indicators of quality of care, they require risk adjustment. As presently derived, a crude overall HAI rate of a hospital provides no means of adjustment for inpatients' intrinsic or extrinsic risks and is meaningless. Thus, CDC has stated categorically that such a rate should not be used for interhospital comparison [24].

Definitions of HAIs

HAI definitions usually involve clinical, laboratory, and imaging parameters. If they involve only laboratory or imaging parameters, there may be no clinical relevance to the event. One may not know that the patient really had an HAI because nearly all laboratory tests have false negatives. Alternatively, there may be no single laboratory test for the event. However, if only clinical parameters are used,

for example, a doctor's note or diagnosis, there may be too much subjective variation for the event to be useful to examine across hospitals. Finding and documenting events in hospitals (i.e., case-finding) such as mortality can occasionally be straightforward. However, finding HAIs requires considerable training before an HCW can reliably and accurately determine whether a patient has the infection. Medical record abstractors have consistently performed poorly at HAI case-finding compared with ICPs or electronic data capture methods [25].

The NNIS system has definitions for 13 major anatomic sites, each with 1–8 specific site codes. Each site code has ≥1 criteria that may include various combinations of the defining parameters as outlined earlier. Experience in the NNIS system has confirmed that targeted surveillance is better than hospitalwide surveillance for three main reasons [26]. First, case-finding is more accurate if targeted in a specific area, for example, a surgical ICU or other specialized units. Second, in practical terms, targeting a specialized unit is more efficient for the ICP and the allocation of limited resources. Third, risk adjustment is much more feasible for patients in targeted units [6].

With increasing numbers of patients currently being managed at home for malignant neoplasms that require intravenous chemotherapy, autoimmune conditions that require immunosuppressive therapy, SSI care following hospital discharge, chronic infections (e.g., osteomyelitis or endocarditis) that require long-term antimicrobial therapy, chronic urinary problems or renal failure with in-dwelling urinary catheters or ambulatory peritoneal dialysis, HAIs associated with the respective indwelling devices or surgical wounds commonly ensue. In addition, increasing numbers of LTCFs have established high dependency units to manage critically ill residents, who inevitably acquire infections once they become exposed to invasive devices or procedures. Notwithstanding the recognition of an increasing problem with infections associated with home healthcare, there are still too few guidelines for uniform standards and definitions of infections acquired in the home or LTCFs. Moreover, formal documentation of infections in these settings remains limited, largely because few facilities have designated surveillance personnel or, if they do, the designated personnel are unsure about what numerator or denominator data to collect. Infections in outpatients and ambulatory care settings are common. However, problems that preclude institution of surveillance activities for infections in these settings include the obvious queries: What infections to survey? What definitions to use? Who would be responsible for surveillance data collection? Where should the data be sent for aggregation and analyses? One of the few successes has been in the area of ambulatory hemodialysis centers. In 1999, CDC established the Dialysis Surveillance Network (DSN), a voluntary national system to monitor and prevent infections in patients undergoing hemodialysis [27,28]. With >100 participating hemodialysis centers, the DSN collects and reports outcome events, including vascular access site infections to CDC.

Rates by Site of HAI

HAIs involve diverse anatomic sites. However, the relative frequencies of these infections vary by site and by pathogen. Among all NNIS ICUs *combined*, the most common HAIs stratified by anatomic site are ventilator-associated pneumonia (VAP)(29%), UTIs (23%), BSIs (17%), and SSIs (7%) (Figure 29-1). However, the overall HAI rates and relative frequencies of different sites of HAIs tend to vary by type of ICU [16]. For example, among adult medical ICUs, the most common HAIs are UTIs (31%), VAP (27%), or primary BSIs (19%) [29]. The corresponding rates for NNIS pediatric ICUs are 15%, 21%, and 28%, respectively [30]. Moreover, the distribution of infection sites and pathogens in pediatric ICU patients differs with age and from those reported from adult ICUs [30]. In 2004, the median rate of VAP per thousand ventilator-days in NNIS hospitals ranged from 2.9 in pediatric ICUs to 15.2 in trauma ICUs [16].

Unlike ICU infections where one risk factor (medical devices) predominates, the risk of SSIs among patients who have undergone surgical procedures is related to a number of factors, which include the operative procedure performed, the experience of the surgeon, the degree of microbiologic contamination of the operative field, duration of operation, and the intrinsic risk of the patient [19,31–33]. An SSI risk index that effectively adjusts SSI rates for most operations was developed by CDC for NNIS hospitals [34]. This risk index is based on a system that scores each operation on a scale of 0–3 by counting the number of risk factors present from among the following three: (1) a patient with an American Society of Anesthesiologists (ASA) preoperative assessment score of 3, 4, or 5, (2) an operation classified as contaminated or dirty-infected, and (3) an operation lasting over T hours, where T is the approximate 75th percentile of the duration of surgery for the respective operative procedures reported to the NNIS data base. T, of course, will depend on the operative procedure being performed. The NNIS risk index is a better predictor of SSI risk than the traditional wound classification system, performs well across a broad range of operative procedures, and predicts varying SSI risks within a wound class. This suggests that all clean operations do not necessarily carry the same risk of SSI. Thus, SSI rates should be stratified by risk categories before comparisons are made among institutions and surgeons or across time. Exceptions are spinal fusion, craniotomy, ventricular shunts, and caesarean section operations in which SSI risk is not predicted by the risk index.

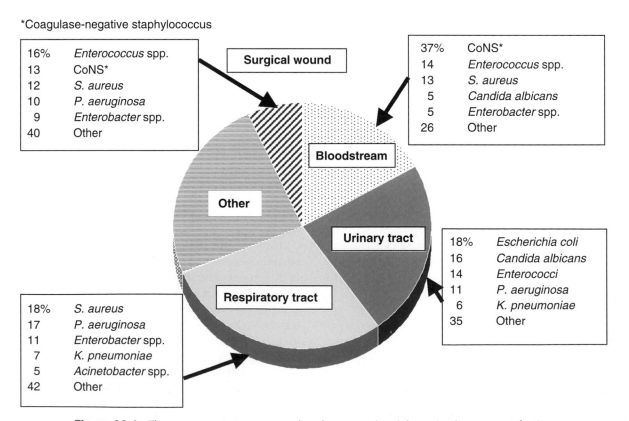

Figure 29-1 The most common nosocomial pathogens isolated from the four major infection sites, intensive care unit component, National Nosocomial Infections Surveillance system (NNIS) hospitals, 1990–1998.

Nosocomial BSIs cause substantial morbidity and mortality with at least 250,000 confirmed BSIs occurring each year in United States hospitals [35]. BSIs are either primary or secondary. The former are culture-documented BSIs in which no other site of infection was found to be seeding the bloodstream and usually ensue following direct infection. Of nosocomial BSIs reported to NNIS, approximately 64% are primary. Intravascular catheter use is the major cause of primary BSI. The microbiologic features of primary BSI have changed since the early 1980s. In 2004, CDC reported the highest mean rates (number BSIs per 1000 central line-days) of central venous catheter-associated BSIs (CVC-BSIs) in trauma ICUs (7.4), followed in descending order by burn ICUs (7.0), pediatric ICU (6.6), and medical ICUs (5.0); the lowest BSI rates (2.7) were found in cardiothoracic units [16].

On the basis of its microbiologic features, the pathogenesis of secondary BSIs (not included in Figure 29-1) appears to be different from primary BSIs. The risk of secondary BSI is highest after lower respiratory infections (7.8%), SSIs (6.6%), or UTIs (4.4%). Complications of infection by secondary BSI are most common on the cardiac surgery service (9.0%), followed by general surgery service (6.5%), the high-risk nursery (6.4%), the burn or trauma service (5.6%), and the urology service (4.9%). Secondary BSI was least likely on the otolaryngology service (2.6%), the orthopedic service (2.5%), and the gynecology service (2.3%). Secondary BSIs also are more likely in teaching hospitals. The organisms most commonly associated with secondary BSIs include *Staphylococcus aureus* (20.9%), *Escherichia coli* (11.3%), *Pseudomonas aeruginosa* (9.6%), and *Enterococcus* spp (9.2%).

Among the few investigations that have characterized BSIs outside the acute inpatient setting, three epidemiologic studies implicated the use of needleless devices as risk factors for acquisition of BSIs in home healthcare settings [36–39]. Associated risk factors included receipt of total parenteral nutrition and use of a multilumen catheter. DSN data from 109 participating hemodialysis centers reported that during 1999 through 2001, the vascular access infection rate per 100 patient-months was 3.2 overall and varied by type of vascular access: 0.6 for native arteriovenous fistulas, 1.4 for synthetic arteriovenous grafts, 8.4 for cuffed catheters, and 12.0 for noncuffed catheters [40].

HAI Rates by Pathogen

CDC data indicate that eight pathogens account for approximately 70% of HAIs in U.S. hospitals (Table 29-1); compounding the problem, all eight pathogens demonstrate antimicrobial resistance to ≥ 1 commonly used antimicrobials [41]. For example, the incidence and prevalence rates of resistance among isolates of *S. aureus* resistant to methicillin group penicillins (MRSA), *Enterococcus* spp. to vancomycin (VRE), and *Klebsiella pneumoniae* to third-generation cephalosporins have been increasing significantly over the past two decades; these rate increases are more marked in the ICU vs. non-ICU inpatient settings [41]. The percentage of MRSA among *S. aureus* HAIs in NNIS ICUs increased from 2.4% in 1975 to >55.0% in 2001; during 1989 to 2003, the proportion of ICU *Enterococcus* spp. HAIs reported to NNIS that were caused by VRE increased from 0.4% to >28.0%. This rate increase, in particular, is of enormous clinical importance because

TABLE 29-1

EIGHT MOST COMMON PATHOGENS ASSOCIATED WITH NOSOCOMIAL INFECTION (BY SITE) IN INTENSIVE CARE UNITS, NATIONAL NOSOCOMIAL INFECTIONS SURVEILLANCE SYSTEM, JANUARY 1989–JULY 1998

	Relative Percentage by Site of Infection					
Pathogen	All Sites (%) N = 235,758	Bloodstream (%) N = 50,091	Pneumonia (%) N = 64,056	Urinary Tract (%) N = 47,502	Surgical Site (%) N = 22,043	Other (%) N = 52,066
CoNS	14.3	39.3	2.5	3.1	13.5	15.4
Staphylococcus aureus	11.4	10.7	16.8	1.6	12.6	13.7
Pseudomonas aeruginosa	9.9	3.0	16.1	10.6	9.2	8.7
Enterococcus spp.	8.1	10.3	1.9	13.8	14.5	5.9
Enterobacter spp.	7.3	4.2	10.7	5.7	8.8	6.8
Escherichia coli	7.0	2.9	4.4	18.2	7.1	4.0
Candida albicans	6.6	4.9	4.0	15.3	4.8	4.3
Klebsiella pneumoniae	4.7	2.9	6.5	6.1	3.5	3.5
Others	30.7	21.8	37.1	25.6	26	37.7
Total	100	100	100	100	100	100

From: Fridkin S, and Gaynes RP. Antimicrobial resistance in intensive care units. *Clin Chest Med* 1999; 20:303–316; with permission.

the documentation during the 1990s suggested that at least 83% of VRE isolates were resistant to most of the available antimicrobials [42,43]. Although newer agents (e.g., daptomycin or linezolid) have proven effective against VRE, treatment options for patients with VRE-HAIs remain limited, often to unproven combinations of other antimicrobials or experimental compounds. That *Enterococcus* spp. infections now present a serious challenge for physicians is underscored by the fact that this is the most common SSI pathogen and the second most common BSI pathogen after coagulase-negative staphylococcus in all NNIS ICUs combined (Table 29-1) [41].

Of the microorganisms that predominate among the four major infection sites (BSI, SSI, VAP, or UTI), *Enterococcus* spp. are the most common cause of SSIs (16%), followed by coagulase-negative staphylococcus (13%), *S. aureus* (12%), and *P. aeruginosa* (10%) (Figure 29-1). Although coagulase-negative staphylococcus remains the most commonly reported cause of nosocomial BSIs (37%), this rate of occurrence is probably inflated largely because coagulase-negative staphylococcus is a common blood culture contaminant in hospitals and, not infrequently, a single blood culture that yields growth of coagulase-negative staphylococcus is deemed clinically significant when in fact it is not. That said, coagulase-negative staphylococcal BSIs remain the best marker of intravascular device-related infections in ICUs. Tokars et al. have shown that for blood cultures positive for coagulase-negative staphylococcus, the positive predictive value for clinical significance was 55% for 1 positive culture result of 1 culture performed, 20% for 1 positive result of 2 performed, and only 5% for 1 positive result of 3 performed [44]. In addition, he showed that for 2 positive culture results of 2 cultures performed, the positive predictive value is 98%, if both samples were obtained through the vein [44]. Further studies like this one and improvements in surveillance definitions and laboratory techniques are needed to further clarify the roles of coagulase-negative staphylococci, anaerobic bacteria, and viruses whose true roles as causes of HAIs have not yet been fully characterized.

NNIS data confirm that in addition to coagulase-negative staphylococcus, other common nosocomial BSI in descending order of frequency include *Enterococcus* spp. (14%), *S. aureus* (13%), *Candida albicans* (5%), and *Enterobacter* spp. (5%). Data from the Surveillance and Control of Pathogens of Epidemiological Importance (SCOPE) study, a multicenter surveillance system for BSIs in the United States, have established that gram-positive organisms are associated with 65.0% of nosocomial BSIs while gram-negative organisms and fungi cause 25.0% and 9.5%, respectively [45]. The frequencies of BSI pathogens in the SCOPE study were as follows: coagulase-negative staphylococcus (31%), *S. aureus* (20%), *Enterococcus* spp. (9%), and *Candida* spp. (9%)—similar to NNIS data.

The increasing role of gram-negative pathogens as important causes of HAIs has been highlighted in a relatively recent editorial [46]. For example, gram-negative BSIs predominate in patients with malignancies, burn patients with catheters, and patients with needleless intravascular devices [38]. Although *S. aureus* remains the most common (18%) cause of nosocomial pneumonia in NNIS hospitals, the next four most common causes are gram-negative microorganisms: *P. aeruginosa* (17%), *Enterobacter* spp. (11%), *K. pneumoniae* (7%), and *Acinetobacter* spp. (5%). In a recent NNIS analysis, Gaynes et al. found that gram-negative bacilli are still commonly associated with HAIs in ICUs and that during 1986 through 2003 were associated with 24% of BSIs, 65% of pneumonias, 34% of SSIs, and 71% of UTIs [47]. In addition, they found that the percentage of BSIs or SSIs associated with gram-negative bacilli decreased from 33.2% in 1986 to 23.8% in 2003 and from 56.5% in 1986 to 33.8% in 2003, respectively. Although the percentages of pneumonias and UTIs associated with gram-negative bacilli remained constant during the study period, the proportion of *Acinetobacter* spp. associated with ICU pneumonias increased from 4.0% in 1986 to 7.0% in 2003 [47].

Risk Factors and Determinants Associated with HAIs

The strongest determinants of HAI risk are the characteristics and exposures of patients that predispose them to infection and the complex interactions of agent (microorganism causing infection), host (susceptible patient), and environment (e.g., hospital ICU, outpatient, hemodialysis center, or home). Agent, host, and environment make up a triad that is a useful model for the characterization of infectious disease epidemiology in healthcare and other settings [48]. In this model, the environment is the backdrop against which a microorganism interacts with a susceptible patient to cause infection. The success of this process depends on both the microorganism and the host: it is increased in the nonimmunized or immunocompromised host and depends on the intrinsic properties (infectivity, pathogenicity, and virulence) of the microorganism. Other factors that are important to the production of disease include the infecting dose, the microorganism's ability to produce toxins, its immunogenicity and ability to resist or overcome the human immune defense system, and its ability to replicate only in certain type of cells, tissues, or patients. Other intrinsic and genetically determined properties of a microorganism may be important for it to survive in the host or environment. In the inpatient setting, these include the organism's response to the effects of heat, drying, disinfection or sterilization, or antimicrobials; its ability to compete with other microorganisms within the host or the environment; and its ability to independently multiply in the environment [48].

For transmission and infection to occur, the microorganism must remain viable in a reservoir or the environment until direct or indirect transfer to a susceptible host and contact with the host has been sufficiently long enough to cause infection and disease. The entire transmission process constitutes a chain of infection. If this chain of infection remains unbroken, the size of the reservoir may increase in the continuing chain of transmission. Examples of reservoirs that allow the agent to survive or multiply include HCW carriage of *S. aureus* in the anterior nares, *P. aeruginosa* under false fingernails, *Serratia marcescens* in soap preparations or damp areas around sinks, *Legionella* spp. in central humidifiers of air conditioning systems that disseminate the organism through the air in droplet nuclei, dialysis fluids that are intrinsically contaminated at the manufacturer, multidose vials that become contaminated during access with a needle and syringe (this becomes a major problem if numerous patients receive fluid from a single contaminated multidose vial), or sterile infusates that become extrinsically contaminated in the hospital pharmacy [49–53].

Indirect-contact transmission is the most common mechanism of transfer of the microorganisms that cause HAIs and commonly occurs via HCW hands. Other examples of indirect contact transmission include contaminated inanimate objects (fomites), work surfaces, and biological fluids (e.g., respiratory, salivary, gastrointestinal, or genital secretions; blood; urine; or stool). Medical devices contaminated with bloodborne pathogens (e.g., hepatitis B and C viruses, cytomegalovirus, or human immunodeficiency virus [HIV]) are sources of infection for both patients and HCWs in hospitals, outpatients, LTCFs, or the home. In pediatric populations, fecal-oral spread is an important means of indirect-contact transmission of a variety of bacterial, viral, and parasitic diseases. The mechanisms are commonly stool-to-hand-to-mouth or stool-object-mouth. Thus, in the United States, rotaviruses account for approximately 50% of all cases of nosocomial gastroenteritis in pediatric patients [54]. The airborne transfer of droplet nuclei is the principal route of transmission of *Mycobacterium tuberculosis*, varicella (chicken pox), measles or *Legionella* spp.

Patient factors (e.g., age, state of debilitation, immune or nutritional status, device usage, invasive procedures, or antimicrobial therapy) play important roles in determining whether or not a patient will acquire an HAI. Special units for intensive medical or surgical care and for extensive burns, trauma, transplantation, and cancer chemotherapy frequently house patients who are susceptible to infection and disease caused by endemic organisms. In these patients, reduced inocula of pathogens may cause infection and disease, and nonpathogenic agents (e.g., coagulase-negative staphylococcus) may cause serious disease or death. Frequent opportunistic infections in these patients require repeated, broad, and extended therapy with multiple antimicrobials, leading to increasingly resistant resident microbial populations. Commensal microorganisms can become opportunistic pathogens under appropriate conditions. Patients with immunosuppression (e.g., patients

with hematology conditions or HIV infection or who have had solid organ or bone marrow transplants or are receiving antineoplastic drugs) are at high risk of opportunistic bacterial, fungal, or protozoal infections.

Whether an infecting agent produces clinical or subclinical infections also depends on the agent and certain host factors, e.g., age and immune status. For example, *P. aeruginosa*, a ubiquitous pathogen that thrives in aquatic environments, soil, and vegetation, seldom causes disease in healthy populations. However, in debilitated populations, such as those with burns, malignancies, leukemia, critical care patients with multiple *in situ* invasive medical devices, or children with cystic fibrosis, this pathogen remains a significant cause of nosocomial pneumonia and BSIs [29,30].

Over the past three decades, much epidemiologic and clinical research have been carried out, either through formal studies or outbreak investigations, to characterize the risk factors associated with the occurrence of HAIs in various U.S. healthcare settings. It has not always been clear whether identified risk factors are merely associations with infection but not necessarily the underlying cause, or are indeed the true cause of the HAI. Undoubtedly, some risk factors will be the true cause of infection while others will be only coincidentally associated with infection because they follow infection, occur along with the truly causal factors, or are merely surrogate markers for the true risk factors. Complicating matters further is the fact that ≥ 2 independent risk factors often occur simultaneously in the same patient, sometimes exerting additive or even synergistic effects. Such risk factors are strongly intercorrelated.

NNIS data show increased HAI rates in ICUs [26,55–59]. The reasons for this increase include (1) increased ICU patient census due to greater need for intensive care, (2) a greater number of susceptible patients (e.g., the very young or elderly, and those with severe underlying disease, burns, malnourishment, or immunosuppression) being admitted to ICUs, (3) increased use of invasive medical devices in ICUs, or (4) HAIs due to lapses in infection control (IC) crowding, decreased nurse-to-patient ratio in the ICU, or increased presence of nosocomial pathogens in the environment [13,60–64].

Environmental factors, the third component of the triad, facilitate the transmission and acquisition of HAI through three principal modes of interaction with agent and host that determine infection or disease (i.e., agent-host, agent-environment, and host-environment interactions). The relative contribution of each of these interactions to acquisition of infection or disease is rendered complex because of the wide variety of infectious agents, hosts, environmental factors, and variability of parameters that make up each of these components. For example, NNIS data suggest that the ICU is currently the area of highest risk for the transmission of HAIs [26]. Moreover, MRSA, VRE, and *P. aeruginosa* already are endemic in many NNIS ICUs [26,65]. A complex interaction of factors, such as a pathogenic microorganism that is endemic in the ICU environment, a population of susceptible patients, inadequate hand hygiene or infection control practices among HCWs, fluctuating staffing levels, unexpected increases in patient census relative to staffing levels in the ICU, or an unexpected increase in the number of severely ill patients with multiple invasive devices could all concomitantly contribute to HAI acquisition caused by these endemic organisms [13,63]. Adding to the complexity of the process would be the transmission of the agent from host to HCW, HCW to HCW, and host to environment. Thus, acceptable HAI prevention and control measures dictate that the hospital epidemiologist looks at and analyzes the interrelationships among all components of the triad of agent, host, and environment.

It is well known that the social environment is extremely important in determining human behavior that affects the direct transmission of agents (e.g., artificial nails worn by HCWs in ICUs) [49]. Equally relevant is the impact of other social factors (e.g., distribution of and access to medical resources) use of preventive services or enforcement of infection control practice recommendations, acceptance of advice or guidelines on the appropriate use of antimicrobials, or appreciation by relatives, patients, and HCWs and personnel alike that patients who are aged, severely ill, born prematurely, or have congenital abnormalities, have numerous indwelling medical devices or have had multiple invasive procedures or surgery will be especially susceptible to HAIs. Finally, there must be a willingness of all involved to appreciate the limitations of medical technology and antimicrobials when all other clinical evidence and experience suggest that the condition of the sick person is irreversible.

To design strategies for preventing HAIs, it is important to differentiate among coincidental indicators of risk, independent causal factors, and synergistic interactions of causal factors. In a study of 169,526 patients who made up a representative sample of patients admitted to acute care U.S. hospitals in 1975 and 1976, population estimates of HAI rates for each of the four major types of infection were calculated within each category of exposure to between 10 and 20 separate risk factors [4,66,67]. A striking finding was that all of the risk factors were associated with HAI at all four major anatomic sites. At first, this seems surprising because one would not expect a direct causal association between mechanical ventilation, for example, and acquiring a urinary tract infection. The explanation, of course, is that some of the associations indicate direct causal relationships; others indicate partial causal relationships, potentiated or diminished by other concurrent influences; and others (such as that between respirators and urinary tract infection) represent largely coincidental associations (most patients on respirators also have indwelling urinary catheters that predispose them to UTI).

The two factors that appeared to exert the strongest causal influences in all four sites of infection were indicators of the degree of the patient's underlying illness: (1) in surgical patients, the duration of the patient's operation, and (2) an index of the number and type of distinct diagnoses and surgical procedures recorded (intrinsic risk index). After these, several factors were strongly associated with infections at one or two sites but not with all four. Having a combined thoracoabdominal operation was strongly associated with pneumonia and SSI; undergoing a "dirty" (or contaminated) operation was associated with SSI; having an indwelling urinary catheter was linked to UTI; being on a respirator, with VAP or BSI; previous HAI, with BSI; and receiving immunosuppressive therapy with BSI. Examples of risk factors that had weaker associations with all four sites were age, gender, previous community-acquired infection, and length of preoperative hospitalization.

Multivariate modeling has demonstrated that the risk of HAI is primarily determined by definable causal factors reflecting the patient's underlying susceptibility to infection or the degree to which microorganisms have access to vulnerable body sites. Modification of ≥ 1 of these factors can alter a patient's risk. Multivariate statistical models can be developed to predict accurately a patient's HAI risk from measurable risk factors.

Colonization is the presence of a microorganism in or on a host with growth and multiplication but without any overt clinical expression or detected immune reaction in the host at the time the microorganism is isolated. In a colonized patient, an infectious agent may establish itself as part of a patient's flora in multiple or specific anatomic sites or may cause low-grade chronic disease after an acute infection. Under suitable conditions, various patient populations who are colonized with *S. aureus* are at an increased risk of developing infection and disease [68,69]. For example, nasal colonization with *S. aureus* may be a risk factor for SSI in pediatric patients undergoing heart operations or for catheter-related infections in pediatric patients on chronic peritoneal dialysis [70,71]. HCW hands, colonized with gram-negative pathogens such as *S. marcescens* or *P. aeruginosa*, may become potential sources of outbreaks in neonatal ICUs [49,50].

Severity of Illness

In the NNIS system, the validity of HAI rates from ICUs, adjusted for extrinsic risk factors, would be enhanced if they were better adjusted with a direct measurement of patients' severity of illness. Otherwise, hospitals providing care for patients with a greater severity of illness may have higher HAI rates. Properties of a severity of illness score should include specificity for a particular HAI and site of infection.

CDC researchers performed a search of the medical literature to identify a severity of illness scoring system (SISS) that would be useful for further adjusting ICU HAI rates [72]. Eleven studies reported use of an SISS; four correlated SISS with all HAI sites but did not meet with success; six showed some predictive value between SISS and nosocomial pneumonia. The Acute Physiology and Chronic Health Evaluation (APACHE II) score was the most commonly used SISS but performed inconsistently and may not be available in many ICUs. Thus, although existing scores predict mortality and resource use, none are presently available for prediction of HAI risk. Until such measures are available, comparative HAI rates will be limited in their use as definitive indicators of quality of care.

Pediatric/Neonatal Populations

The major HAI risk factors in pediatric or neonatal populations include intrinsic host factors that are important to the development and severity of infection or disease. These include gestational age, gender, birth weight, congenital abnormalities, age at infection, race, nutritional status, genetically determined immune status, immunosuppression associated with other infections, therapy, and vaccination status or previous exposure to the relevant microorganism. Extrinsic factors for adults are similar and include invasive medical or surgical procedures, use of medical devices, such as intravenous catheters or mechanical ventilators, duration of hospitalization, or exposure to HCWs [73].

The risk of acquisition and transmission of infectious diseases among pediatric populations in healthcare settings are better characterized if the patients' immune status or immune response is known. Immunization is the most effective method of individual and community protection against epidemic diseases and plays an important role in the prevention and control of certain HAIs acquired by inpatient pediatric populations. As the proportion of a population immunized by previous exposure to the agent or by vaccination increases, the probability and opportunity for transmission of the agent within that population declines. Viruses are a frequent cause of HAI, morbidity, and mortality in pediatric populations [54,59]. Both symptomatic and asymptomatic patients with viral infections can be a source of transmission [74]. At present, the influenza vaccine is the only vaccine available to prevent infection caused by respiratory viruses. Children at high risk for severe influenza infection who should be vaccinated include those with chronic lung disease, congenital heart disease associated with significant hemodynamic disturbances, hemoglobinopathies (e.g., sickle cell disease), and children being treated with immunosuppressive agents [54,59].

Seasonality and Secular Trends of HAIs

Seasonality
The occurrence of HAIs is a dynamic process. Changes are constantly occurring in the types of patients admitted to hospitals, risk factors to which they are exposed, character of the pathogens predominating in the hospital milieu, quality of patient care, thrust of infection control efforts, and other important factors. Two indicators of the dynamic nature of the problem are the seasonality of certain types of HAIs and the long-term secular trends that may occur. Analyses of NNIS data repeatedly have shown seasonal variations in the occurrence of HAIs involving certain gram-negative bacteria [75–78]. The report of the 1980 to 1982 results showed clear seasonal peaks of infections in the summer and early fall for *Klebsiella*, *Enterobacter*, *Serratia*, *Acinetobacter* species, and *P. aeruginosa*; staphylococcal and streptococcal infections show no significant seasonal variation in the hospital. No seasonal variation was observed for infections caused by other common pathogens, such as *E. coli*, *Enterococcus* spp., *Enterobacter* spp., or anaerobes. More recent analyses have confirmed that the frequency of *Acinetobacter* spp. infections is increasing in critical care units in NNIS hospitals and are seasonal in nature [78]. Seasonal variation in the occurrence of *Acinetobacter* spp. HAIs is thought to be associated with changes in climate: summer weather increases the number of *Acinetobacter* spp. in the natural environment and may affect the hospital environment, promoting nosocomial transmission [79]. Nosocomial viral respiratory infections occur mostly during the seasons in which they occur in the community (e.g., influenza and respiratory syncytial virus infections in the winter and early spring) [80,81].

Clostridium difficile-associated diarrhea currently is the major nosocomial gastrointestinal infection and is endemic in many U.S. general hospitals [82,83]. During 1987–2001, there was overall seasonal variation in the occurrence of *C. difficile*-associated diarrhea in NNIS hospitals: Higher rates were documented during the winter months (January–March) vs. the nonwinter months [84]. Reasons for this variation include persistence of viable spores during the winter months and increased patient census or reduced nurse to patient ratios resulting in overcrowding in the ICUs during the winter. Also, because hospitals tend to admit higher numbers of patients with respiratory infections during winter months, one would naturally expect a parallel rise in antimicrobial use, a major risk factor for *C. difficile*-associated diarrhea, during this time of the year. However, the magnitude of the difference between winter and nonwinter rates varied by year [84]. Thus, factors other than climatic conditions (e.g., variation in antimicrobial use, staffing, or severity of illness on admission) may be playing additional roles in the seasonal occurrence of *C. difficile*-associated diarrhea in hospitals [84].

Secular Trends of HAIs
In prevalence studies performed over several decades, the relatively small sample sizes have hampered the detection of secular changes. An analysis of secular trends in the NNIS System from 1970 to 1979 suggested that SSIs decreased slightly over the decade, BSIs might have increased, while other HAI types remained unchanged [75]. NNIS data indicate changes in the entire distribution of HAI rates

following the dissemination of comparative HAI rates back to clinicians. Since 1987, when NNIS began reporting device-associated, device-day rates, there has been a 7% to 10% annual reduction in mean rates for device-associated infections in ICUs [85]. During 1980–1989, however, coagulase-negative staphylococci emerged as one of the most frequently occurring BSI pathogens [86]. During 1990–1999, risk-adjusted rates for BSI, VAP, and UTI decreased significantly in NNIS medical ICUs [87]. NNIS adult and pediatric ICU surveillance data from 1987 through 1996 show a downward trend in the rate of *Acinetobacter* spp. infections *overall* (cf., the increase in ICU pneumonia caused by *Acinetobacter* spp. from 4% in 1986 to 7% in 2003) [47]. The exact reasons for the decreases in risk-adjusted rates for BSI, VAP, or UTI have not been well studied but might be secondary to more hospitals participating in organized, surveillance systems that stimulated infection-prevention efforts [88].

During 1980–1990, the rate of nosocomial fungal infections increased at all four major anatomic sites of infection. Patients with BSIs who had a central intravascular catheter were more likely to have a fungal pathogen isolated than were other patients with BSI [89]. NNIS data from January 1989 through December 1999 have shown a significant decrease in the incidence of *C. albicans* BSIs; however, during the same time, the incidence of *Candida glabrata* BSIs increased [90]. The decrease in *C. albicans* BSIs is likely a reflection of the overall decrease in BSI rates associated with bacterial and fungal pathogens in NNIS hospitals over the past decade and potentially the increased use of antifungal prophylaxis [14].

In 2004, a CDC report confirmed that the incidence of *C. difficile*-associated disease steadily increased from 1987 through 2001 [84]. This report also confirmed that the incidence rate of *C. difficile*-associated disease during this 15-year period increased significantly in the ICUs of hospitals with >500 beds and that the major independent risk factors were longer duration of patient ICU stay, mechanical ventilators, intravascular devices, or urinary catheters. This upward trend in *C. difficile* rates could be due to three major factors: increasing antimicrobial use in U.S. hospitals, increasing ICU patient census, or increased frequency and sensitivity of diagnostic testing.

Although there was a general decrease in the total number of beds in NNIS hospitals during the 1990s, the number of ICU beds increased during the same period [26]. This increase in the numbers of ICU beds would have meant a potentially higher number of patients admitted to ICUs, higher numbers of severely ill patients, and increased antimicrobial use. More recently, Kyne et al. have established that patients who acquired *C. difficile*-associated disease were significantly more likely to have a higher severity of illness score at admission [91]. This, combined with the obvious prolongation of ICU stay and increase in use of invasive medical devices and antimicrobial use that one would expect in the ICU, would be obvious risk

factors for acquiring *C. difficile*-associated disease as was subsequently confirmed in the CDC report [84].

Rates by Service

HAI rates differ by service and specialty areas. The accuracy of HAI rates would be enhanced if better adjusted with, for example, direct measurement of severity of illness or service specialty. The SENIC project showed that surgery patients were not only at highest risk of SSI but compared with medical service patients also were at higher risk of VAP (four times higher), UTI, and BSI (one and one-half times higher). These results, however, reflecting combined data from the ICU and hospitalwide components, were not risk adjusted, and, therefore, were not valid for inter- or intrahospital comparison. By the early 1990s, CDC had begun to report HAI rates that had been adjusted for service. For example, NNIS data during 1990–1994 showed a stepwise decrease in HAI rates (calculated as the number of infections per 1,000 patient-days) by service as follows: burn or trauma service (15.0), cardiac surgery service (12.5), neurosurgery service (12.0), high-risk nursery (9.8), general surgery service (9.2), and oncology service (7.0). Lowest rates were found on the pediatric service (3.3), the well-baby nursery (1.7), and the ophthalmology service (0.6). In the most recent NNIS report summary (January 1992 through June 2004), rates are risk adjusted for device use and type of ICU [16]. CDC data also have shown that medical service inpatients appear to be at greater risk of contracting *C. difficile*-associated disease compared with inpatients on the surgical, pediatric, or obstetrics and gynecology services [84].

Because of this variability with service, risk adjustment according to service is mandatory when conducting inter- or intrahospital HAI rate comparisons. The importance of risk adjusting by service is underscored by the disparate device-associated infection rates in the urinary tract, bloodstream, or respiratory tract reported in the most recent NNIS surveillance report (Table 29-2).

Rates by Hospital Type and Geographic Region

It has long been apparent that, overall, HAI rates differ substantially from one hospital to another. In the mid-nineteenth century, Sir James Y. Simpson found that the rate of death from infection of amputated extremities varied directly with the size of the hospital in which the operation was performed (with larger hospitals having higher rates), a phenomenon he called "hospitalism" [92]. The average HAI rates of NNIS hospitals were reported to vary from 1.7% in small community hospitals to >11.0% in chronic disease hospitals [93]. However, as discussed earlier in this chapter, overall HAI rates like these are meaningless.

Among the numerous NNIS data analyses conducted over the years, characteristics consistently found to be

TABLE 29-2

POOLED MEANS OF THE DISTRIBUTION OF DEVICE-ASSOCIATED INFECTION RATES, BY TYPE OF ICU, ICU COMPONENT, NATIONAL NOSOCOMIAL INFECTIONS SURVEILLANCE SYSTEM, CENTERS FOR DISEASE CONTROL AND PREVENTION, JANUARY 1992 THROUGH JUNE 2004

	Urinary Catheter-Associated UTI Rate[a]	Central Line-Associated BSI Rate[b]	Ventilator-Associated Pneumonia Rate[c]
Coronary	4.5	3.5	4.4
Cardiothoracic	3.0	2.7	7.2
Medical	5.1	5.0	4.9
Medical-surgical			
Major teaching	3.9	4.0	5.4
All others	3.3	3.2	5.1
Neurosurgical	6.7	4.6	11.2
Pediatric	4.0	6.6	2.9
Surgical	4.4	4.6	9.3
Trauma	6.0	7.4	15.2
Burn	6.7	7.0	12.0
Respiratory	6.4	4.8	4.9

UTI, urinary tract infection; BSI, bloodstream infection.

[a] $\frac{\text{Number of urinary catheter-associated UTIs}}{\text{Number of urinary catheter days}} \times 1,000$

[b] $\frac{\text{Number of central line-associated BSIs}}{\text{Number of central line-days}} \times 1,000$

[c] $\frac{\text{Number of ventilator associated pneumonias}}{\text{Number of ventilator days}} \times 1,000$

associated with higher HAI rates include affiliation with a medical school (i.e., teaching vs. nonteaching), size of the hospital and ICU categorized by the number of beds (large hospitals and larger ICUs generally had higher HAI rates), type of control or ownership of the hospital (municipal, nonprofit, investor owned), and region of the country [94]. These relationships were consistent for each of the four major anatomic sites of infection. In addition, within these four hospital groups, rates of UTI, SSI, or BSI were generally higher in the northeast and north-central regions, whereas VAP rates were higher in the west. More recent NNIS data show increased rates of *C. difficile* or *Acinetobacter* spp. infections in the northeast [78,84]. For *C. difficile*, the lowest rates were in nonteaching hospitals, and intermediate rates in teaching hospitals with <500 beds; highest rates were observed in teaching hospitals with ≥500 beds.

Various analyses of the SENIC and NNIS data have found that indices of patients' risk factors explained the greatest part of the interhospital differences. After controlling for patients' risk factors, average length of stay, and measures of the completeness of diagnostic workups for infection (e.g., culturing rates), the differences in the average HAI rates of the various hospital groups virtually disappeared. These

findings suggest that much of the difference in observable HAI rates of various types of hospitals is due to differences in the intrinsic degree of illness of their patients, related factors (e.g., age, co-morbid conditions), and whether or not the hospital has a functioning HAI surveillance system. For these reasons, the overall HAI rate per se usually gives little insight into whether the hospital's infection control efforts are effective.

Trends in HAI Rates vs. Antimicrobial Resistance Rates Associated with Nosocomial Pathogens

Failure to fully apply infection control precautions may result in unmitigated spread of HAI pathogens in ICUs, especially where there is already heavy invasive device use, empiric antimicrobial prescribing, a population of critically ill patients who are more susceptible to overgrowth of endogenous resistant pathogens, high patient census, and numerous opportunities for cross-transmission due to frequent close contacts between the various HCWs who work in such units and patients. A combination of all of these factors with failure to fully identify those patients who are colonized or infected with antimicrobial-resistant pathogens and with the fact that there has been a significant increase in numbers of U.S. ICUs might be the reason for the upward secular trends in antimicrobial resistance among HAI pathogens. Although patients admitted to ICUs in U.S. hospitals are at greatest risk of acquiring HAIs, NNIS data suggest that overall rates of device-associated HAIs are decreasing while rates of HAIs caused by antimicrobial-resistant pathogens continue to increase.

EPIDEMIC HAIS

Incidence, Recognition, and Control

Each year, numerous publications describe the investigation of HAI outbreaks at individual institutions, the findings and inferences of these investigations, and the resulting prevention and control measures that ensue. However, there is a paucity of published data on the frequencies of the underlying causes of these epidemics or on the comparative nature of HAI outbreaks among institutions. The earliest study on this subject was the CDC's CHIP study in the early 1970s [95]. Among seven community hospitals participating in CHIP during 12 months in 1972 to 1973, a computerized threshold program screened the regularly reported episodes of HAI for clusters of infection that might indicate an outbreak, and a CDC epidemiologist analyzed the data to eliminate purely coincidental clusters. Next, CDC personnel visited the hospitals that had potential outbreaks to confirm the nature of the problem and recommend control measures if needed. From these data it was estimated that one true outbreak occurred for every 10,000 hospital admissions and that HAI outbreaks accounted for approximately 2.0% of all documented HAIs. Wenzel et al. estimated that 3.7% of HAIs in a large, university-affiliated referral hospital occurred in outbreaks [96]. Although confined to a relatively small number of hospitals, these estimates appear to confirm the prevailing view that HAI outbreaks account for a fairly small proportion of HAIs in healthcare institutions [95,96]. Other data have indicated that >90% of HAIs do not occur in recognized epidemics [97].

The CHIP investigations also demonstrated that 40% of the outbreaks likely resolved spontaneously whereas the remaining 60% continued until control measures were instituted [95]. Half of the outbreaks that continued were controlled by measures taken by the hospitals' IC staff and the other half completely resolved only after implementation of measures recommended by outside investigators. This relatively high rate of spontaneous resolution might explain the underlying argument against surveillance expressed by some people. However, if these figures are representative of community hospitals in general—and it should be borne in mind that these were hospitals with active HAI surveillance systems—then a large number of outbreaks may be going unrecognized and uncontrolled despite the advanced state of IC programs.

HAI Outbreaks

Investigation of HAI outbreaks requires a systematic approach that includes ascertainment that an epidemic does indeed exist, formulation of an appropriate case definition, and implementation of epidemiologic methods to identify risk factors and determine whether the relation between the factor and infection is associative or causative, which is essential for understanding the mechanisms of infection acquisition and transmission and for implementing appropriate control and preventive measures. This process assumes some previous knowledge of the usual or endemic rate of occurrence of the infection or disease under study. Moreover, for this determination, one must have an understanding of the epidemiology of the infection or disease (i.e., the possible common sources, putative modes of transmission, usual reservoirs, incubation periods, and the microbiology of the microorganism of concern, including pathogenicity and virulence). This information is essential for the formulation of hypotheses and the design of relevant epidemiologic, observational, and microbiologic studies necessary for confirming the hypothesis.

Many factors influence the types of investigations of HAI outbreaks conducted by CDC. These include the types of outbreaks that are recognized, the expertise of the personnel who request CDC's assistance, whether outbreaks are of sufficient potential public health importance (e.g., attributable morbidity or mortality) to warrant CDC's involvement, investigator availability, and whether a CDC investigation might add to infection control knowledge to

help prevent or control similar outbreaks in the future. Thus, CDC outbreak investigations often reflect problems that are unique, urgent, perplexing to ascertain, or difficult to control.

From 1956 to 1979, CDC carried out 252 hospital outbreak investigations; these have been summarized by Stamm and co-workers [97]. In the ensuing 16 years through 1995, CDC assisted in another 193 outbreak investigations. In the early years (1956–1962), the two most common problems investigated were epidemics of gastrointestinal disease, primarily due to *Salmonella* species or enteropathogenic *E. coli*, or staphylococcal infections; both types of epidemics were most frequently encountered in newborn nurseries. In the early 1960s, the investigation of staphylococcal infections abruptly decreased and was followed in the 1970s by a decrease in the number of gastrointestinal outbreak investigations in healthcare settings. This likely reflected a decrease in the incidence of such outbreaks because of improved understanding of the epidemiology and control of such infections or the improved ability of IC personnel to recognize and control such outbreaks without CDC's assistance.

From the late 1960s through the 1980s, there was an increase in the number of investigations of nosocomial BSI outbreaks, SSI, and problems related to ICUs, newly introduced medical devices, and various surgical and invasive medical procedures. Many of these outbreaks were associated with gram-negative pathogens. During the 1970s, outbreaks of BSIs in healthcare settings were the most common types of investigations carried out by CDC. However, increasing numbers of HAI outbreaks were associated with anatomic sites other than the bloodstream, respiratory tract, urinary tract, and surgical wounds or medical devices: These included outbreaks of hepatitis A virus or hepatitis B virus infections; necrotizing enterocolitis in nurseries; sternal wound infections after open heart surgery, particularly those caused by rapidly growing mycobacteria; and nosocomial Legionnaires' disease. Also during this period, CDC recorded increasing numbers of outbreaks associated with microorganisms resistant to multiple antimicrobials, particularly aminoglycoside-resistant *Enterobacteriaceae* and non fermentative gram-negative bacilli, and MRSA.

In a review of outbreak investigations in healthcare settings conducted by CDC during 1980 through 1990, Jarvis documented a total of 125 on-site epidemiologic investigations of HAI outbreaks across the United States [98]. Among these 125 outbreaks, 77 (62%) were caused by bacterial pathogens, 11 (9%) by fungi, 10 (8%) by viruses, and five (4%) by mycobacteria; 22 (18%) were caused by toxins or other organisms. In addition, BSIs predominated, followed by SSIs and pneumonia. Many of the BSI outbreaks resulted from inadequately disinfected transducers in ICU patients or improper reprocessing of dialyzers [99–101]. Although gram-negative organisms accounted for >50% of the outbreaks during the first half of the 1980s, from 1985 to 1990, outbreak investigations increasingly involved gram positive organisms, fungi, viruses, or mycobacteria. During this decade, no outbreaks of UTIs were investigated, <10% of the outbreaks involved nosocomial pneumonia, and rapidly growing mycobacteria were recognized as causes of SSIs, chronic otitis media, and hemodialysis-associated infections [102–104]. Several outbreak investigations implicated noninfectious causes, such as vitamin E toxicity in neonates in ICUs and pyrogenic reactions and chemical toxin exposures in hemodialysis centers (e.g., chloramine, hydrogen peroxide) [105–107].

The characteristics of the investigations conducted throughout the 1980s likely reflected the increasing use of invasive procedures and devices and the introduction of an ever-increasing number of products. Approximately 33% of the outbreaks investigated occurred in ICU settings, and nearly 25% involved patients who had undergone surgery. Fourteen (11%) outbreaks were device related, 16 (13%) were procedure related, and 28 (22%) were product related. The proportion of outbreaks involving products, procedures, or devices increased from 47% during 1980–1985 to 67% between 1986 and July 1990. For example, nine episodes of *Yersinia enterocolitica* sepsis were associated with transfusion of contaminated packed red blood cells [108, 109]. Each of these independent events was traced to mildly symptomatic or asymptomatic infection in the blood donor. Prolonged storage of the blood cells allowed the proliferation of the *Y. enterocolitica*, which resulted in sepsis or endotoxin shock when the blood was transfused [108]. In another outbreak investigation, separate episodes of BSI, SSI, or endophthalmitis were traced to extrinsic contamination of a newly introduced anesthetic agent [110–112]. The manufacturer of this soybean oil–based product, which did not contain a preservative, did not recommend refrigeration. Laboratory studies demonstrated that when contaminated with low numbers of microorganisms, rapid microbial proliferation ensued [110].

In a more recent review of CDC outbreak investigations in healthcare settings carried out during January 1990 through December 1999, Jarvis documented 114 on-site investigations [113]. These outbreaks occurred in 39 states or territories and reflected the increasing use of invasive procedures and devices, the introduction of an ever-increasing number of products within and outside the traditional acute care hospital setting: 81 (71%) occurred in the hospital inpatient setting, 15 (12%) in dialysis centers, 9 (8%) in the outpatients, 6 (5%) in LTCFs, and 5 (4%) in home healthcare settings [37,113]. Of the outbreaks that occurred in the inpatient setting, 23 (28%) occurred in ICUs and 58 (72%) in non-ICU areas. Overall, 44 (39%) of the 114 outbreaks involved BSIs, 17 (15%) the respiratory tract, 10 (9%) SSIs, and 3 (3%) the gastrointestinal tract; the remaining 34% involved ≥2 systems.

Throughout the 1990s, 93 (82%) of the outbreaks were associated with infections: bacteria (61; 53%), mycobacteria (12; 11%), fungi (10; 9%), viruses (8; 7%), or parasites (2; 2%) [113]. The remaining 21 (18%) outbreaks were associated with endotoxin or noninfectious agents: The noninfectious disease outbreaks included aluminum toxicity in dialysis patients, anaphylactic reactions associated with latex hypersensitivity, and carbon monoxide poisoning in surgical patients [114–116]. Viral infection outbreaks included hepatitis A virus transmitted among HCWs in a bone marrow transplant unit, hepatitis B virus infection among LTCF residents or dialysis patients, hepatitis C virus transmission associated with intramuscular immune globulin, and (HIV) transmitted through inadvertent injection of HIV-contaminated material or during dialysis [113,117–119].

Fifty-two (46%) of the 114 outbreaks were associated with either an invasive device or invasive procedure. Dialyzers (10; 43%) were the most common invasive devices associated with outbreaks followed by needleless intravascular device use among patients in inpatient, outpatient, or home care settings (7, 29%) [36–38,120,121]. The most common invasive procedures were surgery (21; 50%), dialysis (16; 37%), or cardiac catheterization (3; 7%). Twenty (17.5%) of the 114 outbreak investigations were associated with contaminated products, including intravenous anesthetics (9; 8.0%), parenteral solutions (5; 4.4%), or blood products (2; 1.8%). Twenty-one (28.6%) of the infectious disease outbreaks were associated with multidrug resistant organisms, including multidrug-resistant *M. tuberculosis*; VRE; *S. aureus* with reduced susceptibility to vancomycin, vancomycin-resistant *Staphylococcus epidermidis*, or extended spectrum beta-lactamase producing *E. coli* and *K. pneumoniae* [113,122–137].

The anatomic sites of infection involved in CDC HAI epidemic investigations differ markedly from those involved in endemic infections (Table 29-3). Of the epidemics investigated by CDC in the 1980s, BSIs predominated, followed by SSIs and pneumonia. Among endemic infections documented during this period, UTIs predominated, followed by SSIs, pneumonia, and BSIs. In addition, the distribution of pathogens associated with epidemic and endemic infections varied markedly. In the 1980s, *Pseudomonas* or *Serratia* spp., *S. aureus*, and *Candida* species were the most common organisms associated with epidemics, whereas *E. coli*, coagulase-negative staphylococci, and *S. aureus* were the predominant endemic HAI pathogens in U.S. hospitals.

During the 1990s, CDC assisted in increased numbers of outbreak investigations caused by *M. tuberculosis*, *Enterococcus* spp., *Aspergillus* spp., and *Enterobacteriaceae*. In addition, seminal outbreak investigations during that decade heralded the emergence of *Enterococcus* spp. that were completely resistant to vancomycin and of *S. aureus* with reduced susceptibility to vancomycin [129,130,136]. Endemic HAI pathogens in NNIS hospitals during the 1990s included *S. aureus*, *E. coli*, coagulase-negative staphylococci, *Enterococcus* spp., *P. aeruginosa*, *Enterobacter* spp., and *K. pneumonia*; these seven pathogens alone were associated with two-thirds of reported HAIs at NNIS hospitals.

TABLE 29-3

COMPARISON OF TYPES OF INFECTIONS AND PATHOGENS INVOLVED IN ENDEMIC AND EPIDEMIC INFECTIONS

		Epidemic Investigations (%)	
	Endemic Infections (%)[a]	Jan 1983–July 1990[b]	Jan 1990–Dec 1999[c]
Site of infection			
Pulmonary	29	12	15
Urinary tract	23	5	<1
Bloodstream	17	20	39
Surgical wound	7	10	9
Central nervous system		5	2
Cutaneous		13	2
Gastrointestinal tract		18	3
Liver (hepatitis)		7	6
Other	24	10	13
Total	100	100	100
Pathogen			
Staphylococcus aureus	13	5	6
Escherichia coli	12	<1	<1
Coagulase-negative staphylococcus	11	<1	2
Enterococcus spp.	10	<1	7
Pseudomonas spp.	9	16	<1
Enterobacter spp.	6	4	4
Klebsiella pneumoniae	5	2	3
Proteus spp.		<1	0
Group A streptococcus		3	<1
Serratia marcescens		5	5
Salmonella spp.	<1	2	<1
Hepatitis	<1	<1	4
Candida species	<1	5	<1
Aspergillus spp.	<1	0	4
Mycobacterium spp.	<1	5	11
Other gram-negative pathogens			13
Other	34	48	36
Total	100	100	100

[a]Centers for Disease Control and Prevention, National Nosocomial Infections Surveillance System, 1990–1998.
[b]Source of data for 1980–1990: Jarvis WR. Nosocomial outbreaks: the Centers for Disease Control's Hospital Infections Program experience, 1980–1990. *AM J Med 1991*;91(suppl 3B):101S.
[c]Source of data for 1990–1999: Jarvis WR. Hospital Infections Program, Centers for Disease Control and Prevention On-Site Outbreak Investigations, 1990–1999. *Semin Infect Control 2001*;1:74–84.

CDC HAI outbreak investigations during the 1990s were essentially similar to the outbreaks of the 1980s: BSIs predominated as before; however, pneumonia moved up to the second place in frequency followed in descending order by SSIs, gastrointestinal infections, and meningitis; among the outbreaks associated with procedures, surgery and hemodialysis predominated. In contrast to the 1980s, the order of occurrence of endemic HAIs reversed during the 1990s with BSIs predominating, followed by pneumonia, and SSIs in that order (Table 29-3).

Epidemic infections commonly involved more unusual organisms, such as multidrug-resistant *M. tuberculosis* (described earlier), *Ewingella americana*, *Tsukamurella* spp., *Rhodococcus bronchialis*, *Nocardia facinica*, *Enterobacter*

hormaechei, *Acremonium kiliense*, *Malassezia pachydermatis*, *Ochrabactrum anthropi*, various nontuberculous mycobacterai, viruses, and fungi [98,138–144]. The profile of these outbreaks likely reflected the facts that HAIs vary by service or location (i.e., ICU vs. non-ICU) and that clusters of infections caused by unusual organisms or usual organisms with unusual antimicrobial susceptibility profiles are more easily recognized, whereas clusters of infections caused by common organisms with unremarkable antimicrobial susceptibility patterns are less likely to be recognized as significant. Also, these differences reflect the fact that unusual outbreaks are more likely to be investigated as are outbreaks in which a common-source or personnel carrier is involved than the more common problem of direct or indirect contact transmission of endemic infections in which organisms are commonly transferred from patient to patient, patient to HCW, or HCW to patient, via the hands, fomites, or the environment.

A number of selection biases influence which outbreaks are investigated by CDC. First, a problem must be recognized at the institutional (e.g., hospital, outpatients, home) level. Once an outbreak is recognized, the degree of available local expertise influences whether CDC assistance will be sought or requested. Second, if a problem at the hospital level is recognized and brought to the attention of the state health department, interest or expertise at the state level might determine whether the state concurs with the hospital's request for CDC's assistance. CDC is not a regulatory agency. Thus, any request for its assistance to conduct an onsite investigation requires an invitation by the facility's administration and IC and the local and state health departments. Finally, if CDC is invited to assist in an on-site epidemiologic investigation, several factors will determine CDC's response to the invitation. First is the potential public health importance of the problem and its implications for patient safety. For example, if an outbreak is potentially product related or is associated with substantial morbidity or mortality, all efforts will be made to respond. Second is whether the outbreak appears to be caused by an unusual pathogen or a common pathogen with unusual characteristics (e.g., an unusual or uncommon reservoir or mode of transmission), third is the availability of trained personnel to travel to the facility, and fourth is whether the field of healthcare epidemiology can be advanced by the investigation.

All investigations are conducted as collaborative efforts, and close working relationships with local, state, and federal personnel are desirable. These and other selection biases undoubtedly contribute to the profile of epidemic HAIs described in this chapter. Of greatest value to IC is the knowledge gained by an investigation regarding the most common sources and modes of transmission of various pathogens in outbreaks. These data help ICPs focus their preventive interventions on the areas most likely to result in containment of ongoing outbreaks.

In general, the mode of transmission of an outbreak pathogen can be categorized into one of the several groups outlined earlier in this chapter: (1) common source, (2) human reservoir (carrier), (3) cross-infection (person to person), (4) airborne, (5) other environmental (e.g., fomites, extrinsic or intrinsic contamination of medications, or introduction of a new type of medical device), or (6) uncertain modes of transmission. In a recent report, Diekema et al. opined that outbreaks are, by definition, "special cause" events and should be preventable, and almost always reflects poorly on IC practice in a hospital [145]. However, the reason why outbreaks occur is more complex than the above categorization and opinion would suggest, especially as the final occurrence of infection and disease involves multifaceted interactions between the patient, the pathogen, and the environment (the healthcare setting). A review of CDC outbreaks in healthcare settings suggests that although poor IC almost always play a role, outbreaks invariably occur when a series of events (including IC practices) go wrong at the same time. Thus, complex occurrences or failure of ≥2 factors, including unsatisfactory hand hygiene and IC practices among HCWs; fluctuating staffing levels; an unexpected increase in patient census relative to staffing levels in the ICU; an unexpected increase in the number of severely ill patients with multiple invasive devices; immunosuppression caused by illness, therapy, or disease; failure to conduct quality control in the laboratory; failure of engineering to maintain negative pressure differential in an operating room that should have been kept at positive pressure; inadvertent contamination (intrinsic or extrinsic) of soaps, medications, vials, allograft tissues, or devices; poor surgical technique; inadvertent bacteriostasis when conducting quality assurance cultures; or even misinterpretation of existing IC guidelines could all contribute to the transmission of an organism that is already endemic in the healthcare facility, a colonizer of patients, staff, or even relatives, or recently introduced into the facility [13,26,50,51,53,63,146–148]. Thus, when outbreaks are classified in terms of mode of transmission, various site-pathogen combinations, often specific to certain patient groups, will almost certainly become apparent and knowledge of these site-pathogen combinations can facilitate *initial* investigative efforts by focusing on the most likely source or modes of transmission and hypothesis development.

The danger, of course, is for a hospital epidemiologist to make premature inferences regarding association or causation based previous knowledge of site-pathogen combinations. For example, although nosocomial *Salmonella* spp. infections can be transmitted from person to person and previous salmonella outbreaks in healthcare settings have indeed been linked to common-source food, salmonella in ICUs has been traced to IC practices and device use [113]. Clusters of *Pseudomonas cepacia* infections should certainly alert IC personnel to the possibility of contaminated solutions, including antiseptics such as povidone–iodine solution [149]; however, *Pseudomonas* spp. infection has been traced to other very different sources (e.g., external ventricular devices in neurosurgical patients) [150]. Although nontuberculous mycobacteria infection associated with endoscopic procedures should certainly lead one to review endoscope disinfection/sterilization practices, sources of tap water, and causes of endoscope washer reservoir contamination, this class of mycobacteria has been associated with other modes of transmission including liposuction and pedicures or foot baths in nail salons [144,151–155]. Similarly, Group A streptococcal SSIs almost always are traced to an HCW carrier, and carriage can involve the rectum, vagina, scalp, or other sites [156]; thus, the underlying reason for transmission must certainly be ascertained. Outbreaks of gram-negative BSIs have been traced to myriad causes, including inadequately disinfected intra-arterial pressure-monitoring transducers, platelet transfusions, soap, contaminated multidose vials, the compounding machine in a hospital pharmacy, and even to staffing levels [13,50,51,53,99,101,157]. Thus, in any HAI outbreak investigation, knowledge of site-pathogen combinations has to be evaluated in the context of the epidemiologic findings during the investigation. Epidemiologic methods should be used to investigate and relate causal factors to an outbreak and are essential for understanding the mechanisms of infection acquisition and transmission and identifying putative risk factors.

The preceding site-pathogen discussion does not lessen the importance of using knowledge of site-pathogen combinations as precedent during the conduct of an outbreak investigation. For example, clusters of *Legionella* spp. pulmonary infections or invasive *Aspergillus* spp. SSIs, especially in immunocompromised patients, should stimulate a search for an environmental source for airborne transmission [158,159]. Clusters of patients with nosocomial acquisition of *M. tuberculosis* or HCWs with tuberculin skin test conversions should lead to an evaluation of tuberculosis patient identification and isolation practices, pressure differentials in isolation rooms, and review of HCW respiratory protective device use [122,123,126,128,160,161]. Recognition of patients infected or colonized with vancomycin-resistant enterococci should lead to an evaluation of IC, hand hygiene, and isolation practices and procedures, antimicrobial use, and whether current recommendations are being fully implemented [129].

The most common cause of both endemic and epidemic infections is cross-infection, whereby organisms are transmitted from HCWs to patients, HCWs to HCWs, patient-to-patient, or patient-to-HCWs. Although almost any organism can be transmitted by cross-infection, gram-negative organisms and *S. aureus* are the most commonly recognized. Nosocomial viral infections, which frequently occur in pediatric patients, also are often transmitted by cross-infection. Thus, acceptable prevention and control measures of HAIs dictate that the hospital epidemiologist look at and analyze the interrelationships between all components of the triad of agent, host, and environment. What must be understood to be equally relevant is an appreciation by relatives, patients, lawyers, administrators, and HCWs alike that patients who were born very prematurely or are elderly, are debilitated, have severe congenital abnormalities, diabetes or end-stage respiratory, liver, renal, or cardiac disease, have numerous indwelling medical devices or have undergone a major surgical procedure or other invasive procedures will be particularly susceptible to HAIs.

Multihospital Epidemics

As hospitals become more and more specialized, the possibility of multiple hospital outbreaks becomes a greater concern. This occurs most commonly by interhospital spread or movement of patients from LTCFs to hospitals and less commonly through the national distribution of products that cause or predispose to infection. First, a pathogen implicated in an epidemic in one healthcare facility may be introduced into a patient population at another facility, usually via one of three modes of transmission: (1) transfer of colonized or infected patients, particularly those with burns or decubitus ulcers, (2) transfer or movement of colonized or infected HCWs, including medical house staff and nursing personnel, between facilities, and (3) transient colonization of hands of HCWs who rotate among different hospitals and other healthcare facilities. Because the transfer of house staff and seriously ill patients occurs primarily among large, university-affiliated, tertiary referral hospitals, interhospital spread appears to occur most frequently in these facilities and less commonly among smaller community hospitals [98,113]; in fact, almost two-thirds of CDC outbreak investigations during 1990–1999 involved inpatients in acute care hospitals [113]. However, the blurring of the interface between the acute care hospital, free-standing specialty units, LTCFs, and home care and the increasing trend of "floating" nurses and technicians, "moonlighting" physicians, and various other ancillary medical personnel toward working for healthcare systems whose business model includes all of these facilities in one region undoubtedly increase interfacility spread or transfer of HAI pathogens among patients or residents in any of these facilities.

It used to be perceived not infrequently that interhospital transmission of HAI pathogens occurred mainly in epidemics involving one of the many pathogens with antimicrobial-resistant profiles. This is certainly true for various resistant pathogens (e.g., multiresistant *Serratia* spp., *Enterobacteriaceae* resistant to aminoglycosides and third-generation cephalosporins, VRE, MRSA, multidrug-resistant *M. tuberculosis*, and extended spectrum beta–lactamase producing *K. pneumoniae*) through genetic colinkage of intrinsic antimicrobial resistance properties with factors that facilitate spread, such as the sharing of genetic information that confers resistance to important antimicrobial agents. Similarly, the diversity of strain types involved in epidemiologically clear outbreaks of MRSA or VRE infections suggests the spread of genetic information among different strains that have strong predispositions for causing infections in hospital patients. Alternatively, the association could be due merely to the fact that resistance provides a dramatic marker that increases the likelihood that an epidemic will be recognized and investigated. If so, as IC personnel in hospitals initiate surveillance activities and develop more sensitive means for recognizing outbreaks and clusters of infections and more effectively share surveillance data with their counterparts in other local hospitals (e.g., through areawide surveillance systems supported by local health departments), interhospital transmission of infection will likely be more readily recognized and controlled. The main drawback is the uncharacterized confounding variables of LTCFs and home care.

In the second type of multiple-hospital involvement, a widely distributed product used in patient care may cause infections in many hospitals simultaneously because of either intrinsic contamination of the product in the factory (e.g., hemolysis in hemodialysis patients traced to faulty blood tubing sets or intrinsic contamination of peritoneal dialysis solution [162]) or design flaws or common usage errors that encourage in-use contamination in the hospitals [36,163]. In-use contamination is a far more common explanation for infections related to newly introduced products and devices [98,113]. Although intrinsic contamination is still recognized, extrinsic contamination of products during manipulation is much more common [98,113].

In the 1980s, the widespread use of an unlicensed intravenous vitamin E preparation in neonates led to a nationwide problem of unusual illness with high fatality in these patients [105]. The recognition of this new syndrome in several neonatal ICUs in some states led to the identification of the source and U.S. Food and Drug Administration (FDA) recall of the product. Similarly, an outbreak of BSIs or SSIs in five states led to the identification of a newly introduced intravenous anesthetic as the source [110,111]. Although only one species of organism was involved in each outbreak, different institutions had different pathogens, including S. aureus, Enterobacter spp., Moraxella species, and C. albicans. On-site epidemiologic investigations at each hospital identified contamination of the product during preparation by anesthesia personnel. This led the FDA and the manufacturer to alert users of this product of the need for strict aseptic handling during preparation. The outbreaks of BSIs in home infusion therapy patients demonstrate that as a new approach to patient care (i.e., home infusion) evolves, it is essential that the introduction of new techniques, such as needleless devices to reduce HCW blood contacts, be evaluated for their risk of patient complications [36,120]. Furthermore, such studies may document the need for new infection control recommendations (e.g., more frequent end cap changes) [36,120]. These experiences highlight the fact that IC personnel should remain alert to the possibility of infections or toxic reactions associated with newly introduced products or procedures. Suspicion of such problems should immediately be reported through the state health department to the CDC and FDA.

Pseudoepidemics

Not all clusters of reported HAIs constitute true epidemics of disease. HAI pseudo-outbreaks occur when there are an increased number of positive tests in the laboratory that do not correlate with clinical findings, a change in the surveillance system, or an improvement in laboratory methods [164,165]. Weinstein defined pseudo-outbreaks as a real clustering of false infections or artifactual clustering

of real infections [166]. Of 181 HAI outbreaks investigated by CDC during 1956 through 1975, 20 (11%) were pseudo-outbreaks [167]. Approximately one-half of these were attributed to processing errors in the microbiology laboratory. The remaining pseudo-epidemics were traced to systematic errors or changes in the definition of infection that resulted in clinical misdiagnosis of infection or surveillance artifacts associated with reporting of infection.

From 1980 to 1990, 6.0% of outbreaks investigated by CDC were pseudo-epidemics. Of these, 75.0% were traced to contaminated products, 12.5% were traced to environmental contamination, and 12.5% were traced to contamination of the culture during laboratory processing. From 1990 through 1994, only one (1.5%) of the epidemics investigated was a pseudo-epidemic; this involved Mycobacterium abscessus contamination of bronchoscopes traced to a contaminated endoscope washer reservoir [152]. In a more recent review of CDC pseudo-outbreak investigations, Manangan and Jarvis reported that of 104 HAI outbreaks that CDC personnel investigated onsite during 1990–2000, 11 (11%) were pseudo-outbreaks of infections involving Mycobacterium abscessus, Tsukamurella paurometabolum, E. cloacae, P. cepacia, Enterococcus durans, or Mycobacterium gordonae [165]. Among the 20 pseudo-outbreaks that occurred during 1956 to 1975 and reviewed by Weinstein and Stamm, the most common sites of suspected infection were the blood (20%), respiratory tract (20%) or gastrointestinal tract (20%), tissues (15%), liver (10%), or central nervous system (5%) [166]. Of the 66 pseudo-outbreaks reviewed by Cunha and Klein during 1976 to 1989, the most common sites of suspected infection were blood (53%), respiratory tract (20%), central nervous system (11%), or tissues (4%) [167]. Manangan and Jarvis found that during 1990 to 2000, the most common sites associated with the 86 pseudo-outbreaks they reviewed were the respiratory tract (37%), multiple sites or sterile fluids (24%), or blood (23%) [165]. In the United States, pseudo-outbreaks of respiratory tract infections now exceed pseudo-outbreaks of BSIs [165].

The two most common causes of HAI pseudo-outbreaks of BSIs are either intrinsic or extrinsic contamination of specimens and faulty procedures or misinterpretation of laboratory tests [165]. Cunha and Klein found that the most common microorganisms associated with pseudo-BSIs were Bacillus spp., Pseudomonas spp., or Streptococcus spp. [167]. Maki described four scenarios when a pseudo-outbreak of BSIs should be suspected: (1) when there is a cluster of blood cultures that are positive for new or unusual pathogens, (2) when affected patients do not consistently show signs or symptoms consistent with a BSI, (3) when the putative epidemic BSIs are primary (i.e., not isolated from likely sites of local infection), and (4) when the BSI is inexplicably high grade [168].

The most common causes of pseudo-outbreaks of respiratory tract infections have been contaminated equipment and use of automated reprocessing systems for endoscopes or bronchoscopes [167]. In several of these pseudo-outbreaks, the underlying cause included user error, washer malfunction, or contamination of the reservoir or lens [165]. Manangan and Jarvis suggested that users of these devices should carefully read the manufacturers' recommendations for use and for disinfection of these machines. In addition, CDC has published guidelines for cleaning, disinfecting, and inspecting these devices and for monitoring unusual clusters of organisms [169].

All nine reported pseudo-outbreaks of infections in tissues during 1990 through 2000 occurred in North America. Five of them involved contamination of specimen transport media, specimen tubes, or solutions used for processing the specimens; two involved tuberculin skin testing with purified protein derivative (PPD): one linked to manufacturer's error and the other caused by an incorrect dose of PPD [165].

Most of the 21 pseudo-outbreaks of infection at multiple sites or sterile body fluids reported during 1990 to 2000 involved contamination of blood or cerebrospinal fluid with wide range of microorganisms. Seven were caused by contamination of specimen during collection, transport, or processing; five were associated with malfunctioning of hardware or software in the laboratory [165].

Generally, pseudo-epidemics are associated with systematic errors, changes in the definition of infection used for surveillance, misdiagnosis of infection, and inaccuracy in the reporting of infection by infection surveillance staff. In addition, many can be traced to contaminated equipment or their processing and cleaning solutions; contamination of microbiology specimens during specimen collection, transport, or processing; and other errors in the microbiology laboratory which could be accidental, associated with glitches in newly introduced computer software and hardware, or linked to quality control problems in antimicrobial susceptibility testing. Because of the added costs (human and financial) and anxiety involved with investigating pseudo-epidemics, it is imperative that ICPs and hospital epidemiologists be familiar with the ascertainment, investigation, control, and prevention of pseudo-epidemics and to be aware that they may be due to diagnostic and reporting errors, contaminated equipment, or errors in the microbiology laboratory as reflected in the CDC investigations.

CONSEQUENCES OF HAIs

The reader of the scientific literature on HAIs is struck by the disproportionately vast number of articles on the adverse consequences associated with these infections. They include protracted duration of hospital stay, extra hospital costs or charges, additional inpatient care requirements, costly alternative antimicrobials, potential costs, lost productivity, long-term sequelae, untreatable infections, and death. The blurring of the borders between the acute hospital setting, LTCFs, and homecare has rendered the problem and its solutions even more complex. The importance of these

studies stems from two factors: first, in contrast to most other healthcare provision services, hospitals have not traditionally been able to charge patients or their insurance carriers directly for the costs of HAI surveillance and control programs. Second, it has been difficult to demonstrate how many HAIs these programs prevent and the cost effectiveness of these programs. Consequently, it has been necessary, or at least very helpful, in many hospitals to estimate the magnitude of adverse effects of HAIs on patients to justify the expenditures of mounting and sustaining a preventive program. The adverse outcomes most often studied are deaths and costs attributable to infection.

Although CDC data confirm that incidence rates of HAIs involving the four major anatomic sites are decreasing in hospitals across the United States, the looming downside is the concomitant increase in the incidence rates of HAIs occurring in LTCFs and homecare and in the rates of infections associated with antimicrobial-resistant pathogens. Nationwide estimates of the number of deaths attributable to HAIs have been increasing over the past three decades up from 19,000 reported in the 1970s (unpublished CDC data) to at least 90,000 deaths annually at the onset of the new millennium [3]. In view of the new strategies of prospective reimbursement for hospital care, the unequivocal evidence for the efficacy of infection surveillance and control programs, and the increasing body of evidence in the medical literature that the cost of implementing HAI surveillance and infection control programs for problem pathogens is substantially offset by savings involved in the reductions of HAIs, healthcare administrations seem loathe to commit fully—both philosophically and financially—to the idea of a total preventive package involving screening and surveillance of HAI pathogens. Home care is now the fastest growing component of healthcare: approximately 34 million people currently receive home care, supported by an increasing outlay of financial resources ($2 billion in 1988 versus $20 billion in 1999) by the Center for Medicare and Medicaid Services. With increasing movement and dynamic interaction of patients and HCWs between home care, LTCFs, outpatient services, and the acute hospital setting, and the fact that few home healthcare companies have designated surveillance personnel, any significant or realistic reduction in HAI rates in the United States is not going to be achieved anytime soon unless there is a concerted effort by healthcare companies and administrators in hospitals, LTCFs, and home care to completely finance evidence-based preventive measures such as those recommended by the Society of Healthcare Epidemiology of American (SHEA), the Association of Professionals in Infection Control (APIC), and CDC [170].

CONTROL AND PREVENTION OF HAIs

That endemic and epidemic HAIs are preventable has periodically been reaffirmed by milestone reports dating back to Semmelweis; to the myriad of studies published over the past two decades dealing with the unequivocal effect of hand hygiene, proper care of urinary catheters, respirators, intravascular catheters, and surgical wounds; numerous evidence-based IC guidelines published by CDC; and position papers issued by SHEA, APIC, and the Infectious Diseases Society of America.

Although overall HAI rates at the main anatomic sites have been falling, infections caused by resistant pathogens have been increasing. Thus, control of antimicrobial-resistance in the 2000s remains inextricably linked to the control of transmission of HAI antimicrobial-resistant pathogens and the infections they cause. The seriousness of the problem was underscored in a recent editorial by Muto, who made the point that "for as long as CDC has measured the prevalence of hospital-acquired infections caused by multidrug-resistant organisms, it has been increasing" [171].

So, what do we do? Indeed, there is little doubt that we would not be where we are today had more attention been paid to the published evidence-based data regarding which interventions have been effective in controlling the transmission of nosocomial, antimicrobial-resistant pathogens. For example, the Hospital Infection Control Practices Advisory Committee (HICPAC) guidelines to prevent and control vancomycin resistance were published in 1995 [172]. Although implementation of these guidelines following VRE outbreak investigations played no small part in the resolution of these outbreaks, no published outcome studies show how implementation of the HICPAC guidelines might have resulted in HAI rate reduction in facilities across the nation, especially for those HAIs caused by resistant pathogens [132,173].

After decades of discussing control of antimicrobial-resistant HAI pathogens in the medical literature, there is little evidence of control of HAIs caused by resistant pathogens in most healthcare facilities. The myriad of articles published have in effect helped explain this failure because much of the published data on HAIs has been carried out in hospitals that had implemented untried control programs or had substantially ineffective programs. Moreover, despite all of the resources put into surveillance activities for HAIs in facilities across the country, there remains substantial variation in surveillance activities from one medical center to another, inconsistent use of effective control measures (e.g., surveillance cultures not being performed as recommended), or failure of hospitals to use effective measures due to lack of commitment by healthcare companies and administrators alike to initiate and sustain these measures. In addition, there appears to be moderate compliance with goals to optimize antimicrobial use and to detect, report, and control the spread of antimicrobial-resistant pathogens. In 1996, Goldmann et al. found that national guidelines seldom are studied thoroughly by physicians, and, if they are read, rarely are incorporated into everyday practice [174]. They go on to

say that "success depends on the hospital leadership—members of the board, the executive administrative staff, and physician opinion leaders—making the campaign against antimicrobial resistance a strategic priority...under the aegis of the hospital's overall efforts to improve quality" [174].

Numerous reports presented at the SHEA annual meetings for each of the years 2003–2005 have repeatedly shown control of endemic or epidemic MRSA and/or VRE infections through implementation of the SHEA guidelines with more emphasis on contact precautions and less on standard precautions (25 such reports in the past two SHEA annual meetings). In fact, CDC has not provided any evidence-based data that show standard precautions and passive surveillance have started to control the spread of MRSA and VRE [175].

The tenets of the SHEA guidelines are based on identification and containment of spread through (1) active surveillance cultures to identify the reservoir for spread, (2) routine hand hygiene, (3) barrier precautions for patients known or suspected to be colonized or infected with epidemiologically important antimicrobial-resistant pathogens, such as MRSA or VRE, (4) implementation of an antimicrobial stewardship program, and (5) decolonization or suppression of colonized patients [170]. The importance of active screening cultures was underscored by data presented at the 2003 annual SHEA meeting, which showed that most patients colonized with MRSA at the time of admission to the surgical unit of a Veterans Administration Hospital had no prior evidence of MRSA colonization. These data also suggested that screening cultures may be necessary to identify the majority of MRSA-colonized patients at the time of admission. Other studies have since established that identification of MRSA-colonized patients at admission may enhance implementation of interventions to decrease infection [176]. There is now growing evidence that active surveillance cultures reduce the incidence of MRSA and/or VRE infections and that programs described in the SHEA Guidelines are effective and cost effective [135,175,177].

In conclusion, active surveillance cultures for resistant pathogens in ICUs with isolation of colonized patients is a highly effective strategy for control of HAIs. Isolation purely on the basis of history of previous detection, at least for VRE or MRSA, appears to be of little benefit. Standard precautions and isolation of the occasional patient recognized to be colonized through routine clinical cultures are minimally effective. The onus is now on healthcare professionals and healthcare administrators to invest intelligently in prevention programs, to enhance existing surveillance activities in targeted areas, and to avoid regarding death and morbidity as inevitable. However, hospital epidemiologists and CDC also have a responsibility to evaluate the effectiveness and cost benefit of the programs described in the SHEA Guidelines for gram-positive and gram-negative pathogens and fungi in the acute care hospitals. Enormous challenges remain for controlling transmission of HAI pathogens in acute care hospitals and conducting similar evaluations and strategies in LTCFs and the home care setting. These challenges include development of uniform surveillance definitions and protocols and a non-punitive reporting system for HAIs in LTCFs and home care; identification of high-risk infections (e.g., BSI, pneumonia, or SSI) that need to be focused on in these settings; and determination of relevant numerators and denominators for calculating device-specific rates for infections in these settings. These challenges are likely to be tempered by the fact that by focusing on specific, albeit high-risk, infections, the true magnitude of home HAIs will remain unknown for some time to come.

REFERENCES

1. Garner JS, Jarvis WR, Emori TG, et al. CDC definitions for nosocomial infections, 1988. *Am J Infect Control* 1988;16:128–140.
2. National hospital discharge survey. National Center for Health Statistics, 2004. Washington, D.C.
3. Centers for Disease Control and Prevention. Public health focus: surveillance, prevention, and control of nosocomial infections. *MMWR* 1992;41:783–787.
4. Haley RW, Culver DH, White JW, et al. The efficacy of infection surveillance and control programs in preventing nosocomial infections in US hospitals. *Am J Epidemiol* 1985;121:182–205.
5. Deming WE. *Out of the crisis.* Cambridge, MA: Center for Advanced Engineering Study, 1986.
6. Archibald LK, Gaynes RP. Hospital-acquired infections in the United States: the importance of interhospital comparisons. *Infect Dis Clin North Am* 1997;11:245–255.
7. Green J, Wintfield N, Sharkey P. The importance of severity of illness in assessing hospital mortality. *JAMA* 1990;263:241–246.
8. Jencks SF, Daley J, Draper D, et al. Interpreting hospital mortality data: the role of clinical risk adjustment. *JAMA* 1988;260:3611–3616.
9. Freeman J, McGowan JE Jr. Methodologic issues in hospital epidemiology. III. Investigating the modifying effects of time and severity of underlying illness on estimates of cost of nosocomial infection. *Rev Infect Dis* 1984;6:285–300.
10. Eickhoff TC, Brachman PW, Bennett JV, Brown JF. Surveillance of nosocomial infections in community hospitals. I. Surveillance methods, effectiveness, and initial results. *J Infect Dis* 1969;120:305–317.
11. Thoburn R, Fekety FR Jr., Cluff LE, Melvin VB. Infections acquired by hospitalized patients: an analysis of the overall problem. *Arch Intern Med* 1968;121:1–10
12. Kislak JW, Eickhoff TC, Finland M. Hospital-acquired infections and antibiotic usage in The Boston City Hospital—January 1964. *N Engl J Med* 1964;271:834–835.
13. Archibald LK, Manning ML, Bell LM, et al. Patient density, nurse-to-patient ratio and nosocomial infection risk in a pediatric cardiac intensive care unit. *Pediatr Infect Dis J* 1997;16:1045–1048.
14. Centers for Disease Control and Prevention. Monitoring hospital-acquired infections to promote patient safety—United States, 1990–1999. *MMWR* 2000;49:149–153.
15. Emori TG, Culver DH, Horan TC, et al. National Nosocomial Infections Surveillance (NNIS) system: description of surveillance methods. *Am J Infect Control* 1991;19:19–35.
16. Centers for Disease Control and Prevention. National Nosocomial Infections Surveillance (NNIS) system report, data summary from January 1992 through June 2004, issued October 2004. *Am J Infect Control* 2004;32:470–485.
17. Tokars JI, Richards C, Andrus M, et al. The changing face of surveillance for health care–associated infections. *Clin Infect Dis* 2004;39:1347–1352.
18. Haley RW, Quade D, Freeman HE, Bennett JV. Study on the efficacy of nosocomial infection control (SENIC Project): summary of study design. *Am J Epidemiol* 1980;111:472–485.
19. Haley RW, Culver DH, White JW, et al. The nationwide nosocomial infection rate: a new need for vital statistics. *Am J Epidemiol* 1985;121:159–167.
20. Fuchs PC. Will the real infection rate please stand? *Infect Control* 1987;8:235–236.
21. Haley RW. Surveillance by objective: a new priority-directed approach to the control of nosocomial infections: the National Foundation for Infectious Diseases lecture. *Am J Infect Control* 1985;13:78–89.
22. Joint Commission on Accreditation of Hospitals. The Joint Commission's agenda for change. Oakbrook Terrace, Illinois: Joint Commission on Accreditation of Hospitals, 1986.
23. Haley R. JCAHO infection control indicators, part 1. JCAHO Infection Control Indicators Task Force report. *Infect Control Hosp Epidemiol* 1990;11:545–546.
24. Nosocomial infection rates for interhospital comparison: limitations and possible solutions: a report from the National Nosocomial Infections Surveillance (NNIS) system. *Infect Control Hosp Epidemiol* 1991;12:609–621.
25. Massanari RM, Wilkerson K, Streed SA, Hierholzer WJ Jr. Reliability of reporting nosocomial infections in the discharge abstract and implications for receipt of revenues under prospective reimbursement. *Am J Public Health* 1987;77:561–564.
26. Archibald L, Phillips L, Monnet D, et al. Antimicrobial resistance in isolates from inpatients and outpatients in the United States: increasing importance of the intensive care unit. *Clin Infect Dis* 1997;24:211–215.
27. Tokars JI. Description of a new surveillance system for bloodstream and vascular access infection in outpatient hemodialysis centers. *Semin Dial* 2000;13:97–100.
28. Tokars JI, Miller ER, Stein G. New national surveillance system for hemodialysis-associated infections: initial results. *Am J Infect Control* 2002;30:288–295.
29. Richards MJ, Edwards JR, Culver DH, Gaynes RP. Nosocomial infections in medical intensive care units in the United States. National Nosocomial Infections Surveillance system. *Crit Care Med* 1999;27:887–892.
30. Richards MJ, Edwards JR, Culver DH, Gaynes RP. Nosocomial infections in pediatric intensive care units in the United States. National Nosocomial Infections Surveillance system. *Pediatrics* 1999;103:e39.
31. Cruse PJ, Foord R. The epidemiology of wound infection: a 10-year prospective study of 62,939 wounds. *Surg Clin North Am* 1980;60:27–40.
32. Ehrenkranz NJ. Surgical wound infection occurrence in clean operations: risk stratification for interhospital comparisons. *Am J Med* 1981;70:909–914.
33. Hooton TM, Haley RW, Culver DH, et al. The joint associations of multiple risk factors with the occurrence of nosocomial infection. *Am J Med* 1981;70:960–970.
34. Culver DH, Horan TC, Gaynes RP, et al. Surgical wound infection rates by wound class, operative procedure, and patient risk index. National Nosocomial Infections Surveillance system. *Am J Med* 1991;91:152S–157S.
35. Pittet D, Li N, Woolson RF, Wenzel RP. Microbiological factors influencing the outcome of nosocomial bloodstream infections: a 6-year validated, population based model. *Clin Infect Dis* 1997;24:1068.
36. Danzig LE, Short LJ, Collins K, et al. Bloodstream infections associated with a needleless intravenous infusion system in patients receiving home infusion therapy. *JAMA* 1995;273:1862–1864.
37. Kellerman S, Shay DK, Howard J, et al. Bloodstream infections in home infusion patients: the influence of race and needleless intravascular access devices. *J Pediatr* 1996;129:711–717.
38. Do AN, Ray BJ, Banerjee SN, et al. Bloodstream infection associated with needleless device use and the importance of infection-control practices in the home health care setting. *J Infect Dis* 1999;179:442–448.
39. Tokars JI, Cookson ST, McArthur MA, et al. Prospective evaluation of risk factors for bloodstream infection in patients receiving home infusion therapy. *Ann Intern Med* 1999;131:340–347.

40. Tokars JI, Frank M, Alter MJ, Arduino MJ. National surveillance of dialysis-associated diseases in the United States, 2000. *Semin Dial* 2002;15:162–171.
41. Fridkin SK, Gaynes RP. Antimicrobial resistance in intensive care units. *Clin Chest Med* 1999;20:303–316.
42. Frieden TR, Munsiff SS, Low DE, et al. Emergence of vancomycin-resistant enterococci in New York City. *Lancet* 1993;342:76–79.
43. Centers for Disease Control and Prevention. Nosocomial enterococci resistant to vancomycin—United States, 1989–1993. *MMWR* 1993;42:597–599.
44. Tokars JI. Predictive value of blood cultures positive for coagulase-negative staphylococci: implications for patient care and health care quality assurance. *Clin Infect Dis* 2004;39:333–341.
45. Wisplinghoff H, Bischoff T, Tallent SM, et al. Nosocomial bloodstream infections in US hospitals: analysis of 24,179 cases from a prospective nationwide surveillance study. *Clin Infect Dis* 2004;39:309–317.
46. Archibald LK. Gram-negative, hospital-acquired infections: a growing problem. *Infect Control Hosp Epidemiol* 2004;25:809–811.
47. Gaynes R, Edwards JR. Overview of nosocomial infections caused by gram-negative bacilli. *Clin Infect Dis* 2005;41:848–854.
48. Archibald LK, Hierholzer W. Principles of infectious diseases epidemiology. In: Mayhall CG, ed. *Hospital epidemiology and infection control*. 3rd ed. New York: Lippincott Williams & Wilkins, 2004.
49. Moolenaar RL, Crutcher JM, San Joaquin VH, et al. A prolonged outbreak of *Pseudomonas aeruginosa* in a neonatal intensive care unit: did staff fingernails play a role in disease transmission? *Infect Control Hosp Epidemiol* 2000;21:80–85.
50. Archibald LK, Corl A, Shah B, et al. *Serratia marcescens* outbreak associated with extrinsic contamination of 1% chlorxylenol soap. *Infect Control Hosp Epidemiol* 1997;18:704–709.
51. Archibald LK, Ramos M, Arduino MJ, et al. *Enterobacter cloacae* and *Pseudomonas aeruginosa* polymicrobial bloodstream infections traced to extrinsic contamination of a dextrose multidose vial. *J Pediatr* 1998;133:640–644.
52. Jarvis WR. Recommended precautions for patients with Legionnaires' Disease. *Infect Control* 1982;3:401–402.
53. Selenic D, Dodson DR, Jensen B, et al. *Enterobacter cloacae* bloodstream infections in pediatric patients traced to a hospital pharmacy. *Am J Health Syst Pharm* 2003;60:1440–1446.
54. Aitken C, Jeffries DJ. Nosocomial spread of viral disease. *Clin Microbiol Rev* 2001;14:528–546.
55. Jarvis WR. The epidemiology of colonization. *Infect Control Hosp Epidemiol* 1996;17:47–52.
56. Jarvis WR. Epidemiology of nosocomial infections in pediatric patients. *Pediatr Infect Dis J* 1987;6:344–351.
57. Jarvis WR, Cookson ST, Robles MB. Prevention of nosocomial bloodstream infections: a national and international priority. *Infect Control Hosp Epidemiol* 1996;17:272–275.
58. Jarvis WR, Edwards JR, Culver DH, et al. Nosocomial infection rates in adult and pediatric intensive care units in the United States. National Nosocomial Infections Surveillance system. *Am J Med* 1991;91:185S–191S.
59. Jarvis WR, Robles B. Nosocomial infections in pediatric patients. *Adv Pediatr Infect Dis* 1996;12:243–295.
60. Weber DJ, Raasch R, Rutala WA. Nosocomial infections in the ICU: the growing importance of antibiotic-resistant pathogens. *Chest* 1999;115:34S–41S.
61. File TM Jr. Overview of resistance in the 1990s. *Chest* 1999;115:3S–8S.
62. Freeman J, McGowan JE Jr. Risk factors for nosocomial infection. *J Infect Dis* 1978;138:811–819.
63. Manning ML, Archibald LK, Bell LM, et al. *Serratia marcescens* transmission in a pediatric intensive care unit: a multifactorial occurrence. *Am J Infect Control* 2001;29:115–119.
64. Gross PA, Beyt BE Jr., Decker MD, et al. Description of case-mix adjusters by the Severity of Illness Working Group of the Society of Hospital Epidemiologists of America (SHEA). *Infect Control Hosp Epidemiol* 1988;9:309–316.
65. Monnet DL, Archibald LK, Phillips L, et al. Antimicrobial use and resistance in eight US hospitals: complexities of analysis and modeling. Intensive Care Antimicrobial Resistance Epidemiology Project and National Nosocomial Infections Surveillance System Hospitals. *Infect Control Hosp Epidemiol* 1998;19:388–394.
66. Haley RW, Culver DH, Morgan WM, et al. Identifying patients at high risk of surgical wound infection: a simple multivariate index of patient susceptibility and wound contamination. *Am J Epidemiol* 1985;121:206.
67. Haley RW, Hooton TM, Culver DH, et al. Nosocomial infections in U.S. hospitals, 1975–1976: estimated frequency by selected characteristics of patients. *Am J Med* 1981;70:947–959.
68. Nguyen MH, Kaufman D, Goodman RP, et al. Nasal carriage of and infection with *Staphylococcus aureus* in HIV-infected patients. *Ann Intern Med* 1999;130:221–225.
69. Yu VL, Goetz A, Wagener MM, et al. *Staphylococcus aureus* nasal carriage and infection in patients on hemodialysis: efficacy of antibiotic prophylaxis. *N Engl J Med* 1986;315:91–96.
70. Ruef C, Fanconi S, Nadal D. Sternal wound infection after heart operations in pediatric patients associated with nasal carriage of *Staphylococcus aureus*. *J Thorac Cardiovasc Surg* 1996;112:681–686.
71. Oh J, von Baum H, Laus G, Schaefer F. Nasal carriage of *Staphylococcus aureus* in families of children on peritoneal dialysis. European Pediatric Peritoneal Dialysis Study Group (EPPS). *Adv Perit Dial* 2000;16:324–327.
72. Keita-Perse O, Gaynes RP. Severity of illness scoring systems to adjust nosocomial infection rates: a review and commentary. *Am J Infect Control* 1996;24:429–434.
73. Parvez FM, Jarvis WR. Nosocomial infections in the nursery. *Sem Pediatr Infect Dis* 1999;10:119–129.
74. Goldwater PN, Martin AJ, Ryan B, et al. A survey of nosocomial respiratory viral infections in a children's hospital: occult respiratory infection in patients admitted during an epidemic season. *Infect Control Hosp Epidemiol* 1991;12:231–238.
75. Allen JR, Hightower AW, Martin SM, Dixon RE. Secular trends in nosocomial infections: 1970–1979. *Am J Med* 1981;70:389–392.
76. Hughes JM, Culver DH, White JW, et al. Nosocomial infection surveillance, 1980–1982. *MMWR CDC Surveill Summ* 1983;32:1SS–16SS.
77. Retailliau HF, Hightower AW, Dixon RE, Allen JR. *Acinetobacter calcoaceticus*: a nosocomial pathogen with an unusual seasonal pattern. *J Infect Dis* 1979;139:371–375.
78. McDonald LC, Banerjee SN, Jarvis WR. Seasonal variation of *Acinetobacter* infections: 1987–1996. National Nosocomial Infections Surveillance system. *Clin Infect Dis* 1999;29:1133–1137.
79. Kalina GP. Bacteria of the genus *Acinetobacter*: their systematics and ecological analysis. *Zh Mikrobiol Epidemiol Immunobiol* 1986;6:20–26.
80. Hall CB. Nosocomial viral respiratory infections: perennial weeds on pediatric wards. *Am J Med* 1981;70:670–676.
81. Graman PS, Hall CB. Nosocomial viral respiratory infections. *Semin Respir Infect* 1989;4:253–260.
82. Gerding DN, Johnson S, Peterson LR, et al. *Clostridium difficile*-associated diarrhea and colitis. *Infect Control Hosp Epidemiol* 1995;16:459–477.
83. Johnson S, Gerding DN. *Clostridium difficile*—associated diarrhea. *Clin Infect Dis* 1998;26:1027–1034.
84. Archibald LK, Banerjee SN, Jarvis WR. Secular trends in hospital-acquired *Clostridium difficile* disease in the United States, 1987–2001. *J Infect Dis* 2004;189:1585–1589.
85. Gaynes RP, Solomon S. Improving hospital-acquired infection rates: the CDC experience. *Jt Comm J Qual Improv* 1996;22:457–467.
86. Banerjee SN, Emori TG, Culver DH, et al. Secular trends in nosocomial primary bloodstream infections in the United States, 1980–1989. National Nosocomial Infections Surveillance system. *Am J Med* 1991;91:86S–89S.
87. Simonds DN, Horan TC, Kelley R, Jarvis WR. Detecting pediatric nosocomial infections: how do infection control and quality assurance personnel compare? *Am J Infect Control* 1997;25:202–208.
88. Richards C, Emori TG, Peavy G, Gaynes R. Promoting quality through measurement of performance and response: prevention success stories. *Emerg Infect Dis* 2001;7:299–301.
89. Beck-Sague C, Jarvis WR. Secular trends in the epidemiology of nosocomial fungal infections in the United States, 1980–1990.

National Nosocomial Infections Surveillance system. *J Infect Dis* 1993;167:1247–1251.

90. Trick WE, Fridkin SK, Edwards JR, et al. Secular trend of hospital-acquired candidemia among intensive care unit patients in the United States during 1989–1999. *Clin Infect Dis* 2002;35:627–630.

91. Kyne L, Sougioultzis S, McFarland LV, Kelly CP. Underlying disease severity as a major risk factor for nosocomial *Clostridium difficile* diarrhea. *Infect Control Hosp Epidemiol* 2002;23:653–659.

92. Simpson JY. Our existing system of hospitalism and its effect. *Edinburgh Medical Journal* 1869;14:816.

93. Bennett JV, Scheckler WE, Maki DG, Brachman PS. Current national patterns: United States. In: *Proceedings of the International Conference on Nosocomial Infections* American Hospital Association: Chicago, 1971:42–49.

94. Haley RW, Morgan WM, Culver DH, Schaberg DR. Differences in nosocomial infection rates by type of hospital: the influence of patient mix and diagnostic medical practices. Presented at the Interscience Conference on Antimicrobial Agents and Chemotherapy, Miami, Florida. October 4, 1982.

95. Haley RW, Tenney JH, Lindsey JO, et al. How frequent are outbreaks of nosocomial infection in community hospitals? *Infect Control* 1985;6:233–236.

96. Wenzel RP, Thompson RL, Landry SM, et al. Hospital-acquired infections in intensive care unit patients: an overview with emphasis on epidemics. *Infect Control* 1983;4:371–375.

97. Stamm WE, Weinstein RA, Dixon RE. Comparison of endemic and epidemic nosocomial infections. *Am J Med* 1981;70:393–397.

98. Jarvis WR. Nosocomial outbreaks: the Centers for Disease Control's Hospital Infections Program experience, 1980–1990. Epidemiology Branch, Hospital Infections Program. *Am J Med* 1991;91:101S–106S.

99. Beck-Sague CM, Jarvis WR. Epidemic bloodstream infections associated with pressure transducers: a persistent problem. *Infect Control Hosp Epidemiol* 1989;10:54–59.

100. Beck-Sague CM, Jarvis WR, Bland LA, et al. Outbreak of gram-negative bacteremia and pyrogenic reactions in a hemodialysis center. *Am J Nephrol* 1990;10:397–403.

101. Beck-Sague CM, Jarvis WR, Brook JH, et al. Epidemic bacteremia due to *Acinetobacter baumannii* in five intensive care units. *Am J Epidemiol* 1990;132:723–733.

102. Lowry PW, Jarvis WR, Oberle AD, et al. *Mycobacterium chelonae* causing otitis media in an ear-nose-and-throat practice. *N Engl J Med* 1988;319:978–982.

103. Lowry PW, Beck-Sague CM, Bland LA, et al. *Mycobacterium chelonae* infection among patients receiving high-flux dialysis in a hemodialysis clinic in California. *J Infect Dis* 1990;161:85–90.

104. Safranek TJ, Jarvis WR, Carson LA, et al. *Mycobacterium chelonae* wound infections after plastic surgery employing contaminated gentian violet skin-marking solution. *N Engl J Med* 1987;317:197–201.

105. Martone WJ, Williams WW, Mortensen ML, et al. Illness with fatalities in premature infants: association with an intravenous vitamin E preparation, E-Ferol. *Pediatrics* 1986;78:591–600.

106. Gordon SM, Tipple M, Bland LA, Jarvis WR. Pyrogenic reactions associated with the reuse of disposable hollow-fiber hemodialyzers. *JAMA* 1988;260:2077–2081.

107. Tipple MA, Bland LA, Favero MS, Jarvis WR. Investigation of hemolytic anemia after chloramine exposure in a dialysis center. *ASAIO Trans* 1988;34:1060.

108. Arduino MJ, Bland LA, Tipple MA, et al. Growth and endotoxin production of *Yersinia enterocolitica* and *Enterobacter agglomerans* in packed erythrocytes. *J Clin Microbiol* 1989;27:1483–1485.

109. Tipple MA, Bland LA, Murphy JJ, et al. Sepsis associated with transfusion of red cells contaminated with *Yersinia enterocolitica*. *Transfusion* 1990;30:207–213.

110. Centers for Disease Control and Prevention. Postsurgical infections associated with an extrinsically contaminated intravenous anesthetic agent—California, Illinois, Maine, and Michigan, 1990. *MMWR* 1990;39:426–433.

111. Bennett SN, McNeil MM, Bland LA, et al. Postoperative infections traced to contamination of an intravenous anesthetic, propofol. *N Engl J Med* 1995;333:147–154.

112. McNeil MM, Lasker BA, Lott TJ, Jarvis WR. Postsurgical *Candida albicans* infections associated with an extrinsically contaminated intravenous anesthetic agent. *J Clin Microbiol* 1999;37:1398–1403.

113. Jarvis WR. Hospital Infections Program, Centers for Disease Control and Prevention On-site Outbreak Investigations, 1990–1999. *Semin Infect Control* 2001;1:74–84.

114. Burwen DR, Olsen SM, Bland LA, et al. Epidemic aluminum intoxication in hemodialysis patients traced to use of an aluminum pump. *Kidney Int* 1995;48:469–474.

115. Kelly KJ, Pearson ML, Kurup VP, et al. A cluster of anaphylactic reactions in children with spina bifida during general anesthesia: epidemiologic features, risk factors, and latex hypersensitivity. *J Allergy Clin Immunol* 1994;94:53–61.

116. Pearson ML, Levine WC, Finton RJ, et al. Anesthesia-associated carbon monoxide exposures among surgical patients. *Infect Control Hosp Epidemiol* 2001;22:352–356.

117. Burkholder BT, Coronado VG, Brown J, et al. Nosocomial transmission of hepatitis A in a pediatric hospital traced to an anti-hepatitis A virus-negative patient with immunodeficiency. *Pediatr Infect Dis J* 1995;14:261–266.

118. Centers for Disease Control and Prevention. Outbreaks of hepatitis B virus infection among hemodialysis patients—California, Nebraska, and Texas, 1994. *MMWR* 1996;45:285–289.

119. Velandia M, Fridkin SK, Cardenas V, et al. Transmission of HIV in dialysis centre. *Lancet* 1995;345:1417–1422.

120. Cookson ST, Ihrig M, O'Mara EM, et al. Increased bloodstream infection rates in surgical patients associated with variation from recommended use and care following implementation of a needleless device. *Infect Control Hosp Epidemiol* 1998;19:23–27.

121. McDonald LC, Banerjee SN, Jarvis WR. Line-associated bloodstream infections in pediatric intensive-care-unit patients associated with a needleless device and intermittent intravenous therapy. *Infect Control Hosp Epidemiol* 1998;19:772–777.

122. Edlin BR, Tokars JI, Grieco MH, et al. An outbreak of multidrug-resistant tuberculosis among hospitalized patients with the acquired immunodeficiency syndrome. *N Engl J Med* 1992;326:1514–1521.

123. Beck-Sague C, Dooley SW, Hutton MD, et al. Hospital outbreak of multidrug-resistant *Mycobacterium tuberculosis* infections. Factors in transmission to staff and HIV-infected patients. *JAMA* 1992;268:1280–1286.

124. Jereb JA, Klevens RM, Privett TD, et al. Tuberculosis in health care workers at a hospital with an outbreak of multidrug-resistant *Mycobacterium tuberculosis*. *Arch Intern Med* 1995;155:854–859.

125. Pearson ML, Jereb JA, Frieden TR, et al. Nosocomial transmission of multidrug-resistant Mycobacterium tuberculosis: a risk to patients and health care workers. *Ann Intern Med* 1992;117:191–196.

126. Coronado VG, Beck-Sague CM, Hutton MD, et al. Transmission of multidrug-resistant Mycobacterium tuberculosis among persons with human immunodeficiency virus infection in an urban hospital: epidemiologic and restriction fragment length polymorphism analysis. *J Infect Dis* 1993;168:1052–1055.

127. Zaza S, Beck-Sague CM, Jarvis WR. Tracing patients exposed to health care workers with tuberculosis. *Public Health Rep* 1997;112:153–157.

128. Zaza S, Blumberg HM, Beck-Sague C, et al. Nosocomial transmission of *Mycobacterium tuberculosis*: role of health care workers in outbreak propagation. *J Infect Dis* 1995;172:1542–1549.

129. Shay DK, Maloney SA, Montecalvo M, et al. Epidemiology and mortality risk of vancomycin-resistant enterococcal bloodstream infections. *J Infect Dis* 1995;172:993–1000.

130. Morris JG Jr., Shay DK, Hebden JN, et al. Enterococci resistant to multiple antimicrobial agents, including vancomycin: establishment of endemicity in a university medical center. *Ann Intern Med* 1995;123:250–259.

131. Beltrami EM, Singer DA, Fish L, et al. Risk factors for acquisition of vancomycin-resistant enterococci among patients on a renal ward during a community hospital outbreak. *Am J Infect Control* 2000;28:282–285.

132. Jochimsen EM, Fish L, Manning K, et al. Control of vancomycin-resistant enterococci at a community hospital: efficacy of

patient and staff cohorting. *Infect Control Hosp Epidemiol* 1999;20:106–109.

133. Singer DA, Jochimsen EM, Gielerak P, Jarvis WR. Pseudo-outbreak of *Enterococcus durans* infections and colonization associated with introduction of an automated identification system software update. *J Clin Microbiol* 1996;34:2685–2687.

134. Trick WE, Kuehnert MJ, Quirk SB, et al. Regional dissemination of vancomycin-resistant enterococci resulting from interfacility transfer of colonized patients. *J Infect Dis* 1999;180:391–396.

135. Ostrowsky BE, Trick WE, Sohn AH, et al. Control of vancomycin-resistant enterococcus in health care facilities in a region. *N Engl J Med* 2001;344:1427–1433.

136. Smith TL, Pearson ML, Wilcox KR, et al. Emergence of vancomycin resistance in *Staphylococcus aureus*. Glycopeptide-Intermediate *Staphylococcus aureus* Working Group. *N Engl J Med* 1999;340:493–501.

137. Garrett DO, Jochimsen E, Murfitt K, et al. The emergence of decreased susceptibility to vancomycin in Staphylococcus epidermidis. *Infect Control Hosp Epidemiol* 1999;20: 167–170.

138. Fridkin SK, Kremer FB, Bland LA, et al. *Acremonium kiliense* endophthalmitis that occurred after cataract extraction in an ambulatory surgical center and was traced to an environmental reservoir. *Clin Infect Dis* 1996;22:222–227.

139. Richet HM, Craven PC, Brown JM, et al. A cluster of *Rhodococcus (Gordona) bronchialis* sternal-wound infections after coronary-artery bypass surgery. *N Engl J Med* 1991;324:104–109.

140. Richet HM, McNeil MM, Edwards MC, Jarvis WR. Cluster of *Malassezia furfur* pulmonary infections in infants in a neonatal intensive-care unit. *J Clin Microbiol* 1989;27:1197–1200.

141. Tokars JI, McNeil MM, Tablan OC, et al. *Mycobacterium gordonae* pseudoinfection associated with a contaminated antimicrobial solution. *J Clin Microbiol* 1990;28:2765–2769.

142. Chang HJ, Christenson JC, Pavia AT, et al. *Ochrobactrum anthropi* meningitis in pediatric pericardial allograft transplant recipients. *J Infect Dis* 1996;173:656–660.

143. Chang HJ, Miller HL, Watkins N, et al. An epidemic of *Malassezia pachydermatis* in an intensive care nursery associated with colonization of health care workers' pet dogs. *N Engl J Med* 1998;338:706–711.

144. Meyers H, Brown-Elliott BA, Moore D, et al. An outbreak of *Mycobacterium chelonae* infection following liposuction. *Clin Infect Dis* 2002;34:1500–1507.

145. Diekema DJ, BootsMiller BJ, Vaughn TE, et al. Antimicrobial resistance trends and outbreak frequency in United States hospitals. *Clin Infect Dis* 2004;38:78–85.

146. Kainer MA, Keshavarz H, Jensen BJ, et al. Saline-filled breast implant contamination with *Curvularia* species among women who underwent cosmetic breast augmentation. *J Infect Dis* 2005;192:170–177.

147. Kainer MA, Linden JV, Whaley DN, et al. *Clostridium* infections associated with musculoskeletal-tissue allografts. *N Engl J Med* 2004;350:2564–2571.

148. Mangram AJ, Archibald LK, Hupert M, et al. Outbreak of sterile peritonitis among continuous cycling peritoneal dialysis patients. *Kidney Int* 1998;54:1367–1371.

149. Centers for Disease Control and Prevention. Contaminated povidone-iodine solution, Texas. *MMWR* 1989;38:133–134.

150. Trick WE, Kioski CM, Howard KM, et al. Outbreak of *Pseudomonas aeruginosa* ventriculitis among patients in a neurosurgical intensive care unit. *Infect Control Hosp Epidemiol* 2000;21:204–208.

151. Montecalvo MA, Shay DK, Patel P, et al. Bloodstream infections with vancomycin-resistant enterococci. *Arch Intern Med* 1996;156:1458–1462.

152. Maloney S, Welbel S, Daves B, et al. *Mycobacterium abscessus* pseudoinfection traced to an automated endoscope washer: utility of epidemiologic and laboratory investigation. *J Infect Dis* 1994;169:1166–1169.

153. Redbord KP, Shearer DA, Gloster H, et al. Atypical *Mycobacterium furunculosis* occurring after pedicures. *J Am Acad Dermatol* 2006;54:520–524

154. Vugia DJ, Jang Y, Zizek C, et al. Mycobacteria in nail salon whirlpool footbaths, California. *Emerg Infect Dis* 2005;11:616–618.

155. Gira AK, Reisenauer AH, Hammock L, et al. Furunculosis due to *Mycobacterium mageritense* associated with footbaths at a nail salon. *J Clin Microbiol* 2004;42:1813–1817.

156. Mastro TD, Farley TA, Elliott JA, et al. An outbreak of surgical-wound infections due to group A streptococcus carried on the scalp. *N Engl J Med* 1990;323:968–972.

157. Zaza S, Tokars JI, Yomtovian R, et al. Bacterial contamination of platelets at a university hospital: increased identification due to intensified surveillance. *Infect Control Hosp Epidemiol* 1994;15:82–87.

158. Buffington J, Reporter R, Lasker BA, et al. Investigation of an epidemic of invasive aspergillosis: utility of molecular typing with the use of random amplified polymorphic DNA probes. *Pediatr Infect Dis J* 1994;13:386–393.

159. Burwen DR, Lasker BA, Rao N, et al. Invasive aspergillosis outbreak on a hematology-oncology ward. *Infect Control Hosp Epidemiol* 2001;22:45–48.

160. Maloney SA, Pearson ML, Gordon MT, et al. Efficacy of control measures in preventing nosocomial transmission of multidrug-resistant tuberculosis to patients and health care workers. *Ann Intern Med* 1995;122:90–95.

161. Wenger PN, Otten J, Breeden A, et al. Control of nosocomial transmission of multidrug-resistant *Mycobacterium tuberculosis* among healthcare workers and HIV-infected patients. *Lancet* 1995;345:235–240.

162. Duffy R, Tomashek K, Spangenberg M, et al. Multistate outbreak of hemolysis in hemodialysis patients traced to faulty blood tubing sets. *Kidney Int* 2000;57:1668–1674.

163. Grohskopf LA, Roth VR, Feikin DR, et al. Serratia liquefaciens bloodstream infections from contamination of epoetin alfa at a hemodialysis center. *N Engl J Med* 2001;344:1491–1497.

164. Wendt C, Herwaldt LA. Epidemics: identification and management. In: Wenzel RP, ed. *Prevention and control of nosocomial infections*. Baltimore, MD: Williams and Wilkins, 1997: 175–213.

165. Manangan LP, Jarvis WR. Healthcare-associated pseudo-outbreaks. *Semin Infect Control* 2001;1:102–110.

166. Weinstein RA, Stamm WE. Pseudoepidemics in hospital. *Lancet* 1977;2:862–864.

167. Cunha BA, Klein NC. Pseudoinfections. *Infect Dis Clin Practice* 1995;4:95–103.

168. Maki DG. Through a glass darkly. Nosocomial pseudoepidemics and pseudobacteremias. *Arch Intern Med* 1980;140:26–28.

169. Centers for Disease Control and Prevention. Bronchoscopy-related infection and pseudoinfections—New York, 1996 and 1998. *MMWR* 1999;48:557–560.

170. Muto CA, Jernigan J, Ostrowsky BE, et al. SHEA guideline for preventing transmission of multidrug-resistant strains of *Staphylococcus aureus* or *Enterococcus* in Healthcare settings. *Infect Control Hosp Epidemiol* 2003; 24:362–386.

171. Muto CA. Why are antibiotic-resistant nosocomial infections spiraling out of control? *Infect Control Hosp Epidemiol* 2005;26:10–12.

172. Hospital Infection Control Practices Advisory Committee (HICPAC). Recommendations for preventing the spread of vancomycin resistance. *Am J Infect Control* 1995; 23:87–94.

173. Shay DK, Goldmann DA, Jarvis WR. Reducing the spread of antimicrobial-resistant microorganisms. Control of vancomycin-resistant enterococci. *Pediatr Clin North Am* 1995;42: 703–716.

174. Goldmann DA, Weinstein RA, Wenzel RP. Strategies to prevent and control the emergence and spread of antimicrobial resistant microorganisms in hospitals: a challenge to hospital leadership. *JAMA* 1996;275:234–240.

175. McGeer AJ. News in antimicrobial resistance: documenting the progress of pathogens. *Infect Control Hosp Epidemiol* 2004;25:97–98.

176. Davis KA, Stewart JJ, Crouch HK, et al. Methicillin-resistant *Staphylococcus aureus* (MRSA) nares colonization at hospital admission and its effect on subsequent MRSA infection. *Clin Infect Dis* 2004;39:776–782.

177. Perencevich EN, Fisman DN, Lipsitch M, et al. Projected benefits of active surveillance for vancomycin-resistant enterococci in intensive care units. *Clin Infect Dis* 2004;38:1108–1115.

Urinary Tract Infections

30

Carol E. Chenoweth and Sanjay Saint

Urinary tract infection (UTI) is the most frequently reported healthcare-associated infection (HAI), accounting for up to 40% of all HAIs [1–4]. The vast majority of nosocomial UTIs is associated with urinary catheters. Urinary catheters are widely used in health care today, especially in the intensive care units (ICU), in postsurgical patients, in long-term care facilities, and increasingly in home care patients [5–8]. Up to 25% of patients have a urinary catheter placed at some time during their hospital stay [9,10]. Worldwide, approximately 96 million urethral catheters are sold every year; nearly a quarter of these in the United States. Like other indwelling catheters, urinary catheters disrupt the normal host immune mechanisms and allow for the formation of biofilm [3,11,12]. Urinary catheter-related infection results in substantial morbidity and significantly increases hospital costs [13,14]. This chapter reviews the pathogenesis, epidemiology, and preventive measures for catheter-associated urinary tract infections (CA-UTIs).

PATHOGENESIS

Urinary catheters readily develop a biofilm composed of clusters of microbial organisms on the internal and external catheter surface surrounded by an extracellular matrix made up of primarily polysaccharide materials [12,15–17]. The biofilm allows for microbial attachment and adherence to catheter surfaces. Microorganisms gain access to the catheter and attach to the biofilm via one of two routes, extraluminally or intraluminally (Figure 30-1). Extraluminal organisms are primarily endogenous, originating from the patient's gastrointestinal tract and colonizing the patient's perineum. Organisms ascend the catheter by direct

inoculation at the time of catheter insertion or by migration in the mucous sheath surrounding the external aspect of the catheter [16,18,19]. Approximately 70% of episodes of bacteriuria in catheterized women are felt to occur through extraluminal entry of organisms [18]. In a recent prospective study of 173 CA-UTIs, 115 (66%) were likely acquired through the extraluminal route [19].

Microorganisms also enter the catheter intraluminally when organisms gain access to the internal lumen of the catheter through failure of a closed drainage system or contamination of the collection bag [16,19,20]. These organisms, usually introduced from exogenous sources, are often the result of cross-transmission of organisms on the hands of healthcare workers (HCWs) [16,20–22]. Intraluminal contamination of the collecting system was recently found

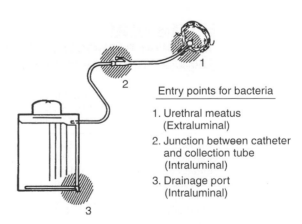

Entry points for bacteria

1. Urethral meatus (Extraluminal)
2. Junction between catheter and collection tube (Intraluminal)
3. Drainage port (Intraluminal)

Figure 30-1 Entry points for bacteria causing catheter-associated urinary tract infection.

to account for 34% of CA-UTIs [19]. Once microorganisms attach and multiply, the resultant sheet of organisms secretes an extracellular matrix of bacterial glycocalyces, imbedding the microorganisms [11,12,15,19,23,24].

Bacteria within the biofilm grow much more slowly than planktonic bacteria and secrete chemical signals that mediate population density–dependent gene expression [11,12,15,19,23,24]. The migration of the biofilm over the inner surface of the catheter to the bladder occurs within 1–3 days or more quickly by swarming organisms, such as *Proteus mirabilis* [11,23–25]. Most biofilms are composed of single organisms; however, biofilms may contain a mixture of up to five organisms [16,26]. Some organisms, such as *Providencia stuartii*, *Pseudomonas* sp., enterococci, or *Proteus* sp., persist in the urine for up to 10 weeks while other organisms appear to spontaneously cycle in and out [16,26]. Several studies suggest that planktonic bacteria found in cultures obtained from the catheter may not reflect bacterial population growing within the biofilm [3,26]. *Proteus* sp., *Pseudomonas aeruginosa*, *Klebsiella pneumoniae*, and *Providencia* sp. have the ability to hydrolyze urea in the urine to free ammonia. The resulting increase in local pH allows precipitation of minerals such as hydroxyapetite or struvite. Mineral deposition within the catheter biofilm causes encrustations that are unique to biofilms formed on urinary catheters [24,27,28]. Encrustations on the inner surface of the catheter can build to completely block catheter flow or act as a nidus for formation of renal calculi [29,30].

The urinary biofilm provides a protective environment from the activity of antimicrobial agents [31,32]. First, the extracellular matrix may prevent the penetration of antimicrobials into the biofilm. For example, both ciprofloxacin and tobramycin have poor diffusion into biofilms. Secondly, organisms growing at a slower rate within the biofilm are more resistant to the effects of antimicrobial agents that require active growth [31–33]. Finally, chemical signaling from organisms growing within the biofilm appears to regulate genes that alter the

molecular targets of antimicrobials [33]. The features of biofilm as described have important implications for both prevention and treatment of CA-UTIs.

EPIDEMIOLOGY

Microbial Etiology

Enterobacteriaceae, including *Escherichia coli*, *Klebsiella* sp., and *Enterobacter* sp., are the most common pathogens associated with HAI CA-UTIs (Table 30-1). Other pathogens, more common in the ICU setting, include *Pseudomonas aeruginosa*, enterococci and *Candida* sp. [6,7,34,35]. European hospitals report a similar spectrum of bacteria associated with nosocomial UTIs, except for *Pseudomonas* sp., which were isolated in only 7% of urine cultures [36]. While 80% of infections associated with short-term indwelling urinary catheters are due to single organisms, infections in long-term catheters are frequently polymicrobial. UTI in long-term catheters are associated with ≥2 organisms in 77–95% of episodes, and 10% have >5 species of organisms present [16,26].

Enterococci emerged as a significant cause of nosocomial UTIs between 1975 and 1984 [37]. Enterococcal UTIs may derive from an endogenous source such as the patient's fecal flora or may be acquired exogenously [38–40]. The emergence and spread of antimicrobial-resistant strains have compounded the problem in many centers. *Candida* spp. are prevalent in the ICU setting where 25% of UTI are associated with *Candida* spp. [6,7]. Risk factors for candiduria include prolonged catheterization and use of broadspectrum antimicrobials. Most candida UTIs are asymptomatic, but candidemia may result in the setting of urinary tract abnormalities or procedures. Other potential complications include fungus balls of the bladder or kidney, renal abscesses, or disseminated candidiasis [41]. Coagulase-positive staphylococci (CPS) are an infrequent

TABLE 30-1

MICROBIAL PATHOGENS ASSOCIATED WITH CATHETER-RELATED URINARY TRACT INFECTIONS [6,7,34,35]

	Hospitalwide 10/1986–12/1990 (%)	Medical-Surgical ICUs 1992–1998 (%)	Pediatric ICUs 1992–1997 (%)	NNIS ICUs 2003 (%)
Escherichia coli	26.0%	18.5%	19.0%	26.0%
Candida sp.	9.0	24.8	21.1	—
Enterococci sp.	16.0	14.3	10.0	17.4
Pseudomonas aeruginosa	12.0	10.3	13.1	16.3
Klebsiella pneumoniae	6.4	5.2	7.3	9.8
Enterobacter sp.	—	4.0	10.3	6.9

cause of CA-UTI [6,7], but when CPS UTIs occur, secondary bacteremia may result [42]. Conversely, CPS bacteremia or endocarditis may result in secondary infection of the urinary tract. In one study, 27% of CPS bacteremias were associated with secondary bacteriuria [43]. The presence of CPS in the urine should prompt consideration of coinciding bacteremia and endocarditis [42,43].

Incidence of Catheter-Associated Urinary Tract Infection

In hospitalwide data, UTIs have accounted for approximately 40% of all HAIs [1,44], but UTIs make up a smaller proportion of HAIs occurring in the ICU setting. UTIs account for 15–21% of HAIs in pediatric ICU patients, 23% of HAIs in adult U.S. ICU patients, and 18% of ICU infections in the European EPIC study [6,7,45,46].

The prevalence of UTI varies by ICU type; rates of CA-UTIs reported through the Centers for Disease Control and Prevention's (CDC) National Nosocomial Infections Surveillance (NNIS) system between January 2002 and June 2004 ranged from 3.0 infections/1,000 catheter-days in cardiothoracic ICUs to 6.7 infections/1,000 catheter-days in burn or neurosurgical ICUs [47]. The rate of UTI in pediatric ICUs was 4.0 infections/1,000 catheter-days, lower than the rate seen in an equivalent adult medical ICU population of 5.1 infections/1,000 catheter-days [47]. Nosocomial UTI is infrequently identified in neonatal ICUs [47–49]. In data collected in a non-ICU setting in 42 German hospitals, the rate of infection was similar, 6.8 infections per 1,000 urinary-catheter days [50].

Risk Factors

The most important and consistent risk factor for bacteriuria is the duration of urinary catheterization (odds ratio [OR] = 2.3–22.4, depending on duration) [51–56]. Urinary catheters are associated with the vast majority of nosocomial UTI; up to 97% of UTIs in ICUs are associated with a urinary catheter [6,13]. Bacteriuria occurs quickly and frequently in catheterized patients with an average daily risk of 3–10% per day [57–59]. In patients with a catheter indwelling for 2–10 days, 26% will develop bacteriuria. Nearly all patients catheterized for a month will have bacteriuria, making this the dividing line between short-term and long-term catheterization [3,26].

Females have a higher risk of bacteriuria than males (relative risk [RR] = 1.7–3.7) [51–54,56,60]. Systemic antibiotics have a protective effect on bacteriuria; therefore, the absence of systemic antimicrobials increases the risk of bacteriuria (RR = 2.0–3.9) [51–54,56,60]. Non adherence to catheter care recommendations has been associated with increased risk of bacteriuria [20,51,53]. Other risk factors identified in >1 studies include rapidly fatal underlying illness (RR = 2.5) [51]; age >50 years (RR = 2) [51,54]; nonsurgical disease (RR = 2.2) [51]; hospitalization on an

TABLE 30-2

RISK FACTORS ASSOCIATED WITH THE DEVELOPMENT OF CATHETER-ASSOCIATED BACTERIURIA

Risk Factor

Increasing duration of catheterization
Not receiving systemic antibiotic therapy
Female sex
Diabetes mellitus
Older age
Rapidly fatal underlying illness
Nonsurgical disease
Faulty aseptic management of the indwelling catheter
Bacterial colonization of drainage bag
Azotemia (serum creatinine concentration greater than 2.0 mg/dl)
Catheter not connected to a urine meter
Periurethral colonization with uropathogens

orthopedic (RR = 51) or urological service (RR = 4) [55]; catheter insertion after the sixth day of hospitalization (RR = 8.6) [55]; catheter inserted outside the operating room (RR = 5.3) [53]; diabetes mellitus (OR = 2.3) [53]; or serum creatinine >2 mg/dL at the time of catheterization (OR = 2.1) [53]. Heavy periurethral colonization with bacteria also has been associated with increased risk of bacteriuria [61]. Significant risk factors for CA-UTI are summarized in Table 30-2.

Risk factors for UTI-related bacteremia are less clearly defined than for catheter-related bacteriuria because catheter-related bacteremia occurs infrequently (<4% of patients with catheter-related bacteriuria develop bacteremia) [62–64]. In a 23-month prospective study by Krieger et al., 1,233 patients with nosocomial UTI were identified [63]. BSIs from a urinary tract origin were found in 32 patients (2.6%). Univariate analysis identified risk factors for secondary nosocomial blood stream infection (BSI) due to *Serratia marcescens*, compared with other organisms (RR = 3.5) and male sex (RR = 2.0) [63]. No other factors (e.g., age, race, underlying disease, hospital service) were found to significantly predispose to bacteremia [63].

CLINICAL MANIFESTATIONS

CA-UTI presents clinically with a spectrum from asymptomatic bacteriuria to urosepsis and death [3,14,57,64]. Only 10–32% of patients with catheter-associated bacteriuria experience symptoms attributable to infection; thus, most patients can be classified as asymptomatic bacteriuria [3,14,57,64]. In a study of 235 patients with nosocomial catheter-related bacteriuria, approximately 90% of infections were asymptomatic [64]. Patients, with and without infection, had no significant differences in fever, dysuria, urgency, flank pain, or leukocytosis.

When present, local symptoms of UTI include lower abdominal discomfort, dysuria, urgency, frequency, or hematuria [14]. Fever, flank pain, or other clinical manifestations of pyelonephritis develop in <1% of patients with catheter-associated bacteriuria [62,65,66]. Clinically recognized infections, including prostatitis, epididymitis, seminal vesiculitis, or renal infection, may arise from bacteriuria originating during catheterization, but the frequency of such infections remains ill defined [62,65,66]. In general, these complications arise primarily in patients with long-term indwelling catheters and are rare in patients whose catheterization lasts <10 days. Signs and symptoms of sepsis, including fever, hypotension, mental status changes, or organ system dysfunction may be associated with secondary bacteremia, especially those due to gram-negative bacilli.

SEQUELAE

From the short-term clinical perspective, most CA-UTIs appear benign. Few patients with catheter-associated bacteriuria have undergone localization studies, and thus the proportion of patients with bladder, prostate, or kidney infections has not been determined. Patients with bacteriuria who die have had autopsy findings of acute pyelonephritis, renal calculi, or perinephric abscesses [62,65,66].

The major systemic complication of catheter-associated bacteriuria is secondary bacteremia. Secondary bacteremia occurs only infrequently (0.4–3.9%) in patients with nosocomial UTI [57,62–64,67]. Bacteremia is less likely to occur with asymptomatic bacteriuria and is more likely to be associated with major underlying disease and comorbidities [64]. Reflecting how often urinary catheters are used in hospitalized patients, the urinary tract is the source of 11–40% of nosocomial BSI [68–70]. A series of hospitalized patients with gram-negative BSI demonstrate that 30–40% of all gram-negative BSI acquired in the hospital originate in the urinary tract [63,68], making this the most commonly recognized source of gram-negative sepsis. Interestingly, the onset of bacteremia usually occurs within 24 hours of the onset of bacteriuria except for *Serratia marcescens* infections, in which bacteremias most commonly originate days after the onset of bacteriuria [63].

Nosocomial UTI is associated with a mortality rate of 14-19% in prospective studies [14,67,71]. Patients with UTI are nearly 3 times more likely to die during hospitalization than patients without infection [67,71]. UTI-related nosocomial BSIs have an attributable case-fatality rate of approximately 12.7% [62], with severely ill patients at highest risk of death. The use of a urinary catheter alone has been independently associated with an increased risk of death in an elderly population residing in long-term care facilities [72,73].

Recent evidence indicates that hospital stay associated with nosocomial UTI is increased by approximately 1 day, with an average cost of infection between $558 and $676 [14,74]. In a retrospective study of adults in acute care hospitals in the United States, Haley et al. estimated that nosocomial UTI occurred in 2.39 patients per 100.00 admissions, prolonged hospitalization 1 day, and cost $593 [44,75]. In another study conducted almost three decades ago, nosocomial UTI resulted in an average increase in length of stay of 2.4 days and an associated cost of $558 [76]. More recent studies suggest that an episode of bacteriuria increases costs by $676 and that urinary catheter-related BSI increases costs $2,836 per episode [14].

DIAGNOSIS

The terms bacteriuria and UTI are often used interchangeably in published reports of CA-UTI. The term bacteriuria or candiduria implies the presence of a significant number of microorganisms in quantitative urine cultures [59,64,77]. Low levels of *Candida* sp. or bacteria in urine grow within 72 hours to concentrations of $>10^5$ cfu/mL unless antibiotic therapy is administered [59]. Therefore, most studies of CA-UTI use bacteriuria as the primary outcome, and growth of $\geq 10^2$ cfu/mL of a predominant pathogen from a catheterized urine specimen collected aseptically from a sampling port is a standard definition for CA-bacteriuria [20,78].

The CDC has developed surveillance definitions for identifying nosocomial UTI that allow for interhospital comparison of infection rates [6,7,79]. The definitions differentiate symptomatic (presence of fever, urgency, frequency, dysuria, or suprapubic tenderness) from asymptomatic infection but do not allow for classification of asymptomatic bacteriuria with $<10^5$ CFU/mL.

Pyuria is an important indicator of UTI in the non-catheterized patient; in the catheterized patient, however, pyuria is not strongly correlated with UTI [77,80]. In one study, pyuria was uniformly present with bacteriuria in catheterized men, but pyuria also was present in 30% of catheterized patients without bacteriuria [80]. A recent prospective study of 761 catheterized patients found that pyuria was most strongly associated with infection caused by gram-negative bacilli; infections caused by coagulase-negative staphylococci, enterococci, or yeast were less frequently associated with pyuria [77]. Urinary white blood cell (WBC) counts >5/high-power field had a specificity of 90% for predicting infections but had a sensitivity of <37% [77].

Neither urinalysis nor urine cultures are reliable tests for diagnosing symptomatic UTI in patients with long-term indwelling urinary catheters [81]. Cultures from these catheters are universally positive and may not reflect bladder cultures [26,82]. Fever and chills are the most consistent symptom of CA-UTI [65,66,83]. UTI in patients with spinal cord lesions may be particularly difficult to diagnose because of the inability of the patient to sense localizing symptoms [83].

TREATMENT

Most patients with CA-bacteriuria are asymptomatic and do not require treatment unless the patient is at high risk for complications (e.g., BSI or renal infection [64,84]. Treatment of asymptomatic bacteriuria may be useful in patients with neutropenia, renal transplants, pregnancy or if the patient is undergoing transurethral resection of the prostate or other urological procedures likely to induce bleeding [84]. In most patients without such complicating clinical features, bacteriuria often resolves spontaneously with removal of the catheter. After catheter removal, the patient can be observed and subsequently treated if the bacteriuria does not resolve spontaneously after 48 hours [84]. The latter may be particularly useful in elderly women in whom the risk of development of symptomatic infection is particularly high [85]. Because the antimicrobial susceptibility patterns of strains causing CA-bacteriuria vary widely, choice of a specific antimicrobial agent should be guided by the *in vitro* antimicrobial susceptibilities of the infecting organism(s).

Treatment with the catheter in place often results in emergence of resistant strains, and eradication of bacteriuria in the presence of an indwelling catheter has been largely unsuccessful [31,86,87]. A recent prospective, randomized, controlled trial of patients with symptomatic UTI found that patients who underwent indwelling catheter replacement before initiation of antibiotic therapy had a significant decrease in bacteriuria and improved clinical outcome when compared with patients who had no catheter replacement [87] Their findings support the recommendation that catheters present for at least one week before onset of CA-infection should be replaced (or removed if no longer required) before antimicrobial therapy [17,88].

PREVENTION

Despite existence and knowledge of guidelines emphasizing the use of aseptic technique and closed urinary drainage for the prevention of nosocomial UTI [89,90], adherence with guidelines varies among institutions. Errors in compliance with guidelines were found in 11% of catheter-days and overall in 29% of catheterized patients at one institution [91]. Surveillance and feedback of nosocomial UTI rates to staff may be useful as an adjunct for improving compliance with recommendations [44,92,93]. Several measures for the prevention of CA-UTI are discussed next (Table 30-3).

Avoidance of Use of Indwelling Catheters

Because as many as 80% of nosocomial UTIs and 97% of UTIs in ICUs are associated with a urinary catheter, the most important prevention strategy is decreasing the

TABLE 30-3
METHODS FOR PREVENTION OF CATHETER-ASSOCIATED INFECTIONS

Avoid catheterization
Decrease duration of catheterization
Insert and care for catheters aseptically
Use a closed sterile drainage system
Maintain gravity drain
Use systemic antimicrobials in selected patient populations
Consider anti-infective catheters in selected populations

use of urinary catheters [4,16,63]. Data from the NNIS system between January 1992 and June 2004 reveal urinary catheter utilization in participating ICUs ranging from 0.30 to 0.91 urinary catheter-days/patient-days. Utilization was highest in trauma, neurosurgical, and cardiothoracic ICUs (0.91, 0.85, and 0.84 catheter-days/patient-days, respectively) and lowest in pediatric ICUs, 0.30 catheter-days/patient-days [47]. The duration of catheterization varies by hospital ward and patient population, but the mean and median durations in acute care hospitals are 2 and 4 days, respectively. Catheters are removed within 7 days in 70% of patients [94].

Overall, urinary catheters are overutilized, and documentation surrounding catheterization is inconsistent [2,95–100]. In recent prospective studies of catheterized patients, the indication for catheterization was judged to be inappropriate 21% to 50% of the time [2,95,97,99,100]. Furthermore, a written order or procedure note was frequently not documented in the medical record [96,97]. A study conducted at four different institutions found that 28% of HCWs were unaware that their patient had an indwelling urinary catheter. Lack of awareness increased with the level of training and correlated with inappropriate catheter use. The authors found that 22% of interns, 28% of residents, and 38% of attending physicians were unaware of catheters in their patients [2].

In addition, urinary catheters may be unpleasant and restrictive to patients. Elderly men at a Veterans Affairs medical center more frequently responded that a condom catheter was comfortable (86%) compared to patients with an indwelling urethral catheter (58%, $P = 0.04$) [101]. Patients also felt that condom catheters were less painful or restrictive of activities of daily living (24% vs. 61%, $P = 0008$) [101]. Another survey of patients and family of residents in long-term care facilities revealed that 85% preferred diapers and 77% preferred prompted voiding to indwelling urinary catheterization [102].

Nevertheless, urinary catheters are important for patients requiring drainage of anatomic or physiologic outlet obstruction, patients undergoing surgery of the genitourinary tract, patients requiring accurate urinary output measurements, and patients with sacral or perineal

TABLE 30-4

APPROPRIATE INDICATIONS FOR SHORT-TERM INDWELLING URINARY CATHETER USE [2,4,90,99,103]

Monitoring of urine output required
  Frequent or urgent monitoring is needed, as for critically ill patients.
  Patient is unable or unwilling to collect urine.
Urinary incontinence (without obstruction)
  Patient has an open sacral or perineal wound.
  At patient request.
  Patient is unable to wear condom catheter.
Bladder outlet obstruction
  Temporary relief of anatomical or functional obstruction.
  Longer term drainage if surgical correction is not indicated.
Prolonged surgical procedures with general or spinal anesthesia

wounds [2,99,103] (Table 30-4). However, limiting urinary catheter use to appropriate indications has important implications. Initial efforts at decreasing unnecessary catheterization have been promising [104–107]. Cornia et al. evaluated a computerized reminder, which shortened the duration of catheterization by 3 days (approximately 30% reduction in catheter days) while not affecting recatheterization rates [104]. Huang et al. evaluated a nurse-based reminder system in the adult ICU of a large hospital in Taiwan and found that nurse reminders to remove unnecessary catheters significantly reduced the duration of catheterization (7 days vs 4.6 days; $P < 0.001$) and UTI (11.5 vs 8.3 per 1000 catheter-days; $P = .009$) [105]. Finally, Saint et al. completed a pilot study in which a nurse-based reminder after 48 hours of catheterization significantly reduced the proportion of time patients were catheterized [106].

Use of Aseptic Insertion and Catheter Care Techniques

Proper aseptic technique, including aseptic insertion and maintenance of the catheter and drainage bag, is another essential strategy for preventing CA-UTI [20,51,89,90]. Cleansing the meatus at urinary catheter insertion has been widely recommended but has not been well studied. A recent randomized study comparing water with 0.1% chlorhexidine cleansing of the periurethral area before catheter insertion revealed no difference in the development of bacteriuria [108]. In addition, routine meatal cleaning of catheterized patients has shown no benefit [109,110]. The collection bag should always remain below the level of the bladder to prevent reflux of urine (and bacteria introduced into the bag) into the bladder. Proper hand hygiene and use of gloves for insertion and manipulation of catheters is critical to prevent introduction of exogenous pathogens [21,22,111–113].

Use of Closed Drainage Systems

An important advance in the prevention of CA-UTI was the introduction of the closed catheter drainage system that includes the use of sealed urinary catheter junctions [58,71,114–117]. A recent evaluation of two closed drainage systems compared a complex system (including a pre attached catheter, antireflux valve, drip chamber, and povidone iodine–releasing cartridge) with a two-chamber system. The authors found no difference in the rate of bacteriuria between the two systems [118]. Improper catheter care and breaches of the closed system remain an important risk factor for the development of bacteriuria [51,91].

Other Catheter Care Practices

Other interventions, such as irrigating the bladder or instilling antibacterial solutions into the urinary collecting bag, have not been shown to have benefit when used on closed urinary collecting systems [119–123]. These practices allow for flow of organisms colonizing the catheter into the bladder and require opening the closed system and are therefore not routinely recommended [124–126]. In addition, use of meatal lubricants and creams (both antibacterial and nonantibacterial) [127–131] or urinary catheters that have been coated with heparin [132] or polymer have not shown benefit for prevention of UTIs [133].

Use of Anti-Infective Urinary Catheters

Several studies support the use of anti-infective (latex-based silver alloy or nitrofurazone impregnated) urinary catheters as adjunct to the preceding proven methods of prevention in patients at high risk for CA-UTI [134–140]. A recent prospective trial of a silicone-based, silver-coated urinary catheter, however, showed no effect in preventing UTIs when compared to a silicone-based hydrogel catheter [141]. Recent analysis of the clinical and economic consequences of urinary catheters indicates that latex-based silver alloy catheters, which cost substantially more than standard catheters, may provide both clinical and economic benefits in patient populations receiving indwelling catheterization for 2–10 days, including the critically ill [10,142]. Al-Habdan et al. evaluated a nitrofurazone-impregnated urinary catheter among 100 postoperative and trauma patients in a hospital in Saudi Arabia. In this randomized trial, patients given the nitrofurazone-impregnated catheter were significantly less likely to develop bacteriuria compared to those given regular latex urinary catheters (12% vs 0%; $P = 0.028$) [143]. Anti-infective urinary catheters thus appear to be a promising method of reducing bacteriuria in the catheterized patient, especially in those patients at highest risk of either bacteriuria or complications associated with bacteriuria. The effect anti-infective urinary catheters will have on the more important clinical outcomes of urinary catheter-related BSI and mortality is not clear [10,135,142].

Use of Systemic Antimicrobials

Systemic antimicrobial therapy may lower the risk of developing a CA-UTI [51–53,55]. However, most experts do not recommend routine use of prophylactic antibiotics for catheterized patients because of their cost, potential adverse effects, and potential for selection of antibiotic-resistant organisms [16,17,144]. Several studies have demonstrated that antibiotic prophylaxis increases the rate of isolation of antibiotic-resistant organisms in catheterized patients [26,145–147]. Prophylaxis with trimethoprim-sulfamethoxazole (TMP/SMX) has been shown to be beneficial for the prevention of UTI after renal transplantation [148,149]. Antibiotic prophylaxis is justifiable for men undergoing transurethral resection of the prostate, especially in those with an indwelling catheter or bacteriuria preoperatively [150].

Methenamine, available as a salt of mandelate or hippurate, has been used for preventing CA-UTI for >30 years [4]. Its breakdown products, hippuric acid and formaldehyde, acidify the urine and have antibacterial properties. In small studies, oral methenamine hippurate therapy (2–6 grams daily) has been found to reduce the incidence of bacteriuria [151,152], symptomatic UTI [153], or pyuria [152]. In recent studies in patients undergoing gynecological surgery, prophylactic treatment with methenamine hippurate significantly reduced the incidence of post operative bacteriuria and symptomatic UTI [154,155]. While methenamine hippurate is not currently recommended, randomized controlled trials evaluating this intervention should be considered [4].

REFERENCES

1. Haley RW, Hooton TM, Culver DH, et al. Nosocomial infections in U.S. hospitals, 1975–1976: estimated frequency by selected characteristics of patients. *Am J Med* 1981;70:947–959.
2. Saint S, Wiese J, Amory JK, et al. Are physicians aware of which of their patients have indwelling urinary catheters? *Am J Med* 2000;109:476–480.
3. Saint S, Chenoweth CE. Biofilms and catheter-associated urinary tract infections. *Infect Dis Clin North Am* 2003;17:411–432.
4. Saint S, Lipsky BA. Preventing catheter-related bacteriuria: can we? should we? how? *Arch Intern Med* 1999;159:800–808.
5. Nicolle LE. Urinary tract infection in long-term-care facility residents. *Clin Infect Dis* 2000;31:757–761.
6. Richards MJ, Edwards JR, Culver DH, Gaynes RP. Nosocomial infections in combined medical-surgical intensive care units in the United States. *Infect Control Hosp Epidemiol* 2000;21:510–515.
7. Richards MJ, Edwards JR, Culver DH, et al. Nosocomial infections in pediatric intensive care units in the United States. *Pediatrics* 1999;103:1–7.
8. Sorbye LW, Finne-Soveri H, Ljunggren G, et al. Indwelling catheter use in home care: elderly, aged 65+, in 11 different countries in Europe. *Age Ageing* 2005;34:377–381.
9. Haley RW, Schaberg DR, Crossley KB, et al. Extra charges and prolongation of stay attributable to nosocomial infections: a prospective interhospital comparison. *Am J Med* 1981;70:51–58.
10. Saint S, Veenstra D, Sullivan S, et al. The potential clinical and economic benefits of silver alloy urinary catheters in preventing urinary tract infection. *Arch Intern Med* 2000;160:2670–2675.
11. Donlan RM, Costerton JW. Biofilms: survival mechanisms of clinically relevant microorganisms. *Clin Microbiol Rev* 2002;15:167–193.
12. Dunne Jr. WM. Bacterial adhesion: seen any good biofilms lately? *Clin Microbiol Rev* 2002;15:155–166.
13. Krieger JN, Kaiser DL, Wenzel RP. Nosocomial urinary tract infections: secular trends, treatment and economics in a university hospital. *J Urol* 1983;130:102–106.
14. Saint S. Clinical and economic consequences of nosocomial catheter-related bacteriuria. *Am J Infect Control* 2000;28:68–75.
15. Donlan RM. Biofilms and device-associated infections. *Emerging Infect Dis* 2001;7:1–4.
16. Stamm WE. Catheter-associated urinary tract infections: epidemiology, pathogenesis, and prevention. *Am J Med* 1991;91:65S–71S.
17. item17. Warren JW. Catheter-associated urinary tract infections. *Int J Antimicrob Agents* 2001;17:299–303.
18. Daifuku R, Stamm WE. Association of rectal and urethral colonization with urinary tract infection in patients with indwelling catheters. *JAMA* 1984;252:2028–2030.
19. Tambyah PA, Halvorson KT, Maki DG. A prospective study of pathogenesis of catheter-associated urinary tract infections. *Mayo Clin Proc* 1999;74:131–136.
20. Maki DG, Tambyah PA. Engineering out the risk of infection with urinary catheters. *Emerging Infect Dis* 2001;7:1–6.
21. Schaberg DR, Haley RW, Highsmith AK, et al. Nosocomial bacteriuria: a prospective study of case clustering and antimicrobial resistance. *Ann Intern Med* 1980;93:420–424.
22. Schaberg DR, Weinstein RA, Stamm WE. Epidemics of nosocomial urinary tract infection caused by multiply resistant gram-negative bacilli: epidemiology and control. *J Infect Dis* 1976;133:363–366.
23. Donlan RM. Biofilm formation: a clinically relevant microbiological process. *Clin Infect Dis* 2001;33:1387–1392.
24. Jones BV, Mahenthiralingam E, Sabbuba NA, Stickler DJ. Role of swarming in the formation of crystalline *Proteus mirabilis* biofilms on urinary catheters. *J Med Microbiol* 2005;54:807–813.
25. Sabbuba N, Hughes G, Stickler DJ. The migration of *Proteus mirabilis* and other urinary tract pathogens over Foley catheters. *BJU International* 2002;89:55–60.
26. Warren JW, Tenney JH, Hoopes JM, et al. A prospective microbiologic study of bacteriuria in patients with chronic indwelling urethral catheters. *J Infect Dis* 1982;146:719–723.
27. Choong S, Wood S, Fry C, Whitfield H. Catheter associated urinary tract infection and encrustation. *Int J Antimicrob Agents* 2001;17:305–310.
28. Mathur S, Suller MTE, Stickler DJ, Feneley RCL. Factors affecting crystal precipitation from urine in individuals with long-term urinary catheters colonized with urease-positive bacterial species. *Urol Res* 2006;34:173–177.
29. Stickler DJ, King JB, Winters C, Morris SL. Blockage of urethral catheters by bacterial biofilms. *J Infect* 1993;27:133–135.
30. Stickler DJ, Zimakoff J. Complications of urinary tract infections associated with devices used for long-term bladder management. *J Hosp Infect* 1994;28:177–194.
31. Donlan RM. Role of biofilms in antimicrobial resistance. *ASAIO J* 2000;46:S47–S52.
32. Stickler DJ. Susceptibility of antibiotic-resistant gram-negative bacilli to biocides: a perspective from the study of catheter biofilms. *J Applied Microbiol* 2002;92 (suppl):163S–170S.
33. Choong S, Whitfield H. Biofilms and their role in infections in urology. *BJU International* 2000;86:935–941.
34. Gaynes R, Edwards JR, National Nosocomial Infections Surveillance System. Overview of nosocomial infections caused by gram-negative bacilli. *Healthcare Epidemiol* 2005;41:848–854.
35. Jarvis W, Martone W. Predominant pathogens in hospital infections. *J Antimicrob Chemother* 1992;29:19–24.
36. Bouza E, San Juan R, Munoz P, et al. European perspective on nosocomial urinary tract infections. I. Report on the microbiology workload, etiology and antimicrobial susceptibility (ESGNI-003 study). *Clin Microbiol Infect* 2001;7:523–531.
37. Morrison AJ, Wenzel RP. Nosocomial urinary tract infections due to enterococcus. *Arch Intern Med* 1986;146:1549–1551.
38. Gross P, Harkavy L, Barden G, Flower M. The epidemiology of nosocomial enterococcal urinary tract infection. *Am J Med Sci* 1976;272:75–81.
39. Murray BE. Vancomycin-resistant enterococcal infections. *N Engl J Med* 2000;342:710–721.

40. Wong AH, Wenzel RP, Edmond MB. Epidemiology of bacteriuria caused by vancomycin-resistant enterococci—a retrospective study. *Am J Infect Control* 2000;28:277–281.
41. Sobel JD, Kauffman CA, McKinsey D, et al. Candiduria: a randomized, double-blind study of treatment with fluconazole and placebo. *Clin Infect Dis* 2000;30:19–24.
42. Muder RR, Brennen C, Rihs JD, et al. Isolation of *Staphylococcus aureus* from the urinary tract: association of isolation with symptomatic urinary tract infection and subsequent staphylococcal bacteremia. *Clin Infect Dis* 2006;42:46–50.
43. Demuth PJ, Gerding DN, Crossley K. *Staphylococcus aureus* bacteriuria. *Arch Intern Med* 1979;139:78–80.
44. Haley RW, Culver DH, White JW, et al. The nationwide nosocomial infection rate: a new need for vital statistics. *Am J Epidemiol* 1985;121:159–167.
45. Singh-Naz N, Sprague BM, Patel KM, Pollack MM. Risk factors for nosocomial infection in critically ill children: a prospective cohort study. *Crit Care Med* 1996;24:875–878.
46. Vincent JL, Bihari DJ, Suter PM, et al. The prevalence of nosocomial infection in intensive care units in Europe: results of the European Prevalence of Infection in Intensive Care (EPIC) Study. *JAMA* 1995;274:639–644.
47. National Nosocomial Infectious Surveillance (NNIS) System report, data summary from January 1992 through June 2004. *Am J Infect Control* 2004;32:470–485.
48. Gaynes RP, Edwards JR, Jarvis WR, et al. Nosocomial infections among neonates in high-risk nurseries in the United States. *Pediatrics* 1996;98:357–361.
49. Langley JM, Hanakowski M, LeBlanc JC. Unique epidemiology of nosocomial urinary tract infection in children. *Am J Infect Control* 2001;29:94–98.
50. Vonberg R-P, Behnke M, Geffers C, et al. Device-associated infection rates for non-intensive care unit patients. *Infect Control Hosp Epidemiol* 2006;27:357–361.
51. Garibaldi RA, Burke JP, Dickman ML, Smith CB. Factors predisposing to bacteriuria during indwelling urethral catheterization. *N Engl J Med* 1974;291:215–219.
52. Hustinx WN, Mintjes de Groot AJ, Verkooyen RP, Verbrugh HA. Impact of concurrent antimicrobial therapy on catheter-associated urinary tract infection. *J Hosp Infect* 1991;18:45–56.
53. Platt R, Polk BF, Murdock B, Rosner B. Risk factors for nosocomial urinary tract infection. *Am J Epidemiol* 1986;124:977–985.
54. Riley DK, Classen DC, Stevens LE, Burke JP. A large randomized clinical trial of a silver-impregnated urinary catheter: lack of efficacy and staphylococcal superinfection. *Am J Med* 1995;98:349–356.
55. Shapiro M, Simchen E, Izraeli S, Sacks TG. A multivariate analysis of risk factors for acquiring bacteriuria in patients with indwelling urinary catheters for longer than 24 hours. *Infect Control* 1984;5:525–532.
56. Tissot E, Limat S, Cornette C, Capellier G. Risk factors for catheter-associated bacteriuria in a medical intensive care unit. *Eur J Clin Microbiol Infect Dis* 2001;20:260–262.
57. Garibaldi RA, Mooney BR, Epstein BJ, Britt MR. An evaluation of daily bacteriologic monitoring to identify preventable episodes of catheter-associated urinary tract infection. *Infect Control* 1982;3:466–470.
58. Kunin CM, McCormack RC. Prevention of catheter-induced urinary-tract infections by sterile closed drainage. *N Engl J Med* 1966;274:1155–1161.
59. Stark RP, Maki DG. Bacteriuria in the catheterized patient: what quantitative level of bacteriuria is relevant? *N Engl J Med* 1984;311:560–564.
60. Johnson JR, Roberts PL, Olsen RJ, et al. Prevention of catheter-associated urinary tract infection with a silver oxide-coated urinary catheter: clinical and microbiologic correlates. *J Infect Dis* 1990;162:1145–1150.
61. Garibaldi RA, Burke JP, Britt MR, et al. Meatal colonization and catheter-associated bacteriuria. *N Engl J Med* 1980;303:316–318.
62. Bryan CS, Reynolds KL. Hospital-acquired bacteremic urinary tract infection: epidemiology and outcome. *J Urol* 1984;132:494–498.
63. Krieger JN, Kaiser DL, Wenzel RP. Urinary tract etiology of bloodstream infections in hospitalized patients. *J Infect Dis* 1983;148:57–62.
64. Tambyah PA, Maki DG. Catheter-associated urinary tract infection is rarely symptomatic: a prospective study of 1,497 catheterized patients. *Arch Intern Med* 2000;160:678–682.
65. Warren JW, Damron D, Tenney JH, et al. Fever, bacteremia, and death as complications of bacteriuria in women with long-term urethral catheters. *J Infect Dis* 1987;155:1151–1158.
66. Warren JW, Muncie HL Jr., Hebel JR, Hall-Craggs M. Long-term urethral catheterization increases risk of chronic pyelonephritis and renal inflammation. *J Am Geriatr Soc* 1994;42:1286–1290 [see comments].
67. Platt R, Polk B, Murdock B, Rosner B. Mortality associated with nosocomial urinary-tract infection. *N Engl J Med* 1982;307:637–642.
68. Kreger B, Craven D, McCabe W. Gram-negative bacteremia. IV. Re-evaluation of clinical features and treatment in 612 patients. *Am J Med* 1980;68:344–355.
69. Lark RL, Chenoweth CE, Saint S, et al. Four year prospective evaluation of nosocomial bacteremia: epidemiology, microbiology, and patient outcome. *Diagn Microbiol Infect Dis* 2000;38:131–140.
70. Weinstein MP, Towns ML, Quartey SM, et al. The clinical significance of positive blood cultures in the 1990s: a prospective comprehensive evaluation of the microbiology, epidemiology, and outcome of bacteremia and fungemia in adults. *Clin Infect Dis* 1997;24:584–602.
71. Platt R, Polk BF, Murdock B, Rosner B. Reduction of mortality associated with nosocomial urinary tract infection. *Lancet* 1983;1:893–897.
72. Kunin CM, Douthitt S, Dancing J, et al. The association between the use of urinary catheters and morbidity and mortality among elderly patients in nursing homes. *Am J Epidemiol* 1992;135:291–301.
73. Nicolle LE, Henderson E, Bjornson J, et al. The association of bacteriuria with resident characteristics and survival in elderly institutionalized men. *Ann Intern Med* 1987;106:682–686.
74. Jarvis WR. Selected aspects of the socioeconomic impact of nosocomial infections: morbidity, mortality, cost, and preventions. *Infect Control Hosp Epidemiol* 1996;17:552–557.
75. Haley RW, White JW, Culver DH, Hughes JM. The financial incentive for hospitals to prevent nosocomial infections under the prospective payment system: an empirical determination from a nationally representative sample. *JAMA* 1987;257:1611–1614.
76. Givens CD, Wenzel RP. Catheter-associated urinary tract infections in surgical patients: a controlled study on the excess morbidity and costs. *J Urol* 1980;124:646–648.
77. Tambyah PA, Maki DG. The relationship between pyuria and infection in patients with indwelling urinary catheters: a prospective study of 761 patients. *Arch Intern Med* 2000;160:673–677.
78. Stamm WE. Criteria for the diagnosis of urinary tract infection and for the assessment of therapeutic effectiveness. *Infection* 1992;3:S151–S154.
79. Garner J, Jarvis W, Emori T, et al. CDC definitions for nosocomial infections, 1988. *Am J Infect Control* 1988;16:128–140.
80. Musher DM, Thorsteinsson SB, Airola VM II. Quantitative urinalysis: Diagnosing urinary tract infection in men. *JAMA* 1976;236:2069–2072.
81. Steward DK, Wood GL, Cohen RL, et al. Failure of the urinalysis and quantitative urine culture in diagnosing symptomatic urinary tract infections in patients with long-term urinary catheters. *Am J Infect Control* 1985;13:154–160.
82. Bergqvist D, Bronnestam R, Hedelin H, Stahl A. The relevance of urinary sampling methods in patients with indwelling Foley catheters. *Br J Urol* 1980;52:92–95.
83. Biering-Sorensen F, Bagi P, Hoiby N. Urinary tract infections in patients with spinal cord lesions: treatment and prevention. *Drugs* 2001;61:1275–1287.
84. Nicolle LE, Bradley S, Colgan R, et al. Infectious Diseases Society of America Guidelines for the diagnosis and treatment of asymptomatic bacteriuria in adults. *Clin Infect Dis* 2005;40:643–654.
85. Harding GKM, Nicolle LE, Ronald AR, et al. How long should catheter-acquired urinary tract infection in women be treated? *Ann Intern Med* 1991;114:713–719.
86. Butler HK, Kunin CM. Evaluation of specific systemic antimicrobial therapy in patients while on closed catheter drainage. *J Urol* 1968;100:567–572.

87. Raz R, Schiller D, Nicolle LE. Chronic indwelling catheter replacement before antimicrobial therapy for symptomatic urinary tract infection. *J Urol* 2000;164:1254–1258.

88. Stamm WE, Hooton TM. Management of urinary tract infections in adults. *N Engl J Med* 1993;329:1328–1334.

89. No author. Guidelines for preventing infections associated with the insertion and maintenance of short-term indwelling urethral catheters in acute care. *J Hosp Infect* 2001;47:S39–S46.

90. Wong ES. Guideline for prevention of catheter-associated urinary tract infections. *Am J Infect Control* 1983;11:28–36.

91. Burke JP, Larsen RA, Stevens LE. Nosocomial bacteriuria: estimating the potential for prevention by closed sterile urinary drainage. *Infect Control* 1986;7:96–99.

92. Goetz AM, Kedzuf S, Wagener M, Muder RR. Feedback to nursing staff as an intervention to reduce catheter-associated urinary tract infections. *Am J Infect Control* 1999;27:402–404.

93. Haley RW, Schaberg DR, Von Allmen SD, McGowan JE, Jr. Estimating the extra charges and prolongation of hospitalization due to nosocomial infections: a comparison of methods. *J Infect Dis* 1980;141:248–257.

94. Scheckler WE. Nosocomial infections in a community hospital. *Arch Intern Med* 1978;138:1792–1794.

95. Bouza E, Rodriguez-Bouza H, Munoz P, et al. Evaluation of indwelling bladder catheterization in a general hospital. *Infect Dis Clin Pract* 1994;3:358–362.

96. Conybeare A, Pathak S, Imam I. The quality of hospital records of urethral catheterisation. *Ann R Coll Surg Engl* 2002;84:109–110.

97. Gardam MA, Amihod B, Orenstein P, et al. Overutilization of indwelling urinary catheters and the development of nosocomial urinary tract infections. *Clin Perform Qual Health Care* 1998;6:99–102.

98. Hartstein AI, Garber SB, Ward TT, et al. Nosocomial urinary tract infection: a prospective evaluation of 108 catheterized patients. *Infect Control* 1981;2:380–386.

99. Jain P, Parada JP, David A, Smith LG. Overuse of the indwelling urinary tract catheter in hospitalized medical patients. *Arch Intern Med* 1995;155:1425–1429.

100. Munasinghe RL, Yazdani H, Siddique M, Hafeez W. Appropriateness of use of indwelling urinary catheters in patients admitted to the medical service. *Infect Control Hosp Epidemiol* 2001;22:647–649.

101. Saint S, Lipsky BA, Baker PD, et al. Urinary catheters: what type do men and their nurses prefer? *J Am Geriatr Soc* 1999;47:1453–1457.

102. Johnson TM, Ouslander JG, Uman GC, Schnelle JF. Urinary incontinence treatment preferences in long-term care. *J Am Geriatr Soc* 2001;49:710–718.

103. Kunin CM. Can we build a better urinary catheter? *N Engl J Med* 1988;319:365–366.

104. Cornia PB, Amory JK, Fraser S, et al. Computer-based order entry decreases duration of indwelling urinary catheterization in hospitalized patients. *Am J Med* 2003;114:404–406.

105. Huang W-C, Wann S-R, Lin S-L, et al. Catheter-associated urinary tract infections in intensive care units can be reduced by prompting physicians to remove unnecessary catheters. *Infect Control Hosp Epidemiol* 2004;25:974–978.

106. Saint S, Kaufman SR, Thompson M, et al. A reminder reduces urinary catheterization in hospitalized patients. *Jt Comm J Qual Saf* 2005;31:455–462.

107. Topal J, Conklin S, Camp K, et al. Prevention of nosocomial catheter-associated urinary tract infections through computerized feedback to physicians and a nurse-directed protocol. *Am J Med Qual* 2005;20:121–126.

108. Webster J, Hood RH, Burridge CA, et al. Water or antiseptic for periurethral cleaning before urinary catheterization: a randomized controlled trial. *Am J Infect Control* 2001;29:389–394.

109. Burke JP, Garibaldi RA, Britt MR, et al. Prevention of catheter-associated urinary tract infections: efficacy of daily meatal care regimens. *Am J Med* 1981;70:655–658.

110. Burke JP, Jacobson JA, Garibaldi RA, et al. Evaluation of daily meatal care with poly-antibiotic ointment in prevention of urinary catheter-associated bacteriuria. *J Urol* 1983;129:331–334.

111. Larson EL. APIC guidelines for hand washing and hand antisepsis in health-care settings. *Am J Infect Control* 1995;23:251–269.

112. Pittet D. Improving adherence to hand hygiene practice: a multidisciplinary approach. *Emerging Infect Dis* 2001;7:234–240.

113. Sotto A, deBoever CM, Fabbro-Peray P, et al. Risk factors for antibiotic-resistant *Escherichia coli* isolated from hospitalized patients with urinary tract infections: a prospective study. *J Clin Microbiol* 2001;39:438–444.

114. Finkelberg Z, Kunin CM. Clinical evaluation of closed urinary drainage systems. *JAMA* 1969;207:1657–1662.

115. Huth TS, Burke JP, Larsen RA, et al. Clinical trial of junction seals for the prevention of urinary catheter-associated bacteriuria. *Arch Intern Med* 1992;152:807–812.

116. Thornton GF, Andriole VT. Bacteriuria during indwelling catheter drainage. II. Effect of a closed sterile drainage system. *JAMA* 1970;214:339–342.

117. Wolff G, Gradel E, Buchman B. Indwelling catheter and risk of urinary infection: a clinical investigation with a new closed-drainage system. *Urol Res* 1976;4:15–18.

118. Leone M, Garnier F, Dubuc M, et al. Prevention of nosocomial urinary tract infection in ICU patients: comparison of effectiveness of two urinary drainage systems. *Chest* 2001;120:220–224.

119. Bastable JR, Peel RN, Birch DM, Richards B. Continuous irrigation of the bladder after prostatectomy: its effect on postprostatectomy infection. *Br J Urol* 1977;49:689–693.

120. Dudley MN, Barriere SL. Antimicrobial irrigations in the prevention and treatment of catheter-related urinary tract infections. *Am J Hosp Pharm* 1981;38:59–65.

121. Gelman ML. Antibiotic irrigation and catheter-associated urinary tract infections. *Nephron* 1980;25:259 [editorial].

122. Kirk D, Dunn M, Bullock DW, et al. Hibitane bladder irrigation in the prevention of catheter-associated urinary infection. *Br J Urol* 1979;51:528–531.

123. Warren JW, Platt R, Thomas RJ, et al. Antibiotic irrigation and catheter-associated urinary-tract infections. *N Engl J Med* 1978;299:570–573.

124. Gillespie WA, Simpson RA, Jones JE, et al. Does the addition of disinfectant to urine drainage bags prevent infection in catheterized patients? *Lancet* 1983;1:1037–1039.

125. Sweet DE, Goodpasture HC, Holl K, et al. Evaluation of H_2O_2 prophylaxis of bacteriuria in patients with long-term indwelling Foley catheters: a randomized controlled study. *Infect Control* 1985;6:263–266.

126. Thompson RL, Haley CE, Searcy MA, et al. Catheter-associated bacteriuria: failure to reduce attack rates using periodic instillations of a disinfectant into urinary drainage systems. *JAMA* 1984;251:747–751.

127. Butler HK, Kunin CM. Evaluation of polymyxin catheter lubricant and impregnated catheters. *J Urol* 1968;100:560–566.

128. Cohen A. A microbiological comparison of a povidone-iodine lubricating gel and a control as catheter lubricants. *J Hosp Infect* 1985;6:155–161.

129. Huth TS, Burke JP, Larsen RA, et al. Randomized trial of meatal care with silver sulfadiazine cream for the prevention of catheter-associated bacteriuria. *J Infect Dis* 1992;165:14–18.

130. Kunin CM, Finkelberg Z. Evaluation of an intraurethral lubricating catheter in prevention of catheter-induced urinary tract infections. *J Urol* 1971;106:928–930.

131. Weinberg SR, Sanford RS, Myman L, et al. Evaluation of a catheter-care ointment. *J Urol* 1972;108:89–90.

132. Ruggieri MR, Hanno PM, Levin RM. Reduction of bacterial adherence to catheter surface with heparin. *J Urol* 1987;138:423–426.

133. Monson T, Kunin CM. Evaluation of a polymer-coated indwelling catheter in prevention of infection. *J Urol* 1974;111:220–222.

134. Bologna RA, Tu LM, Polansky M, et al. Hydrogel/silver ion-coated urinary catheter reduces nosocomial urinary tract infection rates in intensive care unit patients: a multicenter study. *Urology* 1999;54:982–987.

135. Johnson JR, Kuskowski MA, Wilt TJ. Systematic review: antimicrobial urinary catheters to prevent catheter-associated urinary tract infection in hospitalized patients. *Ann Intern Med* 2006;144:116–126.

136. Karchmer TB, Giannetta ET, Muto CA, et al. A randomized crossover study of silver-coated urinary catheters in hospitalized patients. *Arch Intern Med* 2000;160:3294–3298.

137. Newton T, Still JM, Law E. A comparison of the effect of early insertion of standard latex and silver-impregnated latex Foley

catheters on urinary tract infections in burn patients. *Infect Control Hosp Epidemiol* 2002;23:217–218.

138. Plowman R, Graves N, Esquivel J, Roberts JA. An economic model to assess the cost and benefits of the routine use of silver alloy coated urinary catheters to reduce the risk of urinary tract infections in catheterized patients. *J Hosp Infect* 2001;48:33–42.

139. Rupp ME, Fitzgerald T, Marion N, et al. Effect of silver-coated urinary catheters: efficacy, cost-effectiveness, and antimicrobial resistance. *Am J Infect Control* 2004;32:445–450.

140. Saint S, Elmore J, Sullivan S, Emerson S, Koepsell T. The efficacy of silver alloy-coated urinary catheters in preventing urinary tract infection: a meta-analysis. *Am J Med* 1998;105:236–241.

141. Srinivasan A, Karchmer T, Richards A, et al. A prospective trial of a novel, silicone-based, silver-coated Foley catheter for the prevention of nosocomial urinary tract infections. *Infect Control Hosp Epidemiol* 2006;27:38–43.

142. Saint S, Savel RH, Matthay MA. Enhancing the safety of critically ill patients by reducing urinary and central venous catheter-related infections. *Am J Respir Crit Care Med* 2002;165:1475–1479.

143. Al-Habdan I, Sadat-Ali M, Corea JR, et al. Assessment of nosocomial urinary tract infections in orthopaedic patients: a prospective and comparative study using two different catheters. *Int Surg* 2003;88:152–154.

144. Platt R, Polk BF, Murdock B, Rosner B. Prevention of catheter-associated urinary tract infection: a cost-benefit analysis. *Infect Control Hosp Epidemiol* 1989;10:60–64.

145. Mountokalakis T, Skounakis M, Tselentis J. Short-term versus prolonged systemic antibiotic prophylaxis in patients treated with indwelling catheters. *J Urol* 1985;134:506–508.

146. van der Wall E, Verkooyen RP, Mintjes de Groot J, et al. Prophylactic ciprofloxacin for catheter-associated urinary-tract infection. *Lancet* 1992;339:946–951.

147. Verbrugh HA, Mintjes de Groot AJ, Andriesse R, et al. Postoperative prophylaxis with norfloxacin in patients requiring bladder catheters. *Eur J Clin Microbiol Infect Dis* 1988;7:490–494.

148. Fox BC, Sollinger HW, Belzer FO, Maki DG. A prospective, randomized, double-blind study of trimethoprim-sulfamethoxazole for prophylaxis of infection in renal transplantation: clinical efficacy, absorption of trimethoprim-sulfamethoxazole, effects on the microflora, and the cost-benefit of prophylaxis. *Am J Med* 1990;89:255–274.

149. Tolkoff-Rubin NE, Cosimi AB, Russell PS, Rubin RH. A controlled study of trimethoprim-sulfamethoxazole prophylaxis of urinary tract infection in renal transplant recipients. *Rev Infect Dis* 1982;4:614–618.

150. Amin M. Antibacterial prophylaxis in urology: a review. *Am J Med* 1992;92:114S–117S.

151. Nilsson S. Long-term treatment with methenamine hippurate in recurrent urinary tract infection. *Acta Med Scand* 1975;198:81–85.

152. Norberg A, Norberg B, Parkhede U, et al. The effect of short-term high-dose treatment with methenamine hippurate of urinary infection in geriatric patients with indwelling catheters. II. Evaluation by means of a quantified urine sediment. *Ups J Med Sci* 1979;84:75–82.

153. Norrman K, Wibell L. Treatment with methenamine hippurate in the patient with a catheter. *J Int Med Res* 1976;4:115–117.

154. Schiotz HA, Guttu K. Value of urinary prophylaxis with methenamine in gynecologic surgery. *Acta Obstet Gynecol Scand* 2002;81:743–746.

155. Schiotz HA, Tanbo TG. Postoperative voiding, bacteriuria and urinary tract infection with Foley catheterization after gynecological surgery. *Acta Obstet Gynecol Scand* 2006;85:476–481.

Hospital-Acquired Pneumonia

31

Donald E. Craven, Kathleen Steger Craven, and Robert A. Duncan

INTRODUCTION

Hospital-acquired pneumonia (HAP), ventilator-associated pneumonia (VAP), and healthcare-associated pneumonia (HCAP) remain important causes of morbidity and mortality despite recent advances in antimicrobial therapy, better supportive care modalities, and the use of a wide range of prevention measures [1–3]. HAP is an infectious disease of lung parenchyma that occurs ≥48 hours after admission and was not incubating at the time of admission. VAP refers to pneumonia that arises more than 48–72 hours after endotracheal intubation. HCAP includes patients who were hospitalized in an acute care hospital for ≥2 days within 90 days of the infection, resided in a long-term care facility, and received recent intravenous antibiotic therapy, chemotherapy, or wound care within the past 30 days of the current infection or attended a hospital or hemodialysis clinic. Although this document focuses more on HAP and VAP, many of the principles are relevant to HCAP.

Organisms causing HAP may originate from the host's endogenous flora, other patients, visitors, hospital staff, or environmental sources (Figure 31-1). Aspiration and leakage around the endotracheal tube cuff are major risk factors for bacterial entry into the lower respiratory tract [3,4]. Over the past decade, there has been an increase in HAP caused by multidrug-resistant (MDR) pathogens, such as *Pseudomonas aeruginosa, Klebsiella pneumoniae, Acinetobacter baumannii,* and methicillin-resistant *Staphylococcus aureus* (MRSA) [1–3,5].

This chapter highlights the changing epidemiology, pathogenesis, and treatment of HAP, VAP, and, to a lesser extent, HCAP. Our primary focus is on bacterial pathogens causing HAP in immunocompetent adults. Readers are referred to other chapters for specific information on pulmonary infections related to immunodeficiency, mycobacteria, viruses, and fungal pathogens. Our major emphasis is on patient management (diagnosis and treatment), effective prevention strategies, and improved methods for implementing evidence-based risk reduction strategies to improve patient outcomes. New concepts and publications from the past 5 years are prioritized.

EPIDEMIOLOGY

Each year there are between 5 and 10 episodes of HAP/1,000 hospital admissions [1–3]. HAP accounts for 15%

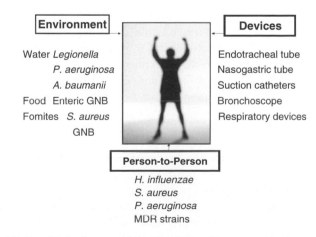

Figure 31-1 Sources of nosocomial respiratory tract pathogens: the environment, invasive devices, patients and hospital staff.

of all healthcare-associated infections (HAIs) and approximately 25% of all intensive care unit (ICU) infections. Clearly, HAP rates are influenced by decreasing lengths of stay and transfers from acute care facilities to other healthcare venues. Rates of HAP tend to be higher in university vs. nonteaching hospitals. Rates of VAP in the Centers for Disease Control and Prevention's (CDC) National Nosocomial Infections Surveillance (NNIS) system varied by type of ICU with a pooled mean of 7.3/1,000 ventilator-days for medical versus 13.2 for surgical ICUs. The 50th percentile (median) was 6.0 for medicine and 11.6/1,000 ventilator-days for surgical ICUs [5].

Crude rates of VAP vary by patient population and method of diagnosis [1–3]. Several studies have demonstrated that rates of VAP increase with the duration of mechanical ventilation, and attack rates have been estimated to be approximately 3% per day during the first 5 days and then 2% per day thereafter [6].

In an era of increased pressure to publicly report and compare HAI rates, Eggimann et al. examined several ways to report HAI rates and suggested some caveats for benchmarking rates of VAP. In a prospective cohort of 1,068 medical ICU patients, 127 episodes of VAP developed in 106 (23.5%) of 451 mechanically ventilated patients [7]. The incidence of first episode of VAP was 22.8/1,000 patient-days; 29.6/1,000 patient-days at risk, 35.7/1,000 ventilator-days, and 44.0/1,000 ventilator-days at risk. When considering all 127 episodes of VAP, infection rates increased from 22.8 to 27.3 episodes/1,000 ICU days and from 35.7 to 42.8 episodes/1,000 ventilator-days. These data demonstrate that, depending on the denominator chosen, the apparent incidence of infection reported by various hospitals may differ by as much as 40–60%. These differences support the use of a standardized calculation of HAI rates among ICUs and hospitals in our current competitive medical environment.

The crude mortality rates for VAP pneumonia range from 20–60%, reflecting, in large part, the severity of underlying disease, organ failure, and specific pathogen(s) and study populations [1–3,8,9]. Estimates of attributable mortality directly related to VAP vary by study design but are approximately 33%. In two major studies of VAP, the mortality rate varied between 4% in patients without prior antibiotic exposure to 73% in those with VAP due to MDR pathogens (e.g., *P. aeruginosa* or *A. baumannii*), and attributable mortality ranged from 6–14% [10,11].

Cost

Prevention programs can be "marketed" to hospital administrators and others involved in resource allocation by demonstrating that preventing VAP results in improved clinical outcomes, significantly reduced costs, and less adverse publicity and liability. In 2002, Rello et al. demonstrated that, on average, an episode of VAP increased

hospitalization by 12 days, mechanical ventilation by 10 days, ventilator days by 6 days, and ICU stay by 6 days at a hospital cost of $40,000; similar results have been reported from a suburban hospital by Warren et al. [9,12]. In addition to these direct savings associated with preventing VAP, the growing trend toward public reporting of institution-specific HAI rates and other outcome data is steadily increasing and may eventually be tied to hospital reimbursement rates.

PATHOGENESIS

Pathogenesis of HAP involves the direct interaction between the pathogen(s) with the host and epidemiologic variables that facilitate this dynamic. There are several mechanisms that contribute to the pathogenesis of HAP, and the relative contribution of each pathway remains controversial and varies by population at risk and the infecting pathogen(s) (Figure 31-2) [1,2]. Microaspiration in nonventilated patients is the primary route of bacterial entry into the lower respiratory tract [1,2]. Dental plaque has also been implicated as a contributing factor. In addition, patients who are sedated, postoperative, or have abnormal swallowing are at higher risk for aspiration [1,2]. Direct inoculation, bacteremic spread, or translocation of bacteria from the gastrointestinal tract are less well documented routes.

High concentrations of bacteria refluxed from the gastric reservoir or infected sinuses may be aspirated and increase levels of bacteria colonizing the oropharynx, but the relative contribution of these sites remains controversial. Bacterial adherence and colonization of the oropharynx clearly is the primary source of bacterial entry into the lung and a conduit for gastric colonization [2,13,14]. The contributory role of the stomach in the pathogenesis of pneumonia may be related to patient position, type of stress ulcer prophylaxis, gastric pH, and underlying gastrointestinal diseases [2,15]. Retrograde colonization of the oropharynx from the stomach may increase the risk of oropharyngeal colonization and lower respiratory tract infection, also known as the "gastropulmonary route of infection."

In the mechanically ventilated patient, inhalation of aerosols, contaminated tubing condensate, and leakage of bacteria and oral secretions around the endotracheal cuff are routes of bacterial entry into the lower respiratory tract (Figure 31-3) [16,17]. In addition, local trauma and inflammation from the endotracheal tube increase tracheal colonization and reduce clearance of organisms and secretions from the lower respiratory tract. The development of biofilm-encased bacteria over time on the endotracheal tube lumen may increase the risk of bacterial embolization into the alveoli following suctioning or bronchoscopy [18].

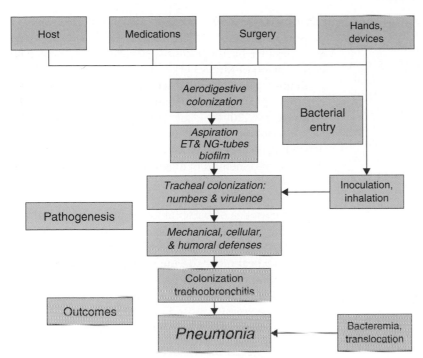

Figure 31-2 Pathogenesis of hospital-acquired pneumonia (HAP) and ventilator-associated pneumonia (VAP) with possible targets for prevention strategies. Stage 1: colonization and invasion of the lower respiratory tract; Stage II: bacterial-host defense interactions (bacterial numbers and virulence versus host mechanical, humoral, and cellular defenses) and Stage III: outcomes (colonization, tracheobronchitis or pneumonia).

Colonization of the Oropharynx

In contrast to healthy people, critically ill patients and those with VAP have high rates of oropharyngeal colonization with bacterial pathogens [1,2]. Colonization with gram-negative bacilli was present in 16% of moderately ill patients vs. 57% of critically ill patients, and rates of pneumonia were increased sixfold in ICU patients with bacterial colonization [13]. Host factors, types of bacteria colonizing the pharynx, and the use of antibiotics may alter colonization and adherence of gram-negative bacilli. Oral epithelial cells rich in fibronectin bind gram-positive organisms, such as streptococci and *S. aureus*; conversely, those poor in fibronectin preferentially bind gram-negative bacilli such as *P. aeruginosa* [19].

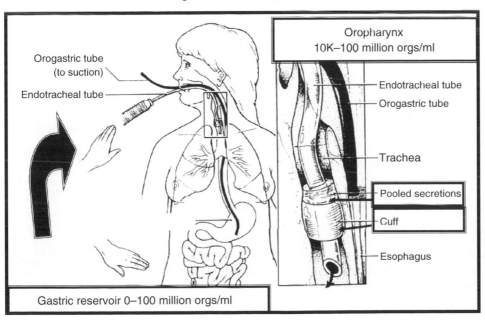

Figure 31-3 An intubated patient with oropharyngeal and gastric colonization; note subglottic secretions pooled above the endotracheal tube cuff. The endotracheal tube prevents mechanical clearance of bacteria and secretions from the trachea and bacteria encased biofilm form in the lumen of the endotracheal tube over time. Endotracheal and gastric tubes are in oropharynx and are potential sources for colonization by multidrug-resistant pathogens.

Gastric Colonization

In mechanically ventilated patients, the stomach and gastrointestinal tract may contribute to oropharyngeal and tracheal colonization with gram-negative bacilli, although some investigators question their importance (Figure 31-3) [2,14,15,20–23]. The stomach often is sterile when the pH is <2 because of the potent bactericidal activity of hydrochloric acid. An increase in gastric colonization occurs with achlorhydria, and various gastrointestinal diseases, malnutrition, or the use of antacids or histamine-2 (H_2) blockers. In mechanically ventilated patients, colonization may reach 1–100 million gram-negative bacilli/ml of gastric juice when the pH is >4 [20].

Immune Defenses in the Lung

The response of pulmonary host defenses to invading microorganisms plays an integral part in the pathogenesis and outcome of infection, yet our understanding is limited and needs further elucidation (Figures 31-2 and 31-3) [1,3,23–25]. Mucociliary and mechanical clearance in the upper airway are important factors in the defense against infection. Bacterial antigens and cytokines that alter the activity and efficacy of ciliary cells in clearing bacteria from the lower airway need further study. The ability of macrophages and polymorphonuclear leukocytes to eliminate bacterial pathogens and the interaction of these cells with inflammatory cytokines probably play important roles in the pathogenesis of pneumonia. Cell-mediated immune response is controlled by a complex array of lipids, peptides, and cytokines, including interleukin-1 and -2, interferons, growth factors, and chemotactic factors. Leukotrienes, complement components, and platelet-activating factor also assist in the inflammatory response and contribute to the pathogenesis of pneumonia. Based on an improved understanding of the molecular interaction between bacteria cell walls, toxins, and host defenses, strategies should be considered to enhance host defenses and supplement current antimicrobial regimens.

Etiologic Agents

The wide spectrum of etiologic agents causing HAP varies with time, by hospital, type of ICU, and patient population studied, emphasizing the importance of current local surveillance data (Table 31-1) [1–3,5,9,26,27]. Bacteria causing HAP may originate from various sources, including the patient's endogenous flora, other patients, staff, contaminated devices, or the environment [4,28,29] (Figure 31-1). Prior hospitalization, exposure to chronic care facilities, and antibiotic therapy also are important predisposing factors for MDR pathogens [30–33]. In the absence of these factors, early onset HAP occurring during the first 5 days of the hospital stay is usually caused by *Streptococcus pneumoniae, Moraxella catarrhalis, Hemophilus influenzae,* or anaerobic bacteria (Table 31-1) [1,3]. In comparison, late onset HAP is commonly caused by MDR gram-negative bacilli (*Klebsiella pneumoniae, A. baumannii, P. aeruginosa*) or MRSA [34].

Gram-negative bacilli have been implicated in >60% of reported episodes of HAP, and *S. aureus* (often MRSA) accounts for 20–40% of episodes and is increasing [2,5,35]. Isolation rates of these bacteria vary considerably, depending on the population at risk, location, hospital size, ICU type, and method of diagnosis. However, overall rates of MDR pathogen infections are increasing in the United States [35–37].

Most episodes of bacterial nosocomial pneumonia are caused by >1 species of bacteria [1–3,9]. The specific etiologies of pneumonia vary by hospital, the presence of an endotracheal tube, and the method used for diagnosis. For example, critically ill patients who often have both acute and chronic underlying diseases are often exposed to numerous invasive procedures and more antibiotics and devices. All of these factors increase the risk of colonization and infection with MDR gram-negative bacilli, MRSA, and vancomycin-resistant or vancomycin-intermediate-resistant (VRSA/VISA) isolates of *S. aureus* [9,36,38–40].

Very few data are available about the bacteriology and risk factors for specific pathogens in patients with HAP and HCAP who are not mechanically ventilated. Unpublished data from a comprehensive hospitalwide surveillance of HAIs at the University of North Carolina described the pathogens causing both VAP and HAP from 2000–2003 (personal communication Dr. David Weber and Dr. William Rutala) [1]. Pathogens were isolated from 92% of mechanically ventilated patients with infection, and 77% of nonventilated patients with infection. Non-ventilated patients had very similar bacteriology to ventilated patients, including infection with MDR pathogens (e.g., MRSA, *P. aeruginosa, Acinetobacter* spp., or *K. pneumoniae*). In fact, MRSA and *K. pneumoniae* were more common in nonventilated than ventilated patients, but MDR gram-negative bacilli (e.g., *P. aeruginosa, Stenotrophomonas maltophilia,* or *Acinetobacter* spp.) were more common in VAP.

More recently, pneumonia due to community-acquired MRSA (CA-MRSA) has emerged in children and adults [39–42]. In contrast to healthcare-associated (HA)-MRSA, CA-MRSA isolates are genetically distinct and almost uniformly carry the Panton-Valentine leukocidin (PVL) that may be associated with greater virulence. These strains also have been identified as an emerging source of infection spreading within hospitals. There also is concern over the evolution of VISA/GISA isolates of *S. aureus* that have been increasing [38,39]. Although a smaller number of VRSA isolates have been reported to date, rates may increase with the lowering of the vancomycin minimum inhibitory concentrations (MICs) from 4 mcg/ml to 2 mcg/ml.

TABLE 31-1
COMMON PATHOGENS CAUSING HAP

Pathogen	Multidrug Resistant (MDR)	Comments
Gram-Positive Cocci		
Staphylococcus aureus	Methicillin-resistant S. aureus (MRSA)	MRSA is increasing in hospitals: community-acquired MRSA (CA-MRSA) isolates are rapidly emerging and less resistant; inducible resistance to clindamycin has been reported
	Vancomycin or Glycopeptide-intermediate S. aureus (VISA,GISA)	New definitions of vancomycin sensitivity (MICs) may increase prevalence of GISA, VISA isolates; currently rare
	Vancomycin-resistant S. aureus (VRSA)	VRSA currently rare
	Linezolid-resistant S. aureus (LRSA)	LRSA strains are rare but may increase with more prescribing
Streptococcus pneumoniae (pneumococcus)	Penicillin-resistant S. pneumoniae (PRSP) and multidrug resistant S. pneumoniae	Usually early onset HAP; PRSP strains increasing: resistant serotypes changing with use of protein-polysaccharide vaccine in children
Gram-Negative Bacilli		
Escherichia coli	Extended-spectrum beta-lactamase (ESBL)+ E. Coli	Not a common HAP pathogen
Klebsiella pneumoniae	ESBL++ K. pneumoniae	ESBL + strains are increasing in the United States
Enterobacter species		Resistance to cephalosporins may develop on therapy
Serratia marcescens		Some resistant isolates reported
	Pseudomonas aeruginosa	Common MDR-pathogen; resistant spectrum common
	Acinetobacter species	Variable; may cause outbreaks of VAP
	Burholderia cepacia	Uncommon
	Stenotrophomonas maltophilia	Uncommon
Gram-Negative Coccobacilli		
Hemophilus influenzae		Early onset HAP; more common chronic lung disease patients; resistant strains usually β-lactamase +
Moraxella catarrhalis		Some resistant strains reported
Special Pathogens		
Legionella pneumophilia		Check hospital water supply; cooling towers (airborne)
Bordetella pertussis		

COMMON PATHOGENS

Streptococcus pneumoniae and Haemophilus influenzae

S. pneumoniae and H. influenzae usually cause early onset HAP. Many strains of S. pneumoniae are penicillin resistant (PRSP) and a smaller number are also resistant to cephalosporins, macrolides, tetracyclines, and clindamycin [1]. Generally, patients with low and moderate levels of resistance to penicillin have clinically improved [43]. All of the MDR-strains in the United States are currently sensitive to vancomycin and linezolid, and most isolates remain sensitive to third- and fourth-generation quinolones. Resistance of H. influenzae to antibiotics other than penicillin and ampicillin is rare.

Klebsiella, Enterobacter, and Serratia Species

Klebsiella spp. are intrinsically resistant to ampicillin and other aminopenicillins and can acquire resistance to cephalosporins and aztreonam by the production of extended-spectrum β-lactamases (ESBLs) [1]. Plasmids encoding ESBLs often carry resistance to aminoglycosides and other drugs, but these usually remain susceptible to carbapenems. Enterobacter spp. has a chromosomal AmpC β-lactamase that is inducible and easily expressed at a high level by mutation with consequent resistance to oxyimino-β-lactams and α-methoxy-β-lactams, such as cefoxitin and cefotetan, but continued susceptibility to carbapenems. Citrobacter and Serratia spp. have the same inducible AmpC β-lactamase and the same potential for resistance development. Plasmid-mediated resistance, such as ESBL production, is a more common mechanism for β-lactam resistance in HAI isolates and is increasingly recognized, not only in isolates of *K. pneumoniae* and *E. coli* but also *Enterbacter* spp.

Pseudomonas aeruginosa

P. aeruginosa, the most common MDR gram-negative bacterial pathogen causing HAP/VAP, has intrinsic resistance to many antimicrobial agents [1]. This resistance is mediated by multiple efflux pumps, which may be expressed continuously or may be up-regulated by mutation. Resistance to piperacillin, ceftazidime, cefepime, other oxyimino-β-lactams, imipenem and meropenem, aminoglycosides, or fluoroquinolones is increasing in the United States. Decreased expression of an outer membrane porin channel (OprD) can cause resistance to both imipenem and meropenem or specific resistance to imipenem but not to other ß-lactams. Although currently uncommon in the United States, there is concern for the acquisition of plasmid-mediated metallo-β-lactamases active against carbapenems and antipseudomonal penicillins and cephalosporins. Currently, some MDR isolates of *P. aeruginosa* are susceptible only to polymyxin B.

Acinetobacter baumannii, Stenotrophomonas maltophilia, Burkholderia cepacia

Although generally less virulent than *P. aeruginosa*, *Acinetobacter* spp. have nonetheless become problem pathogens because of increasing resistance to commonly used antimicrobial agents [1,44]. More than 85% of isolates are susceptible to carbapenems, but resistance is increasing due either to IMP-type metallo-enzymes or carbapenemases of the OXA-type. An alternative for therapy is sulbactam, usually employed as an enzyme inhibitor, but with direct antibacterial activity against *Acinetobacter* spp. *S. maltophilia*, which shares with *B. cepacia* a tendency to colonize the respiratory tract rather than cause invasive disease, is uniformly resistant to carbapenems because of a ubiquitous, metallo-β-lactamase. *S. maltophilia* and *B. cepacia* are most likely to be susceptible to trimethoprim/sulfamethoxazole, ticarcillin/clavulanate, or a fluoroquinolone. *B. cepacia* usually is susceptible to ceftazidime and carbapenems.

MRSA

In the United States, >50% of the ICU infections caused by *S. aureus* are methicillin-resistant organisms [35,36]. MRSA produces a penicillin-binding protein with reduced affinity for β-lactam antibiotics that is encoded by the *mecA* gene, which is carried by one of a family of four mobile genetic elements [1]. Strains with mecA are resistant to all commercially available β-lactams and many other antistaphylococcal drugs with considerable geographic variability worldwide. Although VISA with a minimal inhibitory concentration (MIC) of 8–16 μg/ml and high-level VRSA with MIC ≥32-1024 μg/ml have been isolated from clinical specimens, all of these isolates have been sensitive to linezolid [38,39]. Although linezolid

resistance has emerged in *S. aureus*, it is currently rare. Daptomycin resistance has also been reported, but this drug is not indicated for treatment of pneumonia because of its inactivation by lung surfactant. MRSA now accounts for >50% of the ICU-acquired staphylococcal HAIs in the United States [45]. MRSA is associated with significant morbidity and mortality, making it a challenge for infection control. The introduction of new virulence factors from CA-MRSA strains into HA-MRSA strains may have important clinical and infection control consequences [46].

A recent outbreak of VISA infections in a French ICU may be a harbinger of future problems for other hospitals [38]. Aggressive antibiotic stewardship must focus on more judicious use of all antibiotics, especially fluoroquinolones, which have been shown to increase the chance of acquisition of MRSA three to fivefold. Also, more aggressive infection control measures, such as active surveillance cultures, patient isolation, and eradication of MRSA or "a search and destroy" strategy may be needed [40,41,47].

Legionella pneumophila

Rates of HAP due to *L. pneumophila* vary among hospitals but are increased in immunocompromised patients (e.g., organ transplant recipients or patients with human immunodeficiency virus [HIV] disease) and in those with diabetes mellitus, underlying lung disease or end-stage renal disease [2,48,49]. Serotype 1 is most common and can be cultured on special media but may be more rapidly diagnosed by urinary antigen testing. HAP due to *Legionella* spp. is more common in hospitals where the organism is present in the water supply or may surge during construction. Due to the widespread use of Legionella urinary antigen rather than culture for the diagnosis of Legionella, infection due to serotypes other than serotype 1 may be underdiagnosed. Detailed strategies for prevention of *Legionella* spp. infection and eradication procedures for *Legionella* spp. in cooling towers and the hospital water supply are outlined elsewhere [2] (see Chapter 44).

DIAGNOSIS

Accurate data regarding etiologic agents, epidemiology, and treatment of HAP are limited by the lack of a diagnostic gold standard. Although clinical criteria and semiquantitative criteria for the diagnosis of HAP are the current standard for most U.S. hospitals, there are concerns about lack of diagnostic specificity [1,3,50–55]. Atelectasis, pulmonary edema, pulmonary emboli, neoplastic processes, and some autoimmune diseases can mimic the clinical presentation of HAP. In addition, chest radiographic changes may be difficult to evaluate due to adult respiratory disease syndrome (ARDS) or congestive heart failure, making the clinical diagnosis of pneumonia more difficult. The use of a computerized tomographic (CT) scan may provide improved imaging, but obtaining quality sputum samples for Gram stain and culture is of paramount importance. Finally, sputum may be produced spontaneously, induced by nebulized saline or obtained by bronchoscopy in the nonintubated patient or by endotracheal aspirates, bronchoscopy, or non-bronchoscopic methods in the intubated patient.

For mechanically ventilated ICU patients, there has been considerable controversy regarding the benefits and risks of clinical diagnosis, use of semiquantitative endotracheal aspirates, or use of quantitative diagnosis with either bronchoscopic bronchoalveolar lavage (B-BAL) or protective specimen brush (B-PSB) or "blind" non-bronchoscopic methods (NB-BAL or NB-PSB). The two diagnostic approaches for HAP discussed in detail in the recent American Thoracic Society (ATS)–Infectious Diseases Society of America (IDSA) Guideline are briefly summarized next [1].

Clinical-Semiquantitative Approach

The clinical diagnosis of pneumonia is defined as the presence of a new or progressive radiographic infiltrate plus at least 2 of 3 clinical features (fever >38°C, leukocytosis or leukopenia, and purulent secretions). While sensitivity for the presence of pneumonia is increased if only one criterion is used, specificity is reduced, leading to significantly increased antibiotic administration. Requiring all three clinical criteria is too insensitive, resulting in underprescribing for patients with HAP.

The clinical approach uses semiquantitative cultures of endotracheal aspirates or sputum with initial microscopic examination. Most microbiology laboratories report sputum culture results in a semiquantitative fashion, describing growth as light, moderate, or heavy. Moderate to heavy growth is most consistent with a diagnosis of HAP. It is rare that a sputum culture or tracheal aspirate culture does not contain a pathogen(s) found by invasive methods, but endotracheal aspirates consistently have more microorganisms than quantitative cultures (less specificity) (Table 31-2), frequently resulting in unnecessary treatment and excessive antibiotic use.

Careful examination of a Gram stain is of critical importance to improve diagnostic accuracy, both quantifying polymorphonuclear leukocytes, macrophages, and squamous epithelial cells and looking at the morphology and staining of bacteria. Findings should then be correlated with culture results. Conversely, a negative tracheal aspirate (absence of bacteria or inflammatory cells) in a patient without a recent (within 72 hours) change in antibiotics has a strong negative predictive value (94%) for VAP. A reliably performed Gram stain of tracheal aspirates should reduce the incidence of inappropriate, initial empiric antibiotic therapy and may be helpful in monitoring response to treatment.

TABLE 31-2
RECOMMENDATIONS FOR INITIAL, BROAD-SPECTRUM, EMPIRIC THERAPY FOR PATIENTS WITH SUSPECTED PNEUMONIA

Potential MDR-Pathogens	Combination Therapy
MDR Gram-negative bacilli	
Pseudomonas aeruginosa	**Anti-pseudomonal cephalosporin** e.g., cefepime, ceftazidime
	OR
	Anti-pseudomonal carbapenem (imipenem or meropenem)
	OR
Escherichia coli	**Anti-pseudomonal penicillin** (piperacillin-tazobactam)
	PLUS
	Anti-pseudomonal fluoroquinolone (ciprofloxacin or levofloxacin)
Klebsiella pneumoniae	**OR**
	Aminoglycoside (amikacin, gentamicin, or tobramycin)
ESBL+ Klebsiella pneumoniae*	**Carbapenem**
Acinetobacter species	**Carbapenem + Aminoglycoside**
Non-MDR Gram-negative Bacilli	
Legionella pneumophila	**Fluoroquinolone or Macrolide**
	(ciprofloxacin, Levofloxacin or Azithromycin)
MDR Gram-positive cocci	
Methicillin-resistant	**Vancomycin or Linezolid**
Staphylococcus aureus (MRSA)	

*If Legionella pneumoiae use fluoroquinolone.
Adapted from American Thoracic Society & Infectious Diseases Society of America Guideline Committee.
Guidelines for the management of adults with hospital-acquired, ventilator-associated, and healthcare-associated pneumonia. 2005;171:388–415.

Use of the clinical strategy for diagnosis allows prompt empiric therapy for all patients suspected of having HAP and prevents delays in initiating appropriate antibiotic therapy, which may increase mortality. Therapy can be modified or de-escalated based on clinical response at days 2 and 3 and on the results of semiquantitative cultures. Thus, the clinical approach is easy, inexpensive, and reduces delays in initiating therapy. The major limitation is overuse of antibiotics because semiquantitative cultures do not reliably separate pathogens from colonizers.

In an effort to improve the specificity of clinical diagnosis, Pugin et al. developed the clinical pulmonary infection score (CPIS), which combines clinical, radiographic, physiologic (Pao_2/FiO_2) and microbiologic data into a single numerical result [34]. When the CPIS score was >6, good correlation was found with the presence of pneumonia as defined by quantitative cultures of nonbronchoscopic BAL [50]. Singh et al. used a modified CPIS score that did not rely on culture data to guide clinical management [51]. Patients with a low clinical suspicion of VAP (CPIS ≤6) were randomized to therapy with ciprofloxacin compared to conventional therapy. The ciprofloxacin group had antibiotics discontinued after 3 days if there was no deterioration in their clinical status or CPIS score [51]. The modified CPIS score appears to be an objective measure to define patients who can receive shorter courses of therapy (3 days), achieving better overall outcomes.

Quantitative Approach

The bacteriologic approach uses quantitative cultures of lower respiratory secretions (endotracheal aspirates, BAL, or PSB collected with or without a bronchoscope) to define both the presence of HAP and the specific etiologic agent(s) [1,3]. Growth above the defined threshold concentration (moderate to heavy) is required to diagnose HAP/VAP whereas growth below the threshold is assumed to be due to colonization or contamination. The quantitative approach has been used to guide decisions about initiating antibiotic therapy, targeting specific pathogens, selecting antimicrobial therapy, and determining whether to continue therapy.

The quantitative approach avoids overtreatment with antibiotics by trying to delineate between colonizing and infecting pathogens. As a result, compared to the clinical approach, this method has consistently led to reduced numbers of bacteria treated, use of a narrower spectrum of antibiotics, and reduced numbers of patients treated [53]. For patients with negative cultures, a search for other diagnoses can be initiated. Furthermore, the use of quantitative measures may provide a better standard for comparison of VAP rates among hospitals.

The major limitations of the quantitative approach are that a false-negative culture can lead to a failure to treat and that the results may not always be consistent and reproducible [1]. A major factor causing false-negative quantitative cultures is recent initiation or a change in antibiotic therapy, especially in the preceding 24 hours but also up to 72 hours. Therefore, for BAL, the use of a threshold one log lower than usual may avoid some false-negative results in patients given antibiotics before culturing.

Finding a "Gold Standard"

A major problem with all studies of HAP is the absence of a "gold standard" to which diagnostic results can be compared. Some clinicians are concerned about the safety of withholding therapy in some patients until quantitative results are available [1,3,54]. Thus, most clinicians believe that patients with signs of infection, especially those who are clinically unstable, should receive early, appropriate, and adequate antibiotic therapy as outlined here.

To date, three randomized single-center studies have demonstrated no differences in mortality when invasive techniques (PSB and/or BAL) were compared to either quantitative or semiquantitative endotracheal aspirate culture techniques [1,54]. However, these studies included few patients, and antibiotics were continued in all patients, even those with negative cultures, thereby negating one of the potential advantages of the bacteriologic strategy. Several prospective studies have concluded that antibiotics can be safely stopped in patients with negative quantitative cultures with no adverse impact on mortality.

In one large, prospective, randomized trial of 413 patients with suspected VAP, patients receiving invasive management compared to those managed clinically had a lower mortality rate at day 14 (16% and 25%; $p = 0.02$, but not at day 28), lower mean sepsis-related organ failure assessment scores ($p = 0.04$), and significantly more antibiotic-free days (11 ± 9 vs. 7 ± 7; $p < 0.001$) [53]. Multivariate analysis demonstrated significantly reduced mortality (hazards ratio, 1.54 [CI, 1.10 to 2.16]; $p = 0.01$). Although a high percentage of patients received in both arms adequate initial antibiotics, more patients in the invasive group received adequate therapy than in the clinical group, and the impact of this difference on the observed mortality is of concern. This study suggests that the quantitative approach is safe, leads to less antibiotic use, and may potentially reduce mortality, but use of antibiotics was variable, and it is notable that approximately 10% of the patients managed with a quantitative strategy received antibiotic therapy regardless of bronchoscopic findings because of clinical instability or signs of sepsis.

On the contrary, a recent randomized study by the Canadian Critical Care Trials group compared quantitative and semi-quantitative techniques for diagnosing VAP in 740 patients who were randomized to specifically target antibiotic therapy [55]. Although there were many patients excluded from the study, including those with MRSA and *P. aeruginosa* colonization, the clinical outcomes in terms of length of stay in the hospital/ICU and the 28-day mortality were similar between the two groups.

Currently, clinical signs of pneumonia (fever, leukocytosis and purulent sputum with the presence of more than 50% neutrophils on analysis of lower respiratory tract secretions and the presence of a new and persistent infiltrate on chest x-ray coupled with a pathogen having moderate to heavy growth on a semiquantitative culture of an endotracheal aspirate or quantitative BAL with $>10^4$ CFU/ml or protected specimen brush sample with $>10^3$ CFU/ml provides the most diagnostic sensitivity and specificity for VAP [50,52].

Antimicrobial Management Using Early, Appropriate, and Adequate Initial Empiric Antibiotic Therapy

The 2005 ATS/IDSA Guidelines for the management of HAP are outlined in Figure 31-3 and Table 31-2 [1]. New principles of therapy include the use of initial empiric, broadspectrum antibiotic therapy that is likely effective against the infecting pathogen(s) and then de-escalating or streamlining therapy, and limiting the duration of therapy to 7 to 8 days [1].

Choosing an initial, appropriate intravenous antibiotic regimen depends on the likelihood of infection with MDR pathogens, such as *P. aeruginosa*, *A. baumannii.*, ESBL+ *K. pneumoniae*, or MRSA (Figure 31-3). Risk factors for MDR pathogens include prior hospitalization, late onset infection, prior antibiotic therapy, chronic dialysis, residents of chronic care facilities, and immunocompromised patients.

Patients without MDR risk factors and early onset HAP or VAP usually can be treated with a more limited spectrum of antibiotics, such as ceftriaxone plus azithromycin, a third- or fourth-generation quinolone, such as levofloxacin or moxifloxacin or ampicillin-sulbactam (Table 31-3). Those with known risk factors for MDR pathogens often need broader initial antibiotic coverage. The selection of empiric antibiotics for MDR-pathogens may vary with the patient's risk factors, medical history, and the prevalence and types of endemic MDR-pathogens present in the healthcare facility or specific ICU. For example, patients with no known risk factors for MRSA or those in facilities with a low prevalence of MRSA may not require initial treatment with vancomycin or linezolid. It is important to use doses of antibiotics that will achieve adequate concentrations in the lung parenchyma that are outlined in the ATS/IDSA Guideline [1].

Assessing Clinical Response, Cultures, and Streamlining Therapy

While initial antibiotic coverage should be liberal and broad enough to cover all suspected pathogens, de-escalation or streamlining antibiotic therapy based on the patient's clinical response and microbiologic data is of critical importance to improve patient outcomes by minimizing unnecessary exposure to antibiotics (Figure 31-4) [1,51,56]. Patients without evidence of HAP or VAP, such as those

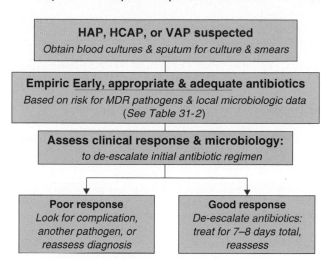

Figure 31-4 Approach to initial antibiotic therapy and management. Appropriate therapy is associated with improved outcomes in terms of morbidity and mortality. Adapted from American Thoracic Society & Infectious Diseases Society of America Guideline Committee. Guidelines for the management of adults with hospital-acquired, ventilator-associated, and healthcare-associated pneumonia. 2005;171:388–415.

without quantitative microbiologic evidence of infection, should have their antibiotics stopped, and if necessary, further workup and treatment for other sources of fever should be pursued.

Limiting Duration of Therapy

In a recent randomized trial of patients with VAP, patients randomized to 8 days of antibiotic therapy had fewer recurrences and less resistance overall than those randomized to 15 days of therapy [58]. No significant differences were noted in mortality or clinical response parameters, but rates of recurrence for those patients with VAP due to *P. aeruginosa* infection were higher in the group treated for 8 rather than 15 days. The ATS/IDSA Guideline recommends 7–8 days of therapy for uncomplicated HAP or VAP with close follow-up for any signs of relapse, especially for patients with HAP or VAP due to *P. aeruginosa* (Figure 31-4) [1]. Evaluation of procalcitonin kinetics may be helpful in determining patients who may need further therapy [60].

PREVENTION

Detailed, evidence-based prevention measures are well summarized in the 2004 CDC (Healthcare Infection Control Prevention Advisory Committee [HICPAC]) and ATS/IDSA Guidelines, as well as several review articles and in Table 31-3 [1,2,61,62]. Unfortunately, prevention programs have often taken a back seat to diagnosis and treatment strategies. Prevention is cost effective, and use of a model team led by a champion is shown in Figure 31-5.

TABLE 31-3

SELECTED VAP PREVENTION STRATEGIES ABSTRACTED FROM RECENT GUIDELINES; MORE DETAILED DISCUSSION AND REFERENCES IN TEST

Intervention/Strategy	Support/Evidence	Comments
Infrastructure		
Multidisciplinary team	Programs developed by team consensus more effective	Input by critical care staff and respiratory therapists crucial
"Champion" of the cause	Recognized leader/expert increases "buy-in" by staff and hospital administration	Leadership needed to set benchmarks, maintain efforts, and secure resources
Targeted staff education	Staff education/awareness programs shown to reduce VAP	Such programs are adaptable to local needs and are cost effective
Infection control	Data support importance in reducing spread of multidrug organisms	Coordinate with quality improvement efforts; feedback data to staff
Antibiotic control	Reduces inappropriate antibiotic use and associated costs	Designated pharmacist optimal; computer programs good alternative
Adequate staffing	Critical for maintaining patient safety and adherence to protocols	Particularly important in critical care units; current nursing shortages exist
Benchmarking/quality	Current recommendations from ICHI and local multidisciplinary teams	Benchmarks should be evaluated routinely and data communicated
Patient care		
Sedation vacation	Supported by clinical data; accessible and feasible	Implement standard protocols
Semi-upright position	Supported by early data; recent data suggest lower elevation target indicated	Few outcome data; poor compliance with strategy; further studies needed
Noninvasive positive pressure ventilation	Supported by several clinical trials in recent review by Cochrane	Experience with technique is suggested for patients with COPD and CHF
Oral care	Evidence is limited, but risk and cost are low	Further studies are needed
Stress bleeding prophylaxis	Data support use of proton pump inhibitors (PPIs) and histamine, type 2 (H2) blockers; limit to high risk patients	PPIs and H2 are more effective than sucralfate in preventing bleeding
Deep vein thrombosis prophylaxis	Evidence supportive	Recommended in the VAP 100,000 Lives Campaign VAP "bundle"
Standardized protocols for weaning and enteral feedings	Rates of VAP lowered by reduced duration of intubation and enteral feeding	Protocols help standardize implementation and provide standards for monitoring
Chlorhexidine +/-colistin	Randomized controlled trials (RCTs) demonstrate efficacy	More data needed
Selective decontamination of the digestive tract	VAP and mortality decreased with intravenous + topical antibiotics	Concerns about antibiotic resistance limit "routine" use
Orotracheal intubation and use of orogastric tubes	Several small clinical trials report decreased sinusitis	Recommended; limited impact on VAP
Continuous aspiration of subglottal secretions	Decreased VAP shown in at least 4 RCT's	Optional; cost and impact on staffing are of concern
Heat moisture exchangers	Trend toward decreased VAP	Recommended; eliminates condensate but decreases humidity
No change of ventilator circuits	Several RCTs support this intervention	Recommended; positive cost and staffing impact
Early tracheostomy	Reports from 3 RCTs; methodological concerns	Optional; further data from rigorous studies needed
Closed endotracheal suctioning	3 RCTs showed no effect on VAP, but probably reduces environmental contamination	Optional, may reduce environmental spread of MDR pathogens
Discharge Issues		
Vaccination	Pneumococcal and influenza vaccination reduce hospitalizations	Recommended; poor routine vaccination rates of high-risk populations
Smoking cessation	Smoking cessation has been demonstrated to reduce morbidity and mortality	Recommended; instructions and referrals should be documented
Nutritional counseling	Obesity is a known risk factor for comorbidities associated with pneumonia	Recommended; instructions and referrals should be documented
Prevention of aspiration	Aspiration is a major risk factor for pneumonia	Check sedation, head of the bed; do speech and swallow studies if indicated

Adapted from Craven DE. Preventing ventilator-associated pneumonia: Sowing seeds of change. *Chest* 2006;130:251–260

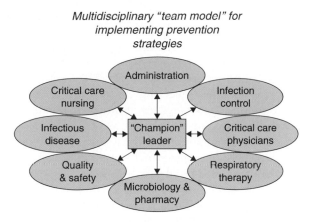

Multidisciplinary "team model" for implementing prevention strategies

Figure 31-5 Possible "model" multidisciplinary team to formulate goals for prevention of HAP and VAP. Adapted from Craven DE. Preventing ventilator-associated pneumonia: Sowing seeds of change. *Chest* 2006;130:251–260.

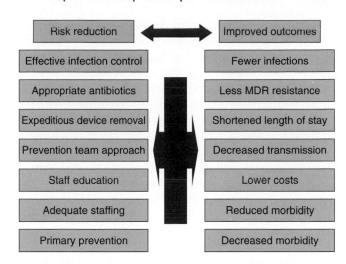

Figure 31-7 Summary of risk-reduction strategies and their potential impact patient outcomes.

Furthermore, some essential ingredients and evidence-based prevention strategies are shown in Table 31-3 and Figures 31-6 and 31-7.

General Prevention Strategies

Staff Education

Staff education is needed for all clinicians and staff who manage HAP and VAP. The ICU should be the cornerstone for initial efforts to reduce the incidence of VAP. Zack et al. initially reported a successful VAP educational prevention program carried out in five ICUs [63]. The program developed by a multidisciplinary team targeted respiratory care providers and ICU nurses who completed a self-study module on risk factors for VAP with evaluation

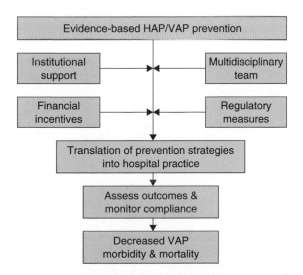

Figure 31-6 Evidence-based hospital-acquired pneumonia (HAP) and ventilator-associated pneumonia (VAP) prevention program aimed at preventing infection and improving patient outcomes. Adapted from Craven DE. Preventing ventilator-associated pneumonia: Sowing seeds of change. *Chest* 2006;130:251–260.

both at baseline and after the program interventions. In-service teaching programs were coordinated with ICU staff meetings, and fact sheets and posters were placed in the ICU and Respiratory Care departments. Rates of VAP dropped nearly 58% to 5.7/1,000 ventilator days, and cost savings were estimated to be between $425,606 to >$4,000,000. Using an extension of this program in an Integrated Health Care System involving four hospitals, Babcock et al. reported a 46% reduction in VAP over an 18-month period [64].

Staffing Levels

Perhaps one of the most important and underappreciated prevention strategies is adequate staffing, particularly in ICUs [2,65]. Staffing must be sufficient to allow patient care to be provided while ensuring that staff are able to comply with essential infection control practices and other prevention strategies [64,66].

In a study of abdominal aortic surgery patients by Dang et al., decreased nursing staff was associated with significantly higher rates of respiratory and cardiac complications than in patients who had higher intensity nursing care [67]. Currently, this is of critical importance due to severe nursing shortages and staffing reductions because of budget constraints. Nurse-to-patient ratios should be 1:1 for high-risk, complicated ICU patients or 2:1 for patients with lower disease acuity. Currently, efforts to establish legislation that would cap the number of patients per nurse are underway in some states.

Infection Control

Effective targeted surveillance for high-risk patients coupled with staff education, the use of proper isolation techniques, and effective infection control practices are cornerstones for prevention of HAP [2,4,66]. Previous studies have indicated that hospitals with effective surveillance and infection control programs have rates of pneumonia 20% lower than hospitals without such programs (see Chapters 3, 5).

Infection control programs have repeatedly demonstrated efficacy in reducing infection and colonization due to MDR-organisms [2,28,65,68–70]. Unfortunately, staff compliance with proven infection control measures, such as hand hygiene, remains inconsistent in many hospitals. Thus, staff education on infection control must be inclusive, frequent, and reiterative. Special attention should be directed toward house staff, students, volunteers, and visitors, and compliance should be monitored periodically.

Surveillance of ICU infections to identify and quantify endemic and new MDR-organisms with timely feedback of data is critical [7,59,68,71,72]. Timely communication of current data among clinicians, laboratory, pharmacy, and infection control staff is essential. Organism-specific strategies for specific MDR-pathogens may be appropriate. For MRSA, VISA (or GISA) isolates, active surveillance cultures and isolation are recommended along with more aggressive eradication methods [38,40,73].

Cross-colonization and cross-infection are important mechanisms in the pathogenesis of HAI [2,4,68] (Figure 31-1). Gram-negative bacilli and *S. aureus* often are present in high concentrations as indigenous flora in critically ill patients, the hospital environment, and on the hands or gloves of hospital personnel [4,74]. Hand washing before and after patient contact is an effective means of removing transient bacteria, but because of the inadequacy of hand-washing practices among hospital personnel, some investigators have advocated the use of barrier precautions (gloves and gowns) for contact with all patients. This practice has been associated with significantly decreased HAI rates in pediatric ICUs [1]. If gloves are used, care must be taken to change them between patients.

Nasal carriage of *S. aureus* is common among healthcare workers (HCWs), and outbreaks are often associated with HCWs with dermatitis or nasal or rectal colonization [2]. Bassetti et al. emphasize the importance of viral respiratory tract infections in the transfer of airborne MRSA from a physician to patients in an ICU [75]. Molecular typing was performed to confirm the source of the outbreak, and experimental induction of rhinovirus infection and its role in airborne dispersion of bacteria was demonstrated (the "cloud adult"). Without the use of surgical masks, the dispersal of *S. aureus* increased transmission 40-fold. These data underscore the importance of upper respiratory tract infection in the dissemination of *S. aureus* and the importance of masks in preventing transmission.

Antibiotic Stewardship Strategies

Antibiotic stewardship programs play an extremely important role in the overall effort to control healthcare-associated infections, reduce emergence of MDR-organisms, and control spiraling healthcare costs. For example, reduced use of fluoroquinolones has been associated with reduced rates of MRSA infection [47]. Antibiotic stewardship is complex and should be focused, dynamic, and carefully monitored and may vary by type of MDR-pathogen. For example, control of specific types of MDR Gram-negative bacilli may require "squeezing the balloon at multiple sites" to prevent the emergence of other MDR-pathogens, as nicely summarized by Rahal et al [22,76]. Adding an infectious disease pharmacist to the ICU team or a computerized decision support program to optimize drug regimens should be considered [1,2].

Data from antibiotic cycling or rotation programs are difficult to evaluate, but this approach has been advocated by some for reducing MDR-pathogens [1,76–79]. In theory, a class of antibiotics or a specific antibiotic is withdrawn from use for a defined time period and re-introduced at a later point in time in an attempt to limit bacterial resistance to the cycled antimicrobial agents.

When outbreaks of infection with a specific strain of resistant bacteria have occurred, restricted access to specific antibiotics has successfully managed the problem with generally no impact on the overall frequency of resistance. However, if disproportionate use of another antibiotic results, resistance rates may be affected. Rahal et al. restricted use of third-generation cephalosporins to combat an outbreak of ESBL (+) *Klebsiella* infections [76]. Restriction of cephalosporins was accompanied by a 44% reduction in infection and colonization with the ESBL (+) *Klebsiella*. However, the use of imipenem increased by 140% during the intervention year and was associated with a 69% increase in the incidence of imipenem-resistant *P. aeruginosa* throughout the medical center. The clinical impact of shifting resistance from one pathogen to another was not assessed.

Gerding et al. evaluated cycling of aminoglycosides over 10 years at the Minneapolis Veterans Affairs Medical Center, cycling amikacin and gentamicin. Using cycle times of 12 to 51 months, these investigators found significantly reduced resistance to gentamicin when amikacin was used [80]. Gentamicin resistance recurred with the rapid re-introduction of gentamicin while subsequent more gradual re-introduction of gentamicin occurred without increased levels of resistance. This experience suggests that cycling antibiotics within the same drug class in some circumstances could be an effective strategy for curbing antimicrobial resistance.

Gruson et al. observed a reduction in the incidence of VAP after introducing an antimicrobial program that consisted of supervised rotation and restricted use of ceftazidime and ciprofloxacin [81]. The antibiotic selection was based on monthly reviews of the pathogens isolated from the ICU and their antibiotic susceptibility patterns. The decreased incidence of VAP was primarily due to a reduction in the number of episodes attributed to antibiotic-resistant jGram-negative bacteria including *P. aeruginosa*, *B. cepacia*, *S. maltophilia*, and *A. baumanii*, which was sustained over a 5-year time period [82].

Environmental Issues

MDR bacteria are commonly found in the environment (Figure 31-1) [38,66]. Although it is widely appreciated that the environment is swarming with microorganisms, this does not necessarily directly result in infection; therefore, widespread routine environmental sampling is not recommended. For example, despite studies showing that Legionella spp. can be recovered from 12–70% of hospital water systems, this source of nosocomial outbreaks remains underappreciated [49].

Studies are beginning to implicate the inanimate environment as an indirect contributor to pathogen acquisition [66]. Special interventions, including targeted environmental sampling and more aggressive environmental disinfection, may be indicated during outbreaks, particularly those involving MDR-organisms or organisms that are more resistant to routine cleaning [74].

MODIFIABLE RISK FACTORS

Risk factors for the development of HAP can be differentiated into modifiable and nonmodifiable conditions. Some modifiable strategies that are feasible, effective, and cost effective have been recommended and are discussed here.

Aspiration, the primary route of bacterial entry into the lung, is commonly increased during hospitalization, with sedation, neuromuscular blockers, head trauma, intubation, enteral feeding, and following surgery [2,83–87]. Supine patient positioning may facilitate aspiration, which can be decreased by maintaining a semirecumbent patient position. With the use of radioactive-labeled enteral feeding, cumulative numbers of endotracheal radioactivity counts were higher when patients were placed in a completely supine position (0°) as compared to a semirecumbent position (45°) [88,89]. One randomized trial demonstrated a threefold reduction in the incidence of ICU-acquired VAP in patients kept in a semirecumbent position vs. supine [90]. VAP rates reached 50% in patients maintained in the supine position while receiving enteral nutrition. These data support maintaining patients in semirecumbent positions, particularly during enteral feeding. In contrast to rotational beds, semirecumbent patient position is a low-cost, easily accessible intervention and may be a more practical and more tolerable approach than rotational beds or prone body position [91,92].

Maintaining mechanically ventilated and/or enterally fed patients in a 30° to 45° semirecumbent position, particularly during enteral feeding, continues to be strongly recommended [1,2,90]. However, recent studies have not only questioned the results of previous studies but also suggested that maintaining semiupright patient position may not be practical, at least at the levels currently recommended. A study by van Nieuwenhoven et al. in which mechanically ventilated patients were randomly assigned to backrest elevation of 45° vs. the standard of 10°

demonstrated barriers to implementing this strategy [93]. Backrest elevation was measured continuously during the first week of ventilation with a monitoring device. The targeted backrest elevation of 45° was not reached; the actual achieved difference was 28° vs. 10°, which did not reduce VAP. Similarly, Grap et al. monitored patient position in ICU patients using a bed frame elevation gauge or electronic bed readout and found very low compliance with maintaining semirecumbent patient position with a mean backrest elevation of only 19.2° with 70% of subjects maintained in a supine position [94,95]. Perhaps further studies measuring the impact of maintaining ventilated and/or enterally fed patients in a semirecumbent position may needed to evaluate more attainable targets. Until this issue is resolved, prevention guidelines recommend elevating the head of the bed for ventilated and/or enterally fed patients.

Enteral Feeding Issues

Enteral nutrition has been considered a risk factor for the development of HAP, mainly secondary to the increased risk of aspiration of gastric contents [2,96]. Parenteral nutrition is associated with a higher risk of intravascular-device associated infection, complications from central venous catheter insertion, higher costs, and loss of intestinal villous architecture, which may facilitate enteral microbial translocation. Some have advised feeding critically ill patients enterally as early as possible, but early (day 1 of intubation and ventilation) enteral feeding was associated with a higher risk of VAP when compared to later enteral feeding (day 5 of intubation) [97].

Seven studies have evaluated the risks for ICU-acquired HAP in patients randomized to either gastric or postpyloric feeding [98]. Although significant differences were not demonstrated in any individual study, a meta-analysis demonstrated that postpyloric feeding was associated with a significant reduction in ICU acquired HAP (relative risk = 0.76, 95% confidence interval 0.59 to 0.99) [99].

Accurate assessment of the patient's nutritional status and the use of enteral feeding, rather than parenteral nutrition, appear to reduce the risk of HAP [2,98]. Early initiation of enteral feeding may help maintain the gastrointestinal epithelium and prevent bacterial translocation, but it is not without risk. Because enteral feedings can be contaminated during preparation, we recommend the routine use of aseptic technique and sterile water for their preparation and for nasogastric tube flushes because we are concerned that tap water may be a source of legionellae and other nosocomial Gram-negative bacilli (see section on *Legionella pneumophila*) [2,49].

Enteral feeding protocols have been suggested to reduce complications [65,100]. Bowman et al. instituted an evidence-based, enteral feeding protocol in which 78–85% of patients reached their enteral feeding goal. Aspiration pneumonia rates decreased from 6.8 to 3.2/1,000 patient-days [100]. Such protocols should be reviewed by multidisciplinary committees to standardize enteral nutrition protocols and risk reduction for VAP.

Early gastrostomy for enteral feedings has been suggested as a strategy to reduce VAP in patients with head injury and stroke [101]. In a small, randomized clinical trial of 20 patients with gastrostomy vs. 21 controls, rates of VAP were reduced (10% vs. 38%, respectively) and most of the VAP episodes were late onset VAP (>5 days). Additional studies with higher enrollment are needed to further assess this strategy in these high-risk patients.

MODULATION OF BACTERIAL COLONIZATON

Oral Care

Oral care has been studied and recommended to prevent VAP [102–105]. In a recent study, Mori et al. compared rates of VAP in a nonrandomized group compared to historic controls [106]. The incidence of VAP in the oral care group was 3.9 episodes/1,000 days vs. 10.4 in the control group. Although there are concerns about the study design, oral care has intuitive benefits and limited cost, but more randomized controlled studies are needed.

Antibiotic Prophylaxis with Selective Decontamination of the Digestive Tract (SDD)

Modulation of oropharyngeal colonization by combinations of oral antibiotics, with or without systemic therapy (selective decontamination of the digestive tract) also is effective in significantly reducing the frequency of HAP, although the methodologic study quality, specific regimens used, study populations, and clinical impact differ widely among studies [1,2,14,102,107,108].

In two recently published prospective randomized trials, SDD was associated with a higher ICU survival among patients [109,110]. In the first study, a subpgroup of patients with a mid-range acute physiology and chronic health evaluation (APACHE) II score on admission had a lower ICU mortality, although ICU mortality rates of all included patients did not differ significantly [109]. In the largest study performed so far, SDD administered to 466 patients in one unit was associated with relative risk for ICU mortality of 0.65 and of hospital mortality of 0.78 when compared to 472 patients admitted in a control ward [110]. In addition, infections due to antibiotic-resistant microorganisms occurred more frequently in the control ward. Importantly, levels of antibiotic-resistant pathogens were low in both wards with complete absence of MRSA. Moreover, a small pre-existing difference in outcome between two wards and the absence of a crossover design warrant confirmation of these beneficial effects of SDD.

In two meta-analyses and one additional study, decreased mortality was demonstrated in critically ill surgical patients receiving SDD, including both systemic and local

prophylactic antibiotics [107,109,111], raising questions about the relative importance of systemic rather than nonabsorbed antibiotics.

The preventive effects of SDD for HAP and VAP also have been considerably lower in ICUs with high endemic levels of MDR-pathogens [2]. Although SDD reduces HAP, routine prophylactic use of antibiotics should be undertaken cautiously, especially in hospital settings where there are high levels of antibiotic resistance [112,113].

Moreover, antibiotics clearly predispose patients to subsequent colonization and infection with antibiotic-resistant pathogens [30,114]. In contrast, prior antibiotic exposure conferred protection (risk ratio 0.37, 95% CI 0.27–0.51) for ICU-acquired HAP in another study [6]. Preventive effects of intravenous antibiotics were evaluated in only one randomized trial: administration of cefuroxime for 24 hours at the time of intubation, which reduced the incidence of early onset HAP in patients with closed head injury [115]. The role of the gastrointestinal tract in the pathogenesis of VAP and the clinical evidence for the efficacy of SDD were recently reviewed by Kallet and Quinn [116] and in a Cochrane review by Liberati et al. [107]. In the latter study, the authors conclude that for topical and systemic antibiotic prophylaxis, 5 patients would need to be treated to prevent one infection, and 21 patients would need to be treated to prevent one death. No recommendation was made for topical prophylaxis. In a recent large study of SDD by de Jonge et al in 2003, SDD was highly effective in preventing pneumonia without an increase in antibiotic resistance [110]. However, citing concerns over rapid increases in antimicrobial resistance in the hospital setting coupled with the association between MDR-pathogens and poorer patient outcomes, recent guidelines have suggested that SDD should be considered for selected ICU populations and in targeted clinical scenarios but not employed "routinely" for VAP prevention [1,2,112].

Antiseptics

Oropharyngeal colonization is the primary source of pathogens causing HAP and VAP, and thus reducing levels of colonization or eliminating potential pathogens is an obvious risk reduction strategy. In a randomized trial, DeRiso et al. demonstrated that the use of the oral antiseptic chlorhexidine (CHX) significantly reduced rates of HAI in patients undergoing coronary artery bypass graft surgery [117]. Although topical antiseptics, such as CHX, provide an attractive alternative to antibiotics, the initial reported success in cardiac surgery patients could not be confirmed by other studies. A recent study by Koeman et al. provides important data from a multicenter, double-blind, randomized, clinical trial of VAP outcomes for subjects treated with 2% CHX paste vs. patients randomized to 2% CHX + 2% colistin (COL) paste to provide more activity against Gram-negative bacilli compared to placebo [118]. Compared to the placebo group, the daily risk of VAP was reduced by 65% in the CHX group ($p = 0.01$) and 55% in the CHX-COL group ($p < 0.03$). This impressive result for an inexpensive, nontoxic, topically applied modality warrants further attention but is difficult to reconcile with the absence of effect on ventilator-days, length of stay, or mortality. It is important to measure how prophylactic use of CHX and CHX-COL complement other effective prevention strategies, and resistance could become an important issue over time.

Colonization Blockers—Protegrins

Iseganan, a topical antimicrobial peptide active against aerobic and anaerobic Gram-positive and Gram-negative bacteria and yeasts, was evaluated in a randomized, double-blind trial to prevent VAP [119]. Although there was a significant reduction in colonization in the treatment group, the rates of VAP among survivors (16% vs. 20%) and 14-day mortality were similar (22% vs. 18%). Although protegrins are ubiquitous antimicrobial peptides and in human trials were able to reduce oral colonization by two logs, these results raise several questions about iseganan efficacy and why it failed.

Probiotics—Lactobacillus GG (LGG)

Interesting data from a double-blind pilot study of subjects randomized to oral and gastric LGG (2×10^9 colony forming units twice daily) ($n = 19$) versus placebo ($n = 21$) were presented by Morrow et al. at the 2005 American Thoracic Society Annual Meeting Symposium [120]. Demographics and APACHE II scores were similar in the two groups, but the LGG group had significantly higher rates of colonization with normal flora ($p < 0.03$), fewer oral pathogens, less clinical VAP (26% vs. 45%, $p = 0.20$), lower microscopic VAP (11% vs. 33%, $p = 0.08$), and a lower mortality rate (0% vs. 10%, $p = 0.17$). Further studies are in progress.

MECHANICAL VENTILATION AND ASSOCIATED DEVICES

Several devices have been identified as risk factors for HAP. Many of these devices are used in mechanically ventilated patients and increase the risk of VAP; intervention strategies are summarized in several review articles and in Table 31-3 [1,2,121].

Noninvasive Positive Pressure Ventilation (NPPV)

NPPV provides ventilatory support without the need for intubation and for earlier removal of the endotracheal tube to reduce complications related to prolonged intubation. NPPV using a face mask is an attractive alternative for patients with acute exacerbations with chronic obstructive pulmonary disease (COPD), acute hypoxemic respiratory failure, for some immunosuppressed patients with pulmonary infiltrates and respiratory failure [1,2]. In a recent Cochrane review, Burns et al reported significant benefits: decreased mortality (RR 0.41, 95% CI 0.22–0.76), lower rates of VAP (RR 0.28, 95% CI 0.90 to 0.85), decreased length of ICU and shorter hospital stays, and lower duration of mechanical support [122]. The impact of NPPV is greater in patients with COPD exacerbations or congestive heart failure than for patients with VAP. Recent data also indicate that NPPV may not be a good strategy to avoid re intubation after initial extubation and is recommended for hospitals with staff who are experienced in this technique [123].

Ventilator Management: Sedation and Weaning

Attention to the specific type of endotracheal tube, its maintenance, and the site of insertion also may be valuable. The use of oral endotracheal and orogastric tubes rather than nasotracheal or nasogastric tubes can reduce the frequency of nosocomial sinusitis and possibly HAP, although causality between sinusitis and HAP has not been firmly established [124]. Efforts to reduce the likelihood of aspiration of oropharyngeal bacteria around the endotracheal tube cuff into the lower respiratory tract include limiting the use of sedative and paralytic agents that depress cough and other host protective mechanisms and maintaining endotracheal cuff pressure at >20 cm H_2O [125]. Re-intubation should be avoided, if possible, because it increases the risk of VAP [126]. Efforts to reduce acute lung injury by using smaller tidal volumes and lower pressures have been suggested [127].

Other strategies to reduce the duration of mechanical ventilation include improved methods of sedation and the use of protocols to facilitate and accelerate weaning [2,128–130]. These interventions clearly depend on adequate ICU staffing [131,132]. Dries et al., using a standardized weaning protocol, reduced the proportion of days of mechanical ventilation (total ICU days) from 0.47% to 0.33%, number of patients failing extubation (25 vs. 43), and rates of VAP (15% to 5%) [133]. Schweickert et al. evaluated seven complications in 128 patients receiving mechanical ventilation and continuous infusions of sedative drug who were randomized to daily interruption of sedative infusions ($N = 66$) vs. sedation directed by the MICU team without this strategy ($N = 60$) [49,128]. Daily interrupted sedative infusions reduced ICU length of stay (6.2 days vs. 9.9, $p < 0.01$), duration of mechanical ventilation (4.8 vs. 7.3 days, $p < 0.003$) and the incidence of complications per patient (13/12 patients vs. 26/19 patients, $p < 0.04$).

Subglottic Secretion Drainage

Continuous aspiration of subglottic secretions (CASS) through the use of especially designed endotracheal tubes with a wider, elliptic hole helps facilitate drainage (Figure 31-3) and has significantly reduced the incidence of early onset VAP in several studies[1,2], In a recent metaanalysis, CASS reduced the incidence of VAP by half (risk ratio 0.51, 95% CI 1.7 to 2.3), shortened ICU stay by 3 days (95% CI 2.1 to 3.9), and delayed the onset of VAP by 6 days. CASS also was cost effective saving $4,992/episode of VAP prevented or $1,872/patient, but mortality was not affected [134]. However, when CASS was combined with semirecumbent positioning, no clinical benefit was observed, underscoring the importance of interactive prevention strategies [135].

Ventilator Circuits, Condensate and Heat Moisture Exchangers

VAP also may be related to colonization of the ventilator circuit tubing (Figure 31-8) [136]. Frequency of circuit changes do not prevent VAP, an area for substantial cost savings [120,137]. Condensate collecting in the ventilator circuit can become contaminated from patient secretions or by opening the circuit; vigilance is needed to prevent inadvertently flushing the condensate into the lower airway or in-line nebulizers at the bedside and during patient transport [136,138]. Furthermore, metered dose inhalers (MDI) may be safer for the delivery of bronchodilators than nebulizers, which, if contaminated, may produce bacterial aerosols [17]. In addition, high-level disinfection of tubing temperature sensors is recommended to prevent cross-contamination between patients [2].

There have been conflicting reports on the use and benefits of heat moisture exchangers (HME) compared to heated humidifiers for preventing VAP [2,137]. Heat moisture exchangers reduce the risk of contaminated condensate entering the lower airway but may not provide sufficient humidity or may become occluded by secretions in some patients. A recent meta-analysis by Kola et al. demonstrated a reduction in the relative risk of developing VAP in the HME group (relative risk 0.7) but may have been affected by the large difference in outcomes in one of the studies [139]. For patients with a mean ventilation of >7 days, the relative risk for VAP fell to 0.57 in the HME group (95% CI = 0.38–0.83). A more recent, large, randomized study by Lacherade et al. found no benefit for the HME group. In another study of HMEs using historic controls, patients who were ventilated >2 days reported a significant reduction in VAP ($p = 0.01$) [140].

Bronchoscopy

Mechanically ventilated patients may undergo bronchoscopy for diagnostic purposes or for removal of mucus plugs or excessive secretions. In one study, bronchoscopy was identified as a risk factor for HAP [2]. This could be related to several factors, including the use of large volumes of BAL that impede the host's removal of bacteria in the lower airway and the introduction of HAI pathogens into the lower airway by releasing bacteria encased in biofilm on the endotracheal tube. As discussed previously, when bacteria encased in biofilm embolize to different areas of the lung, they may be particularly difficult for host defenses to clear effectively. Although these pathogenic mechanisms are hypothetical, they are of concern.

Miscellaneous Strategies

Intensive Insulin Therapy

Hyperglycemia, relative insulin deficiency, or both may directly or indirectly increase the risk of complications and

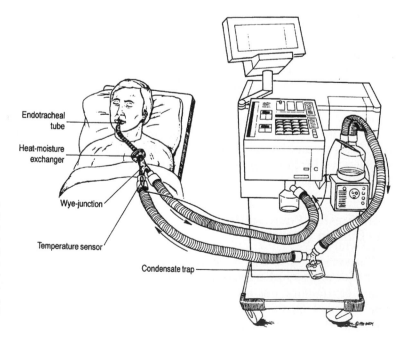

Figure 31-8 Mechanically ventilated patient in the upright position. Humidified air is carried through the inspiratory tubing to the patient's lower respiratory tract. Contaminated condensate may form in the ventilator circuit and should not be allowed to relux into the patient's endotracheal tube. Use of a heat–moisture exchanger (HME) eliminates humidifier and circuit condensate. Adapted from Craven DE, Steger KA. Hospital-acquired pneumonia: perspective for the epidemiologist. *Infect Control Hosp Epidemiol* 1997;18:783–795, with permission.

Labels in figure:
Endotracheal tube
Heat-moisture exchanger
Wye-junction
Temperature sensor
Condensate trap

poor outcomes in critically ill patients. Van den Berghe et al. randomized surgical ICU patients to receive either intensive insulin therapy to maintain blood glucose levels between 80 and 110 mg per deciliter or to receive conventional treatment [141]. The group receiving intensive insulin therapy had reduced mortality (4.6% vs. 8%, $p < 0.04$), and the difference was greater in patients who remained in the ICU >5 days (10.6% vs. 20.2%, $p = 0.005$). When compared to the control group, those treated with intensive insulin therapy had a 46% reduction of bloodstream infections, 41% decreased frequency of acute renal failure requiring dialysis, fewer antibiotic treatment days, and significantly shorter length of mechanical ventilation and ICU stay. While the same degree of benefit may not be seen in VAP as in other populations, aggressive treatment of hyperglycemia has both theoretical and clinical support for SICU patients.

For each prevention strategy, it is critical to assess the risk-benefit ratio. Using a retrospective outcome study, Egi et al. reported that hypoglycemia in surgical ICU patients receiving intensive insulin therapy varied from 1.4–2.7% and estimated that the number of patients needed to be treated to save one life varied from 38 to 113, whereas the rate of hypoglycemia (number needed to harm) varied from 7 to 13 patients [142].

A recent study of intensive insulin therapy in 1,200 medical ICU patients did not significantly reduce overall hospital mortality and actually increased mortality in patients with ICU stays <3 days [143]. However, the intensive insulin therapy group had reduced acquired renal failure, duration of mechanical ventilation, and length of ICU and hospital stay. Unfortunately, predicting length of stay is difficult; coupled with concerns about the risks of hypoglycemia and with increased resource implications, the benefit of intensive insulin therapy for specific hospital or MICU patients will require further evaluation.

Stress Bleeding Prophylaxis

Histamine type 2 (H_2)-antagonists and antacids have been identified as independent risk factors for ICU-acquired HAP. Sucralfate has been used for stress bleeding prophylaxis because it does not increase intragastric acidity or gastric volume but is less effective in preventing gastrointestinal bleeding [1,2]. Numerous randomized trials using different doses and various study populations have provided controversial results on the benefits of specific stress bleeding prophylaxis agents in relation to the increased risk of VAP and bleeding [20,144]. One large randomized trial comparing antacids, H2 blockers, and sucralfate reported no differences in rates of early onset VAP, but rates of late onset VAP were lower in patients treated with sucralfate [20]. More recently, Bornstain et al. examined risk factors for early onset VAP (from 3–7 days) in 747 patients [145]. Several different variables were identified in the univariate analysis, but only sucralfate used in the first 48 hours of ICU stay and unplanned extubation were predictors of VAP in the multivariate analysis, and

antibiotics were protective. In an earlier multicenter study of VAP in patients with ARDS, sucralfate and duration of exposure to sucralfate were associated with an increased risk of VAP [146].

A recent, large, double-blind, randomized trial comparing ranitidine to sucralfate demonstrated a trend toward lower rates of VAP with sucralfate, but clinically significant gastrointestinal bleeding was 4% higher in the sucralfate group [144]. Data indicate that H2 blockers and protein pump inhibitors are associated with lower rates of gastrointestinal bleeding when compared to sucralfate, which may be doubly important because transfusion also is a possible risk factor for VAP.

Transfusion Risk

A landmark prospective randomized trial comparing liberal and conservative "triggers" to transfusion in ICU patients not exhibiting active bleeding and without underlying cardiac disease demonstrated that awaiting a hemoglobin level of 7.0 g per deciliter as opposed to a level of 9.0 g per deciliter for initiating transfusion resulted in fewer transfusions and no adverse effects on outcome [147]. In fact, in those patients less severely ill, as judged by low APACHE II scores, mortality was improved in the "restricted transfusion" group, a result thought to be related to immunosuppressive effects of non-leukocyte depleted red blood cell units with a consequent increased risk of infection. Multiple studies have identified exposure to allogeneic blood products as a risk factor for postoperative infection and postoperative pneumonia, and the length of time of blood storage was another factor modulating risk [1]. In one prospective randomized control trial, the use of leukocyte-depleted red blood cell transfusions resulted in a lower incidence of postoperative infections and specifically a reduced incidence of pneumonia in patients undergoing colorectal surgery [148]. Routine red blood cell transfusion should therefore be conducted with a restricted transfusion trigger policy. Whether leukocyte-depleted red blood cell transfusions will further reduce the incidence of pneumonia in broad populations of patients at risk remains to be determined.

Supporting data were reported in a secondary analysis from a recent, large study of transfusions in which transfusion was identified as an independent risk factor for VAP [149]. These data suggest that transfusion may be a more important modifiable risk factor than previously appreciated. Furthermore, a recent study by Levy et al. reported that mechanically ventilated patients received transfusions at a higher pretransfusion hemoglobin level than nonventilated patients (8.7 vs. 8.2, $p < .0001$) [150].

Secondary Prevention Strategies at Discharge

The focus of prevention has been on ICU patients while in the ICU, but these patients are also at increased risk for relapse or re-infection during their rehabilitation. Therefore, efforts should be directed at risk reduction at discharge, such as routine vaccinations and patient education aimed at health promotion, such as smoking cessation, exercise, and weight control (Table 31-3).

Translating Prevention Guidelines into Practice Barriers

Prevention efforts for HAP should be evidence based and cost effective (Table 31-3) [1,2,61,151]. It may be more prudent to focus initially on a limited number of feasible, cost-effective strategies as suggested by the Institute for Healthcare Improvement (IHI) 100,000 Lives Campaign. IHI has challenged hospitals to adopt a series of measures to reduce HAIs [151]. The VAP or "ventilator bundle" initiative includes five components: elevation of the head of the bed to between 30° and 45°, daily "sedation vacation," daily assessment for readiness to extubate, and prophylaxis for peptic ulcer disease and deep vein thrombosis and oral care. Some of the participating hospitals using this approach have reported no episodes of VAP over sustained periods of time [Donald Berwick, IHI National Forum, December 13, 2005]. Peer-reviewed publications of these dramatic results are needed. However, IHI's principles and approach have been major forces for stimulating interest and drawing national attention to HAIs and the need to place more emphasis on prevention.

Multidisciplinary Team Approach

Prevention efforts targeting VAP must be part of an evidence-based, multidisciplinary prevention program that has a "core" team with an agenda focused on patient safety and quality improvement (Figures 31-5 and 31-6) [61]. Optimally, the team should be led by a "champion" of the cause and include interested clinicians, respiratory care staff, administrators, risk management staff, and other stakeholders as "core" team members (Figure 31-5). This group's responsibilities include setting prevention benchmarks, establishing goals and timelines, providing appropriate education and training, and performing audits with feedback to the staff, all while continually updating themselves on the relevant clinical and prevention strategies (Figures 31-6 and 31-7). Prevention programs should be "marketed" to hospital administrators and others involved in resource allocation by demonstrating that preventing VAP results in improved clinical outcomes and significantly reduced costs.

SUMMARY

Despite rapid technologic and treatment advances in medicine, dramatic reductions in rates of VAP, and effective use of complex prevention and management guidelines remain elusive [1,2]. Prevention outcomes are directly related to reducing risk in the areas suggested in Figure 31-7 and Table 31-4. Investing in prevention can pay great dividends in improved quality of life and reduced morbidity and mortality [61]. In addition, prevention can

have a huge impact in reducing length of hospital stay and healthcare costs during acute care. Spreading the seeds of prevention into chronic care and rehabilitation facilities also is vitally needed in our increasing diversity of healthcare settings.

As described in a recent commentary by Berwick et al, the laudable goal set forth by the IHI to reduce deaths among hospitalized patients in the United States by 100,000 over 18 months through improving patient quality and safety set a very high bar [151]. Each of the six 100,000 Lives Campaign interventions that include VAP prevention is conceptually simple and feasible. Notably, each strategy included in the "VAP bundle" is not new or expensive.

The IHI's 100,000 Lives Campaign may be the call to action that is needed to disseminate prevention and safety information and to implement prevention guidelines consistently and broadly [151]. Preliminary data suggest that the campaign exceeded its goal by saving 122,000 lives and enrolled more than half of the nation's hospitals in this effort. This campaign provides a valuable infrastructure for sowing and disseminating seeds that will grow into trees and for measuring outcomes. This infrastructure coupled with endorsements of government agencies, such as **Joint Commission on Accreditation of Healthcare Organizations (JCAHO)** and Medicare, as well as medical, nursing, and public health groups translates into powerful lobby for the advancement of patient safety and quality care, and for obtaining the necessary resources to incorporate prevention into practice [152].

REFERENCES

1. Weber DJ, Rutala WA, Sickbert-Bennett EE, et al. Microbiology of ventilator-associated pneumonia compared with that of hospital-acquired pneumonia. *Infect Cont Hosp Epid* 2007;28: In Press (July 2007).
2. Tablan OC, Anderson LJ, Besser R, et al. Guidelines for preventing health care–associated pneumonia, 2003: recommendations of CDC and the Healthcare Infection Control Practices Advisory Committee. *MMWR Recomm Rep* 2004;53(RR-3):1–36.
3. Chastre J, Fagon JY. Ventilator-associated pneumonia. *Am J Respir Crit Care Med* 2002;165(7):867–903.
4. Safdar N, Crnich CJ, Maki DG. The pathogenesis of ventilator-associated pneumonia: its relevance to developing effective strategies for prevention. *Respir Care* 2005;50(6):725–739.
5. National Nosocomial Infections Surveillance (NNIS) System Report, data summary from January 1992 through June 2004, issued October 2004. *Am J Infect Control* 2004;32(8):470–485.
6. Cook DJ, Walter SD, Cook RJ, et al. Incidence of and risk factors for ventilator-associated pneumonia in critically ill patients. *Ann Intern Med* 1998; 129(6):433–440.
7. Eggimann P, Hugonnet S, Sax H, et al. Ventilator-associated pneumonia: caveats for benchmarking. *Intensive Care Med* 2003;29(11):2086–2089.
8. Craven DE, Kunches LM, Kilinsky V, et al. Risk factors for pneumonia and fatality in patients receiving continuous mechanical ventilation. *Am Rev Respir Dis* 1986;133(5):792–796.
9. Rello J, Ollendorf DA, Oster G, et al. Epidemiology and outcomes of ventilator-associated pneumonia in a large US database. *Chest* 2002;122(6):2115–2121.
10. Fagon JY, Chastre J, Domart Y, et al. Mortality due to ventilator-associated pneumonia or colonization with Pseudomonas or Acinetobacter species: assessment by quantitative culture of

samples obtained by a protected specimen brush. *Clin Infect Dis* 1996;23(3):538–542.

11. Heyland DK, Cook DJ, Griffith L, et al. The attributable morbidity and mortality of ventilator-associated pneumonia in the critically ill patient: the Canadian Critical Trials Group, Part 1. *Am J Respir Crit Care Med* 1999;159(4):1249–1256.

12. Warren DK, Shukla SJ, Olsen MA, et al. Outcome and attributable cost of ventilator-associated pneumonia among intensive care unit patients in a suburban medical center. *Crit Care Med* 2003;31(5):1312–1317.

13. Johanson WG, Pierce AK, Sanford JP. Changing pharyngeal bacterial flora of hospitalized patients: emergence of gram-negative bacilli. *N Engl J Med* 1969;281(21):1137–1140.

14. Bergmans DC, Bonten MJ, Gaillard CA, et al. Prevention of ventilator-associated pneumonia by oral decontamination: a prospective, randomized, double-blind, placebo-controlled study. *Am J Respir Crit Care Med* 2001; 164(3):382–388.

15. Niederman MS, Craven DE. Devising strategies for preventing nosocomial pneumonia—should we ignore the stomach? *Clin Infect Dis* 1997;24(3):320–323.

16. Craven DE, Steger KA. Nosocomial pneumonia in mechanically ventilated adult patients: epidemiology and prevention in 1996. *Semin Respir Infect* 1996;11(1):32–53.

17. Craven DE, Lichtenberg DA, Goularte TA, et al. Contaminated medication nebulizers in mechanical ventilator circuits: source of bacterial aerosols. *Am J Med* 1984;77(5):834–838.

18. Inglis TJ, Lim EW, Lee GS, et al. Endogenous source of bacteria in tracheal tube and proximal ventilator breathing system in intensive care patients. *Br J Anaesth* 1998;80(1):41–45.

19. Niederman MS. Gram-negative colonization of the respiratory tract: pathogenesis and clinical consequences. *Semin Hospir Infect* 1990;5(3):173–184.

20. Prod'hom G, Leuenberger P, Koerfer J, et al. Nosocomial pneumonia in mechanically ventilated patients receiving antacid, ranitidine, or sucralfate as prophylaxis for stress ulcer: a randomized controlled trial. *Ann Intern Med* 1994;120(8):653–662.

21. Bonten MJ, Gaillard CA. Ventilator-associated pneumonia: do the bacteria come from the stomach? *Neth J Med* 1995;46(1).1–3.

22. Li HY, He LX, Hu BJ, et al. [The impact of gastric colonization on the pathogenesis of ventilator-associated pneumonia]. *Zhonghua Nei Ke Za Zhi* 2004;43(2):112–116.

23. Millo JL, Schultz MJ, Williams C, et al. Compartmentalisation of cytokines and cytokine inhibitors in ventilator-associated pneumonia. *Intensive Care Med* 2004;30(1):68–74.

24. Determann RM, Millo JL, Gibot S, et al. Serial changes in soluble triggering receptor expressed on myeloid cells in the lung during development of ventilator-associated pneumonia. *Intensive Care Med* 2005;31(11):1495–1500.

25. Gibot S, Cravoisy A, Levy B, et al. Soluble triggering receptor expressed on myeloid cells and the diagnosis of pneumonia. *N Engl J Med* 2004;350(5):451–458.

26. Torres A, Aznar R, Gatell JM, et al. Incidence, risk, and prognosis factors of nosocomial pneumonia in mechanically ventilated patients. *Am Rev Respir Dis* 1990;142(3):523–528.

27. Rello J, Lorente C, Diaz E, et al. Incidence, etiology, and outcome of nosocomial pneumonia in ICU patients requiring percutaneous tracheotomy for mechanical ventilation. *Chest* 2003;124(6):2239–2243.

28. Bonten MJ, Weinstein RA. Infection control in intensive care units and prevention of ventilator-associated pneumonia. *Semin Respir Infect* 2000;15(4):327–335.

29. Weinstein RA. Epidemiology and control of nosocomial infections in adult intensive care units. *Am J Med* 1991;91(3B):179S–184S.

30. Trouillet JL, Chastre J, Vuagnat A, et al. Ventilator-associated pneumonia caused by potentially drug-resistant bacteria. *Am J Respir Crit Care Med* 1998;157(2):531–539.

31. Kollef MH, Shorr A, Tabak YP, et al. Epidemiology and outcomes of health-care-associated pneumonia: results from a large US database of culture-positive pneumonia. *Chest* 2005;128(6):3854–3862.

32. Craven DE. What is healthcare-associated pneumonia, and how should it be treated? *Curr Opin Infect Dis* 2006;19(2):153–160.

33. El Solh AA, Aquilina AT, Dhillon RS, et al. Impact of invasive strategy on management of antimicrobial treatment failure in institutionalized older people with severe pneumonia. *Am J Respir Crit Care Med* 2002;166(8):1038–1043.

34. Pugin J, Auckenthaler R, Mili N, et al. Diagnosis of ventilator-associated pneumonia by bacteriologic analysis of bronchoscopic and nonbronchoscopic "blind" bronchoalveolar lavage fluid, part 1. *Am Rev Respir Dis* 1991;143(5):1121–1129.

35. Richards MJ, Edwards JR, Culver DH, Gaynes RP. Nosocomial infections in medical intensive care units in the United States. National Nosocomial Infections Surveillance system. *Crit Care Med* 1999;27(5):887–892.

36. Fridkin SK. Increasing prevalence of antimicrobial resistance in intensive care units. *Crit Care Med* 2001;29(suppl 4):N64–N68.

37. Mylotte JM. Nursing home-acquired pneumonia. *Clin Infect Dis* 2002;35(10):1205–1211.

38. de Lassence A, Hidri N, Timsit JF, et al. Control and outcome of a large outbreak of colonization and infection with glycopeptide-intermediate Staphylococcus aureus in an intensive care unit. *Clin Infect Dis* 2006;42(2):170–178.

39. Craven DE, Shapiro DS. Staphylococcus aureus: times, they are a-changin'. *Clin Infect Dis* 2006;42(2):179–180.

40. Muto CA. Methicillin-resistant Staphylococcus aureus control: we didn't start the fire, but it's time to put it out. *Infect Control Hosp Epidemiol* 2006;27(2):111–115.

41. Nijssen S, Bonten MJ, Weinstein RA. Are active microbiological surveillance and subsequent isolation needed to prevent the spread of methicillin-resistant Staphylococcus aureus? *Clin Infect Dis* 2005;40(3):405–409.

42. Moellering RC Jr. The growing menace of community-acquired methicillin-resistant Staphylococcus aureus. *Ann Intern Med* 2006;144(5):368–370.

43. Mandell LA, Bartlett JG, Dowell SF, et al. Update of practice guidelines for the management of community-acquired pneumonia in immunocompetent adults. *Clin Infect Dis* 2003;37(11):1405–1433.

44. Garnacho-Montero J, Ortiz-Leyba C, Fernandez-Hinojosa E, et al. Acinetobacter baumannii ventilator-associated pneumonia: epidemiological and clinical findings *Intensive Care Med* 2005;31(5):649–655.

45. Kuehnert MJ, Hill HA, Kupronis BA, et al. Methicillin-resistant Staphylococcus aureus hospitalizations, United States. *Emerg Infect Dis* 2005;11(6):868–872.

46. Klevens RM, Edwards JR, Tenover FC, et al. Changes in the epidemiology of methicillin-resistant Staphylococcus aureus in intensive care units in US hospitals, 1992–2003. *Clin Infect Dis* 2006;42(3):389–391.

47. Madaras-Kelly KJ, Remington RE, Lewis PG, Stevens DL. Evaluation of an intervention designed to decrease the rate of nosocomial methicillin-resistant Staphylococcus aureus infection by encouraging decreased fluoroquinolone use. *Infect Control Hosp Epidemiol* 2006;27(2):155–169.

48. Park DR. The microbiology of ventilator-associated pneumonia. *Respir Care* 2005;50(6):742–763.

49. Safdar N, Crnich CJ, Maki DG. The pathogenesis of ventilator-associated pneumonia: its relevance to developing effective strategies for prevention. *Respir Care* 2005;50(6):725–739.

50. Koenig SM, Truwit JD. Ventilator-associated pneumonia: Diagnosis, treatment and prevention. *Clin Micro Rev* 2006;19:637–57.

51. Singh N, Rogers P, Atwood CW, et al. Short-course empiric antibiotic therapy for patients with pulmonary infiltrates in the intensive care unit: a proposed solution for indiscriminate antibiotic prescription, part 1. *Am J Respir Crit Care Med* 2000;162(2):505–511.

52. Klompas M. Does this patient have ventilator-associated pneumonia?. *JAMA* 2007;297:1583–93.

53. Fagon JY, Chastre J, Wolff M, et al. Invasive and non-invasive strategies for management of suspected ventilator-associated pneumonia: a randomized trial. *Ann Intern Med* 2000;132(8):621–630.

54. Torres A, Ewig S. Diagnosing ventilator-associated pneumonia. *N Engl J Med* 2004;350(5):433–435.

55. Canadian Clinical Trials Group. A randomized trial of diagnostic techniques for ventilator-associated pneumonia. *N Engl J Med* 2006;355:2619–30.

56. de Jesus CT, File TM, Jr. Ventilator-associated pneumonia: gearing towards shorter-course therapy. *Curr Opin Infect Dis* 2006;19(2):185–188.

57. Dennesen PJ, van der Ven AJ, Kessels AG, et al. Resolution of infectious parameters after antimicrobial therapy in patients with ventilator-associated pneumonia. *Am J Respir Crit Care Med* 2001;163(6):1371–1375.

58. Chastre J, Wolff M, Fagon JY, et al. Comparison of 8 vs 15 days of antibiotic therapy for ventilator-associated pneumonia in adults: a randomized trial. *JAMA* 2003;290(19):2588–2598.

59. Ibrahim EH, Ward S, Sherman G, et al. Experience with a clinical guideline for the treatment of ventilator-associated pneumonia. *Crit Care Med* 2001;29(6):1109–1115.

60. Luyt CE, Guerin V, Combes A, et al. Procalcitonin kinetics as a prognostic marker of ventilator-associated pneumonia. *Am J Respir Crit Care Med* 2005;171(1):48–53.

61. Craven DE. Preventing ventilator-associated pneumonia: sowing seeds of change. *Chest* 2006;130:251–260.

62. Dodek P, Keenan S, Cook D, et al. Evidence-based clinical practice guideline for the prevention of ventilator-associated pneumonia. *Ann Intern Med* 2004;141(4):305–313.

63. Zack JE, Garrison T, Trovillion E, et al. Effect of an education program aimed at reducing the occurrence of ventilator-associated pneumonia. *Crit Care Med* 2002;30(11):2407–2412.

64. Babcock HM, Zack JE, Garrison T, et al. An educational intervention to reduce ventilator-associated pneumonia in an integrated health system: a comparison of effects. *Chest* 2004;125(6):2224–2231.

65. Kollef MH. Prevention of hospital-associated pneumonia and ventilator-associated pneumonia. *Crit Care Med* 2004;32(6):1396–1405.

66. Crnich CJ, Safdar N, Maki DG. The role of the intensive care unit environment in the pathogenesis and prevention of ventilator-associated pneumonia. *Respir Care* 2005;50(6):813–836.

67. Dang D, Johantgen ME, Pronovost PJ, et al. Postoperative complications: does intensive care unit staff nursing make a difference? *Heart Lung* 2002;31(3):219–228.

68. Eggimann P, Pittet D. Infection control in the ICU. *Chest* 2001;120(6):2059–2093.

69. Rosenthal VD, Guzman S, Crnich C. Impact of an infection control program on rates of ventilator-associated pneumonia in intensive care units in 2 Argentinean hospitals. *Am J Infect Control* 2006;34(2):58–63.

70. Crnich CJ, Proctor RA. Ventilator-associated pneumonia: does surveillance have a role in its management? *Crit Care Med* 2003;31(9):2411–2412.

71. L'Heriteau F, Alberti C, Cohen Y, et al. Nosocomial infection and multidrug-resistant bacteria surveillance in intensive care units: a survey in France. *Infect Control Hosp Epidemiol* 2005;26(1):13–20.

72. Vandenbroucke-Grauls C, Schultsz C. Surveillance in infection control: are we making progress? *Curr Opin Infect Dis* 2002;15(4):415–419.

73. Vos MC, Ott A, Verbrugh HA. Successful search-and-destroy policy for methicillin-resistant Staphylococcus aureus in The Netherlands. *J Clin Microbiol* 2005;43(4):2034–2035.

74. Carling PC, Briggs JL, Perkins J, Highlander D. Improved cleaning of patient rooms using a new targeting method. *Clin Infect Dis* 2006;42(3):385–388.

75. Bassetti S, Sherertz RJ, Pfaller MA. Airborne dispersal of Staphylococcus aureus associated with symptomatic rhinitis allergica. *Ann Intern Med* 2003;139(3):W–W60.

76. Rahal JJ, Urban C, Segal-Maurer S. Nosocomial antibiotic resistance in multiple gram-negative species: experience at one hospital with squeezing the resistance balloon at multiple sites. *Clin Infect Dis* 2002;34(4):499–503.

77. Warren DK, Hill HA, Merz LR, et al. Cycling empirical antimicrobial agents to prevent emergence of antimicrobial-resistant Gram-negative bacteria among intensive care unit patients. *Crit Care Med* 2004;32(12):2450–2456.

78. Isakow W, Kollef MH. Preventing ventilator-associated pneumonia: an evidence-based approach of modifiable risk factors. *Semin Respir Crit Care Med* 2006;27(1):5–17.

79. Kollef MH, Vlasnik J, Sharpless L, et al. Scheduled change of antibiotic classes: a strategy to decrease the incidence of ventilator-associated pneumonia, part 1. *Am J Respir Crit Care Med* 1997;156(4):1040–1048.

80. Gerding DN, Larson TA, Hughes RA, et al. Aminoglycoside resistance and aminoglycoside usage: ten years of experience in one hospital. *Antimicrob Agents Chemother* 1991;35(7):1284–1290.

81. Gruson D, Hilbert G, Vargas F, et al. Rotation and restricted use of antibiotics in a medical intensive care unit: impact on the incidence of ventilator-associated pneumonia caused by antibiotic-resistant gram-negative bacteria, part 1. *Am J Respir Crit Care Med* 2000;162(3):837–843.

82. Gruson D, Hilbert G, Vargas F, et al. Strategy of antibiotic rotation: long-term effect on incidence and susceptibilities of Gram-negative bacilli responsible for ventilator-associated pneumonia. *Crit Care Med* 2003;31(7):1908–1914.

83. Parker CM, Heyland DK. Aspiration and the risk of ventilator-associated pneumonia. *Nutr Clin Pract* 2004;19(6):597–609.

84. Pneumatikos J, Koulouras B, Frangides C, et al. Cisapride decreases gastric content aspiration in mechanically ventilated patients. *Crit Care* (London) 1999;3(1):39–43.

85. Cook D, Mandell L. Endotracheal aspiration in the diagnosis of ventilator-associated pneumonia. *Chest* 2000;117(4 suppl 2):195S–197S.

86. Smith G, Ng A. Gastric reflux and pulmonary aspiration in anaesthesia. *Minerva Anestesiol* 2003;69(5):402–406.

87. Kallel H, Chelly H, Bahloul M, et al. The effect of ventilator-associated pneumonia on the prognosis of head trauma patients. *J Trauma* 2005;59(3):705–710.

88. Orozco-Levi M, Torres A, Ferrer M, et al. Semirecumbent position protects from pulmonary aspiration but not completely from gastroesophageal reflux in mechanically ventilated patients, part 1. *Am J Respir Crit Care Med* 1995;152(4):1387–1390.

89. Torres A, Serra-Batlles J, Ros E, et al. Pulmonary aspiration of gastric contents in patients receiving mechanical ventilation: the effect of body position. *Ann Intern Med* 1992;116(7):540–543.

90. Drakulovic MB, Torres A, Bauer TT, et al. Supine body position as a risk factor for nosocomial pneumonia in mechanically ventilated patients: a randomised trial. *Lancet* 1999;354(9193):1851–1858.

91. Hess DR. Patient positioning and ventilator-associated pneumonia. *Respir Care* 2005;50(7):892–898.

92. Wang JY, Chuang PY, Lin CJ, et al. Continuous lateral rotational therapy in the medical intensive care unit. *J Formos Med Assoc* 2003;102(11):788–792.

93. van Nieuwenhoven CA, Vandenbroucke-Grauls C, van Tiel FH, et al. Feasibility and effects of the semirecumbent position to prevent ventilator-associated pneumonia: a randomized study. *Crit Care Med* 2006;34(2):396–402.

94. Grap MJ, Munro CL, Bryant S, Ashtiani B. Predictors of backrest elevation in critical care. *Intensive Crit Care Nurs* 2003;19(2):68–74.

95. Grap MJ, Munro CL. Quality improvement in backrest elevation: improving outcomes in critical care. *AACN Clin Issues* 2005;16(2):133–139.

96. Pingleton SK, Fagon JY, Leeper KV Jr. Patient selection for clinical investigation of ventilator-associated pneumonia: criteria for evaluating diagnostic techniques. *Chest* 1992;102(5 suppl 1):553S–556S.

97. Ibrahim EH, Mehringer L, Prentice D, et al. Early versus late enteral feeding of mechanically ventilated patients: results of a clinical trial. *JPEN J Parenter Enteral Nutr* 2002;26(3):174–181.

98. Heyland DK, Drover JW, Dhaliwal R, Greenwood J. Optimizing the benefits and minimizing the risks of enteral nutrition in the critically ill: role of small bowel feeding. *JPEN J Parenter Enteral Nutr* 2002;26(6 suppl):S51–S55.

99. Heyland DK, Drover JW, MacDonald S, et al. Effect of postpyloric feeding on gastroesophageal regurgitation and pulmonary microaspiration: results of a randomized controlled trial. *Crit Care Med* 2001;29(8):1495–1501.

100. Bowman A, Greiner JE, Doerschug KC, et al. Implementation of an evidence-based feeding protocol and aspiration risk reduction algorithm. *Crit Care Nurs Q* 2005;28(4):324–333.

101. Kostadima E, Kaditis AG, Alexopoulos EI, et al. Early gastrostomy reduces the rate of ventilator-associated pneumonia in stroke or head injury patients. *Eur Respir J* 2005;26(1):106–111.

102. van Nieuwenhoven CA, Buskens E, Bergmans DC, et al. Oral decontamination is cost-saving in the prevention of ventilator-associated pneumonia in intensive care units. *Crit Care Med* 2004;32(1):126–130.

103. Munro CL, Grap MJ. Oral health and care in the intensive care unit: state of the science. *Am J Crit Care* 2004;13(1):25–33.

104. Brennan MT, Bahrani-Mougeot F, Fox PC, et al. The role of oral microbial colonization in ventilator-associated pneumonia. *Oral Surg Oral Med Oral Pathol Oral Radiol Endod* 2004;98(6):665–672.

105. Cutler CJ, Davis N. Improving oral care in patients receiving mechanical ventilation. *Am J Crit Care* 2005;14(5):389–394.

106. Mori H, Hirasawa H, Oda S, et al. Oral care reduces incidence of ventilator-associated pneumonia in ICU populations. *Intensive Care Med* 2006;32(2):230–236.

107. Liberati A, D'Amico R, Pifferi et al., Antibiotic prophylaxis to reduce respiratory tract infections and mortality in adults receiving intensive care. *Cochrane Database Syst Rev* 2004;(1):CD000022.

108. Silvestri L, Petros AJ, Viviani M, et al. Selective decontamination of the digestive tract and ventilator-associated pneumonia, part 1. *Respir Care* 2006;51(1):67–69.

109. Krueger WA, Unertl KE. Selective decontamination of the digestive tract. *Curr Opin Crit Care* 2002;8(2):139–144.

110. de Jonge E, Schultz MJ, Spanjaard L. Effects of selective decontamination of digestive tract on mortality and acquisition of resistant bacteria in intensive care: a randomised controlled trial. *Lancet* 2003;362(9389):1011–1016.

111. Nathens AB, Marshall JC. Selective decontamination of the digestive tract in surgical patients: a systematic review of the evidence. *Arch Surg* 1999;134(2):170–176.

112. Kollef MH. Selective digestive decontamination should not be routinely employed *Chest* 2003;123(5 suppl):464S–468S.

113. Kollef MH. Ventilator-associated pneumonia: a multivariate analysis. *JAMA* 1993;270(16):1965–1970.

114. Kollef MH. Antibiotic management of ventilator-associated pneumonia due to antibiotic-resistant gram-positive bacterial infection. *Eur J Clin Microbiol Infect Dis* 2005;24(12):794–803.

115. Sirvent JM, Torres A, El Ebiary M, et al. Protective effect of intravenously administered cefuroxime against nosocomial pneumonia in patients with structural coma. *Am J Respir Crit Care Med* 1997;155(5):1729–1734.

116. Kallet RH, Quinn TE. The gastrointestinal tract and ventilator-associated pneumonia. *Respir Care* 2005;50(7):910–921.

117. DeRiso AJ, Ladowski JS, Dillon TA, et al. Chlorhexidine gluconate 0.12% oral rinse reduces the incidence of total nosocomial respiratory infection and nonprophylactic systemic antibiotic use in patients undergoing heart surgery. *Chest* 1996;109(6):1556–1561.

118. Koeman M, van der Ven AJ, Hak E, et al. Oral decontamination with chlorhexidine reduces incidence of ventilator-associated pneumonia. *Am J Respir Crit Care Med* 2006;171:1348–1345.

119. Kollef M, Pittet D, Sanchez GM, et al. A randomized double-blind trial of iseganan in prevention of ventilator-associated pneumonia. *Am J Respir Crit Care Med* 2006;173(1):91–97.

120. Ibid.

121. Hess DR, Kallstrom TJ, Mottram CD, et al. Care of the ventilator circuit and its relation to ventilator-associated pneumonia. *Respir Care* 2003;48(9):869–879.

122. Burns KE, Adhikari NK, Meade MO. A meta-analysis of noninvasive weaning to facilitate liberation from mechanical ventilation. *Can J Anaesth* 2006;53(3):305–315.

123. Esteban A, Frutos-Vivar F, Ferguson ND, et al. Noninvasive positive-pressure ventilation for respiratory failure after extubation. *N Engl J Med* 2004;350(24):2452–2460.

124. Holzapfel L, Chastang C, Demingeon G, et al. A randomized study assessing the systematic search for maxillary sinusitis in nasotracheally mechanically ventilated patients: influence of nosocomial maxillary sinusitis on the occurrence of ventilator-associated pneumonia. *Am J Respir Crit Care Med* 1999;159(3):695–701.

125. Cook D, De Jonghe B, Brochard L, Brun-Buisson C. Influence of airway management on ventilator-associated pneumonia: evidence from randomized trials. *JAMA* 1998;279(10):781–787.

126. Torres A, Gatell JM, Aznar E, et al. Re-intubation increases the risk of nosocomial pneumonia in patients needing mechanical ventilation. *Am J Respir Crit Care Med* 1995;152(1):137–141.

127. Dreyfuss D, Ricard JD. Acute lung injury and bacterial infection. *Clin Chest Med* 2005;26(1):105–112.

128. Schweickert WD, Gehlbach BK, Pohlman AS, et al. Daily interruption of sedative infusions and complications of critical illness in mechanically ventilated patients. *Crit Care Med* 2004;32(6):1272–1276.

129. Kress JP, Pohlman AS, O'Connor MF, Hall JB. Daily interruption of sedative infusions in critically ill patients undergoing mechanical ventilation. *N Engl J Med* 2000;342(20):1471–1477.

130. Marelich GP, Murin S, Battistella F, et al. Protocol weaning of mechanical ventilation in medical and surgical patients by respiratory care practitioners and nurses: effect on weaning time and incidence of ventilator-associated pneumonia. *Chest* 2000;118(2):459–467.

131. Needleman J, Buerhaus P, Mattke S, et al. Nurse-staffing levels and the quality of care in hospitals. *N Engl J Med* 2002;346(22):1715–1722.

132. Thorens JB, Kaelin RM, Jolliet P, Chevrolet JC. Influence of the quality of nursing on the duration of weaning from mechanical ventilation in patients with chronic obstructive pulmonary disease. *Crit Care Med* 1995;23(11):1807–1815.

133. Dries DJ, McGonigal MD, Malian MS, et al. Protocol-driven ventilator weaning reduces use of mechanical ventilation, rate of early reintubation, and ventilator-associated pneumonia. *J Trauma* 2004;56(5):943–951.

134. Dezfulian C, Shojania K, Collard HR, et al. Subglottic secretion drainage for preventing ventilator associated pneumonia: a meta-analysis. *Am J Med* 2005;118(1):11–18.

135. Girou E, Buu-Hoi A, Stephan F, et al. Airway colonisation in long-term mechanically ventilated patients: effect of semi-recumbent position and continuous subglottic suctioning. *Intensive Care Med* 2004;30(2):225–233.

136. Craven DE, Goularte TA, Make BJ. Contaminated condensate in mechanical ventilator circuits: a risk factor for nosocomial pneumonia? *Am Rev Respir Dis* 1984;129(4):625–628.

137. Branson RD. The ventilator circuit and ventilator-associated pneumonia. *Respir Care* 2005;50(6):774–785.

138. Kollef MH, Von Harz B, Prentice D, et al. Patient transport from intensive care increases the risk of developing ventilator-associated pneumonia. *Chest* 1997;112(3):765–773.

139. Kola A, Eckmanns T, Gastmeier P. Efficacy of heat and moisture exchangers in preventing ventilator-associated pneumonia: meta-analysis of randomized controlled trials. *Intensive Care Med* 2005;31(1):5–11.

140. Lacherade JC, Auburtin M, Cerf C. Impact of humidification systems on ventilator-associated pneumonia: a randomized, multicenter trial. *Am J respir Crit Crare Med* 2005;172:276–282.

141. Van den BG, Wouters P, Weekers F, et al. Intensive insulin therapy in the critically ill patients. *N Engl J Med* 2001;345(19):1359–1367.

142. Egi M, Bellomo R, Stachowski E, et al. Intensive insulin therapy in postoperative intensive care unit patients: a decision analysis. *Am J Respir Crit Care Med* 2006;173(4):407–413.

143. Van den BG, Wilmer A, Hermans G, et al. Intensive insulin therapy in the medical ICU. *N Engl J Med* 2006;354(5):449–461.

144. Cook D, Guyatt G, Marshall J, et al. A comparison of sucralfate and ranitidine for the prevention of upper gastrointestinal bleeding in patients requiring mechanical ventilation. *N Engl J Med* 1998;338(12):791–797.

145. Bornstain C, Azoulay E, de Lassence A, et al. Sedation, sucralfate, and antibiotic use are potential means for protection against early-onset ventilator-associated pneumonia. *Clin Infect Dis* 2004;38(10):1401–1408.

146. Markowicz P, Wolff M, Djedaini K, et al. Multicenter prospective study of ventilator-associated pneumonia during acute respiratory distress syndrome: incidence, prognosis, and risk factors. *Am J Respir Crit Care Med* 2000;161(6):1942–1948.

147. Hebert PC, Wells G, Blajchman MA, et al. A multicenter, randomized, controlled clinical trial of transfusion requirements in critical care. *N Engl J Med* 1999;340(6):409–417.

148. Jensen LS, Kissmeyer-Nielsen P, Wolff B, Qvist N. Randomised comparison of leucocyte-depleted versus buffy-coat-poor blood transfusion and complications after colorectal surgery. *Lancet* 1996;348(9031):841–845.

149. Corwin HL, Gettinger A, Pearl RG, et al. The CRIT Study: anemia and blood transfusion in the critically ill—current clinical practice in the United States. *Crit Care Med* 2004;32(1): 39–52.

150. Levy MM, Abraham E, Zilberberg M, MacIntyre NR. A descriptive evaluation of transfusion practices in patients receiving mechanical ventilation. *Chest* 2005;127(3):928–935.

151. Berwick DM, Calkins DR, McCannon CJ, Hackbarth AD. The 100,000 lives campaign: setting a goal and a deadline for improving health care quality. *JAMA* 2006;295(3):324–327.

152. Pauker SG, Zane EM, Salem DN. Creating a safer health care system: finding the constraint. *JAMA* 2005;294(22):2906–2908.

Tuberculosis

32

William R. Jarvis

Tuberculosis (TB) is a major cause of morbidity and mortality throughout the world with an estimated 8 million people contracting disease and 3 million dying annually. Worldwide, the prevalence of TB is increasing, in part due to the human immunodeficiency virus (HIV) epidemic. In the mid-1980s, the incidence of TB reversed its downward trend in the United States and, possibly secondary to the HIV epidemic and increased immigration from countries with a high incidence of TB, began to increase [1–6]. In the 1990s, the increasing trend continued, hospital outbreaks occurred, and additional federal and state TB resources and funding were provided. Subsequently, the increasing trend has been reversed.

As *Mycobacterium tuberculosis* emerged in the late 1980s and early 1990s, an increase in the number of *Mycobacterium tuberculosis* outbreaks, particularly multidrug-resistant strains (MDR-TB; i.e., resistant to at least two first-line antituberculous agents), began to be reported in U.S. healthcare facilities [7].

PATHOGEN AND PATHOGENESIS

TB is caused by bacteria in the *M. tuberculosis* complex, of which *M. tuberculosis* is the most important [2,4]. The primary mode of transmission is by airborne droplet nuclei, which may be produced when people with pulmonary or laryngeal tuberculosis cough, sneeze, speak, or sing. In addition, aerosols can be produced and transmission occurs during manipulation or irrigation of TB lesions or when tissues or secretions from a person with TB are being obtained or processed. The actual sizes of the airborne droplet nuclei are not known but are estimated to be between 1–5μ; such particles are light enough to be carried long distances by ambient air currents. When such airborne droplet nuclei are inhaled, they may traverse the body's defenses and become implanted in the respiratory bronchiole or alveoli. Despite capture by macrophages, the bacilli may replicate within the cell or be carried directly or by macrophages through the lymphatics to regional lymph nodes or the bloodstream, or they may disseminate. Cell-mediated immunity usually limits further multiplication or spread, and lesions resolve. The risk of infection with *M. tuberculosis* varies, depending on the concentration of droplet nuclei in the air and the duration of exposure to the contaminated air. After inhalation, the bacilli remain viable; this condition of latent *M. tuberculosis* infection is asymptomatic and is not contagious. In immunocompetent individuals, a tuberculin skin test (TST) applied 2 to 10 weeks after initial infection is positive; this is secondary to hypersensitivity to *M. tuberculosis* cell wall components. In addition, in immunocompetent individuals, a blood assay for *M. tuberculosis* (BAMT) such as the QuantiFERON-TB Gold test (QFT-G) will be positive [8,9]. In ~10% of infected immunocompetent individuals, the organism begins to multiply and causes active disease in their lifetime. In ~5% of these individuals, this occurs within the first 1 to 2 years after infection, and in the remaining 5%, disease occurs >2 years after infection. Those with immunocompromising conditions are at a >10% risk for development of active TB annually.

TUBERCULOSIS IN THE UNITED STATES

From 1953 through 1984, the number of people in the United States each year with active TB decreased by ~6% per year, from 84,304 to 22,201 [3]. However, from 1985 through 1992, the reported number of people with TB increased by ~20% to 26,673 [4]. Thus, from 1985 through 1992, ~52,000 excess episodes of TB were reported above what would have been expected based on the 1953 to 1984 trend. In addition, the proportion of people infected with MDR-TB increased. Factors contributing to this increase in TB include the HIV epidemic, the increase in the number of people immigrating from countries with a high TB prevalence, adverse social conditions, and inadequate infection control practices in healthcare facilities, all of which facilitate transmission. The combination of an increasing TB prevalence, HIV-infected people, and MDR-TB resulted in an increase in hospitalization of people with infectious TB and an increased risk of *M. tuberculosis* transmission in healthcare facilities to both patients (nosocomial acquisition) and healthcare workers (HCWs) (occupational acquisition). With increased emphasis in hospital- and community-based TB control programs, the reported incidence of TB decreased by 5.2% in 1993 and by another 3.7% in 1994 [5,6]. In the late 1990s and the early 2000s, there has been a reversal of the previous upward trend. In 2001, 15,989 active TB patients were reported to the Centers for Disease Control and Prevention (CDC) representing a 2% decrease from 2000 and a 40% decrease since 1992.

Of the 25,287 people reported with tuberculosis in the United States in 1993, 65% were male, 71.5% were racial and ethnic minorities, 38% were 25 to 44 years of age, and 29% were born in a country other than the United States. In 1993, 64% of the reported episodes of tuberculosis were reported from seven states: California, New York, Texas, Florida, Illinois, New Jersey, and Georgia. In 2001, 62% (9,943) of TB patients were men and 38% (6,045) were women. The rate of TB for men (7.1 per 100,000) was almost double that of women (4.2 per 100,000). The TB rates were dramatically higher for Asians/Pacific Islanders (32.7 per 100,000), African Americans (13.8 per 100,000), Hispanics (11.9 per 100,000), and American Indians/Alaska natives (11.0 per 100,000) than for whites (1.6 per 100,000). There were 4,796 African Americans reported as having TB disease; 3,357 whites; 4,001 Hispanics; 3,552 Asians/Pacific Islanders; and 233 American Indians/Alaskan natives. Factors in reversing the increasing trend in TB in the United States include the successful implementation of recommended TB control programs, including directly observed therapy and improved implementation of hospital infection control practices [10].

DIAGNOSIS OF TUBERCULOSIS

Prevention of transmission of *M. tuberculosis* depends on a high index of suspicion of TB and knowledge of the clinical signs and symptoms and the appropriate diagnostic workup. The initial symptoms of TB may be nonspecific and insidious in onset and include fatigue, anorexia, fever, chills, myalgia, sweating, and weight loss. Pulmonary TB is the most common form and the one usually associated with transmission in healthcare facilities. In pulmonary TB, the nonspecific symptoms are accompanied by an insidious cough that gradually progresses over a period of weeks to months to a productive cough with mucopurulent sputum

or hemoptysis. Hoarseness or a sore throat suggests possible laryngeal involvement; laryngeal TB usually is accompanied by pulmonary disease, large numbers of acid-fast bacilli (AFB) in sputum, and a high degree of contagion. The infectivity of the patient with TB depends on the site of infection, the presence of AFB-positive sputum, the number of organisms expelled into the air, the presence of pulmonary cavitary or endobronchial lesions, the duration of effective therapy, and whether the person remains in isolation or covers his or her mouth when coughing. Extrapulmonary TB without pulmonary or laryngeal involvement usually is not contagious. However, irrigation or manipulation of TB lesions can produce infectious aerosols and transmit *M. tuberculosis*. The appropriate diagnostic workup of a patient with signs or symptoms consistent with TB should include a chest radiograph. With initial infection, parenchymal infiltration with ipsilateral lymph node enlargement may be seen whereas in reactivation, apical or posterior segment lesions in the upper lobes are most common. In all patients, particularly those who are immunocompromised, such as those with HIV infection, the chest radiograph findings may range from normal to miliary in appearance [11]. In those with possible pulmonary TB, respiratory secretions should be obtained promptly for AFB smears and culture; in pediatric patients, gastric aspirates may be needed for those who do not cough. Specimens should be transported to the laboratory promptly and the most rapid laboratory diagnostic methods should be used including fluorescent microscopy and radiometric methods for species identification and drug susceptibility testing [12]. Because the AFB smear is the most rapid presumptive diagnostic test and provides an important assessment of the patient's infectivity, AFB smears using fluorescent microscopy should be promptly performed. The development of genetic probes facilitates the rapid identification of *M. tuberculosis* (see Chapter 10). The initial isolate from people with TB and subsequent isolates from any person not responding to appropriate treatment should be tested for anti-TB drug susceptibility. Anti-TB drug susceptibility results provide the clinician important information for choosing an effective therapeutic regime. Furthermore, the use of genetic probes and nucleic acid amplification techniques can further shorten the time required to determine the species identification. Data show that from 1992 to 1995, the proportion of U.S. hospital laboratories in which the recommended methods were used for AFB smears, primary culture, *M. tuberculosis* identification, and anti-TB drug susceptibility testing has increased [13].

During the initial evaluation, either a TST or QFT-G test should be performed. If a TST is performed, it should be applied to the surface of the patient's forearm using the Mantoux method and read at 48 to 72 hours. Despite the limitations of the TST (<100% sensitivity and specificity; positive predictive value correlates with the TB prevalence), it remains the most practical screening method for identifying people with *M. tuberculosis* infection (i.e., latent TB infection [LTBI]) in most countries. Only the presence or absence of and the extent of induration (not erythema) transverse to the long axis of the forearm should be measured.

The cut point used for defining a positive TST varies depending on the risk of *M. tuberculosis* exposure. For people with HIV infection, people in close contact with a person with infectious TB or with a chest radiograph consistent with pulmonary TB, a TST reaction of ≥ 5 mm is considered positive [14–18]. For people not meeting these criteria but who have other risk factors for TB, a reaction of ≥ 10 mm is considered positive. These factors include people born in countries with a high prevalence of TB; medically underserved populations with a high prevalence of TB; people with conditions predisposing to TB (e.g., gastrectomy, jejunoileal bypass, $\geq 10\%$ below ideal body weight, chronic renal insufficiency, immunosuppressive therapy, some malignancies, diabetes mellitus, gastrectomy, or silicosis); residents of long-term care facilities; or other people identified as at high risk for TB. For others, including those who have received the bacille Calmette-Guérin (BCG) vaccine, a reaction of ≥ 5 mm is considered positive.

The QFT-Gold is a blood test in an *ex vivo* assay that measures the release of interferon-γ in whole blood in response to stimulation by antigens that are more specific for *M. tuberculosis* than tuberculin purified protein derivative. This test does not cause boosting when repeated. If one uses the QFT-Gold test rather than the TST, it should be used in all circumstances in which the TST is currently used, including sequential surveillance testing for infection control [8,9]. Negative tests should be interpreted with caution, particularly in those recently exposed to TB or who are immunocompromised. One must work closely with the laboratory to ensure that the blood specimen arrives at the qualified testing laboratory within 12 hours of being obtained (incubation must occur while the blood cells are viable). A single negative QFT-Gold test is sufficient evidence that the person probably is not infected with *M. tuberculosis*. A person with a positive test does not need to be retested. If doing serial QFT-Gold testing, conversion from negative to positive should be considered in a person with newly diagnosed TB infection.

Periodic TST or QFT-G tests are valuable methods for identifying new *M. tuberculosis* infection in those exposed to people with infectious TB. For people <35 years of age and most HCWs, an increase in TST induration of ≥ 10 mm within 2 years should be considered a TST conversion. For people ≥ 35 years or HCWs with infrequent TB exposure, an increase in TST induration of ≥ 15 mm in 2 years should be considered a TST conversion. Those with TST conversions should be promptly evaluated for active TB disease and placed on preventive therapy (if active disease is ruled out).

Repeated TST of noninfected individuals does not lead to hypersensitivity to tuberculin. However, in individuals with delayed hypersensitivity to tuberculin from either past infection with mycobacteria or BCG vaccination, reactivity may wane over time. In these individuals, the TST may stimulate the hypersensitivity and result in an initial negative TST followed by a subsequent positive TST when tested from 1 week to 1 year or longer after the initial TST (i.e., the "booster phenomenon"). To avoid the booster phenomenon and reduce the likelihood of interpreting a booster reaction as representing recent infection, TSTs should be conducted periodically with the first test being a two-step test. In the two-step test, the individual first has a TST. If negative, a second TST is performed 1 to 3 weeks later. If the second test is positive, it is probably a booster reaction. Other factors that can alter the individual's ability to react to tuberculin include (1) host factors, such as concomitant infection (e.g., viral or bacterial infections), metabolic abnormalities (e.g., chronic renal failure), nutritional factors (e.g., severe protein calorie malnutrition), lymphoid organ abnormalities (e.g., malignancy, sarcoidosis), immunosuppressive agents, age (e.g., newborns or elderly), and stress (e.g., surgery, burns); (2) factors related to the tuberculin used, such as improper storage, improper dilution, chemical degradation, or contamination; (3) factors related to the TST administration method (e.g., injection of too little antigen or delay in administration after drawing up the tuberculin); or (4) factors related to reading the TST, such as an inexperienced reader or misreading. In these situations, use of the QFT-G may be an attractive alternative, particularly in those who have received BCG or have tuberculin sensitivity [8,9].

Once a presumptive diagnosis of TB is established based on clinical findings plus or minus radiologic and laboratory findings, the patient should be placed on appropriate empiric therapy that can be modified once drug susceptibility results are available [14–18]. If the results of anti-TB susceptibility testing indicate resistance to agents being used or the patient fails to respond to the empiric therapy, the therapeutic regime should be modified.

M. TUBERCULOSIS TRANSMISSION IN HOSPITALS

Several factors influence whether *M. tuberculosis* is transmitted to either patients or HCWs in a hospital or other healthcare facility. These include the likelihood that they will be exposed to *M. tuberculosis*, that they will become infected, and that the infection will progress to disease. The risk of exposure in the healthcare setting is influenced by the number of infectious TB patients admitted and the infection control practices implemented in the healthcare facility, including the methods for identifying infectious patients, the type of isolation in which infectious patients are placed, the type of respiratory protection used by the HCW, and the environmental and engineering controls used. Several studies have shown that if the number of TB patients admitted or cared for is low, the risk of exposure to *M. tuberculosis* is low [19–23]. The risk that HCWs or patients will become infected is influenced by the concentration of airborne droplet nuclei they are exposed to, the type and duration of the exposure, and the efficacy of the infection control measures implemented; although immunocompromising conditions increase the risk of disease given infection, they do not appear to increase the risk of infection. The risk that, once infected, a person will progress rapidly from infection to disease depends on the prevalence of conditions in the HCW or patient populations that decrease immunity (e.g., HIV infection, malignancy, or diabetes).

Surveillance for *M. tuberculosis* Infection/Disease in Healthcare Workers

There is no national surveillance system for *M. tuberculosis* infection/disease in U.S. HCWs. Before 1993, the national TB surveillance system did not collect occupational data on those reported with TB. In data reported since 1993, HCWs accounted for 0 to 6% of those reported with TB; however, this system does not provide further investigative data to determine whether the TB was occupationally or community acquired [5]. TST conversion data (LTBI) are not collected in this or any other national surveillance system. In studies conducted at individual institutions, the incidence of TB infection in HCWs ranged from 0.1% to 10.0% [17–44] (Table 32-1).

Several national surveys show that in hospitals with HCW TST programs, overall TST conversion rates range from 0.33% to 5.50% [19–53] (Table 32-1). Several studies have shown that HCWs originating from foreign countries or with a history of BCG have a higher prevalence of TST positivity [43,44,50–53]. Furthermore, in some regions of the country, HCWs have a high prevalence of TST positivity at the time of employment [14–16,42,50–54]. For these reasons, it has been recommended that a two-step TST be performed at the time of employment followed by periodic TST based on the risk of exposure [9,14,50–56] or a BAMT such as the QFT-Gold test [8,9].

Few studies have assessed the risk of TB disease in HCWs. Although U.S. HCWs in general are at low risk of TST conversion or TB, selected HCW groups—those with the closest contact with infectious TB patients or those working in hospitals with *M. tuberculosis* outbreaks—may be at greater risk [57]. In two surveys of physicians affiliated with medical schools, active TB appeared to be more common than in the community population [38,58]. Barrett-Conner found that 3.5% of physicians at one medical center had been treated for active TB, 75.0% of active disease occurred within 10 years after beginning medical school, and 62.0% occurred after infection after the beginning of medical school [33]. In the 1938 to 1981 graduates of the University of Illinois Medical School, active TB was more common than in the general population, and >66% of the episodes occurred ≤6 years after graduation [56]. Twelve studies, most based on either registries or questionnaires,

have assessed the risk of TB disease in HCWs: in five, the risk was estimated to be greater than in the general population; in three, the risk was estimated as less than in the general population; and in four, the risk was not compared with that of the general population [23]. In more recent data from New York state, 2.5% of TB cases in 1994 and 2.0% of cases in 2002 were HCWs; 50.0% of HCWs with TB were foreign born [59].

Nosocomial *M. tuberculosis* Transmission

Before 1989, reports of nosocomial *M. tuberculosis* outbreaks were infrequent [58–65]. The sparsity of such reports may reflect either infrequent transmission or the failure to detect such transmission. Only 5%–10% of immunocompetent people exposed to an infectious TB patient contract TB in their lifetime, and such development would occur months to years after the exposure. Because the patient may not be readmitted to the same facility, the possibility of nosocomial acquisition might not be considered; such disease would not be linked to a prior hospitalization, and nosocomial acquisition would not be documented. Thus, unless there is a large group of immunocompetent or immunocompromised patients with newly diagnosed TB or patients infected with a strain of *M. tuberculosis* with an unusual antimicrobial susceptibility pattern, nosocomial transmission may not be suspected, detected, or reported. Hence, nosocomial patient-to-patient transmission of *M. tuberculosis* may occur more frequently than recognized or reported.

In contrast, occupational acquisition of *M. tuberculosis* infection and disease has been a well-documented risk to U.S. HCWs since the early 1930s. In the mid- to late 1930s, Israel et al. followed a cohort of 637 nursing students during their hospital training [63]. At study entry, 360 (57%) nurses were TST negative and 277 (43%) were TST positive. During their training, 100% of the TST-negative nursing students had TST conversions, and active TB developed in 68/637 (11%). Additional studies in the 1930s and 1940s documented high (79% to 85%) TST conversion rates among nurses [63–66]. Furthermore, during this period, studies documented that the risk of active TB disease among medical school students was >3 times higher than that of the general population [66]. Risk factors for disease among the medical students included exposure to unrecognized TB patients, treating patients in the men's TB ward, and presence in the autopsy room.

Despite these studies suggesting both nosocomial and occupational transmission of *M. tuberculosis*, efforts to introduce appropriate infection control interventions were slow. Many hospitals opened TB wards, sanitaria (or entire hospitals for TB patients) were common, and, in many hospitals, obtaining routine chest radiographs at the time of patient admission to identify the previously unrecognized infectious TB patient was initiated. Concomitantly, increased suspicion of TB by clinicians,

TABLE 32-1

HEALTHCARE WORKER (HCW) TUBERCULIN SKIN TEST (TST) CONVERSION RATES, UNITED STATES, 1960–1999

Reference	State	Study Period	Study Population	Annual TST Conversion Rate (%)
Levine [24]	New York	1960–1967	Nursing students	1.1%
Weiss [25]	Pennsylvania	1962–1971	Nursing students	4.2
Atuk & Hunt [26]	Virginia	1968–1969	HCWs	1.9
Gregg et al. [27]	South Carolina	1969–1973	HCWs	4.1
Berman et al. [28]	Maryland	1971–1976	HCWs	1.4
Craven et al. [29]	Virginia	1971–1973	HCWs	0.5
Vogeler & Burke [30]	Utah	1972–1975	HCWs	0.2
Ruben et al. [31]	Pennsylvania	1973–1975	HCWs	3.1
Ktsanes et al. [32]	Louisiana	1972–1981	HCWs	1.0
Barrett-Conner [33]	California	1974–1975	Physicians	0.4–1.8
Weinstein et al. [34]	New York	1974–1981	Medical students	0.1
Chan & Tabak [35]	Florida	1978–1981	Physicians	4.0
Bass & Serio [36]	Alabama	1979	HCWs	2.9
Thompson et al. [37]	Multiple[a,b]	1979	HCWs	2.9
Kantor et al. [38]	Illinois	1979–1986	HCWs	0.9
Price et al. [39]	North Carolina[a]	1980–1984	HCWs	1.1
Aiken et al. [40]	Washington[a]	1982–1984	HCWs	0.9
Malasky et al. [22]	Multiple[a,b]	1984–1986	Pulmonary fellow	5.7
Raad et al. [41]	Florida	1984–1987	HCWs	0.1
Raad et al. [41]	Florida	1985–1987	HCWs	0.4
Ramirez et al. [42]	Kentucky	1986–1991	HCWs	0.7
Ikeda et al. [43]	New York	1989–1990	HCWs	0.8
Condos et al. [44]	New York	1988–1992	HCWs	1.0
Redwood et al. [45]	New York	1990–1992	HCWs	10.0
Cocchiarella et al. [46]	Illinois	1991	HCWs	16.2, 4.8[c]
Adal et al. [47]	Virginia	1992	HCWs	0.2
Panlilio et al. [48],	Multiple[a,b]	1994–1995	HCWs	1.4
National/state survey				
Manangan et al [49]	Texas[a] (151)[d]	1989–1991	HCWs	0.6–0.9
Sinkowitz et al. [21]	Multiple[a,b] (1,494)[d]	1989–1992	HCWs	0.4–0.5
Fridkin et al. [19,20]	Multiple[a,b] (359)[d]	1992–1993	HCWs	0.2–1.9
Silva et al. [50]	Brazil	1995–1999	Medical students	4.6–16.2
Kassim et al. [51]	Cote d'Ivoire	1996–1997	HCWs	79%
Yanai et al. [52]	Thailand	1995–1996	HCWs	2.2%–9.3%[e]
Roth et al. [53]	Brazil[a,b]	1998–1999	HCWs	10.7[f]

[a]Multiple hospitals.
[b]Multiple states.
[c]High-risk and low-risk HCWs, respectively.
[d]Number of hospitals reporting.
[e]Per 100 person-years.
[f]Per 100 person-months.

improvements in diagnostic and therapeutic modalities, and the identification of effective preventive anti-TB therapy resulted in a dramatic reduction in the incidence of TB in the United States from the mid-1940s until the mid-1980s [1].

Despite the fact that numerous studies have documented that HCWs are at increased risk of occupational acquisition of *M. tuberculosis*, no formal surveillance system for HCW TST conversion or disease has been established. Thus, even today there are few specific data on the risk of acquisition of TB among HCWs in the United States and limited data on HCWs in the developing world where the risk may be even greater because of larger numbers of patients with TB; the presence of large, open wards; and minimal or absent infection control precautions. A questionnaire administered to graduates of the University of Illinois School of Medicine from 1938 to 1981 found that in most years, the incidence of TB in the graduates exceeded that in the general population [58]. In another survey of medical school–affiliated physicians in California, 3.5% of physicians had been treated for TB; 75.0% of active disease had occurred <10 years after beginning medical school [33]. However, data from the North Carolina TB control program show that in 1983 and 1984, hospital personnel had similar or lower rates of TB than the general population [39]. More recently, surveys have shown that many hospitals do not have active HCW TST programs, that nurses and administrative personnel are more likely to be included in the TST program than are physicians, that HCW TST positivity rates at hire can be high and are related most likely to community TB prevalence, and that HCW (primarily nursing staff) TST conversion rates range from 0% to 27% [19–21,67,68].

Nosocomial *M. tuberculosis* in Human Immunodeficiency Virus–Infected Patients

TB is a common infection in HIV-infected patients [14–17,69,70] (see Chapter 42). Most of these episodes of TB are thought to be due to reactivation of latent *M. tuberculosis* infection. In 1985, the incidence of TB began to rise in the United States; it is unclear how much of this rise was due to HIV-infected people who are at increased risk for both reactivation of latent infection and new, primary infection [1]. Nevertheless, between 1985 and 1992, ~52,000 excess episodes of TB occurred above what would have been expected in the United States had the downward trend in TB been maintained; much of this increase was thought to be in HIV-infected people [1]. Thus, the interaction of the HIV and TB outbreaks has resulted in a major public health challenge. In the late 1980s, nosocomial outbreaks of multidrug-resistant *M. tuberculosis* (MDR-TB) began to occur in U.S. hospitals [7]. In 1989, Dooley et al. investigated an outbreak of TB among patients on an HIV ward of a hospital in Puerto Rico [71]. They found that HIV ward patients with exposure to an infectious TB patient were 11 times more likely to contract TB than were HIV ward patients without such an exposure. In addition, nurses (i.e., those with patient care responsibilities) working on the HIV or internal medicine wards were significantly more likely to have a positive TST than clerical staff (i.e., those without direct patient care responsibilities) working on other wards at that hospital. This investigation documented that HIV-infected patients sharing a room with an HIV-infected patient with infectious TB were at increased risk of nosocomial acquisition of *M. tuberculosis*, that the incubation period was most consistent with primary infection, that the risk for development of active disease given exposure to an infectious TB patient was high, and that the duration from *M. tuberculosis* infection to disease (i.e., incubation period) was shortened in HIV-infected patients. These findings were consistent with those from another outbreak investigation that documented increased risk of nosocomial transmission of *M. tuberculosis* among hospitalized, HIV-infected patients [72].

Nosocomial *M. tuberculosis* Outbreaks

As with HCW TB infection or disease, there is no national surveillance or reporting system specifically for nosocomial *M. tuberculosis* outbreaks. Thus, our knowledge of such outbreaks is based on published reports. From 1960 through 1996, more than 20 nosocomial outbreaks in the United States were reported [2,38,48,61,62,71,73–87]. All of the reported outbreaks involved adults and airborne transmission. These outbreaks primarily occurred at acute care general medical–surgical facilities, but outbreaks at a hospice and a health department clinic also have been reported [75,76]. In the healthcare facility, outbreaks have involved the emergency department, inpatient medical wards, inpatient HIV wards, inpatient renal transplant ward, inpatient prison ward, intensive care units, surgical or radiology suites, the outpatient HIV clinic, and an autopsy suite. Most of the reports in the 1960s to 1980s involved patient-to-HCW *M. tuberculosis* transmission, and patient-to-patient transmission was infrequently detected or reported. In contrast, most of the reports in the 1980s and 1990s involved immunocompromised patients and have included both patient-to-patient and patient-to-HCW *M. tuberculosis* transmission. Since the late 1990s, additional reports of nosocomial TB outbreaks have been reported from a large number of international settings.

Nosocomial Multidrug-Resistant *M. tuberculosis* Outbreaks

In the late 1980s and early 1990s, numerous nosocomial TB outbreaks occurred in the United States caused by strains of *M. tuberculosis* resistant to ≥2 anti-TB agents, most commonly isoniazid and rifampin. In 1990, Edlin et al. investigated an outbreak of MDR-TB among acquired immunodeficiency syndrome (AIDS) patients at a New York City hospital [79]. From 1989 through 1990, 18 AIDS patients had acquired infections with *M. tuberculosis* strains resistant to isoniazid and streptomycin; in contrast, only 3 patients had had such infections in the preceding 3 years. Compared with 30 AIDS patients with TB caused by drug-susceptible strains of *M. tuberculosis*, the 18 MDR-TB AIDS patients were significantly more likely to be homosexual men, to have had AIDS for a longer period, or to have been hospitalized at the outbreak hospital within the 6 months preceding diagnosis of their TB. Furthermore, the MDR-TB patients were significantly more likely than AIDS patients infected with drug-susceptible strains of *M. tuberculosis* to have been hospitalized during their exposure period on the same ward at the same time as another patient with infectious MDR-TB. Compared with a group of AIDS patients infected with drug-susceptible strains of *M. tuberculosis* and similar durations of hospitalization, the MDR-TB AIDS patients were more likely to have occupied rooms closer to the room of an infectious MDR-TB patient. Restriction fragment length polymorphism (RFLP) analysis of the strains of 16 MDR-TB AIDS patients showed that 13 had an identical pattern. Thus, this investigation provided both epidemiologic and laboratory data supporting nosocomial acquisition of *M. tuberculosis* by these MDR-TB AIDS patients. The attack rate was 21/346 (6.1%) among all AIDS patients and 18/189 (9.5%) among AIDS patients hospitalized no more than two rooms away from an infectious MDR-TB AIDS patient's room. The estimated period from exposure to the development of active disease (i.e., incubation period) was estimated at 1.5 to 6.0 months. An environmental evaluation showed that only 1/16 patients' rooms had negative pressure. A TST survey conducted at the time of the investigation identified TST conversions (from documented negative to positive) in 11/60 (18.3%) HCWs; those with a follow-up TST >2 years before their baseline negative TST had a TST conversion rate of 9/31 (29.0%), whereas those with a follow-up TST of ≤2 years after their negative baseline had a TST conversion rate of 2/29 (6.9%) [88]. The *M. tuberculosis* strain from the one HCW with active MDR-TB had an RFLP pattern identical to that of the MDR-TB AIDS patient's strain.

At about the same time as the aforementioned outbreak, another MDR-TB outbreak, caused by a strain of *M. tuberculosis* resistant to isoniazid and rifampin, was occurring at a hospital in Florida [80,81,87]. From 1988 through 1990, 25 MDR-TB patients were identified among HIV-infected patients admitted to the hospital's HIV ward. Compared with HIV ward patients with TB caused by drug-susceptible strains, the MDR-TB patients were more likely to have had an opportunistic infection before being diagnosed with TB, to have been exposed to an AFB sputum smear-positive MDR-TB patient during their hospitalization preceding the diagnosis of TB, to have failed to respond to anti-TB therapy, or to have died. MDR-TB patients remained AFB sputum smear positive for a significantly longer proportion of their hospitalization than did HIV-infected patients with TB caused by drug-susceptible strains 375/860 (44%) vs. 197/1445 (14%) person-days. Exposure to AFB sputum smear-positive, culture-positive patients was significantly more likely to result in transmission of *M. tuberculosis* than was exposure to AFB sputum smear-negative, culture-positive patients. Exposures to infectious MDR-TB patients occurred both on the HIV ward and the HIV outpatient clinic. Patients who attended the HIV clinic to receive aerosolized pentamidine were at higher risk for development of MDR-TB than were those attending the clinic but not receiving aerosolized pentamidine. All of the available 13 MDR-TB patient *M. tuberculosis* isolates had one of two RFLP patterns. HCWs on the HIV ward and clinic were significantly more likely than HCWs on a comparison ward to have a TST conversion during the study period (13/39 vs. 0/15). There was a strong correlation between risk for HCW *M. tuberculosis* infection and the number of days that an AFB sputum smear-positive MDR-TB patient was hospitalized on the HIV ward. Six of the 23 AFB isolation rooms were found to have positive pressure. In the HIV clinic, the aerosolized pentamidine administration rooms had positive pressure compared with the treatment room, which was positive pressure relative to the discharge waiting room; also, air from the patient treatment rooms was recirculated back into the clinic.

From 1990 through 1992, the CDC conducted nine nosocomial MDR-TB outbreak investigations [7,43,57,79–85,87–89] (Table 32-2). These outbreaks all occurred between 1988 and 1992 and involved 8 to 42 (median, 18) patients at each facility. Seven of nine outbreaks occurred in New York state, with six of these in New York City hospitals. In all of the outbreaks, the *M. tuberculosis* strain transmitted was resistant to isoniazid; in eight outbreaks, the strain also was resistant to rifampin. Depending on the outbreak, the strains were also resistant to streptomycin, ethambutol, ethionamide, kanamycin, or rifabutin. In two outbreaks, some of the infecting strains were resistant to seven anti-TB agents [43,57]. The proportion of patients in these outbreaks who had HIV infections ranged from 12.5% to 100.0%; most of these outbreaks occurred either on HIV wards or on wards where most of the patients admitted had HIV infection. Mortality ranged from 12.5% to 93.0% (median, 83.0%). The interval from TB diagnosis until death ranged from 4 to 16 (median, 4) weeks. Subsequent nosocomial TB outbreaks in the United States and throughout the world have had similar findings.

Risk Factors for Nosocomial Transmission of Drug-Susceptible or Multidrug-Resistant *M. tuberculosis*

A wide variety of factors was responsible for patient-to-patient or patient-to-HCW *M. tuberculosis* transmission in these outbreaks (Table 32-3). These included factors affecting the likelihood of exposure, of infection given exposure, and of active disease given infection. Patient risk factors included having HIV or AIDS, prior hospitalization at the outbreak hospital, the close proximity of AFB sputum smear-positive (i.e., infectious) TB patients and patients with HIV infection or AIDS, or exposure to an infectious TB patient either because of close proximity of the rooms or exposures outside the patient's room. Other risk factors included delayed recognition of TB in the patient because of nonclassic signs, symptoms, or chest radiograph; low index of suspicion by physicians; delayed recognition of infecting MDR-TB strains because of delayed laboratory identification or communication to the clinicians; and delayed institution of effective antituberculosis therapy. In addition, a number of inadequate infection control practices were identified, including delayed initiation of appropriate AFB isolation; isolation rooms without at least six air changes per hour, negative pressure, or air exhausted to the outside; failure to isolate TB patients until they were no longer infectious; lapses in AFB isolation such as allowing infectious patients in isolation to leave their rooms without wearing a mask or for nonmedical reasons (e.g., to attend group social events, to walk the halls, go to common bathrooms, or visit the lounge or television areas); leaving AFB isolation room doors open; inadequate duration of AFB isolation; and inadequate precautions during aerosol-generating procedures such as sputum

TABLE 32-2

CHARACTERISTICS OF CENTERS FOR DISEASE CONTROL AND PREVENTION-INVESTIGATED NOSOCOMIAL MULTIDRUG-RESISTANT *MYCOBACTERIUM TUBERCULOSIS* OUTBREAKS, 1988–1992

Hospital	Outbreak Period	Number of Case-Patients	Number HIV-Positive Case-Patients (%)	Outbreak Ward	Mortality Number (%)	Infecting Strain Resistance Pattern[a]	RFLP Type	Number Healthcare Worker TST Conversions (%)	Number Isolation Rooms Negative Pressure (%)	References
1	1988–1989	25	25(100%)	HIV	21 (84%)	INH, RIF	Two strains	13/39 (33%)	17/23 (74%)	[80,81]
2	1988–1990	18	18(100)	Medicine	10 (56)	INH, SM	One strain	11/60 (18)	1/16 (6)	[79,88]
3	1989–1991	17	16(94)	Medicine	14 (82)	INH, RIF, SM	One strain	88/352 (25)[b]	None	[57]
4	1990–1991	23	21(91)	HIV	19 (83)	INH, RIF	One strain	6/12 (50)	None	[82]
5	1991–1991	8	1(12.5)	Medicine	1 (12.5)	INH, RIF, EMB, ETA, KM, SM, RTB	One strain	46/696 (6.6)	None	[43]
6	1990–1991	16	14(88)	Medicine	14 (88)	INH, RIF, SM	One strain	Unknown	None	[84]
7	1990–1992	13	13(100)	Infectious disease	11 (85)	INH, RIF	One strain	5/10 (50)	None	[83]
8	1991–1992	37	35(96)	HIV	34 (93)	INH, RIF	One strain	Unknown	None	[87]
9	1990–1992	42	41(98)	Prison	32 (79)	INH, RIF	One strain	N/A	None	[89]

[a]HIV, human immunodeficiency virus; RFLP, restriction fragment length polymorphism; TST, tuberculin skin test; INH, isoniazid; RIF, rifampin; EMB, ethambutol; ETA, ethionamide; KM, kanamycin; SM, streptomycin; RBT, rifabutin; N/A, not applicable.

[b]Eleven healthcare workers with active tuberculosis.

TABLE 32-3
RISK FACTORS FOR NOSOCOMIAL TRANSMISSION OF DRUG-SUSCEPTIBLE AND MULTIDRUG-RESISTANT *M. TUBERCULOSIS*

Patient risk factors
  Human immunodeficiency virus infection
  Acquired immunodeficiency syndrome
  Low CD4 T-lymphocyte count
  Prior hospital admission
    Admission to a room near (<3 rooms) an infectious MDR-TB
      patient
    Exposure to an AFB sputum smear-positive MDR-TB patient
Clinical risk factors
  Delayed diagnosis
    Nonclassic signs/symptoms
    Nonclassic chest radiograph
    Low index of suspicion of tuberculosis by physicians
    Delays in laboratory results (identification and susceptibility)
  Delayed patient isolation
    Low index of suspicion of tuberculosis
    Delayed recognition of MDR-TB
    Inadequate number of isolation rooms
  Delayed institution of effective therapy
    Delayed recognition of MDR-TB
    Delayed laboratory susceptibility data
Infection control factors
  Inadequate isolation
    Isolation rooms
    Positive pressure
      <6 Air changes per hr
      Air recirculated
      Doors open
    Infectious patients leave rooms
      For nonmedical reasons (social, smoking, TV)
      Premature discontinuation of isolation
  Inadequate precautions during aerosol generating procedures
  Inadequate microbiologic methods
    AFB smears not done
    Slow turnaround of identification and susceptibility testing
    Rapid methods not performed for
      Culture
      Identification
      Antimicrobial susceptibility testing
    Delayed communication of results from referral laboratories
    Delayed communication of results to clinicians
    Failure to monitor *M. tuberculosis* antimicrobial
      susceptibility results
    Failure to maintain or analyze results/records of
      M. tuberculosis identification or susceptibility testing

MDR-TB, multidrug-resistant tuberculosis; AFB, acid-fast bacilli.

induction or aerosolization of pentamidine. Last, delay in institution of effective therapy contributed to prolonged infectiousness and increased the risk of transmission of MDR-TB strains.

In these and other MDR-TB outbreaks, the failure to rapidly identify and appropriately isolate infectious patients combined with the prolonged infectiousness of these patients secondary to delays in diagnosis and treatment led to exposure of other patients and HCWs. In each outbreak, the major risk factor for MDR-TB or for a TST conversion was exposure to an infectious MDR-TB patient. A low index of suspicion for TB in HIV-infected patients with pulmonary symptoms and the fact that many of the MDR-TB patients did not present with classic TB signs, symptoms, or chest radiographs (i.e., cavitary or miliary patterns) may have contributed to delayed identification of infectious MDR-TB patients [13,85,86]. In some instances, neither TSTs nor AFB sputum smears were performed on potentially infectious patients. Most MDR-TB patients had abnormal chest radiographs; however, they usually had interstitial patterns rather than classic miliary or cavitary patterns. When cultures were obtained, the results of the cultures or antituberculosis susceptibility testing were not available for a median of 7 weeks because the most rapid methods were not used; in some instances, the results were not available for 6 months. These delays in diagnosis resulted in delays in recognition of MDR-TB, in instituting effective anti-TB therapy, and in appropriate patient isolation; in turn, these lapses resulted in prolonged periods of exposure of infectious TB patients to other patients and HCWs. Although in most of the outbreaks infectious TB patients were the source, outbreaks have been associated with an HCW with infectious TB and with irrigation or manipulation of an undiagnosed tuberculous skin abscess or ulcer [57,75,76,78,85,86].

Molecular Typing of Multidrug-Resistant *M. tuberculosis* Outbreak Isolates

A critical element in confirming the epidemiologic evidence of nosocomial *M. tuberculosis* transmission in each of the MDR-TB outbreak investigations was the molecular typing of the infecting strains (see Chapter 10). In the early 1990s, a new method to type *M. tuberculosis* isolates, RFLP, was developed [90,91]. Thus, in each MDR-TB outbreak, available isolates from patients and HCWs with active TB disease were obtained and RFLP typed. Although occasionally a similar strain was identified at more than one facility, particularly in New York City where patients may have either had contact in or outside of the hospital, in most instances, one or more unique strains was documented to have been transmitted within each facility (see Table 32-2). In one instance, use of a newly developed polymerase chain reaction–based RFLP method was necessary because the source-case isolate was no longer viable [87,91]. The combination of epidemiologic and molecular typing data conclusively proved that MDR-TB strains were being transmitted within these facilities. Future application of RFLP and other molecular typing techniques should facilitate further elucidation of nosocomial and community transmission of *M. tuberculosis*. On the other-hand, depending only on RFLP typing to confirm an outbreak without supporting epidemiologic data can lead to erroneous conclusions.

Risk for Tuberculosis Infection in Healthcare Workers

In each outbreak, occupational acquisition of TB was suspected. However, conclusive documentation was difficult because in most instances, the HCWs had infection but not disease. Furthermore, at a number of the outbreak hospitals, the HCW TST program was inadequate; often, the HCWs had not had either a baseline two-step TST or a routine TST within the past 1 to 2 years [80,82,86,88]. At one MDR-TB outbreak hospital, 18% of HCWs in whom a TST was applied during the investigation had a positive TST; MDR-TB developed in one HCW, and the infecting isolate had the same RFLP pattern as that recovered from MDR-TB outbreak patients [79,88]. In one investigation, HCWs with or without TST conversions on the outbreak ward were similar in age, race, sex, duration of employment on the outbreak ward, occupation, and shift worked [80]. However, compared with HCWs on control wards where TB patients were not admitted, outbreak ward and clinic HCWs were at significantly greater risk for TST conversion. Risk for TST conversion was associated with exposure to MDR-TB patients who were AFB sputum smear positive rather than to drug-susceptible TB patients; HCW infection risk was significantly lower (although not zero) when they had exposure to AFB sputum smear-negative, culture-positive patients. In three MDR-TB outbreak hospitals, adequate TST data were available to assess HCW TST conversion risk; at these institutions, 22% to 50% of HCWs had TST conversions during the outbreak periods [79,80,82–86]. At the time of these investigations, at least 16 HCWs had contracted active MDR-TB; 7 were HIV positive, 7 were HIV negative, and 2 were of unknown HIV status [85]. Five of the 16 (31.2%) HCWs died; 80.0% were known to be HIV infected. In many if not most instances, HCWs were not wearing the 1990 CDC TB guideline-recommended respiratory protection (i.e., particulate [dust-mist, dust-fume-mist, or high-efficiency particulate air filter [HEPA]] respirators); often, the HCWs either wore no or improperly wore respiratory protection [53].

TUBERCULOSIS INFECTION CONTROL PROGRAMS IN THE UNITED STATES

The aforementioned nosocomial MDR-TB outbreaks raised considerable concern about the status of TB infection control programs at U.S. hospitals. Several surveys have been conducted to assess these programs. In 1992, the American Hospital Association (AHA) in collaboration with the CDC conducted a survey of all U.S. municipal, Veterans Administration, and university hospitals, and a 20% random sample of private hospitals [67]. Responses were received from 763 (71%) of the 1,076 surveyed hospitals; of the 763 respondents, 178 (25%) hospitals in 39 states admitted MDR-TB patients. Among the

763 hospitals, the number of AFB isolation rooms meeting 1990 CDC TB guidelines recommendations ranged from 0–60 (median, 7); 219 (29%) hospitals had no AFB isolation rooms meeting the CDC criteria. HCW TST programs varied widely. Fifteen (2%) reported nosocomial transmission of M. tuberculosis to patients, and 91 (13%) reported TB transmission to HCWs.

In 1993, the Society of Healthcare Epidemiology of America (SHEA) in collaboration with the CDC conducted a survey of the SHEA membership, most of whom are at medical school–affiliated teaching hospitals [19,20]. From 1989 through 1992, the number of SHEA member hospitals admitting MDR-TB patients increased from 10/166 (10%) to 49/166 (30%). During this period, the median HCW TST positivity rate at the time of hire increased from 0.54% to 0.81%; in contrast, the median HCW TST conversion rate remained stable at ~0.34% during the period (range, 0.35% to 0.33%). AFB isolation rooms meeting CDC 1990 TB guideline recommendations were reported at 113/181 (62%) hospitals responding to the question. During the study period, the proportion of 191 respondent hospitals in which surgical submicron masks or dust-mist or dust-fume-mist respirators were used increased from 9 (5%) to 85 (43%).

In another survey, conducted in 1993 by the Association for Professionals in Infection Control and Epidemiology (APIC) in collaboration with the CDC and covering the same period, most of the 1,494 respondents were smaller community hospitals, and the proportion of hospitals admitting drug-susceptible tuberculosis or MDR-TB patients increased from 46.4% to 56.6% and 0.8% to 4.5%, respectively [21]. From 1989 through 1992, the HCW pooled mean TST positivity rate at hire rose from 0.95% to 1.14%, and the TST conversion rate increased from 0.4% to 0.5%. In 1992, rooms compliant with the CDC 1990 TB guideline recommendations for AFB isolation were reported at 66% of the hospitals, and at 64% of the hospitals' HCWs still used surgical masks for respiratory protection; from 1989 through 1992, the number of hospitals in which particulate respirators were used increased from 0.4% to 13.8%.

Nosocomial transmission of M. tuberculosis is a particular concern in emergency departments where a wide variety of patients, many of whom have fever and cough, seeks care. Moran et al. found that among patients with active pulmonary TB at an urban emergency department, TB was often not suspected, and isolation of these infectious patients was delayed [92]. In 1993, Moran et al. conducted a survey of infection control practices in emergency departments at a sample of the hospitals responding to the AHA/CDC survey [93]. Of the 446 emergency departments surveyed, 298 returned completed questionnaires. The proportion of emergency departments in which TB patients were seen daily, weekly, monthly, or less frequently was 12.6%, 17.2%, 23.3%, and 46.9%, respectively. The proportion in which TB isolation rooms meeting CDC 1990

TB guideline recommendations were available in triage or waiting rooms or in the emergency department itself was 1.7% and 19.6%, respectively. One or more HCWs had TST conversions in 16.1% of the surveyed emergency departments in 1991 and 26.9% in 1992. Prevention and control of M. tuberculosis in emergency departments depends on (1) education of the staff about the high-risk groups for and signs and symptoms of TB so that they will suspect and promptly identify infectious patients; (2) ensuring that emergency departments have adequate isolation facilities for infectious TB patients; (3) rapid isolation of screened patients who may have infectious TB; and (4) a comprehensive HCW TST program.

The microbiology laboratory plays a critical role in the rapid identification of infectious TB patients (see Chapter 10). However, the microbiologic methods used in many laboratories are not the most rapid, and communication between the laboratories and the clinicians often is inadequate [13,19–21,67,94]. In one survey of U.S. hospital based laboratories, rapid methods were used for AFB microscopy in 47%, primary culture in 72%, M. tuberculosis identification in 38%, and drug susceptibility testing in 13% of the laboratories surveyed [67]. Approximately 46% of hospitals surveyed and an estimated 30% of laboratories at all U.S. hospitals with ≥100 beds performed the minimal number of mycobacterial cultures deemed necessary to maintain competence [12,13]. Fortunately, since 1992, there has been a significant improvement in compliance with recommended methods for AFB smear, culture, and antimicrobial susceptibility testing [13].

These outbreak and survey data show that the emergence of MDR-TB as a major public health problem was associated with the incomplete implementation of the CDC TB guideline recommendations [9,55,56]. Many hospitals do not have the recommended patient isolation facilities, HCW TST or respiratory protection programs, or laboratory processing practices. Although the APIC/CDC survey shows that as many as 50% of community hospitals do not admit TB patients routinely and few admit MDR-TB patients, the SHEA/CDC and AHA/CDC surveys show that urban, larger hospitals and those with a medical school affiliation routinely admit TB or MDR-TB patients [19–21,67]. Data from the SHEA/CDC and APIC/CDC surveys show that there continues to be improvement in the degree of implementation of CDC TB guideline recommendations since the initial AHA/CDC survey. Many, if not most, of the inadequate TB infection control practices reported in the United States exist in healthcare facilities throughout the world. More recently, Manangan et al. in another survey of U.S. hospitals confirmed that from 1992 through 1996, there was continued implementation of the 1994 CDC TB Guideline recommendations and a decreased in HCW TST conversion [95]. In a 1995 survey in Belgium, Ronveaux et al. found that many of the conditions facilitating M. tuberculosis transmission (failure to detect and isolate patients, mixing of HAV and TB patients in the same unit,

HCWs not wearing appropriate respiratory protection, and failing to monitor HCW TSTs) were common and that TB infection control practices needed improvement. [96]

Efficacy of the CDC Tuberculosis Guidelines Recommendations

The nosocomial TB and especially the MDR-TB outbreaks raised concern in the infectious disease, infection control, occupational medicine, and industrial hygiene communities about the effectiveness of the CDC TB guideline recommendations [9,55,56]. To assess the efficacy of these control measures, follow-up investigations were conducted at three of the hospitals where MDR-TB outbreaks had occurred and at one where a drug-susceptible M. tuberculosis outbreak occurred. In each MDR-TB hospital, a wide variety of infection control measures, similar to those in the CDC 1990 and 1994 TB guideline, was implemented (Tables 32-4 and 32-5). Because same-ward exposure to an infectious MDR-TB patient was identified as the most significant risk factor in the initial MDR-TB outbreak investigations, this was assessed as a measure of nosocomial or occupational acquisition of TB in the follow-up studies. In the first follow-up investigation at an MDR-TB outbreak hospital in New York City, Maloney et al. documented that the proportion of patients with MDR-TB strains decreased, the proportion of MDR-TB patients with same-ward exposures decreased, and the TST conversion rates of HCWs assigned to the outbreak wards were lower in the follow-up or intervention period than in the outbreak period [97]. In the second follow-up investigation, Wenger et al. showed that, after implementation of control measures on the MDR-TB outbreak HIV ward, no episodes of MDR-TB could be traced to contact with infectious MDR-TB patients and that HCW TST conversions were terminated [98]. In the third follow-up study, Stroud et al. documented that, after implementation of recommended CDC TB infection control measures, the MDR-TB attack rate for AIDS patients decreased from 19/216 (8.8%) to 5/193 (2.6%) [99]. Blumberg et al. conducted a fourth follow-up investigation at a hospital in which a drug-susceptible M. tuberculosis outbreak had occurred [86,100]. Their study documented that, after the hospital introduced mostly administrative controls—more rapid identification of infectious TB patients, isolation of infectious patients in rooms with increased air exhaust, and improved HCW respiratory protection—a decrease occurred in the number of exposures to infectious TB patients (4.4 to 0.6 per month), cumulative number of days per month that infectious TB patients were not in isolation (35.4 to 3.3), and HCW TST conversions (3.3% to 0.4%) [100].

Despite the fact that none of these interventions was a randomized controlled trial or that each of the individual components was independently assessed, each of these studies shows that with more complete implementation of administrative and engineering/environmental controls

TABLE 32-4

EVALUATION OF PREVENTIVE INTERVENTIONS ON PATIENT-TO-PATIENT MDR-TB TRANSMISSION AT THREE MDR-TB OUTBREAK HOSPITALS

Hospital	Initial Period	Intervention Period	Number of Case-Patients			Proportion of Patients with MDR-TB[a]		Mortality		Nosocomial MDR-TB Exposure	
			Outbreak Period	Intervention Period	Total	Outbreak Period	Intervention Period[a]	Outbreak Period	Intervention Period	Outbreak Period	Intervention Period
1	Jan. 90–May 90	Jun. 90–Jun. 92	15	11	26	26/180	28/498[b] (TB)	—	—	12	0
2	Jan. 89–Mar. 90	Apr. 90–Sep. 92	16	22	38	19/216	9/277 (A)	6	8	11	5[c]
4	Jan. 90–Jun. 91	Jul. 91–Aug. 92	30	10	40	30/95	10/70[c] (O)	25	4	20	1[d]

MDR-TB, multidrug-resistant tuberculosis.

[a] All tuberculosis patients (TB), all outbreak ward patients (O), or all AIDS patients (A).

[b] $p < 0.01$.

[c] Four patients were exposed on HIV ward in initial period, $p = 002$.

[d] $p = 0.003$.

TABLE 32-5

EVALUATION OF PREVENTIVE INTERVENTIONS ON PATIENT TO HEALTHCARE WORKER MDR-TB TRANSMISSION AT THREE MDR-TB OUTBREAK HOSPITALS

Hospital	Initial Period	Intervention Period	Susceptible HCWs		Number of HCWs with Tuberculin Skin Test Conversion		Number of HCWs with Active TB		Total
			Initial Period	Intervention Period	Initial Period	Intervention Period	Initial Period	Intervention Period	
1	Jan. 90–May 90	Jun. 90–Jun. 92	25	27	7	3[a,b]	1	0	1
2	Jan. 89–Mar. 90	Apr. 90–Sep. 92	60	29	11	5	4	0	4
4	Jan. 89–Jun. 91	Jul. 91–Aug. 92	90	78	15	4[c]	1	1	2

MDR-TB, multidrug resistant tuberculosis; HCW, healthcare worker.
[a]All had been exposed to unknown infectious MDR-TB patient.
[b]$p < 0.01$.
[c]$p < 0.02$.

and use of respiratory protective devices for HCWs, *M. tuberculosis* outbreaks can be terminated and further *M. tuberculosis* transmission from patient to patient or patient to HCW can be either terminated or reduced to background TB rates seen on wards where TB patients are not admitted routinely [89]. These data document that the CDC TB guidelines work if they are fully implemented.

CDC Tuberculosis Guidelines

In 1990, the CDC published *Guidelines for Preventing the Transmission of Tuberculosis in Health Care Settings, with Special Focus on HIV-Related Issues* [53]. In 1994, CDC published *Guidelines for Preventing the Transmission of Tuberculosis in Health-Care Facilities, 1994* [56]. Most recently, the 1994 guideline has been updated, in *Guidelines for Preventing the Transmission of Mycobacterium tuberculosis in Health-Care Settings, 2005* [9]. These guidelines provide the elements of an infection control program to prevent the transmission of *M. tuberculosis* in healthcare facilities. Emphasis is placed on methods to prevent the generation of infectious airborne droplet nuclei, early identification of infectious TB patients, preventing the spread of *M. tuberculosis* through source controls, air disinfection to reduce microbial contamination of the air, disinfection and sterilization, and surveillance for TB infection or disease in HCWs. Recommendations for patient AFB isolation rooms included having six or more air changes per hour, negative pressure in relation to other rooms or corridors, and exhausting the air from the room directly to the outside. The guidelines also recommend the use of particulate respirators as respiratory protection for HCWs.

As a result of the nosocomial TB outbreaks and in response to requests for changes or clarifications in the CDC 1990 TB guidelines, the CDC revised these guidelines and published the *Guidelines for Preventing the Transmission of Mycobacterium tuberculosis in Health-Care Facilities, 1994* and then updated them in 2005 [9,56] (Table 32-6). The 1994 and 2005 CDC TB guidelines include a recommendations section followed by extensive supplement material. The recommendations include sections on assignment of responsibility, risk assessment, development of the TB infection control program, and periodic risk assessment; identifying, evaluating, and initiating treatment for patients who may have active TB; management of patients in ambulatory care settings or emergency departments who may have active TB; management of hospitalized patients who have confirmed or suspected TB; engineering control recommendations; HCW protection; cough-inducing and aerosol-generating procedures; education and training of HCWs; HCW counseling, screening, and evaluation; problem evaluation; coordination with the Public Health Department; and additional considerations for selected areas in healthcare facilities and other healthcare settings. The supplements include discussion of determining the infectiousness of a TB patient, diagnosis and treatment of both latent infection and active TB disease, engineering controls (i.e., ventilation and ultraviolet germicidal irradiation), respiratory protection, and decontamination (i.e., cleaning, disinfecting, and sterilizing of patient care equipment).

The major differences in the 2005 Guideline compared to the 1994 Guideline are:

- The risk assessment process includes the assessment of additional aspects of infection control.
- The term "tuberculin skin tests" (TSTs) is used instead of purified protein derivative (PPD).

TABLE 32-6

BASIC ELEMENTS OF AN EFFECTIVE TUBERCULOSIS (TB) INFECTION CONTROL PROGRAM[a]

I. Assignment of responsibility
   A. Assign responsibility for the TB infection control program to qualified people.
   B. Ensure that people with expertise in infection achieve at least 6 air changes per hr for existing control, occupational health, administration, and facilities and at least 12 air changes per hr for engineering are identified and included.

II. Risk assessment, TB infection control plan, and periodic reassessment
   A. Make initial risk assessments.
      1. Obtain information concerning TB in the community.
      2. Evaluate data concerning TB patients in the facility.
      3. Evaluate data concerning PPD tuberculin skin test conversions among HCWs in the facility.
      4. Rule out evidence of person-to-person transmission.
   B. Develop written TB infection-control program.
      1. Select initial risk protocol(s).
      2. Develop written TB infection control protocols.
   C. Repeat risk assessment at appropriate intervals.
      1. Review current community and facility surveillance data and PPD tuberculin skin test results.
      2. Review records of TB patients.
      3. Observe HCW infection control practices.
      4. Evaluate maintenance of engineering controls.

III. Identification, evaluation, and treatment of TB patients
   A. Screen patients for signs and symptoms of active TB
      1. On initial encounter in emergency department or ambulatory care setting.
      2. Before or at the time of admission.
   B. Perform radiologic and bacteriologic evaluation of patients who have signs and symptoms suggestive of TB.
   C. Promptly initiate treatment.
   D. Periodically reevaluate response to therapy; modify regimen if no improvement.

IV. Management of outpatients who have possible infectious TB
   A. Promptly initiate TB precautions.
   B. Place patients in separate waiting areas or TB isolation rooms.
   C. Give patients a surgical mask or box of tissues and instructions regarding the use of these items.
   D. Instruct patients to cover their mouth and nose with tissue when coughing or sneezing.

V. Management of inpatients who have possible infectious TB
   A. Promptly isolate patients who have suspected or known infectious TB.
   B. Monitor the response to treatment.
   C. Follow appropriate criteria for discontinuing isolation.

VI. Engineering recommendations
   A. Design local exhaust and general ventilation in collaboration with people who have expertise in ventilation engineering.
   B. Use a single-pass air system or air recirculation after HEPA filtration in areas where infectious TB patients receive care.
   C. Use additional measures, if needed, in areas where TB patients may receive care.
   D. Design TB isolation rooms in health care facilities to new or renovated facilities.
   E. Regularly monitor and maintain engineering controls.
   F. TB isolation rooms that are being used should be monitored daily to ensure they maintain negative pressure relative to the hallway and all surrounding area.
   G. Exhaust TB isolation room air to outside or, if absolutely unavoidable, recirculate after HEPA filtration.

VII. Initiation of respiratory protection
   A. Respiratory protective devices should meet recommended performance criteria.
   B. Respiratory protection should be used by people entering rooms in which patients with known or suspected infectious TB are being isolated, by HCWs when performing cough-inducing or aerosol-generating procedures on such patients, and by people in other settings where administrative and engineering controls are not likely to protect them from inhaling infectious airborne droplet nuclei.
   C. A respiratory protection program is required in all facilities in which respiratory protection is used to protect health care workers.

VIII. Use of cough-inducing procedures
   A. Do not perform such procedures on TB patients unless absolutely necessary.
   B. Perform such procedures in areas that have local exhaust ventilation devices (e.g., booths or special enclosures) or, if this is not feasible, in a room that meets the ventilation requirements for TB isolation.
   C. After completion of procedures, TB patients should remain in the booth or special enclosure until their coughing subsides.

IX. Implementation of HCW TB training and education
   A. All HCWs should receive periodic TB education appropriate for their work responsibilities and duties.
   B. Training should include the epidemiology of TB in the facility.
   C. TB education should emphasize concepts of the pathogenesis of and occupational risk for TB.
   D. Training should describe work practices that reduce the likelihood of transmitting *M. tuberculosis*.

TABLE 32-6
(CONTINUED)

   X. Implementation of HCW counseling and screening
      A. Counsel all HCWs regarding TB and TB infection.
      B. Counsel all HCWs about the increased risk to immunocompromised people for development of active TB.
      C. Perform PPD skin tests on HCWs at the beginning of their employment, and repeat PPD tests at periodic intervals.
      D. Evaluate symptomatic HCWs for active TB.
   XI. Evaluation of HCW PPD test conversions or blood assay for *M. tuberculosis* test and possible nosocomial transmission of *M. tuberculosis*.
  XII. Coordination of efforts with public health department

PPD, purified protein derivative; HCW, healthcare worker; HEPA, high-efficiency particulate air.
[a]A program such as this is appropriate for healthcare facilities in which there is a high risk for transmission of *M. tuberculosis*.
Adapted from Centers for Disease Control and Prevention. Guidelines for preventing the transmission of *Mycobacterium tuberculosis* in health-care facilities, 1994. *MMWR Moth Mortal Wkly Rep* 1994;43(RR1–13); and Guidelines for preventing the transmission of *Mycobacterium tuberculosis* in health-care facilities, 2005. *MMWR Moth Mortal Wkly Rep* 2005;54(RR–17).

- The whole-blood interferon gamma release assay (IGRA), QuantiFERON® TB Gold test (QFT-G) (Cellestis Limited, Carnegie, Victoria, Australia), an FDA-approved *in vitro* cytokine-based assay for cell-mediated immune reactivity to *M. tuberculosis* that can be used instead of TST in TB screening programs for HCWs. This IGRA is an example of a blood assay for *M. tuberculosis* (BAMT).
- The frequency of TB screening for HCWs has been decreased in various settings, and the criteria for determination of screening frequency have been changed.
- The scope of settings in which the guidelines apply has been broadened to include laboratories and additional outpatient and nontraditional facility-based settings.
- Criteria for serial testing for *M. tuberculosis* infection of HCWs are more clearly defined. In certain settings, this change will decrease the number of HCWs who need serial TB screening.
- These recommendations usually apply to an entire healthcare setting rather than areas within a setting.
- New terms—airborne infection precautions (airborne precautions) and airborne infection isolation room (AII room)—are introduced.
- Recommendations for annual respirator training, initial respirator fit testing, and periodic respirator fit testing have been added.
- The evidence of the need for respirator fit testing is summarized.
- Information on ultraviolet germicidal irradiation (UVGI) and room-air recirculation units has been expanded.
- Additional information regarding MDR TB and HIV infection has been included.

Hierarchy of Controls

The 1994 and 2005 CDC TB guidelines emphasize the importance of understanding the hierarchy of TB control measures; these include administrative controls to identify infectious TB patients promptly and to reduce HCW and patient exposure to such patients, engineering controls to reduce the generation and spread of airborne droplet nuclei, and respiratory protective devices to protect HCWs from inhalation of infectious airborne droplet nuclei. Although each of these measures was discussed in the 1990 CDC TB guidelines, the 1994 CDC TB guidelines highlight the importance of these measures. The first and most critical TB control measure is the use of administrative controls to reduce the risk of patient or HCW exposure to people with infectious TB. Compliance with this recommendation requires the development of effective written policies and protocols and implementation of these into practice to ensure that clinicians maintain a high index of suspicion for TB in patients with respiratory symptoms and conduct an appropriate diagnostic workup of patients suspected of having TB; that rapid laboratory techniques (fluorescence stains for AFB smears, radiometric methods for species identification and susceptibility testing, or genetic probes for species identification) are used; that laboratory results are rapidly communicated to clinicians; and that infectious TB patients are promptly isolated to minimize exposure to other patients or unprotected HCWs [9,55,56].

Administrative source controls are essential for preventing *M. tuberculosis* transmission. A critical element of any TB control program is education of HCWs about the epidemiology of TB, the importance of suspecting TB particularly in patients with HIV infection, the importance of HCW TST and respiratory protection programs, the need for clinicians to know the susceptibility of prevalent *M. tuberculosis* strains in the hospital and community, the importance of rapidly and appropriately isolating TB patients, and the importance of initiating an effective treatment regimen in infectious TB patients.

The next level of the hierarchy is the use of engineering/environmental controls to prevent the generation and spread of airborne droplet nuclei and to reduce the concentration of these infectious particles. These include (1) direct source control using local exhaust ventilation, (2) controlling the direction of air flow to prevent contamination of air in adjacent areas, (3) dilution and removal of contaminated air by general ventilation, and (4) air disinfection by air filtration or ultraviolet germicidal irradiation.

The third and last level of the hierarchy is the use of personal respiratory protective devices by HCWs in areas where the risk of exposure to infectious droplet nuclei and resultant occupational acquisition of *M. tuberculosis* is suspected to be higher than normal (e.g., AFB isolation rooms and where cough-inducing or aerosol-producing procedures are performed).

The outbreak investigations, the follow-up studies at outbreak hospitals, and the surveys have not documented the independent importance of these different measures. Furthermore, because the control measures recommended in the CDC TB guidelines are intended to be implemented as a group, neglecting any one measure could lead to the failure of the others to eliminate or reduce nosocomial transmission of *M. tuberculosis*. Most of the nosocomial or occupational acquisition of TB results from exposure to an unsuspected or undetected infectious TB patient.

Risk Assessment

Another important element of the 1994 and 2005 CDC TB guidelines is the introduction of the concept of conducting a risk assessment. The purpose of the risk assessment is to identify healthcare facilities or areas within those facilities in which the risk of exposure to infectious TB patients and subsequent patient-to-patient or patient-to-HCW *M. tuberculosis* transmission is minimal, very low, low, intermediate, or high. In this way, the TB control program can be individualized for a specific area or hospital so that high- or low-risk facilities would not need to comply with the same recommendations; greater flexibility could be given both between and within institutions. This risk assessment is used to determine the frequency of HCW TST, repeat risk assessment, and ventilation evaluation and to suggest supplemental engineering/environmental interventions.

Tuberculosis Control Program

The basic elements of the TB control program are applicable to all types of healthcare facilities (Table 32-6). These elements emphasize the following:

- Use of rapid laboratory methods to facilitate rapid diagnosis of TB patients.
- The recommendation that smear results be available within 24 hours of specimen collection.
- The importance of considering tuberculosis in HIV-infected patients even if another pathogen is identified.
- The importance of rapid evaluation and triage of infectious patients in outpatient settings.

- The importance of directly observed therapy.
- That patient TB isolation rooms (i.e., private room, negative pressure, ≥6 air changes per hour, air exhausted directly outside) can have recirculation of air to the same patient's room or general ventilation if the air is passed through a HEPA filter in the ventilation system.
- That all infectious TB patients (drug susceptible or MDR-TB strains) remain in isolation until clinically improved *and* have negative AFB sputum smears on 3 consecutive days (because the decision to remove from isolation is usually made before susceptibility results are available).
- That consideration should be given to keeping MDR-TB patients in AFB isolation for their entire hospitalization.
- That discharge should be coordinated with the community's public health department and private clinicians so that compliance with therapy is ensured and to avoid exposure of individuals to an infectious TB patient outside of the healthcare setting.

Respiratory Protection

The 1990 CDC TB guidelines recommended particulate respirators, which include dust-mist, dust-fume-mist, or HEPA filter respirators, for use as respiratory protection against TB. However, the 1994 CDC TB guidelines established new criteria for respiratory protection: (1) the ability to filter particles 1 μm in size (in the unloaded state) with a filter efficiency of 95% or better (i.e., filter leakage <5%), given flow rates of up to 50 liters/minute, (2) the ability to be qualitatively or quantitatively fit tested in a reliable way, (3) the ability to be adequately fit checked before each use in a reliable way, and (4) the ability to fit HCWs with different facial sizes and characteristics, which can usually be met by the availability of at least three sizes of respirator. The criteria were based on the characteristics thought to be most desirable in a respirator and on the in-use experience at drug-susceptible or MDR-TB outbreak hospitals where patient-to-HCW *M. tuberculosis* transmission was terminated by using submicron masks or dust-mist respirators with implementation of the 1990 CDC TB guidelines recommendations [97–101].

When the 1990 CDC TB guidelines first recommended particulate respirators to protect HCWs from occupational acquisition of *M. tuberculosis*, it became clear that the use of respirators was for protection of HCWs from patient infections, not vice versa. This area then came under the jurisdiction of the U.S. Occupational Safety and Health Administration (OSHA) [101,102]. Thereafter, no matter which respirator was recommended, the law required an HCW respirator training, education, and fit testing program. Also, OSHA requires that, in the United States when HCWs wear a respiratory protective device to protect them from disease, they must use a National Institute for Occupational Safety and Health (NIOSH)–certified respirator. Therefore, in 1992, OSHA asked NIOSH to assess and recommend which respirator would be required to protect HCWs from occupational *M. tuberculosis* acquisition. Because of a lack of data about the concentration of *M. tuberculosis* in airborne droplet nuclei, what the minimal infectious dose is, the exact size and size distribution of airborne droplet nuclei particles, the potential of mortality given infection, the risk of toxic reaction from anti-TB prophylactic or therapeutic agents, and the NIOSH/OSHA interest in providing a zero-risk environment, NIOSH recommended a powered air-purifying respirator (PAPR) with a HEPA filter for moderate exposures and a positive-pressure, air-line respirator with a tight-fitting half-mask respirator for high-risk exposures [92]. By law, NIOSH may not consider either cost or practicality in making its recommendation. During 1992 and 1993, various OSHA regions made respirator recommendations ranging from dust-mist respirators to PAPRs. Subsequent to the publication of the 1994 TB Guideline, NIOSH recommended that a respirator providing protection equal to or greater than an N-95 (i.e., that it would be certified to filter at least 95% of particles of ≥ 1 μm) was required.

To understand the complexity involved in arriving at an appropriate respirator recommendation for HCWs to prevent occupational acquisition of *M. tuberculosis*, it is important to understand the relationship between OSHA and NIOSH and the laws specific to the United States [101]. OSHA requires that any respiratory protective device used to protect HCWs must be NIOSH certified [103]. Before 1995, the existing NIOSH respirator certification process did not adequately test the efficacy of dust-mist or dust-fume-mist respirators against low-concentration aerosols in the size range of *M. tuberculosis* droplet nuclei (best estimated at 1 to 5 μm). Subsequently, studies documented that there was wide variability in penetration of dust-mist or dust-fume-mist respirators when challenged by either 1-μm particles or *M. chelonae* aerosols [104]. Although some manufacturers' dust-mist or dust-fume-mist respirators prevented $\geq 95\%$ of these particles from penetrating, other manufacturers' respirators allowed up to 40% penetration. Thus, in contrast to HEPA filter respirators (equivalent to the current N-95 respirators), all of which are certified to prevent penetration of <0.03% of 0.3 μm particles, the efficacy of dust-mist and dust-fume-mist respirators varied widely, was not certified by NIOSH, and thus could not be ensured. For this reason, the 1994 CDC TB guidelines indicated that although some dust-mist or dust-fume-mist respirators would meet the new guidelines criteria, only HEPA-filtered (now N-95) respirators always meet these criteria and were certified by NIOSH to do so [56,101,105].

In 1996, NIOSH implemented a new respirator certification process that tests respirators with a 0.3 μm test particle and designates them into different classes of respirator based on 99.95%, 99.00%, or 95.00% filtration efficacy [106]. All three classes of respirators surpass the minimum filter criteria recommended in the 1994 CDC TB guidelines (i.e., the ability to filter 95% of 1 μm particles). These 95% filtration efficiency respirators, designated N-, P-, or R-95s, are available for use to protect HCWs

from occupational exposure to *M. tuberculosis*. Because of the 1994 TB guidelines recommendations and this new NIOSH respirator certification process, a greater variety of respirators and respirator sizes has become available at lower cost to protect HCWs from *M. tuberculosis*. Follow-up data at several of the MDR-TB outbreak hospitals show that use of submicron surgical masks or dust-mist respirators by HCWs together with implementation of recommendations similar to those in the 1990 CDC TB guidelines terminated patient-to-HCW *M. tuberculosis* transmission on outbreak wards [97–101]. Furthermore, survey data have shown that at healthcare facilities with >6 TB patients or with >200 beds, respirators with submicron filter capability reduce the risk of HCW TST conversion [19,20]. In addition, studies show that some dust-mist or dust-fume-mist respirators filter >95% of particles with a mean size of 0.8 μm, smaller than the estimated particle size of *M. tuberculosis* droplet nuclei [105]. The new NIOSH respirator certification process permits the use of respirators similar to those shown to be effective in outbreak settings and reduces some of the controversy surrounding the use of respirators in healthcare facilities to protect HCWs from *M. tuberculosis*.

Respirator education and fit-test programs are integral parts of the U.S.-required HCW respiratory protection program. These are mandated by OSHA for any HCW potentially exposed to *M. tuberculosis*. Factors to consider when selecting a respirator include face-seal leakage and the ability to fit test and fit check the respirator. HCWs with facial hair (e.g., beards) will not be able to get an adequate face seal with the new N-95 or older particulate respirators. For these HCWs, particularly those performing very high-risk procedures on infectious TB patients, PARPs may be an alternative. In the United States, filtering face-piece respirators used for protection against *M. tuberculosis* must be selected from those approved by CDC/NIOSH under the provisions of 42 CFR 84 (**www.cdc.gov/niosh/npptl/part84.pdf**) [107]. A listing of CDC/NIOSH-approved disposable particulate respirators (filtering face pieces) is available at **www.cdc .gov/niosh/npptl/topics/respirators/disp_part**. On October 17, 1997, OSHA published a proposed standard for occupational exposure to *M. tuberculosis*. On December 31, 2003, OSHA announced the termination of rulemaking for a TB standard. Previous OSHA policy permitted the use of any Part 84 particulate filter respirator for protection against infection with *M. tuberculosis*. Respirator usage for TB had been regulated by OSHA under CFR Title 29, Part 1910.139 (29 CFR 1910.139) and compliance policy directive (CPL) 2.106 (Enforcement Procedures and Scheduling for Occupational Exposure to Tuberculosis). In addition, the 1994 and 2005 CDCTB guidelines recommend annual fit testing for HCWs. However, in 2004, the U.S. Congress passed the Fiscal Year (FY) 2005 Omnibus Spending Bill, which was signed by the President George W. Bush, prohibiting OSHA from enforcing the annual fit testing mandate for occupational exposure to *M. tuberculosis* in U.S. healthcare facilities for FY 2005.

Healthcare Worker Education/Problem Evaluation

Another new section in the 1994 (and expanded in 2005) CDC TB guidelines is on education and training of HCWs. All HCWs with possible *M. tuberculosis* exposure should be taught the epidemiology of TB; the potential for occupational exposure; the principles of TB infection control; the importance of routine and periodic HCW TST or, new to the 2005 guideline, QTF-G testing; the principles of preventive therapy; the importance of seeking evaluation if the HCW has TB symptoms; and the higher risk of disease given infection in those who are immunocompromised, particularly those infected with HIV. In addition, counseling of HCWs and options for voluntary work reassignment should be provided. The guidelines also emphasize the importance of the two-step Mantoux TST or QFT-G for all HCWs at the time of hire and that periodic TST or QFT-G should be performed based on the HCW's risk assessment. Furthermore, a section on evaluating problems provides guidance on investigation of TST conversions or active disease in HCWs or possible patient-to-patient TB transmission. In one nosocomial TB outbreak, an HCW was the source. Both the HCW's lack of recognition of symptoms as consistent with TB and the occupational health department's delay in recognition of TB in other HCWs with TST conversions and abnormal chest radiographs contributed to the outbreak [86,100].

Guideline Supplements

The 1994 and 2005 Guidelines have supplements that provide extensive details on the rationale, methods, and guidance for implementation of various elements of the TB control program. For example, the supplement on diagnosis and treatment provides a table on TST or blood assay for *M. tuberculosis* interpretation, treatment options, and drug dosages. The supplement on engineering controls discusses the basis for current science on ventilation and use of ultraviolet germicidal irradiation, and the supplement on respiratory protection discusses the factors to consider when choosing a respirator, including the key components of a respirator training program and the advantages and disadvantages of the various respirator types.

Cost of Tuberculosis Control Measures

Much of the debate about recommendations for the control of *M. tuberculosis* transmission in healthcare facilities has involved concerns about the cost of these measures. To facilitate identification of the extent of the infection control program that would be necessary at low-risk vs. high-risk hospitals, the 1994 and 2005 TB guidelines recommend conducting a risk assessment. Restricting the admission of infectious TB patients to selected areas of the facility may significantly reduce the cost of the control program by limiting the area requiring environmental/engineering modifications and the number of HCWs requiring respirator education and fit testing and

frequent TST monitoring. The major TB infection control measure costs are related to environmental/engineering modifications of existing older facilities to improve the number of air exchanges or to make the room have negative pressure. Although these costs can be substantial, the modifications are long term, and the costs can be amortized over the life of the equipment. Recent estimates of the cost of such environmental changes at MDR-TB outbreak hospitals varied widely (median, $229,000; range, $70,000–$559,000), depending on the extent and type of modifications required [108].

Most of the concerns about costs of the TB control program have centered around the cost of the respirators and respirator education and fit testing program. Several authors have estimated the cost of respirators or respirator education and fit testing programs based on the number of HCWs at the facility. Nettleman et al. estimated that the use of HEPA-filtered respirators would cost $7 million per case of TB prevented and $100 million per life saved [109]. Adal et al. estimated that at $7.51 to $9.08 per HEPA-filtered respirator, it would cost $1.3 to $18.5 million to prevent one episode of occupational acquisition of *M. tuberculosis* [110]. Both of these estimates come from institutions with a very low TB incidence. Furthermore, these estimates made a number of assumptions, such as single rather than repeated use of the respirator, admission of TB patients throughout the facility, and inclusion of all HCWs at the institution in the respiratory protection program, which may have artificially inflated the estimates. Kellerman et al. found that actual costs of respirators and respiratory education and fit testing programs were substantially less than these estimates at several of the MDR-TB hospitals; the median annual cost of respirators at four MDR-TB outbreak hospitals was $109,000 (range, $70,000–$223,000), and the median annual cost of respirator education and fit testing programs was $10,000 (range, $3,700–$19,700) [108].

Bacille Calmette-Guerin (BCG) Vaccination

Because of concern about occupational acquisition of *M. tuberculosis* by HCWs, the use of BCG vaccination as a protective measure has been questioned. Although in many other countries BCG has been given routinely to all infants for >60 years, routine BCG administration in any age group has never been implemented in the United States. In 1988, the U.S. Advisory Committee on Immunization Practices (ACIP) removed the HCW category from the list of people for whom BCG vaccination should be considered. The MDR-TB outbreaks in the late 1980s and 1990s resulted in a revisiting of this issue. Meta-analyses of the efficacy of BCG found that the data were inadequate (methodologic flaws) to evaluate the effectiveness of BCG in protecting HCWs [111,112]. Furthermore, the situation in the United States would be different from that in countries in which BCG is given in infancy. In the United States, if protecting HCWs were the goal, such vaccination would have to be given to adults. No data are available on how effective BCG administered only in adulthood would be. Furthermore, BCG is unlikely to provide protection for immunocompromised HCWs and might lead to disseminated BCG disease. Many of the countries in which BCG is routinely administered have a very high prevalence of TB in their populations, suggesting that BCG does not prevent pulmonary disease although it may decrease the risk of disseminated disease, particularly in the very young. In such countries with HIV and TB outbreaks, the HCWs still may be at risk for occupational acquisition of *M. tuberculosis*. Few of these countries have either HCW TB infection or disease surveillance programs; thus, there are few data on current rates of TB in BCG-vaccinated HCW populations in areas with high prevalence of HIV or TB, or both. As a result of these and other factors, the ACIP and the American Committee for the Elimination of Tuberculosis decided to maintain their recommendation that use of BCG should be made on an individual basis but that it is not recommended in low-risk areas and in healthcare facilities with effective infection control programs [113].

Pediatric Settings

There has been similar controversy about the need for the CDC TB guidelines recommendations in pediatric settings. Many believe that because most pediatric patients have primary disease, poor or absent cough, and infrequent bronchial and laryngeal TB, transmission is unlikely [114]. Although the risk for such transmission may be less, it is not zero, as illustrated by the nosocomial outbreaks caused by adults visiting children at pediatric facilities [115] or outbreaks in neonatal units as described by Lee et al. [116]. Furthermore, there are few data to document the lack of risk to HCWs in these settings. One survey of pediatric facilities showed that of 158 hospital respondents, 62 (40%) had a TB infection control policy specific for children, 147 (93%) reported admitting <6 tuberculosis patients, and 104 (66%) reported admitting no TB patients [117]. At 141/154 (92%) hospitals, a TB isolation policy existed; most isolated pediatric patients with positive AFB smears (139/143; 97%), evidence of cavitary TB on chest radiograph (141/145; 97%), or an AFB-positive gastric aspirate (107/140; 76%). At 10/154 (6.5%) facilities, clusters of >2 HCWs with similar occupational exposures had TST conversions in the preceding 5 years. Thus, like adults, pediatric patients should be evaluated at the time of admission for possible TB. Those with possible TB should be evaluated for potential infectiousness (i.e., positive sputum AFB smears). Those considered infectious should be placed in appropriate TB isolation. Recently, Berkowitz et al. have developed a decision analysis for initiation of TB prophylaxis in newborns in a nursery [118].

Nosocomial Transmission of *M. tuberculosis* in International Settings

With the worldwide epidemics of HIV and TB, many countries throughout the world are admitting large numbers of patients with HIV infection, TB, or HIV infection and TB to their healthcare facilities. In many of these countries, overall infection control programs are minimal, and TB infection control programs are nonexistent; such facilities often have no HCW TST programs, no TB isolation rooms meeting the CDC-recommended criteria, and minimal laboratory diagnostics for TB (i.e., no rapid AFB smear, culture, or susceptibility capability). In such facilities, *M. tuberculosis* transmission from patient to patient and patient to HCW undoubtedly occurs. It is incumbent on such facilities to conduct a risk assessment and determine the risk of such transmission to both their HCWs and patients. In these situations, simple control measures, such as enhanced administrative controls, HCW respiratory protection, separation of infectious patients, and improved ventilation or ultraviolet germicidal irradiation may be useful in reducing the risk of *M. tuberculosis* transmission.

REFERENCES

1. Centers for Disease Control and Prevention. Expanded tuberculosis surveillance and tuberculosis morbidity: United States, 1993. *MMWR Morb Mortal Wkly Rep* 1994;43:361–366.
2. Kochi A. The global tuberculosis situation and the new controls strategy of the World Health Organization. *Tubercle* 1991;72:1–6.
3. Centers for Disease Control and Prevention. Tuberculosis, final data: United States, 1986. *MMWR Morb Mortal Wkly Rep* 1988;36:387–389, 395.
4. Cantwell MF, Snider DE Jr, Cauthen GM, Onorato IM. Epidemiology of tuberculosis in the United States, 1985 through 1992. *JAMA* 1994;272:535–539.
5. Centers for Disease Control and Prevention. Expanded tuberculosis surveillance and tuberculosis morbidity: United States, 1993. *MMWR Morb Mortal Wkly Rep* 1994;43:361–366.
6. Centers for Disease Control and Prevention. Tuberculosis morbidity: United States, 1994. *MMWR Morb Mortal Wkly Rep* 1995;44:387–389, 395.
7. Centers for Disease Control and Prevention. Nosocomial transmission of multidrug-resistant tuberculosis among HIV-infected person: Florida and New York, 1988–1991. *MMWR Morb Mortal Wkly Rep* 1991;40:585–591.
8. Mazuerk GH, Jereb J, Lobue P, et al. Guidelines for using the QuantiFERON-TB Gold test for detecting Mycobacterium tuberculosis infection, United States. *MMWR Morb Mort Weekly Report* 2005;54(RR-15):1–37.
9. Jensen PA, Lambert LA, Iademarco MF, Ridzon R. Guidelines for preventing the transmission of Mycobacterium tuberculosis in health-care settings, 2005. *MMWR Recomm Rep* 2005;54(RR-7):1–141.
10. Frieden TR, Fujiwara PI, Washko RM, Hamburg MA. Tuberculosis in New York City: turning the tide. *N Engl J Med* 1995;333:229–233.
11. Coronado VG, Beck-Sague CM, Pearson ML, et al. Clinical and epidemiologic characteristics of multidrug-resistant Mycobacterium tuberculosis among patients with human immunodeficiency virus (HIV) infection. *Infect Dis Clin Pract* 1993;2:297–302.
12. Tenover FC, Crawford JT, Huebner RE, et al. Guest commentary: the resurgence of tuberculosis: is your laboratory ready? *J Clin Microbiol* 1993;31:767–770.

13. Tokars JI, Rudnick JR, Kroc K, et al. U.S. hospital mycobacteriology laboratories: status and comparison with state public health department laboratories. *J Clin Microbiol* 1996;34:680–685.

14. Centers for Disease Control and Prevention. Screening for tuberculosis and tuberculosis infection in high-risk populations, and the use of preventive therapy for tuberculosis infection in the United States: recommendations of the Advisory Committee for Elimination of Tuberculosis. *MMWR Morb Mortal Wkly Rep* 1990;39(RR-8):1–7.

15. Centers for Disease Control and Prevention. Treating opportunistic infections among HIV-infected adults and adolescents. *MMWR* 2004;53 (RR-15).

16. Centers for Disease Control and Prevention. Treating opportunistic infections among HIV-exposed and infected children. *MMWR* 2004; 53 (RR-14).

17. Centers for Disease Control and Prevention. Notice to readers: Updated guidelines for the use of rifamycins for the treatment of tuberculosis among HIV-infected patients taking protease inhibitors or nonnucleoside reverse transcriptase inhibitors. *MMWR* 2004; 53(2).

18. Centers for Disease Control and Prevention. Management of persons exposed to multidrug-resistant tuberculosis. *MMWR Morb Mortal Wkly Rep* 1992;41(RR-11):59–71.

19. Fridkin SK, Manangan L, Bolyard E, et al. SHEA-CDC TB survey, part I: status of TB infection control programs at member hospitals, 1989–1992. *Infect Control Hosp Epidemiol* 1995;16:129–134.

20. Fridkin SK, Manangan L, Bolyard E, et al. SHEA-CDC survey, part II: efficacy of TB infection control programs at member hospitals, 1992. *Infect Control Hosp Epidemiol* 1995;16:135–140.

21. Sinkowitz R, Fridkin S, Manangan L, et al. Status of tuberculosis infection control programs at U.S.hospitals, 1989–1992. *Am J Infect Control* 1996;24:226–234.

22. Malasky C, Jordan T, Potulski F, Reichman LB. Occupational tuberculosis infections among pulmonary physicians in training. *Am Rev Respir Dis* 1990;142:505–507.

23. Menzies D, Fanning A, Yuan L, Fitzgerald M. Tuberculosis among healthcare workers. *N Engl J Med* 1995;332:92–98.

24. Levine I. Tuberculosis risk in students of nursing. *Arch Intern Med* 1968;121:545–548.

25. Weiss W. Tuberculosis in student nurses at Philadelphia General Hospital. *Am Rev Respir Dis* 1973;107:136–139.

26. Atuk NO, Hunt EH. Serial tuberculin testing and isoniazid therapy in general hospital employees. *JAMA* 1971;218:1795–1798.

27. Gregg D, Gibson M. Employee TB control in a predominantly tuberculosis hospital. *J S C Med Assoc* 1975;71:160–165.

28. Berman J, Levine ML, Orr ST, Desi L. Tuberculosis risk for hospital employees: analysis of a five-year tuberculin skin testing program. *Am J Public Health* 1981;71:1217–1222.

29. Craven RB, Wenzel RP, Atuk NO. Minimizing tuberculosis risk to hospital personnel and students exposed to unsuspected disease. *Ann Intern Med* 1975;82:628–632.

30. Vogeler DM, Burke JP. Tuberculosis screening for hospital employees: a five year experience in a large community hospital. *Am Rev Respir Dis* 1978;117:227–232.

31. Ruben FL, Norden CW, Schuster N. Analysis of a community hospital employee tuberculosis screening program 31 months after its inception. *Am Rev Respir Dis* 1977;115:23–28.

32. Ktsanes VK, Williams WL, Boudreaux VV. The cumulative risk of tuberculin skin test conversion for five years of hospital employment. *Am J Public Health* 1986;76:65–67.

33. Barrett-Conner E. The epidemiology of tuberculosis in physicians. *JAMA* 1979;241:133–138.

34. Weinstein RS, Oshins J, Sacks HS. Tuberculosis infection in Mount Sinai medical students: 1974–1982. *Mt Sinai J Med* 1984;51:283–286.

35. Chan JC, Tabak JI. Risk of tuberculous infection among house staff in an urban teaching hospital. *South Med J* 1985;78:1061–1064.

36. Bass JB, Serio RA. The use of repeat skin tests to eliminate the booster phenomenon in serial tuberculin testing. *Am Rev Respir Dis* 1981;123:394–396.

37. Thompson NJ, Glassroth JL, Snider DE Jr, Farer LS. The booster phenomenon in serial tuberculin testing. *Am Rev Respir Dis* 1979;119:587–597.

38. Kantor HS, Poblete R, Pusateri SL. Nosocomial transmission of tuberculosis from unsuspected disease. *Am J Med* 1988;84:833–838.

39. Price LE, Rutala WQ, Samsa GP. Tuberculosis in hospital personnel. *Infect Control* 1987;8:97–101.

40. Aitken ML, Anderson KM, Albert RK. Is the tuberculosis screening program of hospital employees still required? *Am Rev Respir Dis* 1987;136:805–807.

41. Raad I, Cusick J, Sheretz RJ, et al. Annual tuberculin skin testing of employees at a university hospital: a cost-benefit analysis. *Infect Control Hosp Epidemiol* 1989;10:465–469.

42. Ramirez JA, Anderson P, Herp S, Raff MJ. Increased rate of tuberculin skin test conversion among workers at a university hospital. *Infect Control Hosp Epidemiol* 1992;13:579–581.

43. Ikeda RM, Birkhead GS, DiFerdinando GT Jr, et al. Nosocomial tuberculosis: an outbreak of a strain resistant to seven drugs. *Infect Contr Hosp Epidemiol* 1995;16:152–159.

44. Condos R, Scluger N, Lacouture R, Rom W. Tuberculosis infections among housestaff at Bellevue Hospital in an epidemic period [Abstract]. *Am Rev Respir Dis* 1993;147(suppl):Al24.

45. Redwood E, Anderson V, Felton CP, Findley S, Ford JG. Tuberculin conversions in hospital employees in a high tuberculosis prevalence area [Abstract]. *Am Rev Respir Dis* 1993; 147(Suppl):A119.

46. Cocchiarella LA, Cohen RAC, Conroy L, Wurtz R. Positive tuberculin skin testing reactions among house staff at a public hospital in the era of resurgent tuberculosis. *Am J Infect Control* 1996;24:7–12.

47. Adal KA, Anglim AM, Palumbo CL, et al. The use of high-efficiency particulate air-filter respirators to protect hospital workers from tuberculosis: a cost-effectiveness analysis. *N Engl J Med* 1994;331:169–173.

48. Panlilio AL, Burwen DR, the TB Infection Surveillance Project. Tuberculosis skin testing surveillance of healthcare workers [Abstract]. *Infect Control Hosp Epidemiol* 1996;17:P17.

49. Manangan LP, Perrotta DM, Banerjee SN, et al. Status of tuberculosis infection control programs at Texas hospitals, 1989–1991. *Am J Infect Control* 1997;25:229–235.

50. Silva VM, Cuhna AJ, Oliveira JR, et al. Medical students at risk of nosocomial transmission of *Mycobacterium tuberculosis*. *Int J Tuberc Lung Dis* 2000;4:420–426.

51. Kassim S, Zuber P, Wiktor SZ, et al. Tuberculin skin testing to assess the occupational risk of *Mycobacterium tuberculosis* infection among health care workers in Abidjan, Cote d'Ivoire. *Int J Tuberc Lung Dis* 2000;4:321–326.

52. Yanai H, Limpakarnjanarat K, Uthaivoravit W, et al. Risk of *Mycobacterium tuberculosis* infection and disease among health care workers, Chiang Rai, Thailand. *Int J Tuberc Lung Dis* 2003;7:36–45.

53. Roth VR, Garrett Do, Laserson KF, et al. A multicenter evaluation of tuberculin skin test positivity and conversion among health care workers in Brazilian hospitals. *Int J Tuberc Lung Dis* 2005;9:1335–1342.

54. Sepkowitz KA, Fella P, Rivera P, et al. Prevalence of PPD positivity among new employees at a hospital in New York City. *Infect Control Hosp Epidemiol* 1995;16:334–337.

55. Centers for Disease Control and Prevention. Guidelines for preventing the transmission of tuberculosis in health-care settings, with special focus on HIV-related issues. *MMWR Morb Mortal Wkly Rep* 1990;39(RR-17).

56. Centers for Disease Control and Prevention. Guidelines for preventing the transmission of *Mycobacterium tuberculosis* in health-care facilities, 1994. *MMWR Morb Mortal Wkly Rep* 1994;43(RR1-13).

57. Jereb JA, Klevens RM, Privett TD, et al. Tuberculosis in healthcare workers at a hospital with an outbreak of multidrug-resistant *Mycobacterium tuberculosis*. *Arch Intern Med* 1995;155:854–859.

58. Geisler PJ, Nelson KE, Crispin RJ, Moses VK. Tuberculosis in physicians: a continuing problem. *Am Rev Respir Dis* 1986;133:773–778.

59. Driver CR, Stricok RL, Granville K, et al. Tuberculosis in health care workers during declining tuberculosis incidence in New York State. *Am J Infect Control* 2005;33:519–526.

60. Pope AS. An outbreak of tuberculosis in infants due to hospital infection. *J Pediatr* 1942;40:297–300.

61. Ehrenkranz JN, Kicklighter LJ. Tuberculosis outbreak in a general hospital: evidence for airborne spread of infection. *Ann Intern Med* 1972;77:377–382.

62. Alpert ME, Levison ME. An epidemic of tuberculosis in a medical school. *N Engl J Med* 1965;272:718–721.

63. Israel HL, Hetherington HW, Ord JG. A study of tuberculosis among students of nursing. *JAMA* 1941;117:839–844.

64. Brandy L. Immunity and positive tuberculin reaction. *Am J Public Health* 1941;31:1040–1043.

65. Badger TL, Ayvazian LE. Tuberculosis in nurses: clinical observations on its pathogenesis as seen in a fifteen year follow-up of 745 nurses. *Am Rev Tubercule* 1949;60:305–327.

66. Abruzzi WA, Hummel RJ. Tuberculosis: incidence among American medical students, prevention and the use of BCG. *N Engl J Med* 1953;248:722–729.

67. Rudnick JR, Kroc K, Manangan L, et al. Are U.S. hospitals prepared to control nosocomial transmission of tuberculosis? Presented at the First World Congress on Tuberculosis, Rockville, Maryland, November 15–18, 1992.

68. Ramaswamy R, Corpuz M, Hewlett D. Tuberculosis surveillance of community hospital employees: a recommended strategy. *Arch Intern Med* 1995;155:1637–1639.

69. Barnes PF, Bloch AB, Davidson PT, Snider DE Jr. Tuberculosis in patients with human immunodeficiency virus infection. *N Engl J Med* 1991;324:1644–1650.

70. Selwyn PA, Hartel D, Lewis VA, et al. A prospective study of the risk of tuberculosis among intravenous drug users with human immunodeficiency virus infection. *N Engl J Med* 1989;320:545–550.

71. Dooley SW, Villarino ME, Lawrence M, et al. Tuberculosis in a hospital unit for patients infected with the human immunodeficiency virus (HIV): evidence of nosocomial transmission. *JAMA* 1992;267:2632–2634.

72. Di Perri G, Cruciani M, Danzi MC, et al. Nosocomial epidemic of active tuberculosis among HIV-infected patients. *Lancet* 1989;2:1502–1504.

73. Cantanzaro A. Nosocomial tuberculosis. *Am Rev Respir Dis* 1982;125:559–562.

74. Haley CE, McDonald RC, Rossi L, et al. Tuberculosis epidemic among hospital personnel. *Infect Control Hosp Epidemiol* 1989;10:204–210.

75. Hutton MD, Stead WS, Cauthen GM, et al. Nosocomial transmission of tuberculosis associated with a draining abscess. *J Infect Dis* 1990;161:286–295.

76. Calder RA, Duclos P, Wilder MH, et al. *Mycobacterium tuberculosis* transmission in a health clinic. *Bulletin of the International Union for Tuberculosis and Lung Disease* 1991;66:103–106.

77. Pierce JR Jr, Sims SL, Holman GH. Transmission of tuberculosis to hospital workers by a patient with AIDS. *Chest* 1992;101:581–582.

78. Frampton MW. An outbreak of tuberculosis among hospital personnel caring for a patient with a skin ulcer. *Ann Intern Med* 1992;117:312–313.

79. Edlin BR, Tokars JI, Grieco MH, et al. An outbreak of multidrug-resistant tuberculosis among hospitalized patients with the acquired immunodeficiency syndrome: epidemiologic studies and restriction fragment length polymorphism analysis. *N Engl J Med* 1992;326:1514–1522.

80. Beck-Sague CM, Dooley SW, Hutton MD, et al. Outbreak of multidrug-resistant tuberculosis among persons with HIV infection in an urban hospital: transmission to staff and patients and control measures. *JAMA* 1992;268:1280–1286.

81. Fischl MA, Uttamchandani RB, Daikos GL, et al. An outbreak of tuberculosis caused by multiple-drug-resistant tubercle bacilli among patients with HIV infection. *Ann Intern Med* 1992;117:177–183.

82. Pearson ML, Jereb JA, Frieden TR, et al. Nosocomial transmission of multidrug-resistant *Mycobacterium* tuberculosis: a risk to hospitalized patients and health-care workers. *Ann Intern Med* 1992;117:191–196.

83. Coronado VG, Valway S, Finelli L, et al. Nosocomial transmission of multidrug-resistant *Mycobacterium tuberculosis* among intravenous drug users with human immunodeficiency virus infection. In: *Abstracts of the third annual meeting of the Society for Hospital Epidemiology of America*, Chicago, April 18–20, 1993. *Infect Control and Hosp Epidemiol.*

84. Coronado VG, Beck-Sague CM, Hutton MD, et al. Transmission of multidrug-resistant *Mycobacterium tuberculosis* among persons with human immunodeficiency virus infection in an urban hospital: epidemiologic and restriction fragment length polymorphism analysis. *J Infect Dis* 1993;168:1052–1055.

85. Jarvis WR. Nosocomial transmission of multidrug-resistant *Mycobacterium tuberculosis*. *Res Microbiol* 1993;144:117–122.

86. Zaza S, Blumberg HM, Beck-Sague C, et al. Occupational risk of infection with *Mycobacterium tuberculosis*: patients and healthcare workers as a source of infection. *J Infect Dis* 1995;172:1542–1549.

87. Centers for Disease Control and Prevention. Outbreak of multidrug-resistant tuberculosis at a hospital: New York City, 1991. *MMWR Morb Mortal Wkly Rep* 1993;42:427–434.

88. Tokars JI, Jarvis WR, Edlin BR, et al. Tuberculin skin testing of hospital employees during an outbreak of multidrug-resistant tuberculosis in human immunodeficiency virus (HIV)-infected patients. *Infect Control Hosp Epidemiol* 1992;13:509–510.

89. Valway SE, Greifinger RB, Papania M, et al. Multidrug-resistant tuberculosis in the New York State prison system, 1990–1991. *J Infect Dis* 1994;170:151–156.

90. Cave MD, Eisenbach KD, McDermott PF, et al. IS6110. conservation of sequence in the *Mycobacterium tuberculosis* complex and its utilization in DNA finger printing. *Mol Cell Probes* 1991;5:73–80.

91. Haas WH, Butler WR, Woodley CL, Crawford JT. Mixed-linker polymerase chain reaction: a new method for rapid fingerprinting of the *Mycobacterium tuberculosis* complex. *J Clin Microbiol* 1993;31:1293–1298.

92. Moran GJ, McCabe F, Morgan MT, Talan DA. Delayed recognition and infection control for tuberculosis patients in the emergency department. *Ann Emerg Med* 1995;26:290–295.

93. Moran GJ, Fuchs MA, Jarvis WR, Talan DA. Tuberculosis infection control practices at emergency departments in the United States, 1993–1994. *Ann Emerg Med* 1995;26:283–289.

94. Huebner RE, Good RC, Tokars JI. Current practices in mycobacteriology: results of a survey of state public health laboratories. *J Clin Microbiol* 1993;31:771–775.

95. Manangan LP, Bennett CL, Tablan N, et al. Nosocomial tuberculosis prevention measures among two groups of U.S. hospitals, 1992 to 1996.

96. Ronveaux O, Jans B, Wanlin M, and Hydebrouck M. Prevention of transmission of tuberculosis in hospitals: a survey of practices in Belgium, 1995. *J Hosp Infect*, 1997;37:15–207.

97. Maloney SA, Pearson ML, Gordon MT, et al. Efficacy of control measures in preventing nosocomial transmission of multidrug-resistant tuberculosis to patients and healthcare workers. *Ann Intern Med* 1995;122:90–95.

98. Wenger PN, Otten J, Breeden A, et al. Control of nosocomial transmission of multidrug-resistant *Mycobacterium tuberculosis* among healthcare workers and HIV-infected patients. *Lancet* 1995;345:235–240.

99. Stroud LA, Tokars JI, Grieco MH, et al. Evaluation of infection control measures in preventing the nosocomial transmission of multidrug-resistant *Mycobacterium tuberculosis* in a New York City hospital. *Infect Control Hosp Epidemiol* 1995;16:141–147.

100. Blumberg HM, Watkins DL, Berschling JD, et al. Preventing the nosocomial transmission of tuberculosis. *Ann Intern Med* 1995;122:658–663.

101. Jarvis WR. Nosocomial transmission of multidrug-resistant *Mycobacterium tuberculosis*. *Am J Infect Control* 1995;23:146–151.

102. Jarvis WR, Bolyard EA, Bozzi CJ, et al. Respirators, recommendations, and regulations: the controversy surrounding protection of healthcare workers from tuberculosis. *Ann Intern Med* 1995;122:142–146.

103. Occupational Safety and Health Administration. OSHA 29DFR-OSH. 29 CFR 1910.134—Occupational safety and health standards, personal protective equipment, respiratory protection. *Code of Federal Regulation*. Washington, DC: U.S. Government Printing Office, Office of the Federal Register, 1972;37:1910–1934.

104. Leidel NA, Mullan RJ. *NIOSH recommended guidelines for personal respiratory protection of workers in health-care facilities potentially*

exposed to tuberculosis. Atlanta: U.S. Department of Health and Human Services, Public health Service, Centers for Disease Control and Prevention, National Institute for Occupational Safety and Health, 1992.

105. Chen SK, Vesley D, Brosseau LM, et al. Evaluation of single-use masks and respirators for protection of healthcare workers against mycobacterial aerosols. *Am J Infect Control* 1994;22: 65–74.

106. National Institute for Occupational Safety and Health. NIOSH 30CFR-NIOSH. 30 CFR, part II: Respiratory protective devices; tests for permissibility, fees. *Code of Federal Regulations.* Washington, DC; U.S. Government Printing Office, Office of the Federal Register, 1972;37:6243–6271.

107. U.S. Department of Health and Human Services. 42 CFR Part 84: Respiratory protective devices; proposed rule. *Federal Register* 1994;59:26849–26889.

108. Kellerman S, Tokars JT, Jarvis WR. The costs of complying with CDC tuberculosis guidelines at hospitals with a history of multidrug-resistant *Mycobacterium* tuberculosis outbreaks [Abstract]. *Infect Control Hosp Epidemiol* 1996;17:17.

109. Nettleman MD, Fredriskson M, Good NL, Hunter SA. Tuberculosis control strategies: the cost of particulate respirators. *Ann Intern Med* 1994;121:37–40.

110. Adal KA, Anglim AM, Palumbo CL, et al. The use of high-efficiency particulate air-filter respirators to protect hospital workers from tuberculosis: a cost-effectiveness analysis. *N Engl J Med* 1994;331:169–173.

111. Brewer TF, Colditz GA. Bacille Calmette-Guerin vaccination for the prevention of tuberculosis in healthcare workers. *Clin Infect Dis* 1995;20:136–142.

112. Brewer TF, Colditz GA. Relationship between bacille Calmette-Guerin (BCG) strains and the efficacy of BCG vaccine in the prevention of tuberculosis. *Clin Infect Dis* 1995;20: 126–135.

113. Centers for Disease Control and Prevention. The role of BCG vaccine in the prevention and control of tuberculosis in the United States. *MMWR Morb Mortal Wkly Rep* 1996;45(RR-4): 1–18.

114. Christie CD, Constantinou P, Marx ML, et al. Low risk for tuberculosis in a regional pediatric hospital: nine-year study of community rates and the mandatory employee tuberculin skin-test program. *Infect Control Hosp Epidemiol* 1998;19: 168–174.

115. Munoz FM, Ong LT, Seavy D, et al. Tuberculosis among adult visitors of children with suspected tuberculosis and employees at a children's hospital. *Infect Control Hosp Epidemiol* 2002;23:568–572.

116. Lee EH, Graham PL III, O'Keefe M, et al. Nosocomial transmission of Mycobacterium tuberculosis in a children's hospital. *Int J Tuberc Lung Dis* 2005;9:689–692.

117. Kellerman S, Simonds D, Jarvis W, Lee T. Tuberculosis infection control policies and procedures at hospitals caring for children: the APIC-CDC survey. In: Twenty-third annual meeting of the Association for Professions in Infection Control and Epidemiology, Inc.; Atlanta, Georgia, June 2–6, 1996. *Am J Infect Control* 1996;24:93.

118. Berkowitz FE, Severens JL, and Blumberg HM. Exposure to tuberculosis among newborns in a nursery: Decision analysis for initiation of prophylaxis. *Infect Control Hosp Epidemiol* 2006;27:604–611.

Infectious Gastroenteritis*

Rebecca H. Sunenshine, Eileen L. Yee, and L. Clifford McDonald

INTRODUCTION

Diarrhea has been variably defined in a number of ways (e.g., ≥ 6 watery stools over 36 hours, ≥ 3 unformed stools over 24 hours for ≥ 2 consecutive days, or ≥ 8 unformed stools over 48 hours) and is a common condition among patients within healthcare facilities and among home healthcare patients [1]. Many, if not most, episodes of diarrhea that occur in hospitalized patients are related to therapeutic interventions. For example, drug side effects are a common cause of diarrhea, nausea, and vomiting. The increased osmotic load of enteral tube feedings on the large intestine is a common cause of diarrhea among patients in some long-term care settings. However, despite the frequency of such noninfectious etiologies, episodes of infectious gastroenteritis account for a significant proportion of all patients in healthcare settings who develop diarrhea with or without nausea and vomiting.

When evaluating one or more patients who develop gastrointestinal symptoms following admission to a healthcare facility, several clues point to an infectious etiology. These include not only associated findings, such as fever or elevated white blood cell (WBC) count, but also the disease course and spread within a population with specific risk factors. For example, antimicrobial agents are not only among the most common drugs responsible for diarrhea without an apparent infectious etiology (i.e., antibiotic-associated diarrhea) but also are the most common risk factor for

disease caused by *Clostridium difficile* [2]. Thus, *C. difficile* in particular should be sought to explain either individual patients or clusters of patients who develop diarrhea following receipt of antimicrobial agents for unrelated conditions. Likewise, clusters of patients who develop diarrhea, nausea, and vomiting lasting only a few days, accompanied by symptomatic healthcare workers should lead to seeking a viral etiology, especially norovirus [3]. The most important aspect of pathogens responsible for infectious gastroenteritis is their ability to be rapidly transmitted in healthcare settings among patients who often are highly susceptible. Such outbreaks can be devastating and lead to significant increased costs, patient morbidity, and, in some instances, mortality.

The focus and scope of this chapter are the three most important infectious etiologies of gastroenteritis acquired in healthcare setting: *C. difficile*, norovirus, and rotavirus. Although there is no evidence that parasitic causes of gastroenteritis pose a significant threat for healthcare transmission, other bacterial agents, such as *Salmonella* and *Shigella* spp. are infrequently transmitted in such settings [4-8]. In the case of nontyphi *Salmonella* spp., Chapter 21 addresses food-borne transmission of infectious agents of gastroenteritis. However, there now are several concerning reports of nonfood-borne transmission in healthcare facilities of multidrug resistant, nontyphi *Salmonella* spp. [4,6]. These organisms act like other multidrug-resistant gram-negative bacteria, which are often transmitted via the hands of healthcare workers (HCWs) and are responsible for a variety of infections of sites ranging from the urinary tract to bloodstream; under such circumstances, patients and healthcare workers only occasionally develop gastrointestinal infection. Partly due

---

*The findings and conclusions in this report are those of the author(s) and do not necessarily represent the views of the Centers for Disease Control and Prevention.

to their very low infectious dose, *Shigella* spp. remain an important cause of infectious gastroenteritis in day care settings where child-to-child transmission occurs and can involve staff [9,10]. However, for reasons not entirely clear but likely include overall better infection control practices, outbreaks of shigellosis have been relatively infrequent in healthcare settings.

CLOSTRIDIUM DIFFICILE

C. difficile is a gram-positive, spore-forming anaerobic bacillus that was first associated with disease in 1978 when it was identified as the causative agent of pseudomembranous colitis (PMC) [11,12]. The organism has been associated with gastrointestinal infections ranging in severity from asymptomatic colonization to severe diarrhea, PMC, toxic megacolon, intestinal perforation, and death [13–15]. The primary virulence factors of *C. difficile* are toxins A and B, which are responsible for inflammation, fluid and mucous secretion, and mucosal damage leading to diarrhea or colitis [16]. A recently identified strain of *C. difficile* that has caused numerous outbreaks of clinically severe disease in North America and Europe produces 16-fold more toxin A and 23fold more toxin B than do other strains [17–19]. In addition, a third toxin, known as *binary toxin*, is associated with this strain, although its significance is unknown. The antimicrobial susceptibility pattern of this strain demonstrates increased resistance to the fluoroquinolones over both historical and contemporary nonoutbreak strains [18]. Reports of outbreaks of severe disease caused by this epidemic strain have heightened clinicians' awareness of *C. difficile*–associated disease (CDAD), emphasizing the importance of early recognition and appropriate treatment.

Epidemiology

C. difficile toxins are isolated from stools of 15–25% of patients with antibiotic-associated diarrhea and more than 95% of patients with PMC [20]. Although CDAD is not a nationally reportable condition, data from the Centers for Disease Control and Prevention's (CDC) National Nosocomial Infections Surveillance (NNIS) system hospitals indicated an average of 12.2 episodes of CDAD per 10,000 patient-days from 1987 to 1998 [21]. Rates were significantly higher in NNIS teaching versus nonteaching hospitals (13.0 vs. 11.7 episodes per 10,000 patient-days) and in medical versus surgical services with higher rates in winter months than nonwinter months. Other data from the CDC reveal that hospitalizations with a discharge diagnosis of CDAD significantly increased per 100,000 population from 31 in 1996 to 61 in 2003 [22]. Healthcare-associated CDAD (HA-CDAD) has been identified as the direct or indirect cause of death in 0.6–1.5% of affected patients [23,24] and estimated to cost an additional $3,669.00

to $7,234.00 per patient hospitalization [25,26]. In addition to the recent increase in disease incidence suggested by hospital discharge statistics, reports indicate that the severity of observed disease is increasing with attributable 30-day mortality of nearly 7% and one-year mortality approaching 17% [19,27].

Multiple risk factors for CDAD are cited in the literature, most notably prior antimicrobial use; with more than 90% of healthcare-associated *C. difficile* infections occurring after or during antimicrobial therapy [2,28]. Almost all antimicrobial agents, with the exception of aminoglycosides, have been associated with the development of CDAD. However, data suggest that broad-spectrum antimicrobial agents, which have a greater influence on the normal intestinal flora, are more likely to be associated with CDAD [2]. Results of several recent studies indicate that fluoroquinolones have emerged as the most important antimicrobial risk factor in CDAD outbreaks, superseding other antimicrobial agents, including clindamycin and β-lactam/β-lactamase inhibitors [19,29,30]. Receipt of multiple antimicrobial agents and longer courses of antimicrobials also are risk factors [2].

At least three studies have identified the following additional risk factors for healthcare-associated CDAD: age >65, severity of underlying illness, presence of a nasogastric tube, antiulcer medications, and duration of hospital stay [2]. Conflicting evidence exists regarding the contribution of stomach acid–suppressing medications, such as proton-pump inhibitors and histamine-2 blockers in the development of CDAD [29,31,32].

Specific populations appear to be at greater risk for developing CDAD than the general population. The majority of CDAD occurs in healthcare facilities [16] as do the majority of CDAD outbreaks [33,34]. This is likely due to the concentration in these facilities of affected patients who serve as reservoirs for infectious spores. These can be transmitted among patients via the fecal/oral route, often following contamination of the patient-care environment and/or the HCW's hands. Among hospitalized patients, medical patients are at significantly higher risk of CDAD than are surgical patients [21,31]. In addition, *C. difficile* is the most common infectious cause of acute diarrheal illness in long-term care facilities (LTCF) [35,36]. In nonoutbreak settings, the prevalence of *C. difficile* colonization in LTCF ranges from 4–20% [36] compared to a rate of <3% reported in healthy adults [20,28]. The LTCF population is associated with several other known CDAD risk factors including increased antimicrobial use, older age, and increased use of stomach acid–suppressing medications. These additional risk factors make determining which factors contribute most to the increased CDAD risk in LTCFs difficult.

Neonates represent another population with increased *C. difficile* colonization with rates ranging from 5–70% [28]. Ironically, despite these high carriage rates, neonates are much less likely to develop CDAD than are adults. Based on observations in rabbits, this is thought to be due to the lack of receptors to toxin A in the immature enterocytes of neonates [37].

Two events appear as prerequisites in the pathogenesis of CDAD: The colon's normal flora must be disrupted, as with antimicrobials, and *C. difficile* must be ingested, although not necessarily in that order [28]. Only toxigenic strains of *C. difficile* produce clinical disease, but toxin production does not guarantee symptomatic progression [16]. Other host factors can influence the clinical presentation, such as pre-existing colonization with *C. difficile* and the presence of humoral immunity. It has been suggested that colonization with *C. difficile* can actually protect against the development of symptomatic disease [38] which could be due to the development of immunity. Kyne et al. demonstrated that patients who became asymptomatic carriers had significantly greater antibody responses to toxin A than those who developed HA-CDAD [39]. This pathogen–host interaction, in which new exposure to the organism confers greater risk of developing disease than chronic colonization highlights the importance of exogenous over endogenous sources of infection in HA-CDAD.

Clinical Presentation

The incubation period between new exposure or, more specifically, ingestion of *C. difficile* and the manifestation of disease has not been well established. One study of serial stool cultures for *C. difficile* performed in hospitalized patients suggested that this interval is in most instances less than 7 days [38]. In a recent study of cancer outpatients however, the median interval between discharge from an inpatient healthcare facility where exposure was likely to have occurred and CDAD diagnosis was 20.3 days, ranging from 2–60 days [40]. This suggests a longer incubation period than had been previously thought. Distinct from the interval between exposure and symptom onset is the duration of increased susceptibility following exposure to an antimicrobial. Although symptoms can develop immediately after beginning antimicrobial therapy, their onset can be delayed up to 6–8 weeks after therapy is completed [16]. This reflects the alteration in bowel flora that can persist for several weeks following completion of some forms of antimicrobial therapy; during this time, a patient remains at increased risk for the development of CDAD whenever exposure to *C. difficile* occurs.

The clinical presentation of *C. difficile* is a continuum that includes asymptomatic carriage, diarrhea, colitis, PMC, and fulminant colitis [16]. It most commonly presents as mild to moderate nonbloody diarrhea, sometimes accompanied by low abdominal cramping. Systemic symptoms are typically absent, and physical exam is remarkable only for mild abdominal tenderness. Colitis, in contrast, tends to present with more severe symptoms, including profuse watery diarrhea, abdominal pain, and distention. Fever, nausea, and dehydration often are present. Occult blood can occur in the stool, but hematochezia is rare. Colonoscopy reveals a characteristic membrane with adherent yellow plaques usually in the distal colon, although occasionally it can be confined to the proximal colon and can be missed on exam.

Patients with severe colitis are at an increased risk of developing paralytic ileus and toxic megacolon [16], which can lead to a paradoxical decrease in diarrhea. Such severe cases can also present as fulminant colitis with acute abdomen and systemic symptoms such as fever and tachycardia. The presence of any of these complications requires an immediate surgical consult. A review of 11 patients with toxic megacolon revealed that 64% required corrective surgery, and once the patients underwent surgery for complications of CDAD, the mortality rate rose from 32% to 50% [41].

Recurrence is one of the most frustrating and challenging complications of CDAD. There is no universal agreement on a clinical definition of CDAD reinfection versus relapse. One strategy defines *relapse* as recurrent symptoms occurring within 2 months following CDAD diagnosis and a *reinfection* as symptoms that develop after 2 months [42–44]. However, studies of patients who have "relapsed" within 2 months of a previous CDAD episode indicate that 48–56% of such patients are actually reinfected with a different strain of *C. difficile* [43,44]. Whether caused by a reinfection versus true relapse, 12–24% of patients develop a second episode of CDAD within 2 months of the initial diagnosis. If a patient has two or more prior episodes of CDAD, the risk of additional recurrences increases to 50–65% [41]. These statistics highlight the importance of the prevention strategies discussed later.

Diagnosis

C. difficile can occur up to several months after antimicrobial agents are discontinued [36,40] and should be suspected in any adult with antimicrobial-associated diarrhea. Due to high rates of colonization, only watery or loose stools should be tested for *C. difficile* to avoid decreased specificity [1]. Suspicion of CDAD in the presence of intestinal ileus, which occurs in <1% of patients, is the primary exception to this rule. Because most laboratories will not accept solid stool for *C. difficile* testing, a clinician should notify the laboratory of the specific patient's circumstances. In general, empiric therapy without testing for *C. difficile* is inappropriate because only 30% of hospitalized patients with diarrhea will have CDAD, even in an epidemic setting. An exception includes a severely ill or rapidly deteriorating patient at high risk for CDAD for whom empiric therapy while awaiting test results may be appropriate.

A variety of methods to detect *C. difficile* exists from tissue culture assays to enzyme immunoassays, each of which has advantages and disadvantages (Table 33-1). Most clinical laboratories use enzyme immunoassays that have a rapid turnaround time and require less technical expertise than tissue culture does. Although the negative predictive value hinges on the sensitivity of the particular

TABLE 33-1

ADVANTAGES AND DISADVANTAGES OF DIAGNOSTIC TESTING METHODS FOR *C. DIFFICILE*

Diagnostic Test	Turnaround Time (Hours)	Sensitivity	Advantages	Disadvantages
Endoscopy	2 h	51%	Diagnostic of PMC	Has low sensitivity
Anaerobic culture	72 h	89–100%	Results useful for molecular typing	Does not distinguish toxin-producing strains
Tissue cytotoxic assay	48 h	94–100%	Detects A⁻ B⁺ strains; "Gold standard"	Gives false positives; Results vary with experience of technologist
Common antigen	0.25–0.75 h	58–92%	Detects A⁻ B⁺ strains; easy to use	Does not distinguish toxin-producing strains; Cross-reacts with other anaerobes
ELISA—Toxin A	2 h	80–95%	Easy to use	Does not detect A⁻ B⁺ strains
ELISA—Toxin A + B	2 h		Detects A⁻ B⁺ strains	Has increased sensitivity for low-level toxin production
Immunochromato-graphic Toxin A	<1 h	60–85%	Simple to use; rapid	Does not detect A⁻ B⁺ strains

assay, in most instances one negative result is enough to rule out CDAD. Nonetheless, a high clinical suspicion can warrant repeat testing. Due to its cost and turnaround time of approximately 72 hours, anaerobic bacterial culture is the method employed least by hospitals to diagnose CDAD [45]. This method's accuracy also varies considerably by institution due to the use of nonstandardized methods and culture media. The primary advantage of anaerobic culture is that it lends itself to molecular typing of strains, which can be useful in an outbreak setting. (Table 33-1).

Treatment

Discontinuation of the inciting antibiotic is the most important step in the initial treatment of CDAD [43]. In addition, 10 days of appropriate oral antimicrobial therapy is recommended [46,47]. In a large study of 189 patients with CDAD, 97% of them responded to initial antibiotic therapy [48]. Although this study was based on treatment predominantly with oral vancomycin, several older studies comparing oral metronidazole to oral vancomycin for the treatment of CDAD indicate that metronidazole has been, at least historically, as effective and less expensive than oral vancomycin [49,50]. In addition, the use of metronidazole avoids the increased risk of promoting vancomycin resistance that could result from the widespread use of oral vancomycin. For these reasons, most experts have recommended metronidazole as the first-line antimicrobial therapy for CDAD [46,51]. A recent prospective observational study reported a 78% response rate to therapy with metronidazole [52], which is significantly lower than previously published response rates to both oral vancomycin and metronidazole. Coupled with the emergence of a more virulent strain, this study has led to a slightly different treatment strategy. For the majority of CDAD patients, metronidazole remains appropriate first-line treatment provided that the clinician

is vigilant about following the patient for response to therapy [47]. However, alternative first-line therapy, such as oral or intraluminal vancomycin, should be considered for patients who present with moderate or severe disease.

In addition, it is important to realize that mild disease caused by *C. difficile* can quickly progress to moderate or severe disease and that these distinctions are not always easy to make. Specific symptoms that suggest moderate disease severity include fever, profuse diarrhea, abdominal pain, and leukocytosis [46]. Severe disease is said to occur when complications of colitis arise, such as sepsis, volume depletion, electrolyte imbalance, hypotension, peritonitis, paralytic ileus, or toxic megacolon. Other authors include a white blood cell (WBC) of >20,000 cells/millimeter (mm)^3 and elevated creatinine as indicators of severe disease [47,53]. Because of possible disease progression despite appropriate therapy, the treating clinician should follow a patient treated for CDAD closely for symptom improvement within 1–2 days of initial therapy [47]. Fever should subside within 24–48 hours, and diarrhea should resolve within 2–5 days [47,48]. If the disease progresses after initiation of treatment, additional or alternative therapeutic options should be considered, including a surgical consult for any signs of toxic megacolon, peritonitis, or sepsis (Table 33-2). However, in the absence of clinical deterioration, a slow clinical response should not lead to the conclusion that a patient has failed treatment before 6–7 days of therapy [54]. Finally, therapeutic response should be based purely on clinical signs and symptoms; performance of a repeat toxin assay as a "test of cure" should be discouraged because patients can remain colonized with toxin-producing strains following recovery [55].

Prevention and Infection Control Strategies

Two approaches to reducing *C. difficile* rates have been described: (1) interruption of horizontal spread of the

TABLE 33-2

THERAPEUTIC OPTIONS FOR
C. DIFFICILE-ASSOCIATED DISEASE (46;99)

Disease/Host Characteristics	Recommended Therapy
Mild disease: absence of systemic symptoms with only mild diarrhea	Metronidazole 250 mg PO qid *or* 500 mg PO tid for 10 days
Moderate disease: presence of fever, profuse diarrhea, abdominal pain, and leukocytosis	Vancomycin 125 mg–500 mg PO qid × 10 days
Severe disease (paralytic ileus, toxic megacolon, dehydration or sepsis)	Surgical consult plus intraluminal vancomycin
Inability to take PO	Intraluminal vancomycin+/− IV metronidazole

organism within healthcare facilities and (2) reduction of the individual's risk of acquiring the disease once exposed to the organism [1]. Because prior antimicrobial use is associated with the vast majority of patients who develop HA-CDAD, restriction of antimicrobial use is potentially an important infection control strategy to reduce patient risk. However, with the exception of clindamycin [56,57] and cephalosporin restrictions [58,59], there remain relatively few reports demonstrating success by reducing the use of a specific class of agents to control CDAD. Vancomycin has been studied for the eradication of asymptomatic colonization in patients; however, its effects are not sustained, and patients can be at increased risk for prolonged carriage after treatment is discontinued. For this reason, experts do not recommend the treatment of patients colonized with *C. difficile* as an infection control strategy [1]. Significant intraluminal levels of metronidazole are achieved only in the presence of diarrhea, which renders the drug ineffective for patients with asymptomatic colonization [43].

Spread of *C. difficile* in healthcare facilities has been well documented in the literature; spread occurs primarily via infected humans (both symptomatic and asymptomatic) and contamination of the patient-care environment [1,60]. The most effective means of decreasing horizontal spread of *C. difficile* has been the combination of vigilant hand hygiene and isolation precautions. The literature contains both direct and indirect evidence for contamination of HCWs' hands in endemic and outbreak settings. The 1994 Hospital Infection Control Practices Advisory Committee (HICPAC) guideline for isolation precautions in hospitals recommends contact precautions for symptomatic patients which includes placing them in a private room or cohorting them with other symptomatic patients, as well as using gowns and gloves upon entering the patient's room [61]. One hospital reported a 60% decrease of CDAD after instituting a more stringent infection control program including increased enforcement of contact precautions, a monthly educational program, triclosan-containing hand soap, and increased environmental cleaning [62].

It is recognized that alcohol is not effective in killing *C. difficile* spores [63]. This information has led infection control personnel to be concerned that the recent increased incidence of CDAD is due to the rise in the use of alcohol-based hand rubs (ABHR) in healthcare facilities. To investigate this hypothesis, Boyce et al. evaluated the trends of ABHR use and the percentage of positive *C. difficile* toxin assays from 2000 to 2003 in a 500-bed tertiary care hospital [64]. These authors calculated a 10fold rise in the use of ABHRs while the percentage of all hand-hygiene episodes performed using soap and water decreased from 90% in 2001 to 15% at the end of 2003. During that period, the proportion of positive *C. difficile* toxin assays also decreased from 10.3% in 2000 to 7.4% in 2003. These data suggest that factors other than increased use of alcohol-based hand-hygiene products are responsible for the recent rise in HA-CDAD. Despite this, if a hospital is experiencing an outbreak, it is prudent for HCWs to hand wash exclusively with soap and water after glove removal in the care of known CDAD patients [63].

Environmental contamination due to *C. difficile* is exacerbated by the persistence of spores that can be highly resistant to routine disinfection and survive on dry surfaces for up to 6 months [65,66]. The rate of surface contamination increases in proportion to the *C. difficile* status, severity of diarrhea, and incontinence of patients in the area [1]. Although asymptomatic carriers of *C. difficile* can serve as reservoirs for disease transmission within healthcare facilities, epidemiologic studies suggest that they appear less contagious than do symptomatic patients. Furthermore, the degree of environmental contamination surrounding asymptomatic carriers is lower than that of surrounding patients with symptomatic disease. Patient-care items such as reusable electronic rectal thermometers have been implicated in outbreaks; and dedication of single-use items to individual patients can eliminate this source of contamination [1,33]. "High-touch" surfaces in patients' bathrooms (e.g., light switches) also have been implicated in outbreaks and should be targeted for enhanced environmental cleaning.

No well-controlled trials of disinfectant use in environmental control strategies for *C. difficile* have been conducted; however, the use of both unbuffered and phosphate-buffered hypochlorite solutions (bleach) has been shown to effectively decrease rates of *C. difficile* contamination, and some studies suggest that cleaning with bleach can lower CDAD rates [65,67–69]. Moreover, these studies suggest that environmental contamination is highest and therefore the likelihood of success of environmental cleaning strategies is greatest when CDAD rates are at their highest. Although there are no Environmental Protection Agency (EPA)–registered disinfectants with a claim for *C. difficile* spore inactivation, the CDC/HICPAC Guideline for Environmental Infection Control in Healthcare Facilities recommends "meticulous cleaning followed by disinfection using hypocholorite-based germicides as appropriate" [65]. When used as part of a cleaning strategy to reduce environmental contamination with *C. difficile* spores, household bleach should be diluted 1:10 to make a final working concentration of sodium-hypochlorite of at least 5,000 parts per million. The bleach solution should be prepared daily. After applying the solution to visibly clean surfaces, it should be allowed to remain moist for at least a 10-minute contact time and then be wiped off to prevent buildup of hypochlorite residual. Unfortunately, sodium-hypochlorite solutions at this concentration can cause respiratory irritation and will cause many surfaces to deteriorate; these solutions can "pit" stainless steel and aluminum and discolor several other materials. Many medical devices, especially electronics, are incompatible with chlorine-based cleaners, highlighting the need to develop other methods to reliably eradicate *C. difficile* spores in healthcare settings. Conducting an infection control risk assessment to identify practices and procedures that facilitate fecal contamination of environmental surfaces is one approach to minimizing contamination, thereby making the problem more manageable.

Surveillance

In light of recent reports of increasing rates and severity of CDAD in the United States, Canada, and parts of Europe, all associated with a more virulent strain of *C. difficile*, the surveillance for CDAD should be conducted in all healthcare facilities providing care to patients at increased risk for disease. Although there are currently no widely accepted surveillance definitions for CDAD, simply tracking the number of patients with new positive *C. difficile* laboratory tests over time could lead to earlier detection of either outbreaks or increasing disease trends. If an increase is noted, consideration should be given to tracking outcomes. Evidence suggests that if increased severe outcomes are noted, measures to more rapidly diagnose CDAD and escalate therapy (e.g., empowering nonphysician personnel to order tests, alerting clinicians to patients with signs of early severe disease) could reduce these severe outcomes [47].

Other principles of surveillance for HA-CDAD include considering the disease to be community acquired in patients who are symptomatic at the time of admission or in those who become symptomatic within a short period (e.g., ≤48 hours) following admission. However, because there is increasing recognition that patients exposed to *C. difficile* while hospitalized can develop symptoms within 1–2 months following discharge [40], consideration should be given to including such recently discharged patients with community-onset CDAD in an institution's definition of HA-CDAD. Finally, because the risk of being exposed to and acquiring *C. difficile* increases in proportion to the duration of hospitalization, rates of CDAD should be expressed as cases per 10,000 patient-days.

Outbreak Management

Whether an outbreak or an increasing trend in HA-CDAD rates is noted, specific steps should be undertaken. First, isolation precautions for CDAD patients should be reinforced by paying particular attention to placing them in single rooms or cohorting them with other CDAD patients and ensuring that CDAD patients do not share bathroom facilities with non-CDAD patients. The appropriate and consistent use of barrier precautions as part of contact precautions should be reinforced, and personnel should be instructed to wash their hands with soap and water after removal of gloves while leaving the CDAD patient room.

Policies and practices surrounding the reuse of patient care equipment for both CDAD and non-CDAD patients should be reevaluated. As noted, for example, reusable electronic rectal thermometers should be replaced throughout the facility with single-use, dedicated-use, or nonrectal thermometers, and the cleaning and reprocessing of all bedside commodes should be reviewed. If sodium hypochlorite was not already part of the institution's cleaning and disinfection strategy for CDAD patients, it should be introduced in recognition of the limitations outlined earlier. If bleach cleaning is already used, the frequency of cleaning in CDAD patients' rooms should be increased if possible with priority given to regular terminal cleaning. If increased rates continue despite these measures, additional attention should be given to the appropriateness of antimicrobial prescribing. Several institutions reporting successful control of the epidemic strain have achieved this success only after both enhancing infection control measures and reducing overall antimicrobial prescribing including fluoroquionlones [19,70].

ROTAVIRUS

Rotaviruses are RNA virus members of the family *Reoviridae*. They were discovered in 1973 by Bishop and colleagues, who performed electron microscopy on duodenal biopsies from children hospitalized in Australia during an outbreak of acute gastroenteritis. These viruses were named for their characteristic "wheel-like" appearance; they are the most common cause of severe gastroenteritis among children less than 5 years old and have caused outbreaks in daycare centers among young children and occasionally in nursing homes for the elderly. The rotavirus genome consists of 11 segments of double-stranded RNA; 6 of these encode for structural proteins and 5 for nonstructural proteins enclosed in a triple-layer, nonenveloped, icosahedral capsid that is 70 nm in diameter. The seven major groups of rotavirus are identified as Groups A through G. Human infections are primarily caused by Groups A, B, and C. Within these groups, specific serotypes are further classified by their outer viral capsid protein (VP), known as VP7 (a glycoprotein, or G-protein) and VP4 (a protease-activated protein, or P-protein). VP7 and VP4 also are the proteins targeted for vaccine development because they induce neutralizing antibodies. Another important structural protein is VP6, which determines the group specificity (A though G), and provides the basis for commercial immunoassay testing.

Epidemiology

The highest incidence of rotavirus infections is reported in children between the ages of 6 to 23 months. By the age of 5, most children will have been infected with it. The first rotavirus infection usually is the most severe and subsequent infections tend to be milder due to stimulated immunity. In the United States, community-acquired rotavirus infections are estimated to cause 2.7 millions diarrheal episodes, approximately 410,000 physician visits, 205,000–272,000 emergency department visits, 55,000–70,000 hospitalizations, and approximately 20–60 deaths each year [71,72].

Rotavirus infections have a predictable winter peak in incidence in the temperate climate of the continental United States. In the Southwest, rotavirus lasts from October to December whereas in the Northeast, it occurs from March to May [73]. However, in tropical climates, rotavirus infections tend to occur throughout the year.

Primary transmission of rotavirus is through the fecal-oral route. Spread also occurs through person-to-person contact and contamination of fomites, environmental surfaces, water, and food. Transmission through either large droplets or airborne particles has been hypothesized on the basis of viral RNA detected in air samples collected from rooms of hospitalized children. Infected persons can shed large quantities (10^7 to 10^{12}/gram) of virus in their stools with a duration of 4 days; however, there have been reports of immunosuppressed patients shedding rotavirus for up to one month even after resolution of symptoms [74]. The typical incubation period for rotavirus infection ranges from 1–3 days after an infectious dose as small as 10 virions [75].

Although the highest incidence of rotavirus infections occurs in young children, sporadic rotavirus infections have also occurred among the elderly and adults in close contact with infected children. Infections in neonates may occur; however, they often are asymptomatic because neonates are likely to be initially protected by maternal antibodies [76]. Rotavirus outbreaks have been well documented in hospitals, neonatal intensive care units, pediatric oncology wards, day care centers, and nursing homes [76–79]. Although it can be difficult to differentiate between infections acquired in hospitals versus in the community but responsible for hospitalization, approximately 55,000–70,000 hospitalizations per year are associated

with rotavirus infection [80,81]. Healthcare-associated rotavirus infections can increase length of hospital stay from 2 to 6 days, directly impacting health care costs [76,82]. Contaminated fomites (i.e., toys) and asymptomatic HCWs carrying rotovirus are speculated to play a role in transmitting healthcare-associated rotavirus.

The survival of rotavirus on hands and environmental surfaces ranges from a few days on hands to 2 weeks on inanimate objects. Rotavirus has been found on the hands of more than 70% of HCWs involved in the care of children with community-acquired rotavirus infection and on the hands of 20% of HCWs not in direct contact with these children [76]. Patient risk factors for healthcare-associated rotavirus infection include prolonged hospital stay, exposure to hospital visitors with gastroenteritis (i.e., infected sibling) and underlying conditions such as prematurity, low birth weight, compromised immunity, and malnutrition [76,81]. Institutional factors associated with outbreaks include failure to isolate patients and implement contact precautions, poor hand hygiene, and use of inadequate disinfection procedures.

Both in the United States and across the globe, serotypes G1, G2, G3, G4, and P[8] account for more than 90% of the circulating rotaviruses. Surveillance for rotavirus strains in the United Stats is conducted by the National Rotavirus Strain Surveillance System at the CDC, which was established in 1996 among 11 voluntary hospital laboratories [83].

Clinical Presentation

Persons infected with rotavirus generally present with acute vomiting followed by watery, nonbloody, and profuse diarrhea with or without fever [84]. Because the disease process is more severe as a first infection, children tend to have episodes that are more severe. Although many adults also are susceptible to rotavirus, they tend to be either asymptomatic or have milder infections. Elderly and immunocompromised persons can also be more vulnerable to complications of dehydration resulting from rotavirus infection.

Diagnosis and Treatment

Laboratory confirmation is achieved by the detection of viral antigen in the stool or an increase in antibody titers in paired sera. Most hospitals use a commercial, monoclonal antibody, enzyme immunoassay (EIA) for stool testing of group A rotaviruses. Further laboratory testing for other rotavirus groups, such as group C, is limited to research laboratories.

Currently, no specific antiretroviral therapy is available for rotavirus illnesses. Supportive therapy is the mainstay of treatment using oral rehydration fluids or intravenous fluids [85]. Passive immunoglobulin therapy, such as hyperimmune bovine colostrum or intravenous gamma globulin, has been used and should be considered for immunocompromised patients with severe gastroenteritis; however, this treatment remains experimental.

Prevention and Control

In early 2006, the Advisory Committee on Immunization Practices (ACIP) recommended routine use of the recently FDA-approved rotavirus vaccine, RotaTeq® (Merck, Blue Bell, Pennsylvania), to prevent rotavirus gastroenteritis in children. Use of trade names and commercial sources is for identification only and does not imply endorsement by the Centers for Disease Control and Prevention or the U.S. Department of Health and Human Services. RotaTeq® vaccine is a live, oral vaccine prepared from five bovine-human reassortment rotaviruses (G1, G2, G3, G4, and P[8]). The recommended administration schedule is at 2, 4, and 6 months of life. Vaccine safety and efficacy studies have included more than 60,000 children worldwide. This vaccine is 74% effective in preventing G1–G4 rotavirus infections of any severity through the first rotavirus season following vaccination (95% confidence interval, 66.8 to 77.9%) and 98% effective in preventing severe G1–G4 rotavirus gastroenteritis (95% confidence interval, 88.3 to 100.0%) [86]. Another rotavirus vaccine, Rotarix® (GlaxoSmithKline Biologics, Rixensart, Begium), which is an attenuated human rotavirus strain of serotype G1P[8], also has been developed but has not yet been licensed. Both vaccines were tested in large clinical trials of more than 60,000 to ensure safety; no evidence was found that either vaccine was associated with intussusception. Breast-feeding could have some effect in preventing rotavirus infections in infants, but more research is needed. The use of probiotics, such as Lactobacillus, has been reported but lacks substantial evidence for effectiveness.

Control measures during outbreaks of rotavirus have consisted of isolating or cohorting ill patients, using contact precautions to prevent secondary transmission, cleaning and disinfecting contaminated surfaces and fomites (i.e., toys, diaper-changing areas, and medical devices), strictly enforcing work restrictions for symptomatic HCWs until 24–48 hours following symptom resolution, encouraging proper hand-hygiene practices, educating staff regarding rotavirus infection, and restricting patients and visitors with gastroenteritis from entering playrooms. The most effective environmental control strategy to inactivate rotavirus is cleaning and disinfecting surfaces [65]. General categories of hard surface disinfectant chemicals that are effective against rotavirus include, but are not limited to, preparations with a high alcohol content (i.e., quarternary ammonium or phenolic preparations with 79–95% ethanol) and chlorine-based products that contain at least 800 parts per million sodium hypochlorite (e.g., a 1:50 dilution of household bleach) [65,74,87]. Also, products with EPA—registered label claims for effectiveness against rotavirus can be used. Heating to temperatures of more than 60°C (i.e., heat pasteurization) is also effective rotavirus inactivation.

NOROVIRUS

Noroviruses are single-stranded RNA viruses from the *Calicivirdae* family; they were discovered in 1972 by Kapikian and colleagues from stools collected in 1968 during an outbreak of gastroenteritis in an elementary school in Norwalk, Ohio. Formally referred to as "Norwalklike viruses" or "small, round-structured viruses," noroviruses are nonenveloped, icosahedral, and small (27 nm in diameter). They are genetically diverse and have been identified in both humans and animals. Noroviruses have been classified into several different genogroups, GI to GV, which can be further divided into more than 25 genetic clusters through sequencing. Only strains within genogroup GI, GII, and GIV are known to affect humans.

Epidemiology

In the United States, norovirus infections are estimated to cause 23 million illnesses a year. Infection can occur year-round but has been referred to as the "winter-vomiting" disease because of its winter predilection and number of patients who present with vomiting.

Noroviruses can be transmitted by multiple routes, such as contaminated food/water and environmental surfaces/fomites, and direct contact, and airborne vomitus droplets [88,89]. The ability of noroviruses to cause infection in persons exposed to less than 100 viral particles with an incubation period of less than 2 days spread through multiple routes persists in the environment on both porous and nonporous surfaces and its relative resistance to inactivation with common cleaning agents, such as quaternary ammonium and phenolic compounds, allow this virus to cause widespread outbreaks with high attack rates.

Norovirus outbreaks have been frequently reported in LTCFs, hospitals, camps, cruise ships, and other areas where crowding occurs [3,90,91]. In 1982, Kaplan and colleagues created a set of criteria for identifying suspected norovirus outbreaks without laboratory confirmation based on clinical and epidemiologic observations because laboratory tests were still being developed at that time [92]. These criteria include vomiting reported in more than 50% of affected persons, median incubation period of 24–48 hours, median duration of illness lasting from 12–60 hours, and no other bacterial or parasitic agents identified in stool specimen. Reevaluation of the Kaplan criteria indicated a sensitivity of 68% and specificity of more than 99% in identifying norovirus outbreaks, proving it to be a useful diagnostic tool, especially since laboratory tests are not widely available [93]. Few documented healthcare-associated outbreaks of norovirus have been reported in the United States; however, data from other regions that conduct surveillance for these events, such as Europe and Australia, indicate that norovirus is the most common agent causing healthcare-associated outbreaks of acute gastroenteritis.

Surveillance data from the United Kingdom and Wales during 1990–1995 suggest that 39% of all norovirus outbreaks occurred in hospitals and 37% in LTCFs [94]. The economic impact of these healthcare-associated outbreaks was estimated to have direct costs of $184 million dollars annually [94]. Other than the strong association between close proximity to other patients with active vomiting and an increased risk for norovirus infection, risk factors for healthcare-associated outbreaks remain unclear [95]. In the United States, the predominant genotypes responsible for both community- and healthcare-associated infections are GII (79%) followed by GI (19%) [96].

Clinical Presentation

The incubation period for norovirus infection ranges from 24–48 hours with a median of 33 hours. Infected persons generally present with acute onset, explosive vomiting, and nonbloody diarrhea with or without fever. Recent studies suggest a genetic component to susceptibility of persons to norovirus infection because volunteer studies have demonstrated a proportion of volunteers infected with norovirus who remain asymptomatic [97]. Other symptoms can include abdominal cramps, nausea, and occasionally a low-grade fever; however, illness usually is self-limiting and should resolve in 3–7 days. Dehydration, especially in those who are very young or elderly, can require prompt medical attention. Because of the large genetic diversity of noroviruses and the lack of protective cross-immunity induced by different strains reinfections with norovirus are frequent with no observable long-term immunity.

Diagnosis and Treatment

Diagnosis of individual patients or outbreaks of norovirus infection require that stool (preferred) and/or vomitus samples be collected and sent to a state health department or research laboratory for detection of viral RNA using the reverse-transcription (RT) polymerase chain reaction (PCR), or RT-PCR. Samples can then be sequenced at standardized regions of the viral genome to allow for typing of isolates; comparison of such genotypes could unmask related and unrelated events during an outbreak. In addition, the Kaplan criteria can be used while awaiting laboratory results or in the absence of available testing. At present, no antiretroviral medications are available to treat norovirus infections. Management involves providing supportive care, including rest and rehydration with oral or intravenous fluids [85].

Prevention and Control

No vaccines are currently available to prevent norovirus infection. Although noroviruses are common and highly contagious and require only a small inoculum for infection, the risk of infection can be reduced by frequent and appropriate hand hygiene, avoidance of potentially contaminated food and/or water, and adequate disinfection of contaminated environmental surfaces and/or fomites [63,65].

Strategies successfully used in the past to manage healthcare-associated norovirus outbreaks include the early detection and/or suspicion of norovirus infections; control measures, such as isolating or cohorting patients using contact precautions; and, in some instances of ongoing widespread outbreaks, closure of wards or units to new admissions. Because nonenveloped viruses such as norovirus can require a higher concentration of alcohol for inactivation than is commonly available in some ABHRs [63] if outbreaks occur and persist while using the ABHR, it is prudent to perform hand washing with soap and water.

Other interventions to reduce secondary transmission include educating of HCWs and patients regarding the risks related to and prevention of norovirus transmission, reinforcing appropriate hand-hygiene measures, and promptly cleaning and containing body fluid spills. Disinfecting of contaminated surfaces/fomites with chlorine-based products (e.g., a 1:50 dilution of household bleach) or EPA registered disinfectants with label claims for norovirus or its test surrogate (feline calcivirus [FCV]) also should be used [65]. If outbreaks continue despite this level of disinfection employing an even higher level disinfection with a 1:10 dilution of household bleach as recommended for *C. difficle* outbreaks could be beneficial. Ill HCWs involved in direct patient care and handling of hospital food should refrain from working until 24–48 hours after symptoms resolve [98]. Use of proper personal equipment such as gowns, masks, and gloves when cleaning up body fluid spills and disinfecting contaminated surfaces/fomites is recommended [65].

ACKNOWLEDGMENT

The authors wish to thank Lynne Sehulster, Ph.D., for her review of the manuscript with regard to environmental disinfection strategies and Marc-Alain Widdowson, VetMB, MA, MSc for his review of the manuscript with regard to rotavirus and norovirus epidemiology, clinical presentation, diagnosis, and control.

REFERENCES

1. Gerding DN, Johnson S, Peterson LR, et al. Clostridium difficile-associated diarrhea and colitis. *Infect Control Hosp Epidemiol* 1995;16:459–477.
2. Bignardi GE. Risk factors for Clostridium difficile infection. *J Hosp Infect* 1998;40:1–15.
3. Lopman BA, Reacher MH, Vipond IB, et al. Clinical manifestation of norovirus gastroenteritis in health care settings. *Clin Infect Dis* 2004;39:318–324.
4. Olsen SJ, DeBess EE, McGivern TE, et al. A nosocomial outbreak of fluoroquinolone-resistant salmonella infection. *N Engl J Med* 2001;344:1572–1579.

5. Vaagland H, Blomberg B, Kruger C, et al. Nosocomial outbreak of neonatal Salmonella enterica serotype Enteritidis meningitis in a rural hospital in northern Tanzania. *BMC Infect Dis* 2004; 4:35.

6. Yong D, Lim YS, Yum JH, et al. Nosocomial outbreak of pediatric gastroenteritis caused by CTX-M-14-type extended-spectrum beta-lactamase-producing strains of Salmonella enterica serovar London. *J Clin Microbiol* 2005;43:3519–3521.

7. Korpela J, Karpanoja P, Taipalinen R, Siitonen A. Subtyping of Shigella sonnei for tracing nosocomial transmission. *J Hosp Infect* 1995;30:261–266.

8. Pillay DG, Karas JA, Pillay A, Sturm AW. Nosocomial transmission of Shigella dysenteriae type 1. *J Hosp Infect* 1997;37:199–205.

9. Day care-related outbreaks of rhamnose-negative Shigella sonnei—six states, June 2001–March 2003. *MMWR Morb Mortal Wkly Rep* 2004;53:60–63.

10. Mohle-Boetani JC, Stapleton M, Finger R, et al. Communitywide shigellosis: control of an outbreak and risk factors in child day-care centers. *Am J Public Health* 1995;85:812–816.

11. Larson HE, Price AB, Honour P, Borriello SP. Clostridium difficile and the aetiology of pseudomembranous colitis. *Lancet* 1978;1:1063–1066.

12. Bartlett JG, Chang TW, Gurwith M, et al. Antibiotic-associated pseudomembranous colitis due to toxin-producing clostridia. *N Engl J Med* 1978;298:531–534.

13. Lyerly DM, Krivan HC, Wilkins TD. Clostridium difficile: Its disease and toxins. *Clin Microbiol Rev* 1988;1:1–18.

14. Gerding DN. Disease associated with Clostridium difficile infection. *Ann Intern Med* 1989;110:255–257.

15. McFarland LV, Stamm WE. Review of Clostridium difficile-associated diseases. *Am J Infect Control* 1986;14:99–109.

16. Kelly CP, Pothoulakis C, LaMont JT. Clostridium difficile colitis. *N Engl J Med* 1994;330:257–262.

17. Warny M, Pepin J, Fang A, et al. Toxin production by an emerging strain of Clostridium difficile associated with outbreaks of severe disease in North America and Europe. *Lancet* 2005;366:1079–1084.

18. McDonald LC, Killgore GE, Thompson A, et al. An epidemic, toxin gene-variant strain of Clostridium difficile. *N Engl J Med* 2005;353:2433–2441.

19. Loo VG, Poirier L, Miller MA, et al. A predominantly clonal multi-institutional outbreak of Clostridium difficile-associated diarrhea with high morbidity and mortality. *N Engl J Med* 2005;353:2442–2449.

20. Bartlett JG. Clostridium difficile: History of its role as an enteric pathogen and the current state of knowledge about the organism. *Clin Infect Dis* 1994;18 (suppl 4):S265–S272.

21. Archibald LK, Banerjee SN, Jarvis WR. Secular trends in hospital-acquired Clostridium difficile disease in the United States, 1987–2001. *J Infect Dis* 2004;189:1585–1589.

22. McDonald LC, Owings M, Jernigan D. *Clostridium difficile* infection in patients discharged from U.S. short-stay hospitals, 1996–2003. *Emerg Infect Dis* 2005;12:409–415.

23. Olson MM, Shanholtzer CJ, Lee JT Jr., Gerding DN. Ten years of prospective Clostridium difficile-associated disease surveillance and treatment at the Minneapolis VA Medical Center, 1982–1991. *Infect Control Hosp Epidemiol* 1994;15:371–381.

24. Miller MA, Hyland M, Ofner-Agostini M, et al. Morbidity, mortality, and healthcare burden of nosocomial Clostridium difficile-associated diarrhea in Canadian hospitals. *Infect Control Hosp Epidemiol* 2002;23:137–140.

25. Kyne L, Hamel MB, Polavaram R, Kelly CP. Health care costs and mortality associated with nosocomial diarrhea due to Clostridium difficile. *Clin Infect Dis* 2002;34:346–353.

26. Wilcox MH, Cunniffe JG, Trundle C, Redpath C. Financial burden of hospital-acquired Clostridium difficile infection. *J Hosp Infect* 1996;34:23–30.

27. Pepin J, Valiquette L, Cossette B. Mortality attributable to nosocomial Clostridium difficile-associated disease during an epidemic caused by a hypervirulent strain in Quebec. *CMAJ* 2005;173:1037–1042.

28. Barbut F, Petit JC. Epidemiology of Clostridium difficile-associated infections. *Clin Microbiol Infect* 2001;7:405–410.

29. Pepin J, Saheb N, Coulombe MA, et al. Emergence of fluoroquinolones as the predominant risk factor for Clostridium difficile-associated diarrhea: A cohort study during an epidemic in Quebec. *Clin Infect Dis* 2005;41:1254–1260.

30. Gaynes R, Rimland D, Killum E, et al. Outbreak of Clostridium difficile infection in a long-term care facility: association with gatifloxacin use. *Clin Infect Dis* 2004;38:640–645.

31. Dial S, Alrasadi K, Manoukian C, et al. Risk of Clostridium difficile diarrhea among hospital inpatients prescribed proton pump inhibitors: cohort and case-control studies. *CMAJ* 2004;171:33–38.

32. Dial S, Delaney JA, Barkun AN, Suissa S. Use of gastric acid-suppressive agents and the risk of community-acquired Clostridium difficile-associated disease. *JAMA* 2005;294:2989–2995.

33. Brooks SE, Veal RO, Kramer M, et al. Reduction in the incidence of Clostridium difficile-associated diarrhea in an acute care hospital and a skilled nursing facility following replacement of electronic thermometers with single-use disposables. *Infect Control Hosp Epidemiol* 1992;13:98–103.

34. McNulty C, Logan M, Donald IP, et al. Successful control of Clostridium difficile infection in an elderly care unit through use of a restrictive antibiotic policy. *J Antimicrob Chemother* 1997;40:707–711.

35. Simor AE, Yake SL, Tsimidis K. Infection due to Clostridium difficile among elderly residents of a long-term-care facility. *Clin Infect Dis* 1993;17:672–678.

36. Simor AE, Bradley SF, Strausbaugh LJ, et al. Clostridium difficile in long-term-care facilities for the elderly. *Infect Control Hosp Epidemiol* 2002;23:696–703.

37. Eglow R, Pothoulakis C, Itzkowitz S, et al. Diminished Clostridium difficile toxin A sensitivity in newborn rabbit ileum is associated with decreased toxin A receptor. *J Clin Invest* 1992;90:822–829.

38. Shim JK, Johnson S, Samore MH, et al. Primary symptomless colonisation by Clostridium difficile and decreased risk of subsequent diarrhoea. *Lancet* 1998;351:633–636.

39. Kyne L, Warny M, Qamar A, Kelly CP. Asymptomatic carriage of Clostridium difficile and serum levels of IgG antibody against toxin A. *N Engl J Med* 2000;342:390–397.

40. Palmore TN, Sohn S, Malak SF, et al. Risk factors for acquisition of Clostridium difficile-associated diarrhea among outpatients at a cancer hospital. *Infect Control Hosp Epidemiol* 2005;26: 680–684.

41. McFarland LV. Alternative treatments for Clostridium difficile disease: What really works? *J Med Microbiol* 2005;54:101–111.

42. Pepin J, Alary ME, Valiquette L, et al. Increasing risk of relapse after treatment of Clostridium difficile colitis in Quebec, Canada. *Clin Infect Dis* 2005;40:1591–1597.

43. Barbut F, Richard A, Hamadi K, et al. Epidemiology of recurrences or reinfections of Clostridium difficile-associated diarrhea. *J Clin Microbiol* 2000;38:2386–2388.

44. Wilcox MH, Fawley WN, Settle CD, Davidson A. Recurrence of symptoms in Clostridium difficile infection—relapse or reinfection? *J Hosp Infect* 1998;38:93–100.

45. Wilkins TD, Lyerly DM. Clostridium difficile testing: After 20 years, still challenging. *J Clin Microbiol* 2003;41:531–534.

46. Malnick SD, Zimhony O. Treatment of Clostridium difficile-associated diarrhea. *Ann Pharmacother* 2002;36:1767–1775.

47. Gerding DN. Metronidazole for Clostridium difficile-associated disease: Is it okay for mom? *Clin Infect Dis* 2005;40:1598–1600.

48. Bartlett JG. Treatment of antibiotic-associated pseudomembranous colitis. *Rev Infect Dis* 1984;6 (suppl 1):S235–S241.

49. Teasley DG, Gerding DN, Olson MM, et al. Prospective randomised trial of metronidazole versus vancomycin for Clostridium-difficile-associated diarrhoea and colitis. *Lancet* 1983;2:1043–1046.

50. Wenisch C, Parschalk B, Hasenhundl M, et al. Comparison of vancomycin, teicoplanin, metronidazole, and fusidic acid for the treatment of Clostridium difficile-associated diarrhea. *Clin Infect Dis* 1996;22:813–18.

51. Recommendations for preventing the spread of vancomycin resistance: Recommendations of the Hospital Infection Control Practices Advisory Committee (HICPAC). *MMWR Recomm Rep* 1995;44:1–13.

52. Musher DM, Aslam S, Logan N, et al. Relatively poor outcome after treatment of Clostridium difficile colitis with metronidazole. *Clin Infect Dis* 2005;40:1586–1590.

53. Pepin J, Valiquette L, Alary ME, et al. Clostridium difficile-associated diarrhea in a region of Quebec from 1991 to 2003: A changing pattern of disease severity. *CMAJ* 2004;171:466–472.

54. Wilcox MH, Howe R. Diarrhoea caused by Clostridium difficile: Response time for treatment with metronidazole and vancomycin. *J Antimicrob Chemother* 1995;36:673–679.

55. Poutanen SM, Simor AE. Clostridium difficile-associated diarrhea in adults. *CMAJ* 2004;171:51–58.

56. Climo MW, Israel DS, Wong ES, et al. Hospital-wide restriction of clindamycin: Effect on the incidence of Clostridium difficile-associated diarrhea and cost. *Ann Intern Med* 1998;128:989–995.

57. Pear SM, Williamson TH, Bettin KM, et al. Decrease in nosocomial Clostridium difficile-associated diarrhea by restricting clindamycin use. *Ann Intern Med* 1994;120:272–277.

58. Thomas C, Stevenson M, Williamson DJ, Riley TV. Clostridium difficile-associated diarrhea: Epidemiological data from Western Australia associated with a modified antibiotic policy. *Clin Infect Dis* 2002;35:1457–1462.

59. Wilcox MH, Freeman J, Fawley W, et al. Long-term surveillance of cefotaxime and piperacillin-tazobactam prescribing and incidence of Clostridium difficile diarrhoea. *J Antimicrob Chemother* 2004;54:168–172.

60. McFarland LV, Mulligan ME, Kwok RY, Stamm WE. Nosocomial acquisition of Clostridium difficile infection. *N Engl J Med* 1989;320:204–210.

61. Garner JS. Guideline for isolation precautions in hospitals: The Hospital Infection Control Practices Advisory Committee. *Infect Control Hosp Epidemiol* 1996;17:53–80.

62. Zafar AB, Gaydos LA, Furlong WB, et al. Effectiveness of infection control program in controlling nosocomial Clostridium difficile. *Am J Infect Control* 1998;26:588–593.

63. Boyce JM, Pittet D. Guideline for hand hygiene in health-care settings: Recommendations of the Healthcare Infection Control Practices Advisory Committee and the HICPAC/SHEA/APIC/IDSA Hand Hygiene Task Force. *Infect Control Hosp Epidemiol* 2002;23:S3–S40.

64. Boyce JM, Ligi C, Kohan C, et al. Lack of association between the increased incidence of Clostridium difficile-associated disease and the increasing use of alcohol-based hand rubs. *Infect Control Hosp Epidemiol* 2006;27:479–483.

65. Sehulster L, Chinn RY. Guidelines for environmental infection control in health-care facilities. Recommendations of CDC and the Healthcare Infection Control Practices Advisory Committee (HICPAC). *MMWR Recomm Rep* 2003;52:1–42.

66. Martirosian G. Recovery of Clostridium difficile from hospital environments. *J Clin Microbiol* 2006;44:1202–1203.

67. Kaatz GW, Gitlin SD, Schaberg DR, et al. Acquisition of Clostridium difficile from the hospital environment. *Am J Epidemiol* 1988;127:1289–1294.

68. Mayfield JL, Leet T, Miller J, Mundy LM. Environmental control to reduce transmission of Clostridium difficile. *Clin Infect Dis* 2000;31:995–1000.

69. Wilcox MH, Fawley WN, Wigglesworth N, et al. Comparison of the effect of detergent versus hypochlorite cleaning on environmental contamination and incidence of Clostridium difficile infection. *J Hosp Infect* 2003;54:109–114.

70. Muto CA, Pokrywka M, Shutt K, et al. A large outbreak of Clostridium difficile-associated disease with an unexpected proportion of deaths and colectomies at a teaching hospital following increased fluoroquinolone use. *Infect Control Hosp Epidemiol* 2005;26:273–280.

71. Glass RI, Kilgore PE, Holman RC, et al. The epidemiology of rotavirus diarrhea in the United States: surveillance and estimates of disease burden. *J Infect Dis* 1996;174 Suppl 1:S5–S11.

72. Zahn M, Marshall GS. Clinical and epidemiological aspects of rotavirus infection. *Pediatr Ann* 2006;35:23–28.

73. Turcios RM, Curns AT, Holman RC, et al. Temporal and geographic trends of rotavirus activity in the United States, 1997–2004. *Pediatr Infect Dis J* 2006;25:451–454.

74. Dennehy PH. Transmission of rotavirus and other enteric pathogens in the home. *Pediatr Infect Dis J* 2000;19:S103–S105.

75. Ward RL, Bernstein DI, Young EC, et al. Human rotavirus studies in volunteers: Determination of infectious dose and serological response to infection. *J Infect Dis* 1986;154:871–880.

76. Gleizes O, Desselberger U, Tatochenko V, et al. Nosocomial rotavirus infection in European countries: A review of the epidemiology, severity and economic burden of hospital-acquired rotavirus disease. *Pediatr Infect Dis J* 2006;25:S12–S21.

77. Rogers M, Weinstock DM, Eagan J, et al. Rotavirus outbreak on a pediatric oncology floor: Possible association with toys. *Am J Infect Control* 2000;28:378–380.

78. Ratner AJ, Neu N, Jakob K, et al. Nosocomial rotavirus in a pediatric hospital. *Infect Control Hosp Epidemiol* 2001;22:299–301.

79. Edmonson LM, Ebbert JO, Evans JM. Report of a rotavirus outbreak in an adult nursing home population. *J Am Med Dir Assoc* 2000;1:175–179.

80. Fischer TK, Bresee JS, Glass RI. Rotavirus vaccines and the prevention of hospital-acquired diarrhea in children. *Vaccine* 2004;22 (suppl 1):S49–S54.

81. Dennehy PH, Peter G. Risk factors associated with nosocomial rotavirus infection. *Am J Dis Child* 1985;139:935–939.

82. Matson DO, Estes MK. Impact of rotavirus infection at a large pediatric hospital. *J Infect Dis* 1990;162:598–604.

83. Griffin DD, Kirkwood CD, Parashar UD, et al. Surveillance of rotavirus strains in the United States: Identification of unusual strains. *J Clin Microbiol* 2000;38:2784–2787.

84. Staat MA, Azimi PH, Berke T, et al. Clinical presentations of rotavirus infection among hospitalized children. *Pediatr Infect Dis J* 2002;21:221–227.

85. King CK, Glass R, Bresee JS, Duggan C. Managing acute gastroenteritis among children: Oral rehydration, maintenance, and nutritional therapy. *MMWR Recomm Rep* 2003;52:1–16.

86. Vesikari T, Matson DO, Dennehy P, et al. Safety and efficacy of a pentavalent human-bovine (WC3) reassortant rotavirus vaccine. *N Engl J Med* 2006;354:23–33.

87. Sattar SA, Jacobsen H, Rahman H, et al. Interruption of rotavirus spread through chemical disinfection. *Infect Control Hosp Epidemiol* 1994;15:751–756.

88. Becker KM, Moe CL, Southwick KL, MacCormack JN. Transmission of Norwalk virus during a football game. *N Engl J Med* 2000;343:1223–1227.

89. Sawyer LA, Murphy JJ, Kaplan JE, et al. 25- to 30-nm virus particle associated with a hospital outbreak of acute gastroenteritis with evidence for airborne transmission. *Am J Epidemiol* 1988;127:1261–1271.

90. Centers for Disease Control and Prevention. Norovirus activity—United States, 2002. *JAMA* 2003;289:693–696.

91. Outbreak of acute gastroenteritis associated with Norwalk-like viruses among British military personnel—Afghanistan, May 2002. *Morb Mortal Wkly Rep.* 2002;51:477–479.

92. Kaplan JE, Gary GW, Baron RC, et al. Epidemiology of Norwalk gastroenteritis and the role of Norwalk virus in outbreaks of acute nonbacterial gastroenteritis. *Ann Intern Med* 1982;96:756–761.

93. Turcios RM, Widdowson MA, Sulka AC, et al. Reevaluation of epidemiological criteria for identifying outbreaks of acute gastroenteritis due to norovirus: United States, 1998–2000. *Clin Infect Dis* 2006;42:964–969.

94. Lopman BA, Reacher MH, Vipond IB, et al. Epidemiology and cost of nosocomial gastroenteritis, Avon, England, 2002–2003. *Emerg Infect Dis* 2004;10:1827–1834.

95. Chadwick PR, McCann R. Transmission of a small round structured virus by vomiting during a hospital outbreak of gastroenteritis. *J Hosp Infect* 1994;26:251–259.

96. Blanton LH, Adams SM, Beard RS, et al. Molecular and epidemiologic trends of caliciviruses associated with outbreaks of acute gastroenteritis in the United States, 2000–2004. *J Infect Dis* 2006;193:413–421.

97. Parashar U, Quiroz ES, Mounts AW, et al. "Norwalk-like viruses": public health consequences and outbreak management. *MMWR Recomm Rep* 2001;50:1–17.

98. Bolyard EA, Tablan OC, Williams WW, et al. Guideline for infection control in healthcare personnel, 1998. *Infect Control Hosp Epidemiol* 1998;19:407–463.

99. Apisarnthanarak A, Khoury H, Reinus WR, et al. Severe Clostridium difficile colitis: the role of intracolonic vancomycin? *Am J Med* 2002;112:328–329.

Central Nervous System Infections

34

Christopher C. Moore, Barry M. Farr, and W. Michael Scheld

Healthcare-associated infections (HAIs) of the central nervous system (CNS) are a rare but serious occurrence in the modern hospital. As with other types of HAIs, infection of the CNS most often follows a procedure that provides access for microbes to bypass normal host barriers. While a majority of episodes follow neurosurgery (NS), other neuroinvasive procedures (e.g., lumbar puncture or placement of an epidural catheter) occasionally can infect the CNS [1,2]. Nosocomial CNS infections that are not due to microbial contamination during procedures generally affect neonates who possess an immature blood-brain barrier that may be more easily crossed during bacteremia and the immunosuppressed. Nosocomial CNS infections range from superficial surgical site infections (SSIs) as the result of neurosurgery to meningitis, meningoencephalitis, or focal suppurations including brain abscess, subdural empyema, or epidural abscess.

INCIDENCE

Data from the Centers for Disease Control and Prevention's (CDC) National Nosocomial Infections Surveillance (NNIS) program, which were collected in 163 U.S. hospitals between 1986 and 1993, document 5.6 NS nosocomial CNS infections for every 100,000 patients discharged [3]. This rate is approximately half of what it was a quarter of a century ago (1/10,000 discharges) [4]. Meningitis is the most common CNS infection, accounting for 91% of the total, followed by intracranial abscesses in 8% and spinal abscesses in only 1%.

Somewhat higher rates of CNS infection have been observed among the immunosuppressed, ranging from 20 per 100,000 discharges for cancer patients [5] to 5–12 per 100 discharges among transplant patients [6]. Meningitis has constituted 71% of CNS infections among cancer patients, followed by brain abscess and encephalitis (making up 27% and 2% of episodes, respectively) [5]. Brain abscess appears to be more common among transplant patients (see Chapter 45), accounting for ~40% of CNS infections after heart and heart-lung transplants [7]. The highest rate of infection for a hospital service has been 45 per 100,000 discharges for the newborn nursery, according to NNIS data collected between 1986 and 1990 [8].

The incidence of CNS infection is relatively high among NS patients compared with other groups of patients. Among patients with American Society of Anesthesiology (ASA) scores <3, an operative duration <75th percentile, and a wound classification of "clean" or "clean contaminated," infection rates in the NNIS program have been 0.56/100 craniotomies, 0.70/100 spinal fusions, and 3.85/100 ventricular shunts [9]. Among patients with higher ASA scores (i.e., greater severity of underlying illnesses), longer durations of the procedure, and/or contamination of the wound, higher rates were observed [9]. The most common infection following NS procedures has been superficial SSI, accounting for 60% of SSIs after craniotomy and 75% after laminectomy, according to NNIS data [3]. According to updated NNIS data from January 1992 through June 2004, the rate of SSI after craniotomy was 2.40/100 operations when patients had a risk index category of 2 or 3. This rate was reduced to 1.72/100 operations and 0.91/100 operations when the risk index category was 1 or 0, respectively. Ventricular shunt placement resulted in SSI in 5.35/100 operations with a risk factor index of 1–3 compared to 4.42/100 operations with a risk factor index of 0 [10]. Meningitis is the second most common CNS infection after craniotomy, accounting for 22% of episodes, and it is the most common form of CNS infection after ventricular shunt placement, accounting for 76% of episodes.

RISK FACTORS

The most obvious risk factor for nosocomial CNS infection has been NS. Skin flora, which usually cannot be cultured from the operative site immediately after antiseptic preparation, regrow during the operation and can be cultured from a majority of operative sites just before closure [11]. As with other types of surgery, it is thus likely that most infections occur during the procedure while the wound is open, becoming contaminated from regrowth of the patient's own skin flora at the margins of the wound or occasionally by organisms from the operative team introduced on contaminated gloves or instruments or settling from the air into the wound. Infection at another body site also is a risk factor for infection of the NS wound. In an outbreak of meningitis due to *Klebsiella* spp., for example, colonization and/or infection of the respiratory or urinary tracts appeared to precede CNS infection [12]. Another study found that in 70% of NS patients with meningitis, there was antecedent or simultaneous isolation of the same organism from another body site [13]. A review of 15,200 NS procedures performed at one tertiary care center from January 1986 to December 2001 revealed an infection rate of 0.28% (35/12,980) after craniotomy and 1.20% (27/2,220) after ventriculostomy or ventriculoperitoneal shunt insertion, with an overall infection rate of 0.40% [14]. Another comprehensive review of 51,133 patients admitted to a NS service from 1993 and 2002 revealed 51 episodes of nosocomial meningitis, all of which were associated with NS intervention. Ventriculoperitoneal shunt procedures, either insertion or revision, accounted for 26 of the episodes. The next largest group consisted of patients undergoing surgery for an intracranial mass [15]. A total of 74% of bacterial meningitis in 61 patients aged 17–40 years identified in Taiwan had a postneurosurgical state as an underlying condition [16].

Factors that amplify the risk of postcraniotomy infection have included duration of the operation, external drainage, re-exploration, and operation through a paranasal sinus [17]. The risk factors contributing to the development of meningitis/ventriculitis after placement of a ventriculostomy have included intracerebral hemorrhage, other NS operations, drainage for >5 days, an air-vented system, irrigation of the system, and intracranial pressure >20 mm Hg [17,18]. The risk for infection of cerebrospinal fluid (CSF) shunts is increased by the duration of the procedure, thrombosis of the catheter, externalization of the shunt, inexperience on the part of the surgeon, and type of shunt (ventriculoatrial carrying a higher risk than

ventriculoperitoneal shunting) [17]. A persistent CSF leak after surgery heightened the risk of infection 13-fold in one study [19]; concurrent infection at a remote site increased the risk of CNS infection 6-fold.

Korinek et al. prospectively evaluated every adult patient undergoing craniotomy in 10 NS units during a 15-month period. Of the 2,944 patients studied, 117 patients developed SSIs. Independent SSI risk factors were postoperative CSF leakage (odds ratio, 145; 95% confidence interval, 72–293) and subsequent operation (odds ratio, 7; 95% confidence interval, 4–12). Independent predictive risk factors were emergency surgery, clean-contaminated and dirty surgery, an operative time >4 hours, and recent NS. Absence of antibiotic prophylaxis was not a risk factor. The investigators also found that the NNIS risk index was effective in identifying at-risk patients [20].

Placement of an intracranial pressure monitor is associated with different rates of infection, depending on where the monitor is positioned. One study found a 7.5% infection rate with a subarachnoid screw, a 14.9% rate with a subdural cup catheter, and a 21.9% rate for a ventriculostomy catheter [21]. Another study found a 0.6% rate for epidural monitors, a 3.0% rate for a subdural bolt, and a 4.0% rate for intraventricular or parenchymal brain monitors [22].

In June 2002, a manufacturer of cochlear implants used to enhance the perception of sounds in patients with severe to profound hearing loss notified the Food and Drug Administration (FDA) of 15 reports of post-implantation bacterial meningitis in patients who received its implants. This led to a cohort study to determine the incidence of bacterial meningitis among children with cochlear implants and a nested case-control study to examine risk factors for meningitis. The incidence of all episodes of meningitis in the cohort was 239.3/100,000 person-years (95% confidence interval, 156.4–350.6). Perioperative meningitis occurred at a rate of 2.1 episodes per 1,000 procedures. On multivariate modeling, the use of a positioner was significantly associated with meningitis (OR, 4.5; 95% CI, 1.3–17.9), as was inner-ear malformation with a CSF leak (OR, 9.3; 95% CI, 1.2–94.5) [23].

Gliadel wafers (1,3-bis [2-chloroethyl]-1-nitosurea) are approved for the treatment of malignant gliomas. These dime-sized disks contain carmustine, the primary chemotherapeutic agent used to treat glioblastoma multiforme. Initial studies reported an SSI rate of <5% with wafer insertion, but subsequent reports revealed infection rates of 15–23%. A 2003 review of 32 patients who received a Gliadel wafer identified 9 patients who developed an SSI. Among these 9 patients, there were four episodes of brain abscess, four of bone flap osteitis, two of epidural abscess, and one each of cellulitis and subgaleal abscess associated with wafer insertion [24].

Patients with head trauma are at increased risk of CNS infection, especially meningitis. CSF fistula raises the risk of infection in this population. A CSF leak was found to be present in 13% of episodes of nosocomial meningitis after head trauma in one series [25]. Infection of the paranasal sinuses may be followed by CNS infection in these patients [26].

Premature birth also appears to be an important risk factor because neonates cared for in neonatal intensive care units have had the highest rates of CNS infection according to NNIS data [8]. This finding seems to be related to the high risk of bacteremia from critical care instrumentation coupled with an increased risk of secondary meningitis from bacteremia stemming from the neonate's immature blood-brain barrier. Immunosuppression is another important risk factor for nonsurgical CNS infection, usually due to hematogenous spread.

ETIOLOGIC AGENTS

Staphylococci and gram-negative bacilli accounted for almost 70% of CNS infections documented in the NNIS hospitals between 1986 and 1992 [3]. During this time, *Staphylococcus aureus* was the most common pathogen after both craniotomy and laminectomy, followed by coagulase-negative staphylococci. These organisms were followed by enterococci, *Streptococcus* spp., *Pseudomonas aeruginosa*, *Acinetobacter* spp., *Citrobacter* spp., *Enterobacter* spp., *Klebsiella pneumoniae*, *Escherichia coli*, miscellaneous other gram-negative bacilli, and yeast, each of which accounted for <10% of episodes. After shunt procedures, *S. aureus* remained the most common pathogen causing superficial SSIs, but coagulase-negative staphylococci were more typical causes of deeper SSIs; gram-negative bacilli were responsible for 19% of deeper SSIs related to shunts [3]. *S. pneumoniae* was the predominant pathogen in the cohort of children with bacterial meningitis as a complication of cochlear implants (15/24) and Staphylococcal spp. were predominantly isolated after infectious complications of Gliadel wafer insertion [23,24].

If all CNS infections are considered, coagulase-negative staphylococci were the most frequent pathogens, making up 31% of episodes compared with 27% for gram-negative bacilli, 11% for *S. aureus*, 18% for streptococcal spp., 4% for yeast, and 9% for others [3]. For meningitis, the most frequently encountered CNS infection, coagulase-negative staphylococci, accounted for 32% followed by gram-negative bacilli (29%), *Streptococcus* spp. (18%), *S. aureus* (10%), yeast (4%), and others (9%) [3]. For intracranial infections, gram-negative bacilli were the cause of 23% of episodes followed by *S. aureus* (19%), coagulase-negative staphylococci (17%), anaerobes (11%), fungi (8%), *Streptococcus* spp. (8%), viruses (4%), yeast (3%), and others (8%). Spinal abscess displayed a dramatically different distribution of etiologic agents: 67% were due to *S. aureus* and 33% were due to coagulase-negative staphylococci [3].

The largest study of nosocomial meningitis from a single hospital was conducted by Durand et al., who reviewed

197 episodes among 151 adult patients at Massachusetts General Hospital during a 27-year period [25]. These nosocomial episodes accounted for 40% of the total of 493 episodes of bacterial meningitis observed during the study period. The proportion of episodes that were HAIs increased during the 27-year period. In this study, gram-negative bacilli were most common, accounting for 38% of episodes, followed by *S. aureus* (9%), coagulase-negative staphylococci (9%), *Streptococcus* spp. (9%), *Haemophilus influenzae* (4%), *Listeria monocytogenes* (3%), and *Enterococcus* spp. (3%) [25]. The microbes responsible for nosocomial gram-negative meningitis in this study were *E. coli* (30%), *Klebsiella* (23%), *Pseudomonas* (11%), *Acinetobacter* (11%), *Enterobacter* (9%), *Serratia* (9%), *Citrobacter* (4%), *Proteus* (2%), coliform types (2%), and nonenteric types (2%) [25]. The higher proportion of gram-negative and lower proportion of staphylococcal isolates in this study than in the more recent NNIS data could be due to the fact that there were only two years of overlap between the 27-year study and the NNIS data.

In Wang's review of 15,200 operative NS procedures from 1986 to 2001, the most frequently isolated pathogen was *S. aureus* (13/62, 21%); 91% of episodes involved a single pathogen with coagulase-negative *Staphylococcus* (7/62, 11%), *Pseudomonas aeruginosa* (5/62, 8%), *Escherichia coli* (5/62, 8%) and *Acinetobacter baumannii* (4/62, 6%) following *S. aureus* in frequency [14]. A review of *S. aureus* meningitis in Denmark over a 16-year period (1984–1999) identified 45 episodes of meningitis and 5 episodes of brain abscesses. Forty-four of these episodes were HAIs and only 6 were community acquired. None of the isolates was methicillin resistant, and 6 were penicillin susceptible [27].

Pathogens most frequently isolated from brain abscesses have been streptococci, Enterobacteriaceae, and anaerobes, together constituting ≤70% of episodes. Among immunocompromised patients, the frequency distribution of etiologic agents is somewhat different; *Toxoplasma gondii* and *Cryptococcus neoformans* are most frequent in patients with the acquired immunodeficiency syndrome, *Aspergillus* and *T. gondii* are the most common after heart and heart-lung transplants, and *Aspergillus* and *C. neoformans* are the most typical after kidney and liver transplants [28]. Among bone marrow transplant recipients, fungi accounted for 92% of episodes in a recent study: *Aspergillus* in 58% of episodes and *Candida* in 33% [28]. A retrospective hospital-based epidemiology study identified 153 patients with brain abscess over a 15-year period (1986–2000). There were 103 community-acquired infections and 20 HAIs. Of the HAIs, 17 occurred in a postneurosurgical state. Overall *Klebsiella pneumoniae* and viridans streptococci were the two most prevalent pathogens, and the addition of *S. aureus* accounted for 47% of post-NS brain abscesses [29].

Outbreaks of CNS infection among neonates or in NS patients most often have involved aerobic gram-negative bacilli [10,30–34]. Such outbreaks sometimes have been linked to a healthcare provider carrying the organism [35]

and at other times to contaminated equipment, such as respirators [36] or a shaving brush used for preoperative hair removal [34]. A review of 30 adult patients with gram-negative bacillary meningitis found that the majority of episodes occurred in men and that *E. coli* was isolated most frequently [37]. Outbreaks due to gram-positive bacteria, such as *Streptococcus* spp. (both groups A and B), *S. aureus*, and *L. monocytogenes*, also have been reported [38–46]. Secondary spread of *Neisseria meningitidis* or *H. influenzae* within the hospital setting appears to be rare [45–47].

CLINICAL MANIFESTATIONS AND DIAGNOSIS

Meningitis

The typical manifestations of meningitis—fever, headache, neck stiffness, and depressed level of consciousness—usually are present with nosocomial CNS infection, but the last three of these symptoms and signs also are frequently present in post-NS patients who do not have meningitis. These findings may stem from the underlying disease or the surgery. For this reason, changes in the degree of these symptoms and signs over time may be more important indications than their mere presence. Meningitis usually begins within 10 days of NS and almost always within a month. Fever is the most reliable single sign because usually it is not seen in postsurgical patients and because it is a component of almost all nosocomial meningitis episodes; 94% of patients with meningitis after NS had fever within the first day of illness in one study [13]. In Wang's review of 15,200 patients undergoing NS, 62 episodes of postsurgical meningitis occurred. Fever occurred in 54 of these patients and all but 13 patients had a disturbance of conscious state [14]. Fever also was a prominent finding in a review of 30 episodes of gram-negative bacillary meningitis (27/30) [37].

These usual clinical manifestations are more diagnostically useful indicators in nonsurgical patients with some exceptions, such as neonates and the immunosuppressed. Neonates with meningitis usually have fever but may fail to manifest other classic findings of meningitis, such as nuchal rigidity or a bulging fontanelle. Instead there may be a weak cry, decreased muscle tone, lack of movement, poor suck, diarrhea, vomiting, dyspnea, or apnea [48]. Likewise, the geriatric patient may not show classic symptoms or signs. High-dose corticosteroid therapy or severe neutropenia may significantly alter the clinical presentation of meningitis [6,49].

Because the clinical picture often is more difficult to interpret for nosocomial than for community-acquired meningitis, CSF analysis is correspondingly more important for confirming the diagnosis. Unfortunately, CSF abnormalities due to underlying disease and/or aseptic inflammation after NS can result in confusion, especially

very early after surgery [50]. Administration of OKT3 has been associated with development of aseptic meningitis in transplant patients with negative culture results for bacteria, fungi, or viruses [51]. The CSF findings most predictive of nosocomial bacterial meningitis have been neutrophilic pleocytosis, with most who are affected having a CSF white blood cell (WBC) concentration >1,000/mm^3 (and almost all having a CSF WBC concentration >100/mm^3), >50% neutrophils, and hypoglycorrhachia (usually <40 mg/dl). Hypoglycorrhachia appears to be the most reliable indicator of infection in the absence of positive results on Gram's stain or culture [13]. CSF lactate has shown some promise as a marker of bacterial meningitis in post-NS patients. When a CSF concentration of 4.0 mmol/L was used as a cut-off value for the diagnosis, the sensitivity was 88%, the specificity was 98%, the positive predictive value was 96%, and the negative predictive value was 94% [54]. Recent guidelines for the management of bacterial meningitis have suggested that empiric antibiotic therapy should be initiated when CSF lactate concentrations are ≥4.0 mmol/L. However, it must be realized that there are many other reasons for an elevated CSF lactate concentration, including cerebral hypoxia or ischemia, anaerobic glycolysis, vascular compromise, and metabolism of CSF leukocytes [55].

Gram's stain confirmed the presence of a pathogen in ~50% and culture in 83% of nosocomial episodes in one large study [25]. After NS, Gram's stain proved *Candida* spp. to be the causative agent in 36% of 18 reported episodes; it is worth noting that *Candida* spp. meningitis resulted in neutrophilic pleocytosis in 62%, with CSF WBC counts ranging from 13 to 8,000/mm^3 and a CSF glucose level of <40 mg/dl in only 12% [52]. False-positive results of Gram's stains reportedly have been due to organisms in stain reagents, on glass slides, in media used for swabs, or in tubes used to centrifuge the CSF [53,56–59]. Culture results often will be rendered negative within 24 hours of starting antibiotic therapy, but changes in glucose, protein, and WBCs usually take days to detect [60]. Antigen detection testing is seldom helpful in nosocomial meningitis but may be useful for detecting *C. neoformans* in immunosuppressed patients [49].

Foreign Body-Associated Infection

Infection of a shunt is classified by the CDCP as an HAI if it occurs <1 year of placement, although most episodes occur within the first 2 months. Pathogens such as *S. aureus* are associated with early onset infections while coagulase-negative staphylococci are associated with a later onset [61]. Fever is the most reliable symptom [62]. Infection of the proximal end of a ventricular shunt often results in symptoms of shunt obstruction (e.g., nausea, vomiting, or headache). Nuchal rigidity is present in one-third [61] of episodes. Symptoms and signs of distal infection of a shunt depend on the location of the tip. With ventriculoperitoneal shunts, peritonitis is the usual manifestation, but intestinal obstruction, intestinal perforation, and intra-abdominal abscesses have each been reported. Aseptic inflammation around the distal end has resulted in development of a peritoneal pseudocyst [63]. A tunnel infection with inflammation along the catheter may be seen.

Ventriculopleural shunts may result in empyema with distal infection while ventriculoatrial catheters can be characterized by symptoms of endocarditis (e.g., lethargy and fever of several weeks' duration). In the cases blood cultures usually are positive, and nephritis may be detected by urinalysis and serum creatinine measurement. When a shunt infection is suspected, aspiration of shunt fluid is indicated for cytology, Gram's stain, and culture. The sensitivity of the Gram's stain is ~50% and of culture ~80% [3]. Nine of 10 patients with shunt infection will have >100 WBCs per mm^3 of CSF. Glucose and protein determinations on CSF from a shunt have not proved useful [64].

In the study of children with cochlear implants, episodes of possible meningitis were associated with a CSF WBC concentration of 300 to 6,115 per cubic millimeter, and in all but one patient, there was a predominance of neutrophils. Nine episodes of bacterial meningitis were perioperative (occurring ≤30 days after surgery); 20 episodes were sporadic and occurred >30 days after surgery. Eight of these 20 patients had evidence of otitis media at presentation. In 11/15 patients with *S. pneumoniae* infection, meningitis was associated with bacteremia, and 1 patient had pneumonia. Two patients had received one dose of 7-valent pneumococcal conjugate vaccine. One other child had received two doses of the same vaccine and had *S. pneumoniae* meningitis caused by serotype 10A, which is not included in the vaccine. Two children had meningitis caused by *H. influenzae* type b (Hib). One child was fully vaccinated against Hib and the other had received 3/4 recommended doses of Hib vaccine [23]. In the four patients who developed brain abscess after Gliadel wafer insertion, the abscesses were diagnosed 22–159 days after implantation. One patient had an unusual presentation that included focal neurological symptoms, an increase in seizure activity, and no symptoms suggestive of infection [24].

Brain Abscess

Brain abscess can occur after NS, sinus infection, sinus surgery, bloodstream infection, or penetrating head trauma (e.g., gunshot wounds) [65–69]. Headache, fever, and focal neurologic abnormalities are the most typical findings while seizures, nuchal rigidity, nausea, vomiting, and papilledema can each be seen in up to half of the patients. Computed tomography scanning or magnetic resonance imaging (MRI) may be useful in confirming the anatomic location and size of lesions. Stereotactic aspiration with computed tomography guidance can be used for therapeutic drainage and for obtaining fluid for cytologic and microbiologic stains and cultures to guide therapy.

Meningoencephalitis

Meningoencephalitis involves inflammation of brain parenchyma and the meninges. Meningoencephalitis has occurred in rare episodes as an HAI after corneal or dural transplants taken from cadavers and after NS using contaminated instruments or electrodes. Both rabies virus and the agent of Creutzfeldt-Jakob Disease (CJD) have been transmitted in this manner. The incubation period for rabies following transplantation was 1 month; for CJD, it was about 18 months [17]. Additionally, there is a report of West Nile Virus being transmitted to a patient via blood products. The patient developed extrapyramidal movement disorders, and MRI images revealed changes in the basal ganglia similar to changes noted in the setting of meningoencephalitis due to other flaviviruses. Although the patient received contaminated blood products, detailed molecular analysis determined that the virus that caused his initial infection and encephalitis was likely acquired naturally from a mosquito [70].

CJD is a rapidly dementing illness with prominent myoclonus. Hypokinesia, rigidity, nystagmus, tremor, or ataxia may each be present in >50% of patients. Seizures occur in 10–20%. The disease generally ends with coma and death after 7–9 months. Rabies begins with a prodrome of nonspecific symptoms (e.g., fever, headache, malaise, anorexia, nausea, vomiting, or diarrhea). The prodrome is followed after 2–20 days by an acute neurologic phase, which may be characterized by hyperactivity and disorientation (furious rabies) or by paralysis. Coma usually supervenes within 10 days of the onset of neurologic symptoms and may last for hours in untreated patients to months in treated patients. The average duration of coma is 7 days in untreated patients and 13 days in patients receiving intensive care. Until 2005, only three recoveries from rabies had been reported. A fourth recovery was recently documented after a phenobarbital coma was induced and the patient was treated with ketamine, midazolam, ribavirin, and amantadine [71].

Spinal Epidural Abscess

The classic stages of an epidural abscess are back pain, radicular pain, radicular weakness, and then paralysis. Other symptoms may include bowel and/or bladder dysfunction, sensory deficits, stiff neck, and altered mental status. Fever usually is present at the time of diagnosis. Laboratory evaluation of peripheral blood usually demonstrates leukocytosis and an elevated erythrocyte sedimentation rate. MRI with gadolinium-DTPA contrast allows the best delineation of an abscess in preparation for surgery, which is done rapidly to preserve or salvage cord function.

Subdural Empyema

Cranial subdural empyema can follow paranasal sinusitis, otitis media, penetrating trauma, or an NS procedure.

Symptoms generally begin with fever and headache followed by seizures, altered mental status, focal neurologic symptoms, nausea, and vomiting. Computed tomography scan or MRI can be used to differentiate empyema from brain abscess. Spinal subdural empyemas have occurred very rarely and show symptoms similar to spinal epidural abscess, but tenderness may be absent on physical exam [3].

PROGNOSIS

CNS infections are regarded as being among the most serious because of the potentially disabling morbidity and mortality. Of 53 deaths among patients with CNS infection in NNIS hospitals between 1988 and 1993, 49 (92%) of the deaths were believed to have been caused or contributed to by the infection rather than a pre-existing illness [3]. The case-fatality rate for nosocomial bacterial meningitis in the study by Durand et al. was 35% compared with 25% for community-acquired bacterial meningitis in adults [25]. In the comprehensive review of 15,200 NS patients, the overall mortality of the 62 patients with meningitis was approximately 34% (21/62). Death was most often associated with sepsis (14/21). Of the 41 surviving patients, 19 were vegetative or had severe neurological deficits [14]. In the study of 30 gram-negative bacillary meningitis patients, death occurred in 11 patients. Inappropriate antibiotics were given in 8 patients, and all 8 patients died [37].

CSF shunt infections were associated with an attributable mortality rate of 23% in a study by Schoenbaum et al. [61]. Walters et al. confirmed the mortality associated with shunt infections and found a doubling of the case-fatality rate, a tripling of the number of additional surgical procedures, and significant prolongation of hospital stay among survivors [72]. The type of therapy appears to have an important effect on outcome. Antimicrobial therapy alone had a 36% success rate in treating shunt infections in one study compared with 65% for antimicrobial therapy and immediate shunt removal and 96% for shunt removal, antibiotic therapy, and ventricular aspirates or external drainage [73]. Mayhall et al. found a case-fatality rate of 100% among untreated patients with ventriculostomy infection [14]. Decline in cognitive ability has been documented following shunt infections [74]. One of the children with cochlear implant associated meningitis died, and three required removal of the implant [23].

Brain abscess is associated with a case-fatality rate of ~10% [65,67] and permanent neurologic side effects in almost 50% of the survivors [66,68]. Adverse prognostic factors include very young or very old age, ventricular rupture, delay of antimicrobial therapy, altered mental status at diagnosis, larger size and greater number of abscesses, or fungal or gram-negative bacillary pathogens [66,68,69]. Spinal epidural abscess was associated with a case-fatality rate of 13% in a review of seven case-series including

188 patients [75], but a more recent study of 43 patients reported only two deaths (5%) [76]. Paralysis was observed in 22% of patients in the review [75] and 20% of patients in the more recent series [76]. Intracranial subdural empyema is associated with a case-fatality rate of 20% to 30% and a high incidence of seizures and other side effects in survivors [77]. The most common CNS infection after NS—superficial SSI—has little effect on mortality but does prolong hospital stay [3].

Prognosis often is related to the specific cause of the CNS infection. In the study by Durand et al., case-fatality rates for the three most common HAI pathogen groups were 36% for gram-negative bacilli, 39% for *S. aureus*, and 0% (0 of 16) for coagulase-negative staphylococci [25]. The etiologic agent has an important effect on prognosis among the immunosuppressed, with case-fatality rates of 84% for gram-negative bacilli, 24% for *S. aureus*, and 37% for *L. monocytogenes* [6,78]. The use of voriconazole has improved survival in the setting of invasive aspergillosis. In one study, voriconazole improved survival at 12 weeks from 57.9% with amphotericin B treatment to 70.8% [79]. The type of underlying illness also affects prognosis in immunosuppressed patients with CNS infection. Case-fatality rates of 90% have been observed among patients with leukemia, compared with 77% for lymphoma and 59% for solid tumors of the head or spine [5,78].

PREVENTION

Because most nosocomial CNS infections are related to surgery, efforts to prevent these infections prominently include general measures for prevention of SSI, which is discussed in detail in Chapter 37. Such measures include strict attention to antiseptic preparation of the skin and aseptic technique, hair removal by depilatory or clipping rather than shaving, and minimizing the duration of operation while avoiding hemorrhage or creation of a CSF fistula, both of which can promote infection. Prophylactic antibiotics reduce the risk of HAI with craniotomy at least threefold. Either cefazolin or vancomycin is acceptable because most infections are caused by staphylococci [80]. Cefazolin would be preferred for hospitals with low rates of methicillin-resistant *S. aureus* (MRSA) infection (see Chapter 41) because high usage of vancomycin appears to select for vancomycin-resistant enterococci (see Chapter 15) within an institution [81]. In hospitals with high rates of MRSA infection, however, vancomycin would be the preferred agent. Due to concern for staphylococcal infection, current guidelines recommend the use of either cefazolin or vancomycin for a patient undergoing craniotomy [82].

For spinal surgery, antibiotic prophylaxis has not been standard because of the perception that infection rates are low without antibiotic prophylaxis. While some studies have documented rates <1% [83–86], others have observed rates from 2.3% to 5.0% [87–90]. One study has shown significant prevention with antibiotic prophylaxis for patients undergoing lumbar laminectomy [91]. It is likely that large randomized trials with adequate statistical power would document benefit as has been demonstrated recently for two other clean surgical procedures with generally low infection rates, herniorrhaphy and breast surgery [92]. Gantz and Godofsky suggested that prophylactic antibiotics are already being used routinely for high-risk situations (e.g., spinal procedures involving fusion or prolonged operations, immunosuppressed patients, and implantation of hardware) [3].

Prevention of infection of a CSF shunt using antibiotic prophylaxis has been difficult to confirm despite 12 randomized trials. Only one of the 12 trials showed significant prevention, but there was very low statistical power in each trial. All but one of the 12 trials showed a trend toward benefit from prophylaxis, which was continued for 24–48 hours in 10 of the 12 trials. To have 80% power to show a statistically significant benefit in the mean reduction of infection in these 12 trials would require a sample size of 790, but the average sample size in the 12 trials was only 113. A meta-analysis of these trials verified a 48% relative reduction in the rate of infection and suggested that this reduction might be beneficial [93]. The infection rate in the treatment group in these trials averaged 6.8%, however, which led the authors of the meta-analysis to suggest that a different strategy (e.g., use of a catheter with antimicrobial or anti-adherence qualities) may be needed for more effective prevention.

Respiratory isolation of patients with suspected meningococcal meningitis in a private room (with clinicians wearing masks) until 24 hours after the start of effective therapy has been associated with only very rare episodes of transmission to other patients [47] or to health care personnel; usually the latter form of transmission has been due to exceptional exposure to the patient's respiratory secretions (e.g., mouth to mouth resuscitation) [94–96]. Chemoprophylaxis of household or other very close contacts of patients with meningitis due to *N. meningitidis* or *H. influenzae* is indicated and may be arranged by the local public health department, which should be contacted promptly after admission of a patient with this disease. Eradication of the organism from the index patient before discharge may require additional therapy with rifampin because many regimens used for therapy of meningitis do not eliminate carriage [8].

REFERENCES

1. Teele DW, Dashefsky B, Rakusan T, Klein JO. Meningitis after lumbar puncture in children with bacteremia. *N Engl J Med* 1981;305:1079–1081.
2. Watanakunakorn C. *Escherichia coli* meningitis and septicemia associated with an epidural catheter. *Clin Infect Dis* 1995;21:713–714.
3. Gantz NM. Nosocomial central nervous system infections. In: Mayhall CG, ed. *Hospital epidemiology and infection control.* Baltimore: Williams & Wilkins, 2004:415–439.
4. Bennett J. Incidence and nature of endemic and epidemic nosocomial infection. In: Bennett J, Brachman P, eds. *Hospital infections.* Boston: Little, Brown, 1979:233–238.
5. Chernik N, Armstrong D, Posner J. Central nervous system infections in patients with cancer. *Medicine* 1973;52:563–581.
6. Hooper D, Pruitt A, Rubin R. Central nervous system infection in the chronically immunosuppressed. *Medicine* 1982;61:166–188.
7. Hall W, Martinez A, Dummer S, et al. Central nervous system infections in heart and heart-lung transplant recipients. *Arch Neurol* 1989;46:173–177.
8. Reingold AL, Broome CV. Nosocomial central nervous system infections. In: Bennett JV, Brachman PS, eds. *Hospital infections.* 3rd ed. Boston: Little, Brown, 1992:673–683.
9. Culver D, Horan T, Gaynes R, et al. Surgical wound infection rates by wound class, operative procedure, and patient risk index. *Am J Med* 1991;91(suppl 3B):152S–157S.
10. National Nosocomial Infections Surveillance. National Nosocomial Infections Surveillance (NNIS) System Report, data summary from January 1992 through June 2004, issued October 2004. *Am J Infect Control* 2004;32:470–485.
11. Bayston R, Lari J. A study of the sources of infection in colonized shunts. *Dev Med Child Neurol* 1974;16(suppl 32):16.
12. Price DJE, Sliehg JD. *Klebsiella meningitis*: report of nine cases. *J Neurol Neurosurg Psychiatry* 1972;35:903.
13. Mangi RJ, Quintiliani R, Andriole VT. Gram-negative bacillary meningitis. *Am J Med* 1975;59:829–836.
14. Wang KW, Chang WN, Huang CR, et al. Post-neurosurgical nosocomial bacterial meningitis in adults: microbiology, clinical features, and outcomes. *J Clin Neurosci* 2005;12:647–650.
15. Palabiyikoglu I, Tekeli E, Cokca F, et al. Nosocomial meningitis in a university hospital between 1993 and 2002. *J Hosp Infect* 2006;62:94–97.
16. Tsai MH, Lu CH, Huang CR, et al. Bacterial meningitis in young adults in Southern Taiwan: clinical characteristics and therapeutic outcomes. *Infection* 2006;34:2–8.
17. Stephens JL, Peacock JE. Uncommon infections: eye and central nervous system. In: Wenzel RP, ed. *Prevention and control of nosocomial infections.* 2nd ed. Baltimore: Williams & Wilkins, 1993:746–775.
18. Mayhall CG, Archer N, Lamb VA, et al. Ventriculostomy-related infections: a prospective epidemiologic study. *N Engl J Med* 1984;310:553–559.
19. Mollman HD, Haines SJ. Risk factors for postoperative neurosurgical wound infection. *J Neurosurg* 1986;64:902–906.
20. Korinek AM. Risk factors for neurosurgical site infections after craniotomy: a prospective multicenter study of 2944 patients. Service Epidemiologie Hygiene et Prevention. *Neurosurgery* 1997;41:1073–1079.
21. Aucoin P, Lotilainen H, Gantz N, et al. Intracranial pressure monitors: epidemiologic study of risk factors and infections. *Am J Med* 1988;80:369–376.
22. Blei A, Olafsson S, Webster S, Levy R. Complications of intracranial pressure monitoring in fulminant hepatic failure. *Lancet* 1993;341:157–158.
23. Reefhuis J, Honein MA, Whitney CG, et al. Risk of bacterial meningitis in children with cochlear implants. *N Engl J Med* 2003;349:435–445.
24. McGovern PC, Lautenbach E, Brennan PJ, et al. Risk factors for postcraniotomy surgical site infection after 1,3-bis (2-chloroethyl)-1-nitrosourea (Gliadel) wafer placement. *Clin Infect Dis* 2003;36:759–765.
25. Durand ML, Calderwood SB, Weber DJ, et al. Acute bacterial meningitis in adults: a review of 493 episodes. *N Engl J Med* 1993;328:21–28.
26. Humphrey MA, Simpson GT, Grindlinger GA. Clinical characteristics of nosocomial sinusitis. *Ann Otol Rhinol Laryngol* 1987;96:687.
27. Norgaard M, Gudmundsdottir G, Larsen CS, et al. Staphylococcus aureus meningitis: experience with cefuroxime treatment during a 16 year period in a Danish region. *Scand J Infect Dis* 2003;35:311–314.
28. Hagensee ME, Bauwens JE, Kjos B, Bowden RA. Brain abscess following marrow transplantation: experience at the Fred

Hutchinson Cancer Research Center, 1984–1992. *Clin Infect Dis* 1994;19:402–408.

29. Lu CH, Chang WN, Lin YC, et al. Bacterial brain abscess: microbiological features, epidemiological trends and therapeutic outcomes. *QJM.* 2002;95:501–509.

30. Sautter RL, Mattman LH, Legaspi RC. *Serratia marcescens* meningitis associated with a contaminated benzalkonium chloride solution. *Infect Control Hosp Epidemiol* 1984;5:223.

31. Parry MF, Hutchinson JH, Brown NA, et al. Gram-negative sepsis in neonates: a nursery outbreak due to hand carriage of *Citrobacter diversus*. *Pediatrics* 1980;65:1105–1109.

32. Goossens H, Henocque G, Kremp L, et al. Nosocomial outbreak of *Hemophilus influenzae* type b meningitis in an enclosed hospital population. *Lancet* 1986;2:146–149.

33. Abrahamsen TG, Finne PH, Lingaas E. *Flavobacterium meningosepticum* infections in a neonatal intensive care unit. *Acta Paediatr Scand* 1989;78:51.

34. Ayliffe GAJ, Lowbury EJL, Hamilton JG, et al. Hospital infections with *Pseudomonas aeruginosa* in neurosurgery. *Lancet* 1965;2:365–369.

35. Burke JP, Ingall D, Klein JO, et al. *Proteus mirabilis* infections in a hospital nursery traced to a human carrier. *N Engl J Med* 1971;284:115–121.

36. Berkowitz FE. *Acinetobacter* meningitis: a diagnostic pitfall: a report of three cases. *S Afr Med J* 1982;61:448.

37. Lu CH, Chang WN, Chuang YC, et al. Gram-negative bacillary meningitis in adult post-neurosurgical patients. *Surg Neurol* 1999;52:438–443.

38. Aber RC, Allen N, Howell JT, et al. Nosocomial transmission of group-B streptococci. *Pediatrics* 1976;58:346–353.

39. Campbell AN, Sill PR, Wardle JK. *Listeria* meningitis acquired by cross-infection in a delivery suite. *Lancet* 1981;2:752.

40. Ho JL, Shands KN, Friedland G, et al. An outbreak of type 4b *Listeria monocytogenes* infection involving patients from eight Boston hospitals. *Arch Intern Med* 1986;146:520–524.

41. Larsson S, et al. *Listeria monocytogenes* causing hospital-acquired enterocolitis and meningitis in newborn infants. *Br Med J* 1978;2:473–474.

42. Nelson KE, et al. Transmission of neonatal listeriosis in a delivery room. *Am J Dis Child* 1985;139:903–905.

43. Schuchat A, et al. Outbreak of neonatal listeriosis associated with mineral oil. *Pediatr Infect Dis J* 1991;10:183–189.

44. Schlech WF, et al. Epidemic listeriosis: evidence for transmission by food. *N Engl J Med* 1983;308:203–206.

45. Glode MP, et al. An outbreak of *Hemophilus influenzae* type b meningitis in an enclosed hospital population. *J Pediatr* 1976;88:36–40.

46. Barton LL, Granoff DM, Barenkamp SJ. Nosocomial spread of *Haemophilus influenzae* type b infection documented by outer membrane protein subtype analysis. *J Pediatr* 1983;102:820.

47. Cohen MS, Steere AC, Baltimore R, et al. Possible nosocomial transmission of group Y *Neisseria meningitidis* among oncology patients. *Ann Intern Med* 1979;91:7–12.

48. Overall JC. Neonatal bacterial meningitis: analysis of predisposing factors and outcome compared with matched control subjects. *J Pediatr* 1970;76:499.

49. Tunkel AR, Scheid M. Central nervous system infection in the immunocompromised host. In: Rubin RH, Young LS, eds. *Clinical approach to infection in the compromised host.* 3rd ed. New York: Plenum Medical Book Company, 1994:163–210.

50. Rahal LJ. Diagnosis and management of meningitis due to gram-negative bacilli in adults. In: Remington JS, Swartz MN. eds. *Current clinical topics in infectious diseases.* New York: McGraw-Hill, 1980:68–84.

51. Martin MA, Massanari RM, Nghiem DD, et al. Nosocomial aseptic meningitis associated with administration of OKT3. *JAMA* 1988;259:2002–2004.

52. Nguyen MH, Yu VL. Meningitis caused by *Candida* species: an emerging problem in neurosurgical patients. *Clin Infect Dis* 1995;21:323–327.

53. Ericsson CD, Carmichael M, Pickering LK, et al. Erroneous diagnosis of meningitis due to false-positive Gram stains. *South Med J* 1978;71:1524.

54. Leib SL, Boscacci R, Gratzl O, et al. Predictive value of cerebrospinal fluid (CSF) lactate level versus CSF/blood glucose ratio for the diagnosis of bacterial meningitis following neurosurgery. *Clin Infect Dis* 1999;29:69–74.

55. Tunkel AR, Hartman BJ, Kaplan SL, et al. Practice guidelines for the management of bacterial meningitis. *Clin Infect Dis* 2004 39:1267–1284.

56. Hoke CH, Batt JM, Mirrett S, et al. False-positive Gram-stained smears. *JAMA* 1979;241:478–480.

57. Musher DM, Schell RF. False-positive Gram stains of cerebrospinal fluid. *Ann Intern Med* 1976;79:603.

58. Peterson E, Thrupp L, Uchiyama N, et al. Factitious bacterial meningitis revisited. *J Clin Microbiol* 1982;16:758.

59. Weinstein RA, Bauer FW, Hoffman RD, et al. Factitious meningitis: diagnostic error due to nonviable bacteria in commercial lumbar puncture trays. *JAMA* 1975;233:878–879.

60. Roos KL, Tunkel AR, Scheid MR. Acute bacterial meningitis in children and adults. In: Scheld MR, Whitely RJ, Durack DT. eds. *Infections of the central nervous system.* New York: Raven Press, 1991:335–409.

61. Schoenbaum SC, Gardner P, Shilito J. Infections of cerebrospinal fluid shunts: epidemiology, clinical manifestations, and therapy. *J Infect Dis* 1975;131:543–552.

62. Gardner P, Leipzig T, Phillips P. Infections of central nervous system shunts: symposium on infections of the central nervous system. *Med Clin North Am* 1985;69:297–314.

63. Parry SW, Schumacher JF, Llwellyn RC. Abdominal pseudocysts and ascites formation after ventriculoperitoneal shunt procedures. *J Neurosurg* 1975;43:476–480.

64. Noetzel MJ, Baker RP. Shunt fluid examination: risks and benefits in the evaluation of shunt malfunction and infection. *J Neurosurg* 1984;61:328–332.

65. Mampalam T, Rosenblum M. Trends in the management of bacterial brain abscesses: a review of 102 cases over 17 years. *Neurosurgery* 1988;23:451–458.

66. Wispelwey B, Dacey R, Scheld W. Brain abscess. In: Scheld W, Whitely R, Durack D. eds. *Infections of the central nervous system.* New York: Raven Press, 1991:457–486.

67. Alderson D, Strong A, Ingham H, et al. Fifteen-year review of the mortality of brain abscess. *Neurosurgery* 1981;8:1–86.

68. Carey ME, Chou SN, French LA. Long-term neurologic residua in patients surviving brain abscess with surgery. *J Neurosurg* 1971;34:652–656.

69. Carey ME, Chou SN, French LA. Experience with brain abscesses. *J Neurosurg* 1972;36:1–9.

70. Solomon T, Fisher AF, Beasley DW, et al. Natural and nosocomial infection in a patient with West Nile encephalitis and extrapyramidal movement disorders. *Clin Infect Dis* 2003 36:E140–145.

71. Willoughby RE Jr, Tieves KS, Hoffman GM, et al. Survival after treatment of rabies with induction of coma. *N Engl J Med* 2005 352:2508–2514.

72. Walters BC, Hoffman JH, Hendrick EB, Humphreys RP. Cerebrospinal fluid shunt infection: influences on initial management and subsequent outcome. *J Neurosurg* 1984;60:1014–1021.

73. Yogev R. Cerebrospinal fluid shunt infections: a personal view. *Pediatr Infect Dis J* 1985;4:113–118.

74. McLone D, Cryzewski D, Raimondi A, et al. Central nervous system infections as a limiting factor in the intelligence of children with myelomeningocele. *Pediatrics* 1982;70:338–342.

75. Danner RL, Hartman BJ. Update on spinal epidural abscess: 35 cases and review of the literature. *Rev Infect Dis* 1987;9:265–274.

76. Darouiche RO, Hamil RJ, Greenberg SB, et al. Bacterial spinal epidural abscess: review of 43 cases and literature survey. *Medicine* 1992;71:369–385.

77. Mauser HW, Tulleken CA. Subdural empyema: a review of 48 patients. *Clin Neurol Neurosurg* 1984;86:255–263.

78. Chernik N, Armstrong D, Posner J. Central nervous system infections in patients with cancer: changing patterns. *Cancer* 1977;40:268–274.

79. Herbrecht R, Denning DW, Patterson TF, et al. Voriconazole versus amphotericin B for primary therapy of invasive aspergillosis. *N Engl J Med* 2002 347:408–415.

80. No author. Antimicrobial prophylaxis in surgery. *Med Lett* 1993;35:91–94.

81. No author. Recommendations for preventing the spread of vancomycin resistance: Hospital Infection Control Practices

Advisory Committee (HICPAC) [Review]. *Infect Control Hosp Epidemiol* 1995;16:105–113.

82. No author. Antimicrobial prophylaxis in surgery. *Med Lett* 2001;43:92–97.
83. Lindholm TS, Pylkkanen P. Discitis following removal of intervertebral disc. *Spine* 1982;7:618–622.
84. El-Gindi S, Aref S, Salama M, Andrew J. Infections of intervertebral discs after operation. *J Bone Joint Surg Br* 1965;58:114–116.
85. Odum G, Hart D, Johnson Smith W, Brown I. A seventeen-year survey of the use of ultraviolet radiation. Presented at the 24th Meeting of the American Academy of Neurologic Surgery. New Orleans, 1962.
86. Puranen J, Makela J, Lande S. Postoperative intervertebral discitis. *Acta Orthop Scand* 1984;56:461–465.
87. Savitz MH, Katz SS. Prevention of primary wound infection in neurosurgical patients: a 10-year study. *Neurosurgery* 1986;18:685–688.
88. Green JR, Kanshepolsky J, Turkian B. Incidence and significance of central nervous system infection in neurosurgical patients. *Adv Neurol* 1974;6:223–228.
89. Quadery LA, Medlery AV, Miles J. Factors affecting the incidence of wound infection in neurosurgery. *Acta Neurochır (Wıen)* 1977;39:133–141.
90. Wright RL. *Craniotomy infections.* Springfield, IL: Charles C Thomas, 1966.
91. Horowitz NH, Curtin JA. Prophylactic antibiotics and wound infections following laminectomy for lumbar disc herniation. *J Neurosurg* 1975;43:727–731.
92. Platt R, Zaleznik DF, Hopkins CC, et al. Perioperative antibiotic prophylaxis for herniorrhaphy and breast surgery. *N Engl J Med* 1990;322:153–160.
93. Langley J, LeBland J, Drake J, Milner R. Efficacy of antimicrobial prophylaxis in placement of cerebrospinal fluid shunts: meta-analysis. *Clin Infect Dis* 1993;17:98–103.
94. Feldman HA. Recent developments in the therapy and control of meningococcal infections. *Dis Mon* 1966:1–30.
95. Centers for Disease Control. Nosocomial meningococcemia—Wisconsin. *MMWR* 1978;27:358.
96. Artenstein MD, Ellis RE. The risk of exposure—avea patient with meningococcal meningitis. *Mil Med* 1968;133:474.

Surgical Site Infections

35

E. Patchen Dellinger, N. Joel Ehrenkranz,
and William R. Jarvis

HISTORICAL BACKGROUND

Until the end of the 19th century, infection was the greatest risk associated with any surgical procedure. Although the practice of surgery had spread rapidly following the introduction of ether at Massachusetts General Hospital in 1846, even relatively minor procedures could be complicated by severe systemic infection and death, which for major procedures was the expected outcome. Increasing knowledge regarding the relationship between bacteria and infection, advanced at the end of the century by such legendary figures as Pasteur, Lister, and Koch, led to a series of discoveries and the development of techniques that ultimately paved the way for modern surgery. Pasteur studied the relationship between bacteria and putrefaction. Lister recognized the role of bacteria in surgical wound infections and in 1867 introduced the practice of spraying antiseptics into wounds to combat bacteria. He gave scant attention, however, to the role of hands in introducing bacteria into surgical wounds. In an early (1878) application of his own postulates concerning microbial pathogens, Koch produced experimental wound infections by the injection of bacteria. Subsequently, in 1881, he verified the superiority of heat over antiseptics for killing bacteria and preventing access of bacteria to wounds [1].

The role of the surgeon's hands in introducing bacteria into wounds was slow to be recognized despite the work of Semmelweis in 1847. In 1882, when Ernst Bergmann arrived at the Ziegelstrasse Clinic in Berlin and was asked what was new in surgery, he replied, "Today we wash our hands *before* operation" [1]. Although rubber gloves were first developed for the use of Halsted's scrub nurse in 1889 to protect her hands from harsh antiseptics, widespread use of rubber gloves in surgical procedures did not become established until well into the 20th century.

In the 20th century, the standardization of aseptic practices in the operating room greatly improved the safety of clean operative procedures, but operations involving anatomic structures with a dense endogenous flora that cannot be eliminated before operation, such as the colon and rectum, continued to carry a very high risk of infection. A major collaborative study organized by the National Research Council (NRC) in 1964 documented the rate of surgical site infection (SSI) following 15,613 operations carried out over 27 months from 1959 to 1962 in 16 operating rooms of five university hospitals [2]. The study was designed to investigate whether the reduction of airborne bacteria in the operating room, accomplished with ultraviolet light irradiation, could achieve a reduction in SSIs. The study found that ultraviolet light produced a significant reduction in airborne bacteria but had no effect on SSIs except in the class of "refined clean" wounds (i.e., those with the lowest probability for contamination by endogenous bacteria). The infection rates in all other classes of wounds—other (clean), clean-contaminated, contaminated, and dirty—were unaffected by ultraviolet irradiation.

The NRC study was one of the earliest and certainly one of the most convincing to document the importance of endogenous bacteria as the primary etiologic agent of SSIs. This report also introduced a system for classifying wounds according to the risk of endogenous contamination (and thus of postoperative wound infection), which provided a basis for comparing SSI statistics. Although more sensitive and specific wound classification systems employing additional risk factors for wound infection have been developed since the NRC study [3,4], all systems continue to incorporate elements of this original scheme. Its NRC report contained results from the largest and most carefully conducted study in its day to examine a host of other factors related to the patient and the environment that influenced the risk of postoperative wound infections.

Multivariate analysis of this large body of data provided convincing evidence of changes in the risk of developing postoperative infections influenced by the patient's age, obesity, steroid administration, malnutrition, presence of remote infection, use of drains, duration of operation, and duration of preoperative hospitalization. It is interesting to note that although diabetic patients had a higher infection rate than did nondiabetics, this apparent difference disappeared after correction for the influence of age.

Although antibiotics were introduced near the end of World War II, their use did not appear to result in a lower infection rate despite early optimism. In fact, some careful observers of surgical practice published articles citing a higher SSI rate with the use of antibiotics than without. This paradox was undoubtedly due to the ineffective (usually postsurgery) use of antibiotics in patients recognized by their surgeons to be at high risk of infection. The effective use of antibiotics for preventing postoperative infection was ultimately made possible by the pioneering studies of John Burke, who used an animal model to demonstrate the critical importance of the timing of prophylactic antibiotic administration [5]. He showed via a guinea pig model that the appropriate antibiotics given before bacterial contamination could cause a significant reduction in the risk of infection while the same antibiotic, given after bacterial contamination, was much less effective. This information was translated into trials demonstrating clinically and statistically significant effects in human patients undergoing scheduled operative procedures, first by Bernard and Cole [6] and then by Polk and Lopez-Mayor [7] in the 1960s. Work on prophylactic antibiotics since that time has focused on defining those procedures and circumstances most likely to benefit from the use of prophylactic antibiotics and on examining the relative efficacy of different drugs and different routes and regimens of administration (see Chapter 13).

As improvements in anesthetic care and understanding of surgical physiology permitted more aggressive and widespread surgical intervention during the second half of the 20th century, the importance of surveillance for infectious complications became more evident. One result of the NRC study cited earlier was the observation of widespread differences in SSI rates among the participating hospitals for similar classes of wounds. This was probably one of the inspirations for the careful analysis of additional factors influencing infection risk that was carried out with that study. Data of this sort encouraged the systematic collection of information regarding postoperative infection rates and factors known to influence these rates.

In the 1970s, the Centers for Disease Control and Prevention (CDC) began the National Nosocomial Infections Surveillance (NNIS) system [8]. Although it included all healthcare-associated infections (HAIs), one component emphasized from the beginning the collection of data on postoperative infections. Data from the NNIS system provide a rich source of information about the relative occurrence of infections at all sites in hospitalized surgical patients [9]. Also, in the 1970s, surgical groups' reports of surveillance of large numbers of incisions validated the relationship between wound class and different risks of infection as well as the beneficial effect of reporting SSI rate data to the operating surgeons [10].

BIOLOGY OF SURGICAL SITE INFECTIONS

SSIs are caused by bacteria, and, in the absence of bacteria, they do not occur. However, surgeons have known for years that many other factors also influence the risk of infection. Burke demonstrated in 1963 that all (50/50) clean surgical incisions contain bacteria at the end of an operation, but only a small number (4% in that report) become infected [11]. An animal study of the relationship between bacterial inoculum and SSI risk showed an increasing danger of infection with increasing numbers of bacteria. This risk was described by a typical sigmoid, biologic curve when inoculum size was graphed against SSI incidence. However, there was no inoculum in that study of 1,028 incisions that resulted in either a zero or a 100% risk of infection [12]. The authors concluded that the development of infection in a surgical incision is "dependent on many factors other than the presence of bacteria." They further predicted that reductions in the incidence of postoperative infection could be achieved both by using techniques to reduce the numbers of bacteria that gain access to surgical wounds and by focusing on methods to increase the efficiency of host defenses in resisting those bacteria that do gain access to the wound. Modern surgical surveillance and surgical infection control must acknowledge both of these areas to achieve the goals of minimum postoperative infection rates.

SURGICAL SURVEILLANCE AND CLASSIFICATION OF SURGICAL WOUNDS

As indicated earlier, the oldest and best-established definitions of surgical wound classes originated with the NRC study of the efficacy of ultraviolet light for reducing wound infections. That study placed all wounds into one of five classes [2]:

1. *Refined-clean*: Clean elective operations, not drained, and primarily closed.
2. *Other (clean)*: Operations that encountered no inflammation and experienced no lapse in technique. In addition, there was no entry into the gastrointestinal or respiratory tract except for incidental appendectomy or transection of the cystic duct in the absence of signs of inflammation. Entrance into the genitourinary tract

or biliary tract was considered clean if the urine and/or bile were sterile.

3. *Clean-contaminated*: Gastrointestinal tract or respiratory tract entered without significant spill. Minor lapse in technique. Entry into the genitourinary tract or biliary tract in the presence of infected urine or bile.

4. *Contaminated*: Major lapse in technique (such as emergency open cardiac massage), acute bacterial inflammation without pus, spillage from the gastrointestinal tract, or fresh traumatic wound from relatively clean source.

5. *Dirty*: Presence of pus, perforated viscus, or traumatic wound that is old or from a dirty source.

All reports since the original NRC report have condensed this system into four groups, combining refined-clean and other (clean) into the one category of clean. Subsequent reports indicate a general consistency of the trends toward decreased overall SSI rates that is most marked in the contaminated and dirty classes of wounds (Table 35-1) [2–4,10,13]. These rates could have been influenced by a variety of factors, including a better understanding of the effective use of prophylactic antibiotics and of the bacteriology of dirty operative procedures and a reduction in the practice of closing the skin in dirty procedures.

Since the NRC study, much effort has focused on understanding which factors other than wound class affect the SSI risk. This trend began with the original analysis of additional risk factors performed with the NRC study. The earliest efforts to control SSI focused on lowering infection rates for clean wounds because these wounds should theoretically have a zero SSI rate if all bacteria could be eliminated from the wound. Thus, efforts focused on aseptic technique for prevention of SSI. Subsequent work found that even clean wounds become contaminated with some bacteria, and evaluation of historical data (Table 35-1) discovered a potential for reducing SSI rates even in high-risk wounds. This provided an incentive to understanding the underlying SSI risk in order to sensibly compare inter- or intrafacility SSI rates.

Another major effort in this area came from the Study of Efficacy of Nosocomial Infection Control (SENIC) project initiated by the CDC in 1974. The SENIC project collected data on SSIs and potential risk factors from 59,352 surgical patients admitted and operated on in 388 representative U.S. hospitals during 1975 and 1976 [3]. Multivariate analysis identified risk factors with roughly equal weight in predicting SSIs: having an abdominal operation, an operation that lasted >2 hours, a contaminated or dirty operation by the traditional NRC definitions, and ≥3 discharge diagnoses. This SENIC risk index was more discriminating than the old NRC classification of wounds (Table 35-2). The range of relative risks of SSI among clean wounds with different SENIC risk indexes is 1:14, and that of clean-contaminated wounds is 1:30; within the SENIC risk index, the range is 1:2.4 among wounds with one risk factor and <1:2 for all other risks. One weakness of the SENIC index was the employment of the number of discharge diagnoses as a factor because this number can be determined accurately only at the time of discharge.

The CDC subsequently developed a simplified risk index based on analyses of NNIS SSI data [4]. In the NNIS SSI risk index, the anesthesiologist's preoperative assessment according to the physical status index of the American Society of Anesthesiology (ASA) [14] is used instead of the number of discharge diagnoses. The ASA index assigns one point for a preoperative assessment score of 3, 4, or 5. Instead of counting any operation lasting >2 hours, a cut point was developed using the 75th percentile for operative duration for most operative procedures. A point is assigned for operative duration >75th percentile. The wound classification of contaminated or dirty is retained as in the SENIC risk index and adds one point to the risk score. The risk factor for abdominal operation is dropped. Thus, the NNIS SSI risk index has a possible score of 0 to 3.

A comparison of the predictive accuracy of the NNIS SSI risk index with the old NRC classification shows that this simpler index retains the increased accuracy and consistency within risk strata of the SENIC index while

TABLE 35-1

INFECTION RATE BY WOUND CLASS, HISTORICAL SERIES

	Years				
	1960–1962	1967–1977	1975–1976	1977–1986	1987–1990
No. of Patients [Reference]	15,613 [2]	62,939 [10]	59,352 [3]	25,919 [13]	84,691 [4]
Wound class					
Clean	5.1	1.5	2.9	1.4	2.1
Clean contaminated	10.8	7.7	3.9	2.8	3.3
Contaminated	16.3	15.2	8.5	8.4	6.4
Dirty	28.0	40.0	12.6	—	7.1

TABLE 35-2

COMPARISON OF SENIC AND NRC RISK PREDICTIONS FOR SURGICAL WOUND INFECTION

NRC Class	SENIC Risk Index						Maximum Ratio[a]
	0	**1**	**2**	**3**	**4**	**All**	
Clean	1.1	3.9	8.4	15.8	—	2.9	14.4
Clean contaminated	0.6	2.8	8.4	17.7	—	3.9	29.5
Contaminated	—	4.5	8.3	11.0	23.9	8.5	5.3
Dirty	—	6.7	10.9	18.8	27.4	12.6	4.1
All	1.0	3.6	8.9	17.2	27.0	4.1	—
Maximum ratio[a]	1.8	2.4	1.3	1.7	1.1	—	—

[a]Ratio of the lowest to the highest infection rate in wound class or in risk index.

being easier to apply (Table 35-3). One can see that the ratio of risks within single NRC wound classes range between 3.9 and 5.4 while all risks within single NNIS risk strata the ratios fall between 1.0 and 2.1. For surveillance programs with limited resources, it can be seen that surveillance of the 53% of patients with ≥1 SSI risk factors would yield data on 75% of all SSIs, thus increasing the efficiency of surveillance efforts [4].

Despite its advantages over the NRC wound classification system as a sole method of estimating SSI risk, the NNIS index, as with all indexes, cannot predict the outcomes for individual patients. In addition, the NNIS index lacks predictive power for certain highly standardized procedures, such as coronary artery bypass grafting [15], cesarean section [16], and craniotomy [17]. Although the NNIS index can accurately distinguish the risk of procedures from different categories of operative procedures, it does a poor job of distinguishing higher- and lower-risk procedures among all patients undergoing the same procedure. In these instances, different risk factors specific to the procedure and to the population become more important. Another potential problem with the NNIS system is

inconsistency in assignment of ASA scores [18]. A comparison of the sensitivity and specificity of ASA scores compared with the presence of ≥3 discharge diagnoses would be of interest. This comparison could probably be carried out on the original data sets used in the studies by Haley et al. [3] and Culver et al. [4].

HOST FACTORS THAT INFLUENCE INFECTION RISK

Many individual host factors influence SSI risk. Several were listed in the discussion of the NRC study earlier in this chapter. Most have been determined in studies like the NRC study in which patients undergoing one procedure or a variety of procedures and stratified by other known risk factors and/or by multivariate analysis have been followed to determine outcomes and the association of postulated risk factors with those outcomes. In most instances, the precise mechanism of action that links the risk factor and the infectious outcome are not known, although plausible explanations often have been provided based on logical reasoning but not on proof. Thus, the increased

TABLE 35-3

COMPARISON OF NNIS AND NRC RISK PREDICTIONS FOR SURGICAL WOUND INFECTION

NRC Class	NNIS Risk Index					Maximum Ratio[a]
	0	**1**	**2**	**3**	**All**	
Clean	1.0	2.3	5.4	—	2.1	5.4
Clean contaminated	2.1	4.0	9.5	—	3.3	4.5
Contaminated	—	3.4	6.8	13.2	6.4	3.9
Dirty	—	3.1	8.1	12.8	7.1	4.1
All	1.5	2.9	6.8	13.0	2.8	—
Maximum ratio[a]	2.1	1.7	1.8	1.0	—	—

[a]Ratio of the lowest to the highest infection rate in wound class or in risk index.

SSI rates observed with advanced age, extreme obesity, weight loss, hypoalbuminemia, or diabetes mellitus have been attributed to nonspecific defects in host defenses. The increased SSI risk observed in patients with anergy is not easily related to other measurable immune functions.

Patients who have an active infection at another body site are at increased risk of postoperative SSI [2]. This finding could relate to the increased risk that significant numbers of bacteria will gain access to the wound during the procedure or to inoculation of the surgical wound by bacteremia [19]. Data from human wounds suggest that the risk of postoperative infection is very great whenever the wound inoculum is $>10^5$ bacteria [20]. Although lymphatics have been suspected as a route of infection in patients with distal infections, evidence is lacking [21]. Patients who have been shaved at the surgical site before the time of operation have a higher risk of infection, which is thought to result from the tiny nicks and cuts caused by the razor and subsequent bacterial proliferation and inflammation in those injuries [22]. In vascular surgery, similar operations have a higher risk of postoperative infection in the groin region than in the arm or neck [23]. This could stem from local vascularity, local differences in bacterial number and type, or both.

INTRAOPERATIVE EVENTS THAT INFLUENCE INFECTION RISK

SSI risk is correlated with several factors that can be measured in the operating room. Other than wound class, one of the most consistently reported factors is the duration of the operative procedure. The precise connection between duration and SSI risk is not known. It is plausible that a prolonged operation results in more desiccation of tissues, potential for hypothermia [24] of the patient, and increased exposure of the wound to bacteria. It also is possible, however, that a longer operative duration is a marker for other, unmeasured factors, such as the underlying difficulty of the procedure, more scarring, larger tumor, patient obesity, or difficulty in exposure. No trial has been, or will be, conducted in which the same surgeon in performing procedures of equal severity deliberately varies the duration of the procedure. An operation that is rushed could heighten the risk of intraoperative contamination or of imperfect hemostasis with subsequent increased SSI risk. Operations should not be prolonged unnecessarily, but emphasis on the speed of operation can be misleading.

Operative technique and skill are widely believed to influence the SSI risk and other operative complications, but direct evidence is wanting. However, it can be shown that gross contamination of the operative field [25], poor hemostasis in the wound [7], and the need for all homologous blood transfusions [26] are associated with a higher incidence of postoperative infection. Surgeons commonly believe that leaving "dead space" or fluid in a wound increases the SSI risk. However, animal models of SSI demonstrate that placing sutures to eliminate dead space [27] or placing drains to close wounds and evacuate fluid [28] amplifies the SSI risk. Few prospective, controlled trials of this type are available for clinical surgery [29]; however, most observational studies demonstrate a greatly increased SSI risk with the use of drains [30,31].

Anything that supports the access of bacteria to the operative wound will increase the SSI risk. As discussed earlier, in intestinal operations, gross spill is associated with a higher SSI rate. In clean operations, a lapse in technique or in the usual protective devices is associated with increased SSI risk. In particular, glove punctures [32,33] or other episodes of contamination of the sterile field [33] raise the SSI rate. While few data directly confirm the value of hand scrubbing by the surgical team, the practice is firmly entrenched and presumably provides some protection against serious bacterial contamination when glove punctures occur. One observational study provides support for the importance of good hand-hygiene techniques [34]. The efficiency of the surgical drapes and gowns in preventing bacterial access to the surgical field also influences SSI risk. Impervious synthetic drapes result in a lower SSI rates in clean wounds when compared with those made of more loosely woven materials [35]. While most bacteria that cause SSIs come from the patient's endogenous flora and a smaller number come by direct contact from the hands and torn gloves of the operating team, occasional SSI epidemics can be traced to a member of the operating team, including a circulating nurse or anesthesiologist who does not have direct contact with the wound [36,37]. Such SSIs can occur without observed breaches of aseptic practice.

Preparation of the Patient and Operative Site

Despite much study, some common practices are of unknown efficacy for preventing SSIs. Different reports indicate reduction in SSIs or no effect from preoperatively bathing the patient with antiseptic soaps [38]. If practical, the lowest SSI rate for clean wounds is associated with no hair removal at the operative site. If hair removal is necessary, depilatory is preferable to clipping, which is preferable to shaving. Any hair removal should be done as close to the time of incision as possible [22]. Several agents are suitable for antiseptic preparation of the operative site. They include chlorhexidine preparations, various iodophor compounds, or tincture of iodine. To be effective, the antiseptic must be allowed to dry naturally before removal. Most operative sites are prepared first by the use of an antiseptic soap followed by an antiseptic preparation without detergent. Various commercial systems that employ foam or adherent plastic drapes with an antiseptic contained within the adhesive also seem to produce acceptable reduction in resident bacteria at the operative site while enhancing convenience or saving time in the operating room.

ANTIMICROBIAL PROPHYLAXIS

Since publication of the first articles [6,7] that cited the effectiveness of perioperative prophylactic antimicrobial administration, literally thousands of other articles covering this topic have been published (see Chapter 13). Recommendations from a recent review sponsored by the Infectious Diseases Society of America and endorsed by the Surgical Infection Society (SIS) are summarized in Tables 35-4, 35-5, and 35-6 [39]. Each recommendation given in these tables is classified according to the strength of the recommendation for or against a particular use and according to the quality of the evidence on which the recommendation is based. These categories are adapted from those published in an article by McGowan et al. [40] and Gross et al. [41].

For most questions, regarding antimicrobial prophylaxis there is a consensus about general principles. The most contentious areas remaining relate to the use of prophylaxis for some clean operative procedures, the specific agent used in some procedures, the duration of antimicrobial administration, and the relative merits of oral antimicrobial agents, parenteral antimicrobial agents, or both for prophylaxis in colorectal procedures. Most practitioners agree that antimicrobial prophylaxis is beneficial for procedures that involve entry into the gastrointestinal tract with resulting exposure of the surgical site to endogenous intestinal bacteria.

In gastric operations, the highly acid gastric contents keep endogenous bacterial numbers very low in patients undergoing elective peptic ulcer operations, and antimicrobial prophylaxis is not considered necessary. With the recent understanding of the role of *Helicobacter pylori* in the pathogenesis of peptic ulcer disease, elective operations for this condition have essentially ceased. Procedures on the stomach for cancer, gastric ulcer, bleeding, obstruction, or perforation are considered high risk because of the higher bacterial densities encountered and the increased risk of postoperative infection; thus, prophylaxis is recommended for these types of surgery. Prophylaxis also is recommended for gastric operations on morbidly obese patients [42–47].

The biliary tract is sterile in healthy persons, and colonization rates are low during elective operations for symptomatic stone disease. Higher rates of colonization and of postoperative infection are encountered in patients >60 years old or who have common duct stones, bile duct obstruction, recent episodes of acute cholecystitis, or previous operations on the biliary tract. Antimicrobial prophylaxis is recommended for patients in these high-risk categories [39,42–47].

Elective colon and rectal procedures are followed by very high SSI rates in the absence of antimicrobial prophylaxis, and such prophylaxis is widely practiced [46,48]. For procedures other than colorectal operations, parenteral administration of the antimicrobial agent is standard. For colorectal procedures, the opportunity exists to use oral (luminal) agents to lower the endogenous bacterial load before operation. Both routes of antimicrobial administration have been found to reduce SSIs when compared with those of a placebo, but the additional benefit of using both together has not been firmly established [48]. Nevertheless, the most common practice in the United States is to achieve mechanical cleansing of the bowel combined with oral administration of antimicrobial agents designed to reduce the luminal bacterial load on the day before the scheduled procedure and to administer parenteral agents in the operating room immediately before the operation [48,49]. The oral regimen that has the best support is the administration of 1 gram (g) each of neomycin and erythromycin base at 19, 18, and 9 hours before the scheduled time for the colon procedure [50].

Some procedures do not enter the gastrointestinal tract but nevertheless have a high rate of postoperative infection without prophylaxis. They include lower-extremity vascular procedures, hysterectomy, primary cesarean section, and craniotomy. Some other procedures do not have excessive SSI rates, but any SSIs that do occur have devastating consequences. These operations include joint replacement or placement of other prosthetic devices, cardiac procedures, and aortic graft placements (see Chapters 38 and 39). These procedures are widely regarded as benefiting from prophylactic antimicrobial administration [39,42–47].

The use of prophylactic antimicrobial agents for clean operations in which the SSI risk is relatively low and the consequences of infection are considered mild is controversial [43,51,52]. When SSI rates are low and the consequences small, the use of antimicrobial agents could expose patients to a drug to prevent a single infection, which could predispose to the development of bacterial resistance and/or an increase in adverse drug reactions in the population being treated. One proposal has been to limit the use of prophylactic antimicrobial agents to those clean procedures that can be demonstrated to carry a high SSI risk using one of the risk indexes discussed previously [46].

Many agents have been found to be effective for perioperative prophylaxis. In recent years, most new antimicrobial agents with any potential for surgical use have been licensed with one or more prophylaxis indications. The primary requirement for a prophylactic antimicrobial agent is that it be active against the pathogens known to be present at the operative site and those typically recovered from SSIs. The agent most commonly recommended for procedures that do not involve the distal ileum, colon, rectum, or appendix, and that, therefore, do not entail much risk of exposure to colonic anaerobes, is cefazolin [39,42–47]. Procedures that do involve these sites require an antimicrobial agent with activity against *Bacteroides fragilis* and other colonic anaerobes and the *Enterobacteriaceae* [48]. Cefoxitin and cefotetan are the two most commonly recommended agents. Newer, so-called advanced-generation agents have

TABLE 35-4

RECOMMENDATIONS FOR PROCEDURES THAT SHOULD RECEIVE PROPHYLACTIC ANTIMICROBIAL AGENTS[a] (MODIFIED FROM [40] AND [41]).

Procedure	Strength of Recommendation	Quality of Evidence
Surgical procedures that enter the gastrointestinal tract	A	I
Esophageal		
Gastric[b]		
Small intestinal		
Biliary[c]		
Colonic[d]		
Appendiceal[e]		
Head and neck procedures that enter the oropharynx	A	I
Abdominal and lower-extremity vascular procedures	A	I
Craniotomy	A	I
Orthopedic procedures with hardware insertion	A	I
Cardiac procedures with median sternotomy	A	I
Hysterectomy	A	I
Primary cesarean section or other cesarean sections involving prolonged rupture of membranes[f]	A	I
Procedures that include the implantation of permanent prosthetic materials[g]	B	III
Optional		
Breast and hernia procedures[h]	B	I
Other "clean" procedures where the clinical setting indicates an increased infection risk[h]	B	III
Initially clean procedures that become contaminated during the conduct of the procedure	C	III
Low risk gastric and biliary procedures[h]	B	III
Not data are currently available to apply these recommendations to so-called minimally invasive procedures, such as laparoscopic cholecystectomy or laparoscopically assisted bowel resections. Pending further data, it seems safest to apply the same standards as would be used for the same procedure done through a traditional incision.	C	III
Open gynecologic and urologic procedures that involve bowel are covered by the same guidelines that have been developed for general surgical procedures. The literature for transurethral procedures is large and controversial. It seems prudent to clear bacteriuria before any urinary tract procedure when clinical circumstances permit. Beyond that, local guidelines for implementation of the standard should reflect local practice.	B	III
It is common practice among pediatric surgeons to employ broad-spectrum antimicrobial prophylaxis for most operative procedures on newborn infants <30 days old.	C	III
No specific data regard the necessity or effectiveness of this practice.		

A-strongly recommended, B-recommended, C-optional; I-evidence from at least one properly randomized, controlled trial, II-evidence from at least one well-designed clinical trial without randomization, cohort or case-controlled analytic studies (preferably from more than one center), multiple time series studies, or dramatic results in uncontrolled experiments; III-evidence from opinions of respected authorities based on clinical experience, descriptive studies, or reports of expert committees.

[a]Specific recommendations are not referred to the original source(s).

[b]"High-risk" patients are those undergoing gastric procedures for cancer, gastric ulcer, bleeding, or obstruction, are morbidly obese, or have iatrogenic or natural suppression of gastric acid secretion.

[c]"High-risk" patients are those over the age of 60 with recent symptoms of acute inflammation, common duct stones, or jaundice or those who have previously had biliary operation.

[d]Oral prophylaxis with neomycin and erythromycin or another proven regimen for 18 hours before surgery is sufficient for scheduled colon operations when effective cleansing of the bowel can be achieved. When cleansing cannot be achieved owing to obstruction or other emergency conditions or the surgeon desires additional prophylactic protection for a high-risk patient, parenteral antimicrobials may also be administered. An agent effective against *Enterobacteriaceae* and *Bacteroides fragilis* group organisms should be used (see Table 35-5).

[e]If the appendix is freely perforated or associated with an abscess, antimicrobial administration is considered therapeutic not prophylactic, for the abdominal cavity and should be continued until an appropriate clinical response is obtained. The preoperative dose could function in a prophylactic manner for the incision, but treatment of established infection in the abdominal cavity requires continuation of the antimicrobial regimen after surgery. An agent effective against *Enterobacteriaceae* and *B. fragilis* group organisms should be included in regimens for both prophylaxis and therapy.

[f]For cesarean section, standard practice is to administer the prophylactic antimicrobial immediately after the cord is clamped.

[g]This standard is widely recommended and practiced, although specific data for the wide range of prosthetic devices in common use are not available. These devices would include various central nervous system shunts, vascular access devices, prosthetic mesh for hernia repair, and many others in addition to specific devices, such as orthopedic hardware and cardiac valves covered under other standards.

[h]Many authorities believe that these patients do not require antimicrobial prophylaxis. Certain clinical contexts increase the risk of postoperative infection and might strengthen the motivation to use prophylactic antimicrobials. These factors include American Society of Anesthesiology (ASA) preoperative assessments of 3, 4, or 5; three or more major preoperative diagnoses; an operation expected to last >2 hours; and an operation that lasts longer than the 75th percentile for that procedure. An undesirable local rate of wound infection could also heighten the benefit achieved from prophylactic antimicrobials, but the underlying cause of such a rate should be sought and corrected.

TABLE 35-5
CHOICE OF ANTIMICROBIAL AGENTS[a] (MODIFIED FROM [40] AND [41]).

Choice of Agent	Strength of Recommendation	Quality of Evidence
Many antimicrobials have been demonstrated to be effective for perioperative prophylaxis. The drug chosen should be active against the pathogens most commonly associated with wound infections that occur after the type of procedure being performed and against the pathogens endogenous to the body region being operated on. For procedures on the distal ileum, colon, and appendix, the antimicrobial(s) used should always be active against both *Enterobacteriaceae* and the common enteric anaerobic species, especially the *Bacteroides fragilis* group. Although infections that occur after gynecologic operations, especially hysterectomy, often involve anaerobic organisms, there has not been a demonstration of superiority by adding specific antianaerobic antibiotics compared with cefazolin alone. A very acceptable choice is to use cefotetan or cefoxitin for operations on the distal ileum, appendix, and colon and to use cefazolin for all other procedures.	A	I
Vancomycin can be given instead of cefazolin for patients who are allergic to cephalosporins or when the infection control committee determines methicillin-resistant *S. aureus* (MRSA) infections to be prevalent. Because vancomycin does not provide any activity against facultative gram-negative rods that can be present in the context of upper-gastrointestinal surgery, lower-extremity vascular surgery, and hysterectomies, another agent with gram-negative activity should be added in these cases. If vancomycin is being given because of concern over MRSA, cefazolin can also be given. If cephalosporin allergy is the concern, aztreonam or an aminoglycoside can be included with vancomycin. An aminoglycoside combined with clindamycin or metronidazole or aztreonam combined with clindamycin can be substituted for cefoxitin or cefotetan in allergic patients scheduled to undergo a colonic procedure. Aztreonam should not be used alone in combination with metronidazole because this combination lacks activity against gram-positive cocci and could lead to an increase in infections caused by *S. aureus*. If this combination is used, an agent with activity against gram-positive cocci must also be included. Unfortunately, data regarding the efficacy of these alternative recommendations are not available.	C	III

A-strongly recommended, B-recommended, C-optional; I-evidence from at least one properly randomized, controlled trial; II-evidence from at least one well-designed clinical trial without randomization, cohort or case-controlled analytic studies (preferably from more than one center), multiple time series studies, or dramatic results in uncontrolled experiments; III-evidence from opinions of respected authorities based on clinical experience, descriptive studies, or reports of expert committees.
[a]Specific recommendations are not referenced to the original source(s).

not been confirmed to be superior to cefazolin, cefoxitin, or cefotetan for the prophylactic indications for which these three drugs have been recommended [47]. Regimens with specific activity against *Enterococcus* spp. have not been shown to achieve superior results in colorectal procedures. Such regimens (ampicillin, amoxicillin, and vancomycin combined with gentamicin) are recommended for prophylaxis against bacterial endocarditis when gastrointestinal or genitourinary procedures are performed on patients with high-risk cardiac conditions [53].

The timing of antimicrobial administration for prophylaxis is important (see Chapter 13). For maximum effectiveness, the agent must have high concentrations in blood and body fluids *before* an incision is made. The original successful reports of prophylaxis specified that drugs were administered to patients "on call" to the operating room [7]. Before then, the practice had been to begin antibiotic therapy in the recovery room after the completion of the procedure. This was ineffective. Recent reports have confirmed the importance of administering prophylactic agents in the immediate preoperative period, usually within 30–60 minutes of the incision (unless vancomycin or quinolones are used, in which instance administration should occur 1–2 hours before the incision) [54,55]. Unfortunately, postoperative initiation of "prophylaxis" is still relatively common [54,56,57].

The necessary duration of antimicrobial prophylaxis has not been established, although analysis of data from some published reports suggests that antimicrobial activity should be present in blood and wound fluids at the time of closure for maximal effectiveness. Most early trials employed administration on a schedule that gave the third and last dose 12 hours after the first preoperative dose. Numerous reports indicate that longer durations and prolonged administration of prophylactic agents are common in clinical practice [54,56,57]. Although a single report suggests better results with longer use of prophylactic therapy in certain high-risk patients undergoing peripheral vascular procedures [58], most published articles support a short duration of antimicrobial prophylaxis [47,59, 60]. Another area of controversy is the prevention of SSI after traumatic injuries that expose the patient to

TABLE 35-6
DOSE, TIMING, AND DURATION OF ANTIMICROBIAL ADMINISTRATION FOR PROPHYLAXIS[a]
(MODIFIED FROM [40] AND [41]).

Antimicrobial Administration	Strength of Recommendation	Quality of Evidence
Dose: Very few reports have ever focused on the appropriate dose to use when administering a prophylactic antimicrobial. The dose used should never be less than the standard therapeutic dose for that drug. Considering the very short duration of administration recommended for prophylaxis and the safety profile of most prophylactic antimicrobial agents, it is reasonable to use a dose on the high side of the usual therapeutic range (1–2 gram (kg) of cefazolin, cefoxitin, or cefotetan for adults and 30–40 mg/kg for children).	C	III
Timing: The goal should be to achieve inhibitory antimicrobial levels at the time of incision and to maintain adequate levels for the duration of the procedure. Parenteral perioperative prophylactic antimicrobials should be administered intravenously during the interval beginning 60 minutes (min) before the incision is made. A time of administration as close as possible to the time of incision is preferred.	A	I
For cesarean section, the antimicrobial should be delayed until the umbilical cord is clamped and then should be administered immediately. Cefazolin, 2 g, is recommended.	A	I
Duration: The optimal duration of antimicrobial administration for perioperative prophylaxis is not known. Many reports document effective prophylaxis when a single dose of drug has been administered. It is likely that no benefit is obtained by administering additional doses after the patient has left the operating room. Thus, pending further data, postoperative dosing is not recommended. Antimicrobials for prophylaxis should be discontinued within 24 hours (hr) of the operative procedure.	B	II
The optimal duration of prophylaxis for cardiac operations is still the subject of debate, and many believe longer durations are needed. However, continuing prophylaxis until all catheters and drains have been removed is not appropriate.	C	III
Repeat doses during the surgical procedure: The necessity of administering additional doses of a prophylactic antimicrobial during an operative procedure of long duration has not been clearly defined. A number of reports, however, cite a reduced effectiveness of prophylactic antimicrobials to prevent infection, either for long-duration procedures or when measurement of serum or tissue levels show low levels of drug during the procedure. Based on current information, additional intraoperative doses of antimicrobial agents should be given at intervals of one or two times the half-life of the drug so that adequate levels are maintained during the entire operation.[b]	C	III

[a]Specific recommendations are not referred to the original source(s).
[b]Representative half-lives (with normal renal function) of the usually recommended prophylactic antimicrobial agents are cefazolin, 1.8 hr; vancomycin, 3–9 hr; cefoxitin, 40–60 min; cefotetan, 3–4.6 hr; aztreonam, 1.6–2.1 hr; aminoglycosides, 2 hr; clindamycin, 2.4–3 hr; and metronidazole, 8 hr.

bacterial contamination before antimicrobial treatment can be initiated. Because prophylactic agents cannot be administered before contamination, some clinicians have termed their use therapeutic rather than prophylactic. However, prophylaxis can be achieved for the operative wounds created in treating the injuries. A number of recent studies have established the fact that even in this context, a short duration of antibiotic treatment is as effective as a prolonged one and probably is preferable [60,61].

Selective Digestive Decontamination

More than 10 years ago, Stoutenbeek et al. proposed a method of selective digestive decontamination (SDD) to lower the infection rate in posttraumatic surgical patients in the intensive care unit (ICU) [62]. The concept holds that potentially pathogenic bacilli reside in an intestinal reservoir and serve as the source for many HAIs. The proposed regimen—tobramycin, polymyxin B, and amphotericin B by nasogastric tube and oral paste for the duration of ICU stay and parenteral cefotaxime for the first 5 days—is supposed to suppress potentially pathogenic microorganisms in the gastrointestinal tract while preserving the useful anaerobic flora that promote colonization resistance. Despite years of study and numerous publications, the concept is still the subject of much controversy. It has many proponents in Europe but has failed to garner much enthusiasm or be put into wide practice in the United States except among some solid organ transplant groups [63]. While many articles report a reduction in nosocomial lower respiratory tract infections, few cite any important differences in mortality rates or duration of ICU stay, and the suspicion arises that what has changed is the diagnosis of pneumonia, a notoriously difficult task in ICU patients (see Chapters 24a, 24b, 31). A number of the articles written about SDD report the early emergence of resistant gram-positive cocci [64,65]. Some recent reviews make clear that the role of SDD is still very controversial [65–67].

SYSTEMIC SURVEILLANCE OF POSTOPERATIVE INFECTION

The basic elements of a successful infection surveillance program include a definition of specific types of postoperative infections, a method for screening patients at risk, and a reliable means of recording and retrieving information (see Chapter 6). The observer who records the presence or absence of infection (infection control professional [ICP] or hospital epidemiologist) should have no conflict of interest in performing these duties. The surgical staff should be aware of methodology for screening and recording SSIs and should accept the definition criteria. It is useful for the observer to make rounds with several surgeons to ensure agreement on the use of definitions. The general criteria put forth by the CDC [68] have recently been updated (Table 35-7). A common definition error is to equate infection with recovery of a bacteria from the wound site. Bacteriologic findings do not distinguish between colonization or infection.

Surveillance objectives should be defined. All SSIs are not necessarily equally important to identify. Highest priority is given to detecting SSIs that lead to death, reoperation, increased intensity of services, or special diagnostic or therapeutic measures (including parenteral administration of antimicrobials, prolongation of hospital stay, or hospital readmission). Lower priority is assigned to finding superficial SSIs that do not lead to the outcomes just cited and that are readily treated on an ambulatory basis without a major increase in therapeutic costs or delay in the patient's return to regular activities. SSIs (especially deep ones complicating operations involving cardiac, vascular, and neurologic structures; bones; joints; stomach; bowel; or rectum) are more likely to compromise a patient's well-being than are similar SSIs complicating hernia repair or uterus, gall bladder, or thyroid operations.

Postoperative infections beyond the operative site may bring about considerable morbidity and should be included in routine systematic surveillance. This is particularly true for pneumonia (see Chapter 31). In special-care surgical units, surveillance of various infections caused by multidrug-resistant bacteria can be especially useful in providing information to surgeons about possible inappropriate antibiotic use and could indicate personnel or environmental transmission of bacteria. Hospitalwide outbreaks of infections due to methicillin-resistant *S. aureus* or vancomycin-resistant enterococci and clusters of diarrhea or colitis due to *Clostridium difficile* can manifest first among postoperative patients (see Chapter 33). Surveillance activities should identify such infections.

Hospital episodes of SSIs and postoperative episodes of bacteremia, pneumonia, and symptomatic urinary tract infection should be identified for the three categories of elective clean, clean-contaminated, and contaminated operations. Whereas patients having dirty operations could acquire a new infection as a complication of the operative procedure, often it is difficult to separate this event from extension of the infection already present at the time of operation. As the surveillance findings from patients undergoing specific types or groups of operations become large enough for meaningful interpretation, SSI rates for various procedures can be established as a baseline and to reflect the specific populations of patients being treated. After a database has been collected, cluster definitions and threshold levels for outbreak investigation could be defined.

The relative sensitivities of various methods for finding HAIs have been reported [69] (see Chapter 6). It may not be possible because of methodologic and interobserver differences and those in groups of patients to directly compare HAI rates complicating specific operations done at different hospitals. At the Florida Consortium for Infection Control, an organization of nonteaching community hospitals, a retrospective medical audit was useful in assessing the accuracy of ICPs in reporting all categories of postoperative infections. The expected ICP sensitivity for detecting SSIs at the operative site is $\geq 80\%$; the specificity is $\geq 97\%$. At the Minneapolis VA Medical Center, the ICP uses the floor nurses who see patients' wounds as part of daily care as sensitive indicators [70]. The nurses have been trained to recognize and to report to the ICPs all clinically suspicious wounds. ICPs personally examine such wounds and determine the wound status. In addition, every nurse on a surgical ward is authorized to send wound fluid for culture without a specific order.

A positive culture is not by itself a sign of infection. Instead, the fact that a culture was sent alerts the ICP that the wound was regarded as suspicious and prompts the ICP to inspect the wound personally. This system allows the ICP to focus his or her efforts on only the most suspicious wounds and provides a complete microbiologic record for those wounds that are determined to be infected [70]. Cardo et al. have reported on the accuracy of a similar system and found that sensitivity varied between 80–90%, depending on the degree of the ICP's experience, and that specificity was >99% [71].

The surveillance methods described here are all labor intensive. Moreover, the ICP's learning period can vary from several months to several years [71,72], depending on the intensity of training. Once a satisfactory level of surveillance sensitivity is achieved, it can be maintained only in direct proportion to the time available for the ICP to conduct surveillance. Yokoe and Platt have outlined a novel screening method in which antibiotic treatment of patients serves as a marker of those with possible SSIs [73]. This method has some promise to be labor efficient.

TABLE 35-7

CDC DEFINITIONS OF NOSOCOMIAL SURGICAL SITE INFECTIONS (SSIs), 1992. (MODIFIED FROM [69]).

Superficial incisional SSIs: Infection occurs within 30 days after the operative procedure *and* involves only skin or subcutaneous tissue of the incision *and* at least *one* of the following signs or symptoms is present:

■ Purulent drainage from the superficial incision

■ Organisms isolated from an aseptically obtained culture of fluid or tissue from the superficial incision

■ At least one of the following signs or symptoms of infection: pain or tenderness, localized swelling, redness, or heat; and superficial incision deliberately opened by the surgeon or attending physician

■ Diagnosis of superficial incisional SSI by the surgeon or attending physician

■ The following are not reported as superficial incisional SSIs: stitch abscess (minimal inflammation and discharge confined to the points of suture penetration), infection of an episiotomy or a neonate's circumcision site,[a] infected burn wound,[a] and incisional SSI that extends into the fascial and muscle layers (see *deep incisional SSI*).

Deep incisional SSIs: Infection occurs within 30 days after the operative procedure if no implant[b] is left in place or within 1 year if implant is in place and the infection appears to be related to the operative procedure *and* involves deep soft tissues (e.g., fascial and muscle layers) of the incision *and* at least *one* of the following signs or symptoms is present.

■ Purulent drainage from the deep incision but not from the organ/space component of the surgical site

■ A deep incision spontaneously dehisced or deliberately opened by a surgeon when the patient has at least one of the following signs or symptoms: fever (>38°C), localized pain, and tenderness unless culture of the incision gives negative results

■ An abscess or other evidence of infection involving the deep incision found on direct examination, during reoperation, or by histopathologic or radiologic examination

■ Diagnosis of a deep incisional SSI by a surgeon or attending physician

Organ/space SSIs: An organ/space SSI involves any part of the anatomy (e.g., organs or spaces) other than the incision opened or manipulated during the operative procedure. Specific sites are assigned to organ/space SSIs to identify the location of the infection. The specific sites that must be used to differentiate organ/space SSIs are listed here. An example is appendectomy with subsequent subdiaphragmatic abscess, which would be reported as an organ/space SSI at the intraabdominal site. Organ/space SSIs must meet the following criteria. Infection occurs within 30 days after the operative procedure if no implant is in place and the infection appears to be related to the operative procedure *and* infection involves any part of the anatomy (e.g., organs or space) other than the incision opened or manipulated during the operative procedure *and* at least *one* of the following is present:

■ Purulent drainage from a drain placed through a stab wound[c] into the organ/space

■ Organisms isolated from an aseptically obtained culture of fluid or tissue in the organ/space

■ An abscess or other evidence of infection involving the organ/space on direct examination, during reoperation, or by histopathologic or radiologic examination

SSIs involving more than one site:

■ Infection that involves *both* superficial and deep incision sites classified as deep incisional SSI

■ Occasional organ/space infection draining through the incision generally not requiring reoperation and considered a complication of the incision; classified as a deep incisional SSI

Specific sites of organ/space SSI:

Arterial or venous infection	Meningitis or ventriculitis
Breast abscess or mastitis	Myocarditis or pericarditis
Disc space	Oral cavity (mouth, tongue, or gums)
Ear, mastoid	Osteomyelitis
Endocarditis	Other infections of the lower respiratory tract
Endometritis	Other infections of the urinary tract
Eye, other than conjunctivitis	Other male or female reproductive tract
Gastrointestinal tract	Spinal abscess without meningitis
Intraabdominal, not specified elsewhere	Sinusitis
Intracranial, brain, or dural infections abscess	Upper respiratory tract, pharyngitis
Joint or bursa	Vaginal cuff
Mediastinitis	

---

[a]Specific criteria are used for infected episiotomy and circumcision sites and for burn wounds.

[b]Implant is defined as a nonhuman-derived implantable foreign body (e.g., prosthetic heart valve, nonhuman vascular graft, mechanical heart, or hip prosthesis) that is permanently placed in a patient during an operation.

[c]If the area around a stab wound becomes infected, it is not an SSI but is considered a skin or soft-tissue infection, depending on its depth.

Any SSI rate determined in such a system is, of course, a minimum estimate of the infection rate because wounds that escape surveillance or that manifest only after discharge will not be counted. A recent consensus paper by the joint Surgical Wound Infection Task Force representing the Society for Hospital Epidemiology of America, Association of Professionals in Infection Control, the CDC, and the SIS has recommended that some form of postdischarge surveillance should be undertaken [74]. Tools to identify postdischarge infections include questionnaires sent to surgeons or to patients, telephone follow-up with surgeons or patients, and systems to detect readmission of patients to hospitals and postoperative antibiotic prescriptions. The best method for accomplishing such surveillance is not known, and some systems appear to be both expensive and insensitive [75]. In addition, postdischarge surveillance can be more useful for some procedures than others. No consensus has been reached on what method of postdischarge surveillance and for what procedures such methods should be used.

Another area that has received very little attention to date is the surveillance of outpatient operative procedures. The NNIS system specifically tracks only inpatients [8,68]. An increasing number of operative procedures are being performed on patients who are not admitted to a hospital, $\geq$50% in many hospitals (see Chapter 28). Preliminary information suggests that SSIs in these patients are less common than in patients having similar procedures as inpatients [76,77]. However, very little systematic information is available. As more and more procedures are performed on an outpatient basis, the usefulness and validity of postdischarge surveillance for SSIs in this population will continue to be debated.

A surveillance worksheet indicating the criteria used for SSI definitions is useful to record important details about an infected patient. Only the minimum information necessary for further tabulation to identify clusters or outbreaks should be included. In general, patients' demographic characteristics and details of operations are readily available on-line or in the medical record and need not be routinely recorded. On infrequent occasions when SSI clusters are found, additional information about host risk factors, technical aspects of surgical procedures, and environmental details concerning the patients' care can be important for stratification during analysis. Computer analysis of surveillance data is helpful only to the extent that the data output is consonant with the previously determined objectives (see Chapter 8).

ANALYSES OF CRUDE DATA: INVESTIGATIONS OF OUTBREAKS AND CLUSTERS

In the workup of an apparent excess frequency of SSIs, acquisition of infection can be evaluated in relation to the sequence of surgical care: preoperative (therapeutic and host factors), intraoperative, and postoperative. Identifying a specific operation as the point of selection rather than as an operator, a wide range of possible contributions to individual infection risks is more likely to be fully explored. Operations should be surveyed for postoperative infections at operative and nonoperative sites.

It is especially important to recognize the potentially pejorative implications of incorrectly interpreting crude data sets of postoperative infections. Dissemination of crude data to an uncritical audience has the power to damage a surgeon or an institution. Access to crude data sets should be restricted to those who have an actual need to know about interval findings of work in progress. The limitations of crude findings of postoperative infections should be identified for those who review them. There also should be constant concern about disseminating interpretations of a single set of data indicating highly unusual findings because of possible sampling or other biases and for type 1 error due to inadequate sample size (see Chapter 7). Failure to identify potential limitations in interpreting crude data and possible sampling errors in small clusters can result in a loss of credibility of the surveillance program, create a climate of suspicion and animosity among the surgical staff, and jeopardize the success of any future efforts. Thus, sound epidemiologic methods and strict confidentiality of records are central to an effective program. However, the recent passage of legislation requiring mandatory reporting of hospital-specific HAI rates, although publicized as beneficial, could lead to efforts to minimize SSI rates and not ultimately lead to reduction of HAIs.

SSI cluster can be sought by grouping infected patients according to characteristics such as time, place, person, infecting organisms, surgeons, types of operations, preoperative host and surgical risk factors, use of various devices, characteristics of critical care, preoperative duration of hospitalization, and postoperative intervals until onset of infection (see Chapter 6). In stratification, the analyst seeks to identify possible commonality in SSI sources. For example, a lengthy preoperative period of hospitalization could indicate patients with unusual or complex manifestations of disease. Relatively long periods from operation to SSI onset can suggest that a postoperative event has played a role. In the latter instance, time periods in >10 to 12 days raise the possibility that postoperative factors (including hematoma, seroma, remote site infection, prolonged or unnecessary use of surgical drains, and postoperative manipulation of the wound) aided in the initiation of infection. An open conduit at the surgical site (e.g., Penrose drain) also could be a factor in permitting infection.

An increase in the incidence of postoperative infection could result from a change in risk characteristics of the patients with the introduction of a population having an increased susceptibility to infection. In small SSI clusters, chance alone can bring about a concatenation of unrelated events, giving the false appearance of a group of SSIs linked by common causation. Alternatively, a small SSI cluster in high-risk patients could indicate a much larger outbreak with a wide array of disease manifestations (see Chapter 6). A systematic search for unreported SSIs, including those arising after hospital discharge, usually is necessary to determine the actual size of such clusters. Case-control analysis, stratified as necessary, is useful when new equipment, procedures, or processes have been introduced.

SURGEON-SPECIFIC SURVEILLANCE

Following the outline of the 1964 NRC study [2], Cruse and Foord [10] devised a program of concurrent observation of surgical wounds in patients undergoing clean operations to provide individual surgeons with SSI rates. This study and others [13] have demonstrated that providing SSI rates to the surgical staff results in a decrease in SSIs. These findings are consonant with the results of the SENIC study [69], in which reduction of SSIs was found to be associated with a strong infection control program that included an effective hospital epidemiologist and a system for reporting specific SSI rates to the specific surgeon. Surgeon-specific SSI rates can be readily determined. Aggregated SSI rates for different classes of operations can be calculated for individual surgeons from NNIS SSI risk index data and compared with a standardized infection ratio [78].

The goal of surgeon-specific surveillance is to lower the SSI rate by making individual surgeons aware of excesses in SSI rates and thereby promote adherence to accepted principles of operative care. Implicit in this approach is the assumption that SSIs can be entirely attributed to flaws in surgical techniques or judgment (including incorrect use of antibiotic prophylaxis). Also implicit is the assumption that any reduction in SSI rates following the provision of information regarding excess rates to an individual surgeon results from improvement in faulty surgical technique, protocols, and/or judgment. Massanari has pointed out some concerns for small sample sizes, validity of methods for risk adjustment, and reliability of data collection methods in this context [79].

Nonetheless, an actual problem in surgical technique could exist for one or several surgeons. This is a thorny issue. There is no methodology to evaluate operative technique as a surveillance activity. Moreover, providing some surgeons with surgeon-specific data could not bring the desired results. In some instances, surgeons in community hospitals with a high rate of postoperative infection have simply moved their practices to other hospitals in which surveillance is less intense.

Lee has suggested that rather than focusing too much attention on absolute SSI rates, the hospital epidemiologist and surgeon should concentrate on classifying each SSI into the dichotomous classes of *potentially avoidable* and *apparently unavoidable infections* [70]. A potentially avoidable SSI is an infection that occurs under circumstances in which any indicated infection-reducing adjuncts were omitted. Such adjuncts would include appropriate use of prophylactic antibiotics (agent, timing, and discontinuing), avoidance of razor shaving on the day before operation, appropriate skin preparation at the operative site, avoiding elective operations in the presence of distant site and active infections, and so on. An apparently unavoidable SSI is one that occurs despite the application of all known appropriate infection-reducing measures. The goal of an SSI surveillance program should be *zero avoidable SSIs* [70]. When a particular infection-reducing strategy is well accepted but not always reliably applied, such as the indicated use of perioperative prophylactic antibiotics, a quality assurance program designed to ensure the reliable application of this method could have a greater effect on SSI rates than could feedback on SSI rates alone [39].

VIRAL INFECTIONS

Studies of patients receiving transplants have confirmed that viral infection is a surgical complication in this context [80] (see Chapter 45). The principal agents are transferred by human tissue organs and blood. Cytomegalovirus, herpesvirus, hepatitis B, hepatitis C, and varicella zoster are the viruses most frequently identified (see Chapter 42). Human immunodeficiency virus is the one most feared (see Chapter 43). Routine methods for surveillance of viral postoperative infections need to be developed.

FUNGAL INFECTIONS

Candida spp. are gaining prominence in consideration as causes of SSI. This is particularly true in the surgical treatment of transplant patients, burn patients, and patients with prosthetic devices (see Chapter 43). Intravenous catheter and urine cultures can yield fungi before systemic involvement, and it is likely that patients are infected from such sources by hematogenous spread. Improved methods to identify and control such infections will become more important as technical advances in surgery lead to treatment of more immunocompromised subjects.

THE COSTS OF SURGICAL INFECTIONS

Postoperative infections in surgical patients can prolong the length of hospitalization for substantial periods, depending on the type of operation, and thereby greatly increase the cost of their care. Cardiothoracic, orthopedic, and gastrointestinal operations are likely to be especially costly in this regard as the result of both pulmonary and operative site infections [81,82]. In addition to the higher direct costs of care, indirect costs should be considered in calculating the consequences of postoperative infection. These costs include the time the patient loses from gainful employment and the possible medicolegal actions that the patient could take against a hospital or the surgical staff (see Chapter 17).

NEW DIRECTIONS IN PREVENTING POSTOPERATIVE INFECTION

As the incidence of SSIs progressively declines, new thinking is required to define the next step in improving the care of patients in relation to controlling postoperative infection. Perioperative colonization with virulent bacteria can be a source of both endogenous infection and cross-infection. The association between nasal carriage of *S. aureus* (or *MRSA*) and postoperative infection is well known [83]. Some evidence exists that topical nasal treatment with mupirocin can reduce endogenous SSIs with *S. aureus* [84–86] and minimize *S. aureus* cross-infection in a surgical ICU (see Chapter 40). Both nasal colonization with *S. aureus* [85] and lower respiratory tract colonization with *Haemophilus* spp. [87] appear to be sources of postoperative pulmonary infection. How to identify and reduce the latter, especially in the preoperative treatment of the patient with traumatic injury, remains to be established. Before, during, and after surgery, a number of additional potential measures for controlling SSIs [88–93], such as intravenous administration of immunoglobulins, could lessen the frequency of postoperative acquisition of bloodstream infection or pneumonia. Aggressive and consistent infection control activities will be important in further reducing the incidence of postoperative infections.

Recently, the Center for Medicare and Medicaid Services (CMS) initiated a national SSI prevention initiative [94–96]. This effort focused on the appropriate use of prophylactic antibiotics in selected surgical patients. The major initial focus was on evaluating the appropriateness of antibiotic prophylaxis; this study documented that the correct drug was given at the correct time and stopped correctly in only 38% of patients [97]. The Surgical Infection Prevention Project (SIPP) has evolved to the Surgical Care Improvement Project (SCIP). In the second phase, prospective improvements in prophylactic antibiotic use, glucose control, and normothermia in selected surgical patients will be initiated. These projects can be the forerunners to CMS's paying for performance; those who have high compliance with performance indicators will be paid more and those who have lower rates will be paid less.

REFERENCES

1. Wangensteen OH, Wangensteen SD. *The rise of surgery: From empiric craft to scientific discipline.* Minneapolis: University of Minnesota Press, 1978:785.
2. Howard JM, Barker WF, Culbertson W, et al. Postoperative wound infections: The influence of ultraviolet irradiation on the operating room and of various other factors. *Ann Surg* 1964;160(suppl 2): 1–196.
3. Haley RW, Culver DH, Morgan WM, et al. Identifying patients at high risk of surgical wound infection: A simple multivariate index of patient susceptibility and wound contamination. *Am J Epidemiol* 1985;121:206–15.
4. Culver DH, Horan TC, Gaynes RP, et al. Surgical wound infection rates by wound class, operative procedure, and patient risk index: National Nosocomial Infections Surveillance System. *Am J Med* 1991;91(3B):152S–57S.
5. Burke J. The effective period of preventive antibiotic action in experimental incisions and dermal lesions. *Surgery* 1961;50:161–68.
6. Bernard H, Cole W. The prophylaxis of surgical infection: The effect of prophylactic antimicrobial drugs on the incidence of infection following potentially contaminated operations. *Surgery* 1964;56:151–57.
7. Polk HC Jr, Lopez-Mayor JR. Postoperative wound infection: A prospective study of determinant factors and prevention. *Surgery* 1969;66(1):97–103.
8. Emori TG, Culver DH, Horan TC, et al. National Nosocomial Infections Surveillance System (NNIS): Description of surveillance methods. *Am J Infect Control* 1991;19(1):19–35.
9. Gaynes RP, Culver DH, Horan TC, et al. Surgical site infection (SSI) rates in the United States, 1992–1998: The National Nosocomial Infections Surveillance System basic SSI risk index. *Clin Infect Dis* 2001;33:S69–77.
10. Cruse PJ, Foord R. The epidemiology of wound infection: A 10-year prospective study of 62,939 wounds. *Surg Clin North Am* 1980; 60(1):27–40.
11. Burke JF. Identification of the source of staphylococci contaminating the surgical wound during operation. *Ann Surg* 1963; 158(5):898–904.
12. Morris PJ, Barnes BA, Burke JR. The nature of the "irreducible minimum" rate of incisional sepsis. *Arch Surg* 1966;92(3):367–70.
13. Olson MM, Lee JT Jr. Continuous, 10-year wound infection surveillance: Results, advantages, and unanswered questions. *Arch Surg* 1990;125(6):794–803.
14. (No author). New classification of physical status. *Anesthesiology* 1963;24:111.
15. Morales EA, Embrey RP, Herwaldt LA, et al. A new severity of underlying illness scale to predict postoperative wound infections following coronary artery bypass surgery. *Infect Control Hosp Epidemiol* 1995;16 (suppl 4, part 2):43 [abstract].
16. Horan TC, Culver DH, Gaynes RP. Risk factors for surgical site infections following C-section: Preliminary results of a multicenter study. *Infect Control Hosp Epidemiol* 1995;16 (suppl 4, part 2):22 [abstract].
17. The Neurosurgical Infections Study Group, France. Risk factors for surgical wound infections in craniotomy: A multicenter study in 2,944 patients. Paper presented at the 35th Interscience Conference on Antimicrobial Agents and Chemotherapy of the American Society for Microbiology, San Francisco, September 17–20, 1995 [abstract].
18. Salemi CS, Anderson D, Flores D. Surgical site infection NNIS risk indexing: A problem with anesthesia department ASA scoring. *Infect Control Hosp Epidemiol* 1995;16(suppl 4, part 2):21 [abstract].
19. Howe CW. Experimental wound sepsis from transient *Escherichia coli* bacteremia. *Surgery* 1969;66(3):570–74.
20. Robson M, Krizek T, Heggers J. Biology of surgical infection. *Curr Probl Surg* 1973;3:2–62.
21. Josephs LG, Cordts PR, DiEdwardo CL, et al. Do infected inguinal lymph nodes increase the incidence of postoperative groin wound infection? *J Vasc Surg* 1993;17(6):1077–80.
22. Alexander JW, Fischer JE, Boyajian M, et al. Influence of hair-removal methods on wound infections. *Arch Surg* 1983;118: 347–52.
23. Kaiser AB, Clayson KR, Mulherin JL Jr., et al. Antibiotic prophylaxis in vascular surgery. *Ann Surg* 1978;188(3):283–89.
24. Kurz A, Sessler DI, Lenhardt R. Perioperative normothermia to reduce the incidence of surgical-would infection and shorten hospitalization. Study of wound infection and temperature group. *N Engl J Med* 1996;334(19):P1209–15.
25. Hojer H, Wetterfors J. Systemic prophylaxis with doxycycline in surgery of the colon and rectum. *Ann Surg* 1978;187:362–68.
26. Ford CD, VanMoorleghem G, Menlove RL. Blood transfusions and postoperative wound infection. *Surgery* 1993;113(6):603–7.

27. DeHoll D, Rodeheaver G, Edgerton MT, et al. Potentiation of infection by suture closure of dead space. *Am J Surg* 1974; 127(6):716–20.

28. Magee C, Rodeheaver G, Golden G, et al. Potentiation of wound infection by surgical drains. *Am J Surg* 1976;131:547–49.

29. Monson JR, Guillou PJ, Keane FB, et al. Cholecystectomy is safer without drainage: The results of a prospective, randomized clinical trial. *Surgery* 1991;109(6):740–46.

30. Cerise E, Pierce W, Diamond D. Abdominal drains: Their role as a source of infection following splenectomy. *Ann Surg* 1970;171:764–69.

31. Simchen E, Rozin R, Wax Y. The Israeli study of surgical infection of wound infection in operations for hernia. *Surg Gynecol Obstet* 1990;170(4):331–37.

32. Le Gallou F, Fleury M, Baranger F, et al. Could surgical gloves play a role in the perioperative transmission of methicillin-resistant *Staphylococcus aureus*? Paper presented at the 35th Interscience Conference on Antimicrobial Agents and Chemotherapy of the American Society for Microbiology. San Francisco, September 17–20, 1995:J156.

33. Roy M-C, Stephens D, Herwaldt LA, et al. Risk factors for surgical site infections. Paper presented at the 35th Interscience Conference on Antimicrobial Agents and Chemotherapy of the American Society for Microbiology. San Francisco, September 17–20, 1995 [abstract].

34. Grinbaum RS, de Mendonca JS, Cardo DM. An outbreak of hand scrubbing-related surgical site infections in vascular surgical procedures. *Infect Control Hosp Epidemiol* 1995;16:198–202.

35. Moylan JA, Kennedy BV. The importance of gown and drape barriers in the prevention of wound infection. *Surg Gynecol Obstet* 1980;151(4):465–70.

36. Berkelman RL, Martin D, Graham DR, et al. Streptococcal wound infections caused by a vaginal carrier. *JAMA* 1982; 247(19):2680–82.

37. Beck-Sague CM, Chong WH, Roy C, et al. Outbreak of surgical wound infections associated with total hip arthroplasty. *Infect Control Hosp Epidemiol* 1992;13(9):526–34.

38. Lynch W, Davey PG, Malek M, et al. Cost-effectiveness analysis of the use of chlorhexidine detergent in preoperative whole-body disinfection in wound infection prophylaxis. *J Hosp Infect* 1992;21(3):179–91.

39. Dellinger EP, Gross PA, Barrett TL, et al. Quality standard for antimicrobial prophylaxis in surgical procedures. *Clin Infect Dis* 1994;18:422–27.

40. McGowan JE Jr, Chesney PJ, Crossley KB, et al. Guidelines for the use of systemic glucocorticoids in the management of selected infections. *J Infect Dis* 1992;165:1–13.

41. Gross PA, Barrett TL, Dellinger EP, et al. Purpose of quality standards for infectious diseases. *Clin Infect Dis* 1994;18:421.

42. Kaiser AB. Antimicrobial prophylaxis in surgery. *N Engl J Med* 1986;315:1129–38.

43. Meakins JL. Prophylactic antibiotics. In: Wilmore DW, Brennan MF, Harken AH, et al., eds. *American College of Surgeons: Care of the surgical patient*, vol. 2. New York: Scientific American Medicine, 1991: (section 6)1–10.

44. Nichols RL, Condon RE, Barie PS. Antibiotic prophylaxis in surgery—2005 and beyond. *Surg Infect (Larchmt)* 2005;6:349–61.

45. Polk HC Jr, Malangoni MA. Chemoprophylaxis of wound infections. In: Howard RJ, Simmons RL, eds. *Surgical infectious diseases*, 2nd ed. Norwalk: Appleton & Lange, 1988:351–61.

46. Page CP, Bohnen JMA, Fletcher JR, et al. Antimicrobial prophylaxis for surgical wounds: Guidelines for clinical care. *Arch Surg* 1993; 128:79–88.

47. ASHP Commission on Therapeutics. ASHP therapeutic guidelines on antimicrobial prophylaxis for surgery. *Clin Pharm* 1992; 11:483–513.

48. Gorbach SL. Antimicrobial prophylaxis for appendectomy and colorectal surgery. *Rev Infect Dis* 1991;13(suppl 10):S815–20.

49. Solla JA, Rothenberger DA. Preoperative bowel preparation: A survey of colon and rectal surgeons. *Dis Colon Rectum* 1990; 33:154–59.

50. Clarke JS, Condon RE, Bartlett JG, et al. Preoperative oral antibiotics reduce septic complications of colon operations: Results of prospective, randomized, double-blind clinical study. *Ann Surg* 1977;186(3):251–59.

51. Platt R, Zaleznik DF, Hopkins CC, et al. Perioperative antibiotic prophylaxis for herniorrhaphy and breast surgery. *N Engl J Med* 1990;322:253–60.

52. Hopkins CC. Antibiotic prophylaxis in clean surgery: Peripheral vascular surgery, noncardiovascular thoracic surgery, herniorrhaphy, and mastectomy. *Rev Infect Dis* 1991;13 (suppl 10):S869–73.

53. Dajani AS, Bisno AL, Chung KJ, et al. Prevention of bacterial endocarditis: Recommendation by the American Heart Association. *JAMA* 1990;264:2919–92.

54. Classen DC, Evans RS, Pestotnik SL, et al. The timing of prophylactic administration of antibiotics and the risk of surgical-wound infection. *N Engl J Med* 1992;326(5):281–86.

55. DiPiro JT, Vallner JJ, Bowden TA, et al. Intra-operative serum and tissue activity of cefazolin and cefoxitin. *Arch Surg* 1985;120:829–32.

56. Crossley K, Gardner LC. Task Force on Prophylactic Antibiotics in Surgery. Antimicrobial prophylaxis in surgical patients. *JAMA* 1985;245:722–26.

57. Currier JS, Campbell H, Platt R, et al. Perioperative antimicrobial prophylaxis in middle Tennessee, 1989–1990. *Rev Infect Dis* 1991;12(suppl 10):S874–78.

58. Richet HM, Chidiac C, Prat A, et al. Analysis of risk factors for surgical wound infections following vascular surgery. *Am J Med* 1991;91(suppl 3B):170s–72s.

59. DiPiro J, Cheung R, Bowden T Jr. Single dose systemic antibiotic prophylaxis of surgical wound infections. *Am J Surg* 1986; 152:552–59.

60. Dellinger EP. Antibiotic prophylaxis in trauma: Penetrating abdominal injuries and open fractures. *Rev Infect Dis* 1991;13 (suppl 10):S847–57.

61. Fabian TC, Croce MA, Payne LW, et al. Duration of antibiotic therapy for penetrating abdominal trauma: A prospective trial. *Surgery* 1992;112:788–95.

62. Stoutenbeek CP, van-Saene HK, Miranda DR, et al. The effect of selective decontamination of the digestive tract on colonisation and infection rate in multiple trauma patients *Intensive Care Med* 1984;10(4):185–92.

63. Wiesner RH, Hermans P, Rakela J, et al. Selective bowel decontamination to prevent gram-negative bacterial and fungal infection following orthotopic liver transplantation. *Transplant Proc* 1987;19(1):2420–23.

64. Blair P, Rowlands BJ, Lowry K, et al. Selective decontamination of the digestive tract: A stratified, randomized, prospective study in a mixed intensive care unit. *Surgery* 1991;110(2):303–9.

65. Kollef MH. The role of selective digestive tract decontamination on mortality and respiratory tract infections: A meta-analysis. *Chest* 1994;105(4):1101–8.

66. Brun-Buisson C. Selective decontamination in critical care: Interpreting the synthesized evidence. *Chest* 1994;105(4):978–80.

67. Heyland DK, Cook DJ, Jaeschke R, et al. Selective decontamination of the digestive tract: An overview. *Chest* 1994;105(4):1221–29.

68. Horan TC, Gaynes RP, Martone WJ, et al. CDC definitions of nosocomial surgical site infections, 1992: A modification of CDC definitions of surgical wound infections. *Am J Infect Control* 1992;20:271–74.

69. Haley RW, Culver DH, White JW, et al. The efficacy of infection surveillance and control programs in preventing nosocomial infections in U.S. hospitals. *Am J Epidemiol* 1985;121(2):182–205.

70. Lee JT. Surgical site infection surveillance: Accomplishments and pitfalls. *Surg Infect (Larchmt)* 2006;7:s43–55.

71. Cardo DM, Falk PS, Mayhall CG. Validation of surgical wound surveillance. *Infect Control Hosp Epidemiol* 1993;14(4):211–15.

72. Ehrenkranz NJ, Sultz JM, Richter E. Recorded criteria as a "gold standard" for sensitivity and specificity estimates of surveillance of nosocomial infection: A novel method to measure job performance. *Infect Control Hosp Epidemiol* 1995;16:697–702.

73. Yokoe DS, Platt R. Surveillance for surgical site infections: The uses of antibiotic exposure. *Infect Control Hosp Epidemiol* 1994;15(11):717–23.

74. Sherertz RJ, Garibaldi RA, Marosok RD, et al. Consensus paper on the surveillance of surgical wound infections. *Am J Infect Control* 1992;20:263–70.

75. Manian FA, Meyer L. Comparison of patient telephone survey with traditional surveillance and monthly physician questionnaires

in monitoring surgical wound infections. *Infect Control Hosp Epidemiol* 1993;14:216–18.

76. Audry G, Johanet S, Achrafi H, et al. The risk of wound infection after inguinal incision in pediatric outpatient surgery. *Eur J Pediatr Surg* 1994;4(2):87–89.

77. Zoutman D, Pearce P, McKenzie M, et al. Surgical wound infections occurring in day surgery patients. *Am J Infect Control* 1990;18(4):277–82.

78. Culver D, Horan T, Gaynes R. Comparing surgical site infection (SSI) rates using the NNIS SSI index and the standardized infection ratio. *Am J Infect Control* 1994;22:102.

79. Massanari RM. Profiling physician practice: A potential for misuse. *Infect Control Hosp Epidemiol* 1994;15(6):394–96.

80. Lubbers MJ. Infection in organ transplant recipients: problems and solutions. *Curr Opin Surg Infect* 1993;1:53–56.

81. Wenzel RP, Osterman CA, Hunting KJ. Hospital-acquired infections. II. Infection rates by site, service and common procedures in a university hospital. *Am J Epidemiol* 1976;104(6):645–51.

82. Penin GB, Ehrenkranz NJ. Priorities for surveillance and cost-effective control of postoperative infection. *Arch Surg* 1988;123(11):1305–8.

83. Wenzel RP, Pert TM. The significance of nasal carriage of *Staphylococcus aureus* and the incidence of postoperative wound infection. *J Hosp Infect* 1995;31:13–24.

84. Kluytmans JA, Mouton JW, Ijzerman EP, et al. Nasal carriage of *Staphylococcus aureus* as a major risk factor for wound infections after cardiac surgery. *J Infect Dis* 1995;171(1):216–19.

85. Talon D, Rouget C, Cailleaux V et al. Nasal carriage of *Staphylococcus aureus* and cross-contamination in a surgical intensive care unit: *Efficacy of mupirocin ointment. J Hosp Infect* 1995;30(1):39–49.

86. Perl TM, Cullen JJ, Wenzel RP, et al. Intranasal mupirocin to prevent postoperative Staphylococcus aureus infections. *N Engl J Med* 2002;346:1871–77.

87. Morran GG, McNaught W, McArdle CS. The relationship between intraoperative contamination of the lower respiratory tract and postoperative chest infection. *J Hosp Infect* 1995;30(1):31–37.

88. Webster J, Osborne S. Meta-analysis of preoperative antiseptic bathing in the prevention of surgical site infection. *Br J Surg* 2006;93:1335–41.

89. Ives CL, Harrison DK, Stansby GS. Tissue oxygen saturation, measured by near-infrared spectroscopy, and its relationship to surgical-site infections. *Br J Surg* 2007;94:87–91.

90. O'Reilly M, Talsma A, VanRiper S, et al. An anesthesia information system designed to provide physician-specific feedback improves timely administration of prophylactic antibiotics. *Anesth Analg* 2006;103:908–12.

91. Dellinger EP. Roles of temperature and oxygenation in prevention of surgical site infection. *Surg Infect (Larchmt)* 2006;7(suppl 3):s27–32.

92. Leaper D. Effects of local and systemic warming on postoperative infections. *Surg Infect (Larchmt)* 2006; 7 (suppl 2):S101–3.

93. Ehrenkranz NJ. Control of surgical infections. *Curr Opin Surg Infect* 1994;2:103–9.

94. Bratzler DW, Houck PM. Surgical Infection Prevention Guideline Writers Workgroup. Antimicrobial prophylaxis for surgery: An advisory statement from the National Surgical Infection Prevention Project. *Am J Surg* 2005;189:395–404.

95. Bratzler DW, Hunt DR. The surgical infection prevention and surgical care improvement projects: National initiatives to improve outcomes for patients having surgery. *Clin Infect Dis* 2006; 43:322–30.

96. Dellinger EP, Hausmann SM, Bratzler DW, et al. Hospitals collaborate to decrease surgical site infections. *Am J Surg* 2005; 190:9–15.

97. Bratzler DW, Houck PM, Richards C, et al. Use of antimicrobial prophylaxis for major surgery: Baseline results from the National Surgical Infection Prevention Project. *Arch Surg* 2005;140:174–82.

Infections of Burn Wounds*

36

David W. Mozingo, Albert T. McManus, and Basil A. Pruitt, Jr.

Infection, the risk of which is proportional to the extent of injury, continues to be the predominant determinant of outcome in thermally injured patients despite improvements in overall care in general and wound care in particular. The control of invasive burn wound infection through the use of effective topical chemotherapy, prompt surgical excision, and timely closure of the burn wound has resulted in unsurpassed survival rates. Even so, infection remains the most common cause of death in these severely injured patients.

ETIOLOGY OF BURN INJURY

Burns are estimated to affect 1.25 million people in the United States annually [1]. Of this number, 50,592–68,488 patients require hospital admission, 20,000–25,000 of whom have injuries of such significance that care is best undertaken in a burn center. House and structure fires are responsible for >70% of the yearly 3,785 burn-related deaths, 75% of which result from smoke inhalation or asphyxiation and 25% are due to burns. However, these fires are responsible for only 4–5% of burn admissions. Injuries due to contact with flame or ignition of clothing are the most common cause of burn in adults whereas scald burns are most common in children. The majority of patients sustain burns of such limited severity and extent (>80% of burns involve <20% of the body surface) that they can be treated on an outpatient basis. Approximately 170–230 patients per million population per year require hospital admission owing to the extent of their burns or to other complicating factors. Approximately 33% of patients who require in-hospital care have a major burn injury—as defined by the American Burn Association on the basis of burn size, causative agent, preexisting disease, and associated injuries—and should be treated in a tertiary care burn center [2].

Changes in wound care over the past 40 years, including the use of effective topical antimicrobial chemotherapy and excision of the burned tissue to achieve timely closure of the burn wound, have significantly reduced the occurrence of invasive burn wound infection and its related morbidity and mortality. Regular collection of cultures from patients permits early identification of the causative pathogens of those infections that do arise. Moreover, infection control procedures, including strict enforcement of patient and staff hygiene and use of patient isolation methods, have been effective in controlling the spread of resistant organisms and eliminating them from the burn center. These advances and the improvements in the general care of critically ill burn patients have resulted in markedly improved survival rates. However, as a manifestation of the systemic immunosuppressive effects of burn injury, infection at other sites, predominantly the lungs, remains the most typical cause of morbidity and death in these severely injured patients (Figure 36-1).

HOST IMMUNE FUNCTION

Thermal injury initiates a deleterious pathophysiologic response in every organ system with the extent and duration of organ dysfunction proportionate to the size of the

---

*The views of the authors contained herein do not purport to reflect the positions of the Department of the Army or the Department of Defense.

FREQUENCY OF INFECTION IN BURN PATIENTS

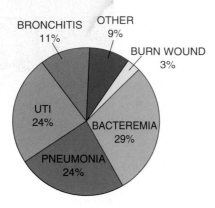

Figure 36-1 The frequency of infection by site expressed as a percentage of all infections complicating thermal injury. (From United States Army Institute of Surgical Research, 1991–1995.)

burn. Direct cellular damage is manifested by coagulation necrosis with the depth of tissue destruction determined by the duration of contact and the temperature to which the tissue is exposed. Following a burn, the normal skin barrier to microbial penetration is lost, and the moist, protein-rich avascular eschar of the burn wound provides an excellent culture medium for microorganisms. While destruction of the mechanical barrier of the skin contributes to the increased susceptibility to infection, postburn alterations in immune function also could be of significant importance. Every component of the humoral and cellular limbs of the immune system appears to be affected after thermal injury; the magnitude and duration of dysfunction are proportional to the extent of injury.

During the first weeks after injury, the total white blood cell count is elevated, but peripheral blood lymphocyte counts decrease. Alterations in lymphocyte subpopulations, including reversal of the normal ratio of T-helper cells to T-suppressor cells, have been described [3,4]. Delayed hypersensitivity reactions and peripheral blood lymphocyte proliferation in the mixed lymphocyte reaction are both inhibited following burns. Alterations in interleukin-2 (IL-2) production and IL-2 receptor expression by lymphocytes have been observed with burn injury; a direct correlation has been established between the extent of the burn and the decline of IL-2 production by peripheral lymphocytes [5].

Increased numbers of circulating B lymphocytes are evident early in the postburn course; however, serum immunoglobulin G (IgG) levels decline after burn injury and gradually return to normal over the succeeding 2 to 4 weeks. The association of higher numbers of circulating B cells but reduced serum levels of IgG suggests a defect in the ability of B cells to generate a normal response after burn injury [6]. Similar findings have been observed in IgM-producing cells isolated from murine mesenteric lymph nodes and spleens following burns [7]. Exogenous administration of IgG to burn patients has been shown

to promptly restore normal IgG levels but exerts no demonstrable effect on the incidence or outcome of infections [8].

Burn injury induces a severity-related shift in the maturity of circulating granulocytes that continues for several weeks after injury. Alterations in granulocyte function, including those of chemotaxis, adherence, degranulation, oxygen radical production, and complement receptor expression, have been identified [9]. Granulocytes isolated from burn patients exhibit increased cytosolic oxidase activity and greater than normal oxidase activity after in vitro stimulation, suggesting that these neutrophils are primed and capable of producing more tissue and organ injury [10]. Recent investigations have verified elevations of F-actin content and impaired ability to polymerize F-actin in the granulocytes of burn patients when compared with those of controls [11]. These alterations can in part be responsible for the observed changes in chemotaxis and migration after thermal injury.

ETIOLOGY OF BURN WOUND INFECTION

Both the nature of the burn wound and microorganism-specific factors influence the rate of microbial proliferation in and penetration of the burn eschar. Burn tissue, rich in coagulated protein and well hydrated by the transeschar movement of fluid and serum, creates an excellent microbial culture medium. The eschar is avascular owing to thermal thrombosis of nutrient vessels, limiting both the delivery of systemically administered antibiotics and the migration of phagocytic cells into the burned tissue. Bacterial proliferation in the wound also can be enhanced by such factors as wound maceration, pressure necrosis, and wound desiccation with neoeschar formation. In addition, secondary impairment of blood flow to the wound could further predispose the patient to invasive infection by curtailing the delivery of oxygen, nutrients, and phagocytic cells to the viable subeschar tissue.

The character of the microbial flora of the burn wound changes with time. The gram-positive organisms that predominate in the early postburn period are replaced by gram-negative organisms by the second week. Without the application of topical antimicrobial agents, the density of bacteria grows progressively, and the microorganisms penetrate the eschar by migration along sweat glands and hair follicles until they reach the eschar/nonviable tissue interface. Additional microbial proliferation occurs in the subeschar space, enhancing the lysis of denatured collagen and sloughing the eschar. If the density and invasiveness of the microorganisms exceed the host's defense capacity, proliferating organisms in the subeschar space can invade the underlining viable tissue, leading to invasive burn wound infection and even systemic spread to remote tissues and organs. Bacterial invasion is uncommon unless the number of microorganisms exceeds 10^5/grams (g) of biopsy tissue.

Certain strain-specific factors also appear to be important in the pathogenesis of invasive burn wound infection. The production of enzymes, such as collagenase, elastase, protease, and lipase, can enhance the organisms' ability to penetrate the eschar. Moreover, bacterial motility and antibiotic resistance appear to be important in the development of invasive infection. Effective topical antimicrobial chemotherapy limits intraeschar bacterial proliferation and the attendant risk of invasive infection.

HISTOLOGIC STAGING OF BURN WOUND COLONIZATION AND INFECTION

The presence of microorganisms in the nonviable burned tissue, termed *colonization*, is a distinctly different entity from the presence of microorganisms in viable tissue beneath the burn eschar, termed *invasive burn wound infection*. Histologic examination of a biopsy of the burn wound and underlying viable tissue is the most rapid and reliable method for differentiating microbial colonization from invasive infection [12]. Burn wound biopsy is performed as an intensive care unit or ward procedure.

An elliptical biopsy (0.5×1.0 centimeters), which includes the subjacent unburned viable tissue, is obtained by scalpel dissection from an area of burn wound suspected of being infected. Hemostasis is easily achieved by the application of direct pressure or by electrocoagulation. One-half of the specimen is cultured to identify microorganisms and their antibiotic sensitivities. The remaining half is submitted to the pathology laboratory for histologic examination. Using the rapid section technique, results are available in 3–4 hours, whereas a frozen-section technique can yield a diagnosis in 30 minutes, albeit with an attendant 4% falsely negative diagnosis rate [13]. The presence of microorganisms in viable tissue confirms the diagnosis of invasive burn wound infection (Figure 36-2). When the organisms are confined to the necrotic eschar or there is suppuration in the subeschar space separating nonviable from viable tissue, the wound is considered to be colonized, not infected (Figure 36-3). Table 36-1 presents a histologic staging scheme for burn wound colonization and infection.

Surface cultures of the burn eschar cannot distinguish colonization from invasive infection. Although commonly used in clinical practice, quantitative bacteriologic cultures of the burn wound correlate poorly with the presence of invasive burn wound infection. When bacteriologic counts are <10^5/g of biopsy tissue, invasive burn wound infection rarely is present; however, even when quantitative

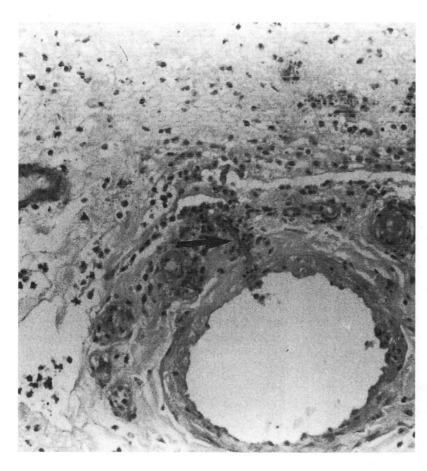

Figure 36-2 Photomicrograph of a burn wound biopsy specimen showing hyphae typical of *Aspergillus* species present in unburned tissue. The perivascular location of the hyphal element indicates stage IIC invasion.

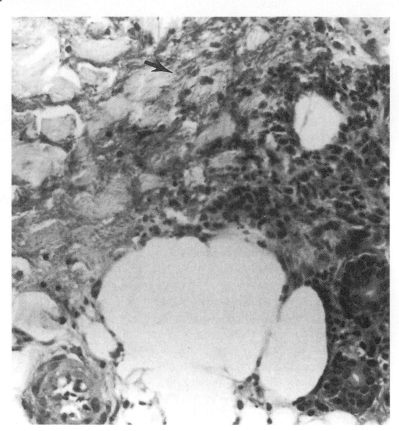

Figure 36-3 Photomicrograph of a burn wound biopsy specimen showing dense inflammatory cell accumulation at the interface of the viable tissue to the right and the nonviable tissue to the left. Branched hyphal elements are localized in this area, indicating stage IC colonization (arrow).

counts exceed 10^5 organisms/g, histologic examination confirms the presence of invasive infection in <50% of such specimens. Burn wound biopsies can at times yield misleading results but less commonly than wound cultures. Failing to include viable subeschar tissue in the biopsy specimen or sampling of a noninfected area can limit the usefulness of this technique. Negative biopsy results in the presence of clinical deterioration necessitate reexamination

---

HISTOLOGIC STAGING OF BURN WOUND COLONIZATION AND INVASION

Stage I: Colonization
  Superficial: sparse microbial population on surface of burn wound
  Penetration: microorganisms present in variable thickness of eschar
  Proliferation: dense population of microorganism at the interface of viable and nonviable tissue
Stage II: Invasion
  Microinvasion: microscopic foci of organisms in viable tissue immediately subjacent to subeschar space
  Generalized: widespread penetration of microorganisms deep into viable subcutaneous tissues
  Microvascular: involvement of lymphatics and microvasculature

---

of the burn wound and procurement of biopsy material from other areas when other sources of systemic infection have been discounted.

BURN WOUND MICROBIAL FLORA

Over the past 20 years, significant changes in the microbial ecology of the burn wound have been noted. The recovery of *Pseudomonas* and other gram-negative bacteria, which were once the most common organisms causing burn wound infection, has markedly declined with improvements in the isolation of patients [14]. Consequently, invasive *Pseudomonas* burn wound infection has essentially disappeared as a complication of burn patients treated in tertiary burn centers [15]. Tables 36-2 and 36-3 review all burn wound biopsy results in general and those demonstrating invasive burn wound infection in particular, respectively, during a recent 5-year period at the U.S. Army Institute of Surgical Research and confirm this fact. Patients who have received broad-spectrum antibiotics for perioperative coverage or treatment of septic complications and whose wounds remain open for many days owing to the extent of the burn are at increased risk of burn wound colonization and infection by yeasts, fungi, and multiple antibiotic-resistant bacteria. The true fungi have replaced bacteria as the most common microbes causing burn wound infection in recent years [16]. This predominance of fungal wound infections

TABLE 36-2

MICROORGANISMS CAUSING BURN WOUND INFECTION (FROM U.S. ARMY INSTITUTE OF SURGICAL RESEARCH, 1991–1995)

Type	No.
Aspergillus species	12
Mucor species	3
Enterobacter cloacae	1
Aeromonas hydrophila	1
Enterococcus faecalis	1
Total	18

must be viewed in the context of the marked overall decline in wound infections. Moreover, improperly cared for and neglected burn wounds have the same high risk of bacterial infection as was common in this country several decades ago.

Viral burn wound infections are relatively uncommon and usually are caused by herpes simplex virus type 1 (see Chapter 42) [17]. Recently healed or healing partial-thickness burns, particularly those in the nasolabial area, are most frequently affected. The appearance of serrated crusted lesions, particularly on the lips, is characteristic of viral infection. Diagnosis is made by histologically examining biopsy material or scrapings from the cutaneous lesions. Applications of topical 5% acyclovir ointment every 3 hours for 1 week has been reported to shorten the time to heal these lesions, the duration of associated pain, and the duration of viral shedding. Even without treatment, these infections usually are self-limited and of little or

TABLE 36-3

ORGANISMS ISOLATED FROM BURN WOUND BIOPSY SPECIMENS (FROM U.S. ARMY INSTITUTE OF SURGICAL RESEARCH, 1991–1995)

Gram-negative species		
Pseudomonas aeruginosa	174	
Other species	270	
Total		444 (29.1%)
Gram-positive species		
Staphylococcus aureus	157	
Other species	271	
Total		428 (28.0%)
Nonbacterial pathogens		
Mold species (principally *Aspergillus*)	557	
Candida albicans	71	
Other yeasts	26	
Total		654 (42.9%)
Total		1,526

no systemic consequence. However, if systemic signs and symptoms of disseminated infection are present, such as unexplained sepsis and/or unrelenting fever, the diagnosis of disseminated viral infection should be entertained.

PREVENTION OF BURN WOUND INFECTION

Progress in the general care of the critically burned patient emphasizes preventing infectious complications. These efforts have focused mainly on the areas of environmental control (through single-bed rooms and other forms of isolation) and topical antimicrobial prophylaxis of the burn wound. Effective infection control programs are essential to reduce the exposure of patients in critical care units to healthcare-associated infection (HAI) pathogens. Such control includes strictly enforced hand hygiene, gowning, and gloving policies. When new endemic microbial strains are identified, prevention of patient-to-patient spread and unit environmental contamination can be accomplished using patient cohorting (see Chapters 13 and 26). Cohorting, which entails the assignment of patient care personnel in teams to provide care for only a specific patient or only patients colonized or infected with a targeted organism limits the spread of and can even eliminate antibiotic-resistant endemic organisms [18].

Effective infection control programs for burn centers should include scheduled microbial surveillance of colonization of patients, environmental hygiene–monitoring procedures (see Chapter 20), biopsy assessment of the microbial status of the burn wound as necessary, monitoring of the incidence and causes of infection, and timely review of culture and clinical data by the infection control team (see Chapter 5). The patient colonization surveillance program typically includes thrice weekly cultures of sputum and the burn wound surface and twice weekly cultures of urine and stool. The determination of a panel of antibiotic sensitivities for the predominant isolated organisms or targeted organisms aids in the recognition of problems with cross-contamination and introduction of multiply resistant bacterial strains into the unit's usual flora. Strict criteria for the definition and identification of infections that occur in burn patients are necessary to avoid nonessential and inappropriate antibiotic use. To minimize the emergence of microbial resistance, antibiotics are used in general only for specific indications. Effective infection control policies require continual reevaluation of surveillance culture results and correlation with the sites and treatment of infections. Prompt institution of effective infection control practices is required when cross-contamination and/or other breaches in infection control are identified through these surveillance programs.

Patient isolation in single-bed rooms has been shown to lower the incidence of cross-contamination and subsequent infections complicating the hospital course of burn patients [19]. In general, the air flow patterns of the isolation rooms are probably not as important as the prevention of patient-to-patient contact. However, positive air flow design can delay colonization by HAI flora. Negative air flow rooms in burn centers are generally reserved for patients with infections spread by the airborne route (e.g., *Mycobacterium tuberculosis*) that could be hazardous to other patients and hospital staff members (see Chapter 33).

BURN WOUND HYGIENE AND TOPICAL ANTIMICROBIAL THERAPY

Care of the burn wound begins at the accident scene by covering it with clean sheets or blankets to preserve body temperature and prevent continued environmental exposure. In the absence of gross contamination, burn wounds can be treated safely without topical antimicrobial agents for the first 24–48 hours. When a burn patient arrives at the definitive care facility, initial burn wound debridement should be performed. General anesthesia is not necessary; intravenous analgesia is sufficient for pain control during this procedure. The burns are gently cleansed with a surgical detergent disinfectant, and nonviable epidermis is debrided. Bullae should be excised and body hair shaved from the area of thermal injury beyond the margin of normal skin. The patient is placed in a clean bed, and bulky dressings can be positioned beneath the burned parts to absorb the often copious serous exudate. These dressings should be changed when they become saturated or soiled, and patients should be turned frequently to prevent maceration of burned and unburned skin. The initial debridement and daily cleansing with an antimicrobial-containing surgical scrub is best performed in a shower area using a handheld shower head with the patient lying on a disposable plastic sheet-covered litter or specially designed shower cart. Alternatively, the patient can be placed on a slanted plinth suspended over a physical therapy tank. Immersion hydrotherapy is not necessary and can serve only to disseminate the fecal flora or other contaminating organisms over the entirety of the burn wound. For patients whose general condition is too critical to permit movement to a shower area, daily wound care can be carried out at the bedside. Following cleansing and debridement, the topical antimicrobial agent of choice is applied.

Mafenide acetate (Sulfamylon), silver sulfadiazine (Silvadene), and silver nitrate are the three most commonly employed topical antimicrobial agents for burn wound care. Each agent has specific limitations and advantages with which the physician must be familiar to ensure the patient's safety and optimal benefit. Mafenide acetate and silver sulfadiazine are available as topical creams to be applied directly to the burn wound whereas silver nitrate is applied as a 0.5% solution in occlusive dressings. Either cream is applied in a 1/8-inch layer to the entire burn wound in an aseptic manner after initial debridement and reapplied at 12-hour intervals or as required to maintain continuous topical coverage. Once daily, all of the topical agents should be cleansed from the patient using a surgical detergent disinfectant solution and the burn wounds examined by the attending physician. Silver nitrate is applied as a 0.5% solution in multilayered occlusive dressings that are changed twice each day.

Mafenide acetate burn cream is an 11.1% suspension in a water-soluble base. This compound diffuses freely into the eschar owing to its high degree of water solubility. Sulfamylon is the preferred agent if the patient has heavily contaminated burn wounds or has had burn wound care delayed by several days. Sulfamylon has the added advantage of being highly effective against gram-negative organisms, including most *Pseudomonas* species. Physicians using this agent must be aware of several potential clinical limitations associated with its use. Hypersensitivity reactions occur in 7% of patients, and pain or discomfort of 20–30 minutes duration is common when it is applied to partial-thickness burn wounds. This agent also inhibits carbonic anhydrase, and a diuresis of bicarbonate often is observed after its use. The resultant metabolic acidosis could accentuate postburn hyperventilation, and significant acidemia could develop if compensatory hyperventilation is impaired. Inhibition of this enzyme rarely persists for >7 to 10 days, and the severity of the acidosis can be minimized by alternating applications of Sulfamylon with silver sulfadiazine cream every 12 hours.

Silver sulfadiazine burn cream is a 1% suspension in a water-miscible base. Unlike Sulfamylon, Silvadene has limited solubility in water and, therefore, limited ability to penetrate into the eschar. The agent is most effective when applied to burns soon after injury to minimize bacterial proliferation on the wound's surface. This agent is painless upon application, and its use does not affect serum electrolytes and acid-base balance. Hypersensitivity reactions are uncommon; an erythematous maculopapular rash subsides on discontinuation of the agent. Silver sulfadiazine occasionally induces neutropenia by a mechanism thought to involve direct bone marrow suppression; white blood cell counts usually return to normal following discontinuation [20]. With continual use, resistance to the sulfonamide component of silver sulfadiazine is common, particularly in certain strains of *Pseudomonas* and many *Enterobacter* species. However, the continued sensitivity of microorganisms to the silver ion of this compound has maintained its effectiveness as a topical antimicrobial agent.

A 0.5% silver nitrate solution has a broad spectrum of antibacterial activity imparted by the silver ion. This agent does not penetrate the eschar because the silver ions are rapidly precipitated on contact with any protein or cationic material. Use of this agent is not associated with more intense wound pain except from the mechanical action required for dressing changes. The dressings, which are changed twice daily, are moistened every 2 hours with the silver nitrate solution to prevent evaporation from increasing the silver nitrate concentration to cytotoxic levels within the dressings. Transeschar leaching of sodium, potassium, chloride, and calcium should be anticipated, and these chemical constituents should be appropriately replaced. Hypersensitivity to silver nitrate has not been described. Mafenide acetate, silver sulfadiazine, and 0.5% silver nitrate are effective in preventing invasive burn wound infection; however, because of their lack of eschar penetration, silver nitrate soaks and silver sulfadiazine burn cream are most effective when applied soon after burn injury.

Recently, many silver-containing dressings have become available and are marketed as antimicrobial barrier dressings. Some have the indication to be used on second degree burns. Also, most of these dressings can be left on the wounds for several days. Like silver nitrate, the bacteriocidal properties of silver are responsible for the antimicrobial nature of these dressings but are not indicated for use on full-thickness burns. There is no indication that silver is absorbed significantly into the burn. When using dressings that can be left in place for more than 1–2 days, it is essential to ascertain that the wounds indeed are partial thickness in nature and that healing would be expected to occur within 1–3 weeks. A serious burn wound infection could occur beneath an occlusive dressing left in place for an extended period on a full-thickness burn.

The acceptance and widespread appliance of prompt burn wound excision in the early care of burn patients also has contributed to the decreased incidence of bacterial burn wound infection. Surgical excision and split-thickness skin grafting of burns diminish the time during which the wound is at risk of invasive infection. In patients with burns of <40% of the total body surface, excision is associated with shorter hospital stays, and the burn wounds can be definitively grafted in one or two surgical procedures [21]. In patients with burns over ≥40% of the total body surface, burn wound excision can shorten the duration and magnitude of injury-related physiologic stress and the subsequent degree of immunologic impairment. As soon as the initial burn resuscitation is complete and the patient is physiologically stable, burn wound excision can be initiated in staged procedures so that the entirety of the full-thickness or deep partial-thickness wounds can be removed within several weeks. When skin donor sites are not available for complete grafting of these wounds, a variety of skin substitutes and biologic dressings can be used as a bridge to complete wound coverage. The exact contribution of surgical treatment to the decline in incidence of invasive bacterial burn wound infection has not been well documented; however, the temporal relationship cannot be ignored.

CLINICAL DIAGNOSIS OF BURN WOUND INFECTION

Burn wound infection occurs most commonly in patients in whom the extent of burn exceeds 30% of the body surface

TABLE 36-4
CLINICAL SIGNS OF BURN WOUND INFECTION

- Focal dark brown or black discoloration of wound
- Conversion of second-degree burn to full-thickness necrosis
- Degeneration of wound with neoeschar formation
- Unexpectedly rapid eschar separation
- Hemorrhagic discoloration of subeschar fat
- Violaceous or erythematous edematous wound margin
- Metastatic septic lesions in unburned skin or distant organs

and in those who have suffered skin graft failure that left an open wound. Successful treatment of burn wound infection requires early detection; therefore, it is mandatory that the entire wound be examined daily to detect changes in appearance. The clinical signs of invasive burn wound infection often are indistinguishable from those observed in uninfected hypermetabolic burn patients or in burn patients with other forms of sepsis. These findings can include hyper- or hypothermia, tachycardia, tachypnea, ileus, glucose intolerance, and disorientation. Physical and tinctorial changes in the appearance of the burn wounds are more reliable signs of invasive burn wound infection (Table 36-4). Conversion of an area of partial-thickness burn to full-thickness necrosis and the appearance of focal areas of dark hemorrhagic or black discoloration are the most commonly noted changes indicative of burn wound infection (Figure 36-4). The development of clinical signs and symptoms of sepsis in the thermally injured patient should prompt a thorough examination of the burn wound to identify areas suspected of harboring invasive infection. Confirmation of the diagnosis of burn wound infection is made by histologic examination of a biopsy specimen as previously described.

The emergence of nonbacterial opportunists as the major pathogens invading the burn wound has resulted in changes in the classic clinical presentation of burn wound infection. *Candida* spp. rarely invade the wound to cause systemic infection. However, *Candida* spp. infection can arise in the interstices of a meshed skin graft and in an excised burn wound that remains unclosed as a consequence of the loss of a skin graft or a biologic dressing. Filamentous fungi are more aggressive invaders of the burn wound and could cause severe infection. These fungi rarely traverse fascial planes and remain confined to the subcutaneous tissues. *Aspergillus* spp. can be detected as colonizers and occasionally as invaders of the burn eschar by histopathologic examination of burn wounds at the time of excision and skin grafting. The clinically relevant infections occur, however, relatively late in the hospital course of patients with extensive burns who have already undergone multiple operative procedures (for which they have received perioperative broadspectrum antibiotics) and

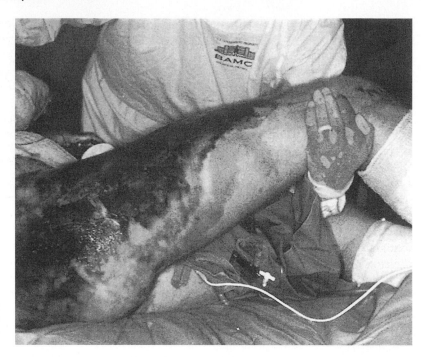

Figure 36-4 Multiple areas of dark discoloration on the thigh and buttocks of this patient, accompanied by unexpectedly rapid eschar separation, characteristic of burn wound infection.

still have unexcised eschar or previously excised, ungrafted open wounds. These infections often resemble a colony of mold with a somewhat fuzzy texture, appearing in a skin graft interstice or an area of open wound. This surface appearance often is accompanied by subcutaneous burrowing tunnels filled with the invading fungus and detected at the time of surgical debridement.

The phycomycetes are typically aggressive, spreading rapidly along tissue plains, traversing fascia, and invading blood vessels and lymphatics [22]. Infections caused by these organisms are characterized by expanding soft-tissue ischemic necrosis with a peripheral edematous rim and, frequently, hematogenous dissemination to remote sites. The diagnosis is confirmed, as with bacterial burn wound infection, by histologic examination of a biopsy specimen.

TREATMENT OF BURN WOUND INFECTION

The treatment of burn wound infection is initiated upon histologic confirmation of the presence of microorganisms in viable tissue. If only colonization (stage 1A to stage 1C) is present, no specific change in antimicrobial therapy is indicated unless serially obtained biopsy specimens document progression of the colonization stage. If stage 2 (invasion) is observed, prompt treatment for invasive burn wound infection should begin. In the case of bacterial burn wound invasion, topical twice-daily applications of mafenide acetate should be used. The eschar-penetrating ability of this agent extends the antimicrobial activity throughout the depth of the burn eschar. Systemic antibiotic therapy is initiated based on previous burn

wound surveillance cultures and burn center organism prevalence. Additional refinements in antibiotic treatment are based on the individual patient's wound culture and sensitivity results. Supportive critical care is employed to maintain hemodynamic and respiratory stability, as it is for other severely ill patients.

Injection of an antibiotic solution into the subcutaneous tissue beneath the eschar (subeschar clysis) is recommended before surgical excision of an infected burn wound to minimize the risk of hematogenous seeding and precipitation of florid septic shock [23]. Half of the daily dose of a broad spectrum antipseudomonal penicillin, such as piperacillin or ticarcillin, delivered in 1 liter of normal saline is infused into the subeschar tissues using a no. 20 spinal needle to minimize the number of injection sites. The patient is prepared and scheduled for surgical excision of the infected tissue within the next 6–12 hours, and the subeschar clysis is repeated immediately before surgery.

Excision of the burn wound to the level of the investing muscle fascia ensures complete removal of all nonviable infected tissue. After excision of the burn, the wound is treated with moist dressings containing an antimicrobial agent, such as 0.5% silver nitrate solution (the authors use a 5% mafenide acetate solution, which is not generally available). Alternatively, a biologic dressing can be applied if all nonviable tissue has been removed and the exposed tissue appears to be uninfected. The patient is returned to the operating room in 24 to 48 hours; at that time, the wound is inspected, and redebridement or split-thickness skin grafting can be performed as needed.

The treatment for candidal or fungal burn wound infection is similar to that of invasive bacterial infection. Infection or new colonization of previously excised or grafted wounds requires treatment by twice-daily application of a topical antifungal agent, such as clotrimazole cream or ciclopiroxolamine cream. Such treatment usually controls surface colonization. However, if the superficial infection continues to extend or the fungal infection is shown to involve deep tissue, such as fascia or muscle, if it has invaded the microvasculature of underlying viable tissue, or if it is associated with systemic signs of sepsis, parenteral administration of amphotericin B should be initiated. The infected tissue must be widely debrided and treated with a topical antifungal agent applied beneath occlusive dressings, which should be changed two to three times daily. The patient is returned to the operating room 24–48 hours later for further debridement and closure of the burn wound by autografting or applying a biologic dressing as dictated by the adequacy of the initial debridement.

INFECTIONS OF SPECIAL CONCERN

Clostridium Tetani

Tetanus, caused by the neurotoxin of *Clostridium tetani*, an anaerobic, gram-positive, spore-forming rod ubiquitous in soil and the gastrointestinal tracts of humans and animals, has been reported as a rare complication of thermal injury. This organism thrives in hypoxic wounds and necrotic tissue, both of which exist in the full-thickness burn. The diagnosis of tetanus is based on characteristic physical findings because wound cultures often fail to detect the causative organism. The usual initial signs and symptoms are severe trismus with stiffness of the paraspinous and abdominal musculature. Localized or generalized muscle spasm, dysphagia, and laryngospasm can develop; the disease can progress to involve more muscle groups, causing generalized rigidity. Ventilation can be impaired by involvement of the diaphragm, chest, and abdominal musculature. Severe episodes require endotracheal intubation and mechanical ventilation. Treatment is mainly supportive and involves aggressive critical care management of the hemodynamic and respiratory systems.

When the diagnosis is made, tetanus immune globulin should be administered immediately to neutralize any circulating free exotoxin. The usual dose is 3,000 to 6,000 (u) given intramuscularly. Intravenous penicillin G (10–40 million u per day) should be given to eradicate the clostridial organisms. Uncontrolled muscle spasms can lead to rhabdomyolysis and skeletal fractures. Morphine, magnesium sulfate, and epidural anesthesia all have been used to reduce muscle spasticity. Sedation with benzodiazepines or barbiturates could be necessary, and, in severe cases, neuromuscular blockade could be required.

Fortunately, tetanus is readily prevented. During the initial care of the burn patient, the patient's tetanus immunization status should be determined. The burn patient who has been immunized against tetanus should be given a booster dose of tetanus toxoid if the last dose was administered > 5 years earlier. Patients with no history or an uncertain history of active immunization should receive tetanus immune globulin in addition to the initial dose of tetanus toxoid. Active immunization is subsequently completed according to the routine dosage schedule.

Staphylococcus aureus

Toxin-producing Staphylococcal spp. have been isolated from both colonized and infected burn wounds and other sites of infection [24,25] (see Chapter 41). The emergence of gram-positive organisms as the predominant flora in burn patients has contributed to a lessening in the impact of infection; the virulence of *Staphylococcus aureus* can be strain specific, and bacteremia resulting from strains possessing the gene for the production of toxic shock syndrome toxin has been associated with episodes of unexplained profound hemodynamic instability. This gene, however, has been identified in staphylococcal strains recovered from patients with wound colonization, bacteremia, and other infections without evidence of profound physiologic disturbance.

The diagnosis of a variant of the toxic shock syndrome should be considered in thermally injured patients with staphylococcal infections who manifest hemodynamic instability that responds poorly to treatment and that is out of proportion to what is usually encountered in gram-positive infections. Initial treatment requires aggressive intravenous fluid resuscitation to restore hemodynamic stability. Vancomycin should be administered intravenously unless the organism is known to be sensitive to methicillin when a β-lactamase-resistant antistaphylococcal antibiotic, such as nafcillin, can be given.

At present, an antitoxin to the toxic shock syndrome toxin 1 is not available. Approximately 90% of the general population has antibodies against the toxin, but nearly all patients with toxic shock syndrome related to menstruation have had undetectable antibodies at the onset of the disease. Although this relationship has not been confirmed in thermally injured patients thought to have the variant toxic shock syndrome, the isolation of a strain of *S. aureus* producing the toxic shock syndrome toxin 1 and the absence of circulating antibodies to the toxin could help establish the definitive diagnosis.

Antibiotic-resistant bacteria of special note and the subject of much controversy are the methicillin-resistant strains of *S. aureus* (MRSA) (see Chapters 15 and 41). Since the 1960s, these strains have been reported and treated as if they were distinct pathogens with more virulence than other methicillin-sensitive strains. Undoubtedly, the emergence of antibiotic-resistant organisms is of concern, and efforts should be made to limit their inroads. However, the unique concern about MRSA in particular has resulted in temporary closure of burn and other intensive care facilities and restriction of patients' movements among levels of care.

The benefits of these practices must always be weighed against their clinical, epidemiologic, and economic value.

The virulence and pathologic significance of MRSA compared with methicillin-sensitive strains causing infections in burn wound patients were evaluated in a 1989 study [26]. Colonization with any strain of staphylococcus was identified in 658 burn patients treated during a 6-year period; of this total, 319 (or nearly half) of these patients were colonized with MRSA. In this group, a total of 253 staphylococcal infections occurred in 178 patients: 58% of infections were pulmonary and 38% were bacteremias. In 58/178 patients, infections were caused by MRSA. The outcomes of patients infected with MRSA and methicillin-sensitive strains of *Staphylococcus aureus* were compared using a multiple logistic regression analysis of mortality. In both groups, all patients were treated with vancomycin, and no differences in the observed and predicted mortality were found between groups. We believe these findings suggest that both MRSA and MSSA in burn patients can lead to serious adverse outcomes. The main concern related to frequent use of vancomycin is the possible development of vancomycin and MRSA resistance prompted by the recent recognition of vancomycin-resistant strains of *S. aureus* and *enterococci* (see Chapter 15). Individual centers should adopt strict criteria for diagnosing specific infections in burn patients and specific indications for antibiotic use based on the prevalence of resistant organisms to avoid inappropriate prescription of vancomycin and other antibiotics.

Aeromonas Species

Human infection with *Aeromonas* spp. most often is associated with either traumatic injuries contaminated with water or soil or with immunosuppression. Infections in burn patients caused by *Aeromonas* spp. are rare; <20 episodes have been reported in the English literature. A recent report by Barillo et al. describes a series of eight thermally injured patients treated over a 35-year period in whom *Aeromonas hydrophila* bacteremia developed during their hospital stays [27]. In 6/8 patients, the organism was isolated from wound cultures as well. Aquatic exposure was known or suspected in only 3 of the patients, and 5 of the 8 patients died. In general, soft-tissue infection with *Aeromonas* spp. has a rapid onset, usually within 48 hours of injury. Subcutaneous abscess formation is common but could not be clinically apparent on initial examination. Infections are usually polymicrobial and accompanied by a foul odor. Aeromonas spp. is particularly destructive of muscle, and necrotizing myonecrosis, resulting in amputation or death, could develop from local infections and hematogenous spread in otherwise healthy individuals. *Aeromonas* spp. infection can mimic *Pseudomonas* spp. infection in the formation of ecthyma gangrenosum and can produce gas in soft-tissue planes similar to that seen with clostridial infection.

The treatment of *Aeromonas* spp. burn wound infection includes systematic antibiotics and surgical intervention. *Aeromonas* spp. produce β-lactamase and are resistant to penicillins and first-generation cephalosporins. Aminoglycosides, aztreonam, ciprofloxacin, and third-generation cephalosporins usually are effective against these organisms. For the management of burn wound infection, surgical debridement should be accomplished expeditiously as outlined previously.

SUMMARY

Despite significant improvements in the survival of burn patients, infectious complications continue to be the major cause of morbidity and mortality. Control of invasive bacterial burn wound infection by effective topical antimicrobial agents and prompt excision and split-thickness skin grafting of the burn wound clearly is possible with modern burn care. In addition, strict isolation techniques and infection control policies have significantly minimized the occurrence of burn wound infections in general and those caused by gram-negative organisms in particular. In those patients in whom a burn wound infection develops, bacterial infection has been largely supplanted by infection caused by nonbacterial opportunists, namely, fungi and yeasts. Scheduled wound surveillance and microbiologic monitoring with the use of wound biopsies to provide histologic confirmation of burn wound infection permits prompt diagnosis of microbial invasion at a stage when timely institution of antibiotic therapy and surgical intervention can save the patient.

REFERENCES

1. Pruitt BA Jr., Wolf SE, Mason AD Jr. Epidemiological, demographic, and outcome characteristics of burn injury. In: Herndon DN, ed. *Total burn care*, Elsevier Inc., 2007:14–32.
2. Resources for optional care of patients with burn injury. In: *Resources for optimal care of the injured patient*. Chicago: Committee on Trauma, American College of Surgeons, 1993:63.
3. Zapata-Sirvent RL, Hansbrough JE. Temporal analysis of human leucocyte surface antigen expression and neutrophil respiratory burst activity after thermal injury. *Burns* 1993;19:5–11.
4. Burleson DG, Vaughn GK, Mason AD Jr, et al. Flow cytometric measurement of rat lymphocyte subpopulations after burn injury and burn injury with infection. *Arch Surg* 1987;122(2):216–20.
5. Wood JJ, Rodrick ML, O'Mahony JB, et al. Inadequate interleukin-2 production: A fundamental immunological deficiency in patients with major burns. *Ann Surg* 1984;200:311–20.
6. Molloy RG, Nestor M, Collins KH. The humoral immune response after thermal injury: An experimental model. *Surgery* 1994;115:341–48.
7. Tabata T, Meyer AA. Effects of burn injury on class-specific B-cell population and immunoglobulin synthesis in mice. *J Trauma* 1993;35:750–55.
8. Shirani KZ, Vaughn GM, McManus AT, et al. Replacement therapy with modified immunoglobulin G in burn patients: Preliminary kinetic studies. *Am J Med* 1984;76:175–80.
9. Cioffi WG, Burleson DG, Pruitt BA Jr. Leukocyte responses to injury. *Arch Surg* 1993;128:1260–67.
10. Cioffi WG Jr, Burleson DG, Jordan BS, et al. Granulocyte oxidase activity after thermal injury. *Surgery* 1992;112:860–65.

11. Drost AC, Cioffi WG Jr, Carrougher GJ, et al. The relationship of granulocyte F-actin levels and infection following thermal injury. Paper presented at The Third International Congress on the Immune Consequences of Trauma, Shock and Sepsis, Munich, March 2–5, 1994.

12. Kim SH, Hubbard GB, Wurley BL, et al. A rapid section technique for burn wound biopsy. *J Burn Care Rehabil* 1985;6:433–35.

13. Kim SH, Hubbard GB, Wurley BL, et al. Frozen section technique to evaluate early burn wound biopsy: A comparison with the rapid section technique. *J Trauma* 1985;25:1134–37.

14. McManus AT, McManus WF, Mason AD Jr, et al. Microbial colonization in a new intensive care bum unit. *Arch Surg* 1985;120:217–23.

15. Pruitt BA Jr, McManus AT. The changing epidemiology of infection in burn patients. *World J Surg* 1992;16:57–67.

16. Mozingo DW, Pruitt BA Jr. Infectious complications after burn injury. *Curr Opin Surg Infect* 1994;2:69–75.

17. Kagan RJ, Maraquis, Matsuda T, et al. Herpes simplex virus and cytomegalovirus infections in burn patients. *J Tauma* 1985;25:40–45.

18. Shirani KZ, McManus AT, Vaughn GM, et al. Effects of environment on infection in burn patients. *Arch Surg* 1986;121:31–36.

19. McManus AT, Mason AD Jr, McManus WF, et al. A decade of reduced gram negative infections on mortality associated with improved isolation of burn patients. *Arch Surg* 1994;129:1306–9.

20. Gamelli RL, Paxton TP, O'Reilly M. Bone marrow toxicity by silver sulfadiazine. *Surg Gynecol Obstet* 1993;177:115–20.

21. Muller MJ, Herndon DN. The challenge of burns. *Lancet* 1994;343:216–20.

22. Pruitt BA Jr. Phycomycotic infections. In: Alexander SW, ed. *Problems in general surgery*. Philadelphia: Lippincott, 1984.

23. McManus WF, Goodwin CW Jr, Pruitt BA Jr. Subeschar treatment of burn-wound infection. *Arch Surg* 1983;118:291–94.

24. Egan WC, Clark WR. The toxic shock syndrome in a burned victim. *Burns* 1988;14:135.

25. Frame JD, Eve MD, Hackett MEJ, et al. The toxic shock syndrome in burned children. *Burns* 1986;11:234–41.

26. McManus AT, Mason AD Jr, McManus WF, et al. What's in a name? Is methicillin-resistant *Staphylococcus aureus* just another *S. aureus* when treated with vancomycin? *Arch Surg* 1989;124:1456–59.

27. Barillo DJ, McManus AT, Cioffi WG, et al. *Aeromonas* bacteraemia in burn patients. *Burns* 1996;22:48–52.

Infections Due to Infusion Therapy

37

Dennis G. Maki and Leonard A. Mermel

Reliable intravascular access for administration of fluids and electrolytes, blood products, drugs, and nutritional support, and for hemodynamic monitoring is now one of the most essential features of modern medical care (Table 37-1). Each year in the United States, ~150 million intravascular devices are purchased by hospitals and clinics. The vast majority are peripheral venous catheters; however, >5 million central venous devices of various types are sold in the United States annually.

More than one half of all epidemics of nosocomial bacteremia or candidemia reported in the world literature between 1965 and 1991 derived from vascular access in some form [1,2]. One third to one half of episodes of nosocomial endocarditis have been traced to infected intravascular catheters [3–5], and healthcare-associated intravascular device-related bloodstream infection (IVDR-BSI) is associated with a 12%-28% attributable mortality [6–9]. Yet, infusion therapy generally has an underappreciated potential for producing iatrogenic disease. For example, <50% of the intensive care units (ICUs) in the United Kingdom had a written policy concerning the care of central venous catheters (CVCs) after insertion [10].

Infusion-related BSI is too frequently unrecognized, in great measure due to its relative infrequency. The percentage of infusions identified as producing BSI is sufficiently low—<1% on the average—that an average physician or nurse is unlikely to encounter more than an occasional episode. But even a low incidence of infection applied to the estimated 30 million patients who receive infusion therapy in U.S. hospitals annually translates to an estimated 50,000 to 100,000 BSIs nationwide each year [1,2], with 55,000 due to CVCs in U.S. ICUs [11]. Because neither the device nor the infusate is routinely cultured, the source of the BSI in a large proportion of episodes is never recognized.

Intravascular device-related bloodstream infection is largely preventable. This premise forms the thesis for this review: the primary goal must not be simply to identify and treat these iatrogenic infections, but rather to prevent them. By critically scrutinizing existing knowledge of the pathogenesis and epidemiology of device-related infection the reservoirs of healthcare-associated infection (HAI) pathogens and modes of transmission to patients' infusions—rational and effective guidelines for prevention can be formulated [12].

SOURCES AND FORMS OF INFUSION-RELATED INFLAMMATION AND BLOODSTREAM INFECTION

There are three major sources of BSI associated with any intravascular device: 1) colonization of the cannula wound, 2) colonization of the cannula hub, or 3) contamination of the fluid (i.e., infusate) administered through the cannula. Cannulas, which cause most *endemic* IVDR-BSIs, produce BSI far more frequently than contaminated infusate, the source of most *epidemics* of infusion-associated BSI [1].

It is important to understand the different stages and forms of device-related inflammation or infection, which range from infusion phlebitis—usually unrelated to infection—to asymptomatic colonization of the intravascular device—usually by skin commensals with little intrinsic virulence—to overwhelming septic shock originating from an infected thrombus in a cannulated great central vein or from infusate heavily contaminated by gram-negative bacilli.

TABLE 37-1

APPLICATIONS OF INFUSION THERAPY IN THE 2000S

Fluid and electrolyte replacement
Transfusion therapy
Blood products
Exchange transfusion
Plasmapheresis and apheresis
IV drug administration
Immediate circulatory access for critically ill patients
High blood and tissue levels
Drugs that cause tissue necrosis
Drugs that cause thrombolysis
Hemodialysis
Hemodynamic monitoring
Central venous catheters
Central venous pressure
Pulmonary artery Swan-Ganz catheters
Pulmonary artery pressure
Pulmonary artery occlusion (left atrial filling) pressure
Thermodilution cardiac output
Arterial catheters
Continuous arterial blood pressure
Total parenteral nutrition
Hyperalimentation (central venous catheters)
Peripheral parenteral nutrition (peripheral IV catheters)
Special nutritional support regimens for:
Acute renal failure
Hepatic failure
Cardiac cachexia
Pancreatitis
Acquired immunodeficiency syndrome
Intraarterial cancer chemotherapy

IV, intravenous.

Infusion Phlebitis

Infusion phlebitis, defined as inflammation of the cannulated vein—pain, erythema, tenderness, or an inflamed, palpable, thrombosed vein—is a frequent cause of pain and discomfort to the millions of patients who receive infusion therapy through peripheral intravenous (IV) cannulas each year in U.S. hospitals. Most investigators have concluded that infusion phlebitis is primarily a physicochemical phenomenon, and prospective studies have shown that the cannula material, length, and bore size; operator skill on insertion; the anatomic site of cannulation; the duration of cannulation; the frequency of dressing changes; the character of the infusate; and host factors such as patient age, Caucasian race, female gender, and the presence of underlying diseases significantly influence the risk of infusion phlebitis (Table 37-2).

In a prospective clinical study of 1,054 peripheral IV catheters, the Kaplan-Meier risk for phlebitis exceeded 50% by the fourth day after catheterization. IV antibiotics (relative risk (RR), 2.0), female gender (RR, 1.9), catheterization beyond 48 hours (RR, 1.8), and catheter

material (polyetherurethane (Vialon), tetrafluoroethylenehexafluoropropylene (Teflon), RR, 0.7) were strong predictors of phlebitis in a Cox proportional hazards model (each, $p < 0.003$) [13]. The best-fit model for severe phlebitis identified the same predictors plus catheter-related infection (RR, 6.2), phlebitis with the previous catheter (RR, 1.5), and anatomical site (hand: forearm, RR, 0.7; wrist: forearm, RR, 0.6).

Although not all studies have identified an association between phlebitis and catheter-related infection [14,15], this large, prospective study showed a strong statistical association, as have other studies [16–20]. Phlebitis also can be produced by contaminated infusate. Patients with BSI from intrinsically contaminated fluid in a large nationwide epidemic traced to the contaminated products of one U.S. manufacturer in 1970 to 1971 had a much higher incidence of phlebitis than patients receiving IV fluids who did not develop BSI [21].

Only a small proportion of patients with IV cannula-associated peripheral vein phlebitis have infusion-related infection, and <50% of patients with peripheral IVDR-BSI show phlebitis; however, the presence of phlebitis connotes a substantially increased risk of infection and indicates the need for immediate removal of the catheter to reduce the severity of phlebitis, for symptomatic relief, and to prevent catheter colonization from progressing to BSI.

Cannula-Related Infections

Between 5% and 25% of intravascular devices are *colonized* by skin organisms at the time of removal, as reflected by semiquantitative or quantitative cultures showing large numbers of organisms on the intravascular portion of the removed catheter or its tip. Colonization, which in most instances is asymptomatic, provides the biologic setting for systemic infection to occur and can be considered synonymous with localized infection. However, colonized cannulas are more likely than noncolonized ones to show phlebitis or local inflammation, especially purulence—pus spontaneously draining or expressable from the insertion site—and are far more likely to cause systemic infection (i.e., *cannula-related bacteremia* or *fungemia*) [17,22,23].

One of the most serious forms of intravascular device-related infection occurs when intravascular thrombus surrounding the cannula becomes infected. This causes *septic (suppurative) thrombophlebitis* when it occurs in association with peripheral IV cannulas [24,25], or *septic thrombosis of a great central vein* when associated with centrally placed catheters [26,27]. With suppurative phlebitis, the vein becomes an intravascular abscess, discharging myriads of microorganisms into the bloodstream, even *after the cannula has been removed.* The clinical picture is predictable: overwhelming BSI with high-grade and often unremitting bacteremia or fungemia. This syndrome is most likely to be encountered in burned patients or other ICU patients who have heavy cutaneous colonization and develop a cannula-related infection that goes unrecognized,

TABLE 37-2

RISK FACTORS FOR INFUSION PHLEBITIS IN PERIPHERAL IV THERAPY IDENTIFIED IN PROSPECTIVE STUDIES BY MULTIVARIATE DISCRIMINANT ANALYSIS OR IN PROSPECTIVE, RANDOMIZED, CONTROLLED TRIAL[a]

Catheter material
Polypropylene > Teflon
Silicone elastomer > polyurethane
Teflon > polyetherurethane
Teflon > steel needles
Catheter size
Large bore > smaller bore
8″ > 2″ Teflon
Insertion in emergency room > inpatient units
Disinfection of skin with antiseptic before catheter insertion
Experience, skill of person inserting catheter
House officers, nurses > hospital IV Team
House officers, nurses > decentralized unit IV nurse educator
Increasing duration of catheter placement in site
Subsequent catheters beyond the first infusate
Low-pH solutions (e.g., dextrose-containing)
Potassium chloride
Hypertonic glucose, amino acids, lipid for parenteral nutrition
Antibiotics (especially β-lactams, vancomycin, metronidazole)
High rate of flow of IV fluid (>90 ml/hr)
Disinfection of insertion site before catheter insertion
None > chlorhexidine–alcohol
Frequent IV dressing changes
Daily > every 48 hr
Catheter-related infection
Host factors
"Poor-quality" peripheral veins
Insertion site
Upper arm, wrist > hand
Age
Children: older > younger
Adults: younger > older
Sex
Female > male
Race
White > African American
Underlying medical disease
Individual biologic vulnerability
IV, intravenous.
Factors shown not to increase risk in well controlled, prospective, randomized trials include catheters made of polyethylene versus
  siliconized elastomer or of Teflon versus siliconized elastomer; type of antiseptic solutions used for cutaneous disinfection; use of
  topical antimicrobial ointment or spray on catheter insertion sites; type of dressing (e.g., gauze vs. transparent polyurethane
  dressing); dressing change every 48 hr versus not at all; administration of infusate by gravity flow versus pump; administration of IV
  antibiotics by slow infusion versus "IV push" over 2 min; maintenance of heparinm locks with saline versus heparinized saline); and
  frequency of routine change of IV delivery system.

[a]Denotes significantly greater risk of phlebitis; factors found to be significant predictors of risk in a prospective
study of 1,054 peripheral IV catheters at the University of Wisconsin Hospital and Clinics.
Source: From Maki DG, Ringer M. Risk factors for infusion-related phlebitis with small peripheral venous catheters.
A randomized controlled study. *Ann Intern Med* 1991;114:845–854, with permission.

permitting microorganisms to proliferate to high levels within the intravascular thrombus. The catheter insertion site is devoid of signs of inflammation >50% of the time, and the clinical picture may not present until several days after the catheter has been removed. *In any patient with an IV catheter who develops high-grade BSI that persists after an* *infected cannula has been removed, it is likely the patient has infected thrombus in the recently cannulated vein, and may even have secondary endocarditis or seeding to other distant sites* [28].

The microorganisms most frequently implicated in suppurative phlebitis are predominantly *Staphylococcus aureus,* and *Candida* species [24–27]. Although coagulase-negative staphylococci commonly cause IVDR-BSI, they rarely cause suppurative thrombophlebitis, possible because of their lesser tendency to bind to host-derived protein components of thrombus compared with other pathogens such as *S. aureus* [29,30].

Suppurative phlebitis of peripheral IV catheters is now rare, and the syndrome of IV suppuration is predominantly a complication of CVCs, characteristically catheters that have been left in place for many days in heavily colonized ICU patients.

Bloodstream Infection From Contaminated Infusate

It also is important to recognize that the infusate—parenteral fluid, blood products, or IV medications—administered through an intravascular device also can become contaminated and produce infusion-related BSI, which is more likely than cannula-related infection to culminate in frank septic shock. Contaminated fluid is a rare cause of endemic infection with short-term peripheral IV devices, but the infusate is more commonly associated with infections of catheters used for hemodynamic monitoring, CVCs, and, possibly, surgically implanted cuffed Hickman or Broviac catheters [31–34]. Most nosocomial *epidemics* of infusion-related BSI, however, have been traced to contamination of infusate by gram-negative bacilli, introduced during its manufacture (*intrinsic contamination*) [21] or during its preparation or administration in the healthcare system (*extrinsic contamination*) [1,2,35,36].

DIAGNOSIS OF INFUSION-RELATED BLOODSTREAM INFECTION

Clinical Features

Although meticulous aseptic technique during cannula insertion and good follow-up care greatly reduce the risk of IVDR-BSI, sporadic episodes and even epidemics still can be expected occasionally to occur because of human error, intrinsically contaminated products, or the undue susceptibility to infection of many patients. If affected patients are to survive, the causal relationship between an infusion and the BSI must be recognized as early as possible.

The general clinical features of infusion-related bacteremia or fungemia are nonspecific and indiscernible from BSIs arising from any local site of infection, such as urinary tract infection (UTI) or surgical site infection (SSI) (Table 37-3). There also appears to be a poor correlation between clinical judgment and microbiologic confirmation of IVDR-BSI [37]. Infusion-related BSI occurring in ICU patients can be particularly insidious: bacteremia or fungemia usually is identified by positive blood cultures but is attributed to nosocomial pneumonia, UTI or SSI, or is simply accepted as "cryptogenic" and treated empirically.

Certain clinical, epidemiologic, and microbiologic findings can be extremely helpful to the clinician evaluating a hospitalized patient with a picture of nosocomial BSI or cryptogenic bacteremia or candidemia, and point toward an IVD as the source (Table 37-3):

TABLE 37-3

CLINICAL, EPIDEMIOLOGIC, AND MICROBIOLOGIC FEATURES OF INTRAVASCULAR DEVICE-RELATED BLOODSTREAM INFECTION

Nonspecific	Suggestive of Device-related Etiology
Fever	Patient unlikely candidate for bloodstream infection (e.g., young, no underlying diseases)
Chills, shaking, rigors[a]	Source of bloodstream infection inapparent
Hypotension, shock[a]	No identifiable local infection
Hyperventilation	Intravascular device in place, especially central venous catheter
Respiratory failure	Inflammation or purulence at insertion site
Gastrointestinal[a]	Abrupt onset, associated with shock[a]
Abdominal pain	Bloodstream infection refractory to antimicrobial therapy, or dramatic
Vomiting	improvement with removal of cannula and infusion[a]
Diarrhea	Bloodstream infection caused by staphylococci (especially coagulase-negative
Neurologic[a]	staphylococci), *Corynebacterium* (especially JK-1) or *Bacillus* species, *Candida*,
Confusion	*Trichophyton*, *Fusarium*, or *Malassezia* species
Seizures	

[a]Commonly seen in overwhelming gram-negative bloodstream infection originating from contaminated infusate, peripheral suppurative phlebitis, or septic thrombosis of a central vein.

1. The patient is an unlikely candidate for BSI, being healthy and without underlying predisposing diseases [21,38].
2. No local infection to account for a picture of BSI [21,38].
3. An IVD in place, *especially a CVC*, at the outset of BSI [38].
4. Local inflammation [17,22,23,39], especially purulence at the insertion site [23,39], which while present in only a minority of cases, is strongly suggestive of catheter-related infection.
5. Abrupt onset, associated with fulminant shock—suggestive of massively contaminated infusion [40].
6. Nosocomial BSI caused by staphylococci [38], especially coagulative-negative staphylococci, *Corynebacterium* (especially JK-1) or *Bacillus* spp., or *Candida* [38], *Fusarium, Trichophyton*, or *Malassezia* spp., suggests IVDR-BSI. In contrast, bacteremia caused by streptococci, aerobic gram-negative bacilli—especially *Pseudomonas aeruginosa*—or anaerobes is very unlikely to have originated from an infected IVD [38].
7. BSI refractory to antimicrobial therapy or dramatic improvement with removal of the cannula or discontinuation of the infusion [21,38].

During a large, nationwide outbreak in 1970 to 1971 due to intrinsic contamination of one U. S. manufacturer's products, patients treated with antibiotics to which the epidemic organisms were susceptible remained clinically septic, continued to have positive blood cultures after 24 hours or more of appropriate therapy, and did not improve clinically until their infusions were serendipitously or intentionally removed [21].

Focal retinal lesions—cotton wool spot patches—may be seen in patients with disseminated *Candida spp.* infection deriving from CVCs, even in those without positive blood cultures [41]. Careful ophthalmologic examination should be routinely performed in the evaluation of patients with CVCs with suspected IVDR-BSI, especially patients receiving total parenteral nutrition (TPN). BSI from arterial catheters may be heralded by embolic lesions that manifest as tender, erythematous papules, 5–10 mm in diameter, appearing in the distal distribution of the involved artery, usually in the palm or sole—Osler's nodes [42,43]. Arterial bleeding from the insertion site often is the harbinger of BSI caused by an infected arterial catheter and may denote an infective pseudoaneurysm [42,44,45]. Endocarditis, particularly right sided, is a rare but well documented complication of flow-directed pulmonary artery catheters [46–48].

Blood Cultures

Blood cultures are essential to the diagnosis of IVDR-BSI (see Chapter 9), and in any patient suspected of infusion-related infection, two or three separate 10-ml blood cultures should be drawn [49–51], ideally from peripheral veins, by separate venipunctures. If the patient is receiving antimicrobial therapy, blood cultures obtained immediately before a dose is due to be administered and blood antibiotic levels are likely to be low, may provide a higher yield. Use of resin-containing media to adsorb and remove any antibiotic present in the blood specimen [52], adsorb serum factors detrimental to the growth of Enterobacteriaceae [53], and lyse the cell wall of neutrophils, thereby releasing intracellular pathogens [54], also may increase the yield [55].

The use of a biphasic system, such as the Isolator® (E. I. DuPont, Nemours and Co., Wilmington, DE), or systems with selective high blood volume fungal media (BACTEC; Becton Dickinson Diagnostic Instrument Systems, Sparks, MD) appear to significantly enhance the laboratory detection of fungemia [56,57].

The volume of blood cultured is critical to maximize the yield of blood cultures for diagnosis of bacteremia or candidemia: in adults, obtaining at least 20 ml, ideally 30 ml, per drawing—each specimen containing 10 or 15 ml, inoculated into aerobic and anaerobic media—significantly improves the yield, compared with obtaining only 10 ml at each drawing and culturing a smaller total volume [58,59]. It is rarely necessary to obtain > two 15-ml cultures or three 10-ml cultures in a 24-hour period. If at least 30 ml of blood is cultured, 99% of detectable bacteremias should be identified [58].

It is common practice in many ICUs to draw blood cultures through central venous or arterial catheters or, in neonates, through umbilical catheters. Comparative studies of standard blood cultures drawn through central venous or arterial catheters in adults usually have shown good concordance with cultures drawn by percutaneous peripheral venipuncture [60–62], but rates of false-positive (contaminated) cultures can be considerably higher with catheter-drawn specimens [63]. The practice of drawing non-qualitative blood cultures through indwelling vascular catheters probably ought not to be encouraged because of the risk of introducing contamination during the manipulation [64]. If, however, to preserve dwindling superficial veins it is considered unavoidable to use a vascular catheter to obtain blood cultures, an attempt should be made to use a newly inserted catheter [60–62] and to draw at least every other specimen by percutaneous venipuncture.

If the laboratory is prepared to do pour-plate blood cultures or has available an automated quantitative system for culturing blood, such as the Isolator® system, catheter-drawn blood cultures can permit the diagnosis of IVDR-BSI to be made with reasonable sensitivity and specificity (both in the range of 90%), without removing the catheter [65–71]. With infected catheters, a quantitative blood culture drawn through the catheter usually shows a marked step-up—often >10-fold—in the concentration of organisms compared with quantitative blood cultures drawn at the same time percutaneously through a peripheral vein.

Quantitative catheter-drawn blood cultures probably have their greatest utility in diagnosis of device-related infection with surgically implanted cuffed Hickman or Broviac catheters and subcutaneous central venous ports [65–68].

Finding microbes on Gram stain or acridine orange stain of blood drawn through CVCs has been shown to be highly sensitive and specific for diagnosing IVDR-BSI [73,74]. If confirmed by others using the same and other IVDs, these may be the methods of choice for the rapid diagnosis of serious intravascular catheter-related infections. Intracellular bacteria have been found on Wright-stained peripheral smears in asymptomatic patients with occult CVC-BSI [75].

Microbiology of Intravascular Device-Related Bloodstream Infection

The microbiologic profile of BSI (Table 37-3) can strongly suggest an infusion-related source. Cryptogenic staphylococcal BSI, particularly with coagulase-negative staphylococci, BSI caused by *Bacillus* or *Corynebacterium* (especially JK-1) spp. or *Enterococcus*, or fungemia caused by *Candida, Fusarium, Trichophyton,* or *Malassezia* spp., especially in a patient with a CVC, is most likely to reflect catheter-related infection [1,2,38].

BSIs caused by *Enterobacter cloacae* or, especially, *Pantoea* (formerly *Enterobacter*) *agglomerans, Burkholderia cepacia, Stenotrophomonas maltophilia,* or *Citrobacter* spp., in the setting of infusion therapy, may signal an epidemic and should prompt studies to rule out contaminated infusate [76]. A BSI cluster should mandate a full-scale investigation, which may include culturing of large numbers of in-use infusions and informing the local, state, and Federal public health authorities. Such actions averted a large, nationwide epidemic in 1973, when, prompted by five unexplained BSIs in three hospitals, intrinsic contamination of one U.S. company's products was identified and a recall put into effect so rapidly that the outbreak was limited to the five initially recognized patients [77]. It must be emphasized, however, that for BSI surveillance to be maximally effective, all blood culture isolates must always be fully identified—that is, identified to the genus and species level. Failure to do so during the 1970 to 1971 nationwide epidemic traced to the contaminated products of one U.S. manufacturer resulted in pre-eminent hospitals experiencing large numbers of infections that were recognized as infusion-related only in retrospect [21].

Cryptogenic nosocomial BSI caused by psychrophilic (cold-growing) organisms, such as non-*aeruginosa* pseudomonads, *Ochrobactrum anthropi* (formerly *Achromobacter*) *Flavobacterium, Enterobacter,* or *Serratia* spp. [78,79], or by *Salmonella* [80] or *Yersinia* spp. [81], with a picture of overwhelming BSI, may indicate a contaminated blood product.

Cultures of Intravascular Devices

Some laboratories still culture vascular catheters qualitatively, amputating the tip aseptically and immersing it in liquid media. Unfortunately, a positive culture by this technique is diagnostically nonspecific because a single organism picked up from the skin as the catheter is removed can produce a positive—false-positive—culture [82]. Many IVDR-BSIs derive from local infection of the transcutaneous cannula tract (see discussion later). Culture of the external surface of the withdrawn cannula should reflect the microbiologic status of the wound, and quantitative culture should more accurately distinguish infection from contamination. A standardized, semiquantitative method for culturing vascular cannulas in solid media was developed in 1977 [17]. Colony counts on semiquantitative culture are bimodally distributed, as they are in quantitative urine cultures. The method provides excellent discrimination between colonization and insignificant contamination acquired during catheter removal. Fifteen or more colony-forming units (cfu) growing on a semiquantitative plate is regarded as a positive culture, and denotes significant growth or colonization [17]. Based on experience with >10,000 IVDs, positive cultures found using this technique have shown a 15%-40% association with concordant BSI. Cannulas positive on semiquantitative culture also are strongly associated with local inflammation [17].

Good correlation between high colony counts and IVDR-BSI have been demonstrated with cultures of catheter segments semiquantitatively on solid media [83–85] or quantitatively in liquid media—removing organisms from the catheter by vortexing or sonication [83,86,87]. The latter techniques appear to have the greatest sensitivity and specificity for the diagnosis of vascular catheter-related infection [72,88]. However, a negative catheter culture may not rule out a catheter-related BSI (CR-BSI) [33,37, 72,88,89]. Using >1 catheter culture technique increases the yield [88], as does bedside plating of catheters for semiquantitative culture [90]. Direct Gram stains [91] or acridine orange stains [92] of intravascular segments of removed catheters also show excellent correlation with quantitative techniques for culturing catheters and can permit rapid diagnosis of catheter-related infection.

Given the strong evidence implicating cutaneous microorganisms in the genesis of most BSIs caused by short-term, noncuffed intravascular catheters, a number of studies have shown that a quantitative culture [22,93] or Gram stain [94] of skin at the insertion site also can identify infected catheters with reasonable sensitivity and specificity, greatly exceeding an assessment based solely on clinical signs of infection. The combination of culturing skin both at the insertion site and the catheter hub has been reported to provide even better sensitivity for diagnosis of catheter-related infection, without removing the catheter [33,95,96].

To reliably diagnose infection caused by contaminated infusate requires a sample of fluid to be aspirated from the line and cultured quantitatively [76]. A variety of techniques are now available for culturing or processing parenteral admixtures and fluid medications in the laboratory for microbial contamination [97,98]. Because there is no evidence that anaerobic bacteria can grow in parenteral crystalloid admixtures, anaerobic culture techniques are not necessary unless blood or another biologic product is involved.

Definitions for Infusion-Related Infection

Using the results of semiquantitative or quantitative culture of the catheter and cultures of the hub of the catheter and of infusate aspirated from the line at the time the catheter is removed, and concomitant blood cultures, it is possible to formulate rigorous definitions for intravascular device-related infection [99] (Table 37-4).

The term "catheter sepsis" appears frequently in the literature, but lacks stringent criteria. Although sepsis has been defined by a consensus panel [100], the term as applied to catheter-related infections may be insensitive because many of these infections are due to coagulase-negative staphylococci, and in some studies, only 55%-71% of patients with bacteremia due to this pathogen had leukocytosis [101,102]. Also, the maximal body temperature is <38°C in many patients with coagulase-negative staphylococcal BSI [102,103]. This term should likely not be further promulgated in the literature, especially in those prospective, comparative studies involving IVDs [99].

In addition, the definitions listed previously may be unnecessarily rigorous for use in clinical HAI surveillance because very few clinicians obtain cultures of catheter hubs or infusate, even if the cannula is cultured. Moreover, patients with disseminated candidiasis originating from an infected catheter often have negative blood cultures. It also is important to realize that multiple sites often are colonized when cultures are performed at the time of catheter withdrawal and it may be difficult to distinguish with certainty the source of many catheter-BSIs. Therefore, for routine surveillance, use of the Centers for Disease Control and Prevention (CDC) definitions is recommended [104,105].

TABLE 37-4
DEFINITIONS FOR INTRAVASCULAR DEVICE-RELATED INFECTION

I. Catheter colonization: Significant growth of a microbial pathogen from the catheter tip, subcutaneous segment of the catheter, or catheter hub

II. Localized Intravascular Catheter-Related Infection
  A. Microbiologically Proven Exit Site Infection: Purulent exudate within 2 cm of the catheter exit site, in the absence of concomitant BSI
  B. Clinically Suspected Exit Site Infection: Erythema or induration within 2 cm of the catheter exit site, in the absence of concomitant BSI and without concomitant purulence
  C. Tunnel Infection: Tenderness, erythema, or induration >2 cm from the catheter exit site along the subcutaneous tract of a tunneled (e.g., Hickman or Broviac) catheter, in the absence of concomitant BSI
  D. Pocket Infection: Purulent fluid in the subcutaneous pocket of a totally implanted intravascular catheter that may or may not be associated with spontaneous rupture and drainage or necrosis of the overlying skin, in the absence of concomitant BSI

III. Systemic Infection
  A. IVDR-BSI: Concordant microbial growth between a catheter segment or hub, infusate, or exit site exudate, and percutaneously drawn blood cultures or concordant microbial growth between catheter-drawn and percutaneously drawn quantitative blood cultures (catheter-drawn blood cultures: percutaneously drawn blood cultures ≥4: 1)
    1. Primary Hub-Related BSI: Concordant growth from the catheter hub and a percutaneously drawn culture, regardless of the catheter tip results, with negative cultures or growth of a different microbe from the exit site and/or subcutaneous catheter segment culture by the roll-plate method. A negative culture or discordant growth from the catheter tip by the roll plate method [17] supports the diagnosis
    2. Primary Skin-Related BSI: Concordant growth from the exit site and/or subcutaneous catheter segment by the roll-plate method, and a percutaneously drawn blood culture with negative cultures or growth of a different microbe from the hub and infusate; concordant growth from the catheter tip by the roll-plate method further supports the diagnosis
    3. Primary Infusate-Related BSI: Concordant growth from the infusate and a percutaneously drawn blood culture with negative cultures or discordant growth from the hub, exit site, and/or subcutaneous catheter segment by the roll-plate method
  B. Definite Intravascular Catheter-Related Sepsis: CR-BSI infection in the setting of sepsis-defining symptoms [100]
  C. Probable Intravascular Catheter Sepsis: Sepsis in the setting of negative blood cultures, resolution of sepsis-defining symptoms shortly after catheter withdrawal, and a catheter component with significant growth of a microbial pathogen or growth from purulent material at the exit site or subcutaneous pocket, or erythema and induration extending along the tunnel tract of a Hickman or Broviac catheter

CANNULA-ASSOCIATED INFECTION

Incidence of Cannula-Related Bloodstream Infection

IVDR-BSI is perhaps the least frequently recognized HAI. The true incidence of IVDR-BSI is underestimated in most centers because a catheter often is not suspected as a source of the patient's clinical picture of nosocomial BSI, and is not cultured. Prospective studies in which every device enrolled is cultured at the time of removal clearly indicate that every type of IVD carries some risk of causing BSI, but the magnitude of risk *per device* varies greatly, depending on its type [2].

Table 37-5 shows representative rates of infection for various types of intravascular devices. The lowest rates are with small peripheral IV steel needles and Teflon or polyurethane catheters: large prospective studies have shown rates of approximately 0.2 BSIs per 100 peripheral IV catheters [13–16,19,105–109]; two large, comparative trials have shown that if IV cannulas are inserted under scrupulous aseptic conditions, plastic catheters probably pose no greater risk of device-related bacteremia or candidemia than steel needles [106]. Prospective studies of arterial catheters used for hemodynamic monitoring have found rates of infusion-related bacteremia in the range of 1% [110].

The device that poses the greatest risk of iatrogenic BSI is the CVC in its numerous forms [9,111–113]. Many prospective studies of short-term, noncuffed, single- or multilumen catheters inserted percutaneously into the subclavian or internal jugular vein have found rates of CR-BSI in the range of 2%-5% [9,83,114–119]. Percutaneously inserted, noncuffed CVCs used for hemodialysis have been associated with the highest rates of BSI, >10% [120–122]; however, cuffed hemodialysis catheter use appears to be associated with a lower incidence of BSI [123,124]. *Peripherally inserted* central catheters (PICCs) pose a substantially lower risk of CR-BSI (0.04 to 0.4 per 100 catheter days), comparable to Hickman catheters [125,126]. Swan-Ganz pulmonary artery catheters used for hemodynamic monitoring are associated with a 1% rate of BSI or 0.3 per 100 catheter-days [110]. The lowest rates of infection with CVCs have been with surgically implanted Hickman or Broviac catheters that incorporate a Dacron cuff, which have been associated with rates of infection in the range of 0.1 bacteremias or fungemias per 100 catheter-days [127,128], and surgically implanted subcutaneous central venous ports, associated with a rates of BSI of <0.05 per 100 device-days [127,128]. In prospective studies, the incidence of BSI has been demonstrated to be lower in patients who have subcutaneously implanted ports compared with those with tunneled catheters with a Dacron cuff [129–134].

TABLE 37-5

APPROXIMATE RISKS OF BLOODSTREAM INFECTION ASSOCIATED WITH VARIOUS TYPES OF DEVICES FOR INTRAVASCULAR ACCESS[a]

Type of Device	Representative Rate	Representative Range
Short-term temporary access[b]		
Peripheral IV cannulas		
Winged steel needles	<0.2	0–1
Peripheral IV catheters		
Percutaneously inserted	0.2	0–1
Cutdown	6	0–1
Midline catheters	0.7	0.7–0.8
Arterial catheters	1	—
Central venous catheters		
All-purpose, multilumen	3	1–7
Pulmonary artery	1	0–5
Hemodialysis	10	3–18
Long-term indefinite access[c]		
Peripherally inserted, central venous catheters (PICCs)	0.20	—
Cuffed central catheters (e.g., Hickman, Broviac)	0.20	0.10–0.53
Subcutaneous central venous ports (e.g., Infusaport®), Port-a-cath®, Landmark®)	0.04	0.00–0.10
IV, intravenous.		

[a]Based on data from recently published, prospective studies.
[b]Number of bloodstream infections per 100 devices.
[c]Number of bloodstream infections per 100 device-days.

It has been estimated that 90% of IVDR-BSIs originate from CVCs of various types [2], leading to ~55,000 BSIs in U.S. ICUs each year [11]. Data from the CDC's National Nosocomial Infections Surveillance (NNIS) study have shown that the incidence of secondary BSIs, deriving from identifiable local infections such as UTIs, SSIs, or pneumonias, has remained stable over the past decade; in contrast, the incidence of primary nosocomial BSIs, the largest proportion of which derive from IVDs, has increased more than twofold over this same period [2,135], reflecting the great increase in the use of infusion therapy and, especially, the use of CVCs of all types. It seems clear that the greatest hope for reducing the risk of IVDR-BSI will come from better understanding of infection with CVCs, which will form the basis for more effective strategies for prevention.

Epidemiology

The first and perhaps most important question that must be addressed to develop effective strategies for prevention is to determine the major source or sources of microorganisms that can colonize a percutaneous IVD (Fig. 37-1) and cause invasive infection leading to bacteremia or candidemia. An intravascular catheter can easily become colonized extraluminally by organisms from the patient's cutaneous microflora. Contamination may occur during catheter insertion [136] or shortly thereafter [137]. Microorganisms also can contaminate the catheter hub where the administration set attaches to the catheter, or they may gain access to the fluid column and be infused directly into the patient's bloodstream; the device also can become infected hematogenously from remote sources of local infection; or the device might even be contaminated from its manufacture—which fortunately is very rare.

A large body of clinical and microbiologic data indicates that most IVDR-BSIs caused by *short-term*, percutaneously inserted, noncuffed catheters are caused by extraluminal microorganisms of cutaneous origin that invade the transcutaneous insertion wound at the time the catheter is inserted or in the days after insertion.

Numerous prospective studies of intravascular device-related infection have shown that coagulase-negative staphylococci, the predominant aerobic species on the human skin, are now the most common agents of CR-BSI [1,2,9,48,105 109,111,117,127,135]. The vast majority of vascular CR-BSIs are caused by microorganisms that colonize the skin of hospitalized patients: staphylococci, both coagulase-negative and coagulase-positive (*S. aureus*); *Candida, Corynebacterium,* and *Bacillus* spp.; and, to a lesser degree, aerobic gram-negative bacilli (Table 37-6).

Prospective studies also have shown strong concordance between organisms present on skin surrounding the catheter insertion site and organisms recovered from CVCs producing BSI [22,34,48,93,94,114–116,136]. There appears to be a direct parallel between the level and profile of cutaneous colonization at the insertion sites of short-term central venous, arterial, or peripheral IV catheters and the risk of CR-BSI [138,139].

ICU unit and hemodialysis patients with cutaneous colonization by *S. aureus* experience four- to sixfold higher rates of IVDR-BSI [140,141]. Use of recombinant interleukin-2, with or without lymphokine-activated killer (LAK) cells for cancer immunotherapy, which is associated with frequent dermatotoxicity (desquamation) and heavy cutaneous colonization by *S. aureus*, has been associated with a prohibitively high incidence of CVC-related *S. aureus* BSI [142].

Burned patients, who have huge populations of microorganisms on the skin surface, experience very high rates of CR-BSI [143,144] (see Chapter 38).

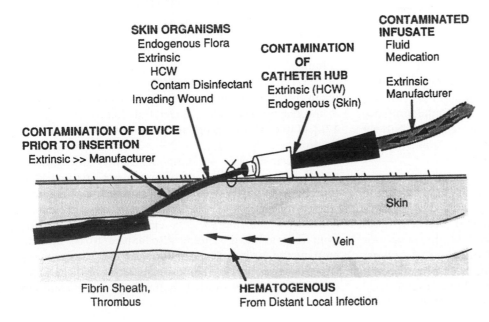

Figure 37-1 Sources of intravascular cannula-related infection. The sources are the skin flora, contamination of the catheter hub, contamination of infusate, and hematogenous colonization of the intravascular device and its fibronectin–fibrin sheath. (HCW, health-care worker).

TABLE 37-6

MICROORGANISMS MOST FREQUENTLY ENCOUNTERED IN VARIOUS FORMS OF INTRAVASCULAR LINE-RELATED INFECTION

Source	Pathogens
Catheter-related	
Peripheral IV catheter	Coagulase-negative staphylococci[a]
	Staphylococcus aureus
	Candida spp[a]
Central venous catheters	Coagulase-negative staphylococci
	S. aureus
	Candida spp
	Corynebacterium spp (especially JK-1)
	Klebsiella and Enterobacter spp
	Mycobacterium spp
	Trichophyton beiglii
	Fusarium spp
	Malassezia furfur[a]
Contaminated IV infusate	Tribe Klebsielleae
	Enterobacter cloacae
	Enterobacter agglomerans
	Serratia marcescens
	Klebsiella spp
	Burkholderia cepacia
	Burkholderia acidivorans, Burkholderia pickettii
	Stenotrophomonas maltophilia
	Citrobacter freundii
	Flavobacterium spp
	Candida tropicalis
Contaminated blood products	E. cloacae
	S. marcescens
	Ochrobactrum anthropi
	Flavobacterium spp
	Burkholderia spp
	Yersinia spp
	Salmonella spp

IV, intravenous.
[a]Also seen with peripheral IV catheters in association with the administration of lipid emulsion for parenteral nutritional support.

Numerous outbreaks of IVDR-BSI have been traced to contaminated cutaneous antiseptics [145–148].

High counts of microorganisms on semiquantitative culture of the external surface of a removed catheter are strongly associated with bacteremia caused by the catheter [17,22,83–85,95,121,143,149].

Microscopic examination of infected CVCs has shown heavy colonization of the external surface [91,92], especially with short-term catheters [150].

Prospective studies have shown that use of a more effective cutaneous antiseptic, e.g., chlorhexidine, for antisepsis of the insertion site at the time of catheter insertion and in follow-up care of the catheter greatly reduces the risk of infusion-related BSI [32,151–153].

Prospective trials have shown that antiseptics or antimicrobials applied topically to the intravascular catheter insertion site can reduce the risk of CR-BSI [122,154].

Surgically implanted Broviac or Hickman catheters, which have a subcutaneous Dacron cuff that becomes ingrown by tissue and poses a mechanical barrier against invasion of the tract by skin organisms, have been associated with considerably lower rates of CR-BSI (∼0.20 episodes per 100 catheter-days) [155–157] than short-term, noncuffed CVCs (0.6 to 1.0 per 100 catheter days) [22,91,111,114,115,117] (Table 37-5). However, in a clinical trial, nonsurgically implanted, non-tunneled, noncuffed Silastic catheters were inserted for prolonged periods of time with a very low risk of infection [125]. These data suggest that with careful follow-up, insertion of noncuffed CVCs with the Seldinger technique outside of the operating room may be an acceptable alternative to Hickman or Broviac cuffed catheters. With one exception [158], prospective, randomized, clinical trials of a subcutaneous silver-impregnated cuff that can be attached to a short-term (<10 to 14 days) CVC at the time of insertion also can reduce the risk of catheter colonization and CR-BSI [115,116,159]. However, with more prolonged catheterization (>14 days), this device does not appear to be efficacious [160–162]. Studies have shown that novel short-term (∼7 days) CVCs with an externally antimicrobial [163,164] or antiseptic or heparin [165–169] greatly reduce the incidence of catheter colonization and, in some instances, CR-BSI. Again, efficacy of these novel devices has not been demonstrated with more prolonged catheterization [170,171]. This may reflect the greater importance of the catheter hub as a source of invading pathogens, compared with the skin at the insertion site, with more prolonged catheterization [72,150]. A number of studies have shown that the colonized hubs of IVDs are an important source of pathogens causing CR-BSIs [34], particularly with more prolonged duration of catheterization [33,72,95,150,172–174].

Central venous and arterial catheters also can become colonized hematogenously, from remote, unrelated sites of infection, but the evidence suggests that this occurs relatively less frequently than colonization from microbes at the insertion site or catheter hub [32,34,48,115,175,176] (Table 37-7), except in patients with short bowel syndrome [177].

Although infusate not infrequently becomes contaminated by small numbers of organisms, mainly skin commensals such as coagulase-negative staphylococci, with the exception of arterial catheters used for hemodynamic monitoring [31,32], endemic BSIs originating from contaminated infusate also appear to be uncommon in the United States, although common in many facilities with limited resources [32,109,115]. In contrast, contaminated infusate is the single most common

TABLE 37-7

POTENTIAL SOURCES OF SWAN-GANZ PULMONARY ARTERY (PA) CATHETER-RELATED BLOODSTREAM INFECTION, BASED ON A PROSPECTIVE STUDY OF 442 SWAN-GANZ PULMONARY ARTERY CATHETERS

	Gauze (2 days)	Conventional Polyurethane (5 days)	Highly Permeable Polyurethane (5 days)	Overall
Total no. of catheter-related bloodstream infections	2	1	2	5
Microbiologic				
Concordance with source				
Intravascular segment of introducer or PA catheter	2	1	2	5
Skin	1	—	1	2
Hub	1	1	1	3
Infusate	1	1	1	3
Extravascular portion of PA catheter, beneath external protective sleeve	—	—	1	1
Hematogenous from remote source	—	1	1	—

Source: From Maki DG, Stolz SS, Wheeler S, Mermel LA. A prospective, randomized trial of gauze and two polyurethane dressings for site care of pulmonary artery catheters: implications for catheter management. Crit Care Med 1994;22:1729–1737.

identified cause of epidemic nosocomial BSI [1,2], caused predictably by microorganisms capable of multiplying in parenteral glucose-containing admixtures, members of the tribe Klebsielleae (*Klebsiella, Enterobacter* and *Serratia*), *B. cepacia, Burkholderia pickettii*, or *Citrobacter* spp. [76]. Nearly 100 epidemics of infusion-related BSI since 1965 have been traced to contaminated infusate or IV medications, with microorganisms most frequently introduced during preparation or administration in the hospital (*extrinsic* contamination) or during its manufacture (*intrinsic* contamination).

Analysis of risk factors predisposing to intravascular catheter-related infection by stepwise logistic regression of data from large, prospective studies of peripheral IV catheters [109], arterial catheters used for hemodynamic monitoring [31], multilumen CVCs used in ICU patients [32], or Swan-Ganz pulmonary artery catheters [175] shows that heavy cutaneous colonization of the insertion site is one of the most powerful predictors of catheter-related infection with all types of short-term, percutaneously inserted catheters (Table 37-8).

Pathogenesis

Examination of an infected IVD by scanning electron microscopy characteristically shows the surface covered by an amorphous film [150,176,189], presumably representing host proteins, with microcolonies of the infecting organism encased in a thick matrix of glycocalyx (slime), all comprising a "biofilm" [190] (Fig. 37-2). Studies of the pathobiology of prosthetic device-related infection have shown considerable differences in the capacity of microorganisms to adhere to various prosthetic materials. In vitro, catheters made of Teflon or polyurethane are more resistant to bacterial adherence, especially by staphylococci, than catheters made of polyethylene, polyvinylchloride, or, especially, silicone [191,192]. These differences are maintained if the experiments are done with previously implanted catheters or catheters precoated with specific plasma procatheters or catheters precoated with specific plasma proteins [193–196].

Initial attachment of *Staphylococcus epidermidis* directly to a catheter is mediated, in part, by the hydrophobicity of the strain [197] and by specific adhesins [198–202]. Initial attachment of *S. aureus* to catheters appears to be more dependent on the presence of preadsorbed plasma or tissue proteins such as fibronectin, thrombospondin, fibrin, vitronectin, and laminin [29,30,196,203]. Because many of these proteins are an integral part of thrombus formation, the presence of thrombus on the catheter surface also appears to promote adherence and catheter-associated infection [88,180,204,205]. Persistence of bacteria and fungi attached to the catheter surface appears to be promoted by surface exoglycocalyx [206,207]. Whereas subtherapeutic levels of antibiotics reduce microbial adherence [195,208], once microorganisms such as coagulase-negative staphylococci colonize a prosthetic surface, host defenses become secondarily impaired and are unable to spontaneously eradicate the infection [209,210]. Moreover, once associated with a foreign surface, microorganisms exhibit increased resistance to antimicrobials [211–216]. It should be no surprise that infections of prosthetic implants are difficult to cure with antimicrobial therapy alone, even with prolonged administration of high doses of bactericidal drugs.

RISK FACTORS FOR INTRAVASCULAR CATHETER-RELATED INFECTION BASED ON MULTIVARIATE ANALYSIS OF DATA FROM LARGE, PROSPECTIVE STUDIES

Type of Catheter [ref.]	No. Catheters Studied	Risk Factors	Relative Risk
Peripheral IV [109]	2,050	Cutaneous colonization of site $>10^2$ cfu	3.9
		Contamination of catheter hub	3.8
		Moisture on site, under dressing	2.5
		Placement >3 days	1.8
		Systemic antimicrobial therapy	0.5
Peripheral IV [153] (pediatric patients)	826	Heavy colonization of insertion site	3.6
		Catheterization for $\geq$72 hr	2.0
		Gestational age $\leq$32 wk	1.8
		Ampicillin infusion	0.4
		Cutaneous antisepsis with chlorhexidine	0.2
Arterial [31]	491	Cutaneous colonization of site $>10^2$ cfu	10.0
		Second catheter in site, placed over guidewire	—
Umbilical artery [178] (pediatric patients)	189	Very low birth weight	
		Prolonged antibiotic therapy	—
		Antibiotic therapy at time of catheter removal	—
Umbilical vein [178] (pediatric patients)	144	High birth weight	—
		Hyperalimentation in high-birthweight patients	—
Central venous [179]	345	Exposure of catheter to unrelated bacteremia	9.4
		Cutaneous colonization of site $>10^2$ cfu	9.2
		Placement >4 days	—
Central venous [193]	188	Catheter-related thrombosis	—
Central venous [181]	1,258	Respiratory tract colonization or infection	—
		Hypoalbuminemia	—
Central venous [182]	76	Heavy insertion site colonization	13.2
		Difficult catheter insertion	5.4
		Female gender	0.2
		Underlying secondary diagnosis	0.2
Central venous [183]	1,212	Internal jugular vein insertion	3.3
		Patient transfer within the hospital	3.0
		Disease of the gastrointestinal tract	2.4
		Prolonged hospital length of stay before catheter insertion	1.0
		Concomitant antibiotic use	0.3
		Polyurethane catheter	0.2
Central venous [22]	140	Insertion site colonized with organisms other than coagulase-negative staphylococci	14.9
		Insertion site erythema	4.4
		Insertion site colonized with >50 cfu of coagulase-negative staphylococci or >1 cfu of any other microbe	6.4
Pulmonary artery [175]	297	Cutaneous colonization of site $>10^3$ cfu	5.5
		Internal jugular vein cannulation	4.3
		Duration >3 days	3.1
		Placement in operating room under less stringent barrier precautions	2.1
Pulmonary artery [184]	86	Catheterization >5 days	14.4
		Antibiotic use	0.2
Hemodialysis [120]	53	Chronic renal failure	7.2
Peripheral, central venous, arterial, and pulmonary artery (pediatric patients) [185]	1,649	Age <1 yr	—
		Dwell time = 3 days	—
		Inotropic support	—
Peripheral, central venous, arterial [186]	353	Distant focus of infection	8.7
		Inappropriate catheter care	5.3
		Prolonged hospitalization >14 days	3.5
Peripheral, central venous, arterial (burn patients) [144]	101	Insertion site colonization at catheter removal	6.2
Peripheral, central venous, pulmonary artery, arterial [174]	623	Duration of catheterization 7–14 days	3.9
		Duration of catheterization >14 days	5.1

(CONTINUED)

Type of Catheter [ref.]	No. Catheters Studied	Risk Factors	Relative Risk
		Coronary care unit	6.7
		Surgery service	4.4
		Second catheterization	7.6
		Insertion site colonization	56.6
		Hub colonization	17.9
Hickman [187]	690	Double-lumen catheter	2.1
		Obesity	1.7
		Granulocytopenia	1.6
Implantable port [188]	1,550	Increased number of line breaks/day	—

cfu, colony-forming units.

BLOODSTREAM INFECTION FROM CONTAMINATED INFUSATE

It took >10 years after the introduction of intravascular plastic catheters before they were ultimately recognized as an important source of serious iatrogenic infection; however, it required >40 years and the occurrence of epidemic gram-negative BSIs in hospitals across the United States in 1970 and 1971 [21] to bring about awareness that fluid given in intravascular infusions—infusate—also was vulnerable to contamination. It has become clear that although the majority of IVDR-BSIs derive from infection of the percutaneous infection wound or contamination of the catheter hub, contamination of infusate is the most common cause of epidemic IVDR-BSI [1]. From 1965 to 1978, 28/30 (85%) reported epidemics of infusion-related

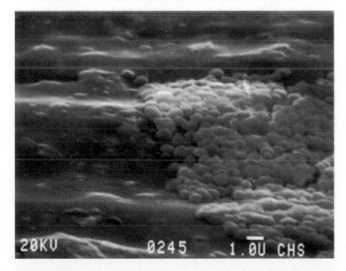

Figure 37-2 Scanning electron micrograph of an infected central venous catheter (x6,000). The amorphous matrix encasing the microcolonies of *Staphylococcus epidermidis* is glycocalyx (slime).

BSI were traced to contaminated infusate, with the organisms introduced during its manufacture (intrinsic contamination, which accounted for 7/20 epidemics) or during its preparation and administration in the hospital (extrinsic contamination, which accounted for the remaining 21 outbreaks) [1,2].

Growth Properties of Microorganisms in Parenteral Fluids

The pathogens implicated in nearly all reported BSIs linked to contaminated infusate have been aerobic gram-negative bacilli capable of rapid growth at room temperature (25°C) in the solution involved [76]: for example, certain members of the family Enterobacteriaceae in 5% dextrose-in-water, and pseudomonads or *Serratia* spp. in distilled water. It must be emphasized that microbial growth in most parenteral solutions—the exception being lipid emulsion—actually is quite limited.

In 1970, we evaluated the ability of 105 clinical isolates from human HAIs, representing 9 genera and 13 species, to grow at room temperature (25°C) in 5% dextrose-in-water, the most frequently used commercial parenteral solution [217]. Of 51 strains of the tribe Klebsielleae—Klebsiella, *Enterobacter*, and *Serratia* spp.— 50 attained concentrations of ≥100,000 cfu/ml within 24 hours, beginning with washed organisms at an initial concentration of 1 cfu/ml. In contrast, only 1/54 strains of other bacteria, including staphylococci, *Escherichia coli*, *P aeruginosa*, *Acinetobacter spp.*, or *Candida* spp., showed any growth in 5% dextrose-in-water. With most microorganisms, even with a level of contamination exceeding 10^6 cfu/ml of fluid, evidence of microbial growth was not visible to the unaided eye.

Review of studies of the growth properties of microorganisms in various commercial parenteral products has shown [76] that rapid multiplication in 5% dextrose-in-water appears limited mainly to the tribe Klebsielleae and *B. cepacia*; in distilled water, *P. aeruginosa, B. cepacia, Acinetobacter spp.,* or *Serratia spp.*; and in lactated Ringer's solution, *P. aeruginosa, Enterobacter,* or *Serratia* spp. Normal (0.9%) sodium chloride solution allows growth of most bacteria while supporting the growth of *Candida* spp. rather poorly. *Candida* spp. can grow in the synthetic amino acid–25% glucose solutions used for total parenteral nutrition (TPN), but only very slowly; most bacteria are greatly inhibited [218]. Most microorganisms grow rapidly in commercial 10% lipid emulsion for infusion (Intralipid®) [219,220]; in a study of 57 strains, we found that 12/13 bacterial species tested and *Candida* spp. multiplied in Intralipid almost as rapidly as in bacteriologic media [219]. Infections with *Malassezia furfur* also have been associated with administration of lipids [221–223]. This is not surprising because this dimorphic, lipophilic yeast cannot synthesize medium- and long-chain fatty acids and uses exogenous lipids, such as those found in supplemented TPN, for growth [220]. Use of TPN supplemented with lipids also has been shown to significantly increase the BSI risk by coagulase-negative staphylococci [224,225]. Epidemics also have been reported due to extrinsic contamination of a lipid-based anesthetic, propofol (Diprivan; Stuart Pharmaceuticals, Wilmington, Delaware, U.S.A.) [36]. This anesthetic agent, which initially did not contain a bacteriostatic agent, supported the exuberant growth of several gram-negative, gram-positive bacteria and *Candida albicans* [226].

The growth properties of most microorganisms in commercial parenteral admixtures and the vast aggregate experience with epidemic or endemic BSIs traced to contaminated infusate have shown that the identity of an organism causing nosocomial BSI can point strongly toward contaminated fluid as the plausible source: *P. agglomerans, E. cloacae, Serratia marcescens, B. cepacia,* or *Citrobacter* spp. cultured from the blood of a patient receiving infusion therapy should prompt strong suspicion of contaminated infusate—parenteral fluid or an IV drug (Table 37-6). Conversely, recovery of organisms, such as *E. coli, Proteus, Acinetobacter,* or staphylococci, all of which grow poorly if at all in parenteral admixtures, suggests strongly that the BSI is unlikely to be due to contaminated infusate.

Mechanisms of Fluid Contamination

As noted, the vast majority of published nosocomial BSIs traced to contaminated infusate occurred in an epidemic setting [1,2]. Parenteral fluids do, however, commonly become contaminated during administration in the hospital. Culture surveys of in-use IV fluids in the hospital have shown contamination rates in the range of 1% to 2% [227–229]. However, most of the organisms recovered from positive in-use cultures are common skin commensals that are generally considered of low virulence and grow poorly, if at all, in the parenteral admixture;

the level of contamination (<10 cfu/ml) usually is far too low to produce clinical illness, even in the most compromised host. When contamination occurs with gram-negative bacilli capable of proliferation in the product to concentrations >10^2 to 10^3 cfu/ml, however, the risk of BSI and even septic shock becomes substantial.

The likelihood of fluid becoming contaminated during use is directly related to the duration of uninterrupted infusion through the same administration set and the frequency with which the set is manipulated. Microorganisms gain access from air entering bottles as they evacuate, from entry points into the administration set—during injections into the line or aspiration of blood specimens from the IVD through the line—or at the junction between the administration set and the catheter hub. Microorganisms capable of growth in fluid, once introduced into a running infusion, may persist in an administration set for many days despite multiple replacements of the bottle or bag and high rates of flow [21]; it appears more likely, however, that the majority of introduced contaminants are rapidly cleared from the running infusion by the continuous flow [227–230], especially if the organisms grow poorly in the fluid.

A healthcare worker may rarely encounter a filmy cloud in a glass IV bottle. Microscopic examination of the material reveals it is a filamentous fungus, such as *Penicillium* or *Aspergillus* spp. Molds usually gain access to glass IV bottles through microscopic cracks long before the bottle is hung for use, and over the course of weeks or months grow to produce visible cloudiness or filmy precipitates. Fortunately, "fungus balls" in IV bottles have rarely resulted in systemic infection in patients receiving a mold-contaminated infusion [233].

The incidence of endemic nosocomial BSI caused by extrinsically contaminated IV fluid is not precisely known, but based on studies of the pathogenesis of device-related infection, is 5- to 10-fold lower than the incidence of endemic cannula-related BSI. Moreover, prospective studies of the optimal interval for periodic replacement of administration sets [227–233] (Table 37-9), which have involved cultures of infusate from large numbers of in-use infusions in an institution, have shown low rates of contamination and a very low risk of related BSI: meta-analysis of five studies in which >9,000 infusions in 5 hospitals were prospectively cultured, with no associated episodes of bacteremia or candidemia identified, yields an incidence of endemic BSI due to contaminated infusate of <1 episode per 2,000 IV infusions. It must be emphasized, however, that IV infusate can be identified as the source of BSI only if it is cultured. Because this rarely occurs in most hospitals, unless there is a cluster of BSIs—an epidemic—occurs, it is likely that most sporadic (endemic) BSIs caused by contaminated fluid go unrecognized or are attributed to the IVD.

Approximately 50% of the BSIs caused by arterial infusions used for hemodynamic monitoring stem from contamination of fluid in the infusion [31], perhaps because

TABLE 37-9

STUDIES OF REPLACING INTRAVENOUS ADMINISTRATION SETS AT PERIODIC INTERVALS AS AN INFECTION CONTROL MEASURE

Reference	Location of Patients	Types of Infusion	No. of Sets Cultured	Prevalence of Contamination in Sets Changed at Intervals			
				24 Hr	48 Hr	72 Hr	Indefinite
[229]	Ward	Mainly peripheral[a]	2,537	0.4	0.6	—	—
[231]	Ward, ICU	Peripheral	694	0.5	1.0	0.7	—
		Central, access[a,b] plus TPN	119	0	0	0	—
[232]	ICU	Peripheral (62%) plus central, access (38%)[a]	676	2.0	4.0		
[230]	Ward	Peripheral	219	—	0.8	—	0.8
[227]	ICU	Peripheral, plus central, access[a]	1,194	—	5.0	4.4	—
[228]	Ward, ICU	Peripheral	878	—	0.2	1.0	—
		Central, access	331	—	1.9	1.2	—
		Central, TPN	165	—	2.7	4.4	—
	Ward	All types	1,168	—	0.5	1.4	—
	ICU	All types	204	—	3.2	1.8	

ICU, intensive care unit; TPN, total parenteral nutrition.

[a]Infusions for TPN excluded; contamination rates with different types of infusions not given.

[b]"Access" refers to a central venous infusion used for administering fluids, blood products, delivery of drugs, or hemodynamic monitoring, but not TPN.

Source: From Maki DG, Botticelli JT, LeRoy ML, Thielke TS. Prospective study of replacing administration sets for intravenous therapy at 48- vs 72-hour intervals: 72 hours is safe and cost effective. JAMA 1987;258:1777–1781.

these infusions consist of a stagnant column of fluid subjected to frequent manipulations, including frequent drawing of blood specimens. However, more recent studies have demonstrated that infusate contamination of hemodynamic pressure monitoring equipment is rare [234]. Over the past 20 years, there have been 28 epidemics of nosocomial BSI traced to contaminated fluid in arterial infusions used for hemodynamic monitoring [235–238]. Nearly all of these epidemics have involved gram-negative bacilli, particularly S. marcescens, pseudomonads, or Enterobacter spp. that are able to multiply rapidly in the 0.9% saline commonly used in these infusions.

Endemic BSIs resulting from transfusion of contaminated blood products have been rare, presumably because most blood products are routinely refrigerated, because contamination is low level, and because of universal awareness that blood products must be used promptly after removal from refrigeration [79,239]. BSI from contaminated whole blood is associated with adverse reactions in 50% of episodes, including fever (80%), rigors (53%), hypotension (37%), and nausea or vomiting (26%), with an associated mortality of 35% [79]. Overwhelming shock usually is due to contamination with massive numbers of psychrophilic (cold-growing) organisms such as Serratia spp., B. cepacia, S. maltophilia, Yersinia spp.,or other uncommon, nonfermentative gram-negative bacilli, e.g.,Flavobacterium species, in the contaminated unit [79–81,241]. Bacteria often have been visible on a direct Gram-stained smear of the product. Blood products should be infused immediately after they are removed from refrigeration. On completion of the transfusion, the entire delivery system should be replaced. If BSI is suspected of being related to a contaminated blood product, the entire infusion should be removed. Aliquots of the remaining product should be cultured aerobically and anaerobically on solid media at both $35°–37°C$ and $16°–20°C$ [76]. Platelet units may be stored at room temperature for 5 days before use and may be more prone to contamination with large numbers of microbial pathogens. As many as 10% of platelet pools used for transfusion are contaminated with bacteria [239]. Although most contaminants are skin flora [242], contamination with gram-negative bacilli has been reported [79,80].

The most important measures to prevent rare sporadic BSIs from contaminated in-use infusate are stringent asepsis during the preparation and compounding of admixtures in the hospital central pharmacy or on individual patient-care units, and good aseptic technique when infusions are handled during use, e.g., during injections of medications or changing bags or bottles of fluids. It also appears that replacing the administration set at periodic intervals can prevent the build-up of dangerous introduced contaminants and further reduce the risk of related BSI; during the large, nationwide U.S. epidemic in 1971 due to the contaminated products of one manufacturer, the empiric recommendations that the entire delivery system be routinely changed every 24 hours and that at every change of the cannula all equipment be totally replaced resulted in a substantial reduction in epidemic BSIs [21]. Since that time, routinely replacing the delivery system at periodic intervals has been practiced in most North American hospitals as an important measure for reducing the hazard of contaminated infusate. However, in some instances, routine replacement at more prolonged intervals may be associated with epidemics, particularly in vulnerable patient populations and when the fluids infused promote microbial growth [243].

EPIDEMIC INFUSION-RELATED BLOODSTREAM INFECTIONS

Outbreaks Due to Intrinsic Contamination

Since 1970, there have been >12 reported epidemics of infusion-related BSI caused by intrinsically contaminated infusate—blood products, IV drugs, or vacutainer tubes (Table 37-10)—illustrating the potential iatrogenic hazards of infusion therapy. The frequency and size of these outbreaks have declined since the late 1980s [2], reflecting appreciation of the importance of stringent quality control during the manufacturing process.

The first and largest epidemic—and the outbreak that more than any other factor brought about wide-scale appreciation of the iatrogenic hazards of infusion therapy—had its onset several years ago when one U.S. manufacturer of large-volume parenterals began to distribute bottles of fluid with a new elastomer-lined screw cap closure [21]. By early 1970, the first episodes of infusion-related BSI caused by biologically characteristic strains of *E. cloacae* and *P. agglomerans* (designated *Erwinia* at the time) were reported to the CDC, although retrospective review subsequently showed that numerous hospitals had been experiencing epidemic BSIs for a number of months. Although it was established very early, virtually at the outset of the investigation, that epidemic BSIs resulted from contaminated IV fluids, the ultimate source of contamination—*intrinsic* contamination of the new closures—was not conclusively established until March, 1971. Between July 1970 and April 1971, 25 U.S. hospitals reported nearly ~400 episodes of infusion-related BSI to the CDC (Fig. 37-3). It is likely that there were >10,000 episodes nationwide. More than 20 microbial species, including *P. agglomerans*, were isolated from the closures of previously unopened bottles. Organisms were readily dislodged from the cap liner and introduced into IV fluid when bottles were handled under conditions duplicating normal in-hospital use. The appearance of epidemic BSIs in individual hospitals paralleled the distribution of the company's product with the new closures, and the epidemic was terminated only by a nationwide product recall in early April 1971.

Since 1975, numerous additional outbreaks have been reported from hospitals in a number of countries, all

REPORTED SOURCES OF EPIDEMICS OF INTRAVASCULAR DEVICE-RELATED BLOODSTREAM INFECTION

Extrinsic contamination
Antiseptics or disinfectants
Arterial pressure monitoring infusate
Disinfectants
Transducers
Heparin
Ice for chilling blood gas syringes
Aneroid pressure calibration device
Hand carriage by medical personnel
Hemodialysis related
Inadequate decontamination of reused dialyzer coils
Contaminated dialysate water
Contaminated disinfectants
Parenteral crystalloid solutions
Lipid emulsion
Hyperalimentation solutions in central pharmacy
IV medications, multidose vials
Theft of fentanyl and replacement by (contaminated) distilled water
Blood products
Whole blood
Platelet packs
Blood donor with silent transient bacteremia
Intravenous radiologic contrast media
Sclerosing solution for injecting esophageal varices
Central venous catheter hubs
Leaking catheter hub administration set connections
Adhesive tape used in IV site dressings
Warming bath for blood products
Green soap
Hand carriage by medical personnel
Heart–lung machines
Intraaortic balloon pumps
Inordinately prolonged intravascular catheterization in intensive care unit patients
Intrinsic (manufacturer-related) contamination
Commercial IV crystalloid solutions, container closures
Blood products
Platelet packs
Human albumin
Plasma protein fraction (PPF)
IV drugs
Vacutainer' tubes

IV, intravenous.

involving gram-negative bacilli and parenteral products shown to have been contaminated during manufacture [76, 77,244–256]. Most have been of national scope. A large outbreak in Greece in 1981 [245] reaffirmed the findings of the large 1970 to 1971 U.S. outbreak [21] that screw-cap closures are not microbiologically safe for fluids used in medical care that must remain sterile. Outbreaks of pyrogenic reactions [248] and epidemic *Pseudomonas* spp. BSI [249] have been traced to intrinsically contaminated normal serum albumin, and an epidemic of BSI with

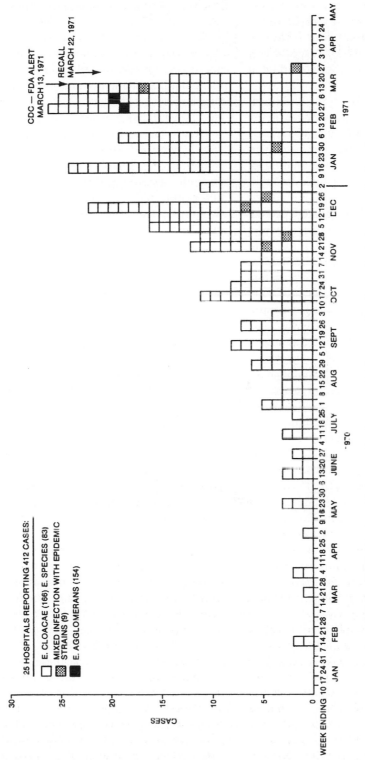

Figure 37-3 Nationwide outbreak of nosocomial bacteremias due to intrinsic contamination of one U.S. manufacturer's large-volume parenteral products. Three hundred ninety-seven cases of IV-associated bloodstream infection in 25 tabulated U.S. hospitals, occurring between July 1, 1970, and April 27, 1971, fulfilled criteria for epidemic cases. The epidemic was curtailed immediately in individual hospitals and nationally by a nationwide recall of the manufacturer's products. (From Maki DG, Rhame FS, Mackel D, Bennett JV. Nationwide epidemic of bloodstream infection caused by contaminated intravenous products. *Am J Med* 1976;60:47–485, with permission.)

Ochrobactrum anthropi has been traced to organisms from contaminated rabbit antithymocyte globulin [250]. Most notably, during the past decade outbreaks of *Pseudomonas* spp. infection have been traced to intrinsic contamination of 10% povidone–iodine [251], an agent widely used worldwide for cutaneous antiseptic for preparation of the CVC insertion site [252]. Dilute chlorhexidine solution, which is increasingly being used for skin antisepsis, [32, 151–153], may support the growth of bacteria, leading to epidemic BSI [148].

All of these outbreaks illustrate how subtle and insidious the factors that influence sterility can be. In many instances, there was no documented failure of the sterilization process. Instead, seemingly minor alterations in the manufacturing process resulted in contamination of individual units in the manufacturing plant after the sterilization stage [253].

Although intrinsic contamination is, fortunately, exceedingly rare, its potential for producing harm is great because of the large numbers of patients in multiple hospitals who may be affected. Also, direct contamination of infusate at the manufacturing level gives contaminants an opportunity to proliferate to dangerously high concentrations.

It seems likely that intrinsic contamination is a continuous source of infusion-related BSI, but of such low magnitude that the resulting BSIs are never identified as related to intrinsic contamination. Only when infusion-associated BSIs occur in epidemic numbers is intrinsic contamination likely to be suspected and proven. A substantial increase in the incidence of cryptogenic infusion-associated BSI, particularly with *Enterobacter* spp., pseudomonads, *Burkholderia* spp., or *Citrobacter* spp., should prompt immediate, in-depth studies to exclude intrinsic contamination. There are no clinical clues reliably to differentiate intrinsic from extrinsic contamination. BSI from contaminated fluid has the same manifestations and signs as CR-BSI and other nosocomial BSIs. The few clues to infusion-related BSI—absence of an obvious source of infection, its common occurrence in patients without a predilection to systemic infection, and the dramatic clinical response to discontinuing the infusion (Table 37-3)—do not differentiate between intrinsic and extrinsic sources of contamination. The distinction must be made epidemiologically.

If intrinsic contamination of a commercially distributed product is identified, or even strongly suspected, especially if clinical infections have occurred as a consequence, the local, state, and Federal (CDC and the Food and Drug Administration (FDA)) public health authorities must be immediately contacted. Unopened samples of the suspect lot or lots should be quarantined and saved for analysis.

Outbreaks Due to Extrinsic Contamination

Even when commercially manufactured products are sterile on arrival in the hospital, circumstances of hospital use can compromise that initial sterility. As previously noted, most sporadic infections resulting from infusion therapy, whether due to the cannula or contaminated infusate, are of extrinsic origin. Similarly, most reported epidemics have originated from exposure of multiple patients' infusions to a common source of contamination in the hospital [2,36,235,254–258].

Numerous outbreaks of infusion-related BSI have been caused by use of unreliable chemical antiseptics, or antiseptics such as aqueous benzalkonium and aqueous chlorhexidine used for cutaneous antisepsis [145–148] or, in more recent years, for decontaminating transducer components used in hemodynamic monitoring [235] (Table 37-10).

Despite the numerous reports of epidemic gram-negative BSIs deriving from contaminated disinfectants used for decontaminating reusable transducer components in hemodynamic monitoring during the 1970s, one third of all nosocomial BSI outbreaks investigated by the CDC between 1977 and 1987 were traced to contamination of infusions used for arterial pressure monitoring [256]. Since 1980, there have been 28 nosocomial BSI outbreaks associated with arterial pressure monitoring reported in the literature, nearly all caused by gram-negative bacilli, most frequently *S. marcescens* or *Burkholderia* spp. [235–238]. Two thirds of these epidemics were linked to failed decontamination of reusable transducer components. Epidemic organisms were most commonly found on metal transducer heads, in the interface between transducers and disposable chamber domes. Eight epidemics were traced to introduction of organisms into closed monitoring systems from external sources of contamination in the hospital, such as contaminated ice used to chill syringes for drawing arterialized blood for blood gas measurements, heparinized saline from multidose vials, and contaminated external devices to calibrate pressure-monitoring systems. The epidemic organisms were found on the hands of healthcare providers in at least nine outbreaks; however, most of the reports do not provide sufficient data to establish the precise mechanism of fluid contamination.

With all forms of infusion therapy, the connection between the administration set and the catheter must be secure. This is especially important with CVCs, where accidental disconnections can result in exsanguination or life-threatening air embolus or blood loss. In TPN, a faulty connection also may increase the risk of iatrogenic infection: one reported outbreak of 23 CR-BSIs caused by different strains of coagulase-negative staphylococci was linked to a manufacturing defect that resulted in hyperalimentation solution leaking from administration set–catheter connections and seeping under dressings, where it resulted in heavy bacterial overgrowth [259]. Another outbreak of coagulase-negative staphylococcal BSIs has been associated with excessive manipulation of a catheter delivery system because of air appearing in the IV pump tubing. This resolved when the IV pump was placed at or below the heart level of the patients and air entry into the tubing ceased [260].

During the 1970s, numerous outbreaks of gram-negative BSI, particularly with pseudomonads other than *P. aeruginosa*, were traced to contamination of dialysate in patients' hemodialysis machines [261] (see Chapter 24); however, improved quality control, the decontamination of reused dialyzer coils, and the widespread use of disposable dialyzers have resulted in a marked decline in the incidence of HAI outbreaks traced to contaminated dialysate [2].

Compounding of admixtures is another important means by which contamination can be introduced [262]. The greatest concern about this mode of contamination, especially if it occurs in the central pharmacy, is that a large number of patients may be exposed. Moreover, the delay between compounding and use provides opportunity for proliferation of introduced microorganisms to levels that can cause overwhelming septic shock when administered. Two large outbreaks of candidemia have been traced to contaminated solutions used for IV hyperalimentation [263,264]; in each outbreak, a vacuum system in the hospital's pharmacy used to evacuate fluid from bottles before introducing other admixture components was shown to be heavily contaminated by the epidemic strain of *Candida* spp. Presumably, organisms refluxed into bottles during compounding of the admixtures. In outbreaks traced to contaminants introducing during compounding, after compounding, bottles were permitted to stand at room temperature for up to 48 hours before use. The necessity for stringent attention to a BSI in central admixture programs cannot be overemphasized. Fluid admixtures should be used within 6 hours or immediately refrigerated.

Investigations of >100 epidemics [1,2] have documented contamination of in-use infusate or contamination of cannula insertion sites, deriving from a myriad of extrinsic sources in the hospital (Table 37-10). In many outbreaks, the hospital reservoir of the epidemic pathogen and even the mode of transmission eluded detection, but the microorganism was found in large numbers on the hands of healthcare providers caring for patients receiving infusion therapy and handling their infusions. Manipulations of the delivery system, especially the administration set, appear to provide a highly effective means for access of microorganisms to in-use infusate, as illustrated by HAI outbreaks across the United States traced to in-use contamination of the IV anesthetic, propofol (Diprivan®). The solution, when initially marketed did not contain a bacteriostatic agent. The anesthetic provided a rich medium for rapid microbial proliferation [226], and outbreaks of primary BSI or SSI with a variety of gram-positive and gram-negative organisms and yeasts were traced to in-use contamination of propofol administered in the operating room, because of poor aseptic technique, storage of opened vials at room temperature, and use of single vials for multiple patients [36,264,265]. Similarly, a veritable explosion of hospital outbreaks of nosocomial candidemia in the past 2–3 decades [265–267], primarily in ICUs, has been linked to carriage of the epidemic strain on the hands

of healthcare providers handling vulnerable patients' IVDs and infusions.

Approach to an Epidemic

If an epidemic is suspected, the epidemiologic approach must be methodical and thorough, yet expeditious. It is directed toward establishing the *bona fide* nature of the putative epidemic infections [269] and existence of an epidemic, defining the reservoirs and modes of transmission of the epidemic pathogens, and, most importantly controlling the epidemic quickly and completely. Control measures obviously are predicated on accurate delineation of the epidemiology of the causative pathogen (see Chapter 6).

The essential steps in dealing with a suspected outbreak of nosocomial BSI can be found in Table 37-11. To illustrate

TABLE 37-11

EVALUATION OF A SUSPECTED EPIDEMIC OF NOSOCOMIAL BLOODSTREAM INFECTIONS

Administrative preparedness
Immediately retrieve putative epidemic blood isolates for confirmation of identity through spaces and subtyping by one or more methods:
Biotyping
Antimicrobial susceptibility pattern (antibiogram)
Serotyping
Phage typing
Bacteriocin typing
SDS-PAGE protein electrophoresis
Polymerase chain reaction
Pulsed-field gel electrophoresis
Immunoblot pattern
Multifocus enzyme electrophoresis
Restriction enzyme digestion and restriction fragment polymorphism patterns
DNA probes
Preliminary evaluations and control measures
Identify and characterize individual cases in time, place, risk factors
Strive to identify source of bloodstream infections
Ascertain if cases represent true bloodstream infections, rather than "pseudobacteremias"
Ascertain if cases represent a true epidemic, rather than a "pseudoepidemic"
Provisional control measures
Intensify surveillance, to detect every new case
Review general infection control policies and procedures
Determine need for assistance, especially extramural (local, state, Centers for Disease Control and Prevention)
Epidemiologic investigations
Clinicoepidemiologic studies, especially case–control studies
Microbiologic studies
Definitive control measures
Confirm control of epidemic by intensified follow-up surveillance
Report the findings
SDS-PAGE, sodium dodecyl sulfate–polyacrylamide gel electrophoresis.

the approach to an epidemic of infusion-related BSI, the epidemiologic investigation of an extraordinary outbreak that occurred in the University of Wisconsin Hospital and Clinics is recounted [35].

During a 2-week period in late March 1985, three patients in our university hospital acquired primary nosocomial BSI with a similar nonfermentative gram-negative bacillus. All three patients had had open heart surgery between March 11 and March 25 and became bacteremic 48–148 hours after operation.

The BSI pathogen in each patient was *B. pickettii* biovariant 1. The organism also was cultured from the IV fluid of two of the patients at the time because, serendipitously, during the outbreak most adult patients in the hospital receiving IV fluids were participating in a study of IV catheter dressings [109]; as part of the study protocol, specimens were routinely obtained from patients' IV fluid when the catheter was removed. Review of nearly 1000 cultures of IV fluid from the infusions of participants in the study since its outset 3 months earlier showed that three additional surgical patients operated on in March had had IV fluid cultures positive for *B. pickettii* biovariant 1, even though none had shown clinical signs of BSI. Molecular subtyping by restriction enzyme digestion and pulsed-field electrophoresis showed all six isolates to be identical. Three more patients who had been operated on in January had had IV fluid cultured positive for a similar nonfermentative gram-negative bacillus; although the three isolates were no longer available, the results of screening by AP-20E biochemical panel (API Analytab, Inc., Plainville, New York, U.S.A.) at the time were identical to those of the six patients with *B. pickettii* contamination of IV fluid, with or without associated BSI.

All of the patients had had multiple positive blood cultures and were in septic shock. *B. pickettii* had not been isolated from any local site of infection, such as the urinary tract, lower respiratory tract, or surgical site, in any of the patients.

Review of nosocomial BSIs over the preceding 7 years showed that *B. pickettii* had not previously been identified in blood cultures from our institution, indicating that the cluster of three episodes and six instances of contaminated infusate without BSI represented a true epidemic, and with the results of the subtyping, a common-source epidemic.

The CDC and the manufacturer were contacted: none of more than 70 NNIS hospitals had reported *B. pickettii* BSIs in the past year, and the manufacturer had never identified contamination with *B. pickettii* in its quality-control microbiologic sampling of fentanyl before distribution, or received any complaints from users about suspected contamination of their fentanyl. Moreover, survey of surrounding hospitals that also used the manufacturer's fentanyl revealed none experiencing nosocomial BSIs with *B. pickettii*.

A case–control study comparing the 9 infected patients, all of whom had had recent surgery, and 19 operated

patients who had had negative IV fluid cultures in the IV dressing study, showed that all 9 cases but only 9/19 operated controls had received fentanyl intravenously in the operating room ($p = 0.05$); the mean total dose given to the 9 case-patients was far greater than that given to control-patients who received the drug (3,080 vs. 840 µg, $p < 0.001$).

At the time, fentanyl was used at the University of Wisconsin Hospital only in the operating rooms (ORs) as part of balanced anesthesia. The drug was received in 20-ml ampules from the manufacturer and each week, one of three pharmacy technicians, by rotation, pre-drew into sterile syringes all fentanyl likely to be needed the following week in the operating rooms. Each day, one of the technicians delivered enough pre-drawn syringes to the ORs to meet the needs of the patients being operated on that day. Cultures of pre-drawn fentanyl in syringes in the central pharmacy, prompted by the findings of the case–control study, showed that 20/50 (40%) 30-ml syringes sampled were contaminated by *B. pickettii* in a concentration $>10^4$ cfu/ml; none of 35 5-ml or 2-ml syringes showed contamination ($p < 0.001$).

Extensive culturing in the central pharmacy was negative for evidence of environmental contamination by *B. pickettii*, with one exception: *B. pickettii* biovariant 1, with an identical antimicrobial susceptibility pattern and restriction enzyme fragment pattern to the epidemic strain recovered from blood cultures or patients' IV infusions, was cultured in a concentration of 28–80 cfu/ml from five specimens of distilled water drawn from a tap in the central pharmacy. The epidemic strain was shown to multiply well in the fentanyl solution, attaining concentrations $>10^4$ cfu/ml within 48 hours.

A second case–control study strongly suggested that the epidemic was caused by theft of fentanyl from 30-ml syringes by a pharmacy staff member and replacement with distilled water that the individual thought was sterile, but that, unfortunately, was contaminated by *B. pickettii*. The pharmacy member resigned early in the investigation. On April 29, the hospital's system for providing fentanyl and other narcotics to the ORs was changed; narcotics were no longer pre-drawn into syringes in the central pharmacy, but were delivered to the ORs in unopened vials or ampules; anesthesiologists' orders for narcotics are filled by a staff pharmacist assigned to the OR. There have been no further *B. pickettii* BSIs since March 25, 1985, and cultures of >6,000 samples of hospitalized patients' IV fluid in research studies since that time have shown no further contamination by *B. pickettii*.

This outbreak illustrates the power of epidemiology, e.g., case–control analyses, to identify the probable cause of an epidemic. It further illustrates the potential for contamination of parenteral drugs or admixtures and the extraordinary range of epidemiologic mechanisms of nosocomial BSI deriving from such contamination.

STRATEGIES FOR PREVENTION

Extensive guidelines for prevention of catheter-related infection have been published [12]. Specific interventions are discussed in the following sections.

Aseptic Technique

To accord it due respect, any device for vascular access must be thought of in fundamental terms as a direct conduit between the external world, with its myriad of microorganisms, and the bloodstream of the patient. Vigorous hand hygiene, ideally with an antiseptic-containing preparation, and gloving always must precede the insertion of a peripheral IV cannula and also should precede later handling of the device or the administration set [270]. Furthermore, sterile gloves should be routinely used during the insertion of peripheral IV cannulas in high-risk patients, such as those with severe burns. Sterile gloves are strongly recommended for placement of all other types of IVDs—arterial and all CVCs—which are associated with a higher risk of associated BSI [12].

Although there has been considerable controversy as to the level of barrier precautions necessary during insertion of a CVC, in a study of Swan-Ganz pulmonary artery catheters, the use of maximal barrier precautions—sterile gloves, a long-sleeved sterile surgical gown, a surgical mask, and a large, sterile sheet drape covering the patient, as contrasted to the use of sterile gloves, a surgical mask, and a small, fenestrated drape—was associated with a twofold lower risk of infection [175]. Despite the fact that Swan-Ganz catheters inserted in the ICU using maximal barrier precautions remained in place an average of 22 hours longer than catheters inserted in the OR (inserted with lesser barrier precautions), were more frequently placed in infected patients, and were used more frequently for TPN, catheters inserted in the ICU using maximal barrier precautions were much less likely to be contaminated under the external protective sheath or infected than catheters inserted in the OR by anesthesiologists using lesser barrier precautions. The efficacy of maximal barrier precautions in the prevention of nontunneled CVC-related infection has been demonstrated [271,272]. In this study, the incidence of CR-BSI was 6.3 times higher in those patients who were prospectively randomized to have their catheters inserted with only sterile gloves and small sterile drapes, compared with those patients whose catheters were inserted with maximal barrier precautions (mask, cap, sterile gloves, gown, and large, sterile drape) [272]. In another study, use of maximal barrier precautions with CVC insertion, in addition to a mandatory 5-minute scrub of the insertion site, reduced the incidence catheter colonization from 36% to 17% [273]. Considering that of all IVDs, CVCs are most likely to produce nosocomial BSI, a strong case can be made for mandating maximal barrier precautions during the insertion of such devices, particularly the use of a long-sleeved surgical gown and large, sterile sheet drape, to minimize touch contamination, in addition to sterile gloves, the use of which should be routine [12,272].

Inappropriate catheter care is an independent risk factor for catheter-related infections [186]. Not surprisingly, the use of special IV therapy teams, consisting of trained nurses or technicians to ensure a high level of aseptic technique during catheter insertion and in follow-up care of the catheter, has been associated with substantially lower rates of catheter-related infection [108,273–282] (Table 37-12). Such teams are highly cost effective, reducing the costs of complications of infusion therapy nearly 10-fold [281,282].

In the absence of a dedicated IV team, some investigators have carried out intensive educational programs in catheter care. In one study, this led to improved care overall and a concomitant reduction of colonization of the catheter insertion site; however, the incidence of catheter hub colonization was unchanged [283]. In some U.S. hospitals, all CVCs, particularly those dedicated to TPN, are cared for by such teams. Other investigators also have shown that institutions can greatly reduce their CR-BSI rate by scrutiny of catheter care protocols and more intensive education and training of nurses and physicians [284]. The importance of adequate staffing of nurses to care for patients with CVCs has recently been demonstrated [286]. After controlling for other risk factors associated with catheter-related infection in a logistic regression model, as the patient-to-nurse ratio doubled due to nurse understaffing in an ICU, the risk of CVC-BSI increased dramatically (OR 62). This seminal observation suggests that in this era of fiscal restraint in healthcare, cost-cutting measures which lead to understaffing of personnel aimed at caring for IVDs will ultimately increase cost and increase the risk of HAIs in today's hospitalized patients.

Cutaneous Antisepsis

Given the evidence for the important role of cutaneous microorganisms in the genesis of many IVDR-infections, measures to reduce cutaneous colonization of the insertion site would seem of the highest priority, particularly the use of chemical antiseptics of the site. Worldwide, an iodophor such as 10% povidone–iodine commonly is used [252]. The lack of published comparative trials of cutaneous antiseptics to prevent catheter-related infection prompted the following prospective investigation: 668 patients' central venous and arterial catheters in a surgical ICU were randomized to 10% povidone–iodine, 70% alcohol, or 2% aqueous chlorhexidine with alcohol for antisepsis of the site before insertion and site care every other day thereafter [32]. Chlorhexidine was associated with the lowest incidence of infection; of the 14 infusion-related BSIs, 1 was in the chlorhexidine group and 13 were in the other two groups (odds ratio, 0.16; $p = 0.04$) (Table 37-13). This study suggests that the use

TABLE 37-12

IMPACT OF A DEDICATED IV TEAM ON THE RATE OF CATHETER-RELATED BLOODSTREAM INFECTION

Type of Study [Reference]	Type of Catheter	Care Given By	No. Catheters	Incidence IV-related Bloodstream Infection (per 100 Catheters)	p-value
		Concurrent but not randomized			
[274]	PIV	House officers	4,270	0.40	
		IV team	470	0.04	<0.001
[275]	CVC-TPN	Ward nurses	33	21.2[a]	
		IV nurses	78	2.3	<0.001
[276]	CVC-TPN	Ward nurses	391	26.2	
		IV team	284	1.3	<0.001
[277]	CVC-TPN	Ward nurses	179	24.0	
		IV team	377	3.5	<0.001
[278]	CVC-TPN	House officers	45	28.8	
		IV nurses	30	3.3	<0.001
		Historical controls			
[279]	CVC-TPN	Ward nurses	335	28.6	
		IV team	172	4.7	<0.001
[280]	CVC-TPN	Ward nurses	51	33.0	
		IV nurses	48	4.0	<0.001
[281][a]	PIV and CVC	House officers	—	—	0.001
		IV team	—	—	
		Randomized, concurrent controls			
[108]	PIV	House officers	427	2.1	
		IV team	433	0.2	<0.05
[282]	PIV	House officers	453	1.5	
		IV team	412	0.0	<0.02

IV, intravenous; PIV, peripheral IV catheter; CVC, central venous catheter; TPN, total parenteral nutrition.
[a]Catheter-related bacteremia with house officers (4.5/1,000 patient discharges) vs. with IV team (1.7/1,000 patient discharges).

TABLE 37-13

RESULTS OF A PROSPECTIVE, RANDOMIZED TRIAL OF THREE CUTANEOUS ANTISEPTICS FOR PREVENTION OF INTRAVASCULAR DEVICE-RELATED BLOODSTREAM INFECTION

Source of Bloodstream Infection	10% Povidone–iodine (n = 227)	70% Alcohol (n = 227)	2% Chlorhexidine (n = 214)
Catheter related	6	3	1
From contaminated:			
Infusate		3	
Hub	1		
All sources (%)	7 (3.1)	6 (2.6)	1 (0.5)[a]

[a]Compared with the other two groups combined, odds ratio, 0.16, p = 0.04.
Source: From Maki DG, Alvarado CJ, Ringer M. A prospective, randomized trial of povidone–iodine, alcohol and chlorhexidine for prevention of infection with central venous and arterial catheters. *Lancet* 1991;338:339–343.

of 2% chlorhexidine, rather than 10% povidone–iodine or 70% alcohol, for cutaneous antispesis before insertion of an IVD and in post-insertion site care can substantially reduce the incidence of IVD-related infection. Other investigators also have found that use of aqueous chlorhexidine to prepare the catheter insertion site is associated with a lower incidence of catheter-related infection compared with povidone–iodine [151–153].

In a historical analysis of the impact on the incidence of CR-BSI of using different antiseptics for site care and disinfection of tubing connections in a home TPN program, 0.58 episodes per catheter-year were observed during use of 10% povidone–iodine as contrasted to 0.26 to 0.28 episodes per catheter-year during use of a 0.5% to 2% tincture of iodine or 0.5% tincture of chlorhexidine [287]. Prospective, randomized studies comparing the blood culture contamination rate using povidone–iodine vs. iodine tincture to prepare the puncture site, use of iodine tincture was associated with a contamination rate one-half that of the povidone–iodine group [288].

"Defatting" the skin with acetone is still widely practiced in many centers as an adjunctive measure for disinfecting CVC sites, especially in TPN; however, it was found to be of no benefit whatsoever in a prospective, randomized trial [114]. In contrast, the use of acetone was associated with greatly increased inflammation and discomfort to the patient.

Topical Antimicrobial Ointments

In theory, application of topical antimicrobial agents to the catheter insertion site should confer some protection against microbial invasion. Clinical trials of topical polyantibiotic ointments (polymyxin, neomycin, and bacitracin) on peripheral venous catheters have shown only moderate or no benefit [154,290], and the use of polyantibiotic ointments has been associated with an increased frequency of *Candida* spp. infections [116,154]. In prospective, randomized trials, application of the topical antibacterial, mupirocin, which is active primarily against gram-positive organisms, to catheter insertion sites has been associated with a significant reduction in CVC colonization, but not arterial or peripheral catheter colonization. Without colonization by *Candida* spp., the impact on CR-BSI could not be assessed [291]. However, widespread use of mupirocin at catheter insertion sites may lead to resistance [292], and for this reason it is not recommended for routine application to the CVC insertion site.

There have been two prospective studies of topical povidone–iodine ointment applied to CVC sites; one large, randomized trial in a surgical ICU showed no benefit [293], but a more recent comparative trial with subclavian hemodialysis catheters showed a fourfold reduction in the incidence of hemodialysis CR-BSI [122].

Dressings

The importance of the cutaneous microflora in the pathogenesis of IVDR infection might suggest that the dressing applied to the catheter insertion site could have considerable influence on the incidence of catheter-related infection. When used on vascular catheters, transparent dressings permit continuous inspection of the site, secure the device reliably, and are generally more comfortable than gauze and tape. Moreover, transparent dressings permit patients to bathe and shower without saturating the dressing. Clinical trials of these dressings have been prompted by the knowledge that cutaneous occlusion with tape or impervious plastic films results in an explosive increase in cutaneous microflora, with overgrowth of gram-negative bacilli and yeasts [293]. Although polyurethane dressings are semipermeable—impervious to extrinsic microbial contaminants and liquid-phase moisture, and variably permeable to oxygen, carbon dioxide, and water vapor—and studies in healthy volunteers have shown little effect of these dressings on the cutaneous flora [294], a meta-analysis has raised concern that these dressings could increase cutaneous colonization and the risk of catheter-related infection [295].

Transparent polyurethane dressings are more expensive than gauze and tape, and to obviate the issue of greater cost and to increase convenience, many users leave transparent dressings on for prolonged periods, for up to 7 days or even longer. It has been questioned whether transparent dressings left on for prolonged periods might increase the risk of catheter-related infection. There have been a number of trials comparing polyurethane dressings with gauze and tape on peripheral venous catheters [14,15,107,109, 296–300]. Three trials [296–298] have found significantly higher rates of catheter colonization with transparent dressings left on indefinitely. Other investigators also found a higher rate in catheters dressed with a transparent dressing, but only during the summer months [107]. In additional studies, however, significant differences were found [14,15,109,299,300]. Rates of catheter colonization in all of these trials have been low with all dressings, in the range of 1.6%-8.5%. Only 3 CR-BSIs were identified among the nearly 4,000 catheters studied in all of the reported trials.

In a prospective, randomized trial of various dressings used with 2,088 Teflon peripheral IV catheters [109], the transparent polyurethane dressing studied, left on for the lifetime of the catheter, was not associated with increased cutaneous colonization under the dressing or an increased rate of catheter colonization, compared with the control gauze and tape dressing; however, there were no CR-BSIs. Cutaneous colonization was not heavier under transparent dressings during the spring and summer months, as previously described [107], perhaps because the hospital was air conditioned. Multivariate analysis showed cutaneous colonization of the insertion site (relative risk of infection, 3.9) and moisture under the dressing (relative risk, 2.5) to be significant risk factors for catheter-related infection (Table 37-8). These data indicate that it is probably not cost effective to redress peripheral IV catheters at periodic intervals, and that for most patients either sterile gauze or a transparent dressing can be used and left on until the catheter is removed [12].

Studies of transparent dressings on short-term, non-cuffed central venous and/or pulmonary artery catheters have yielded conflicting results [34,182,300–308], in part reflecting differences in study protocols (e.g., the use of topical antimicrobial ointments under the dressing in the control gauze group, but not in the transparent dressing group) and different dressings studied. One group of investigators [302] reported a threefold increase in infectious complications associated with subclavian catheters using transparent dressings for ≤7 days compared with gauze replaced three times weekly, but the difference did not achieve statistical significance. Others [182] have found a much higher rate of CR-BSI using transparent dressings compared with gauze and tape (16% vs. 0%). In a similar trial performed in an ICU, there were no significant differences in catheter-related infection with transparent dressings compared with gauze dressings when the transparent dressing was changed every 2 days [305]; however, in these high-risk ICU patients, we observed a significant build-up of skin flora, associated with a 50% increase in catheter-related infection, when transparent dressings were left on for up to 7 days between changes, suggesting that if used on CVCs in ICU patients, the dressing studied may need to be replaced more frequently. Other prospective trials, which in aggregate studied hundreds of CVCs in high-risk patients, many of whom were receiving TPN through the catheter, did not find an increased risk of catheter-related infection associated with transparent dressing left on for a prolonged duration, as compared with gauze and tape replaced more frequently [34,300,301,303,304,306–308]. In a large, prospective, randomized clinical trial, we found no difference in the incidence of catheter colonization or CR-BSI in patients whose catheters were covered with gauze and tape dressing changed every 2 days, conventional polyurethane dressing, or a polyurethane dressing with a high moisture vapor transmission rate, both replaced every 5 days [34]. However, at the time of catheter withdrawal, insertion site colonization was greater under both polyurethane dressings compared with the gauze and tape dressing group. There was no significant difference in colonization between the polyurethane dressing groups. Similarly, the incidence of CVC-BSI was no different for patients whose catheters were dressed with gauze and tape every 2 days compared with transparent dressing every 5 days in a multi-center trial however, colonization was significantly more common in the polyurethane dressing group [308].

Two randomized studies of the use of transparent dressings on surgically implanted, cuffed Hickman or Broviac catheters have been reported in which microbiologic data were provided [305,309]; in both trials, one in renal transplant patients [305] and the other in bone marrow transplant recipients [309], the transparent dressing studied provided satisfactory cover, and even when left on for prolonged periods, for up to 5–7 days, was not associated with a significantly increased risk of exit site or tunnel infection, or of CR-BSI. These studies of central venous, pulmonary artery, or long-term tunneled catheters suggest that either transparent or gauze and tape dressings can be safely used to cover the insertion site of these devices.

There have been only two reported studies of transparent polyurethane dressings with arterial catheters [15,305]. In one prospective study of dressings for arterial catheters used for hemodynamic monitoring in a surgical ICU, the use of the transparent dressing, even replaced every other day, was associated with a fivefold increased incidence of CR-BSI, compared with gauze and tape [305]. The greatly increased risk of infection associated with transparent dressings used on arterial catheters found in this study may reflect the presence of macroscopic blood in the puncture wound, under arterial pressure, which is common under transparent dressings on arterial catheters; if the blood cannot be cleared, it may provide a rich medium for microbial proliferation, which can result in infection of the catheter. As a consequence, gauze and tape is preferred to transparent dressings for arterial catheters.

Changing Catheters Over a Guidewire

The Seldinger technique, in which the vessel is identified and entered percutaneously with a fine-gauge needle and cannulated with a guidewire passed through the needle, after which the cannula is guided into the vessel over the guidewire, has been a major advance, permitting vessels to be cannulated with large catheters with much less risk of vascular injury and, in the case of subclavian or internal jugular CVCs, pneumothorax, and with less manipulation and potential for contamination. To avoid iatrogenic pneumothorax and other mechanical complications associated with percutaneous insertion of a new cannula, particularly a CVC, new catheters are commonly placed over a guidewire in the site of an old catheter [118]. Prospective, randomized clinical trials have shown that routinely replacing CVCs over guidewires is unnecessary [118,158,310]. In the largest of these studies [118], the incidence of CR-BSI per 1,000 catheter days was nearly twofold higher in patients randomized to the guidewire groups, and 75% of CR-BSIs and fungemias occurred within 72 hours of guidewire exchange or catheter insertion. In a study performed in a pediatric ICU, CVCs were left in place without routine guidewire exchange [311]. Despite prolonged catheterization, the incidence density of catheter-related infection did not increase with the duration of time the catheters were left *in situ*. Similar results were found in a study of adult oncology patients whose noncuffed, non-tunneled CVCs were left in place for a mean of 136 days [125]. These data suggest that routine guidewire exchange of CVCs is unnecessary in patients who are without unexplained fever and without induration or drainage from the catheter insertion site. In two prospective studies of central venous and Swan-Ganz pulmonary artery catheters, the incidence of catheter-related infection was not significantly different among patients whose catheters were routinely changed over guidewires or left in place [118,310]. However, the data derived from all prospective clinical trials of Swan-Ganz pulmonary artery catheters demonstrate that the incidence of BSI rises sharply on the fifth day of catheterization [48]. Because of these conflicting results, firm recommendations regarding the safe duration of Swan-Ganz pulmonary artery catheters cannot be made at this time.

One prospective study of arterial catheters found that there was a greater incidence of CR-BSIs when catheters were routinely exchanged over guidewires compared with catheters removed after 7 days and inserted into a new site [31]. Other studies have shown that the incidence density of arterial catheter-related infection did not increase with the duration of time the catheters were left in place [312,313], and in three prospective studies in which the catheters, transducers, and plasticware were not routinely changed [314–316], the incidences of catheter colonization (2.9%) and CR-BSI (0.2%) were quite low and comparable with those in other prospective studies. Therefore, these data suggest that arterial catheters, similar to CVCs, may not need to be replaced at routine intervals as long as signs of localized infection are absent and the patient is without unexplained fever. It is important to remember that all invasive devices, including intravascular catheters of any type, increase the risk of infection, and their need should be assessed on a daily basis. In one study, nearly 20% of patients on medical wards had idle catheters for ≥ 2 consecutive days, and 20% of all patient-days of IV catheter use were idle and unnecessarily increasing the risk of catheter infection in these patients [317]. In a follow-up study, intensive educational efforts reduced the incidence of idle catheters [318].

If it is considered desirable to replace a central venous or arterial catheter because it has been in place for a prolonged period and there is suspicion of infection (e.g., unexplained fever), it is not unreasonable to replace the catheter in the same site over a guidewire *if* the patient has limited sites for new access or would be at high risk for the percutaneous puncture required for placement of a new catheter in a new site (e.g., has coagulopathy or is morbidly obese). However, it is imperative that the same meticulous aseptic technique that should be mandatory during insertion of any new catheter must be employed, including the routine use of sterile gloves and a sterile drape, and for CVCs, a sterile gown as well. After vigorously cleansing the site and the old catheter with the antiseptic solution, inserting the guidewire, removing the old catheter, and cleansing the guidewire and site once more with the antiseptic solution, the operator should *reglove and redrape the site* because the original gloves and drapes are likely to be contaminated from manipulation of the old catheter. After regloving and repreparing the site, the new catheter can be inserted over the guidewire.

It also is important *routinely* to culture the old catheter after guidewire exchange and, if the patient is febrile or shows other signs of BSI, to obtain blood cultures. If these cultures demonstrate that the old catheter was colonized, the new catheter just placed in the old site should be immediately removed to prevent progression to CR-BSI (or perpetuation of ongoing CR-BSI) because the new catheter has been inserted into an infected tract. Need for continued access would mandate placement of a new catheter in a new site. If, on the other hand, culture of the old catheter is negative, it has been possible to preserve access and to examine the initial catheter microbiologically and exclude it as the cause of fever or BSI, without subjecting the patient to the hazards associated with percutaneous insertion of a new catheter.

If the old insertion site is inflamed at the outset, especially if it is purulent, or the patient shows signs of sepsis that might be originating from the catheter, or the catheter recently has been shown to be infected by quantitative blood cultures drawn through the catheter, it is strongly recommended that a new catheter not be inserted over a guidewire into an old, potentially infected site.

The Effect of Subcutaneous Tunnel Insertion of Central Venous Catheters

Subcutaneous tunnel insertion of CVCs has traditionally been carried out in an effort to reduce the risk of catheter-related infection. In a prospective, randomized study in immunocompromised patients, the incidence of CR BSI was the same in those patients whose catheters were tunneled, compared to those whose catheters were not [318]. In a randomized trial of catheters used for administering TPN [279], the incidence of catheter sepsis was reduced with tunneling of catheters before, but not after, a trained IV nurse assumed complete responsibility for catheter care. In a more recent, prospective, randomized study, tunneling CVCs inserted into the internal jugular vein dramatically reduced the incidence of CR-BSI (RR 0.19 [320]). However, this may be difficult to extrapolate to the U.S. experience, since most tunneled catheters in the United States are inserted in the subclavian, rather than the internal jugular vein. Also, no blood was drawn through the catheters in this study, which is common practice in the United States. This may have led to a lower incidence of hub-related BSI, further magnifying the difference in tunneled and non-tunneled catheter groups with regards to BSI. In another study [125], non-tunneled CVCs in immunocompromised patients inserted for prolonged periods of time also had a very low incidence of BSI when the catheters were cared for by specialized IV nurses. Therefore, CVCs cared for by specialized IV nurses may not need to be tunneled in an attempt to reduce the incidence of catheter-related infection. The utility of tunneled subclavian CVCs in situations without specialized IV nursing teams requires further study.

Measures Aimed at the Delivery System

Numerous studies have shown that most CR-BSIs are caused by infections contaminated infusate [1,2]; however, infusate can occasionally become contaminated and cause endemic bacteremia or fungemia [32–34,115,175]. If an infusion runs continuously for an extended period, the cumulative risk of contamination increases, and further, there is increased risk that the contaminants can grow to dangerously high concentrations that will result in BSI in the recipient of the fluid. For nearly 20 years, most U.S. hospitals routinely replaced the entire delivery system of patients' IV infusions at 24- or 48-hour intervals [1,2], to reduce the BSI risk from extrinsically contaminated fluid. Prospective studies (Table 37-9), however, now indicate that IV delivery systems do not need to be replaced more frequently than every 72 hours, including infusions used for TPN or any infusions in ICU patients [227,228,230]; extending the duration of use allows considerable cost savings to hospitals [228]. Other prospective studies have demonstrated that replacement of the IV delivery system every 96–120 hours did not increase the incidence of catheter-related infection [312,321]. It is important to remember that replacement of the IV delivery system at more prolonged intervals may predispose to epidemic BSI, particularly when the fluids infused promote microbial growth [243].

Three clinical settings might be regarded as exceptions to using 72 hours as an interval for routine set change: 1) during administration of blood products or 2) lipid emulsions, or 3) if an epidemic of infusion-related BSI is suspected. In these circumstances, it is most prudent that administration sets be changed routinely at 24- or 48-hour intervals. Minute amounts of blood buffers acidic solutions and provides organic nutrients that greatly enhance the ability of most microorganisms to grow in parenteral fluids [217]. Moreover, most hospital pathogens, including coagulase-negative staphylococci, some gram-negative bacilli, *Candida* spp., or *M. furfur*, grow rapidly in commercial lipid emulsion [219,220,225,243], and BSI outbreaks have been associated with administration of lipid emulsion [243,246,323].

Studies suggest that the infusion system, including the administration set and other delivery components, for hemodynamic monitoring may not need routine replacement as long as the catheter insertion site is without induration or discharge and the patient is without an unresolved source of fever [234,314–316].

The type of infusion pump and delivery system used may affect the incidence of catheter-related infection.

Line breaks associated with some infusion pumps and delivery systems appear to be susceptible to air entry into the tubing, leading to greater manipulation, and at one institution this was associated with an outbreak of coagulase-negative staphylococcal BSI [260]. Some systems require significantly fewer line breaks than others [324], and this may lessen the risk of catheter-related infection because an excessive number of line breaks per day has been demonstrated to be an independent risk factor for catheter-related infection [188].

Needleless IV systems have come into widespread use in an effort to reduce the risk of exposure to bloodborne pathogens. However, the risk of CR-BSI associated with use of these systems has not been systematically addressed in prospective, randomized trials. A number of studies have found that these systems may actually increase the risk of catheter-related infection [258,325–329]. A unifying problem is the inability to clean the inner components of these systems; once they become contaminated, bacteria and fungi can proliferate to large numbers, leading to intraluminal seeding of the blood [325,326]. Prospective studies are needed to determine the safety of needleless systems with regard to needlestick injury, catheter hub colonization, and BSI.

Terminal in-use membrane filters continue to be advocated as a means of reducing the hazard of contaminated infusate. However, filters must be changed at periodic intervals and can become blocked, leading to added manipulations of the system and, paradoxically, greater potential for contamination [330,331]. Some commercial in-line filters may also permit the passage of endotoxin [331,332]. The increased risk for phlebitis associated with the administration of IV antibiotics may be reduced by removing the microparticulates that are associated with compounding these drugs with 0.22 or 0.44 μm in-line filters [334]; however, not all randomized trials have shown a substantial reduction in phlebitis with the use of in-line filters [335]. Moreover, filters are expensive, and their use adds substantially to the costs of phlebitis from microparticulates. Few controlled, prospective clinical trials have been done to assess the effect of in-line filters on the incidence of serious catheter-related infections. In these studies, small numbers of patients were enrolled and the outcomes were variable [336,337]; however, studies carried out in animals suggest that with heavily contaminated infusate, in-line filters reduce mortality [337]. Large, prospective, double-blind clinical studies establishing their efficacy and cost effectiveness are needed before their routine use can be advocated, especially as a control measure for prevention of rare sporadic BSIs resulting from extrinsic contamination of infusate [12].

Innovative Technology

The development and application of novel technology holds the greatest promise for a quantum reduction in the risk of infusion-related BSI, especially infection due to the percutaneous device used for intravascular access: innovations in the design or construction of the infusion apparatus that implicitly deny access of microorganisms to the system or that prevent organisms that might gain access from proliferating to high concentrations or colonizing the implanted cannula can obviate poor aseptic technique or undue patient vulnerability.

In a burn model, silver-coated dressings reduced the tissue penetration of *P. aeruginosa* in animals and may reduce the risk of catheter-related infections [339]. Previous studies of incorporating an antiseptic, namely povidone–iodine into a transparent catheter dressing to suppress cutaneous colonization under the dressing have been disappointing [109]. However, in view of the superiority of chlorhexidine over povidone–iodine for cutaneous antisepsis of vascular catheter sites [32,151–153], incorporation of chlorhexidine into a dressing's adhesive has been prove more effective. A chlorhexidine-impregnated urethane sponge composite (Biopatch; Johnson & Johnson, Arlington, Texas, U.S.A.) has been shown significantly to reduce epidural catheter colonization, from 29% to 4% [340]. In a nonrandomized clinical trial using historical controls, use of the composite sponge reduced the incidence of CVC-BSIs from 21 to 13 per 1,000 catheter-days [341]. In two prospective, randomized studies in pediatric patients, this technology has been shown to significantly reduce skin colonization, be at least equivalent to gauze dressings in preventing CR-BSIs and to reduce local infections [342,343]. In a randomized control trial, we found that this technology in adults reduced both CR-BSIs (2.4% vs 6.1%) and local site infections (16.4% vs. 23.9%) compared to gauze dressings. [344]

A tissue–interface barrier (VitaCuff; Vitafore Corporation, San Carlos, California, U.S.A.) has been developed that incorporates aspects of the technology of Hickman and Broviac catheters; the device consists of a detachable cuff made of biodegradable collagen to which silver ion is chelated (Fig. 37-4). The cuff can be attached to CVCs immediately before insertion. After insertion, subcutaneous tissue grows into the collagenous matrix, anchoring the catheter and creating a barrier against invasive organisms from the skin. The silver ion provides an additional chemical barrier against introduced contamination, augmenting the mechanical barrier. However, this device affords protection against extraluminal, not intraluminal, migration of microbial pathogens into the bloodstream. In most prospective, randomized clinical trials of short-term CVCs, the incidence of catheter colonization and CR-BSI was reduced with use of the cuff [116,117,159] (Table 37-14). The cuff did not confer protection, however, against infection with catheters inserted over a guidewire to old sites [116]. A cost-benefit analysis shows that if an institution's rate of short-term CVC-BSI is in the range of 2%-3%, use of the cuff should prove cost effective [116]. In prospective studies of patients in whom the duration of central venous

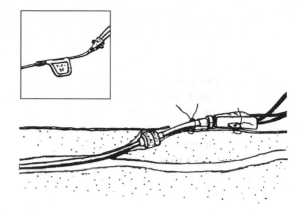

Figure 37-4 Schematic depiction of a silver-impregnated, tissue barrier cuff (VitaCuff) and the cuff attached to a central venous catheter *in situ*. It is important for the cuff to be positioned at least 0.5 to 1.0 cm below the surface of the skin and for the catheter to be well immobilized, preferably with a skin suture, to prevent extrusion. (From Maki DG, Cobb L, Garman JK, Shapiro J, Ringer M, Helgerson RB. An attachable silver-impregnated cuff for prevention of infection with central venous catheters. A prospective randomized multicenter trial. *Am J Med* 1988;85:307–314.)

catheterization was >2 weeks [161,162,346], cuff use was not found to reduce the incidence of catheter colonization or CR-BSI. This may be due to the greater importance of hub colonization as a source of catheter-related infections with more prolonged catheterization [72,150]. Therefore, use of the cuff should be considered in patients with an expected duration of catheterization of <2 weeks.

Given the multiplicity of potential sources for infection of an IVD and the importance of adherence of microorganisms to the catheter surface in the pathogenesis of infection, it would seem logical that the best strategy

TABLE 37-14

EFFICACY OF THE SILVER-IMPREGNATED CUFF (VITACUFF) CATHETER COLONIZATION IN PREVENTING CATHETER-RELATED BLOODSTREAM INFECTION (CRBSI)

Catheter Colonization (%)		CRBSI (%)		
Cuff	Control	Cuff	Control	Reference
9	29[a]	1	4	[115]
8	36[a]	0	14	[116][b]
13	28	—	—	[159][b]
15	18	5	0	[158][b]
5	5	12	14	[346][c]
—	—	36	32	[161][c]
15	20	4	4	[162][c]

[a]p <0.05.
[b]Catheterization (mean) ≤14 days.
[c]Catheterization (mean) ≥14 days.

for prevention might be to develop a catheter material implicitly resistant to colonization. It has been demonstrated that hydrophilic catheters are less likely to become colonized by bacteria in in vitro assays [347,348]. Binding a nontoxic antiseptic or antimicrobial to the catheter surface or incorporating such a substance into the catheter material itself might prove to be the most effective technologic innovation for preventing device-related infection. In a prospective, randomized clinical trial of central venous or arterial catheters in a surgical ICU, catheters coated with cefazolin bonded to the surface with a cationic surfactant were associated with a sevenfold reduction in colonization of the catheter; however, there were no CR-BSIs identified in the study population [163]. More recently, catheters coated with minocycline and rifampin have been shown significantly to reduce the incidence of catheter colonization and CR-BSIs [164]. Widespread use of these devices is also tempered by the risk of the development of resistance to these valuable antibiotics [349]. We have studied a novel CVC in which the catheter material itself, polyurethane, is impregnated with minute quantities of silver sulfadiazine and chlorhexidine (Arrowgard; Arrow International, Reading, Pennsylvania, U.S.A.); in a randomized, comparative trial in 402 patients in a surgical ICU, antiseptic catheters were twofold less likely to be colonized and fourfold less likely to produce BSI [168]. Adverse effects from the test catheter were not seen. In a prospective, randomized study, other investigators also have found that this device reduced the incidence of catheter-related infection [169]; however, with more prolonged catheterization, efficacy appears to wane [170,171] (Table 37-15). Silver-coated catheters also have been shown to reduce the incidence of catheter-related infection [165], as have catheters bound with Benzalkonium or heparin [166,167]. Strategies that hold the greatest promise are those that will change the IVD itself in a novel way that is unlikely to promote resistance to antibiotics or antiseptics. One innovative approach is to apply an electric current to the catheter [350,351]. In vitro studies with these catheters demonstrate that they inhibit the growth of bacteria and fungi [350] and are resistant to colonization, and that application of an electric current sterilizes colonized catheters [350]. In an animal model of S. aureus catheter-related infection, these catheters were more effective in preventing infection than the silver sulfadiazine-chlorhexidine-impregnated catheters [351].

Strategies aimed at reducing hub-related BSI have been devised, and in a clinical trial, a novel hub incorporating an iodine tincture reservoir reduced the incidence of BSI fourfold [352]. Recently, in an in vitro study in which we contaminated the surface of mechanical valve needleless connectors and then disinfected them with alcohol or used a chlorhexidine-impregnated cap, found that the cap was significantly more likely to eliminate contaminants than was alcohol when used for 10 seconds [353]. Although no clinical trials have been performed on the best antiseptic to use for IVD disinfection, it is clear that sufficient contact time (at least 15–30 secs of alcohol) is necessary to insure that contamants are removed.

The addition of a nontoxic, biodegradable or easily metabolized antiseptic to IV fluid or IV admixtures [354–358] might eliminate the hazard of fluid contamination altogether and, further, reduce the risk of hub contamination, obviating the need for periodic replacement of the delivery system. Use of vancomycin containing flushes or catheter/valve dwells have been shown to reduce the risk of CR-BSI and to potentially salvage some contaminated CVCs [359,361]. In hemodialysis patients, the use of EDTA with minocycline reduced CR-BSIs [362]. These solutions have significantly reduced the risk of CR-BSI in high-risk pediatric oncology or neonatal ICU patients.

THE FUTURE

We believe that the future is very hopeful for continued progress in the prevention of device-related infection. A great deal of progress has been made over the past decade, with studies showing reduced rates of infection with the use

---

TABLE 37-15

EFFICACY OF THE CHLORHEXIDINE-SILVER SULFADIAZINE CATHETER (CHSS) [ARROWGARD™] IN PREVENTING CATHETER COLONIZATION AND CATHETER-RELATED BLOODSTREAM INFECTION (CRBSI)

Catheter Colonization (%)		CRBSI (%)		Duration	
CHSS	Control	CHSS	Control	(Days)	Reference
13.5	24.1[a]	1.0	7.6[a]	6	168
18.1	30.8[a]	0	2.6	~8	169
		6.3	7.5	10–11	171
10.9	12.1	8.7	8.1	12–13	170

[a]p <0.05.

TABLE 37-16

CENTRAL VENOUS CATHETER BLOODSTREAM INFECTION (CVC-BSI) PREVENTION BUNDLE

Hand hygiene by catheter inserters

Maximum barrier precautions (gowns, gloves mask, cap)

Chlorhexidine (with alcohol) skin antisepsis of catheter insertion site

Trained catheter inserters

Proper selection of type of catheter and insertion site

Insert catheters only when medically necessary

Have all materials needed for catheter insertion at the bedside before starting insertion

Time-out called if proper procedures are not followed (then start again)

Use of aseptic technique during catheter manipulation (including hub disinfection)

Remove catheters when no longer medically necessary

Executive leadership support for bundle implementation

Frequent feedback of bundle compliance and outcomes (catheter-related infection rates)

---

of more stringent barrier precautions during CVC insertion, with IV teams, with the use of more effective cutaneous antiseptics, and with the results of the first studies of innovative technologies, such as contamination-resistant hubs, attachable cuffs, and catheters with colonization-resistant surfaces. We are optimistic that future IVDs will be highly resistant to thrombosis and infection, and that it will be possible to allow percutaneously inserted catheters safely to remain in place in high-risk patients nearly indefinitely.

In the past several years, studies have demonstrated that we should have zero tolerance for catheter-related infections. Interventions using a "bundle approach", that has included many of the interventions discussed previously, have been able to reduce catheter-related infections (including CVC-BSI) rates in ICUs to very low levels (sometimes zero for many months) (Table 37-16) [363–365]. Current practice in many healthcare facilities falls short of those used in successful prevention programs [366]. As more and more facilities throughout the world implement the bundle approach for catheter-related infection prevention using the most effective measures [367–372], many lives will be saved [363].

REFERENCES

1. Maki DG. Nosocomial bacteremia. *Am J Med* 1981;70:183–196.
2. Maki DG. The epidemiology and prevention of nosocomial blood-stream infections [Abstract]. In: *Program and abstracts of the third international conference on nosocomial infections, August 1990, Atlanta, Georgia.* Centers for Disease Control, The National Foundation for Infectious Diseases and the American Society for Microbiology, 1990:20.
3. Friedland G, von Reyn CF, Levy B, et al. Nosocomial endocarditis. *Infect Control* 1984;5:284–288.
4. Terpenning MS, Buggy BP, Kauffman CA. Hospital-acquired infective endocarditis. *Arch Intern Med* 1988;148:1601–1603.
5. Fang G, Keys TF, Gentry LO, et al. Prosthetic valve endocarditis resulting from nosocomial bacteremia: a prospective, multicenter study. *Ann Intern Med* 1993;111:560–567.
6. Martin MA, Pfaller MA, Wenzel RP. Coagulase-negative staphylococcal bacteremia: mortality and hospital stay. *Ann Intern Med* 1989;110:9–16.
7. Smith RL, Meixler SM, Simberkoff MS. Excess mortality in critically ill patients with nosocomial bloodstream infections. *Chest* 1991;100:164–67.
8. Pittet D. Nosocomial bloodstream infections in the critically ill. *JAMA* 1994;272:1819–1820.
9. Collignon PJ. Intravascular catheter associated sepsis: a common problem. *Med J Aust* 1994;161:374–378.
10. Inglis TJJ, Sproat LJ, Hawkey PM, et al. Infection control in intensive care units: U.K. national survey. *Br J Anaesth* 1992;68:216–220.
11. Mermel LA. Prevention of intravascular catheter-related infections. *Ann Intern Med.* 2000;132:391–402.
12. O'Grady NP, Alexander M, Dellinger EP, Gerberding JL, Heard SO, Maki DG, Masur H, McCormick RD, Mermel LA, Pearson ML, Raad II, Randolph A, Weinstein RA; Healthcare Infection Control Practices Advisory Committee. Guidelines for the prevention of intravascular catheter-related infections. *Infect Control Hosp Epidemiol.* 2002;23:759–69.
13. Maki DG, Ringer M. Risk factors for infusion-related phlebitis with small peripheral venous catheters. *Ann Intern Med* 1991;114:845–854.
14. Gantz NM, Presswood GM, Goldberg R, et al. Effects of dressing type and change interval on intravenous therapy complication rates. *Diagn Microbiol Infect Dis* 1984;2:325–332.
15. Hoffman KK, Western SA, Kaiser DL, et al. Bacterial colonization and phlebitis-associated risk with transparent polyurethane film for peripheral intravenous site dressings. *Am J Infect Control* 1988;16:101–106.
16. Collin J, Collin C, Constable FL, et al. Infusion phlebitis and infection with various cannulas. *Lancet* 1975;2:150–153.
17. Maki DG, Weise CE, Sarafin HW. A semiquantitative culture method for identifying intravenous-catheter-related infection. *N Engl J Med* 1977;296:1305–1309.
18. Smallman L, Burdon DW, Alexander-Williams J. The effect of skin preparation on the incidence of infusion thrombophlebitis. *Br J Surg* 1980;67:861–862.
19. Larson E, Hargiss C. A decentralized approach to maintenance of intravenous therapy. *Am J Infect Control* 1984;12:177–186.
20. Adams SD, Killien M, Larson E. In-line filtration and infusion phlebitis. *Heart Lung* 1986;15:134–140.
21. Maki DG, Rhame FS, Mackel DC, et al. Nationwide epidemic of septicemia caused by contaminated intravenous products. *Am J Med* 1976;60:471–485.
22. Armstrong CS, Mayhall CG, Miller KB, et al. Clinical predictors of infection of central venous catheters used for total parenteral nutrition. *Infect Control Hosp Epidemiol* 1990;2:71–78.
23. Safdar N, Fine JP, Maki DG. Meta-analysis: methods for diagnosing intravascular device-related bloodstream infection. *Ann Intern Med.* 2005;142:451–66.
24. Torres-Rohas JR, Stratton CW, Sanders CV, et al. Candidal suppurative peripheral thrombophlebitis. *Ann Intern Med* 1982;96:431–435.
25. Johnson RA, Zajac RA, Evans ME. Suppurative thrombophlebitis: correlation between pathogen and underlying disease. *Infect Control* 1986;7:582–585.
26. Strinden WD, Helgerson RB, Maki DG. Candida septic thrombosis of the great veins associated with central catheters: clinical features and management. *Ann Surg* 1985;202:653–658.
27. Verghese A, Widrich WC, Arbeit RD. Central venous septic thrombophlebitis: the role of medical therapy. *Medicine* 1985;64:394–400.
28. Raad II, Sabbagh Mouin F. Optimal duration of therapy for catheter-related *Staphylococcus aureus* bacteremia: a study of 55 cases and review. *Clin Infect Dis* 1992;14:75–82.
29. Herrmann M, Vaudaux PE, Pittet D, et al. Fibronectin, fibrinogen, and laminin act as mediators of adherence of clinical staphylococcal isolates to foreign material. *J Infect Dis* 1988;158:693–701.

30. Herrmann M, Suchard SJ, Boxer LA, et al. Thrombospondin binds to Staphylococcus aureus and promotes staphylococcal adherence to surfaces. *Infect Immun* 1991;59:279–288.

31. Maki DG, Ringer M. Prospective study of arterial catheter-related infection: incidence, sources of infection and risk factors [Abstract]. In: *Programs and abstracts of the twenty-ninth interscience conference on antimicrobial agents and chemotherapy, September 1989, Houston, Texas.* Washington, DC: American Society for Microbiology, 1989:284.

32. Maki DG, Alvarado CJ, Ringer M. A prospective, randomized trial of povidone–iodine, alcohol and chlorhexidine for prevention of infection with central venous and arterial catheters. *Lancet* 1991;338:339–343.

33. Segura M, Llado L, Guirao X, et al. A prospective study of a new protocol for *"in situ"* diagnosis of central venous catheter related bacteraemia. *Clin Nutr* 1993;12:103–107.

34. Maki DG, Stolz SS, Wheeler S, et al. A prospective, randomized trial of gauze and two polyurethane dressings for site care of pulmonary artery catheters: Implications for catheter management. *Crit Care Med* 1994;32:1729–1737.

35. Maki DG, Klein BS, McCormick RD, et al. Nosocomial Pseudomonas pickettii bacteremias traced to narcotic tampering: a case for selective drug screening of healthcare personnel. *JAMA* 1991;265:981–986.

36. Bennett SN, McNeil MM, Bland LA, et al. Postoperative infections traced to contamination of an intravenous anesthetic, propofol. *N Engl J Med* 1995;333:147–154.

37. Schmitt S, Hall G, Knapp C, et al. Poor correlation between clinical judgment and microbiologic confirmation of catheter-related bacteremia (CRB) due to coagulase-negative staphylococci (CNS) [Abstract]. In: *Programs and abstracts of the ninety fourth general meeting of the American Society for Microbiology, May 1994, Las Vegas, Nevada.* Washington, DC: American Society for Microbiology, 1994:615.

38. Mermel LA, Velez LA, Zilz MA, et al. Epidemiologic and microbiologic features of nosocomial bloodstream infection (NSBI) implicating a vascular catheter source: a case–control study of 85 vascular catheter-related and 101 secondary NBSIs [Abstract]. In: *Program and abstracts of the thirty-first interscience conference on antimicrobial agents and chemotherapy, October 1991, Chicago, Illinois.* Washington, DC: American Society for Microbiology, 1991:174.

39. Band JD, Maki DG. Infections caused by indwelling arterial catheters for hemodynamic monitoring. *Am J Med* 1979;67:735–741.

40. Maki DG. Sepsis arising from extrinsic contamination of the infusion and measure for control. In: Phillips I, ed. *Microbiologic hazards of infusion therapy.* Lancaster, England: MTP Press, 1977:99–141.

41. Henderson DK, Edwards JE, Montgomerie JZ. Hematogenous Candida endophthalmitis in patients receiving parenteral hyperalimentation fluids. *J Infect Dis* 1981;143:655–661.

42. Maki DG, McCormick RD, Uman SJ, et al. Septic endarteritis due to intra-arterial catheters for cancer chemotherapy: I. Evaluation of an outbreak. IT. Risk factors, clinical features and management. III. Guidelines for prevention. *Cancer* 1979;44:1228–1240.

43. Cohen A, Reyes R, Kirk B, et al. Osier's nodes, pseudoaneurysm formation, and sepsis complicating percutaneous radial artery cannulation. *Crit Care Med* 1984;12:1078–1079.

44. Arnow PM, Costas CO. Delayed rupture of the radial artery caused by catheter-related sepsis. *Rev Infect Dis* 1988;10:1035–1037.

45. Falk P, Scuderi PE, Sherertz RJ, et al. Infected radial artery pseudoaneurysms occurring after percutaneous cannulation. *Chest* 1992;101:490–495.

46. Ehrie M, Morgan AP, Moore FD, et al. Endocarditis with the indwelling balloon-tipped pulmonary artery catheter in burn patients. *J Trauma* 1978;18:664–666.

47. Rowley KM, Clubb KS, Smith GJW, et al. Right-sided infective endocarditis as a consequence of flow-directed pulmonary-artery catheterization: a clinicopathologic study of 55 autopsied patients. *N Engl J Med* 1984;311:1152–1156.

48. Mermel LA, Maki DG. Infectious complications of Swan-Ganz pulmonary artery catheters. *Am J Respir Crit Care Med* 1994;149:1020–1036.

49. Aronson MD, Bor DH. Blood cultures. *Ann Intern Med* 1987;106:246–253.

50. Weinstein MP. Current blood culture methods and systems: clinical concepts, technology, and interpretation of results. *Clin Infect Dis* 1996;23:40–46.

51. Mermel LA, Maki DG. Detection of bacteremia in adults: consequences of culturing an inadequate volume of blood. *Ann Intern Med* 1993;119:270–272.

52. Crepin O, Roussel-Delvallez M, et al. Effectiveness of resins in removing antibiotics from blood cultures. *J Clin Microbiol* 1993;31:734–735.

53. Reimer LG, Barth Reller L, et al. Controlled comparison of a new Becton Dickinson agar slant blood culture system with Roche Septichek for the detection of bacteremia and fungemia. *J Clin Microbiol* 1989;27:2637–2639.

54. Jungkind D, Thakur M, Dyke J. Evidence for a second mechanism of action of resins in BACTEC NR16A aerobic blood culture medium [Abstract]. In: *Programs and abstracts of the eighty-ninth general meeting of the American Society for Microbiology, May 1989, New Orleans, Louisiana.* Washington, DC: American Society for Microbiology, 1989:431.

55. Tegtmeier BR, Vice JL. Evaluation of the BACTEC 16B medium in a cancer center. *Am J Clin Pathol* 1984;81:783–786.

56. Tarrand JJ, Guillot C, Wenglar M, et al. Clinical comparison of the resin-containing BACTEC 26 Plus and the Isolator 10 blood culturing systems. *J Clin Microbiol* 1991;29:2245–2249.

57. Wilson M, Davis TE, Mirrett S, et al. Controlled comparison of the BACTEC high-blood-volume fungal medium, BACTEC Plus 26 aerobic blood culture system for detection of fungemia and bacteremia. *J Clin Microbiol* 1993;31:865–871.

58. Weinstein MP, Reller LB, Murphy HR et al. The clinical significance of positive blood cultures: a comprehensive analysis of 500 episodes of bacteremia and fungemia in adults: I. laboratory and epidemiological observations. *Rev Infect Dis* 1983;5:35–53.

59. Koontz FP, Flint KK, Reynolds JK, et al. Multicenter comparison of the high volume (10 ml) NR Bactec Plus system and the standard (5 ml) NR bactec system. *Diagn Microbiol Infect Dis* 1991;14:111–118.

60. Wormser GP, Onorato IM, Preminger TJ, et al. Sensitivity and specificity of blood cultures obtained through intravascular catheters. *Crit Care Med* 1990;18:152–156.

61. Isaacman DJ, Karasic RB. Utility of collecting blood cultures through newly inserted intravenous catheters. *Pediatr Infect Dis J* 1990;9:815–818.

62. Pourcyrous M, Korones SB, Bada HS, et al. Indwelling umbilical arterial catheter: a preferred sampling site for blood culture. *Pediatrics* 1988;81:821–825.

63. Bryant JK, Strand CL. Reliability of blood cultures collected from intravascular catheter vs. venipuncture. *Am J Clin Pathol* 1987;88:113–116.

64. Maki DG, Hassemer CH. Endemic rate of fluid contamination and related septicemia in arterial pressure monitoring. *Am J Med* 1981;70:733–738.

65. Weightman NC, Simpson EM, Speller DCE, et al. Bacteraemia related to indwelling central venous catheters: prevention, diagnosis and treatment. *Eur J Clin Microbiol Infect Dis* 1988;7:125–129.

66. Flynn PM, Shenep JL, Stokes DC, et al. In situ management of confirmed central venous catheter-related bacteremia. *Pediatr Infect Dis J* 1987;6:729–734.

67. Raucher HS, Hyatt AC, Barzilai A, et al. Quantitative blood cultures in the evaluation of septicemia in children with Broviac catheters. *J Pediatr* 1984;104:29–33.

68. Benezra D, Kiehn T, Gold JWM, et al. Prospective study of infections in indwelling central venous catheters using quantitative blood cultures. *Am J Med* 1988;85:495–498.

69. Ascher DP, Shoupe BA, Robb M, et al. Comparison of standard and quantitative blood cultures in the evaluation of children with suspected central venous line sepsis. *Diagn Microbiol Infect Dis* 1992;15:499–503.

70. Capedevila JA, Planes AM, Palomar M, et al. Value of differential quantitative blood cultures in the diagnosis of catheter-related sepsis. *Eur J Clin Microbiol Infect Dis* 1992;11:403–407.

71. Douard MC, Clementi E, Arlet G, et al. Negative catheter-tip culture and diagnosis of catheter-related bacteremia. *Nutrition* 1994;10:397–404.

72. Siegman-Igra Y, Anglim AM, Shapiro DE, et al. Diagnosis of vascular catheter-related bloodstream infection: a meta-analysis. *J Clin Microbiol* 1997;35:928–936.

73. Rushforth JA, Hoy CM, Kite P, Puntis JW. Rapid diagnosis of central venous catheter sepsis. *Lancet* 1993;342:402–403.

74. Moonens F, EL Alami S, Van Gossum A. Usefulness of Gram staining of blood collected from total parenteral nutrition catheter for rapid diagnosis of catheter-related sepsis. *J Clin Microbiol* 1994;32:1578–1579.

75. Torlakovic E, Hibbs JR, Miller JS, et al. Intracellular bacteria in blood smears in patients with central venous catheters. *Arch Intern Med* 1995;155:1547–1550.

76. Anderson RL, Highsmith AK, Holland BW. Comparison of the standard pour plate procedure and the ATP and Limulus amoebocyte lysate procedures for the detection of microbial contamination in intravenous fluids. *J Clin Microbiol* 1986;23:465–468.

77. Centers for Disease Control and Prevention. Septicemias associated with contaminated intravenous fluids. *MMWR Morb Mortal Wkly Rep* 1973;22:99–114, 124.

78. Braude AI, Carey FJ, Siemienski J. Studies of bacterial transfusion reactions from refrigerated blood: the properties of cold-growing bacteria. *J Clin Invest* 1955;34:311–325.

79. Morduchowicz G, Silvio D, Pitlik D, et al. Transfusion reactions due to bacterial contamination of blood and blood products. *Rev Infect Dis* 1991;3:307–314.

80. Heal JM, Jones ME, Chaudhry A, et al. Fatal Salmonella septicemia after platelet transfusion. *Transfusion* 1987;27:2–5.

81. Centers for Disease Control and Prevention. Red blood cell transfusions contaminated with Yersinia enterocolitica—United States, 1991–1996, and initiation of a national study to detect bacteria-associated transfusion reactions. *MMWR* 1997; 46:553–555.

82. Nahass RG, Weinstein MP. Qualitative intravascular catheter tip cultures do not predict catheter-related bacteremia. *Diagn Microbiol Infect Dis* 1990;13:223–226.

83. Kristinsson KG, Burnett IA, Spencer RC. Evaluation of three methods for culturing long intravascular catheters. *J Hosp Infect* 1989;14:183–191.

84. Gutierrez J, Leon C, Matamoros R, et al. Catheter-related bacteremia and fungemia. *Diagn Microbiol Infect Dis* 1992;15: 575–578.

85. Dooley DP, Garcia A, Kelly JW, et al. Validation of catheter semi-quantitative culture technique for nonstaphylococcal organisms. *J Clin Microbiol* 1996;34:409–412.

86. Brun-Buisson C, Abrouk F, Legrand P, et al. Diagnosis of central venous catheter-related sepsis: critical level of quantitative tip cultures. *Arch Intern Med* 1987;147:873–877.

87. Sherertz RJ, Raad II, Belani A, et al. Three-year experience with sonicated vascular catheter cultures in a clinical microbiology laboratory. *J Clin Microbiol* 1990;28:76–82.

88. Raad II, Sabbagh MF, Rand KH, Sherertz RJ. Quantitative tip culture methods and the diagnosis of central venous catheter-related infections. *Diagn Microbiol Infect Dis.* 1992;15:13–20.

89. Collignon P. Quantitative blood cultures for catheter-associated infections. *J Clin Microbiol* 1989;27:1487–1488.

90. Hnatiuk OW, Pike J, Stoltzfus D, et al. Value of bedside plating of semiquantitative cultures for diagnosis of central venous catheter-related infections in ICU patients. *Chest* 1993;103: 896–899.

91. Cooper GL, Hopkins CC. Rapid diagnosis of intravascular catheter-associated infection by direct gram staining of catheter segments. *N Engl J Med* 1985;18:1142–1150.

92. Zufferey J, Rime B, Francioli P, et al. Simple method for rapid diagnosis of catheter-associated infection by direct acridine orange staining of catheter tips. *J Clin Microbiol* 1988;26:175–177.

93. Raad II, Baba M, Bodey GP. Diagnosis of catheter-related infections: the role of surveillance and targeted quantitative skin cultures. *Clin Infect Dis* 1995;20:593–597.

94. McGeer A, Righter J. Improving our ability to diagnose infections associated with central venous catheters: value of Gram's staining and culture of entry site swabs. *Can Med Assoc J* 1987; 137:1009–1021.

95. Fan ST, Teoh-Chan CH, Lau KF, et al. Predictive value of surveillance skin and hub cultures in central venous catheter sepsis. *J Hosp Infect* 1988;12:191–198.

96. Cercenado E, Ena J, Rodriguez-Creixems M, et al. A conservative procedure for the diagnosis of catheter-related infections. *Arch Intern Med* 1990;150:1417–1420.

97. Mayhall CG, Pierpaoli PG, Hall GO, et al. Evaluation of a device for monitoring sterility of infectable fluids. *Am J Hosp Pharm* 1981;38:1148–1150.

98. Longfield JN, Charache P, Diamond EL, et al. Comparison of broth and filtration methods for culturing of intravenous fluids. *Infect Control* 1982;3:397–400.

99. Mermel LA. Defining intravascular catheter-related infections: a plea for uniformity. *Nutrition* 1996;12:1–3.

100. Bone RC, Balk RA, Cerra FB, et al. American College of Chest Physician/Society of Critical Care Medicine Consensus Conference: definitions for sepsis and organ failure and guidelines for the use of innovative therapies in sepsis. *Crit Care Med* 1992; 20:864–874.

101. Sattler FR, Foderato JB, Aber RC. Staphylococcus epidermidis bacteremia associated with vascular catheters: an important cause of febrile morbidity in hospitalized patients. *Infect Control* 1984;5:279–283.

102. Ponce DeLeon S, Wenzel RP. Hospital acquired bloodstream infections with Staphylococcus epidermidis. *Am J Med* 1984;77: 639–644.

103. Kirchhoff LV, Sheagren JN. Epidemiology and clinical significance of blood cultures positive for coagulase-negative staphylococcus. *Infect Control* 1985;6:479–486.

104. Garner JS, Jarvis WR, Emori TG, et al. CDC definitions for nosocomial infections, 1988. *Am J Infect Control* 1988;16:128–140.

105. Sheretz RJ. Surveillance for infections associated with vascular catheters. *Infect Control Hosp. Epidemiol* 1996;17:746–752.

106. Williams DN, Gibson J, Vos J, et al. Infusion thrombophlebitis and infiltration associated with intravenous cannulae: a controlled study comparing three different cannula types. *NITA* 1982;5:379–382.

107. Craven DE, Lichtenberg A, Kunches LM, et al. A randomized study comparing a transparent polyurethane dressing to a dry gauze dressing for peripheral intravenous catheter sites. *Infect Control* 1985;6:361–366.

108. Tomford JW, Hershey CO, McLaren CE, et al. Intravenous therapy team and peripheral venous catheter-associated complications: a prospective controlled study. *Arch Intern Med* 1984; 144:1191–1194.

109. Maki DG, Ringer M. Evaluation of dressing regimens for prevention of infection with peripheral intravenous catheters. *JAMA* 1987;258:2396–2403.

110. Mermel LA, Maki DG. Infectious complications of Swan-Ganz pulmonary artery catheters and peripheral artery catheters. In: Seifert H, Jansen B, Farr BM, eds. *Catheter related infections.* New York: Marcel Dekker, 1997.

111. Nystrom B, Olesen Larsen S, Dankert J, et al. Bacteraemia in surgical patients with intravenous devices: a European multicentre incidence study. *J Hosp Infect* 1983;4:338–349.

112. Trilla A, Gatell JM, Mensa J, et al. Risk factors for nosocomial bacteremia in a large Spanish teaching hospital: a case–control study. *Infect Control Hosp Epidemiol* 1991;2:150–156.

113. Wey SB, Mori M, Pfaller MA, et al. Risk factors for hospital-acquired candidemia: a matched case–control study. *Arch Intern Med* 1989;149:2349–2353.

114. Maki DG, McCormack KN. Defatting catheter insertion sites in total parenteral nutrition is of no value as an infection control measure. *Am J Med* 1987;83:833–840.

115. Maki DG, Cobb L, Garman JK, et al. An attachable silver-impregnated cuff for prevention of infection with central venous catheters: a prospective randomized multicenter trial. *Am J Med* 1988;85:307–314.

116. Flowers RH III, Schwenzer KJ, Kopel RJ, et al. Efficacy of an attachable subcutaneous cuff for the prevention of intravascular catheter-related infection. *JAMA* 1989;261:878–883.

117. Richet H, Hubert B, Nitemberg G, et al. Prospective multicenter study of vascular-catheter-related complications and risk factors for positive central-catheter cultures in intensive care unit patients. *J Clin Microbiol* 1990;28:2520–2525.

118. Cobb DK, High KP, Sawyer RG, et al. A controlled trial of scheduled replacement of central venous and pulmonary-artery catheters. *N Engl J Med* 1992;327:1062–1068.

119. Pittet D, Hulliger S, Auckenthaler R. Intravascular device-related infections in critically ill patients. *J Chemother.* 1995 Jul;7 Suppl 3:55–66.

120. Almirall J, Gonzalez J, Rello J, et al. Infection of hemodialysis catheters: incidence and mechanisms. *Am J Nephrol* 1989;9:454–459.

121. Rello J, Gatell JM, Almirall J, et al. Evaluation of culture techniques for identification of catheter-related infection in hemodialysis patients. *Eur J Clin Microbiol Infect Dis* 1989;8:620–622.

122. Levin A, Mason AJ, Jindal KK, et al. Prevention of hemodialysis subclavian vein catheter infections by topical povidone–iodine. *Kidney Int* 1991;40:934–938.

123. Schwab SJ, Buller GL, McCann RL. Prospective evaluation of a Dacron cuffed hemodialysis catheter for prolonged use. *Am J Kidney Dis* 1988;11:166–169.

124. Dryden MS, Samson A, Ludlam HA, et al. Infective complications associated with the use of the Quinton "Permcath" for long-term central vascular access in haemodialysis. *J Hosp Infect* 1991;19:257–262.

125. Raad I, Davis S, Becker M, et al. Low infection rate and long durability of nontunneled silastic catheters. *Arch Intern Med* 1993;153:1791–1796.

126. Pauley SY, Vallande NC, Riley EN, et al. Catheter-related colonization associated with percutaneous inserted central catheters. *J Intraven Nurs* 1993;16:50–54.

127. Clarke DE, Raffin TA. Infectious complications of indwelling long-term central venous catheters. *Chest* 1990;97:966–972.

128. Mayhall G. Diagnosis and management of infections of implantable devices used for prolonged venous access. *Curr Clin Top Infect Dis* 1992;12:83–110.

129. Carde P, Cosset-Delaigue MF, LaPlanche A, et al. Classical external indwelling central venous catheter vs. totally implanted venous access systems for chemotherapy administration: a randomized trial in 100 patients with solid tumors. *Eur J Cancer Clin Oncol* 1989;25:939–944.

130. Ingram J, Weitzman S, Greenberg ML, et al. Complications of indwelling venous access lines in the pediatric hematology patient: a prospective comparison of external venous catheters and subcutaneous ports. *American Journal of Pediatric Hematology and Oncology* 1991;13:130–136.

131. Pegues D, Axelrod P, McClarren C, et al. Comparison of infections in Hickman and implanted port catheters in adult solid tumor patients. *J Surg Oncol* 1992;49:156–162.

132. Mueller BU, Skelton J, Callender DPE, et al. A prospective randomized trial comparing the infectious and noninfectious complications of an externalized catheter vs. a subcutaneously implanted device in cancer patients. *J Clin Oncol* 1992;10:1943–1948.

133. Groeger JS, Lucas AB, Thaler HT, et al. Infectious morbidity associated with long-term use of venous access devices in patients with cancer. *Ann Intern Med* 1993;119:1168–1174.

134. Pullyblank AM, Carey PD, Pearce SZ, et al. Comparison between peripherally implanted ports and externally sited catheters for long-term venous access. *Ann R Coll Surg Engl* 1994;76:33–38.

135. Banerjee SN, Emori G, Culver DH, et al. National Nosocomial Infections Surveillance System: secular trends in nosocomial primary bloodstream infections in the United States, 1980–1989. *Am J Med* 1991;91(Suppl 3B):86S–89S.

136. Elliott TSJ, Tebbs SE, Moss HM, et al. Nosocomial infections and surgical infections and related epidemiologic studies [Abstract]. In: *Programs and abstracts of the thirty-fifth interscience conference on antimicrobial agents and chemotherapy, September 1995, San Francisco, California.* Washington, DC: American Society for Microbiology, 1995:257.

137. Cooper GL, Schiller AL, Hopkins CC. Possible role of capillary action in pathogenesis of experimental catheter-associated dermal tunnel infections. *J Clin Microbiol* 1988;26:8–12.

138. Maki DG. Marked differences in insertion sites for central venous, arterial and peripheral IV catheters: the major reason for differing risks of catheter-related infection. In: *Program and abstracts of the thirtieth interscience conference on antimicrobial agents and chemotherapy, October 1990, Atlanta, Georgia.* Washington, DC: American Society for Microbiology, 1990:205.

139. Bertone SA, Fisher MC, Mortensen JE. Quantitative skin cultures at potential catheter sites in neonates. *Infect Control Hosp Epidemiol* 1994;15:315–318.

140. Yu VL, Goetz A, Wagener M, et al. Staphylococcus aureus nasal carriage and infection in patients on hemodialysis: efficacy of antibiotic prophylaxis. *N Engl J Med* 1986;315:91–96.

141. Pujol M, Pena C, Pallares R, et al. Nosocomial Staphylococcus aureus bacteremia among nasal carriers of methicillin-resistant and methicillin-susceptible strains. *Am J Med* 1996;100:509–516.

142. Snydman DR, Sullivan BS, Gill M, et al. Nosocomial sepsis associated with interleukin-2. *Ann Intern Med* 1990;112:102–107.

143. Maki DG, Jarrett F; Sarafin HW. A semiquantitative culture method for identification of catheter-related infection in the burn patient. *J Surg Res* 1977;22:513–520.

144. Franceschi D, Gerding RL, Phillips G, et al. Risk factors associated with intravascular catheter infections in burned patients: a prospective, randomized study. *J Trauma* 1989;29:811–816.

145. Dixon RE, Kaslow RA, Mackel DC, et al. Aqueous quaternary ammonium antiseptics and disinfectants: use and misuse. *JAMA* 1976;236:2415–2417.

146. Frank MJ, Schaffner W. Contaminated aqueous benzalkonium chloride: an unnecessary hospital infection hazard. *JAMA* 1976;236:2418–2419.

147. Kahan A, Philippon A, Paul G, et al. Nosocomial infections by chlorhexidine solution contaminated with Pseudomonas pickettii (biovar VA-I). *J Infect* 1983;7:256–263.

148. Pein F, Lebbar A, Lecointe D, et al. Nosocomial outbreak of catheter related bacteremia due to Pseudomonas pickettii originated from a contaminated antiseptic solution [Abstract]. In: *Programs and abstracts of the thirty-fourth interscience conference on antimicrobial agents and chemotherapy, October 1994, Orlando, Florida.* Washington, DC: American Society for Microbiology, 1994:241.

149. Rello J, Coll P, Prats G. Laboratory diagnosis of catheter-related bacteremia. *Scand J Infect Dis* 1991;23:583–588.

150. Raad I, Costerton W, Sabharwal U, et al. Ultrastructural analysis of indwelling vascular catheters: a quantitative relationship between luminal colonization and duration of placement. *J Infect Dis* 1993;168:400–407.

151. Sheehan G, Leicht K, O'Brien M, et al. Chlorhexidine vs. povidone–iodine as cutaneous antisepsis for prevention of vascular-catheter infection [Abstract]. In: *Programs and abstracts of the thirty-third interscience conference on antimicrobial agents and chemotherapy, October 1993, New Orleans, Louisiana.* Washington, DC: American Society for Microbiology, 1993:414.

152. Mimoz O, Pieroni L, Lawrence C, Edouard A, Costa Y, Samii K, Brun-Buisson C. Prospective, randomized trial of two antiseptic solutions for prevention of central venous or arterial catheter colonization and infection in intensive care unit patients. *Crit Care Med.* 1996;24:1818–23.

153. Garland JS, Buck RK, Maloney P, et al. Comparison of 10% povidone–iodine and 0.5% chlorhexidine gluconate for the prevention of peripheral intravenous catheter colonization in neonates: a prospective trial. *Pediatr Infect Dis J* 1995;14:510–516.

154. Maki DG, Band JD. A comparative study of polyantibiotic and iodophor ointments in prevention of catheter-related infection. *Am J Med* 1981;70:739–744.

155. Fuchs PC, Gustafson ME, King JT, et al. Assessment of catheter-associated infection risk with the Hickman right atrial catheter. *Infect Control* 1984;5:226–530.

156. Press OW, Ramsey PG, Larson EB, et al. Hickman catheter infections in patients with malignancies. *Medicine* 1984;63:189–200.

157. Wurzel CL, Halom C, Feldman JG, et al. Infection rates of Broviac-Hickman catheters and implantable venous devices. *American Journal of Diseases of Children* 1980;142:536–540.

158. Bonawitz SC, Hammell EJ, Kirkpatrick JR. Prevention of central venous catheter sepsis: a prospective randomized trial. *Am Surg* 1991;57:618–623.

159. Rafkin HS, Hoyt JW, Crippen DW. Prevention of central venous catheter related infection with a silver-impregnated cuff. *Chest* 1990;98:117S.

160. Babycos CR, Barrocas A, Webb WR. A prospective randomized trial comparing the silver-impregnated collagen cuff with the bedside tunneled subclavian catheter. *JPEN J Parenter Enteral Nutr* 1993;17:61–63.

161. Groeger JS, Lucas AB, Coit D, et al. A prospective, randomized evaluation of the effect of silver impregnated subcutaneous cuffs for preventing tunneled chronic venous access catheter infections in cancer patients. *Ann Surg* 1993;218:206–210.

162. Dahlberg PJ, Agger WA, Singer JR, et al. Subclavian hemodialysis catheter infections: a prospective, randomized trial of an attachable silver-impregnated cuff for prevention of catheter related infections. *Infect Control Hosp Epidemiol* 1995;16:506–511.

163. Kamal GD, Pfaller MA, Rempe LE, et al. Reduced intravascular catheter infection by antibiotic bonding. *JAMA* 1991;265:2364–2368.

164. Raad I, Darouiche R, Dupuis J, Abi-Said D, Gabrielli A, Hachem R, Wall M, Harris R, Jones J, Buzaid A, Robertson C, Shenaq S, Curling P, Burke T, Ericsson C. Central venous catheters coated with minocycline and rifampin for the prevention of catheter-related colonization and bloodstream infections. A randomized, double-blind trial. The Texas Medical Center Catheter Study Group. *Ann Intern Med.* 1997;127:267–74.

165. Goldschmidt H, Hahn U, Salwender H, et al. Prevention of catheter related infections by silver coated central venous catheters in oncological patients. *Zbl Bakt* 1995;283:215–223.

166. Mermel LA, Stolz SM, Maki DG. Surface antimicrobial activity of heparin-bonded and antiseptic-impregnated vascular catheters. *J Infect Dis* 1993;167:920–924.

167. Applegren P, Ransjo U, Bindsley L, et al. Does surface heparinisation reduce bacterial colonisation of central venous catheters? *Lancet* 1995;345:130.

168. Maki DG, Wheeler SJ, Stolz SM, et al. Clinical trial of a novel antiseptic central venous catheter. In: *Program and abstracts of the thirty-first interscience conference on antimicrobial agents and chemotherapy, September 1994, Chicago, Illinois.* Washington, DC: American Society for Microbiology, 1991:176.

169. Bach A, Schmidt H, Bottiger B, et al. Retention of antibacterial activity and bacterial colonization of antiseptic-bonded central venous catheters. *J Antimicrob Chemother* 1996;37:315–322.

170. Ciresi DL, Albrecht RM, Volkers PA, et al. Failure of antiseptic bonding to prevent central venous catheter-related infection and sepsis. *Am Surg* 1996;62:641–646.

171. Pemberton Beaty L, Ross V, Cuddy P, et al. No difference in catheter sepsis between standard and antiseptic central venous catheters. *Arch Surg* 1996;131:986–989.

172. deCicco M, Chiaradia V, Verones A, et al. Source and route of microbial colonisation of parenteral nutrition catheters. *Lancet* 1989;2:1258–1261.

173. Salzman MB, Isenberg HD, Shapiro JF, et al. A prospective study of the catheter hub as the portal of entry for microorganisms causing catheter-related sepsis in neonates. *J Infect Dis* 1993;167:487–490.

174. Moro LM, Vigano EF, Lepri AC, et al. Risk factors for central venous catheter-related infections in surgical and intensive care units. *Infect Control Hosp Epidemiol* 1994;15:253–264.

175. Mermel LA, McCormick RD, Springman SR, et al. The pathogenesis and epidemiology of catheter-related infection with pulmonary artery Swan-Ganz catheters: a prospective study utilizing molecular subtyping. *Am J Med* 1991;91(Suppl 3B):197S–205S.

176. Anaissie E, Samonis G, Kontoyiannis D, et al. Role of catheter colonization and infrequent hematogenous seeding in catheter-related infections. *Eur J Clin Microbiol Infect Dis* 1995;14:134–137.

177. Kurkchubasche AG, Smith SD, Rowe MI: Catheter sepsis in short-bowel syndrome. *Arch Surg* 1992;127:21–25.

178. Landers S, Moise AA, Fraley JK, et al. Factors associated with umbilical catheter-related sepsis in neonates. *American Journal of Diseases of Children* 1991;145:675–680.

179. Maki DG, Will L. Risk factors for central venous catheter-related infection within the ICU: a prospective study of 345 catheters [Abstract]. In: *Programs and abstracts of the thirtieth interscience conference on antimicrobial agents and chemotherapy, October 1990, Atlanta, Georgia.* Washington, DC: American Society for Microbiology, 1990:205.

180. Timsit JF, Farkas JC, Boyer JM, Martin JB, Misset B, Renaud B, Carlet J. Central vein catheter-related thrombosis in intensive care patients: incidence, risks factors, and relationship with catheter-related sepsis. *Chest.* 1998 Jul;114(1):207–13.

181. Ehrenkranz NJ, Eckert DG, Phillips PM. Sporadic bacteremia complicating central venous catheter use in a community hospital: a model to predict frequency and aid in decision-making for initiation of investigation. *Am J Infect Control* 1989;17:69–76.

182. Conly JM, Grieves K, Peters BA. A prospective, randomized study comparing transparent and dry gauze dressings for central venous catheters. *J Infect Dis* 1989;159:310–319.

183. Pittet D. Intravenous catheter-related infections: current understanding [Abstract]. In: *Programs and abstracts of the thirty-second interscience conference on antimicrobial agents and chemotherapy, October 1992, Anaheim, California.* Washington, DC: American Society for Microbiology, 1992:411.

184. Rello J, Coll P, Net A, et al. Infection of pulmonary artery catheters: epidemiologic characteristics and multivariate analysis of risk factors. *Chest* 1993;103:132–136.

185. Damen J, Van Der Tweel I. Positive tip cultures and related risk factors associated with intravascular catheterization in pediatric cardiac patients. *Crit Care Med* 1988;3:221–228.

186. Ena J, Cercenado E, Martinez D, et al. Cross-sectional epidemiology of phlebitis and catheter-related infections. *Infect Control Hosp Epidemiol* 1992;13:15–20.

187. Newman KA, Reed WP, Schimpff SC, et al. Hickman catheters in association with intensive cancer chemotherapy. *Support Care Cancer* 1993;1:92–97.

188. Duthoit D, Devleeshouwer C, Paesmans M, et al. Infection of totally implantable chamber catheters (TICC) in cancer patients: multivariate analysis of risk factors [Abstract]. In: *Programs and abstracts of the thirty-third interscience conference on antimicrobial agents and chemotherapy, October 1993, New Orleans, Louisiana.* Washington, DC: American Society for Microbiology, 1993:416.

189. Passerini L, Lam K, Costerton JW, et al. Biofilms on indwelling vascular catheters. *Crit Care Med* 1992;20:665–673.

190. Hoyle BD, Jass J, Costerton JW. The biofilm glycocalyx as a resistance factor. *J Antimicrob Chemother* 1990;26:1–6.

191. Sheth NK, Rose HD, Franson TR, et al. In vitro quantitative adherence of bacteria to intravascular catheters. *J Surg Res* 1983;34:213–218.

192. Ashkenazi S, Weiss E, Drucker MM. Bacterial adherence to intravenous catheters and needles and its influence by cannula type and bacterial surface hydrophobicity. *J Lab Clin Med* 1986;107:136–140.

193. Barrett SP. Bacterial adhesion to intravenous cannulae: influence of implantation in the rabbit and of enzyme treatments. *Epidemiol Infect* 1988;100:91–100.

194. Vaudaux P, Pittet D, Haeberli A, et al. Host factors selectively increase staphylococcal adherence on inserted catheters: a role for fibronectin and fibrinogen or fibrin. *J Infect Dis* 1989;160:865–875.

195. Pascual A, Fleer A, Westerdaal NAC, et al. Modulation of adherence of coagulase-negative staphylococci to Teflon catheters in vitro. *Eur J Clin Microbiol* 1986;5:518–522.

196. Vaudaux P, Pittet D, Haeberli A, et al. Fibronectin is more active than fibrin or fibrinogen in promoting Staphylococcus aureus adherence to inserted intravascular catheters. *J Infect Dis* 1993;167:633–641.

197. Hogt AH, Dankert J, De Vries JA, et al. Adhesion of coagulase-negative staphylococci to biomaterials. *J Gen Microbiol* 1983;129:2959–2968.

198. Tojo M, Yamashita N, Goldmann DA, et al. Isolation and characterization of transposon mutants of Staphylococcus epidermidis. *J Infect Dis* 1988;157:713–722.

199. Christensen GD, Barker LP, Mawhinney TP. Identification of an antigenic marker of slime production for Staphylococcus epidermidis. *Infect Immun* 1990;58:2906–2911.

200. Timmerman CP, Fleer A, Besnier JM, et al. Characterization of proteinaceous adhesin of Staphylococcus epidermidis

which mediates attachment to polystyrene. *Infect Immun* 1991;59:4187–4192.

201. Rupp ME, Archer GL. Hemagglutination and adherence to plastic by Staphylococcus epidermidis. *Infect Immun* 1992;60: 4322–4327.

202. Mack D, Siemssen N, Laufs R. Parallel induction by glucose of adherence and a polysaccharide antigen specific for plastic-adherent Staphylococcus epidermidis: evidence for functional relation to intercellular adhesin. *Infect Immun* 1992;60:2048–2057.

203. Herrmann M, Lai QJ, Albrecht RM, et al. Adhesion of Staphylococcus aureus to surface-bound platelets: role of fibrinogen/fibrin and platelet integrins. *J Infect Dis* 1993;167:312–322.

204. Stillman RM, Soliman F, Garcia L, et al. Etiology of catheter-associated sepsis: correlation with thrombogenicity. *Arch Surg* 1977;112:1497–1499.

205. Raad I, Luna M, Khalil SAM, et al. The relationship between the thrombotic and infectious complications of central venous catheters. *JAMA* 1994;271:1014–1016.

206. Muller E, Takeda S, Shiro H, et al. Occurrence of capsular polysaccharide/adhesin among clinical isolates of coagulase-negative staphylococci. *J Infect Dis* 1993;168:1211–1218.

207. Goldmann DA, Pier GB. Pathogenesis of infections related to intravascular catheterization. *Clin Microbiol Rev* 1993;6:176–192.

208. Schadow KH, Simpson WA, Christensen GD. Characteristics of adherence to plastic tissue culture plates of coagulase-negative staphylococci exposed to subinhibitory concentrations of antimicrobial agents. *J Infect Dis* 1988;157:71–77.

209. Zimmerli W, Lew PD, Waldvogel FA. Pathogenesis of foreign body infection: evidence for a local granulocyte defect. *J Clin Invest* 1984;73:1191–1200.

210. Gristina AG. Biomaterial-centered infection: microbial adhesion vs. tissue integration. *Science* 1987;237:1588–1595.

211. Gristina AG, Jennings RA, Naylor PT, et al. Comparative in vitro antibiotic resistance of surface-colonizing coagulase-negative staphylococci. *Antimicrob Agents Chemother* 1989;33:813–816.

212. Widmer AF, Frei R, Rajacic Z, et al. Correlation between *in vivo* and in vitro efficacy of antimicrobial agents against foreign body infections. *J Infect Dis* 1990;162:96–102.

213. Widmer AF Frei R, Rajacic Z, et al. Killing of nongrowing and adherent Escherichia coli determines drug efficacy in device-related infections. *Antimicrob Agents Chemother* 1991;35:741–746.

214. Vergeres P, Blaser J. Amikacin, ceftazidime, and flucloxacillin against suspended and adherent Pseudomonas aeruginosa and Staphylococcus epidermidis in an in vitro model infection. *J Infect Dis* 1992;165:281–289.

215. Chuard C, Vaudaux P, Waldvogel FA, et al. Susceptibility of Staphylococcus aureus growing on fibronectin-coated surfaces to bactericidal antibiotics. *Antimicrob Agents Chemother* 1993; 37:625–632.

216. Gander S. Bacterial biofilms: resistance to antimicrobial agents. *J Antimicrob Chemother* 1996;37:1047–1050.

217. Maki DG, Martin WT. Nationwide epidemic of septicemias caused by contaminated infusion products: IV. Growth of microbial pathogens in fluids for intravenous infusion. *J Infect Dis* 1975;131:267–272.

218. Goldmann DA, Martin WT, Worthington JW. Growth of bacteria and fungi in total parenteral nutrition solutions. *Am J Surg* 1973;126:314–318.

219. Didier ME, Fischer S, Maki DG. Total nutrient admixtures appear safer than lipid emulsion alone as regards microbial contamination: growth properties of microbial pathogens at room temperature. *JPEN J Parenter Enteral Nutr.* 1998 Sep-Oct; 22(5):291–6.

220. Crocker KS, Noga R, Filibeck DJ, et al. Microbial growth comparisons of five commercial parenteral lipid emulsions. *JPEN J Parenter Enteral Nutr* 1984;8:391–394.

221. Redline RW, Redline SS, Boxerbaum B, et al. Systemic Malassezia furfur infections in patients receiving intralipid therapy. *Hum Pathol* 1985;16:815–822.

222. Chang HJ, Miller HL, Watkins N, Arduino MJ, Ashford DA, Midgley G, Aguero SM, Pinto-Powell R, von Reyn CF, Edwards W, McNeil MM, Jarvis WR. An epidemic of Malassezia pachydermatis in an intensive care nursery associated with colonization of health care workers' pet dogs. *N Engl J Med.* 1998; 338:706–11.

223. Shparago NI, Bruno PP, Bennett J. Systemic Malassezia furfur infection in an adult receiving total parenteral nutrition. *J Am Osteopath Assoc* 1995;95:375–377.

224. Freeman J, Goldmann DA, Smith NE, et al. Association of intravenous lipid emulsion and coagulase-negative staphylococcal bacteremia in neonatal intensive care units. *N Engl J Med* 1990;323:301–308.

225. Shiro H, Muller E, Takeda S, et al. Potentiation of Staphylococcus epidermidis catheter-related bacteremia by lipid infusions. *J Infect Dis* 1995;171:220–224.

226. Arduino MJ, Bland LA, McAllister SK, et al. Microbial growth and endotoxin production in the intravenous anesthetic propofol. *Infect Control Hosp Epidemiol* 1991;12:535–539.

227. Snydman DR, Reidy MD, Perry LK, et al. Safety of changing intravenous (IV) administration sets containing burettes at longer than 48 hour intervals. *Infect Control* 1987;8:113–116.

228. Maki DG, Botticelli JT, LeRoy ML, et al. Prospective study of replacing administration sets for intravenous therapy at 48- vs 72-hour intervals. *JAMA* 1987;258:1777–1781.

229. Buxton AE, Highsmith AK, Garner JS, et al. Contamination of intravenous fluid: effects of changing administration sets. *Ann Intern Med* 1979;90:764–768.

230. Josephson A, Gombert ME, Sierra MF, et al. The relationship between intravenous fluid contamination and the frequency of tubing replacement. *Infect Control* 1985;6:367–370.

231. Band JD, Maki DG. Safety of changing intravenous delivery systems at longer than 24-hour intervals. *Ann Intern Med* 1979;91:173–178.

232. Gorbea HF, Snydman DR, Delaney A, et al. Intravenous tubing with burettes can be safely changed at 48-hour intervals. *JAMA* 1984;251:2112–2115.

233. Daisy, JA, Abrutyn EA, MacGregor RR. Inadvertent administration of intravenous fluids contaminated with fungus. *Ann Intern Med* 1979;91:563–565.

234. O'Malley MK, Rhame FS, Cerra FB, et al. Value of routine pressure monitoring system changes after 72 hours of continuous use. *Crit Care Med* 1994;22:1424–1430.

235. Mermel LA, Maki DG. Epidemic bloodstream infections from hemodynamic pressure monitoring: signs of the times. *Infect Control Hosp Epidemiol* 1989;10:47–53.

236. Gahm-Hansen B, Alstrup P, Dessau R, et al. Outbreak of infection with Achromobacter xylosoxidans from contaminated intravascular pressure transducers. *J Hosp Infect* 1988;12:1–6.

237. Hekker TAM, Overhage WV, Schneider AJ. Pressure transducers: an overlooked source of sepsis in the intensive care unit. *Intensive Care Med* 1990;16:511–512.

238. Thomas A, Lalitha MK, Jesudason MV. Transducer related Enterobacter cloacae sepsis in postoperative cardiothoracic patients. *J Hosp Infect* 1993;25:211–215.

239. Goldman M, Blajchman MA. Blood product-associated bacterial sepsis. *Transfus Med Rev* 1991;5:73–78.

240. Heal JM, Jones ME, Forey J, et al. Fatal Salmonella septicemia after platelet transfusion. *Transfusion* 1997;27:2–5.

241. Heltberg O, Skov F, Gerner-Smidt P, et al. Nosocomial epidemic of Serratia marcescens septicemia ascribed to contaminated blood transfusion bags. *Transfusion* 1993;33:221–227.

242. Centers for Disease Control and Prevention. Bacterial contamination of platelet pools. Ohio, 1991. *MMWR Morb Mortal Wkly Rep* 1992;41:36–37.

243. Sherertz RJ, Gledhill KS, Hampton KD, et al. Outbreak of Candida bloodstream infections associated with retrograde medication administration in a neonatal intensive care unit. *J Pediatr* 1992;120:455–461.

244. Roberts LA, Collignon PJ, Cramp VB, et al. An Australia-wide epidemic of Pseudomonas pickettii bacteraemia due to contaminated "sterile" water for injection. *Med J Aust* 1990;152: 652–655.

245. Melin P, Struelens M, Mutsers J, et al. Nosocomial outbreak of Pseudomonas pickettii bacteremia originating from intrinsically contaminated sterile saline [Abstract]. In: *Programs and abstracts of the thirty-fifth interscience conference on antimicrobial agents and chemotherapy, September 1995, San Francisco, California.* Washington, DC: American Society for Microbiology, 1995:266.

246. Fernandez C, Wilhelmi I, Andradas E, et al. Nosocomial outbreak of Burkholderia pickettii infection due to a manufactured

intravenous product used in three hospitals. *Clin Infect Dis* 1996;22:1092–1095.

247. Matsaniotis NS, Syriopolou VP, Theodoridou MC, et al. Enterobacter sepsis in infants and children due to contaminated intravenous fluids. *Infect Control* 1984;5:471–477.

248. Steere AC, Rifaat MK, Seligmann EB Jr, et al. Pyrogenic reactions associated with the infusion of normal serum albumin (human). *Transfusion* 1978;18:102–107.

249. Steere AC, Tenney JH, Mackel DC, et al. Pseudomonas species bacteremia caused by contaminated normal human serum albumin. *J Infect Dis* 1977;135:729–735.

250. Ezzedine H, Mourad M, Van Ossel C, et al. An outbreak of Ochrobactrum anthropi bacteraemia in five organ transplant patients. *J Hosp Infect* 1994;27:35–42.

251. Panlilio AL, Beck-Sague CM, Siegel JD, et al. Infections and pseudoinfections due to povidone–iodine solution contaminated with Pseudomonas cepacia. *Clin Infect Dis* 1992;14:1078–1083.

252. Clemence MA, Walker D, Farr BM. Central venous catheter practices: results of a survey. *Am J Infect Control* 1995;23:5–12.

253. Mackel DC, Maki DG, Anderson RL, et al. Nationwide epidemic of septicemia caused by contaminated intravenous products: mechanisms of intrinsic contamination. *J Clin Microbiol* 1975;2:486–497.

254. Jarvis WR, the Epidemiology Branch, Hospital Infections Program. Nosocomial outbreaks: the Centers for Disease Control's Hospital Infections Program experience, 1980–1991. *Am J Med* 1991;91(Suppl 3B):101S–106S.

255. Beck-Sague CM, Jarvis WR. Epidemic bloodstream infections associated with pressure transducers: a persistent problem. *Infect Control Hosp Epidemiol* 1989;10:54–59.

256. Pergues DA, Carson LA, Anderson RL, et al. Outbreak of Pseudomonas cepacia bacteremia in oncology patients. *Clin Infect Dis* 1993;16:407–411.

257. Goetz A, Muder RR, Rihs JP, et al. An outbreak of infusion-related Klebsiella pneumoniae bacteremia on a liver transplantation service. *Am J Infect Control* 1995;23:103.

258. Chodoff A, Pettis AM, Schoonmaker D, et al. Polymicrobial gram-negative bacteremia associated with saline solution flush used with a needleless intravenous system. *Am J Infect Control* 1995;23:357–363.

259. Deitel M, Krajden S, Saldanha CF, et al. An outbreak of Staphylococcus epidermidis bloodstream infection. *JPEN J Parenter Enteral Nutr* 1983;7:569–572.

260. Jackson S, Colligan M, Bender C. Increased nosocomial line-associated bacteremias in a neonatal intensive care unit related to a change in intravenous therapy administration [Abstract]. *Am J Infect Control* 1994;22:122.

261. Maki DG. Epidemic nosocomial bacteremias. In: Wenzel RR, ed. *Handbook of hospital infection.* West Palm Beach, FL: CRC Press, 1981:371–512.

262. Plouffe JF, Brown DG, Silva J, et al. Nosocomial outbreak of Candida parapsilosis fungemia related to intravenous infusions. *Arch Intern Med* 1977;137:1686–1689.

263. Solomon SL, Khabbaz RF, Parker RH, et al. An outbreak of Candida parapsilosis bloodstream infections in patients receiving parenteral nutrition. *J Infect Dis* 1984;149:98–102.

264. Centers for Disease Control and Prevention. Postsurgical infections associated with an extrinsically contaminated intravenous anesthetic agent: California, Illinois, Maine, and Michigan, 1990. *MMWR Morb Mortal Wkly Rep* 1990;39:426–433.

265. Veber B, Gachot B, Bedos JP, et al. Severe sepsis after intravenous injection of contaminated propofol. *Anesthesiology* 1994;80:712.

266. Solomon SL, Alexander H, Eley JW, et al. Nosocomial fungemia in neonates associated with intravascular pressure-monitoring devices. *Pediatric Infectious Disease* 1986;5:680–685.

267. Burnie JP, Matthews R, Lee W, et al. Four outbreaks of nosocomial systemic candidiasis. *Epidemiol Infect* 1987;99:201–211.

268. Reagan DR, Pfaller MA, Hollis RJ, et al. Characterization of the sequence of colonization and nosocomial candidemia using DNA fingerprinting and a DNA probe. *J Clin Microbiol* 1990; 28:2733–2738.

269. Maki DG. Through a glass darkly: nosocomial pseudoepidemics and pseudobacteremias. *Arch Intern Med* 1980;140:26–28.

270. Maki DG. The use of antiseptics for handwashing by medical personnel. *J Chemother* 1989;1(Suppl 1):3–11.

271. Raad I, Hohn DC, Gilbreath BJ, et al. Prevention of central venous catheter-related infections by using maximal sterile barrier precautions during insertion. *Infect Control Hosp Epidemiol* 1994;15:237–238.

272. Maki DG. Yes, Virginia, aseptic technique is very important: maximal barrier precautions during insertion reduce the risk of central venous catheter-related bacteremia. *Infect Control Hosp Epidemiol* 1994;15:227–230.

273. Bull DA, Neumayer LA, Hunter GC, et al. Improved sterile technique diminishes the incidence of positive line cultures in cardiovascular patients. *J Surg Res* 1992;52:106–110.

274. Bentley DW, Lepper MH. Septicemia related to indwelling venous catheter. *JAMA* 1968;206:1749–1752.

275. Freeman JB, Lemire A, MacLean LD. Intravenous alimentation and septicemia. *Surg Gynecol Obstet* 1972;135:708–712.

276. Nehme AE. Nutritional support of the hospitalized patient: the team concept. *JAMA* 1980;243:1906–1908.

277. Faubion WC, Wesley JR, Khalidi N, et al. Total parenteral nutrition catheter sepsis: impact of the team approach. *JPEN J Parenter Enteral Nutr* 1986;10:642–645.

278. Nelson DB, Kien CL, Mohr B, et al. Dressing changes by specialized personnel reduce infection rates in patients receiving central venous parenteral nutrition. *JPEN J Parenter Enteral Nutr* 1986;10:220–222.

279. Sanders RA, Sheldon GF. Septic complications of total parenteral nutrition: a five year experience. *Am J Surg* 1976;132:214–220.

280. Keohane PP, Jones BJM, Attrill H, et al. Effect of catheter tunneling and a nutrition nurse on catheter sepsis during parenteral nutrition: a controlled trial. *Lancet* 1983;2:1388–1390.

281. Goetz A, Miller J, Squier C, et al. A comparison of nosocomial intravenous-related infections pre and post institution of an intravenous therapy team. *Am J Infect Control* 1993;82:xxx.

282. Tomford JW, Hershey CO: The I.V. therapy team: impact on patient care and costs of hospitalization. *NITA* 1985;8:387–389.

283. Soifer NE, Borzak S, Edlin BR, Weinstein RA. Prevention of peripheral venous catheter complications with an intravenous therapy team: a randomized controlled trial. *Arch Intern Med.* 1998;158:473–7.

284. Parras F, Ena J, Bouza E, del Carmen Guerrero M, et al. Impact of an educational program for the prevention of colonization of intravascular catheters. *Infect Control Hosp Epidemiol* 1994;15:239–242.

285. Puntis JWL, Holden CE, Smallman S, et al. Staff training: a key factor in reducing intravascular catheter sepsis. *Arch Dis Child* 1990;65:335–337.

286. Fridkin SK, Pear SM, Williamson, et al. The role of understaffing in central venous catheter-associated bloodstream infections. *Infect Control Hosp Epidemiol* 1996;17:150–158.

287. Rannem T, Ladefoged K, Hegnhoj J, et al. Catheter-related sepsis in long-term parenteral nutrition with Broviac catheters: an evaluation of different disinfectants. *Clin Nutr* 1990;9:131–136.

288. Strand CL, Wajsbort RR, Sturmann K. Effect of iodophor vs iodine tincture skin preparation on blood culture contamination rate. *JAMA* 1993;269:1004–1006.

289. Little JR, Murray PR, Traynor S, et al. Blood culture contamination rates following venipuncture site disinfection with iodophor vs iodine tincture. *Infect Control Hosp Epidemiol* 1997;18:55.

290. Zinner SH, Denny-Brown BC, Braun P, et al. Risk of infection with intravenous indwelling catheters: effect of application of antibiotic ointment. *J Infect Dis* 1969;120:616–619.

291. Hill RL, Casewell MW. Reduction in the colonization of central venous cannulae by mupirocin. *J Hosp Infect.* 1991 Sep;19 Suppl B:47–57.

292. Zakrzewska-Bode A, Muytjens HL, et al. Mupirocin resistance in coagulase-negative staphylococci after topical prophylaxis for the reduction of colonization of central venous catheters. *J Hosp Infect* 1995;31:189–193.

293. Prager RL, Silva J. Colonization of central venous catheters. *South Med J* 1984;77:458–461.

294. Rhame FS, Feist JF, Mueller CL, et al. Transparent adherent dressings (TADs) do not promote abnormal skin flora. *Am J Infect Control* 1983;11:152.

295. Hoffmann KK, Weber DJ, Samsa GP, et al. Transparent polyurethane film as an intravenous catheter dressing: a meta-analysis of the infection risks. *JAMA* 1992;267:2072–2076.

296. Andersen PT, Herlevsen P, Schaumburg H. A comparative study of "Op-site" and "Nobecutan gauze" dressings for central venous line care. *J Hosp Infect* 1986;7:161–168.

297. Kelsey MC, Gosling M. A comparison of the morbidity associated with occlusive and non-occlusive dressings applied to peripheral intravenous devices. *J Hosp Infect* 1984;5:313–321.

298. Joseph P, Marzouk J. Transparent vs. dry gauze dressings for peripheral IV sites [Abstract]. In: *Program and abstracts of the general meeting of the American Society, for Microbiology, March 1985, Las Vegas, Nevada.* Washington, DC: American Society for Microbiology, 1985:378.

299. McCredie KB, Lawson M, Marts K, et al. A comparative evaluation of transparent dressings and gauze dressings for central venous catheters. *JPEN J Parenter Enteral Nutr* 1984;8:96.

300. Ricard P, Martin R, Marcoux JA. Protection of indwelling vascular catheters: incidence of bacterial contamination and catheter-related sepsis. *Crit Care Med* 1985;13:541–543.

301. Pinheiro SMC, Starling CAF, Couto BRGM. Transparent dressing versus conventional dressing: comparison of the incidence of related catheter infection. *Am J Infect Control* 1997;25:148.

302. Powell C, Regan C, Fabri PJ, et al. Evaluation of opsite catheter dressings for parenteral nutrition: a prospective, randomized study. *JPEN J Parenter Enteral Nutr* 1982;6:43–46.

303. Palidar PJ, Simonowitz DA, Oreskovich MR, et al. Use of Op-Site as an occlusive dressing for total parenteral nutrition catheters. *JPEN J Parenter Enteral Nutr* 1982;6:150–151.

304. Nehme AE, Trigger JA. Catheter dressings in central parenteral nutrition: a prospective randomized comparative study. *Nutrition Support Services* 1984;4:42–43.

305. Maki DG, Will L. Colonization and infection associated with transparent dressings for central venous, arterial, and Hickman catheters: a comparative trial [Abstract]. In: *Program and abstracts of the thirty-fourth interscience conference on antimicrobial agents and chemotherapy, October 1994, Orlando, Florida.* Washington, DC: American Society for Microbiology, 1984:253.

306. Powell CR, Traetow MJ, Fabri PJ, et al. Op-site dressing study: a prospective randomized study evaluating povidone iodine ointment and extension set changes with 7-day op-site dressings applied to total parenteral nutrition subclavian sites. *JPEN J Parenter Enteral Nutr* 1985;9:443–446.

307. Young GP, Alexeyeff M, Russell DM, et al. Catheter sepsis during parenteral nutrition: the safety of long-term OpSite dressings. *JPEN J Parenter Enteral Nutr* 1988;12:365–370.

308. Maki DG, Mermel LA, Martin M, et al. A highly-semipermeable polyurethane dressing does not increase the risk of CVC-related BSI: a prospective, multicenter, investigator-blinded trial [Abstract]. In: *Programs and abstracts of the thirty-sixth interscience conference on antimicrobial agents and chemotherapy, September 1996, New Orleans, Louisiana.* Washington, DC: American Society for Microbiology, 1996:230.

309. Shivnan JC, McGuire D, Freeman S, et al. Comparison of transparent adherent and dry sterile gauze dressings for long-term central catheters in patients undergoing bone marrow transplant. *Oncology Nurses Forum* 1991;18:1349–1356.

310. Eyer S, Brummitt C, Crossley K, et al. Catheter-related sepsis: prospective, randomized study of three methods of long-term catheter maintenance. *Crit Care Med* 1990;18:1073–1079.

311. Stenzel JP, Green TP, Fuhrman BP, et al. Percutaneous central venous catheterization in a pediatric intensive care unit: a survival analysis of complications. *Crit Care Med* 1989;17:984–988.

312. Pinilla JC, Ross DF, Martin T, et al. Study of the incidence of intravascular catheter infection and associated septicemia in critically ill patients. *Crit Care Med* 1983;11:21–25.

313. Leroy O, Billiau V, Beuscart C, et al. Nosocomial infections associated with long-term radial artery cannulation. *Intensive Care Med* 1989;15:241–246.

314. Thomas F, Burke JP, Parker J, et al. The risk of infection related to radial vs. femoral sites for arterial catheterization. *Crit Care Med* 1983;11:807–812.

315. Shinozaki T, Deane RS, Mazuzan JE Jr, et al. Bacterial contamination of arterial lines. *JAMA* 1983;249:223–225.

316. Furfaro S, Gauthier M, Lacroix J, et al. Arterial catheter-related infections in children: a 1-year cohort analysis. *American Journal of Diseases of Children* 1991;145:1037–1043.

317. Lederle FA, Parenti CM, Berskow LC, et al. The idle intravenous catheter. *Ann Intern Med* 1992;116:737–738.

318. Parenti C, Lederle FA, Impola CL, et al. Reduction of unnecessary intravenous catheter use: internal medicine house staff participate in a successful quality improvement project. *Arch Intern Med* 1994;154:1829–1832.

319. Andrivet P, Bacquer A, Vu Ngoc C, et al. Lack of clinical benefit from subcutaneous tunnel insertion of central venous catheters in immunocompromised patients. *Clin Infect Dis* 1994;18:199–206.

320. Timsit J-F, Sebile V, Farkas J-C, et al. Effect of subcutaneous tunneling on internal jugular catheter-related sepsis in critically ill patients. A prospective randomized multicenter study. *JAMA* 1996;276:1416–1420.

321. Sitges-Serra A, Linares J, Perez JL, et al. A randomized trial on the effect of tubing changes on hub contamination and catheter sepsis during parenteral nutrition. *JPEN J Parenter Enteral Nutr* 1985;9:322–325.

322. Alothman A, Scharf S, Bryce EA. Extending central venous catheters tubing changes to five days: safety and cost effectiveness. *Programs and Abstracts of the Thirty-Fourth Infectious Diseases Society of America Annual Meeting, October 1994, Orlando, FL.* Washington, DC: Infectious Diseases Society of America, 1994: 861.

323. Moro ML, Maffei C, Manso E, et al. Nosocomial outbreak of systemic candidosis associated with parenteral nutrition. *Infect Control Hosp Epidemiol* 1990;11:27–35.

324. Craver D, Hodges L, Hutchenson K, et al. Baxter infusion pumps and needleless tubings/devices have lower infection control risks and costs for intravenous therapy than Abbott infusion pumps and needleless tubings/devices. *Am J Infect Control* 1994;22:104.

325. McDonald LC, Banerjee SN, Jarvis WR. Line-associated bloodstream infections in pediatric intensive-care-unit patients associated with a needleless device and intermittent intravenous therapy. *Infect Control Hosp Epidemiol.* 1998;19:772–7.

326. Danzig LE, Short LJ, Collins K, et al. Bloodstream infections associated with needleless intravenous infusion system in patients receiving home infusion therapy. *JAMA* 1995;273:1862–1864.

327. Vassallo D, Blanc-Jouvan M, Bret M, et al. Staphylococcus aureus septicemia and a needleless system of infusion [Abstract]. In: *Programs and abstracts of the thirty-fifth interscience conference on antimicrobial agents and chemotherapy, September 1995, San Francisco, California.* Washington, DC: American Society for Microbiology, 1995:259.

328. Maragakis LL, Bradley KL, Song X, Beers C, Miller MR, Cosgrove SE, Perl TM. Increased catheter-related bloodstream infection rates after the introduction of a new mechanical valve intravenous access port. *Infect Control Hosp Epidemiol.* 2006;27:67–70

329. Do AN, Ray BJ, Banerjee SN, Illian AF, Barnett BJ, Pham MH, Hendricks KA, Jarvis WR. Bloodstream infection associated with needleless device use and the importance of infection-control practices in the home health care setting. *J Infect Dis.* 1999 Feb;179(2):442–8.

330. Miller RC, Grogan JB. Incidence and source of contamination of intravenous nutritional infusion systems. *J Pediatr Surg* 1973;8:185–190.

331. Freeman JB, Litton AA. Preponderance of gram-positive infections during parenteral alimentation. *Surg Gynecol Obstet* 1974;139:905–908.

332. Baumgartner TG, Schmidt GL, Thakker KM, et al. Bacterial endotoxin retention by inline intravenous filters. *Am J Hosp Pharm* 1986;43:681–684.

333. Holmes CJ, Kundsin RB, Ausman RK, et al. Potential hazards associated with microbial contamination of in-line filters during intravenous therapy. *J Clin Microbiol* 1980;12:725–731.

334. Falchuk KH, Peterson L, McNeil BJ. Microparticulate-induced phlebitis: its prevention by in-line filtration. *N Engl J Med* 1985;312:78–82.

335. Maddox RR, John JF Jr, Brown LL, et al. Effect of inline filtration on postinfusion phlebitis. *Clin Pharm* 1983;2:58–61.

336. Quercia RA, Hills SW, Klimek JJ, et al. Bacteriologic contamination of intravenous infusion delivery systems in an intensive care unit. *Am J Med* 1986;80:364–368.

337. Ginies JL, Joseph MG, Champion G, et al. Etude prospective de l'efficacite des diltres intibacteriens sur la prevention des complications de la nutrition parenterale centrale chez le nouveau-ne. *Agressologie* 1990;31:495–496.

338. Rapp RP, Brack A, Bivins A, et al. Sepsis in rabbits following administration of contaminated infusions through filters of various pore sizes. *Am J Hosp Pharm* 1979;36:1711–1713.

339. Heggers JP, Stabenau J, Listengarten D, et al. A new efficacious Ag-coated dressing: II. *in vivo* assay [Abstract]. *Am J Infect Control* 1995;23:135.

340. Shapiro JM, Bond EL, Garman JK. Use of a chlorhexidine dressing to reduce microbial colonization of epidural catheters. *Anesthesiology* 1990;73:625–631.

341. Keyserling H, Dykes F, Newsome P, et al. Pilot study of a chlorhexidine disc catheter dressing in a neonatal unit. *NAVAN* 1994;1:12–13.

342. Garland JS, Alex CP, Mueller CD, Otten D, Shivpuri C, Harris MC, Naples M, Pellegrini J, Buck RK, McAuliffe TL, Goldmann DA, Maki DG. A randomized trial comparing povidone-iodine to a chlorhexidine gluconate-impregnated dressing for prevention of central venous catheter infections in neonates. *Pediatrics.* 2001;107:1431–6.

343. Levy I, Katz J, Solter E, Samra Z, Vidne B, Birk E, Ashkenazi S, Dagan O. Chlorhexidine-impregnated dressing for prevention of colonization of central venous catheters in infants and children: a randomized controlled study. *Pediatr Infect Dis J.* 2005;24:676–9.

344. Maki DG, Mermel LA, Klugar D, et al. The efficacy of a chlorhexidine impregnated sponge (Biopatch) for the prevention of intravascular catheter-related infection- a prospective randomized controlled multicenter study [Abstract]. Presented at the Interscience Conference on Antimicrobial Agents and Chemotherapy. Toronto, Ontario, Canada: American Society for Microbiology, 2000.

345. Clementi E, Marie O, Arlet G, et al. Usefulness of an attachable silver-impregnated cuff for prevention of catheter-related sepsis (CRS) [Abstract]. In: *Programs and abstracts of the thirty-first interscience conference on antimicrobial agents and chemotherapy, October 1991, Chicago, Illinois.* Washington, DC: American Society for Microbiology, 1991:175.

346. Tebbs SE, Sawyer A, Elliott TSJ. Influence of surface morphology on in vitro bacterial adherence to central venous catheters. *Br J Anaesth* 1994;72:587–591.

347. wFrancois P, Vaudaux P, Mathiue HJ, et al. Effects of surface treatment on the surface chemistry and topography of central venous catheters (CVC) and on protein-d adhesion of Staphylococcus aureus [Abstract]. In: *Programs and abstracts of the thirty-fourth interscience conference on antimicrobial agents and chemotherapy, October 1994, Orlando, Florida.* Washington, DC: American Society for Microbiology, 1994:194.

348. Neu HC. The crisis in antibiotic resistance. *Science* 1992;257:1064–1072.

349. Liu WK, Tebbs SE, Byrne PO, et al. The effects of electric current on bacteria colonising intravenous catheters. *J Infect* 1993;27:261–269.

350. Raad I, 'Hachem R, Zermeno A. Silver iontophoretic catheter: a prototype of a long-term antiinfective vascular access device. *J Infect Dis* 1996;173:495–498.

351. Segura M, Alvarez-Lerma F, Ma Tellado J, et al. A clinical trial on the prevention of catheter-related sepsis using a new hub model. *Ann Surg* 1996;223:363–369.

352. Menyhay SZ, Maki DG. Disinfection of needleless catheter connectors and access ports with alcohol may not prevent microbial entry: the promise of a novel antiseptic-barrier cap. *Infect Control Hosp Epidemiol.* 2006;27:23–7.

353. Freeman R, Holden MP, Lyon R, et al. Addition of sodium metabisulfite to left atrial catheter infusate as a means of preventing bacterial colonization of the catheter tip. *Thorax* 1982;37:142–144.

354. Root JL, McIntyre OR, Jacobs NJ, et al. Inhibitory effect of disodium EDTA upon growth of Staphylococcus epidermidis in vitro: relation to infection prophylaxis of Hickman catheters. *Antimicrob Agents Chemother* 1983;32:1627–1631.

355. Elliot TSJ, Curran A. Effects of heparin and chlorbutol on bacterial colonisation of intravascular cannulae in an in vitro model. *J Hosp Infect* 1989;14:193–200.

356. Wiernikowski JT, Elder-Thornley D, Dawson S, et al. Bacterial colonization of tunneled right atrial catheters in pediatric oncology: a comparison of sterile saline and bacteriostatic flush solutions. *American Journal of Pediatric Hematology and Oncology* 1991;13:137–140.

357. Kropec A, Huebner J, Frank U, et al. In vitro activity of sodium bisulfite and heparin against staphylococci: new strategies in the treatment of catheter-related infection. *J Infect Dis* 1993;168:235–237.

358. Henrickson KJ, Axtell RA, Hoover SM, Kuhn SM, Pritchett J, Kehl SC, Klein JP. Prevention of central venous catheter-related infections and thrombotic events in immunocompromised children by the use of vancomycin/ciprofloxacin/heparin flush solution: A randomized, multicenter, double-blind trial. *J Clin Oncol.* 2000;18:1269–78.

359. Garland JS, Alex CP, Henrickson KJ, McAuliffe TL, Maki DG. A vancomycin-heparin lock solution for prevention of nosocomial bloodstream infection in critically ill neonates with peripherally inserted central venous catheters: a prospective, randomized trial. *Pediatrics.* 2005;116:198–205.

360. Safdar N, Maki DG. Use of vancomycin-containing lock or flush solutions for prevention of bloodstream infection associated with central venous access devices: a meta-analysis of prospective, randomized trials. *Clin Infect Dis.* 2006;43:474–84.

361. Bleyer AJ, Mason L, Russell G, Raad II, Sherertz RJ. A randomized, controlled trial of a new vascular catheter flush solution (minocycline-EDTA) in temporary hemodialysis access. *Infect Control Hosp Epidemiol.* 2005;26:520–4.

362. Berenholtz SM, Pronovost PJ, Lipsett PA, Hobson D, Earsing K, Farley JE, Milanovich S, Garrett-Mayer E, Winters BD, Rubin HR, Dorman T, Perl TM. Eliminating catheter-related bloodstream infections in the intensive care unit. *Crit Care Med.* 2004;;32:2014–20.

363. Wachter RM, Pronovost PJ. The 100,000 lives campaign: A scientific and policy review. *Jt Comm J Qual Patient Saf.* 2006; 32:621–7.

364. Centers for Disease Control and Prevention (CDC). Reduction in central line-associated bloodstream infections among patients in intensive care units–Pennsylvania, April 2001-March 2005. *MMWR Morb Mortal Wkly Rep.* 2005 14;54:1013–6.

365. Braun BI, Kritchevsky SB, Wong ES, Solomon SL, Steele L, Richards CL, Simmons BP; Evaluation of Processes and Indicators in Infection Control Study Group. Preventing central venous catheter-associated primary bloodstream infections: characteristics of practices among hospitals participating in the Evaluation of Processes and Indicators in Infection Control (EPIC) study. *Infect Control Hosp Epidemiol.* 2003;24: 926–35.

366. Maki DG, Kluger DM, Crnich CJ. The risk of bloodstream infection in adults with different intravascular devices: a systematic review of 200 published prospective studies. *Mayo Clin Proc.* 2006;81:1159–71.

367. Safdar N, Maki DG. Risk of catheter-related bloodstream infection with peripherally inserted central venous catheters used in hospitalized patients. *Chest.* 2005;128:489–95.

368. Rosenthal VD, Maki DG. Prospective study of the impact of open and closed infusion systems on rates of central venous catheter-associated bacteremia. *Am J Infect Control.* 2004;32: 135–41.

369. Safdar N, Maki DG. The pathogenesis of catheter-related bloodstream infection with noncuffed short-term central venous catheters. *Intensive Care Med.* 2004;30:62–7.

370. Safdar N, Kluger DM, Maki DG. A review of risk factors for catheter-related bloodstream infection caused by percutaneously inserted, noncuffed central venous catheters: implications for preventive strategies. *Medicine (Baltimore).* 2002;81: 466–79.

371. Crnich CJ, Maki DG. The promise of novel technology for the prevention of intravascular device-related bloodstream infection. I. Pathogenesis and short-term devices. *Clin Infect Dis.* 2002;34:1232–42.

372. Crnich CJ, Maki DG. The promise of novel technology for the prevention of intravascular device-related bloodstream infection. II. Long-term devices. *Clin Infect Dis.* 2002;34:1362–8.

Infections of Implantable Cardiac and Vascular Devices

38

Raymond Chinn

INTRODUCTION

In response to the Centers for Disease Control and Prevention (CDC) report that heart disease is the leading cause of death for both men and women in the United States, strategies to prevent and manage cardiovascular disease have become national healthcare priorities [1]. Significant technological advances have made it possible to circumvent the natural history of cardiovascular disease by providing implantable devices that replace or bypass the failing components of the cardiovascular system. Doing so, these devices can salvage a limb or sustain life by maintaining hemodynamic and electrical stability. Prosthetic valves, permanent pacemakers, implantable cardioverter-defibrillators (ICD), left ventricular assist devices (LVAD), total artificial hearts, vascular stents, vascular patches, and vascular grafts are included in this group of devices.

The incidence of device associated-infection (DAIs) varies and depends on the type of implanted device (Table 38-1). In most instances, DAIs are rare (the notable exception are LVADs with infection rates between 25–75%), but their occurrence is associated with significant morbidity and mortality.

Most patients who develop implantable cardiac or vascular DAIs are in older age groups; have required frequent hospitalizations; have significant comorbid conditions, such as diabetes and renal failure; and often are subjected to intense antibiotic pressure, the latter resulting in colonization and subsequent healthcare-associated infection (HAI) with multidrug-resistant organisms. The implanted devices are made of inert materials with inherent properties to overcome immunologic barrier that would confer a survival advantage for patients. However, exposure of the foreign body to microbes results in the elaboration of a biofilm that contributes to the persistence of DAIs. Mechanical failure, thromboembolic events, and anticoagulation-associated bleeding also compromise DAIs' longevity and functional capabilities and such complication increase with the duration of device use.

This chapter examines the pathogenesis common to all implantable cardiac and vascular DAIs in healthcare settings, reviews specific DAIs, discusses the strategies to prevent HAIs, and identifies further research needs. The chapter does not discuss DAIs related to central lines or vascular access for dialysis settings, which are reviewed elsewhere.

PATHOGENESIS

Following the implantation of a medical device, successful integration occurs when host cells adhere to the surface of the device, multiply, and form granulation tissue that envelops the device and renders it resistant to invasion by microorganisms. However, in a permissive host, this normal event is replaced by adhesion of microbes onto the

TABLE 38-1

INCIDENCE OF IMPLANTABLE CARDIAC AND VASCULAR-ASSOCIATED INFECTIONS [ADAPTED FROM 2–4]

Type of Prosthesis Intracardiac	Incidence of Infection (%; Range, Median)
Prosthetic valves[a]	3.1%–6.4%
Permanent pacemaker	<6%
Implantable defibrillator	<4%
Left ventricular assist device[b]	25–70% (40%)
Coronary stents	Rare
Pledgets, conduits, patches, plugs	Rare
Arterial	
Vascular grafts[c]	1–6% (4%)
Peripheral vascular stents	Rare
Carotid Dacron patches	Rare
Closure devices	≤1.9%

[a]Within the first year, 5–7 years, 15 years
[b]Calculated for various time periods (occurring ≤3 months of implant)
[c]Includes arteriovenous, femoropopliteal, aortic grafts (overall rate)

device. The majority of implanted DAIs are caused by the staphylococci; *Staphylococcus aureus* produces a number of adherence molecules collectively known as the *microbial surface components recognizing adhesive matrix molecules* (MSCRAMM). These molecules bind the microorganisms onto the surface of medical devices after interacting with host plasma proteins such as fibronectin and fibrinogen, a process similar to the implicated pathogenesis for infective endocarditis [2,5,6]. The exposure of host plasma proteins results from increased turbulence due to an alteration of the normal cardiovascular flow and from the physiologic shear rates caused by the implanted device. An in vitro model suggests that the shear stress induces apoptosis of neutrophils, thereby preventing the host's first line of immunologic response from fully activating [7–9]. In this setting, elaboration of microbial virulence factors overcomes the host's immunologic barrier and initiates a cascade of events that culminates in the formation of an intricate extracellular matrix, the biofilm. Within the confines of the biofilm, the microbes reside and create an environment that is relatively impervious to antimicrobials and resistant to the innate host defenses. The presence of an avascular foreign body enhances the risk of surgical site infections (SSIs), by reducing the infecting dose of microorganisms that cause SSIs.

Microorganisms attach to medical devices in the free-floating (plaktonic) form, divide, interact, become embedded in a biofilm and then transforming into the surface-associated form. An adhesive matrix then creates a protective complex that becomes heterogenous with multiple channels providing transporting nutrients and oxygen to the microorganisms within the biofilm. The surface cells divide, and as the thickness of the biofilm increases, the host's normal immune response to microbiologic challenge is blunted, and the capacity of the host neutrophil's ability to phagocytize, affect intracellular killing, and proliferate is diminished. Microorganisms embedded in biofilms are much more resistant than planktonic cells to antimicrobials and can survive despite concentrations 10–1,000 times what is necessary to eradicate plaktonic forms. In a suspended state of activity, these forms become resistant to the cell wall, growth-phase-dependent antimicrobials, such as penicillin, cephalosporins, and vancomycin. In the deeper layers of the biofilm, microorganisms require less nutritional support and are better able to tolerate environments of lower oxygen tension, a characteristic that renders the microorganism resistant to the aminoglycosides, agents maximally effective in aerobic conditions [10,11]. Clinically, the persistence of DAIs caused by *S. aureus* and *Staphylococcus lugdunensis* has been attributed to small colony variant phenotypes that can exchange genetic material codes for an antimicrobial-resistant phenotype that ensures their survival [12,13]. Biofilms have been most studied in *S. aureus*; however, emerging evidence suggests their role in the pathogenesis of DAIs due to coagulase-negative staphylococci (CoNS), *Pseudomonas aeruginosa*, and other gram-negative rods, enterococci, and *Candida albicans* [14–20].

Comorbid conditions, such as diabetes mellitus, have deleterious effects on chemotaxis, phagocytosis, and adherence of granulocytes, components in the initial line of defense against invading microbes [21,22]. Hyperglycemia, especially in the immediate postoperative period, is a risk factor for SSIs as described in the cardiac bypass literature [23–26].

Microbial exposure can occur with intraoperative contamination, as a result of hematogenous seeding from a secondary bloodstream infection (BSI) and from an extension of a local infection as occurs with pacemaker or ICD infections. Whether microbial exposure results in infection depends on microbial virulence factors and the host's response to the implanted device. Once the protective biofilm forms, eradication of the infection requires not only appropriate antimicrobial therapy but also, more importantly, explantation of the implanted cardiac or vascular device.

PROSTHETIC VALVE ENDOCARDITIS

Epidemiology

More than 60,000 patients per year undergo heart valve replacement in the United States [7]. Prosthetic valves are either mechanical that are constructed of carbon alloys, a ball-and-cage, single tilting disk, or bi-leaflet tilting disk (most common) configuration or bioprosthetic valves that include porcine heterografts, bovine pericardium constructed into three cusps mounted on a stent, and the rarely used homografts, that are preserved human aortic valves or pulmonary autografts [28].

Traditionally, prosthetic valve endocarditis (PVE) is classified as early (occurring <60 days of implantation), intermediate (2–12 months), or late (>12 months). CoNS is the pathogen commonly isolated in early PVE and attributed to intraoperative contamination or hematogenous seeding during BSI from other sites such as central venous catheters. However, patients infected with CoNS, a fairly indolent organism, may not have clinical manifestations until the intermediate period. Therefore, for surveillance purposes, the CDC's National Healthcare Safety Network (NHSN; formerly the National Nosocomial Infections Surveillance, or NNIS, system) defines a healthcare-associated postoperative SSI as any SSI that occurs within 1 year of device implantation [29].

The incidence of PVE varies according to the duration of the follow-up period and is estimated to be around 3.1% (data from 1980s) during the first 12 months. The risk of infection is highest within the first 3 months and declines to a fairly constant rate of 0.3–0.6% annually thereafter [30–34]. A recent early PVE study (occurring <12 months after valve surgery) of 77 patients reported decreasing rates comparing two periods, 1.5% in 1992–1994 versus 0.7% in 1995–1997 [35]. A long-term study of the Veterans Affairs population in the 1990s reported the incidence of PVE to increase from 3–5.7% at 5 years to 13% at 15 years [36].

Risk Factors

Risk factors associated with PVE include implantation of multiple prostheses [30], longer cardiopulmonary bypass time [37], valve replacement in the setting of infective endocarditis, New York Heart Association (NYHA) functional class III or IV, alcohol consumption, fever in the intensive care unit, gastrointestinal bleeding, and healthcare-associated blood stream infection (HA-BSI) [32, 37–40]. Three studies reviewed the risk of PVE in patients who developed HA-BSI and reported rates between 11–50%. Investigators of one study of 51 patients reported that approximately half of the patients with a prosthetic valve (PV) or a ring who developed *S. aureus* BSI (SA-BSI) had definite evidence of PVE at the time of the BSI (using the modified Duke criteria [41,42]) and that the risk was independent of the type, location, or age of the PV or ring. The most common source of early (<12 months of valve placement) SA-BSI was SSIs (59%), whereas patients with late SA-BSI (>1 year after valve placement) had an unidentified source of BSI in 48% of patients. Hallmark features of definite PVE in this study were persistent fever and sustained BSI [43]. In the second study of 171 patients with PVs (excluding 33% of patients who had a diagnosis

of PVE at the time of the BSI), 15% of patients developed PVE with a mean of 45 days after documentation of the BSI despite having received antimicrobial therapy. Thirty-three percent was attributed to BSI due to intravascular devices, and skin infections accounted for another 30%; the mitral valve site and Staphylococcal spp. BSI were significantly associated with the development of PVE [44]. The third study describes 37 patients with PV who had no evidence of PVE during the initial 4-week follow-up period after documentation of postoperative candidemia; 11% of patients who had sustained fungemia developed fungal PVE [45]. The studies highlight the importance of preventing BSI and skin infections following PV placement.

Early studies comparing mechanical with bioprosthetic valve and aortic versus mitral site on the incidence of PVE were inconclusive; however, a recent study reported that the incidence of early PVE (occurring <12 months of implantation) was similar in mechanical and bioprosthetic valves. After a longer observation period, the incidence of PVE was higher with bioprosthetic valves due to the platelet-fibrin thrombus deposition on aging leaflets that can become a nidus for infection [31]. In early PVE, infection develops along the suture lines of the prosthesis-annulus interface and perivalvular tissue with resultant dehiscence of sutures. Late infection is similar to native valve endocarditis and begins with platelet-fibrin thrombi deposition on the prosthesis followed by adherence of microorganisms. Early PVE was significantly lower for prosthetic mitral valve than for aortic valve placement [31,35].

Although outbreaks of healthcare-associated PVE are uncommon, they have been described for *Mycobacterium chelonei* due to contamination of the bioprosthetic valve [46]; *Staphylococcus epidermidis* in association with surgical staff carriage [47–49]; *Legionella pneumophila* and *L. dumoffii* from exposure of wounds and chest/mediastinal tubes to tap water in a healthcare facility [50]; and *Candida parapsilosis* possibly related to torn gloves used by the surgical team [51]. Refinements in molecular typing techniques have enabled investigators to link outbreaks to a common source.

In early studies, PVE was associated with mortality rates of 10–70%. Recent reports indicate that the PVE mortality rates are between 4–20% and likely reflect earlier detection, more optimal use of combination antibiotic therapy, and prompt surgical intervention [4]. Risk factors for higher mortality rates resulting from PVE include early PVE (≤1 year of onset), Staphylococcal spp. infection, presentation or development of heart failure, infections involving the aortic valve, and medical management alone. Management of *S. aureus* PVE with surgical intervention was associated with a 28% mortality rate in contrast to 48% in the medical group in one study [52]. American Society of Anethesiology (ASA) class IV and bioprosthetic valves were independent predictors of mortality when subjected to multivariable analysis. A subset of medically treated

TABLE 38-2
ETIOLOGY OF PROSTHETIC VALVE ENDOCARDITIS [ADAPTED FROM 31 AND 35]

| | Number of Cases (%) | |
| | Time of Onset of PVE | |
Organism	<12 months N = 269	>12 months N = 194
Streptococcus (excludes enterococcus)	12 (4%)	61 (31%)
Enterococcus	23 (8%)	22 (11%)
Staphylococcus aureus	48 (18%)	34 (18%)
Coagulase-negative staphylococci	102 (38%)	22 (11%)
Diphtheroids	10 (4%)	5 (3%)
Gram-negative bacilli	24 (9%)	11 (6%)
HACEK[a]	0	11 (6%)
Fungi/yeast	26 (10%)	3 (1%)
Polymicrobial/other	6 (2%)	9 (5%)
Culture negative	9 (3%)	16 (8%)

[a]HACEK, *Haemophilus aphrophilus, Actinobacillus actinomycetemcomitans, Cardiobacterium hominis, Eikenella species, and Kingella species* (fastidious gram-negative rods).

patients characterized by age <50 years, ASA score III, and the absence of cardiac, central nervous system, and systemic complications was cured without surgical intervention.

Microbiology

In early PVE, the predominant organisms (in decreasing order of frequency) are CoNS, *S. aureus*, fungi/yeast, gram-negative bacilli, and enterococci (Table 38-2). In contrast, the nonenterococcal streptococci are the most common pathogens in late PVE, similar to native valve endocarditis (excluding the intravenous drug–using population). In late PVE, CoNS remains a common pathogen while the HACEK bacteria, uncommon in early PVE, emerge as pathogens.

Clinical Manifestations, Diagnosis, and Therapy of Prosthetic Valve Endocarditis

Fever is a common manifestation of PVE, and the presence of sustained fever in a patient with a PV, regardless of the timing of implantation, should prompt a clinical investigation to confirm or exclude the diagnosis. Often it is tempting in clinical practice to attribute fever in the postoperative patient to a urinary tract infection or early pneumonia and initiate empiric antibiotic therapy based on clinical suspicion. However, in patients with PVs, it is a good practice to obtain blood cultures before initiating empiric antibiotics to avoid missing a diagnosis of PVE. Salient clinical features of PVE show similarities with native valve endocarditis and

are determined by the time of onset, the virulence of the pathogen, and host responses. Patients with PVE due a pathogen such as *S. aureus* can present with fulminant sepsis in association with central nervous system emboli and hemorrhagic events with intracardiac manifestations (e.g., acute valvular failure, conduction abnormalities, and progression of perivalvular infection) resulting in rapid cardiac decompensation and with septic peripheral emboli. In contrast, infections caused by the more indolent organisms, such as CoNS, are associated with a subacute presentation characterized by peripheral stigmata of endocarditis (autoimmune arthralgias/arthritis, Osler nodes, Janeway lesions).

In the absence of antibiotic exposure, it is estimated that blood culture would be positive in $\geq$90% of patients with PVE [4]. Isolation of organisms such as *S. aureus* and *Candida* spp. without evidence of a secondary source of infection is likely due to PVE. However, ascertaining the significance of the isolation of skin organisms, such as CoNS and diphtheroids could be difficult unless there is demonstration of persistent BSI with suggestive clinical and echocardiographic features. With refinements of molecular typing techniques, confirmation of the presence of clonality is possible and helpful when it is important to distinguish pathogens from contaminants; however, the possibility of polymicrobial infections also should be considered [4,53].

As with native valve endocarditis, the modified Duke criteria are used to establish a diagnosis of PVE [41,42]. Echocardiographic findings, therapy (need for bactericidal antimicrobial agents, issues with combination therapy, treatment of multidrug-resistant pathogens, and optimal use of pharmacodynamic strategies), and indications for surgical intervention are beyond the scope of this chapter and discussed elsewhere [4,31].

LEFT VENTRICULAR ASSIST DEVICES

Introduction

Heart failure compromises the health of >5,000,000 Americans; 550,000 new patients are diagnosed with this disease each year. Each year, approximately 250,000 persons in the United States develop severe, end-stage heart failure (NYHA Class IV) and are candidates for transplantation. Limited donor availability has narrowed the therapeutic options for this group of patients, estimated to be up to 5,000 at any one time for heart transplantation, a staggering figure when one considers that only about 2,400 heart transplants are performed each year [54].

The introduction of the LVAD catapulted the management of severe end-stage cardiomopathy refractory to ionotropic therapy, intraaortic balloon counterpulsation, or both into a new era. The device was originally approved in 1994 by the Food and Drug Administration as a bridge to transplantation. Subsequent studies demonstrated that the use of the LVAD was associated with improvement in hemodynamic and end-organ function and conferred a meaningful survival benefit in implanted patients as compared with controls managed with medical therapy alone, with an impressive 70% of patients surviving until heart transplantation [55,56]. Furthermore, following transplantation, the survival at 3 years was 95% ± 4% for the LVAD group and 65% ± 10% years for the control group managed with inotropes alone. The survival for LVAD-implanted patients was 95% at 3 years compared with 65% in the control group [57]. Even in the presence of LVAD-associated infections, heart transplantation recipients had similar outcomes when compared with patients without infection [58–60]. A later study detected a doubling of LVAD-support days that could delay transplantation, a trend for longer hospital stays posttransplant and increased early mortality resulting from a newly acquired infection in the cohort with LVAD-related infection [61–63]. The long-term survival was not statistically significant when compared with patients on LVAD support who developed an LVAD-associated infection. These important findings quiet the unease of subjecting LVAD-associated infected patients to intense immunosuppression following their transplants for fear of aggravating their infections [61].

When it became apparent that patients managed with the LVAD had better outcomes compared to their medically treated counterparts, the indications for LVAD implantation broadened to include those ineligible for transplantation (destination therapy). The Randomized Evaluation of Mechanical Assistance for the Treatment of Congestive Heart Failure (REMATCH) trial investigated the use of LVADs for destination therapy: 41% of deaths in the LVAD recipient group resulted from sepsis of any cause; within three months after implantation, the probability of an HAI-related to the LVAD was 28% [56]. The Kaplan-Meier survival analysis did show a 48% reduction in the risk of death from any cause in those patients randomized to LVAD implantation during the first year. However, the aggregate adverse event rate was twice as likely to occur in LVAD patients. By the second year of study, the survival rate of 23% between the two groups was not statistically significant. Those LVAD patients who did not have sepsis had superior survival rates of 60% at 1 year and 38% at 2 years compared with 39% and 8%, respectively, in LVAD patients who developed sepsis. Localized infections such as percutaneous site and pocket infection did not have an adverse impact on survival [64]. An additional 2 years of observation in the REMATCH trial revealed that patients randomized to LVAD implantation in the period after 2000 had a statistically significantly higher survival rate of 59% at 1 year and 38% at 2 years when compared to the 44% and 21% rates, respectively, for the medically treated group. The improved survival rate in patients implanted during the second study period was attributed to the experience gained in areas of patient care and device modifications [65].

A review of 46 patients with LVAD-associated infections (the most common being the driveline site) noted that infections developed at an average of 65 days postimplantation with a mortality rate of 17% (8 patients) with (5/8) infected patients dying from sepsis before transplantation [63]. Postoperative LVAD-associated infections were identified in 46% of 35 patients in whom 36 LVADs were implanted for a mean of 73 days. Deep SSIs were associated with the requirement for postoperative hemodialysis [66].

Epidemiology

The LVAD infection attack rate is about 34% and likely reflects the population studied (Table 38-3).

A report on nosocomial LVAD-associated BSIs in 214 patients revealed an incidence of 38%; the BSI was statistically significantly associated with death (the overall incidence of BSI in recipients of LVADs from any cause was 49%). Fungemia had the highest hazard ratio (10.9) followed by gram-negative (with *Pseudomonas aeruginosa* predominating) and gram-positive bacteremia. The duration of LVAD support before the onset of any BSI was 19.5 days for gram-negative bacilli, 28 days for yeast, and 242 days for gram-positive cocci [62]. Forty-six LVAD-associated infections were described in 50% (38/76) of patients who underwent LVAD implantation as a bridge to transplantation. Twenty-nine LVAD-associated BSIs included 5 LVAD endocarditis and 17 localized LVAD infection (exit site, LVAD pocket infections) [61].

The Jarvik 2000 LVAD designed for permanent use was compared to the more conventional HeartMate® [Thoratec] LVAD; although only 17 patients were studied, implantation of the HeartMate® was associated with a 0.43 device-related infections per 100 patient-days compared with 0.08 device-related infections per 100 patient-days when the Jarvik 2000 was implanted. The authors postulated that the decrease in infection risk could be due to the smaller size of the Jarvik 2000 and the unique power cable that is tunneled to the retroauricular skull area connected to the power supply [67].

TABLE 38-3

LEFT VENTRICULAR-ASSOCIATED DEVICE INFECTIONS/SURGICAL SITE INFECTIONS

Reference	Patients Device Days	Number of Patients	Infected (%)
Gordon, 2001 [69]	17,831	214	53 (25%)[a]
Malani, 2002 [71]	2,565	35	16 (31)
Simon, 2005 [66]	9,466	76	38 (50)

[a]Included only LVAD infections with bacteremia.

Microbiology

The microbiology of LVAD-associated infections is fairly consistent with gram-positive organisms predominating and likely resulting from disruption of the cutaneous barrier with the subsequent biofilm formation. *S. aureus* was the most common organism isolated in one series followed by gram-negative rods, *candida*, *Enterococcus* sp., and CoNS [63]. Another series found that CoNS was the most frequent pathogen isolated in BSIs in LVAD-implanted patients from any cause followed by *S. aureus* (of which 36% were methicillin resistant), *Candida* sp., and *Pseudomonas aeruginosa*. Although the enterococci accounted for only about 8% of BSIs, 50% of the isolates were vancomycin resistant [62].

A recent report of 76 LVAD-patients noted that of 47 isolates, 78% and 19% of LVAD-associated infections were due to gram-positive organisms and gram-negative rods, respectively, with only 1 infection due to yeast. Diabetes mellitus was identified as a risk factor for the 30 BSIs in this cohort. There was a striking incidence of post-transplantation invasive vancomycin-resistant *Enterococcus faecium* (VREF) infections in 6 patients with an associated mortality of 67%. This is in marked contrast to LVAD-support patients who did not develop LVAD-associated infections in whom there was no postoperative invasive VREF [61].

Emerging evidence suggests that LVAD implantation is associated with progressive defects of cellular immunity by inducing an aberrant activation of T-cells, resulting in program CD4 cell death [68–70]. Ankersnitt et al. concluded that defects in cellular immunity predisposes patients to infections caused by *Candida* sp., and the risk of developing disseminated candidiasis in that study was 28% in LVAD recipients compared to 3% of controls [68]. This finding coupled with the fact that advanced age (patients on destination therapy) also is associated with decreased cellular immunity [14] introduces major challenges ahead for mechanical circulatory support [71].

Types of Left Ventricular Assist Device-Associated Infections, Diagnosis, and Management

The components of the LVAD (e.g., HeartMate) consist of an intracorporeal blood pump encased in titanium (placed in the abdominal cavity or preperitoneal pocket), an inflow cannula (inserted into the apex of the left ventricle) an outflow cannula (inserted into the ascending aorta), and porcine valves within the inflow and outflow cannulas to maintain unidirectional flow. Implantation of the LVAD requires an extended median sternotomy. A driveline connects the blood pump to an external power source that exits through the abdominal wall, usually contralateral to the side of the pump (Figure 38-1).

Although the driveline is tunneled before exiting the abdomen, its size and the bulk of the battery pack increase the risk of skin trauma resulting in the loss of the protective skin barrier and permits invasion by microorganisms.

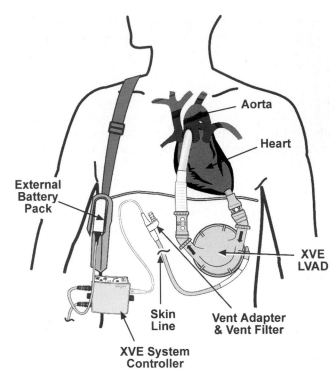

Figure 38-1 HeartMate™ left ventricular assist device (LVAD).

The spectrum of LVAD-associated infections is categorized according to the anatomical site and are not mutually exclusive: (1) driveline exit site (Figure 38-2), (2) pump pocket (Figure 38-3), and the least frequent (3) endocarditis [2,4,61,62]. Pathogens causing LVAD infections can result from intraoperative inoculation from entry through the percutaneous driveline exit site or from hematogenous seeding from central venous catheter-associated BSIs, catheter-associated urinary tract infection, and ventilator-associated

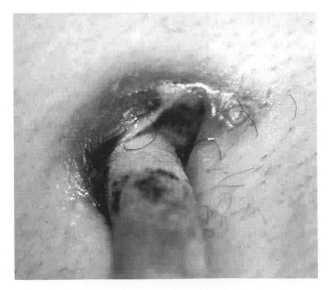

Figure 38-2 Driveline exit site infection.

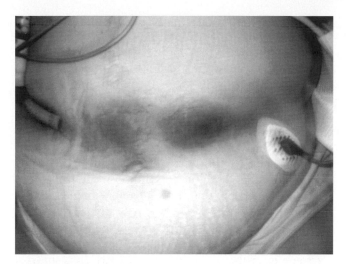

Figure 38-3 Pump pocket infection.

pneumonia. In driveline exit site infections, there often is evidence of localized inflammation at the exit site accompanied by poor tissue healing; seropurulent/purulent drainage can be present with variable systemic manifestations of infection. In the early phases of driveline exit site infection, it could be difficult to differentiate irritation from an inadequately immobilized driveline from infection because pain and erythema are common features to both situations.

Pump pocket infections can result from secondary infection of a localized hematoma and seroma from the operative procedure or inadvertent trauma. The clinical presentation depends on the pathogenicity of the microorganism. Characteristic features of infection could be absent, and infection could be suspected on the basis of unexplained leukocytosis, generalize malaise, and low-grade fevers. In some instances, palpation over the incision can lead to discovery of an abscess [72].

LVAD-associated endocarditis is characterized by involvement of the surface components of the mechanical device that is in contact with blood: the blood pump and the inflow or outflow tracts. It shares many of the clinical features diagnostic of infective endocarditis (i.e., persistent BSI, systemic signs and symptoms [e.g., fever, toxicity, emboli, immune complex disease, valvular incompetence]).

Radiographic studies (e.g., echocardiography, computed tomography, and nuclear imaging for abscess localization) are of limited value in the presence of hardware and the absence of standards for interpretation but could be helpful identifying a fluid collection(s) that could lead to a diagnostic aspiration.

Distinguishing LVAD-related BSI from a non-LVAD-related BSI can be difficult; however, identical microorganisms recovered from the device (e.g., valves, internal pump surface, and pump pocket) and the bloodstream would suggest an LVAD-associated BSI. Single positive blood cultures for cutaneous organisms (e.g., CoNS, diphtheroids) should

be interpreted with caution because these organisms are common causes of pseudobacteremia; therefore, multiple cultures are necessary to interpret results correctly.

Management

The therapy of LVAD-associated infections depends on the infected site. Driveline exit site and pocket infections are managed by (1) aggressive wound care, (2) immobilization of the driveline to avoid further tissue trauma, (3) gentle debridement of devitalized tissue and cleansing of exit site, and (4) exploration of the pump pocket as indicated. Use of polymethylmethacrylate (PMMA) beads containing vancomycin and tobramycin (and potentially other antimicrobial agents) that coat the external surface of the LVAD is an experimental approach to managing pocket infection [72,73], but more research is warranted to determine optimum bead material, size, shape, and positioning. Placement of a KCI vacuum-assisted closure (VAC) device (WoundVac™) is reported to be beneficial after appropriate drainage and debridement of large wounds [74].

LVAD-associated endocarditis usually requires device removal, urgent transplantation, and bactericidal antibiotics [59,75,76]. A report by Nurozler et al. on fungal endocarditis in which early diagnosis, prompt institution of antimicrobials, and device removal and replacement followed by transplantation was associated with a 80% favorable outcome in 5 patients [77].

Culture results dictate the choice of systemic bactericidal antibiotics. Continuous antimicrobial treatment before, during, and after transplantation was associated with fewer relapses when compared to limited courses of antibiotics ($p < .001$). Discontinuing antibiotics after a 2–6 week course was associated with relapse or a secondary infection; however, the survival rates for the two groups at 1 year were similar [61]. Treatment strategies include the use of a suppressive component for destination therapy patients with recalcitrant infections in whom device exchange is associated with prohibitive risks. However, with increasing duration of device utilization, pathogens tend to be multidrug-resistant, and therapy relies on parenteral and potentially nephrotoxic agents.

To minimize the sequelae of intraoperative contamination during device implantation, some centers use a combination of five different perioperative antibiotics including vancomycin, a quinolone, rifampin, fluconazaole, and a β-lactam or a monobactam for 48–72 hours [66]; other institutions recommend a quinolone or β-lactam plus vancomycin [61]. Preoperative colonization (e.g., tracheal aspirates from ventilated patients or wounds) and infection should be considered when choosing preoperative prophylactic agents. The impact of broadspectrum antimicrobial prophylaxis on the emergence of multidrug-resistant organisms has not been formally evaluated but is a perceived risk.

TOTAL ARTIFICIAL HEARTS

The total artificial heart (TAH) was designed to provide the necessary mechanical support for patients with severe biventricular failure that is refractory to inotropic therapy and replaces both native cardiac ventricles and all cardiac valves. Indications for use include aortic insufficiency, severe ventricular arrhythmias, left ventricular thrombus, and calcified left ventricular aneurysm. It is also considered for those patients who are not transplant candidates by virtue of their underlying disease, such as amyloidosis and cardiotoxicity from chemotherapy, diffuse cardiac tumors, failure, heart transplants from graft failed and rejection, the latter group being candidates for destination therapy [78].

Two TAHs, the CardioWest Total Artificial Heart and Abiocor, are currently under investigation. The CardioWest Total Artificial Heart uses pneumatic drives and shares the same characteristics with the LVAD in terms infection risk (i.e., the presence of an external drive line). A bridge to transplantation study of 81 patients reported a 79% survival rate in the study group compared with 46% in the control, medically treated group. The 1-year survival for TAH recipients was 70%. This cohort included 17 driveline infections, 7 BSIs (6 associated with an infusion catheter), and 5 mediastinal infections. In 68 patients, there were no delays to transplantation or deaths due to infection. Transplantation was delayed in 5 patients due to any infection; when further stratified, 3 infections were related to the TAH: 2 drivelines and 1 mediastinum. Seven deaths were attributed to infection from any cause; one was from mediastinitis [79].

The AbioCor TAH, targeted for destination patients, uses an electrohydraulic actuator system. The 30-day survival for the first 7 patients was 71% compared to 13% predicted survival for patients medically treated; at 60 days, the survival was 43%. When reviewed in 2004, two patients were still alive at 234 and 181 days. No DAIs were reported in this small cohort, and it is believed that the absence of a percutaneous external access decreases the risk of infection significantly in eliminating a portal of entry for microorganisms. The large size of this TAH, however, increases the risk for increase thrombosis [80].

CARDIAC RHYTHM MANAGEMENT DEVICE INFECTIONS

Cardiac rhythm management devices (CRMD) include permanent pacemakers and implantable cardioverter defibrillators (ICD) that provide electrical stability to patients with ischemic cardiomopathy or other conditions that place them at risk for fatal ventricular arrhythmias. Implantation of CRMDs involves subcutaneously inserting a generator or defibrillator into the chest (most common) or abdominal wall; lead wires are threaded into the soft tissues, enter at the subclavian vein, and gain access to the right side of the heart; the electrodes are implanted in the right atrium and/or right ventricular endocardium.

It is estimated that 3.25 million pacemakers worldwide and 180,000 cardioverter defibrillators with 300,000 CRMDs are implanted in the United States annually with reported infection rates that vary from 1–7% [2,3,81], the lower rates due to device refinement and improved technique.

A variety of CRMD-associated infections have been described and are not mutually exclusive: (1) device pocket infection that can or cannot involve the lead wires, (2) infection that is limited to the lead wires in the subcutaneous space, and (3) endocarditis that involves the transvenous component of the electrode with consequent infection of the endocardium at the tip of the electrode or at the tricuspid valve [82,83]. In a study of 33 episodes of pacemaker-associated endocarditis, three settings were noted with equal distribution: (1) infection localized to the pacemaker, (2) pacemaker lead infection combined with the involvement of either the right or left side, and (3) infection of the valve independent of the pacemaker leads. In two-thirds of the episodes, endocarditis involved the valvular structures that surprisingly included the left side [84]. Of 123 patients with CRMD-associated infections, 25% occurred in the first 4 weeks, and 42% occurred 1 year following implantation. Infections that develop >60 days tend to be more indolent [81].

Host-related issues, comorbid conditions, and procedure-related challenges associated with pacemaker infections are similar to those described for other cardiovascular surgical procedures and include diabetes mellitus, advanced age, use of steroids/immunosuppressive agents, malnutrition, chronic skin conditions, underlying malignancy, anticoagulant use, and multiple manipulations rather than complicated implantations [2,84,85]. Secondary BSI can seed the implanted device, and localized trauma resulting in hematomas can cause tension along the suture line, disrupt the skin barrier, and expose the implant.

The predominant pathogen causing CRMD-associated infections is *Staphylococci* spp. [83]; other skin pathogens that have been implicated in pocket infections include *Corynebacteria* sp., *Propionibacterium acnes*, and *Micrococcus* which result when the device erodes through the skin. In one series of 87 pacemaker-associated and 36 ICD-associated infections, the most common pathogens were CoNS (68%), *S. aureus* (23%), and enteric gram-negative bacilli (13%) [81]. Instances of *Candida* sp. and fungi such as aspergillus are rare [86–88]. Fungal infections occurred at the rate of 0.1% (3,648 procedures); associated risk factors include abdominal placement, local versus systemic infection, and longer duration from original implant to presentation.

Chamis studied a cohort of patients with CRMD and *S. aureus* BSI (SA-BSI) over a 6-year period. The total number of confirmed CRMD infections was 45.4% (15/33) episodes of SA-BSI. Nine of 12 patients (75%) were

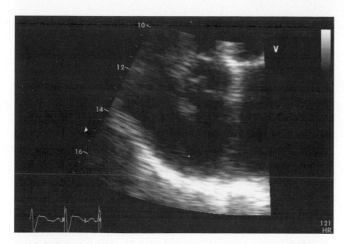

Figure 38-4 Large vegetation on tricuspid valve adjacent to pacemaker wire.

found to have CRMD infection with SA-BSI within a year of CRMD implantation or manipulation; in 6/9 patients, SA-BSI resulted from CRMD infection, and the remaining 3 patients developed CRMD infection as a result of hematogenous seeding. In the 21 patients who developed SA-BSI >1 year following CRMD implantation, the device was rarely implicated as the initial source of SA-BSI; however, as a result of SA-BSI, CRMD infection developed in 28% of the patients [89]. In contrast, a 7-year retrospective cohort study of 49 patients with gram-negative BSI (GN BSI) showed that 6% (3) had definite/possible CRMD GN-BSI at presentation; hematogenous seeding of CRMD was not encountered. Thirty-four patients with retained CRMD were observed for 3 months; only 3% (2) developed relapsing BSI, but alternative sources for the relapse were present [90].

Symptoms of CRMD infection depend on the anatomical area of infection. Localized inflammatory changes over the device pocket are fairly diagnostic, although with indolent pathogens, such as CoNS, signs can be absent even with an exposed device. One series noted that of the patients, <1/3 presented with fever and one-fourth had occult BSI without systemic symptoms. The Duke criteria [41,42] can be used to diagnose CRMD infections; the inclusion of device abnormalities (use of ultrasound or computed tomography [CT] for fluid) and the presence of septic pulmonary emboli by CT increases the diagnostic yield [91]. Blood cultures should be obtained even in the absence of systemic symptoms to detect occult bacteremia. Transesophageal echocardiography (TEE) has a sensitivity of >95% compared to <30% for transthoracic echocardiography (TTE) in identifying vegetations [81] (see Figure 38-4).

Optimal management requires the institution of bactericidal antimicrobials and the removal of the CRMD, but device removal itself can result in complications such as arrhythmias and tearing or perforation of myocardial wall as the lead is removed. An operative mortality of zero was

reported in a series of 123 patients; of these, 95% (117) underwent CRMD removal with an 8% (1/117) relapse rate versus a 50% (3/6) relapse rate in the medically treated group. In a study of 31 patients with CRMD endocarditis, the only prognostic factor identified with failure of therapy or mortality was the absence of surgical intervention; however, the mortality rate despite surgical and medical therapy was still 12.5% (3/24) [92].

A meta-analysis found preoperative antimicrobial prophylaxis to be beneficial in preventing pacemaker infections [93]. A study of 2,564 patients identified no significant impact on CRMD-associated pocket infection rates using local povidone-iodine solution pocket irrigation of the subcutaneous pocket before wound closure [94].

CORONARY ARTERIAL STENTS

In the United States, >700,000 percutaneous transluminal coronary angioplasty (PTCA) procedures are performed annually [2]; coronary artery stents are placed to decrease the risk of restenosis following PTCA. There is a paucity of reports on coronary artery stent–associated infections. To date, only 10 infections occurring between 2 days to 4 weeks following stent placement (age distribution between 38–80 years) have been reported in the world's literature [95] It is notable that all patients had positive blood cultures, with S. aureus recovered in 70% of them, the other pathogens were Pseudomonas aeruginosa in 2 patients and CoNS in 1 patient. Clinical features included fever, chest pain in 50% of patients with 2 patients sustaining myocardial infarction, and multiple systemic septic emboli. Four patients were diagnosed by coronary angiography; 4 false aneurysms were identified, the fatality rate was 40%. Only 1 patient in this series underwent placement of a drug-eluting stent to prevent restenosis by its immunomodulating and antiproliferative effects [96]. Additional reports describe 2 patients who developed DAIs following placement of rapamycin-eluting and paclitaxel-eluting coronary stents [97,98].

ENDOCASCULAR STENTS AND PROSTHETIC VASCULAR GRAFTS

Vascular Prosthetic Grafts

Prosthetic graft infections are uncommon, and their rate of occurrence is determined by the anatomic location of the graft with reported incidences of <1% for abdominal grafts, increasing to 1.5–2% for aortofemoral grafts and to 6% for infrainguinal grafts [99]. Significant morbidity is associated with peripheral graft infection because of the threatened loss of limb and high mortality rates associated with aortic graft infections. Identified risk factors include groin incision, wound complications (e.g., hematoma, wound separation), emergent and repeated procedures, diabetes mellitus or suboptimal glycemic control, obesity, and operative time [4,100–104]. The majority of infrainguinal graft infections occur within 1–2 months postoperatively and therefore are attributed to intraoperative contamination or extension from an adjacent postoperative SSI. Early infections can be marked by inflammatory soft tissue changes over the graft, sinus tract formation, peripheral emboli, development of pseudoaneurysms, and graft malfunction. However, an increasing number of infections are caused by cutaneous organisms such as CoNS, *Corynebactereium* sp. and *Propionibacterium acnes* that result in abdominal graft infections; their indolent course explains their subacute presentation with aortoenteric fistula or enlarging inguinal mass presenting years after implantation [2]. Pounds et al. reported a high number of SSIs following vascular reconstruction surgery including aortic, extraanatomic, and infrainguinal procedures [105]. A retrospective case-control study of 410 procedures identified 45 infections including graft infection in 67% (30/45). Of these patients, 27% (12/45) presented with anastomotic disruption. Multivariate regression analysis identified previous hospitalization, younger age, and groin incision as risk factors. The emergence of methicillin resistant *S. aureus* (MRSA) as the predominant pathogen causing 53% of the SSIs was disturbing a trend also noted by Taylor in vascular surgery infections [106].

Radiographic studies (e.g., ultrasonography, Indium-labeled white cell scan, CT) are used to identify pseudoaneuryms and perigraft fluid and to detect the presence of air beyond what is expected in the early postoperative period [106]. Magnetic resonance imaging (MRI) in patients suspected of having a prosthetic graft infection with CT-negative studies can reveal subtle inflammatory changes [107].

The guiding principles of therapy for vascular graft infections include (1) excision of the foreign body, (2) debridement of infected or devitalized tissue, (3) and establishment and maintenance of vascular supply, and (4) institution of appropriate antibiotic therapy [4,108]. Estimated overall mortality and limb amputation of lower extremeties are 14–58% and 8–52% respectively [102].

The value of preoperative antibiotics in preventing early graft infection has not been studied. Rifampicin bonding to Dacron grafts had no beneficial effect [109].

Peripheral Vascular Stents

It is estimated that >400,000 patients undergo stent placement in the United States as a strategy to prevent vessel restenosis following PTCA for the nonsurgical management of artherosclerotic vascular disease. The reported infection rate is <1/10,000 patients [110]. Potential risk factors include (1) prolonged use of indwelling vascular catheter or sheath and reuse of the sheath after 24 hours, (2) thrombolytic therapy, for patients, (3) recurrent use

of the same femoral artery for vascular access within a week, (4) local hematoma formation, (5) prolonged stent insertion time, (6) use of same site for interventions, and (7) iliac artery access [111]. In addition to death and loss of limb, other complications include pseudoaneurysms, mycotic aneurysms, and cutaneous fistulae [112,113].

A review of 65 aortioiliac stent graft infections involving 50 aortic and 15 iliac artery grafts identified the following: (1) the frequency of infection was 0.43%, (2) 23% had immunodeficiency issues, (3) the male:female ratio was 1.4, (4) 31% of patients had associated aortoenteric fistulae, (5) *S. aureus* was recovered in 54.5% of patients, (6) the overall mortality was 18%; when stratified according to conservative treatment versus surgical treatment, the rates were 36.4% and 14%, respectively, and (7) risk factors were poorly defined [114].

The majority of infections of endovascular stent and stent/grafts implanted through the groins are caused by *S. aureus*. The preponderance of these organisms has been attributed to the high concentration of bacteria harbored within the many eccrine sweat glands within the intertriginous zones of the groin [115].

OTHER VASCULAR DEVICES

Arterial Closure Devices

The discomfort and time necessary to achieve hemostasis at the femoral puncture site accessed for cardiac catheterization by conventional means led to the development of percutaneous arterial closure devices in the 1990s. However, when compared with traditional manual and mechanical compression, there is an increased risk of infection. Although the risk is relatively low, infections related to arterial closure devices require multiple surgical procedures and, at times, amputation of the limb; high mortality rates have been reported [116,117]. In one study, the reported infection rate was 1.6%, 80% (4/5) of which were due to *S. aureus* (2 were methicillin resistant) and resulted in groin abscesses and mycotic aneurysms; the crude mortality rate was 40% [118]. Over a 4-year time period, 46 patients with a mean age of 64 with diabetes mellitus and obesity as comorbidities had a documented mortality rate of 6% were reviewed. Mycotic pseudoaneurysm was encountered in 22 patients, and *S. aureus* accounted for 75% of the isolates [119].

Prosthetic (Dacron) Carotid Patches

Until the introduction of Dacron carotid patches, carotid arterotomies were primarily closed or "patched" with autologous saphenous veins, the purpose of which was to decrease patient morbidities such as thrombosis and restenosis after primary closure. The use of Dacron carotid patches ensured successful closure of arterotomies with ease and predictability, but infectious complications were inherent in their use as they are for any foreign body. Over a period of 4 years, 8 patients were described with an infection rate of 0.5% in 1,258 procedures with no mortality and a zero relapse rate. Gram-positive pathogens were recovered in 7 patients (4 staphylococci, 3 steptococci)[120,121]. A subsequent study that described 4 subacute episodes of pseudoaneursyms (3 related to Dacron) confirmed these observations [122]. Treatment consisted of removing the foreign body, debriding infected tissue, performing autologous saphenous vein patch angioplasty or interposition grafting, and using appropriate antimicrobial therapy.

Cardiac Suture Line Pledget

The 1998 review on infections of the cardiac suture line after left ventricular surgery is the most recent. It describes 3 patients from one institution and includes a literature review on 22 other patients [123]. While distinctly rare and occult in presentation, such infections are associated with a long incubation period, at an average 16 months after surgery. Clinical features include cardiocutaneous fistulae with bleeding, pleuropulmonary symptoms with hemoptysis, chest wall abscess, BSIs that mimick endocarditis, and left ventricular false aneurysms that developed in 60% (15/25) of patients. The most frequent pathogens encountered were the staphylococci and gram-negative bacilli. Optimal treatment included appropriate antibiotics and excision of all infected sutures, pledgets, and infected tissue. The overall survival rate was 79%.

PREVENTION OF CARDIAC AND VASCULAR DEVICE-ASSOCIATED INFECTIONS

The devastating consequences of cardiac and vascular DAIs highlight the importance of implementing prevention strategies. These include (1) the appropriate use of prophylactic antibiotics, (2) a reduction of intraoperative risk by adhering to infection control guidelines, (3) glycemic control, and (5) prevention of secondary BSI.

Prophylactic Antibiotics

While there are data to support the use of perioperative antibiotics for cardiac bypass surgery [124,125], no randomized prospective trials have been conducted to assess whether antimicrobial prophylaxis confers benefit to prevent implantable cardiac and vascular DAIs, meta-analysis of seven randomized trials involving 2,023 patients that showed a reduction of permanent pacemaker-associated infections when prophylactic antibiotics were administered before implantation [93]. No randomized studies

are projected for the future, largely due to the infrequent occurrence of these infections and the large number of patients required to demonstrate benefit [3] as well as some concern as to whether performing such studies is ethical. Despite the absence of direct scientific data, systemic antimicrobial prophylaxis is recommended for implantation of cardiac and vascular devices, and guidance is extrapolated from recommendations for cardiac bypass surgery and orthopedic implants. Included are prosthetic valves, CRMDs, LVADs, TAHs, cardiac pledgets, vascular grafts, and arterial patches [2].

The choice of antibiotics is dictated by epidemiologic data that suggest that intraoperative contamination with cutaneous microorganisms resulted in early infections. Generally, a cephalosporin is recommended to target methicillin-susceptible *S. aureus*; it should be administered within an hour (2 hours if vancomycin is used due to the lengthy infusion time) of incision to ensure therapeutic concentrations at the surgical site and continued no longer than 24–48 hours following the procedure. Intraoperative bleeding >1.5 liters (assuming 25% of blood volume) or operative time >2.5 times the half-life of prophylactic agent(s) require redosing of the antibiotic (for cefazolin, about 3–4 hours) [124,125]. Preoperative colonization (e.g., tracheal aspirates from ventilated patients) and concurrent antibiotic therapy for infection could have an impact on the choice of preoperative prophylactic antibiotics.

Continuing antimicrobial prophylaxis >48 hours in cardiovascular surgery does not confer additional benefits but does increase the development of antimicrobial resistance (isolation of cephalosporin-resistant enterobacteriaceae and vancomycin-resistant enterococci) [124,125]. Prolonged prophylactic antibiotic use also has been associated with *Clostridium difficile*-associated disease [124,125]. The microbiologic landscape of SSIs is ever changing and reflects an increasing number of MRSA isolates [62,105,106] and the emergence of vancomycin-resistant *Enterococcus faecium* as pathogens in LVAD patients [61,62].

The use of secondary antimicrobial prophylaxis (i.e., for dental, respiratory, gastrointestinal, genitourinary cases) is recommended for patients with valvular heart disease [126]; however, because the majority of pathogens causing DAIs originate from the cutaneous flora, secondary prophylaxis is not generally recommended [2].

Clinical practice uses four local antimicrobial measures to prevent implantable DAIs: local irrigation, antimicrobial carriers, dipping of implants in antibiotic solution, and antibiotic coating of prosthesis. Use of such strategies in cardiovascular surgery has not been studied [127]. Antibiotic irrigation of the surgical site is an accepted standard among surgeons. Antimicrobial carriers such as the silver-impregnated dressings (Silverlon®, Argentum Medical LLC,) that provide local antisepsis to LVAD driveline sites are being used to prevent site-associated infection; however, clinical studies are needed to define their utility and efficacy. While antibiotic-coated beads have been used for treatment, their role in prophylaxis has not been studied [73]. Rifampicin bonding to Dacron grafts (dipping in solution before implantation) had no beneficial effect [109]. Studies demonstrating efficacy in the prevention of line-related BSI by using antibiotic-impregnated or antiseptic-coated catheters [128] led to the development of a silver-coated sewing ring for mechanical valves, but clinical trials were terminated due to early paravalvular leaks in the study patients [129].

The impact of intranasal mupirocin on cardiac and vascular device–associated *S. aureus* infections is not well characterized, especially because an estimated 60% of the *S. aureus* infections at surgical sites appear not to have originated from the patient's nose [130]. The conclusions of clinical studies somewhat discordant [131,132]. One study of 3,864 patients undergoing various types of surgical procedures reported that *S. aureus* HAIs were significantly reduced in nasal carriers treated with mupirocin. The study reported a tendency toward lower *S. aureus* SSI rates, but significance was not achieved when compared to those nasal carriers who did not receive mupirocin [133]. A meta-analysis concluded that the use of perioperative mupirocin was associated with a reduction in SSIs in nongeneral surgery patients (i.e., those undergoing cardiothoracic, orthopedic, and neurosurgery) [134]. More studies are needed to better define the role of intranasal mupirocin for SSI prevention, especially related to implantable cardiac and vascular devices; however, conducting such studies could be difficult because of the requirements for a large study sample size. One proposed strategy is to treat *S. aureus* nasal carriers who are to undergo nongeneral surgical procedures (i.e., cardiac surgery and implants).

Glycemic Control

There is ample evidence that strict perioperative glycemic control reduces SSIs in patients undergoing cardiac bypass surgery [23–26]. The favorable impact of this strategy can be applied to patients undergoing implantation of cardiac and vascular devices because some studies indicate that diabetes often is a comorbid condition or is a risk factor for DAIs as discussed previously.

Intraoperative Contamination

The predominance of gram-positive organisms causing early DAIs is attributed to intraoperative contamination. CDC has outlined strategies to decrease the risks of SSIs [29] that include: optimal aseptic technique, appropriate environmental controls, and reduction of the risk of bacterial shedding. Airborne dispersal of MRSA and CoNS of nasal carriers with experimental rhinovirus as a potential transmission means in the nonsurgical setting has been described; surgical masks were reportedly effective in decreasing MRSA shedding but

not CoNS [135,136]. Additionally, individuals with dermatitis shed an increased number of squamous cells that contain cutaneous microorganisms [29].

In-situ air-sampling studies conducted during an 18-month period involving 70 separate vascular surgical procedures; samples obtained from 0.5–4 meters from the surgical wound reported recovery of CoNS and *S. aureus* from 86% and 64% procedures, respectively. Of these, 51% and 39% respectively, were from within 0.5 meters of the surgical wound. Pulse-field gel electrophoresis confirmed that the origin of these isolates was from the surgical team. In separate studies, the surgical mask did not protect against shedding [137]. Another potential source of intraoperative contamination is the vertical air curtain used to provide ultraclean air directed downward toward the patient. In experimental studies during simulated surgical activity, the surgeon shed particles into the wound model, but the number shed decreased when ventilation was directed away from the wound [138].

Prevention of Secondary BSIs

Secondary BSIs, especially those due to *S. aureus*, can result in hematogenous seeding of the implanted device [43,90, 139]; careful attention to CVC insertion practices and site management [128] along with prompt removal of devices, including ventilators and indwelling urinary catheters, reduced BSI risks.

CONCLUSION

Implantable cardiac and vascular devices have been integrated into the fabric of modern medicine and allow for the reconstruction of the heart and vessels. Doing so restores hemodynamic and electrical stability to patients afflicted with valvular heart disease and medically refractory end-stage cardiomyopathy. Improving circulation to limbs of patients with severe peripheral vascular disease is a way to salvage limbs. The incidence of DAIs is relatively low (except for LVADs), but when infections develop, they are associated with considerable morbidity and mortality, especially among the frail and elderly who have a variety of comorbid conditions. Furthermore, cure in conjunction with antimicrobial therapy requires device explantation, and prolonged hospitalization, repeated operations, and substantial costs have significantly adverse impact on quality of life. These observations highlight the importance of adhering to infection prevention strategies to maximize the cost-effective use of these implantable devices and offer the host the advantage in the ongoing conflict between man and microbe.

Areas of future research that could increase the survival benefit of patients with implantable cardiac and vascular devices include (1) nonsurgical treatment of chronic biofilm-associated infections with antimicrobials (experimental in vitro data suggest that certain ones [e.g., rifampin, daptomycin, and linezolid] in a vascular graft model for staphylococci [140], tigercycline for *S. epidermis* [141], and caspofungin for *Candida albicans* could be effective in penetrating the biofilm [142]; (2) introduction of smaller devices and drive lines of LVADs and TAHs or complete internalization of the device and lines, thereby decreasing SSI risk; (3) development of devices that would resist biofilm formation (possibly by incorporating antiseptic/antimicrobials without having a significant impact on the emergence multidrug-resistant microorganisms); (4) the environment as a source of intraoperative contamination; and (5) the reversal of defects of the immune system, specifically CD4 bearing T-lymphocytes that are sequelae of age and implanted devices such as the LVAD.

REFERENCES

1. The presentive services tool kit. (www.cdc.gov/nccdphp/publications/aag/cvh.htm)
2. Baddour LM, Bettmann MA, Bolger AF, et al. Nonvalvular cardiovascular device-related infections. *Circulation* 2003;108:2015–2031.
3. Darouiche RO. Current concepts: Treatment of infections associated with surgical implant. *N Engl J Med* 2004;350:1422–1429.
4. Baddour LM, Wilson WR. Infections of prosthetic valves and other cardiovascular devices. In: Mandell GL, Bennett JE, Dolin R, eds. *Principles and practice of infectious disease.* vol 2. Philadelphia: Churchill Livingstone, 2005.
5. Que YA, Francois P, Haefliger JA, et al. Reassessing the role of *Staphylococcus aureus* clumping factor and fibronectin-binding protein by expression in *Lactococcus lacti*. *Infect Immun* 2001;69:296–302.
6. Moreillon P, Que YA, Bayer AS. Pathogenesis of streptococcal and staphylococcal endocarditis. *Infect Dis Clin North Am* 2002;16:297–318.
7. Shive MS, Salloum MI, Anderson JM. Shear stress-induced apoptosis of adherent neutrophils: A mechanism for persistence of cardiovascular device infections. *Proc Natl Acad Sci USA* 2000;97:6710–6715.
8. Shive MS, Hasan SM, Anderson JM. Shear stress effects on bacterial adhesion, leukocyte adhesion, and leukocyte oxidative capacity on a polyetheurethane. *J Biomed Mater Res* 1999;46:511–519.
9. Fisher AM, Chien S, Barakat AI, et al. Endothelial cellular response to altered shear stress. *Am J Physiol Lung Cell Mol Physiol* 2001;281:L529–33.
10. Donlan RM. Biofilm formation: A clinically relevant microbiological process. *Clin Infect Dis* 2001;33:1387–1392.
11. Jefferson KK. What drives bacteria to produce a biofilm? *FEMS Microbiol Lett* 2004;236:163–173.
12. Seifert H, Oltmanns D, Becker K, et al. *Staphylococcus lugdunensis* pacemaker-related infection. *Emerg Infect Dis* 2005;11:1283–1286.
13. Seifert H, Wisplinghoff H, Schnabel P, von Eiff C. Small colony variants of *Staphylococcus aureus* pacemaker-related infection. *Emerg Infect Dis* 2003;9:1316–1318.
14. Chandra J, Kuhn DM, Mukherjee PK, et al. Biofilm formation by the fungal pathogen *Candida albicans*: Development, architecture, and drug resistance. *J Bacteriol* 2001;183:5385–5394.
15. Bagge N, Ciofu O, Skovgaard LT, Hoiby N. Rapid development *in vitro* and *in vivo* of resistance to ceftazidime in biofilm-growing *Pseudomonas aeruginosa* due to chromosomal β-lactamase. *APMIS* 2000;108:589–600.
16. Stewart PS, Costerton JW. Antibiotic resistance of bacteria in biofilms. *Lancet* 2001;358:135–138.
17. Xu KD, McFeters GA, Stewart, PS. Biofilm resistance to antimicrobial agents. *Microbiology* 2000;146:547–549.
18. von Eiff C, Peters G, Heilmann C. Pathogenesis of infections due to coagulase-negative staphylococci. *Lancet Infect Dis* 2002;2:677–685.
19. Cramton SE, Gerke C, Schnell NF, et al. The intercellular adhesion locus is present in *Staphylococcus aureus* and is required for biofilm formation. *Infect Immun* 1999;67:5427–5433.
20. Baldassarri L, Creti R, Montanaro L, et. al. Pathogenesis of implant infections by enterococci. *Int J Artif Organs* 2005;28:1101–1109.
21. Delamaire M, Maugendre D, Moreno M, et. al. Impaired leukocyte functions in diabetic patients. *Diabet Med* 1997;14:29–34.
22. Hostetter MK. Handicaps to host defense: Effects of hyperglycemia on C3 and *Candida albicans*. *Diabetes* 1990;39:271–275.
23. Latham R, Lancaster AD, Covington JF, et al. The association of diabetes and glucose control with surgical-site infections among cardiothoracic surgery patients. *Infect Control Hospital Epidemiol* 2001;22:607–612.
24. Talbot TR. Diabetes mellitus and cardiothoracic surgical site infections. *Am J Infect Control* 2005;33:353–359.
25. Estrada CA, Young JA, Knifing LW, Chitwood WR Jr. Outcomes and perioperative hyperglycemia in patients with or without diabetes mellitus undergoing coronary artery bypass grafting. *Ann Thorax Surge* 2003;75:1392.
26. Trick WS, Sheckler WE, Tokars JI, et al. Modifiable risk factors associated with deep sternal site infection after coronary artery bypass grafting. *J Thorax Cardiovascular Surge* 2000;119:108.
27. Vongpatanasin W, Hillis LD, Lange RA. Prosthetic heart valves. *N Engl J Med* 1996; 335:407.
28. Thamilarasan M, Griffin B. Choosing the most appropriate valve operation and prosthesis. *Cleve Clin J Med* 2002;69:688–703.
29. Mangram AJ, Horan TC, Pearson ML, et al. Guideline for prevention of surgical site infection, 1999. *Infect Control Hosp Epidemiol* 1999;20:250–280. www.cdc.gov/ncidod/hip/SSI/SSI_guideline.htm
30. Calderwood SB, Swinski LA, Waternaux CM, et al. Risk factors for the development of prosthetic valve endocarditis. *Circulation* 1985;72:31–37.
31. Karchmer AW, Longworth D. Infections of intracardiac devices. *Cardiol Clin* 2003;21:253–271.
32. Agnihotri AK, McGiffin DC, Galbraith AJ, O'Brien MF. The prevalence of infective endocarditis after aortic valve replacement. *J Thorac Cardiovasc Surg* 1995;110:1708.
33. Horstkotte D, Piper C, Niehues R, et al. Late prosthetic valve endocarditis. *Eur Heart J* 1995;16(Suppl B):39.
34. Rutledge R, Kim BJ, Applebaum RE. Actuarial analysis of the risk of prosthetic valve endocarditis in 1,598 patients with mechanical and bioprosthetic valves. *Arch Surg* 1985;120:469.
35. Gordon SM, Serkey JM, Longworth DL, et al. Early onset prosthetic valve endocarditis. The Cleveland Clinic experience 1992–1997. *Ann Thorac Surg* 2000;69.1388–1392.
36. Hammermeister KE, Sethi G, Henderson WE, et al. Outcomes 15 years after valve replacement with a mechanical versus a bioprosthetic valve: Final report of the Veteran Affairs randomized trial. *J Am Coll Cardiol* 2000;36:1152–1158.
37. Ivert TS, Dismukes WE, Cobbs CG, et al. Prosthetic valve endocarditis. *Circulation* 1984; 69:223.
38. Arvay A, Lengyel M. Incidence and risk factors of prosthetic valve endocarditis. *Eur J Cardiothorac Surg* 1998;2:340–346.
39. Grover FL, Cohen DJ, Oprian C, et al. Determinants of the occurrence of and survival from prosthetic valve endocarditis. *J Thorac Cardiovasc Surg* 1994;108:207.
40. Farinas MC, Perez-Vazquez A, Farinas-Alvarez C, et al. Risk factors of prosthetic valve endocarditis: A case-control study. *Ann Thorac Surg* 2006;81:1284–1290.
41. Durack DT, Lukes AS, Bright DK. New criteria for diagnosis of infective endocarditis: Utilization of specific echocardiographic findings. *Am J Med* 1994;96:200.
42. Li JS, Sexton DJ, Mick N, et al. Proposed modifications to the Duke criteria for the diagnosis of infective endocarditis. *Clin Infect Dis* 2000;30:633.
43. El-Ahdab F, Benjamin DK Jr., Wang A. Risk of endocarditis among patients with prosthetic valves and *Staphylococcus aureus* bacteremia. *Am J Med* 2005;118:225–229.
44. Fang G, Keys TF, Gentry LO, et al. Prosthetic valve resulting from nosocomial bacteremia. *Ann Intern Med* 1993;119:560–567.
45. Nasser, RM, Melgar, GR, Longworth, DL, Gordon, SM. Incidence and risk of developing fungal prosthetic valve endocarditis after nosocomial candidemia. *Am J Med* 1997;103:25.

46. Rumisek JD, Albus RA, Clarke JS. Late *Mycobacterium celonei* bioprosthetic valve endocarditis: Activation of implanted contaminant. *Ann Thorac Surg* 1985;39:277–279.

47. Boyce JM, Potter-Bynoe G, Opal SM. A common-source outbreak of *Staphylococcus epidermidis* infections among patients undergoing cardiac surgery. *J Infect Dis* 1990;161:493–499.

48. van den Broek PJ, Lampe AS, Berbee GA, et al. Epidemic of prosthetic valve endocarditis caused by *Staphylococcus epidermidis*. *Br J Med* 1985;291:949–950.

49. Lark RL, VanderHyde K, Deeb GM, et al. An outbreak of coagulase-negative staphylococcal surgical site infections following aortic valve replacement. *Infect Control Hosp Epidemiol* 2001;22:618–623.

50. Tompkins LS, Roessier BJ, Redd SC. Legionella prosthetic-valve endocarditis. *N Engl J Med* 1988;318:530–535.

51. Diekema DJ, Messer SA, Hollis RJ, et al. An outbreak of *Candida parapsilosis* prosthetic valve endocarditis. *Diagn Microbiol Infect Dis* 1997;29:147–153.

52. Sohail MR, Martin KR, Wilson WR, et al. Medical versus surgical management of *Staphylococcus aureus* prosthetic valve endocarditis. *Am J Med* 2006;119:147–154.

53. Breen, JD, Karchmer, AW. Usefulness of pulsed-field gel electrophoresis in confirming endocarditis due to *Staphylococcus lugdunensis*. *Clin Infect Dis* 1994;19:985.

54. *Heart disease and stroke statistics—2004 update*. Dallas: American Heart Association, 2004:244–254.

55. Frazier OH, Rose EA, Oz MC, et al. Multicenter clinical evaluation of the Heartmate vented electric left ventricular assist system in patients awaiting heart transplantation. *J Thorac Cardiovasc Surg* 2001;122:1186–1195.

56. Rose EA, Gelijns AC, Moskowitz AJ, et al. Long-term use of a left ventricular assist device for end-stage heart failure. *N Engl J Med* 2001;345:1435–1443.

57. Aaronson KD, Eppinger MJ, Dyke DB. Left ventricular assist device therapy improves utilization of donor hearts. *J Am Coll Cardiol* 2002;39:1247–1254.

58. Poston RS, Husain S, Sorce D, et al. Left ventricular assist device bloodstream infections: Therapeutic rationale for transplantation after LVAD infection. *J Heart Lung Transplant* 2003;22:914–921.

59. Prendergast TW, Todd B, Beyer AJ, et al. Management of left ventricular assist device infections with heart transplantation. *Ann Thorac Surg* 1997;64:142–147.

60. Argenziano M, Catanese KA, Moazami N, et al. The influence of infection on survival and successful transplantation in patients with left ventricular assist devices. *J Heart Lung Transplant* 1997;16:822–831.

61. Simon D, Fischer S, Grossman A, et al. Left ventricular assist device-related infection: Treatment and outcome. *Clin Infect Dis* 2005;40:1108–1115.

62. Gordon SM, Schmitt SK, Jacobs M, et al. Nosocomial blood stream infections in the patients with implantable ventricular assist devices. *Ann Thorac Surg* 2001;72:725–730.

63. Sivaratnam K, Duggan J. Left ventricular assist device infections: Three case reports and a review of the literature. *ASAIO J* 2002;48:2–7.

64. Holman WL, Park SJ, Long JW, et al. Infection in permanent circulatory support: Experience for the REMATCH trial. *J Heart Lung Transplant* 2004;23:1359–1365.

65. Park SJ, Tector A, Piccioni W, et al. Left ventricular assist devices as destination therapy: A new look at survival. *J Thorac Cardiovasc Surg* 2005;129:9–17.

66. Malani PN, Dyke DBS, Pagani FD, Chenoweth CE. Nosocomial infections in left ventricular assist device recipients. *Clin Infect Dis* 2002;34:1295–1300.

67. Siegenthaler MP, Martin J, Pernice K. The Jarvik 2000 is associated with less infections than the HeartMate left ventricular assist device. *Eur J Cardiothorac Surg* 2003;23:748–754.

68. Ankersnitt HS, Tugulea S, Spanier T, et al. Activation of T-cell death, and immune dysfunction after implantation of left ventricular assist device. *Lancet* 1999;354:550–555.

69. Itescu S, Ankersmit JH, Kocher AA, et al. Immunobiology of left ventricular assist devices. *Prog Cardiovasc Dis* 2000;43:67–80.

70. Erren M, Schlueter B, Fobker M, et al. Immunologic effects of implantation of left ventricular assist devices. *Transplant Proceed* 2001;33:1965–1968.

71. Yoshikawa TT. Perspective: Aging and infectious disease—Past, present, and future. *J Infect Dis* 1997;176:1053–1057.

72. Holman WL, Rayburn BK, McGiffin DC, et al. Infection in ventricular assist devices: Prevention and treatment. *Ann Thorac Surg* 2003;75:S48–S57.

73. McKellar SH, Allred BD, Marks JD, et al. Treatment of infected left ventricular assist device using antibiotic-impregnated beads. *Ann Thorac Surg* 1999;67:554–555.

74. Baradarian S, Stahovich M, Krause S, et al. Case series: Clinical management of persistent mechanical assist device driveline drainage using vacuum-assisted closure therapy. *ASAIO J* 2006;52:354–356.

75. Poston RS, Husain S, Sorce D, et al. Left ventricular assist device bloodstream infections: Therapeutic rationale for transplantation after LVAD infection. *J Heart Lung Transplant* 2003;22:914–921.

76. Vichez RA, McEllistram C, Harrison LH, et al. Relapsing bacteremia in patients with ventricular assist device: An emergent complication of extended circulatory support. *Ann Thorac Surg* 2001;72:96–101.

77. Nurozler F, Argenziano M, Oz MC, Naka Y. Fungal left ventricular assist device endocarditis. *Ann Thorac Surg* 2001;71:614–618.

78. Gray NA, Sezman CH. Current status of the total artificial heart. *Am Heart J* 2006;152:4–10.

79. Copeland JG, Smith RG, Arabia FA, et al. Cardiac replacement with a total artificial heart as a bridge to transplantation. *N Engl J Med* 2004;351:859–867.

80. Dowling RD, Gray LA Jr, Etoch SW, et al. Initial experience with the AbioCor implantable replacement heart system. *J Thorac Cardiovasc Surg* 2004;127:131–141.

81. Chua JD, Wilkoff BL, Lee I, et al. Diagnosis and management of infections involving implantable electrophysiologic cardiac devices. *Ann Intern Med* 2000;133:604.

82. Klug D, Lacroix D, Savoye C, et al. Systemic infection related to endocarditis on pacemaker leads: Clinical presentation and management. *Circulation* 1997;95:2098.

83. Cacoub P, Leprince P, Nataf P, et al. Pacemaker infective endocarditis. *Am J Cardiol* 1998;82:480.

84. Duval X, Selton-Suty C, Alla F, et al. Endocarditis in patients with a permanent pacemaker: A 1-year epidemiological survey on infective endocarditis due to valvular and/or pacemaker infection. *Clin Infect Dis* 2004;39:68.

85. Eggimann, P, Waldvogel, F. *Pacemaker and defibrillator infections*. In: Waldvogel, FA, Bisno, AL, eds. *Infections associated with indwelling medical devices*. Washington, DC: American Society for Microbiology Press, 2000:247.

86. Hindupur S, Muslin AJ. Septic shock induced from an implantable cardioverter-defibrillator lead-associated *Candida albicans* vegetation. *J Interv Card Electrophysiol* 2005;14:55–59.

87. Cook RJ, Orszulak TA, Nkomo VT. Aspergillus infection of implantable cardioverter-defibrillator. *May Clin Pro* 2004;79:549–552.

88. Ho IC, Milan DJ, Mansour MC. Fungal infection of implantable cardioverter-defibrillators: Case series of five patients managed over 22 year. *Heart Rhythm* 2006;3:919–923.

89. Chamis, AL, Peterson, GE, Cabell, CH, et al. *Staphylococcus aureus* bacteremia in patients with permanent pacemakers or implantable cardioverter-defibrillators. *Circulation* 2001;104:1029.

90. Uslan DZ, Sohail MR, Firedman PA. Frequency of permanent pacemaker or implantable cardioverter-defibrillator infection in patients with gram-negative bacteremia. *Clin Infect Dis* 2006;43:731–736.

91. Klug D, Lacroix D, Savoye C, et al. Systemic infection related to endocarditis on pacemaker leads: Clinical presentation and management. *Circulation* 1997;95:2098.

92. del Rio A, Anguera I, Miro JM, et al. Surgical treatment of pacemaker and defibrillator lead endocarditis. *Chest* 2003;124;1451–1459.

93. Da Costa A, Kirkorian G, Cucherat M, et al. Antibiotic prophylaxis of permanent pacemaker implantation: A meta-analysis. *Circulation* 1998;97:1796–1801.

94. Lakkireddy D, Valasareddi S, Ryschon K, et al. The impact of povidone-iodine pocket irrigation use on pacemaker and defibrillator infections. *Pacing Clin Electrophysiol* 2005;28: 789–794.

95. Kaufmann BA, Kaiser C, Pfisterer ME, Bonetti PO. Coronary stent infection: A rare but severe complication of percutaneous coronary intervention. *Swiss Med Wkly* 2005;135:483–487.

96. Costa MA, Simon DI. Molecular basis of restenosis and drug-eluting stents. *Circulation* 2005;111:2257–2273.

97. Alfonso F, Moreno R, Vergas J. Fatal infection after rapamycin eluting coronary stent implantation. *Heart* 2005;91:e51.

98. Marcu CB, Balf DV, Donohue TJ. Post-infectious pseudoaneurysm after coronary angioplasty using drug-eluting stents. *Heart Lung Circ* 2005;14:85.

99. Seeger JM. Management of patients with prosthetic vascular graft infection. *Am Surg* 2000;66:166–177.

100. Vriesendorp TM, Morelis QJ, Devires JH, et al. Early postoperative glucose levels are an independent risk factor for infection after peripheral vascular surgery: A retrospective study. *Eur J Vasc Endovasc Surg* 2004;28:520–528.

101. Oderich GS, Panneton JM. Aortic graft infection: What have we learned during the last decade? *Acta Chir Belg* 2002,102: 7–13.

102. Chang JK, Calligaro KD, Ryan S, et al. Risk factors associated with infection of lower extremity revascularization: Analysis of 365 procedures performed at a teaching hospital. *Ann Vasc Surg* 2003;17:91–96.

103. Lee ES, Santili SM, Olson MM, et al. Wound infection after infrainguinal bypass operation: Multivariate analysis of putative risk factors. *Surg Infect* 2000;1:257–263.

104. Antonios VS, Baddour LM. Intra-arterial device infections. *Curr Infect Dis Rep* 2004;6:263–269.

105. Pounds LL, Montes-Walters M, Mayhall CG, et al. A changing pattern of infection after major vascular reconstruction. *Vasc Endovascular Surg* 2005;39:511–517.

106. Taylor MD, Napolitano LM. Methicillin-resistant *Staphylococcus aureus* infections in vascular surgery: Increasing prevalence. *Surg Infect* 2004;5:180–187.

107. Valentine RJ. Diagnosis and management of aortic graft infections. *Semin Vasc Surg* 2001;14:292–301.

108. Bunt TJ. Vascular graft infections: An update. *Cardiovasc Surg* 2001;9:225–233.

109. Stewart A, Eyers P, Earnsaw J. Prevention of infection in arterial reconstruction. *Cochrane Database Syst Rev* 2006;19(3):CD003073.

110. Myles O, Thomas WJ, Daniels JT, et al. Infected endovascular stents managed with medical therapy alone. *Cath Cardiovasc Interv* 2000;51:471–476.

111. Dosluoglu HH, Curl GR, Doerr RJ, et al. Stent related iliac artery and iliac vein infections: Two unreported presentations and review of the literature. *J Endovasc Ther* 2001;8:202–209.

112. Kaviani A, Ouriel K, Kashyap VS. Infected carotid pseudoaneurysm carotid-cutaneous fistula as a late complication of carotid artery stenting. *J Vasc Surg* 2006;43:379–383.

113. Latham JA, Irvine A. Infection of endovascular stent: An uncommon but important complication. *Cardiovasc Surg* 1999;7:179–182.

114. Ducasse E, Calisti A, Speziale F, et al. Aortoiliac stent graft infection: Current problems and management. *Ann Vasc Surg* 2004;18:521–525.

115. Antonios, AN. Prosthetic graft infections. In: Moore, WE, ed. *Vascular Surgery: A Comprehesive Review.* Philadelphia: WB Sunders, 2002:741–750.

116. Carey D, Martin JR, Moore CA, et al. Complications of femoral artery closure devices. *Catheter Cardiovasc Interv* 2001;52:3–8.

117. Johanning JM, Franklin DP, Elmore JR, et al. Femoral artery infections associated with percutaneous arterial closure devices. *J Vasc Surg* 2001;34:983–985.

118. Smith TP, Cruz CP, Moursi MM, et al. Infectious complications resulting from use of hemostatic puncture closure devices. *Am Thorac Surg* 2001;182:658–662.

119. Sohail MR, Khan AH, Holmes DR, et al. Infectious complications of percutaneous vascular closure devices. *Mayo Clin Proc* 2005;80:1011–1015.

120. Rizzo A, Hertzer NRT, O'Hara PJ et al. Dacron carotid patch infection: A report of eight cases. *J Vasc Surg* 2000;32:602–606.

121. Sternbergh WC III. Regarding "Dacron carotid patch infection: A report of eight cases." *J Vasc Surg* 2001;33:663–664.

122. Borazjani BH, Wilson SE, Fujitani RM, et al. Postoperative complications of carotid patching: Pseudoaneurysm and infection. *Ann Vasc Surg* 2003;17:156–161.

123. McHenry MC, Longworth DL, Rehm SJ, et al. Infections of the cardiac suture line after left ventricular surgery. *Am J Med* 1988;85:292–300.

124. Bratzler DW, Houck PM, Richards C, et al. Use of antimicrobial prophylaxis for major surgery: Baseline results from the National Surgical Infection Prevention Project. *Arch Surg* 2005;140: 174.

125. Bratzler, DW, Houck, PM. Antimicrobial prophylaxis for surgery: An advisory statement from the National Surgical Infection Prevention Project. *Clin Infect Dis* 2004;38:1706.

126. Dajani AS, Taubert KA, Wilson W, et al. Prevention of bacterial endocarditis: Recommendations by the American Heart Association, from the Committee on Rheumatic Fever, Endocarditis, and Kawasaki Disease, Council on Cardiovascular Diseases in the Young. *JAMA* 1997; 277:1794.

127. Darouiche RO. Antimicrobial approaches for preventing infections associated with surgical implants. *Clin Infect Dis* 2003;36:1284–1289.

128. O'Grady NP, Alexander M, Dellinger EP, et al. Guidelines for the prevention of intravascular catheter-related infections. *Infect Control Hosp Epidemiol* 2002;23:759–769.

129. Schaff HV, Carrel TP, Jamieson WRE, el al. Paravalvular leak and other events in Silzone coated mechanical heart valves: A report from AVERT. *Ann Thorac Surg* 2002;73:785–792.

130. Farr BM. Mupirocin to prevent *S. aureus* infections *N Engl J Med* 2002;346:1905.

131. Nicholson MR, Huesman LA. Controlling the usage of mupirocin does impact the rate of *Staphylococcus aureus* deep sternal wound infections in cardiac surgery patients. *Am J Infect Control* 2006;34:44–48.

132. Konvalinka A, Errett L, Fong IW. Impact of treating *Staphylococcus aureus* nasal carrier on wound infections in cardiac surgery. *J Hosp Infect* 2006;64:162–168.

133. Perl TM, Cullen JJ, Wenzel RP, et al. Intranasal mupirocin to prevent postoperative *Staphylococcus aureus* infections. *N Engl J Med* 2002;346:1871.

134. Kallen AJ, Wilson CT, Larson RJ. Perioperative intranasal mupirocin for the prevention of surgical-site infections: Systematic review of the literature and meta-analysis. *Infect Control Hosp Epidemiol* 2005;26:916–922.

135. Sheretz RJ, Reagan DR, Hampton KD, et al. A cloud adult: The *Staphylococcus aureus*-virus interaction revisited. *Ann Intern Med* 1996;124(15):539–547.

136. Bischoff WE, Bassetti S, Bassetti-Wyss BA, et al. Airborne dispersal as a novel transmission route of coagulase-negative staphylococci: Interaction between coagulase-negative staphylococci and rhinovirus infection. *Infect Control Hosp Epidemiol* 2004;25:504–511.

137. Edmiston CE Jr, Seabrook GR, Cambria RA. Molecular epidemiology of microbial contamination in the operating room environment: Is there a risk for infection? *Surgery* 2005;138: 573–579.

138. Persson M, van der Linden J. Wound ventilation with ultraclean air for prevention of direct airborne contamination during surgery. *Infect Control Hosp Epidemiol* 2004;25:297–301.

139. vonEiff C, Becker K, Machka K, et al. Nasal carriage as a source of *Staphylococcus aureus* bacteremia. *N Engl J Med* 2001;344: 11–16.

140. Edmiston CE Jr, Goheen MP, Seabrook GR. Impact of selective antimicrobial agents on staphylococcal adherence to biomedical devices. *Am J Surg* 2006;192:344–354.

141. Pornpen L, Petersen PJ, Bradford PA. *In vitro* activity of tigecycline against *Staphylococcus epidermis* growing in an adherent-cell biofilm model. *Antimicrob Agents Chemother* 2003;47: 3967–3969.

142. Bachmann SP, VandeWalle K, Ramage G, et al. In-vitro activity of caspofungin against *Candida albicans* biofilms. *Antimicrob Agents Chemother* 2002;46:3591–3596.

Infections in Skeletal Prostheses

39

Ilker Uçkay and Daniel P. Lew

INTRODUCTION

Over the past decades, joint replacement has become one of the most common types of prosthetic surgery because of its success in restoring function to disabled arthritic persons [1–4]. More than 200,000 total hip replacements and millions of implants are implemented in the United States each year, and it is estimated that total knee replacement is performed as frequently as total hip replacement [2,5]. The safety and biocompatibility of these devices are good, and only 10% of all patients experience complications during their lifetime. Second to loosening of the prosthesis, infection is the most common complication of orthopedic implant surgery. In the United States, it is estimated that 4% of all implants become infected [5]. The rate of infection after total hip arthroplasty in early surgical series was initially unacceptably high. In Charnley's early series, the infection rate was 7%. Air filtration and prophylactic antibiotics reduced the rate of infection to 0.6% in a later series [6]. At present, the lifetime infection rate is thought to be 0.5–1.0% for total hip arthroplasty, 0.5–2.0% for knee, and <1% for shoulder replacement [2,3,7]. Even though the incidence has fallen steadily, the absolute number is rising because of the increase in the number of orthopedic operations performed. The economic burden to healthcare-associated infection (HAI) with septic prosthetic joints is very high. The cost to treat patients with hip or knee prosthetic osteomyelitis, respectively, has been calculated to be 5.3- and 7.2-fold higher than the primary operations [8].

Musculoskeletal Allografts

The use of human allografts in orthopedic surgery has gained momentum. In 2001, approximately 875,000 musculoskeletal allografts were distributed by U.S. tissue banks compared to 350,000 in 1990 [9]. Processed tissue allografts are not necessarily sterile and may result in viral or bacterial infections. Tomford et al. reported a 5% and a 4% incidence of infection related to the use of allografts in patients who had surgery for bone tumor and revision hip arthroplasty, respectively [10]. Other studies have demonstrated infection rates as high as 12.2% when banked allografts are used for reconstructive surgery [11]. Mankin et al. found in a series of 945 patients who received cadaveric allografts 7.9% primary infections and an additional 4.9% infections related to re-operations [12]. Cadaveric allografts have been shown to be contaminated at a rate of 27% in the study by Ibrahim et al. [13] and other studies.

PATHOGENESIS

According to a proposed classification in the 1970s, prosthetic joint infections can be classified according to the time of onset of infection [3]. By this classification, acute infection (stage 1) is defined as occurring within six months of surgery (≤40% of total infections); they are often evident within the first few weeks. The mechanism involved is the introduction of microorganisms during the operative procedure. *Staphylococcus aureus* is the classic pathogen. The freshly implanted biomaterial is highly susceptible to infection. The majority of joint infections is acquired in the operating room (OR). Reasons for that are the efficacy of perioperative antibiotic prophylaxis, laminar flow in the OR and the similarity of skin flora and the pathogens that cause prosthesis infections. Moreover, during the early postimplantation period, when superficial infections can develop, the fascial layers have not healed, and the deep, periprosthetic tissue is not protected by the usual physical barriers. Any factor or event that delays wound healing increases the risk of infection: ischemic necrosis, hematomas, and, more directly, wound sepsis or suture abscesses [14,15].

Subacute infection (stage 2) develops within 2 years of operation (≤45% of total infections). They are due to low-virulence microorganisms included during surgery (e.g., coagulase-negative staphylococci). Late infections (stage 3) emerge after 2 years of pain-free mobility (≥15% of total infections) and are mostly attributed to hematogenous seeding with selective persistence of the microorganisms in the joint. Dentogingival infections and manipulations, although exceptional, have been described as causes of viridans group streptococcal and anaerobic infections of prostheses. Pyogenic skin processes can cause staphylococcal (S. aureus and S. epidermidis) and streptococcal infections of replaced joints. Genitourinary and gastrointestinal tract surgeries or infections are associated with gram-negative bacillary, enterococcal, and anaerobic infections of prostheses. The use of antibiotic prophylaxis in grade III open fracture procedures has substantially decreased the frequency of bone infections and subsequent surgery.

Infecting Microorganisms

Virtually any microorganism can cause prosthetic joint infection. A single pathogen can be identified in only about two-thirds of patients [16]. The predominant microorganisms are staphylococcal species (~50% in several series), evenly divided between S. epidermidis and S. aureus. Aerobic streptococci are responsible for a significant group of infections (between 10–20% in different series), followed by Gram-positive organisms ordinarily considered culture "contaminants," such as Corynebacteria spp., Propionibacteria spp., and Bacillus spp. Gram-negative aerobic bacilli have been identified in some series in ≤25% of patients, and anaerobes usually do not account for >10% of all pathogens. In up to 10% of patients, no organisms can be detected. Among allografts, Gram-positive bacteria are equally the most frequent infecting pathogens [13]. Recently, organisms such as Clostridium spp. have become a concern. Malinin et al. showed that among 795 donors of allografts in the United States, 8.1% of donor blood, marrow, or donor musculoskeletal samples grew clostridia, mainly C. sordellii [17]. The pathogenicity of this organism is related to its ability to produce lethal factors, which cause local necrosis, edema, and hemorrhage. This said, it should not be forgotten that Clostridia spp. may be involved not only in allograft infections but also in more classical prosthetic joint infections [18,19].

Role of the Foreign Body and Biofilms

Attachment of bacteria to a prosthetic joint is a critical first step in the pathogenesis of virtually all foreign body–associated infections. A foreign body reduces the inoculum of S. aureus required to induce subcutaneous infection from >100,000-fold to as little as 100 colony-forming units [4,20]. In addition, the interaction of neutrophils with the foreign body can induce a neutrophil defect that may enhance the susceptibility to infection [21]. Ultra-high molecular weight polyethylene particles, emitted by prosthesis material, seem to add to the inhibition of the neutrophil antibacterial activity [22]. Bacteria deep within the biofilm that are metabolically inactive or in various stages of dormancy are protected from host defenses such as phagocytes and are highly resistant to antimicrobial agents [23]. The micro-environment within a biofilm may also adversely affect diffusion of antimicrobial agents. Soon after a biofilm is established, the susceptibility of bacteria to antimicrobial agents considerably decreases. With an infection of >1 month duration, it has been postulated that the biofilm has progressed to such a degree that cure with prosthetic retention is less achievable than with removal.

DIAGNOSIS

Clinical Presentation

There are no uniform clinical criteria for the diagnosis of prosthetic joint infections. Most patients experience a long, indolent course of infection characterized by steadily increasing joint pain and the occasional formation of cutaneous draining sinuses. A minority of patients has an acute fulminant illness associated with high fever, severe joint pain, local swelling, and erythema. Patients with late-onset infections due to hematogenous seeding can present with acute onset of symptoms in one or several previously well-functioning joints. The pattern of clinical presentation is determined largely by the nature of the infecting microorganism (i.e., the symptoms are more prominent in S. aureus infections compared with S. epidermidis). Infection must be differentiated from aseptic mechanical problems. Constant joint pain suggests infection whereas mechanical loosening commonly causes pain only with motion and weight bearing. Nevertheless, often it is difficult to differentiate delayed-onset infection from aseptic joint loosening of hip or knee prostheses.

Erythrocyte Sedimentation Rate (ESR) and C-Reactive Protein (CRP) Levels

Persistent elevation of the ESR suggests infection but is neither very sensitive (87%) nor very specific (47%) because it may be due to many other causes [24]. The same is true for leucocytosis or CRP. Combined measurement of the CRP and ESR seems to have an acceptable negative predictive value although it does not completely rule out a prosthetic joint infection. These two parameters also are more appropriate to measure as follow-up during therapy than for diagnosis. The role of pro-Calcitonin in nonsystemic prosthetic infections needs further evaluation, although it seems to be useful at least in pediatric osteomyelitis [25].

Radiology

A plain radiograph can display abnormal lucencies (>2 mm in width) at the bone-cement interface, changes in the position of prosthetic components, cement fractures, periosteal reaction, and motion of components. Periosteal new bone formation suggests infection but is infrequently present because it is the presence of fistula between the joint and soft tissue. When both the distal and proximal components of a prosthetic joint demonstrate radiographic abnormalities, infection is more likely than simple mechanical loosening. In the report of Bernard et al., the sensitivity and the specificity of radiographic anomalies were 73% and 76%, respectively [24]. Magnetic resonance imaging or computed tomography techniques for evaluating prosthetic joints for infection are of little help because metal present in prostheses causes interference. Radioisotopic scans demonstrate increased uptake in areas of bone with enhanced blood supply or increased metabolic activity, but this does not help to diagnose true infection because increased uptake routinely is seen around normal prostheses for several months after arthroplasty. Smith et al. investigated the usefulness of bone scintigraphy between knee replacement surgery and onset of knee pain of 3 years. The pattern of isotope uptake in the abnormal studies was not specific enough to reliably differentiate aseptic from septic loosening [26]. This result was confirmed in a report of 144 patients who underwent revision hip arthroplasty; bone-gallium imaging offered no additional advantage in diagnosis over hip aspiration [27]. According to Bernard, sensitivity and specificity of bone scintigraphy was at best 76% each [24]. Only limited data are available for positron emission tomography (PET). In a report of 35 patients with painful hip replacements, PET scan performed similarly to scintigraphy and was less sensitive and more specific than conventional bone radiography [28]. In conclusion, a normal bone scintigraphy is generally useful to exclude the need for surgical intervention aimed at correcting joint loosening or infection [26].

Joint Aspiration

Laboratory tests and imaging studies may be of value but are usually not diagnostic. As a result, the diagnosis of prosthetic joint infections always requires obtaining samples of joint fluid or tissue [29–31]. The most important step is to isolate the offending organisms so that the appropriate antimicrobial therapy can be chosen.

The importance of the identification of the pathogen cannot be overemphasized. Alternatively, isolation can be achieved by blood culture, generally only in hematogenous osteomyelitis, or by direct biopsy from the involved bone because the joint fluid aspirate may be falsely negative or positive (the latter because of contamination with skin organisms). Whenever biopsy or aspiration is done, the samples should be processed for aerobic and anaerobic cultures. Samples for mycobacterial and fungal cultures should be taken and processed if commonly cultured microorganisms are not present and if the clinical features are compatible. Often culture growth time has to be extended beyond the standard incubation period of 5 days. Tissue specimens also should be submitted for histopathologic study. Special staining techniques may reflect unusual or slowly growing microorganisms.

Hip aspiration arthrography had a sensitivity of 79% for diagnosing the infection and a specificity of 100% [1]. Trampuz et al. reported that a synovial fluid leukocyte differential of >65% neutrophils has a 97% sensitivity and 98% specificity for diagnosis of prosthetic knee infection [31]. A negative Gram's stain is of no value because the reported sensitivity is as low as 12–19% in perioperative specimens.

Histopathologic examination showing acute inflammation (a high number of neutrophils per microscopic field) has a sensitivity of >80% and specificity of >90% [32]. When intra-articular fluid is difficult to obtain, irrigation with sterile normal saline can provide the necessary fluid for culture. However, such cultures may be difficult to interpret if coagulase-negative staphylococci or common contaminants are recovered. When initial cultures indicate a relatively avirulent microorganism (*S. epidermidis*, corynebacteria, propionibacteria, or *Bacillus* spp.), a second aspiration should be considered to confirm the bacteriologic diagnosis and to eliminate the possibility of contamination. Semiquantitative cultures may be useful to distinguish between infection and colonization for indolent microorganisms. Material taken from an open sinus or from joint fluid tract by swabbing will give misleading results because the isolates may include nonpathogenic microorganisms that are colonizing the site [4].

Cultures obtained at operation are diagnostic if the patient has not received antimicrobial therapy before the procedure whereas routine cultures performed during clean orthopedic implant insertion procedure are not useful for predicting postoperative infection [33].

TREATMENT

Treatment of prosthetic joint infections is not standardized due to the variable clinical presentations and the lack of data from randomized, controlled trials. Treatment usually involves both medical and surgical measures [3], depending on the cause and timing of the infection and the condition

TABLE 39-1

ANTIBIOTIC TREATMENT OF PROSTHETIC JOINT INFECTION

Microorganisms Isolated	Parenteral Therapy		Oral Therapy[a]
	Treatment of Choice	Alternatives	
S. aureus or coagulase negative			
Penicillin sensitive	Penicillin G (4 million u every 6 hr)	A cephalosporin II,[b] clindamycin (600 mg every 6 hr), or vancomycin	Amoxicillin (750 mg every 8 hr)
Penicillin resistant	Nafcillin[c] (2 g every 6 hr)	A cephalosporin II,[b] clindamycin (600 mg every 6 hr), or vancomycin	Quinolone[d]-rifampin (600 mg every 24 hr)
Methicillin resistant	Vancomycin (1 g every 12 hr)	Teicoplanin[e] (400 mg every 24 hr, first day every 12 hr)	Fusidic acid-rifampin (600 mg every 24 hr)
Various streptococci (group A or B β-hemolytic, S. pneumoniae)	Penicillin G (4 million u every 4 to 6 hr)	Clindamycin (600 mg every 6 hr), erythromycin (500 mg every 6 hr), or vancomycin	Amoxicillin (750 mg every 8 hr)
Enteric gram-negative rods	Quinolone[d] (initially i.v., followed by early oral switch)	A cephalosporin III[f]	Quinolone[d]
Serratia spp, P. aeruginosa	A cephalosporin III[f,g] or quinolone quinolone (with aminoglycosides)	Piperacillin[g] (4 g every 6 hr) and gentamicin (5 mg/kg/day)	Quinolone[d]
Anaerobes	Clindamycin (600 mg every 6 hr)	Amoxicillin-clavulanic acid (2.2 mg every 8 hr) or metronidazole for gram-negative anaerobes (500 mg every 8 hr)	Clindamycin (600 mg every 6 hr)
Mixed infection (aerobic and anaerobic microorganisms)	Amoxicillin-clavulanic acid (2.2 mg every 8 hr)	Imipenem[h] (500 mg every 6 hr)	Amoxicillin-clavulanic acid (625 mg every 8 hr)

[a]Oral therapy is usually given after 2 to 4 wk of parenteral therapy with the exception of quinolones.
[b]Second generation, such as cefuroxime (1.5 g every 6 hr).
[c]Flucloxacillin in Europe.
[d]Quinolone, such as ofloxacin (200 mg every 8 hr), ciprofloxacin (500–750 mg every 12 hr).
[e]Teicoplanin is presently available only in Europe; it may be given by the intramuscular route.
[f]Third generation, such as ceftazidime (2 g every 8 hr).
[g]Depends on sensitivities; piperacillin/tazobactam and imipenem are useful alternatives.
[h]In cases of aerobic gram-negative microorganisms resistant to amoxicillin-clavulanic acid.

of the host. Treatment should begin immediately after the onset of symptoms because organisms within the biofilm are more resistant to therapy; as a result, antimicrobial therapy often is unsuccessful unless the biofilm is physically disrupted or removed by surgical debridement.

Single-agent chemotherapy usually is adequate for intravenous treatment of prosthetic joint infection. Antibiotics should be chosen based on the susceptibility of the isolated microorganism, bone penetration and, in later stage, the best oral bioavailability. As a general principle, antibiotics should be given parenterally for 2 to 4 weeks, which may be followed by several weeks to months of oral therapy. The conventional choices of antimicrobial agents for the most commonly encountered microorganisms in infections of skeletal prostheses are given in Table 39-1.

Antibiotic Therapy without Prosthesis Removal

Antibiotic treatment alone without the removal of the prosthesis is not considered standard therapy for prosthetic

joint infection and has been associated with a failure rate of >90% [3,4]. However, in selected patients, antibiotic treatment might be an option under the condition that at least one early and careful concomitant surgical debridement is performed and that the prosthesis is not loose. By definition, this approach is possible only in so-called early onset infections and can be curative in a high proportion of cases [34]. There is a greater chance of success when microorganisms are of low virulence and highly susceptible to IV and orally administered antibiotics. Open debridement is necessary in most patients with acute infected hip and knee prostheses.

In a recent review, Zimmerli et al. have published an algorithm [3] showing that debridement with prosthesis retention supplemented by irrigation and antibiotic treatment with a regimen active in biofilms (containing rifampin for staphylococci and a quinolone for gram-negative pathogens) for 3 to 6 months is adequate for early onset or hematogenous infections with symptoms <3 weeks and stable implant under the condition that there are no difficult to treat pathogens, such as MRSA.

The exact duration of antibiotic therapy after debridement is somewhat arbitrary with suggestions ranging from 3 to 6 months (for knee joint replacement), particularly when oral antibiotics are used [3,37]. However, the majority of patients presenting with a chronic or subacute infection associated with prosthesis loosening will not be cured unless the prosthesis is removed. In patients in whom removal of the prosthesis is not feasible (owing to medical and/or surgical contraindication or the patient's refusal to undergo surgery) and the patient tolerates an active drug for prolonged periods, suppressive antimicrobial therapy may be attempted. Careful monitoring is important because of the danger of extension of the septic process, progressive bone resorption, and side effects of a chronic oral antibiotic treatment.

Antibiotic Therapy with Prosthesis Removal and Reimplantation

To achieve a microbiologic cure, it is almost always necessary to remove the prosthesis and all associated cement and completely debride devitalized tissue and bone. Duration of concomitant intravenous antibiotic therapy is at least 6 weeks. Upon removal of the prosthesis, there are several options; they include resection arthroplasty without reimplantation, arthrodesis, or one-stage or two-stage reimplantation of a new prosthesis.

In the absence of a prospective randomized study with prolonged follow-up, it is difficult at present to recommend one- over two-stage arthroplasty [3,4,35]. For hip prosthesis, analysis of published studies does not show any advantage of the one-stage exchange arthroplasty with or without antibiotic cement compared to the two-stage approach. All reports have been retrospective studies, and only a few described the proportion of patients with infected arthroplasties who received one-stage exchange arthroplasty and adequately contrasted their clinical features with patients who received alternative treatments. With one-stage exchange arthroplasty, the infected components are excised, surgical debridement is performed, and a new prosthesis is immediately put in place under antibiotic coverage. It may be suitable in highly selected hip prosthesis patients who have satisfactory soft tissue, no severe coexisting illnesses, no fistula, no need for bone graft, and infection with organisms that are highly susceptible to antimicrobial drugs [35]. Zimmerli et al. believe that one-stage hip replacement arthroplasty is successful in >80% of carefully selected patients [3].

The two-stage approach requires careful surgical removal of all foreign body material and infected tissue followed by prolonged parenteral and oral therapy [3,4]. The advantages of two-stage hip reimplantation arthroplasty are that it allows for additional debridement and optimization of the choice of antibiotic and duration of therapy for more virulent pathogens. The ideal pause between surgeries is not well established but frequently results in considerable economic hardship and morbidity [35]. The shortest duration of antibiotic therapy would be 6 weeks. The disadvantage is that, as a result of scarring, the second intervention is more difficult to perform and can lead to a second perioperative morbidity and mortality risk for patients with advanced age and serious comorbidities. In patients who have experienced extensive bone loss, a third stage, consisting of bone grafting, is required between resection and reimplantation. Reported success rates of >90% are achieved with two-stage replacement arthroplasty for infected hip prostheses with the interim use of antibiotic-loaded cement [36]. Most U.S. centers use two-stage arthroplasty, whereas the one-stage approach in more commonly performed in Europe with a variable intermediate period between excision and reimplantation [3].

Similar results have been reported in patients with infected knee prostheses. Among a total of 1,143 infections treated with one-stage exchange arthroplasty and with antibiotic-impregnated cement, 915 did not recur (80% success rate). The success rate of two-stage arthroplasty (with or without antibiotic-impregnated cement) was slightly higher (85%) among a total of 262 patients analyzed. Most surgeons favor the delayed two-stage exchange arthroplasty, but this position does not reflect a large body of evidence [37]. However, with the two-stage procedure, patients are at risk of scarring, with resultant loss of range of motion after resection, and, thus, the period of parenteral antimicrobial therapy before re-implantation is not prolonged beyond 6 weeks to preserve joint function. For other prosthetic joints (shoulder, elbow), two-stage exchange with the use of antibiotic-impregnated cement is preferred, although this procedure is costly and time consuming.

Close monitoring and normalization of clinical and inflammatory parameters are mandatory. Prosthetic joint infections due to *M. tuberculosis* sometimes can be cured without joint removal if the infection is recognized early [38]. Fungal prosthetic joint infections are difficult to cure with medical therapy alone. As a result, most such patients require prosthesis removal and arthrodesis to resolve their infections [39].

Antibiotic-Impregnated Cement

Antibiotic-impregnated cement is widely used for prophylaxis and therapy of implant surgery infections but still remains controversial [2,40]. Many antibiotics appear to be released from the cement in potentially efficacious amounts, but the duration of time over which these antibiotics continue to be released is less certain. Moreover, the advantage appears minimal in two-stage procedures. Thus, a lowering of the infection rate often is difficult to attribute to the use of antibiotic-impregnated cement alone. It also is worth noting that gentamicin, the most widely used compound, is not the agent of choice to prevent or treat staphylococcal infections and may lead to local development of *S. aureus* small colony variants [41].

Musculoskeletal Allografts

There are no guidelines or consensus for the duration of concomitant antibiotic therapy for musculoskeletal allograft infections.

RISK FACTORS AND PREVENTION

General Preventive Measures

Today, well-established risk factors for surgical site infections (SSIs) in the literature (mostly for cardiovascular surgery) include insufficient perioperative glycemic control, prolonged hospitalization before surgery, malnutrition, preioperative hair shaving instead of clipping, timing of hair removal, lack of perioperative normothermia, concomitant immunosuppressive therapy, inexperienced surgical team, long operating time, lack of a OR with laminar airflow, lack of compliance with hand hygiene, lack of surveillance, feedback of results and infection control policy for SSIs, and appropriate antibiotic prophylaxis. All these are potential and modifiable quality indicators to reduce the incidence of SSIs.

Preventive Measures and Risks for Prosthesis Infections

A case-control study compared 462 first episodes of prosthetic hip or knee infection with controls matched for age, gender, site of prosthesis, and the date of surgery. The major risk factor was an SSI at a site other than the prosthesis (odds ratio 35.9) [42]. Another study found among 4,240 total hip, knee, and elbow arthroplasty procedures the following risk factors: rheumatoid arthritis, perioperative nonarticular infections, prior infection of the joint or adjacent bone, prior surgery on the joint, prolonged duration of surgery, higher number of OR personnel, postoperative bleeding or hematoma formation, and advanced age [43].

Benefits of Antibiotic Prophylaxis and Ultraclean Air Systems

Between 1970 and 1980, several studies suggested that antimicrobial prophylaxis reduces the incidence of deep incisional SSI after total joint replacement. Hill et al. reported that prophylaxis with cefazolin significantly reduced the SSI incidence compared with a placebo [44]. However, when the results were examined according to the type of OR used, differences were found to be significant only among patients whose surgery was performed in a conventional setting. In a "hypersterile" environment, the rates of SSI were the same for cefazolin-treated and placebo-treated groups. Thus, antibiotic prophylaxis and ultraclean air systems appear to be independent factors in limiting the rate of foreign body infection. Cefazolin has generally been used for prophylaxis in total joint replacement and other surgery because of its greater intrinsic activity against staphylococci, narrower side effect profile, and lower cost, but many reports in the surgical literature also have evaluated the newer cephalosporins. For those with skin colonization with methicillin-resistant *S. aureus* (MRSA), vancomycin prophylaxis may be warranted. On the other hand, despite high prevalence of MRSA SSIs within an institution, a meta-analysis failed to show a benefit of vancomycin compared to beta-lactams in cardiac surgery [45]. Contrary to the cardiovascular surgical literature, topical or nasal mupirocin prophylaxis before orthopedic surgery has not been proven efficacious.

Several studies have found that administration of antibiotics for 12–24 hours is as effective as prolonging antibiotic therapy for several days [46]. Patients receiving the prophylaxis within a 2-hour "window" before the initial incision have lower rates of SSI than patients receiving the antibiotic either too early or postoperatively [47].

Some experimental evidence suggests that there is a risk of SSI of joint implants in the context of bacteremia, especially in the early postoperative period. There also is clear evidence that hematogenous infection of prosthetic joints sometimes stems from overt infections elsewhere in the body, particularly those of the urinary tract or the skin. Thus, vigorous treatment of infection elsewhere in the body is required before total joint replacement. The situation with regard to dental procedures is less clear. Analysis of a large number of patients indicates that the incidence of late-stage prosthetic joint infections associated with dental treatment is low (29 to 68 episodes per 10^6 dental visits) [48]. Accordingly, the American Dental Association has published statements that prophylaxis is not mandatory during dental procedure, but it should be considered in patients with increased risk, such as immunocompromised patients, and within one year after implantation. Treatment of severe periodontal disease and abscesses of the teeth and gums, in the presence of a foreign body, certainly requires administration of systemic antibiotics before orthopedic implant surgery [16].

Prophylaxis of Musculoskeletal Allograft Infections

After the death from *Clostridium sordellii* sepsis of a 23-year-old, otherwise healthy man who had received a contaminated allograft for his knee, the Centers for Disease Control and Prevention (CDC) reported in their investigation 0.12% infections among patients who received sports-medicine tissues and 0.36% among those who received femoral condyles in particular. Almost all *Clostridium* spp. infections were traced back to one single tissue bank [9]. Certainly, precautions are taken according to regional and national guidelines to minimize cross-infection of potential recipients. According to British procedures, procurement usually is performed under aseptic techniques and in an OR. The cadavers are draped and the skin is decontaminated with 10% iodine solution. The allografts are taken from the cadavers and passed to a second person working at a separate table. They are washed in normal saline and stripped of their soft tissue, swabbed over the entire surface for aerobic and anaerobic culture, and then placed into broth. Finally, the allografts are wrapped in sterile towels and plastic bags and are stored at −80°C [13]. If the time interval between death and retrieval is >24 hours or when culture results from blood or bone turn out to be positive, bone allografts are furthermore gamma irradiated or discarded. It has to be mentioned, however, that high doses of gamma irradiation may adversely effect the properties of the allografts [9] and that discarding contaminated bone would result in a wastage of resources in the graft banks where there is a shortage of donors, and infection following the implantation of bone allograft is a serious complication.

Despite these precautions, aseptic processing of tissue minimizes but does not eliminate bacterial contamination of spores, especially in tissue that is heavily contaminated at the time of recovery. Current regulations do not require tissue banks to eliminate bacteria present on tissues at the time of recovery or to use processing methods that guarantee tissue sterility. The main risk factor for contamination seems to be increased time between death and tissue excision.

In the CDC investigation mentioned earlier, there were several "system failures" leading to the epidemic of *Clostridial* spp. allograft infections: First, implanted tissues were not processed using methods that achieved sterility or that were sporicidal. Second, no tissues were cultured before being exposed to antimicrobial agents. Third, evidence of *Clostridium* spp. or bowel flora at other anatomical sites or reports of infections in other allograft recipients were not used as criteria for determining the suitability of donor tissues for transplantation [9]. The contamination of the allografts with *Clostridium* spp. is thought to be via hematogenous route of a donor because the interval between the donor's death and refrigeration of the body exceeded the limit recommended by voluntary industry standards (American Association of Tissue Banks [AATB]).

Sterilization methods that do not adversely affect the functioning of transplanted tissue would be best. Improved guidelines for tissue processing and testing, together with monitoring of allograft-associated adverse events, should enhance tissue-transplantation safety. The time interval between death and procurement should be kept as short as possible. The European Association of Musculoskeletal Transplantation (EAMST) and AATB recommend, for example, that harvesting of bone allograft should take place between 12 and 24 hours after death [49]. Finally physicians should have a high index of suspicion because relying on the results of postprocessing cultures alone to identify and discard tissues potentially contaminated with *Clostridium* spp. spores or other bacterial, fungal, or viral contamination is problematic. Recently, because of the underrecognition of allograft-associated infections and the increasing reports of such infections in the United States, the Food and Drug Administration has initiated a reporting system to better determine the extent of these infections.

REFERENCES

1. Brause BD. Infected orthopedic prostheses. In: Bisno AL, Waldvogel FA, eds. *Infections associated with indwelling medical devices.* Washington, DC: American Society for Microbiology, 1989.
2. Widmer AF. New developments in diagnosis and treatment of infection in orthopedic implants. *Clin Infect Dis* 2001;33 (suppl 2):S94–S106.
3. Zimmerli W, Trampuz A, Ochsner PE. Prosthetic joint infections. *N Engl J Med* 2004;351(16):1645–1654.
4. Lew DP, Waldvogel FA. Osteomyelitis. *Lancet* 2004;364(9431): 369–379.
5. Darouiche RO. Treatment of infections associated with surgical implants. *N Engl J Med* 2004;350(14):1422–1429.
6. Charnley J. Postoperative infection after total hip replacement with special reference to air contamination in the operating room. *Clin Orthop* 1972;87:167–187.
7. Sperling JW, Kozak TK, Hanssen AD, Cofield RH. Infection after shoulder arthroplasty. *Clin Orthop Relat Res* 2001;382:206–216.
8. Bengtson S. Prosthetic osteomyelitis with special reference to the knee: risks, treatment and costs. *Ann Med* 1993;25:523–529.
9. Kainer MA, Linden JV, Whaley DN, et al. Clostridium infections associated with musculoskeletal-tissue allografts. *N Engl J Med* 2004;350(25):2564–2571.
10. Tomford WW, Thongphasuk J, Mankin HJ, Ferraro MJ. Frozen musculoskeletal allografts: a study of the clinical incidence and causes of infection associated with their use. *J Bone Joint Surg Am* 1990;72:1137–1143.
11. Sutherland AG, Raafat A, Yates P, Hutchison JD. Infection associated with the use of allograft bone from the north east Scotland bone bank. *J Hosp Infect* 1997;35:215–222.
12. Mankin HJ, Hornicek FJ, Raskin KA. Infection in massive bone allografts. *Clin Orthop Relat Res* 2005;(432):210–216.
13. Ibrahim T, Stafford H, Esler CN, Power RA. Cadaveric allograft microbiology. *Int Orthop* 2004;28(5):315–318.
14. Rasul AT Jr., Tsukayama D, Gustilo RB. Effect of time of onset and depth of infection on the outcome of total knee arthroplasty infections. *Clin Orthop* 1991;98–104.
15. Gordon SM, Culver DH, Simmons BP, et al. Risk factors for wound infections after total knee arthroplasty. *Am J Epidemiol* 1990;131:905–916.
16. Gillespie WJ. Infection in total joint replacement. *Infect Dis Clin North Am* 1990;4:465–484.
17. Malinin TI, Buck BE, Temple HT, et al. Incidence of clostridial contamination in donors' musculoskeletal tissue. *J Bone Joint Surg Br* 2003;85(7):1051–1054.
18. Lazzarini L, Conti E, Ditri L, et al. Clostridial orthopedic infections: case reports and review of the literature. *J Chemother* 2004;16(1):94–97.
19. McCarthy J, Stingemore N. Clostridium difficile infection of a prosthetic joint presenting 12 months after antibiotic-associated diarrhoea. *J Infect* 1999;39(1):94–96.
20. Zimmerli W, Waldvogel FA, Vaudaux P, Nydegger UE. Pathogenesis of foreign body infection: description and characteristics of an animal model. *J Infect Dis* 1982;146:487.
21. Zimmerli W, Lew PD, Waldvogel FA. Pathogenesis of foreign body infection: *evidence for a local granulocyte defect. J Clin Invest* 1984;73:1191.

22. Bernard L, Vaudaux P, Merle C, et al. The inhibition of neutrophil antibacterial activity by ultra-high molecular weight polyethylene particles. *Biomaterials* 2005;26(27):5552–5557.

23. Donlan, RM. Biofilm formation: a clinically relevant microbiological process. *Clin Infect Dis* 2001;33:1387.

24. Bernard L, Lubbeke A, Stern R, et al. Value of preoperative investigations in diagnosing prosthetic joint infection: retrospective cohort study and literature review. *Scand J Infect Dis* 2004;36(6–7):410–416.

25. Butbul-Aviel Y, Koren A, Halevy R, Sakran W. Procalcitonin as a diagnostic aid in osteomyelitis and septic arthritis. *Pediatr Emerg Care* 2005;21(12):828–832.

26. Smith SL, Wastie ML, Forster I. Radionuclide bone scintigraphy in the detection of significant complications after total knee joint replacement. *Clin Radiol* 2001;56:221.

27. Kraemer WJ, Saplys R, Waddell JP, et al. Bone scan, gallium scan, and hip aspiration in the diagnosis of infected total hip arthroplasty. *J Arthroplasty* 1993;8:611.

28. Stumpe KD, Notzli HP, Zanetti M, et al. FDG PET for differentiation of infection and aseptic loosening in total hip replacements: comparison with conventional radiography and three-phase bone scintigraphy. *Radiology* 2004;231:333.

29. Roberts P, Walters AJ, McMinn DJW. Diagnosing infection in hip replacements: the use of fine-needle aspiration and radiometric culture. *J Bone Joint Surg* 1992;74B:265–269.

30. Lopitaux R, Levai JP, Raux P, et al. Value of puncture-arthrography in the diagnosis of infection of total hip arthroplasty [In French]. *Rev Chir Orthop Reparatrice Appar Mot* 1992;78:34–37.

31. Trampuz A, Hanssen AD, Osmon DR, et al. Synovial fluid leukocyte count and differential for the diagnosis of prosthetic knee infection. *Am J Med* 2004;117(8):556–562.

32. Spangehl MJ, Masri BA, O'Connell JX, Duncan CP. Prospective analysis of preoperative and intraoperative investigations for the diagnosis of infection at the sites of two hundred and two revision total hip arthroplasties. *J Bone Joint Surg Am* 1999;81:672.

33. Bernard L, Sadowski C, Monin D, et al. The value of bacterial culture during clean orthopedic surgery: a prospective study of 1,036 patients. *Infect Control Hosp Epidemiol* 2004;25(6):512–514.

34. Wilde AH. Management of infected knee and hip prostheses. *Curr Opin Rheumatol* 1994;6(2):172–176.

35. Bernard L, Hoffmeyer P, Assal M, et al. Trends in the treatment of orthopaedic prosthetic infections. *J Antimicrob Chemother* 2004;53(2):127–129.

36. Hsieh PH, Shih CH, Chang YH, et al. Two-stage revision hip arthroplasty for infection: comparison between the interim use of antibiotic-loaded cement beads and a spacer prosthesis. *J Bone Joint Surg Am* 2004;86-A:1989.

37. Laffer RR, Graber P, Ochsner PE, Zimmerli W. Outcome of prosthetic knee-associated infection: evaluation of 40 consecutive episodes at a single centre. *Clin Microbiol Infect* 2006;12(5):433–439.

38. Spinner RJ, Sexton DJ, Goldner RD, Levin LS. Periprosthetic infections due to Mycobacterium tuberculosis in patients with no prior history of tuberculosis. *J Arthroplasty* 1996;11(2):217–222.

39. Lerch K, Kalteis T, Schubert T, et al. Prosthetic joint infections with osteomyelitis due to Candida albicans. *Mycoses* 2003;46(11–12):462–466.

40. Duncan CP, Masri BA. The role of antibiotic-loaded cement in the treatment of an infection after a hip replacement. *J Bone Joint Surg Am* 1994;76:1742–1751.

41. Vaudaux P, Kelley WL, Lew D. Staphylococcus aureus small colony variants: difficult to diagnose and difficult to treat [Editorial Comment]. *Clin Infect Dis* 2006;43:968–70.

42. Berbari EF, Hanssen AD, Duffy MC, et al. Risk factors for prosthetic joint infection: case-control study. *Clin Infect Dis* 1998;27(5):1247–1254.

43. Poss R, Thornhill TS, Ewalt FC, et al. Factors influencing the incidence and outcome of infection following total joint arthroplasty. *Clin Orthop* 1984;182:117.

44. Hill C, Flamant R, Mazas F, et al. Prophylactic cefazolin versus placebo in total hip replacement: report of a multicentre double-blind randomised trial. *Lancet* 1981;1:795–796.

45. Bolon MK, Morlote M, Weber SG, et al. Glycopeptides are no more effective than beta-lactam agents for prevention of surgical site infection after cardiac surgery: a meta-analysis. *Clin Infect Dis* 2004;38(10):1357–1363.

46. Norden CW. Antibiotic prophylaxis in orthopedic surgery. *Rev Infect Dis* 1991;13:842–846.

47. Classen DC, Evans RS, Pestotnik SL et al. The timing of prophylactic administration of antibiotics and the risk of surgical-wound infection [Comments]. *N Engl J Med* 1992;326:281–286.

48. Jacobson JJ, Schweitzer SO, Kowalski CJ. Chemoprophylaxis of prosthetic joint patients during dental treatment: a decision-utility analysis. *Oral Surg Oral Med Oral Pathol* 1991;72:167–177.

49. European Association of Musculo-Skeletal Transplantation (1994) Standards for tissue banking and current developments. EAMST, Brussels, Belgium.

The Importance of Infection Control in Controlling Antimicrobial-Resistant Pathogens

40

Cassandra D. Salgado and Barry M. Farr

INTRODUCTION

Infection control (IC) programs were created almost four decades ago to control healthcare-associated infections (HAIs) caused by antimicrobial resistant pathogens (ARPs) but have not succeeded in most nations. This chapter discusses the importance of using IC measures to prevent nosocomial spread of two ARPs, methicillin-resistant *Staphylococcus aureus* (MRSA) and vancomycin-resistant *Enterococcus* (VRE). Use of IC measures is important for controlling these pathogens because the measures have prevented both spread and infections [1–131]. An assumption will be made that preventable infections causing serious morbidity and mortality should not be allowed to continue spreading but should be controlled using available data to guide control efforts. MRSA and VRE infections have been associated with more prolonged illness, higher excess costs, and higher risk of death as compared with infections due to antibiotic-susceptible strains of the same species [132–135], and they are two of the most out-of-control pathogens in U.S. healthcare facilities (Figure 40-1) [136].

Epidemiologic Data Regarding the Risk for Colonization or Infection by Antibiotic-Resistant Pathogens

Effective prevention of any illness depends on having reliable data demonstrating modifiable risk factors. Many studies of ARP colonization and infection have identified two primary causes. The first cause appears to be clinical use of an antimicrobial. For example, before clinical use of penicillin began in the mid-1940s, resistance among clinical isolates of *S. aureus* was rare, but after three years of treating infections at the Hammersmith Hospital in London, about half of *S. aureus* clinical isolates had become resistant to penicillin and treating infections caused by them seemed to have no effect. The relationship between the use of an antimicrobial and the development of resistance has varied for different microbe-drug pairs, but clinically important antibiotic resistance usually starts showing up about a year or two after onset of widespread use of an antibiotic. This occurred with resistance to methicillin among clinical isolates of *S. aureus*; however, treating *S. aureus* infection with methicillin (or another antibiotic) will virtually never result in that strain of

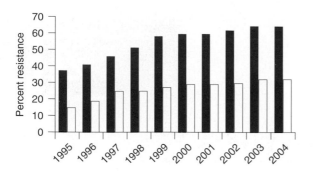

Figure 40-1 Methicillin-resistant *Staphylococcus aureus* (shown in black bars) and vancomycin-resistant *Enterococcus* (shown in white bars) among ICU patients in United States, 1995–2004. Source: Adapted from National Nosocomial Infections Surveillance (NNIS) System report, data summary from January 1992 through June 2004. *Am J Infect Control* 2004;32:470–485.

S. aureus developing resistance to methicillin *de novo*. Also, treating a patient with vancomycin will virtually never result in the patient's own strain of *Enterococcus* developing resistance to vancomycin *de novo* [137,138]. By contrast, treating *M. tuberculosis* infection with isoniazid alone predictably results in treatment failure in about 70% of patients due to a strain with isoniazid resistance [139], the monotherapy not causing mutation to resistance but providing a selective advantage for resistant mutants and favoring their survival. Additionally, surveys have shown that 25–50% of patients in U.S. hospitals and virtually all patients in ICUs receive antimicrobial therapy [140], and many studies have confirmed the importance of exposure to antibiotics as a risk factor for nosocomial ARP colonization or infection [141–144].

The other important cause of ARP colonization or infection has been patient-to-patient spread. Spread of lethal infection via contaminated hands or clothing of healthcare workers (HCWs) has been recognized for more than a century [145,146], and transmission of ARP infections has been documented repeatedly [12,47,117, 147]. Transmission among patients likely often involves transient contamination of HCWs' hands [148–151], apparel [149,152], personal equipment [153], or medical equipment that can recontaminate the HCWs' hands or serve as a fomite vector [114,149,154–161]. Clinicians moving between patients often fail to cleanse their hands [162] and almost never disinfect their clothing or personal or medical equipment between patient contacts.

Studies controlling for antimicrobial therapy have concluded that colonization pressure (i.e., the prevalence of colonization) and spread from other colonized patients is the most important predictor of a patient becoming colonized by MRSA or VRE [163,164]. Similarly, proximity to non-isolated, newly colonized patients was the most important predictor of acquiring VRE in a clonal outbreak; by contrast, proximity to VRE-colonized patients in contact isolation was not a risk factor [117]. Crowding

and decreased nurse-to-patient ratios [45,46] make contamination of HCWs' hands, apparel, or equipment more likely and, thus, transmission more likely. Severe illness necessitates more touching over a longer time and usually antimicrobial therapy, each of which increases risk. In addition to transmitting MRSA or VRE from patient to patient, HCWs sometimes become colonized and transmit the organism to patients without needing to become transiently contaminated by a colonized patient [47,165–167]. This phenomenon has been best studied in Holland where MRSA has been rare and cultures of exposed clinicians have demonstrated that at least transient colonization occurs often enough for colonized HCWs to contribute significantly to MRSA epidemics [166].

The high frequency of antimicrobial therapy in healthcare facilities and frequent nosocomial spread of microbes from person to person give ARPs a selective advantage to survive, proliferate, and spread [11]. This means that without effective IC measures, ARP infections tend to increase to a high prevalence within a ward [45,168,169], hospital [12,19,170,171], region [147,172], and nation [136,173].

IMPORTANCE OF USING INFECTION CONTROL TO CURB ANTIMICROBIAL-RESISTANT PATHOGENS IN REGARD TO EFFECTIVENESS

Effectiveness of Controlling Antibiotic Use to Curb MRSA and VRE

Recommendations to control antibiotic use have been made for decades [174]. This seems attractive because overuse also generates excess pharmacy and nursing costs while potentiating antibiotic resistance. Discontinuation of all antibiotic use would remove the selective advantage for ARP infections, and they likely would dwindle away, but antibiotic therapy currently is perceived as indispensable, so the only control of antibiotic use considered feasible has been limiting it to prudent, judicious usage and sometimes refraining from using one antimicrobial while substituting another. Unfortunately, the former likely still provides sufficient selective advantage to facilitate epidemic spread of ARPs such as MRSA or VRE [11,67,112]. The latter can be associated with at least transient declines in some types of antimicrobial resistance but often is accompanied by off-setting increases in another type of antimicrobial resistance [175], which has been likened to squeezing a balloon.

The Intensive Care Antibiotic Resistance Epidemiology program of the Centers for Disease Control and Prevention (CDC) included 47 hospitals, each claiming to have an antibiotic control program [176], but these hospitals may have been more interested and motivated than average, although their programs were described as less than fully compliant with a prior SHEA–IDSA position paper on antimicrobial control [177]. ARP infections of almost every type increased at these hospitals from 1996 to 1999 [178]. A survey of all hospitals in Virginia and North Carolina revealed that MRSA and VRE were common HAI pathogens despite the fact that about two-thirds of responding hospitals had antibiotic control programs as of 1999 [179].

One hospital used a computer algorithm to educate and advise physicians and found physicians willing to accept advice (and control) when offered by a computer program [180]. Reductions in antibiotic usage and financial savings from lower pharmacy expenditures have been reported by many programs [140,181–183]. Harder to document have been substantial, lasting reductions in ARP HAIs. One hospital reported that antibiotic resistance stopped increasing but did not fall to a low level [140]. Another reported that a control program was associated with a decline in *C. difficile* and VRE but not MRSA [183]. When piperacillin-tazobactam was substituted for ceftazidime, VRE was significantly reduced by about two-thirds in one hospital [184] and in a cancer ward [185]. By contrast, another study reported that increasing use of piperacillin-tazobactam was not consistently associated with reductions in VRE rates in four hospitals [186], and another hospital reported that reducing usage of third-generation cephalosporins by 85% was temporally associated with continually rising VRE rates [187].

Several hospitals have reported at least modest decreases in MRSA with specific changes in antibiotic usage. One switched from a third generation cephalosporin to a first-generation cephalosporin for antimicrobial prophylaxis of surgical site infection (SSI) [188]. The second restricted use of ceftazidime and ciprofloxacin and rotated usage of other beta-lactams [189] while the third also significantly reduced use of third-generation cephalosporins and clindamycin [175]. A fourth hospital reported a significant reduction in MRSA in the first year of an antimicrobial control program [181], but then MRSA and VRE increased substantially despite continuation of the program [190].

In summary, the effects of antibiotic control on MRSA or VRE have tended to be modest as compared with the effects of preventing spread [1–131] and inconsistent from one study to the next although using apparently similar methods. For this reason, despite the cardinal importance of antibiotic use, substantive, sustained control of nosocomial MRSA and VRE infections seems to require a prominent focus on controlling spread.

Effectiveness of Controlling Patient-to-Patient Spread to Curb MRSA and VRE

The most important and indisputable evidence showing that ARP infections can be controlled convincingly comes from multiple nations in Northern Europe and from the state of Western Australia, each using a similar approach to control MRSA HAI to very low levels, in some instances for

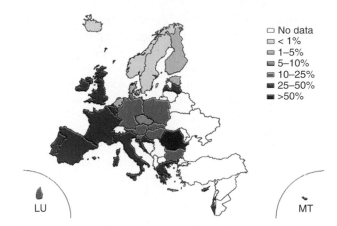

Figure 40-2 Proportion of invasive *Staphylococcus aureus* isolates resistant to oxacillin (or equivalent) in Europe, 2004. Source: EARS Annual Report. Chapter 5. Antimicrobial Resistance in Europe, 2004. ISBN-90-6960-131-1; pg 51.

decades [21,22,28,191–193]. Their approach has involved finding and isolating all patients suspected or known to be MRSA colonized using surveillance cultures and eradicating colonization to reduce further the reservoir for spread. Other countries in Europe and other states in Australia not using these methods routinely [194–197], have had much higher rates of MRSA HAIs (Figure 40-2) [191–193,198]. Also, strain typing has shown that strains considered uncontrollable (e.g., EMRSA16) by some in other European nations are well controlled in Northern European countries [44]. Such strains apparently can be well controlled in countries generally unsuccessful at controlling MRSA if (and for as long as) such measures are applied. For example, a large British hospital demonstrated tight control of MRSA for a decade using such measures [19]. EMRSA16 was introduced into that hospital on six different occasions and controlled each time, never establishing endemicity. After control measures were relaxed because of the perception that they were clinically inconvenient, however, MRSA then became endemic in that hospital and MRSA bloodstream infections (BSIs) increased from 2 and 1 during the two years before relaxation, respectively, to 18 and 74 during the two years after relaxation of control measures [19]. This increase may, in part, have been due to spread throughout the rest of the healthcare system not using such measures that resulted in increasingly frequent transfers and admissions of colonized patients.

Some suggest that Northern European control must be due to having "single payer" national health insurance, but the United Kingdom has this and one of the higher MRSA HAI rates in Europe [191,192,199]. The low rate in Western Australia and much higher rates in other Australian states show that control of MRSA HAIs has more to do with the approach to control used than with a nation's method of financing healthcare [28,193].

Others suggest that prudent antimicrobial usage by Northern European nations may explain their lower

MRSA HAI rates than those in other European nations. Hospital usage rates reportedly have not been publicly available [200], but Denmark and Holland have had the lowest aggregate outpatient antibiotic sales of defined daily doses per 1,000 people in the population while Finland, which at the time had hospital MRSA HAI rates as low as Denmark and Holland [20,21], had a moderate rate of outpatient antibiotic sales, similar to that of the United Kingdom [200], which had a high and growing MRSA HAI rate [191,192,197,201]. If outpatient usage correlates with total antibiotic usage, as implied by the authors, this may suggest that similar measures used to control spread may be more likely to explain the similarity in MRSA HAI rates among Finland, Denmark, and Holland. Other reasons to consider that relatively low antibiotic usage may not be primarily responsible for success in controlling MRSA in Northern Europe include the facts that (1) epidemics of MRSA frequently occur in Holland when colonized patients are not suspected, cultured, and isolated [11,67], (2) nosocomial VRE epidemics can occur in Holland if colonized patients are not suspected, cultured, and isolated despite decades of restricting antibiotic use [112], and (3) methicillin-resistant *S. epidermidis*, not targeted for identification and isolation, has not been controlled to low levels like MRSA despite prolonged antibiotic control [22].

A recent article suggested that the key to controlling MRSA in Northern Europe may be quick eradication therapy [173], but Dutch eradication therapy usually is delayed until conditions are optimal, often after discharge [202]. Nevertheless, eradication of colonization helps prevent MRSA spread because an individual no longer colonized is one less reservoir for nosocomial spread [77,203,204], and a decolonized patient is less likely to acquire an MRSA-HAI [205–209]. Some regimens are more successful than others at eradicating colonization [22,210–213], and some strategies have failed to control MRSA HAIs because they facilitated spread of mupirocin-resistant MRSA strains [214–217]. Giving mupirocin only to the subset with MRSA has been associated with less mupirocin resistance than more widespread application [205,217]. Although most studies show a reduction in *S. aureus* and MRSA infections, these reductions have not always been statistically significant [206,218], in some instances because of transmission to and infection of previously noncolonized patients [219,220] and perhaps because a brief course of intranasal mupirocin in patients colonized at other sites often fails to eradicate colonization [15,211,212].

Eradication of colonization, although helpful, apparently is not essential to dramatically lower nosocomial MRSA spread and HAI rates [12,15,83,91], and data from scores of studies of VRE in Northern Europe, Western Australia, and elsewhere confirm that active detection and isolation of all colonized patients can control spread and infection by an ARP even when eradication is not feasible [112,115,122,221]. In addition to eradication therapy,

Northern European hospitals often close wards at the first signs of epidemic spread, but multiple studies convincingly controlling MRSA or VRE spread without ward closure suggest that this also is not essential [3,33,83,91,126,221].

Are data available from outside Northern Europe and Western Australia supporting the findings cited above? We reviewed 131 studies that reported control of MRSA and/or VRE using active surveillance cultures and contact precautions [1–131]; four reporting simultaneous control of MRSA and VRE using this approach [33,74,81,94]. Multiple institutions reported controlling both MRSA and VRE with this approach but usually in different publications. The majority of the reported successes were not from Northern Europe or Western Australia. Ninety-seven studies described control of MRSA (67 publications in peer-reviewed journals and 30 abstract presentations at national scientific meetings) [1–97]. Among them, at least 50 described control of endemic spread [2–5,10–13,19,22,24,26–30,33–35,37,40,42,45, 48,55,59,65,70,71,73–83,86,87,89–92,94–97], and 52 used MRSA decolonization protocols as an adjunctive control measure [1–3,7–11,14–18,22,24–29,31,34–36,39–48, 52,53,56–59,61–64,68,69,71,72,77,80,84,89,92,93,97]. Thirty-eight studies reported control of VRE [33,74,81,94,98–131]. Among them, 20 described control of endemic spread [33,74,81,94,98–100,104, 107,109–111,115,119,120,125–128,131], and 8 reported using antibiotic control as an adjunctive control measure [101,104,105,109,111,122,123,128]. Two of the 131 studies reported improved control while continuing surveillance cultures and isolation of colonized patients due to apparently improved use of the approach with additional education [5,99], and others reported improved control as compliance increased over time [83,91,126]. Although suboptimal, a measure of control can be achieved even in a single ward [91] or hospital [3,83,111,126] despite surrounding wards/facilities making no intervention to control the spread of MRSA or VRE.

Effectiveness of Hand Hygiene to Control MRSA and VRE

If preventing spread is acknowledged to be key to controlling ARPs such as MRSA and VRE, some may wonder whether better compliance with hand hygiene and/or use of antimicrobial hand cleansers might suffice for this purpose. Hand-hygiene noncompliance has been frequently studied [162,222,223], but the problem persists. Even Boyce and Pittet, primary authors of a guideline recommending alcohol hand-rubs and motivational campaigns to increase clinicians' compliance [224], have admitted that these did not control MRSA in their hospitals and that surveillance cultures [4,14,204] or polymerase chain reaction (PCR) of screening samples [206] and contact isolation of all colonized patients were thus added for control. Huang et al. reported that implementation of alcohol hand rubs for routine HCW hand hygiene between patients and a motivational campaign that increased hand-hygiene compliance from 40 to 80% was not associated with a significant change in MRSA BSI rates [83].

Another problem with the hypothesis that better compliance with hand hygiene and/or use of antimicrobial hand cleansers might suffice to control nosocomial MRSA or VRE to a very low level for a prolonged time is the lack of any examples across geographical areas with long-term control of MRSA or VRE spread with this approach. Although thousands of U.S. hospitals have been required to use standard precautions since 1996, relatively few have reported even modest control using hand hygiene without surveillance cultures and isolation [39,225–228]. By contrast, very few U.S. hospitals have reported using surveillance cultures and contact precautions for all colonized patients [179,229], yet there are many reports of control from U.S. healthcare facilities with their use [1–131]. Another important problem with believing that hand hygiene alone could control MRSA and VRE is that care of a colonized patient often results in contamination of a clinician's clothing [149,152], personal equipment used in the colonized patient's room (e.g., ink pen, notebook, PDA, pager, cell phone) [153], and medical equipment (e.g., stethoscope, tourniquet, sphygmomanometer cuff, reflex hammer, otoscope, ophthalmoscope, electronic thermometers, EKG leads, computer keys) [149] that can transmit contagion directly to another patient or contaminate the HCW's hands and lead to transmission. Touching environmental surfaces near a non-isolated patient often results in contamination of the HCW's hands [148], which can transmit contagion or contaminate equipment [151]. MRSA or VRE sometimes remain viable on cloth or plastic surfaces for weeks to months if not disinfected [230]. Except when a patient has been recognized to be colonized and placed in contact isolation, equipment has not traditionally been disinfected between contacts with different patients. Likewise, rooms contaminated by colonized patients can remain contaminated after routine hospital cleaning methods [231] and may require additional measures to remove contaminants [231,232]. Mathematical models based on epidemiologic data have supported the efficacy of surveillance cultures and isolation and questioned the efficacy of hand hygiene alone for controlling transmission of ARPs [233–235].

Even if hand hygiene cannot be relied on to control such HAIs alone, it nevertheless should help [224], and several studies have suggested better control of MRSA or VRE due to some improvement in hand hygiene although the effects often tended to be modest and control of one microbe was not always associated with control of the other [39,225–228]. For example, Larson et al. reported a significant decline in VRE in a small intervention hospital in association with improved compliance with hand washing with soap and water, but MRSA did not change significantly, and VRE went down a relative 44% in the neighboring,

small, control hospital despite lack of an intervention [225]. Two studies reported control of MRSA in neonatal intensive care units (ICUs) after changing to a different antimicrobial soap for HCW hand hygiene and for antiseptic bathing all neonates in one [39,226], but both reported continuing all other IC measures, including surveillance cultures (and presumably control measures for culture-positive patients) in one [226] and gloves, gowns, cohorting, and surveillance cultures in the other [39]. It was unclear that changing from chlorhexidine to 0.3% triclosan was primarily responsible for control in the latter because only 2 months were allowed before changing to triclosan, and delayed control was also probably due to relatively infrequent surveillance cultures (i.e., only done on admission and discharge) [39]. Three years after switching from use of antimicrobial soap to use of an alcohol handrub at a VA hospital, Gordin reported a 41% relative reduction in patients with any type of new, nosocomial VRE isolate (amounting to 17 fewer patients per year for the hospital) and a 21% relative reduction in patients with new, nosocomial MRSA (amounting to 19 fewer patients per year for the hospital) [227]; because only a small fraction of all colonized patients are detected by clinical cultures, failure to do surveillance cultures made the estimate of the intervention's effect less precise than if they had been done and the reported reductions were modest compared with those achieved using active detection and contact isolation precautions [83,91,126]. Implementing use of an alcohol handrub isn't always associated with improved hand hygiene compliance [236,237]. Pittet et al. reported significantly better control of MRSA after switching to the use of an alcohol hand rub and a motivational campaign resulting in improved compliance [238], but simultaneously implemented surveillance cultures and contact precautions for every colonized patient, making the relative contribution of the changes in hand hygiene difficult to determine [14].

Studies Suggesting Isolation Is not Needed, Does not Work, or Harms Patients

Several recent publications have been used by isolation opponents to suggest that active detection and isolation are not needed to control MRSA or VRE because (1) MRSA reportedly does not spread even when colonized patients are not isolated [239], (2) isolation does not work [169], or (3) isolation harms isolated patients [240]. Nijssen et al. reported a study from an ICU where MRSA was said to be endemic, but no MRSA spread was found over 10 weeks in 2000 from nine colonized, non-isolated patients [239]. Unfortunately, Nijssen et al. failed to specify what precautions (such as standard precautions or universal barrier precautions) they used, making interpretation difficult. They also reported that the rate of clinical MRSA isolates did not change significantly over a 4-year period from 1999 through 2002 in the ICU including the study period, suggesting that MRSA really was not being controlled and that the small 10-week sample was not only statistically imprecise but also misleading. Other recent ICU studies confirm continuing ICU spread despite standard precautions [83,91,136,173,241] and show that MRSA clinical isolates can be significantly reduced after implementing surveillance cultures and contact precautions for all colonized patients [3], one showed a 75% reduction in MRSA BSIs in the 16 months following a phase-in period [83], and another reported continual reduction for 3 years after implementing surveillance cultures and contact precautions for all colonized patients, with the final year showing an MRSA infection rate <10% that of the year in which the intervention began [91]. These data contrast sharply with the lack of improvement over 4 years reported by Nijssen et al. not using identification and isolation [239].

Cooper et al. have authored several publications that have led some to question whether isolation can control ARPs like MRSA [169,242,243]. The first was a structured review of 46 selected studies of MRSA control, which concluded that the studies had not allowed conclusions about the efficacy of individual isolation measures but that "there is evidence that concerted efforts that include isolation can reduce MRSA even in endemic settings and . . .should continue to be applied until further research establishes otherwise"[242]. Then they published another study 4 months later concluding that isolation worked no better than standard precautions to control endemic MRSA [169].

The review said that 6 studies provided "stronger evidence" than the other, generally smaller 40 studies [242], presumably because there could be little question of alpha error or regression to the mean contributing to the observed outcome. Five showed success using surveillance cultures and isolation, but after a decade of control, one of the five failed after relaxing these control measures because they came to be viewed as clinically "inconvenient"[19]. Cooper et al. said that the failure of control was due to a "rise in numbers colonized on admission or change in strain rather than changed [i.e., relaxed] control measures" but offered no rationale for this conclusion [242]. After relaxation of control measures, the numbers of MRSA BSIs increased from 3 during the two years before to 92 during the two years after relaxation, respectively [19]. The sixth study reported control failure despite using surveillance cultures and contact precautions for eight years [244], but Cooper et al. failed to note that most newly identified colonization was from clinical cultures, which suggested that most colonized patients were not being identified and isolated [245]. If this occurred throughout the eight years, it likely could explain the program's failure.

Most of the other studies of surveillance cultures and isolation reported control of MRSA but were dismissed as "intermediate" or "weaker" evidence by Cooper et al., implying that they may have been flawed by chance or biased because they tended to be smaller and lacked randomization and multivariate analysis. The review, which faulted prior reviews for not being systematic and

possibly missing something important, failed to note that MRSA had been controlled to exceedingly low levels in some instances for decades across multiple entire nations and the state of Western Australia, all using a similar approach, and that other European nations [191,192] and Australian states [193] not routinely using this approach had much higher MRSA rates. It also failed to note that virtually all reviewed studies reporting the use of surveillance cultures and isolation of all colonized patients demonstrated success controlling MRSA, the only apparent exceptions being the two mentioned earlier, one after relaxing control measures and the other not identifying and isolating all colonized patients. Cooper et al. suggested that a third study, said to be of "intermediate" strength, also failed to control MRSA, but this was not what the article in question said [25], and a British national guideline disagreed with Cooper, citing the study as an example of success, saying that this and "several other large outbreaks confirm that they often can be controlled and the numbers of patients colonized or infected with MRSA reduced substantially with aggressive management"[201]. It seems unlikely that virtually all of the scores of studies using surveillance cultures and isolation would report success due to some being valid and correct and the rest being invalid and incorrect.

Cepeda et al's. next article began by citing their own review discrediting prior studies reporting success controlling MRSA as "generally undertaken in response to outbreaks rather than within intensive-care units of high endemicity"[169], but many studies have reported control of MRSA using surveillance cultures and contact isolation in settings where it had been endemic for years [2–5,10,24,26,27,30,32–35,37,40,42,45,55, 59,65,70,71,73–83,86,87,89–92,94–97], including multiple settings involving ICUs [3,4,24,26,27,30,70,75,76, 83,91]. Many other supportive studies could be cited showing control with the same measures for endemic VRE [33,74,81,94,98–100,104,107,109–111,115,119,120, 125–128,131], another ARP with similar patterns of spread and a similar selective advantage for proliferation and spread in ICUs; Hill said that "reasoning by analogy" to other conditions was an important way to get at the truth from epidemiologic studies [246].

Cepeda et al. concluded from their brief study that isolation did not reduce MRSA transmission "over and above the use of standard precautions," but this question was not even addressed in the study. Cepeda et al. reported using the same barrier precautions in both study phases (i.e., nurses wearing disposable aprons "throughout each nursing shift" and donning gloves to turn a patient with intact skin) and using dedicated equipment for every patient (i.e., precautions very similar to contact precautions) [169]; Wilson and two of the other authors said in reply to a letter to the editor that the only thing that varied between the two study phases had been whether colonized patients were moved into an isolation room or not [247]. This comparatively small difference between the two study phases (i.e., moving vs. not moving colonized patients) and the brief study period both favored a negative result as did dividing the "move" phase into two separate 3-month blocks. Multiple studies reporting dramatic control with active detection and isolation showed that it took considerably longer than a 6-month intervention to achieve such results [83,91] including one that, like Cepeda, used multivariate analysis adjusting for other predictors of control [30]. Reasons for the lack of trend toward control in either study phase (i.e., despite using barrier precautions for all patients in both study phases) likely included the selection of sleeveless aprons rather than gowns as barriers and leaving HCW colonization uncontrolled in ICUs with a chronic high prevalence, likely contributing to spread in both study phases [47,165–167,203]. The aprons likely allowed contamination of sleeves and probably contributed to spread in both study phases. For example, when a nurse caring for one of the many MRSA patients cross covered for "nurses from adjacent bed spaces" or helped them turn their patients, sleeve contamination could spread MRSA to noncolonized patients even if hands had been washed and contaminated aprons removed, but the nurses' measured hand-hygiene rate was only 21%, and apron removal was not monitored. Nurses reportedly were wearing aprons 99% of the time when monitored, raising concern that they may have worn them "throughout each nursing shift" without removing them appropriately as needed to prevent spread. Multiple prior studies have reported MRSA spread when barriers were left on between patients [5,248,249].

Cepeda et al. called for a randomized trial to confirm their finding that isolation did not work [169], but it should be noted that (1) randomization would not have removed the problems favoring a negative result in Cepeda's study noted earlier and (2) randomization is not needed to provide a representative study sample when the approach is used for the entire patient population as in multiple countries in Northern Europe [22,191,192] and Western Australia [28]. An NIH-supported cluster-randomized trial (RCT) of MRSA and VRE control in U.S. hospitals (**www.ClinicalTrials.gov**, accessed April 13, 2006) is underway but should not be expected to provide definitive results; no single epidemiologic study is ever definitive. Some assume that randomized trials are much more likely to reach accurate, valid results than nonrandomized epidemiologic studies, but recent meta-analyses found that the variability of results for studies of a particular question were usually as large for randomized as for nonrandomized studies [250,251]. The reason for the similarity in variation and error rates between randomized and nonrandomized studies of a particular question may have been that randomization primarily helped prevent selection bias, just 1 of 23 types of bias listed in a recent dictionary of epidemiology, but did nothing to influence many other types of bias, nor did it reduce

the probability of other types of error, such as beta error due to inadequate sample size and statistical power. A prior NIH double-blind RCT of vitamin C as therapy for common colds was believed by its authors to possibly have been biased due to unblinding of study subjects [252]. The NIH RCT of MRSA and VRE control is unblinded and thus more subject to a number of biases for this reason.

The NIH trial protocol chose not to replicate the results of the 131 prior studies showing efficacy of active detection and isolation of MRSA and/or VRE (apparently accepting these results as valid), saying that it instead sought to evaluate a previously unstudied question, comparing the effects of surveillance cultures and contact isolation of colonized patients with the effects of "enhanced standard precautions" (i.e., using alcohol hand rubs and a motivational campaign to increase hand hygiene compliance). However, a study by Huang et al. at Brigham and Women's Hospital recently compared those two approaches and found that active detection and isolation worked better than enhanced standard precautions, reporting no effect of enhanced standard precautions on MRSA BSI rates and a 75% reduction in MRSA BSIs using surveillance cultures and isolation of colonized patients [83]. Huang's study was a nonrandomized, retrospective time-series analysis, but there were multiple important differences other than randomization between the two studies nominally comparing the same measures. For example, Huang's study was much longer and obviously had ample statistical power whereas the NIH trial protocol stated that it would have 80% power only to detect a reduction at least 40% more in the isolation group than the enhanced standard precautions group. This seems inadequate given an intervention period set to last six months and a protocol provision that a study ICU could submit as little as three months of data and have that count as full participation. The lack of such rapid change in recent, eventually dramatically positive studies [30,83,91] makes an intervention period of only 3–6 months in the NIH study seem inadequate to detect a 40% reduction and makes a false negative result seem more likely. Moreover, including only one ICU from a very large hospital, doing admission cultures only on the subset likely to stay >3 days (likely representing a minority of patients in a number of participating ICUs), defining "admission culture" as one done in the first 48 hours, and sending surveillance cultures to an outside laboratory by one-day mail made a negative result seem more likely in the NIH trial than in the Huang study, which sought to culture all patients on admission in all ICUs, thus addressing spread among a much larger fraction of the hospital's high-risk patients. Each of the factors just listed is potentially important and could bias the NIH study toward finding less efficacy of surveillance cultures and isolation of colonized patients with contact precautions; in combination, they could have a major impact on study results.

One nonrandomized study has suggested that patients isolated for MRSA were significantly more likely to suffer decubitus ulcers, falls, or fluid/electrolyte disorders than were nonisolated patients without MRSA [240]. It did not find significant increases in diagnostic, operative, anesthetic, medical procedure or adverse drug events, or mortality. Its authors emphasized that their findings would need confirmation in follow-up studies by others. Opponents of using isolation to control MRSA or VRE have cited this finding as a reason to oppose using isolation for this purpose, but nobody has objected to using isolation to contain other infections like SARS or tuberculosis that infect and kill HCWs, suggesting that they believe isolation to be acceptable for protecting HCW safety. If Stelfox's result is confirmed by additional studies, failure to care properly for isolation patients should not be tolerated by medical management and should be addressed as a quality improvement issue. It should not be used as a reason to refrain from using effective control measures and thus to allow spread of lethal infections.

IMPORTANTANCE OF USING INFECTION CONTROL TO CURB ANTIMICROBIAL-RESISTANT PATHOGENS IN REGARD TO COST EFFECTIVENESS

Multiple studies have documented higher human and financial costs associated with MRSA or VRE HAIs than with infections due to susceptible strains of the same species [1, 132–135,253–257], but some have questioned the cost effectiveness of using surveillance cultures to identify and isolate all colonized patients. Of 12 studies of this question found, each used different approaches, and each concluded that investing in control of spreading infection in this manner was less expensive than taking no effective measures and allowing current rates of endemic or epidemic spread [2,13,33,120,255,257–263]. One concluded that this was cheaper because isolation costs paradoxically declined as surveillance cultures were done to find and isolate all colonized patients because spread was curtailed and fewer patients then required isolation [263]. The other 11 generally found lower costs at least in part because of significantly lower rates of more expensive infections due to MRSA or VRE [2,13,33,120,255,257–262].

SUMMARY

Uncontrolled spread of ARP has resulted in hundreds of thousands of patients suffering HAIs and more than 13,000 deaths in the U.S. healthcare system each year, according to a CDC estimate. Components of a successful control program include education of HCWs regarding the importance of HAIs due to ARPs, encouraging compliance with appropriate hand-hygiene methods using compliance monitoring and feedback, encouraging appropriate use of antibiotics, and, as this chapter has demonstrated, identifying all reservoirs for spread (especially colonized patients) in order to implement appropriate contact precautions. Active surveillance cultures and contact precautions for all colonized individuals have controlled MRSA and VRE infections and saved money. Efficacy has been demonstrated for both endemic and epidemic spread and at the level of the individual hospital unit, hospital, region, and nation.

REFERENCES

1. Rao N, Jacobs S, Joyce L. Cost-effective eradication of an outbreak of methicillin-resistant *Staphylococcus aureus* in a community teaching hospital. *Infect Contrl Hosp Epidemiol* 1988; 9:255–60.
2. West T, Guerry C, Hiott M, et al. Effect of targeted surveillance for control of methicillin-resistant *Staphylococcus aureus* in a community hospital system. *Infect Contrl Hosp Epidemiol* 2006; 27:233–238.
3. Pan A, Carnevale G, Catenazzi P, et al. Trends in methicillin-resistant *Staphylococcus aureus* (MRSA) bloodstream infections: effect of the MRSA "search and isolate" strategy in a hospital in Italy with hyperendemic MRSA. *Infect Contrl Hosp Epidemiol* 2005; 26:127–133.
4. Boyce JM, Havill NL, Kohan C, et al. Do infection control measures work for methicillin-resistant *Staphylococcus aureus?* *Infect Contrl Hosp Epidemiol* 2004; 25:395–401.
5. Poutanen SM, Vearncombe M, McGeer AJ, et al. Nosocomial acquisition of methicillin-resistant *Staphylococcus aureus* during an outbreak of severe acute respiratory syndrome. *Infect Contrl Hosp Epidemiol* 2005; 26:134–137.
6. Andersen BM, Lindemann R, Bergh K, et al. Spread of methicillin-resistant *Staphylococcus aureus* in a neonatal intensive unit associated with understaffing, overcrowding and mixing of patients. *J Hosp Infect* 2002; 50:18–24.
7. Andersen BM, Bergh K, Steinbakk M, et al. A Norwegian nosocomial outbreak of methicillin-resistant *Staphylococcus aureus* resistant to fusidic acid and susceptible to other antistaphylococcal agents. *J Hosp Infect* 1999; 41:123–132.
8. Khoury J, Jones M, Grim A, et al. Eradication of methicillin-resistant *Staphylococcus aureus* from a neonatal intensive care unit by active surveillance and aggressive infection control measures. *Infect Contrl Hosp Epidemiol* 2005; 26:616–621.
9. Saiman L, Cronquist A, Wu F, et al. An outbreak of methicillin-resistant *Staphylococcus aureus* in a neonatal intensive care unit. *Infect Contrl Hosp Epidemiol* 2003; 24:317–321.
10. Cooper CL, Dyck B, Ormiston D, et al. Bed utilization of patients with methicillin-resistant *Staphylococcus aureus* in a Canadian tertiary-care center. *Infect Contrl Hosp Epidemiol* 2002; 23:483–484.
11. Vriens MR, Fluit AC, Troelstra A, et al. Is methicillin-resistant *Staphylococcus aureus* more contagious than methicillin-susceptible *S. aureus* in a surgical intensive care unit? *Infect Control Hosp Epidemiol* 2002; 23:491–494 [erratum appears on *Infect Control Hosp Epidemiol.* 2002;23:579].
12. Thompson RL, Cabezudo I, Wenzel RP. Epidemiology of nosocomial infections caused by methicillin-resistant *Staphylococcus aureus*. *Ann Intern Med* 1982; 97:309–317.
13. Jernigan JA, Clemence MA, Stott GA, et al. Control of methicillin-resistant *Staphylococcus aureus* at a university hospital: one decade later. *Infect Control Hosp Epidemiol* 1995; 16:686–696.
14. Harbarth S, Martin Y, Rohner P, et al. Effect of delayed infection control measures on a hospital outbreak of methicillin-resistant *Staphylococcus aureus*. *J Hosp Infect* 2000; 46:43–49.
15. Back NA, Linnemann CC Jr., Staneck JL, Kotagal UR. Control of methicillin-resistant *Staphylococcus aureus* in a neonatal intensive-care unit: use of intensive microbiologic surveillance and mupirocin. *Infect Control Hosp Epidemiol* 1996; 17:227–231.

16. Murray-Leisure KA, Geib S, Graceley D, et al. Control of epidemic methicillin-resistant *Staphylococcus aureus*. *Infect Control Hosp Epidemiol* 1990; 11:343–350.

17. Nicolle LE, Dyck B, Thompson G, et al. Regional dissemination and control of epidemic methicillin-resistant *Staphylococcus aureus*. *Infect Control Hosp Epidemiol* 1999; 20:202–205.

18. Kotilainen P, Routamaa M, Peltonen R, et al. Eradication of methicillin-resistant *Staphylococcus aureus* from a health center ward and associated nursing home. *Arch Intern Med* 2001; 161:859–863.

19. Farrington M, Redpath C, Trundle C, et al. Winning the battle but losing the war: methicillin-resistant *Staphylococcus aureus* (MRSA) infection at a teaching hospital. *Quart J Med* 1998; 91:539–548.

20. Salmenlinna S, Lyytikainen O, Vuopio-Varkila J. Community-acquired methicillin-resistant *Staphylococcus aureus*, Finland. *Emerg Infect Dis* 2002; 8:602–607.

21. Salmenlinna S, Lyytikainen O, Kotilainen P, et al. Molecular epidemiology of methicillin-resistant *Staphylococcus aureus* in Finland. *Euro J Clin MicrobiolInfect Dis* 2000; 19:101–107.

22. Verhoef J, Beaujean D, Blok H, et al. A Dutch approach to methicillin-resistant *Staphylococcus aureus*. *Euro J Clin Microbiol Infect Dis* 1999; 18:461–466.

23. Campbell JR, Zaccaria E, Mason EO, Jr., Baker CJ. Epidemiological analysis defining concurrent outbreaks of Serratia marcescens and methicillin-resistant *Staphylococcus aureus* in a neonatal intensive-care unit. *Infect Control Hosp Epidemiol* 1998;19:924–928.

24. Cosseron Zerbib M, Roque Afonso AM, Naas T, et al. A control programme for MRSA (methicillin-resistant *Staphylococcus aureus*) containment in a paediatric intensive care unit: evaluation and impact on infections caused by other microorganisms. *J Hosp Infect* 1998;40:225–235.

25. Cox RA, Conquest C, Mallaghan C, Marples RR. A major outbreak of methicillin-resistant *Staphylococcus aureus* caused by a new phage-type (EMRSA-16). *J Hosp Infect* 1995;29:87–106.

26. Girou E, Pujade G, Legrand P, et al. Selective screening of carriers for control of methicillin-resistant *Staphylococcus aureus* (MRSA) in high-risk hospital areas with a high level of endemic MRSA. *Clin Infect Dis* 1998;27:543–550.

27. Souweine B, Traore O, Aublet-Cuvelier B, et al. Role of infection control measures in limiting morbidity associated with multi-resistant organisms in critically ill patients. *J Hosp Infect* 200;45:107–116.

28. Dailey L, Coombs GW, O'Brien FG, et al. Methicillin-resistant *Staphylococcus aureus*, Western Australia. *Emerg Infect Dis* 2005;11:1584–1590.

29. Lugeon C, Blanc DS, Wenger A, Francioli P. Molecular epidemiology of methicillin-resistant *Staphylococcus aureus* at a low-incidence hospital over a 4-year period. *Infect Control Hosp Epidemiol* 1995;16:260–267.

30. Lucet JC, Paoletti X, Lolom I, et al. Successful long-term program for controlling methicillin-resistant *Staphylococcus aureus* in intensive care units. *Inten Care Med* 2005;31:1051–1057.

31. Harberg D. Society for Healthcare Epidemiology of America guideline approach works to control a methicillin-resistant *Staphylococcus aureus* outbreak. *Infect Control Hosp Epidemiol* 2005;26.115–116.

32. Bager F, DANMAP 98. Consumption of antimicrobial agents and occurence of antimicrobials in bacteria from food animals, food and humans in Denmark. www.danmap.org. Accessed May 29, 2007.

33. Calfee DP, Farr BM. Infection control and cost control in the era of managed care. *Infect Control Hosp Epidemiol* 2002;23:407–410.

34. Talon D, Vichard P, Muller A, et al. Modelling the usefulness of a dedicated cohort facility to prevent the dissemination of MRSA. *J Hosp Infect* 2003;54:57–62.

35. Schelenz S, Tucker D, Georgeu C, et al. Significant reduction of endemic MRSA acquisition and infection in cardiothoracic patients by means of an enhanced targeted infection control programme. *J Hosp Infect* 2005;60:104–110.

36. Rashid A, Solomon L, Lewis H, Khan K. Outbreak of epidemic methicillin-resistant *Staphylococcus aureus* in a regional burns unit: management and implications. *Burns* 2006;32:452–457.

37. Mishal J, Sherer Y, et al. Two-stage evaluation and intervention program for control of methicillin-resistant *Staphylococcus aureus* in the hospital setting. *Scan J Infect Dis* 2001;33:498–501.

38. De Lucas-Villarrubia J, Lopez-Franco M, Granizo J, et al. Strategy to control methicillin-resistant *Staphylococcus aureus* post-operative infection in orthopaedic surgery. *International Orthopaedics* 2004;28:16–20.

39. Zafar AB, Butler RC, Reese DJ, et al. Use of 0.3% triclosan (BactiStat) to eradicate an outbreak of methicillin-resistant *Staphylococcus aureus* in a neonatal nursery. *A J I C* 1995;23:200–208.

40. Singh N, Squier C, Wannstedt C, et al. Impact of an aggressive infection control strategy on endemic *Staphylococcus aureus* infection in liver transplant recipients. *Infect Control Hosp Epidemiol* 2006;27:122–126.

41. Valls V, Gomez-Herruz P, Gonzalez-Palacios R, et al. Long-term efficacy of a program to control methicillin-resistant *Staphylococcus aureus*. *Euro J Clin Microbiol Infect Dis* 1994;13:90–95.

42. Blumberg LH, Klugman KP. Control of methicillin-resistant *Staphylococcus aureus* bacteraemia in high-risk areas. *Euro J Clin Microbiol Infect Dis* 1994;13:82–85.

43. Coello R, Jimenez J, Garcia M, et al. Prospective study of infection, colonization and carriage of methicillin-resistant *Staphylococcus aureus* in an outbreak affecting 990 patients. *Euro J Clin Microbiol Infect Dis* 1994;13:74–81.

44. Seeberg S, Larsson L, Welinder-Olsson C, et al. How an outbreak of MRSA in Gothenburg was eliminated: by strict hygienic routines and massive control-culture program. *Lakartidningen* 2002;99:3198–3204.

45. Haley RW, Cushion NB, Tenover FC, et al. Eradication of endemic methicillin-resistant *Staphylococcus aureus* infections from a neonatal intensive care unit. *JID* 1995;171:614–624.

46. Arnow P, Allyn PA, Nichols EM, et al. Control of methicillin-resistant *Staphylococcus aureus* in a burn unit: role of nurse staffing. *J Trauma-Injury Infect Crit Care* 1982;22:954–959.

47. Jernigan JA, Titus MG, Groschel DH, et al. Effectiveness of contact isolation during a hospital outbreak of methicillin-resistant *Staphylococcus aureus*. [erratum appears on 1079]. *Am J Epidemiol* 1996;143:496–504.

48. Linnemann CC Jr., Mason M, Moore P, et al. Methicillin-resistant *Staphylococcus aureus*: experience in a general hospital over four years. *Am J Epidemiol* 1982;115:941–950.

49. Alvarez S, Shell C, Gage K, et al. An outbreak of methicillin-resistant *Staphylococcus aureus* eradicated from a large teaching hospital. *Am J Infect Control* 1985;13:115–121.

50. Selkon JB, Stokes ER, Ingham HR. The role of an isolation unit in the control of hospital infection with methicillin-resistant staphylococci. *J Hosp Infect* 1980;1:41–46.

51. Price EH, Brain A, Dickson JA. An outbreak of infection with a gentamicin and methicillin-resistant *Staphylococcus aureus* in a neonatal unit. *J Hosp Infect* 1980;1:221–28.

52. Duckworth GJ, Lothian JL, Williams JD. Methicillin-resistant *Staphylococcus aureus*: report of an outbreak in a London teaching hospital. *J Hosp Infect* 1988;11:1–15.

53. Mayall B, Martin R, Keenan AM, et al. Blanket use of intranasal mupirocin for outbreak control and long-term prophylaxis of endemic methicillin-resistant *Staphylococcus aureus* in an open ward. *J Hosp Infect* 1996;32:257–266.

54. Shanson DC, Johnstone D, Midgley J. Control of a hospital outbreak of methicillin-resistant *Staphylococcus aureus* infections: value of an isolation unit. *J Hosp Infect* 1985;6:285–292.

55. Jans B, Suetens C, Struelens M. Decreasing MRSA rates in Belgian hospitals: results from the national surveillance network after introduction of national guidelines. *Infect Control Hosp Epidemiol* 2000;21:419.

56. Christensen A, Scheel O, Urwitz K, Bergh K. Outbreak of methicillin-resistant *Staphylococcus aureus* in a Norwegian hospital. *Scand J Infect Dis* 2001;33:663–666.

57. Law MR, Gill ON, Turner A. Methicillin-resistant *Staphylococcus aureus*: associated morbidity and effectiveness of control measures. *Epidemiol & Infect* 1988;101:301–309.

58. Pearman JW, Christiansen KJ, Annear DI, et al. Control of methicillin-resistant *Staphylococcus aureus* (MRSA) in an Australian metropolitan teaching hospital complex. *Med J Aust* 1985;142:103–108.

59. Brady LM, Thomson M, Palmer MA, Harkness JL. Successful control of endemic MRSA in a cardiothoracic surgical unit. *Med J Aust* 1990;152:240–245.

60. Pfaller MA, Wakefield DS, Hollis R, et al. The clinical microbiology laboratory as an aid in infection control. The application of molecular techniques in epidemiologic studies of methicillin-resistant *Staphylococcus aureus*. *Diagnostic MicrobiolInfect Dis* 1991;14:209–217.

61. Walsh TJ, Vlahov D, Hansen SL, et al. Prospective microbiologic surveillance in control of nosocomial methicillin-resistant *Staphylococcus aureus*. *Infect Control* 1987;8:7–14.

62. Ward TT, Winn RE, Hartstein AI, Sewell DL. Observations relating to an inter-hospital outbreak of methicillin-resistant *Staphylococcus aureus*: role of antimicrobial therapy in infection control. *Infect Control* 1981;2:453–459.

63. Jones MR, Martin DR. Outbreak of methicillin-resistant *Staphylococcus aureus* infection in a New Zealand hospital. *New Zealand Med J* 1987;100:369–373.

64. Shanson DC, Kensit JC, Duke R. Outbreak of hospital infection with a strain of *Staphylococcus aureus* resistant to gentamicin and methicillin. *Lancet* 1976;2:1347–1348.

65. Wernitz MH, Swidsinski S, Weist K, et al. Effectiveness of a hospital-wide selective screening programme for methicillin-resistant *Staphylococcus aureus* (MRSA) carriers at hospital admission to prevent hospital-acquired MRSA infections. *Clin Microbiol Infect* 2005;11:457–465.

66. Schlunzen L, Lund B, Schouenborg P, Skov RL. Outbreak of methicillin resistant *Staphylococcus aureus* in a central hospital. *Ugeskrift for Laeger* 1997;159:431–435.

67. Esveld MI, de Boer AS, Notenboom AJ, et al. Secondary infection with methacillin resistant *Staphylococcus aureus* in Dutch hospitals (July 1997–June 1996). *Nederlands Tijdschrift voor Geneeskunde* 1999;143:205–208.

68. Karchmer TB, Adkins C, Gaither B, et al. Use of surveillance cultures to control a methicillin-resistant *Staphylococcus aureus* (MRSA) outbreak in a neonatal intensive care unit (NICU). Abstracts of the 11th Annual Meeting of the Society for Healthcare Epidemiology of America, April 1–3, 2001, Toronto CA. Abstract 109:62–63.

69. Gavin P, Peterson L, Collins S, et al. The use of active surveillance and strict infection control to successfully control an outbreak of MRSA in a neonatal intensive care unit (NICU). Abstracts of the 12th Annual Meeting of the Society for Healthcare Epidemiology of America, April 6–9, 2002, Salt Lake City, UT. Abstract 240:99.

70. Herrera O, Rhoton B, Cantey J. Control of methicillin-resistant *Staphylococcus aureus* (MRSA) in a neonatal intensive care unit using active surveillance: one year follow-up. Abstracts of the 13th Annual Meeting of the Society for Healthcare Epidemiology of America, April 5–8, 2003, Arlington, VA. Abstract 92:74.

71. Garcia C, Manrique A, Basso M, et al. Controlling the spread of methicillin-resistant *Staphylococcus aureus* in a neonatal unit. Abstracts of the 13th Annual Meeting of the Society for Healthcare Epidemiology of America, April 5–8, 2003, Salt Lake City, UT. Abstract 172:91.

72. Gavin P, Vescio T, Fisher A, et al. Successful control of recurrent outbreaks of mupirocin and methicillin-resistant *Staphylococcus aureus* in a neonatal intensive care unit: role of active surveillance. Abstracts of the 13th Annual Meeting of the Society for Healthcare Epidemiology of America, April 5–8, 2003, Salt Lake City, UT. Abstract 254:110.

73. Main C, Griffiths-Turner M, Korver J, et al. Multi-faceted MRSA active surveillance program successfully controls nosocomial MRSA rates. Abstracts of the 13th Annual Meeting of the Society for Healthcare Epidemiology of America, April 5–8, 2003, Salt Lake City, UT. Abstract 256:110.

74. Karchmer TB, Cook E, Lovato J, et al. Active surveillance cultures for methicillin-resistant *Staphylococcus aureus* (M) and vancomycin-resistant enterococci (V) decreased the incidence of new colonization. Abstracts of the 13th Annual Meeting of the Society for Healthcare Epidemiology of America, April 5–8, 2003, Salt Lake City, UT. Abstract 257:110–111.

75. Salgado C, Nobels D, Ruisz M, et al. Control of nosocomial methicillin-resistant *Staphylococcus aureus* (MRSA) using active surveillance cultures and contact precautions. Abstracts of the

76. Karchmer T, Cook E, Adkins C, et al. Active surveillance cultures to identify patients asymptomatically colonized with methicillin-resistant *Staphylococcus aureus* (MRSA) followed by contact precautions decreased the rate of new MRSA colonization and nosocomial infections (NI). Abstracts of the 14th Annual Meeting of the Society for Healthcare Epidemiology of America 2004, April 17–20, Philadelphia. Abstract 43:66–67.

77. Tomic V, Svetina SP, Trinkaus D, et al. Comprehensive strategy to prevent nosocomial spread of methicillin-resistant *Staphylococcus aureus* in a highly endemic setting. *Arch Intern Med* 2004;164:2038–2043.

78. Havill N, Kohan C, Dumigan D, Boyce J. A staged approach to implementing active surveillance cultures for methicillin-resistant *Staphylococcus aureus* (MRSA): Impact on MRSA infections in high risk units. Abstracts of the 14th Annual Meeting of the Society for Healthcare Epidemiology of America, April 17–20, 2004, Philadelphia. Abstract 69:72–73.

79. Clancey M, Wilson M, Johnson J, et al. Active surveillance is effective in reducing methicillin-resistant *Staphylococcus aureus* (MRSA) infection in intensive care units. Abstracts of the 14th Annual Meeting of the Society for Healthcare Epidemiology of America, April 17–20, 2004, Philadelphia. Abstract 72:73.

80. Widmer AF, Tietz A, Frei R. Effective infection control results in low incidence of methicillin-resistant S. aureus bloodstream infections. Abstracts of the 14th Annual Meeting of the Society for Healthcare Epidemiology of America, April 17–20, 2004, Philadelphia. Abstract 176:96.

81. Calfee DP, Salgado CD, Giannetta ET, Farr BM. Effectiveness of surveillance cultures (SC) and contact precautions (CP) for controlling methicillin-resistant S. aureus (MRSA) and vancomycin- resistant *Enterococcus* (VRE) in a non-academic community hospital. Abstracts of the 14th Annual Meeting of the Society for Healthcare Epidemiology of America, April 17–20, 2004, Philadelphia. Abstract 363:128.

82. Muder R, McCray E, Perreiah P, et al. Reducing methicillin-resistant *Staphylococcus aureus* infection rates in a surgical care unit using a systems engineering approach. Abstracts of the 14th Annual Meeting of the Society for Healthcare Epidemiology of America, April 17–20, 2004, Philadelphia. Abstract 366:128–129.

83. Huang SS, Yokoe DS, Hinrichsen VL, et al. Impact of Routine Intensive Care Unit Surveillance Cultures and Resultant Barrier Precautions on Hospital-Wide Methicillin-Resistant Staphylococcus aureus Bacteremia. *Clin Infect Dis* 2006, 43:971–978.

84. Simpson M, Steinmann K, Bennett M, Pfeiffer J. Nosocomial outbreak of methicillin-resistant *Staphylococcus aureus*-USA 300 (MRSA-USA 300) in a burn unit. Abstracts of the 15th Annual Meeting of the Society for Healthcare Epidemiology of America, April 9–12, 2005, Los Angeles CA. Abstract 216:14.

85. Kanerva M, Kolho E, Anttila V, et al. An outbreak of methicillin-resistant *Staphylococcus aureus* (MRSA) and control measures used in a tertiary care hospital in Helsinki, Finland. Abstracts of the 15th Annual Meeting of the Society for Healthcare Epidemiology of America, April 9–12, 2005, Los Angeles. Abstract 209:13.

86. Haile J, Steed L, Fogle P, et al. Significant decrease in nosocomial (N) methicillin-resistant *Staphylococcus aureus* (MRSA) bloodstream infections (BSI) associated with implementation of a active surveillance culture (ASC) program. Abstracts of the 15th Annual Meeting of the Society for Healthcare Epidemiology of America, April 9–12, 2005, Los Angeles. Abstract 206:112.

87. Mermel L, Jefferson J, Monti S, et al. The impact of hospital-wide active surveillance of adult high-risk patients on the incidence of nosocomial MRSA infections. Abstracts of the 15th Annual Meeting of the Society for Healthcare Epidemiology of America, April 9–12, 2005, Los Angeles. Abstract 23:65.

88. Gornick W, Lang D, Glenn L, et al. Nosocomial methicillin-resistant *Staphylococcus aureus* (MRSA) transmission in a NICU; can admission screening cultures help? Abstracts of the 15th Annual Meeting of the Society for Healthcare Epidemiology of America, April 9–12, 2005, Los Angeles. Abstract 10:61.

89. Daha T, Bilkert M. MRSA, the Dutch approach. Abstracts of the 15th Annual Meeting of the Society for Healthcare Epidemiology of America, April 9–12, 2005, Los Angeles. Abstract 2:59.

90. Ridenour G, Wong E, Federspiel J, et al. Prevention of nosocomial transmission of MRSA among ICU patients by selective use of intranasal mupirocin and chlorhexadine bathing. Abstracts of the 15th Annual Meeting of the Society for Healthcare Epidemiology of America, April 9–12, 2005, Los Angeles. Abstract 21:64.

91. Blank M, Haas L, Donahoe M, et al. Sustained effect in reducing methicillin-resistant Staphylococcus aureus (MRSA) hospital-acquired infections (HAIs) using active MRSA surveillance cultures (MSC): three year follow-up. Abstracts of the 15th Annual Meeting of the Society for Healthcare Epidemiology of America, April 9–12, 2005, Los Angeles. Abstract 22:64.

92. Shaikh Z, Bryant K, Miller L, Strelczyk K. "Search and contain" strategy can effectively limit the spread of methicillin-resistant Staphylococcus aureus (MRSA) in the intensive care unit (ICU). Abstracts of the 16th Annual Meeting of the Society for Healthcare Epidemiology of America, March 17–20, 2006, Chicago. Abstract 69:87.

93. Fonseca S, Brandemarte H, Page T, et al. Controlling methicillin-resistant S. aureus (MRSA) in a neonatal intensive care unit (NICU). Abstracts of the 16th Annual Meeting of the Society for Healthcare Epidemiology of America, March 17–20, 2006, Chicago. Abstract 111:98.

94. Gornik W, Lang D, Vaupel-Phillips J, et al. MRSA and VRE: admission screening cultures among high-risk patients in a tertiary pediatric facility. Abstracts of the 16th Annual Meeting of the Society for Healthcare Epidemiology of America, March 18–21, 2006, Chicago. Abstract 279:138.

95. Nouer A, Araujo A, Chebabo A, et al. Control of methicillin-resistant Staphylococcus aureus (MRSA) in an intensive care unit (ICU) after institution of routine screening. Abstracts of the 42nd Annual Meeting of the Interscience Conference on Antimicrobial Agents and Chemotherapy 2002, September 27–30, San Francisco:K–97.

96. Horcajada J, Marco F, Martinez J, et al. Prevalence of methicillin-resistant Staphylococcus aureus colonization at admission in a tertiary hospital: usefulness of early detection. Abstracts of the 42nd Annual Meeting of the Interscience Conference on Antimicrobial Agents and Chemotherapy 2002, September 27–30, San Francisco:K–98.

97. Gerard M, Dediste A, Van Esse R, et al. Cost effectiveness of a policy of methicillin-resistant Staphylococcus aureus (MRSA) screening, decontamination and isolation in a medical ICU. Abstracts of the 42nd Annual Meeting of the Interscience Conference on Antimicrobial Agents and Chemotherapy 2002, September 27–30, San Francisco:K–99.

98. Vernon M, Hayden M, Trick W, et al. Chlorhexadine gluconate to cleanse patients in a medical intensive care unit. Arch Intern Med 2006;166:306–312.

99. Wright MO, Hebden JN, Harris AD, et al. Aggressive control measures for resistant Acinetobacter baumannii and the impact on acquisition of methicillin-resistant Staphylococcus aureus and vancomycin-resistant Enterococcus in a medical intensive care unit. Infect Control Hosp Epidemiol 2004;25:167–168.

100. Dembry LM, Uzokwe K, Zervos MJ. Control of endemic glycopeptide-resistant enterococci. Infect Control Hosp Epidemiol 1996;17:286–292.

101. Rubin LG, Tucci V, Cercenado E, et al. Vancomycin-resistant Enterococcus faecium in hospitalized children. Infect Control Hosp Epidemiol 1992;13:700–705.

102. Golan Y, Doron S, Sullivan B, Snydman DR. Transmission of vancomycin-resistant Enterococcus in a neonatal intensive care unit. Ped Infect Dis J 2005;24:566–567.

103. Boyce JM, Mermel LA, Zervos MJ, et al. Controlling vancomycin-resistant enterococci. Infect Control Hosp Epidemiol 1995;16:634–637. [erratum appears in Infect Control Hosp Epidemiol 1996;17(4):211].

104. Montecalvo MA, Jarvis WR, Uman J, et al. Infection-control measures reduce transmission of vancomycin-resistant enterococci in an endemic setting. Ann Intern Med 1999;131:269–272.

105. Malik RK, Montecalvo MA, Reale MR, et al. Epidemiology and control of vancomycin-resistant enterococci in a regional neonatal intensive care unit. Ped Infect Dis J 1999;18:352–356.

106. Karanfil LV, Murphy M, Josephson A, et al. A cluster of vancomycin-resistant Enterococcus faecium in an intensive care unit. Infect Control Hosp Epidemiol 1992;13:195–200.

107. Silverblatt FJ, Tibert C, Mikolich D, et al. Preventing the spread of vancomycin-resistant enterococci in a long-term care facility. J Am Geriatr Soc 2000;48:1211–1215.

108. Montecalvo MA, Horowitz H, Gedris C, et al. Outbreak of vancomycin-, ampicillin-, and aminoglycoside-resistant Enterococcus faecium bacteremia in an adult oncology unit. AAC 1994;38:1363–1367.

109. Siddiqui AH, Harris AD, Hebden J, et al. The effect of active surveillance for vancomycin-resistant enterococci in high-risk units on vancomycin-resistant enterococci incidence hospital-wide. Am J Infect Control 2002;30:40–43.

110. Price CS, Paule S, Noskin GA, Peterson LR. Active surveillance reduces the incidence of vancomycin-resistant enterococcal bacteremia. Clin Infect Dis 2003;37:921–928.

111. Calfee DP, Giannetta ET, Durbin LJ, et al. Control of endemic vancomycin-resistant Enterococcus among inpatients at a university hospital. Clin Infect Dis 2003;37:326–332.

112. Mascini EM, Troelstra A, Beitsma M, et al. Genotyping and preemptive isolation to control an outbreak of vancomycin-resistant Enterococcus faecium. Clin Infect Dis 2006;42:739–746.

113. Boyce JM, Opal SM, Chow JW, et al. Outbreak of multidrug-resistant Enterococcus faecium with transferable vanB class vancomycin resistance. J Clin Microbiol 1994;32:1148–1153.

114. Livornese LL Jr., Dias S, Samel C, et al. Hospital-acquired infection with vancomycin-resistant Enterococcus faecium transmitted by electronic thermometers. Ann Intern Med 1992;117:112–116.

115. Ostrowsky BE, Trick WE, Sohn AH, et al. Control of vancomycin-resistant Enterococcus in health care facilities in a region. New Engl J Med 2001;344:1427–1433.

116. Hachem R, Graviss L, Hanna H, et al. Impact of surveillance for vancomycin-resistant enterococci on controlling a bloodstream outbreak among patients with hematologic malignancy. Infect Control Hosp Epidemiol 2004;25:391–394.

117. Byers KE, Anglim AM, Anneski CJ, et al. A hospital epidemic of vancomycin-resistant Enterococcus: risk factors and control. Infect Control Hosp Epidemiol 2001;22:140–147.

118. Rupp ME, Marion N, Fey PD, et al. Outbreak of vancomycin-resistant Enterococcus faecium in a neonatal intensive care unit. Infect Control Hosp Epidemiol 2001;22:301–303.

119. Jochimsen EM, Fish L, Manning K, et al. Control of vancomycin-resistant enterococci at a community hospital: efficacy of patient and staff cohorting. Infect Control Hosp Epidemiol 1999;19:106–109.

120. Muto CA, Giannetta ET, Durbin LJ, et al. Cost-effectiveness of perirectal surveillance cultures for controlling vancomycin-resistant Enterococcus. Infect Control Hosp Epidemiol 2002;23:429–435.

121. Armstrong-Evans M, Litt M, McArthur MA, et al. Control of transmission of vancomycin-resistant Enterococcus faecium in a long-term-care facility. Infect Control Hosp Epidemiol 1999;20:312–317.

122. Christiansen KJ, Tibbett PA, Beresford W, et al. Eradication of a large outbreak of a single strain of vanB vancomycin-resistant Enterococcus faecium at a major Australian teaching hospital. Infect Control Hosp Epidemiol 2004;25:384–390.

123. Kohnen W, Ullmann A, Schon-Hoiz K, et al. Early cessation of a vancomycin-resistant enterococci (VRE) outbreak in a hematology-oncology department after implementation of an enhanced infection control intervention: a single center experience. Abstracts of the 16th Annual Meeting of the Society for Healthcare Epidemiology of America, March 18–21, 2006, Chicago. Abstract 307:144.

124. Drews S, Wray R, Freeman R, et al. An aggressive screening program is successful in identifying and containing an outbreak of vancomycin-resistant Enterococcus faecium (VRE) in a children's tertiary-care pediatric hospital. Abstracts of the 16th Annual Meeting of the Society for Healthcare Epidemiology of America, March 18–21, 2006, Chicago. Abstract 106:97.

125. Roth V, Ramotar K, Toye B, et al. Impact of admission screening on the regional spread of vancomycin-resistant enterococci (VRE). Abstracts of the 15th Annual Meeting of the Society for Healthcare Epidemiology of America, April 9–12, 2005, Los Angeles. Abstract 20:4.

126. Muto CA, Posey K, Blank M, et al. Controlling vancomycin resistant enterococci (VRE) using weekly surveillance culturing

(VRESC) and barrier precautions (BP). Abstracts of the 14th Annual Meeting of the Society for Healthcare Epidemiology of America, April 17–20, 2004 Philadelphia. Abstract 365:128.

127. Butcher J, Thronton V, Lockamy K, Kaye K. Control of nosocomial vancomycin-resistant *Enterococcus* (VRE) acquisition through active surveillance of dialysis patients. Abstracts of the 13th Annual Meeting of the Society for Healthcare Epidemiology of America, April 5–8, 2003, Arlington, VA. Abstract 258:111.

128. Shaikh Z, Osting C, Hanna H, Raad I. Effectivness of a multifaceted infection control policy in reducing vancomycin usage and vancomycin-resistant enterococci at a tertiary cancer center. Abstracts of the 11th Annual Meeting of the Society for Healthcare Epidemiology of America, April 1–3, 2001, Toronto. Abstract 165:75.

129. Krystofiak S, Posey K, Nouri K, et al. Active surveillance for VRE-looking below the tip of the iceberg. Abstracts of the 11th Annual Meeting of the Society for Healthcare Epidemiology of America, April 1–3, 2001, Toronto. Abstract 175:77–78.

130. Singh N, Leger MM, Campbell J, et al. Control of vancomycin-resistant enterococci in the neonatal intensive care unit. *Infect Control Hosp Epidemiol* 2005;26:646–649.

131. Salgado CD, Nobels D, Ruisz M, et al. Effect of active surveillance cultures and contact precautions for controlling endemic vancomycin-resistant *Enterococcus*. Abstracts of the 14th Annual Meeting of the Society for Healthcare Epidemiology of America, April 17–20, 2004, Philadelphia. Abstract 364:128.

132. Cosgrove SE, Sakoulas G, Perencevich EN, et al. Comparison of mortality associated with methicillin-resistant and methicillin-susceptible *Staphylococcus aureus* bacteremia: a meta-analysis. *Clin Infect Dis* 2003;36:53–59.

133. Whitby M, McLaws ML, Berry G. Risk of death from methicillin-resistant *Staphylococcus aureus* bacteraemia: a meta-analysis. *Med J Aust* 2001;175:264–267.

134. Salgado CD, Farr BM. Outcomes associated with vancomycin-resistant enterococci: a meta-analysis. *Infect Control Hosp Epidemiol* 2003;24:690–698.

135. DiazGranados CA, Zimmer S, Klein M, Jernigan JA. Comparison of mortality associated with vancomycin-resistant and vancomycin-susceptible enterococcal bloodstream infections: a meta-analysis. *Clin Infect Dis* 2005;41:327–333.

136. National Nosocomial Infections Surveillance System. National Nosocomial Infections Surveillance (NNIS) System report, data summary from January 1992 through June 2004. *Am J Infect Control* 2004;32:470–485.

137. Salgado CD, Giannetta ET, Farr BM. Failure to develop vancomycin-resistant *Enterococcus* with oral vancomycin treatment of *Clostridium difficile*. *Infect Control Hosp Epidemiol* 2004;25:413–417.

138. Bernard L, Vaudaux P, Vuagnat A, et al. Effect of vancomycin therapy for osteomyelitis on colonization by methicillin-resistant *Staphylococcus aureus*: lack of emergence of glycopeptide resistance. *Infect Control Hosp Epidemiol* 2003;24:650–654.

139. Marshall G, Crofton J, Cruickshank R, et al. The treatment of pulmonary tuberculosis with isoniazid. *Br Med J* 1952;2:735–746.

140. Pestotnik SL, Classen DC, Evans RS, Burke JP. Implementing antibiotic practice guidelines through computer-assisted decision support: clinical and financial outcomes. *Ann Intern Med* 1996;124:884–890.

141. McGowan JE Jr. Antimicrobial resistance in hospital organisms and its relation to antibiotic use. *Rev Infect Dis* 1983;5:1033–1048.

142. Fridkin SK, Steward CD, Edwards JR, et al. Surveillance of antimicrobial use and antimicrobial resistance in United States hospitals: project ICARE phase 2. Project Intensive Care Antimicrobial Resistance Epidemiology (ICARE) hospitals. *Clin Infect Dis* 1999;29:245–252.

143. Dancer SJ, Coyne M, Robertson C, et al. Antibiotic use is associated with resistance of environmental organisms in a teaching hospital. *J Hosp Infect* 2006;62:200–206.

144. Kernodle DS, Barg NL, Kaiser AB. Low-level colonization of hospitalized patients with methicillin-resistant coagulase-negative staphylococci and emergence of the organisms during surgical antimicrobial prophylaxis. *AAC* 1988;32:202–208.

145. Holmes O. The contagiousness of puerperal fever. *N Engl Q J Med Surg* 1842;1:501–530.

146. Semmelweis I. *The etiology, the concept, and the prophylaxis of childbed fever:* Pest. CA Hartleben's Verlag-Expedition 1861.

147. Silva Coimbra MV, Silva-Carvalho MC, Wisplinghoff H, et al. Clonal spread of methicillin-resistant *Staphylococcus aureus* in a large geographic area of the United States. *J Hosp Infect* 2003;53:103–110.

148. Bhalla A, Pultz NJ, Gries DM, et al. Acquisition of nosocomial pathogens on hands after contact with environmental surfaces near hospitalized patients. *Infect Control Hosp Epidemiol* 2004;25:164–167.

149. Zachary KC, Bayne PS, Morrison VJ, et al. Contamination of gowns, gloves, and stethoscopes with vancomycin-resistant enterococci. *Infect Control Hosp Epidemiol* 2001;22:560–564.

150. Noskin GA, Stosor V, Cooper I, Peterson LR. Recovery of vancomycin-resistant enterococci on fingertips and environmental surfaces. *Infect Control Hosp Epidemiol* 1995;16:577–581.

151. Duckro AN, Blom DW, Lyle EA, et al. Transfer of vancomycin-resistant enterococci via health care worker hands. *Arch Intern Med* 2005;165(3):302–307.

152. Boyce J, Chenevert C. Isolation gowns prevent health care workers (HCWs) from contaminating their clothing, and possibly their hands, with methicillin-resistant *Staphylococcus aureus* (MRSA) and resistant enterococci. Abstracts of the Eighth Annual Meeting of the Society for Healthcare Epidemiology of America, 1998, Orlando, FL. Abstract S74:52.

153. Singh D, Kaur H, Gardner WG, Treen LB. Bacterial contamination of hospital pagers. *Infect Control Hosp Epidemiol* 2002;23:274–276.

154. Embil JM, McLeod JA, Al Barrak AM, et al. An outbreak of methicillin resistant *Staphylococcus aureus* on a burn unit: potential role of contaminated hydrotherapy equipment. *Burns* 2001;27:681–688.

155. Ackelsberg J, Kostman J. A laboratory and clinical study of stethoscopes as potential fomites of infection. Abstracts of the 33rd Annual Meeting of the Infectious Diseases Society of America 1995, San Francisco CA.

156. Bernard L, Kereveur A, Durand D, et al. Bacterial contamination of hospital physicians' stethoscopes. *Infect Control Hosp Epidemiol* 1999;20:626–628.

157. Breathnach AS, Jenkins DR, Pedler SJ. Stethoscopes as possible vectors of infection by staphylococci. *BMJ* 1992;305:1573–1574.

158. Maki D, Halvorson K, Fisher S. The stethoscope: a medical device with potential for amplifying cross-infection of resistant nosocomial organisms in the hospital. Abstracts of the 36th Annual Meeting of the IInterscience Conference on Antimicrobial Agents and Chemotherapy 1996, New Orleans, LA. Abstract 154:247.

159. Smith MA, Mathewson JJ, Ulert IA, et al. Contaminated stethoscopes revisited. *Arch Intern Med* 1996;156:82–84.

160. Cohen HA, Amir J, Matalon A, et al. Stethoscopes and otoscopes—a potential vector of infection? *Family Practice* 1997;14:446–449.

161. Edmond MB, Ober JF, Weinbaum DL, et al. Vancomycin-resistant *Enterococcus faecium* bacteremia: risk factors for infection. *Clin Infect Dis* 1995;20:1126–1133.

162. Pittet D, Mourouga P, Perneger TV. Compliance with handwashing in a teaching hospital: infection control program. *Ann Intern Med* 1999;130:126–130.

163. Merrer J, Santoli F, Appere d V, et al. "Colonization pressure" and risk of acquisition of methicillin-resistant *Staphylococcus aureus* in a medical intensive care unit. *Infect Control Hosp Epidemiol* 2000;21:718–1723.

164. Bonten MJ, Slaughter S, Ambergen AW, et al. The role of "colonization pressure" in the spread of vancomycin-resistant enterococci: an important infection control variable. *Arch Intern Med* 1998;158:1127–1132.

165. Suh HK, Jeon YH, Song JS, et al. A molecular epidemiologic study of methicillin-resistant Staphylococcus aureus infection in patients undergoing middle ear surgery. *European Archives of Oto-Rhino-Laryngology* 1998;255:347–351.

166. Blok HE, Troelstra A, Kamp-Hopmans TE, et al. Role of healthcare workers in outbreaks of methicillin-resistant *Staphylococcus aureus*: a 10-year evaluation from a Dutch university hospital. *Infect Control Hosp Epidemiol* 2003;24:679–685.

167. Sherertz RJ, Reagan DR, Hampton KD, et al. A cloud adult: the *Staphylococcus aureus*-virus interaction revisited. *Ann Intern Med* 1996;124:539–547.

168. Huang YC, Su LH, Wu TL, Lin TY. Molecular surveillance of clinical methicillin-resistant *Staphylococcus aureus* isolates in neonatal intensive care units. *Infect Control Hosp Epidemiol* 2005;26:157–760.

169. Cepeda JA, Whitehouse T, Cooper B, et al. Isolation of patients in single rooms or cohorts to reduce spread of MRSA in intensive-care units: prospective two-centre study. *Lancet* 2005;365:295–304.

170. Ip M, Lyon DJ, Chio F, Cheng AF. A longitudinal analysis of methicillin-resistant *Staphylococcus aureus* in a Hong Kong teaching hospital. *Infect Control Hosp Epidemiol* 2004;25: 126–129.

171. Pavillard R, Harvey K, Douglas D, et al. Epidemic of hospital-acquired infection due to methicillin-resistant *Staphylococcus aureus* in major Victorian hospitals. *Med J Aus* 1982;1:451–454.

172. Polgreen P, Beekmann S, Chen Y, et al. Epidemiology of methicillin-resistant *Staphylococcus aureus* and vancomycin-resistant *Enterococcus* in a rural state. *Infect Control Hosp Epidemiol* 2006;27:252–256.

173. Klevens R, Edwards J, Tenover F, et al. National Nosocomial Infections Surveillance System: changes in the epidemiology of methicillin-resistant *Staphylococcus aureus* in intensive care units in US hospitals, 1992–2003. *Clin Infect Dis* 2006;42:389–391.

174. Kunin CM, Tupasi T, Craig WA. Use of antibiotics: a brief exposition of the problem and some tentative solutions. *Ann Intern Med* 1973;79:555–560.

175. Landman D, Chockalingam M, Quale JM. Reduction in the incidence of methicillin-resistant *Staphylococcus aureus* and ceftazidime-resistant *Klebsiella pneumoniae* following changes in a hospital antibiotic formulary. *Clin Infect Dis* 1999;28:1062–1066.

176. Lawton RM, Fridkin SK, Gaynes RP, McGowan JE Jr. Practices to improve antimicrobial use at 47 US hospitals: the status of the 1997 SHEA/IDSA position paper recommendations. *Infect Control Hosp Epidemiol* 2000;21:256–259.

177. Shlaes DM, Gerding DN, John JF Jr., et al. Society for Healthcare Epidemiology of America and Infectious Diseases Society of America Joint Committee on the Prevention of Antimicrobial Resistance: guidelines for the prevention of antimicrobial resistance in hospitals. *Clin Infect Dis* 1997;25:584–599.

178. Fridkin SK, Hill HA, Volkova NV, et al. Temporal changes in prevalence of antimicrobial resistance in 23 US hospitals. *Emerg Infect Dis* 2002;8:697–701.

179. Salgado C, Sherertz R, Karchmer T, et al. Public health initiative to control MRSA and VRE in Virginia and North Carolina. Abstracts of the 11th Annual Meeting of the Society for Healthcare Epidemiology of America, April 1–3, 2001, Toronto. Abstract 164:75.

180. Evans RS, Classen DC, Pestotnik SL, et al. Improving empiric antibiotic selection using computer decision support. *Arch Intern Med* 1994;154:878–884.

181. Frank MO, Batteiger BE, Sorensen SJ, et al. Decrease in expenditures and selected nosocomial infections following implementation of an antimicrobial-prescribing improvement program. *Clin Performance & Qual Health Care* 1997;5:180–188.

182. Evans RS, Pestotnik SL, Classen DC, et al. A computer-assisted management program for antibiotics and other antiinfective agents. *New Engl J Med* 1998;338:232–238.

183. Carling P, Fung T, Killion A, et al. Favorable impact of a multidisciplinary antibiotic management program conducted during 7 years. *Infect Control Hosp Epidemiol* 2003;24:699–706.

184. Quale J, Landman D, Saurina G, et al. Manipulation of a hospital antimicrobial formulary to control an outbreak of vancomycin-resistant enterococci. *Clin Infect Dis* 1996;23:1020–1025.

185. Bradley SJ, Wilson AL, Allen MC, et al. The control of hyperendemic glycopeptide-resistant *Enterococcus* spp. on a haematology unit by changing antibiotic usage. *J Antimicrobial Chemotherapy* 1999;43:261–266.

186. Stiefel U, Paterson DL, Pultz NJ, et al. Effect of the increasing use of piperacillin/tazobactam on the incidence of vancomycin-resistant enterococci in four academic medical centers. *Infect Control Hosp Epidemiol* 2004;25:380–383.

187. Lautenbach E, Larosa LA, Marr AM, et al. Changes in the prevalence of vancomycin-resistant enterococci in response to antimicrobial formulary interventions: impact of progressive restrictions on use of vancomycin and third-generation cephalosporins. *Clin Infect Dis* 2003;36:440–446.

188. Fukatsu K, Saito H, Matsuda T, et al. Influences of type and duration of antimicrobial prophylaxis on an outbreak of methicillin-resistant *Staphylococcus aureus* and on the incidence of wound infection. *Arch Surg* 1997;132:1320–1325.

189. Gruson D, Hilbert G, Vargas F, et al. Rotation and restricted use of antibiotics in a medical intensive care unit: impact on the incidence of ventilator-associated pneumonia caused by antibiotic-resistant gram-negative bacteria. *Am J Resp Crit Care Med* 2000;162:837–843.

190. Batteiger BE. *Personal communication.* Indiana University, Indiana 2001.

191. Tiemersma EW, Monnet DL, Bruinsma N, et al. *Staphylococcus aureus* bacteremia, Europe. *Emerg Infect Dis* 2005;11:1798–1799.

192. Tiemersma EW, Bronzwaer SL, Lyytikainen O, et al. Methicillin-resistant *Staphylococcus aureus* in Europe, 1999–2002. *Emerg Infect Dis* 2004;10:1627–1634.

193. Boyce JM, Cookson B, Christiansen K, et al. Methicillin-resistant *Staphylococcus aureus*. *Lancet Infect Dis* 2005;5:653–663.

194. Gastmeier P, Schwab F, Geffers C, Ruden H. To isolate or not to isolate? analysis of data from the German Nosocomial Infection Surveillance System regarding the placement of patients with methicillin-resistant *Staphylococcus aureus* in private rooms in intensive care units. *Infect Control Hosp Epidemiol* 2004;25:109–13.

195. L'Heriteau F, Alberti C, Cohen Y, et al. Nosocomial infection and multidrug-resistant bacteria surveillance in intensive care units: a survey in France. *Infect Control Hosp Epidemiol* 2005;26:13–20.

196. Troche G, Joly LM, Guibert M, Zazzo JF. Detection and treatment of antibiotic-resistant bacterial carriage in a surgical intensive care unit: a 6-year prospective survey. *Infect Control Hosp Epidemiol* 2005;26:161–165.

197. Hails J, Kwaku F, Wilson AP, et al. Large variation in MRSA policies, procedures and prevalence in English intensive care units: a questionnaire analysis. *Inten Care Med* 2003;29:481–483.

198. Zinn CS, Westh H, Rosdahl VT, Sarisa Study Group. An International multicenter study of antimicrobial resistance and typing of hospital *Staphylococcus aureus* isolates from 21 laboratories in 19 countries or states. *Microbial Drug Resistance-Mechanisms Epidemiology & Disease* 2004;10:160–168.

199. Lessing MP, Loveland RC. Isolation of patients with MRSA infection. *Lancet* 2005;365:1303.

200. Cars O, Molstad S, Melander A. Variation in antibiotic use in the European Union. *Lancet* 2001;357:1851–1853.

201. No autho. Revised guidelines for the control of methicillin-resistant *Staphylococcus aureus* infection in hospitals. *J Hosp Infect* 1998;39:253–290.

202. Muto CA, Vos M, Jarvis W, Farr B. Control of nosocomial methicillin-resistant *Staphylococcus aureus* infection. *Clin Infect Dis* 2006;43:387.

203. Boyce JM, Opal SM, Potter-Bynoe G, Mcdeiros AA. Spread of methicillin-resistant *Staphylococcus aureus* in a hospital after exposure to a health care worker with chronic sinusitis. *Clin Infect Dis* 1993;17:496–504.

204. Sax H, Posfay-Barbe K, Harbarth S, et al. Control of a cluster of community-associated, methicillin-resistant *Staphylococcus aureus* in neonatology. *J Hosp Infect* 2006;63:93–100.

205. Sandri A, Dalarosa M, Ruschel de Alcantara L, et al. Reduction in incidence of nosocomial methicillin-resistant *Staphylococcus aureus* (MRSA) infection in an intensive care unit: role of treatment with mupirocin ointment and chlorhexidine baths for nasal carriers of MRSA. *Infect Control Hosp Epidemiol* 2006;27:185–187.

206. Harbarth S, Masuet-Aumatell C, Schrenzel J, et al. Evaluation of a rapid screening and pre-emptive contact isolation for detecting and controlling methicillin-resistant *Staphylococcus aureus* in critical care: an interventional cohort study. *Crit Care* 2006;10:R25.

207. Muller A, Talon D, Potier A, et al. Use of intranasal mupirocin to prevent methicillin-resistant *Staphylococcus aureus* infection in intensive care units. *Crit Care* 2005;9:R246–R250.

208. Kluytmans JA, Mouton JW, VandenBergh MF, et al. Reduction of surgical-site infections in cardiothoracic surgery by elimination of nasal carriage of *Staphylococcus aureus*. *Infect Control Hosp Epidemiol* 1996;17:780–785.

209. Wilcox MH, Hall J, Pike H, et al. Use of perioperative mupirocin to prevent methicillin-resistant *Staphylococcus aureus* (MRSA) orthopaedic surgical site infections. *J Hosp Infect* 2003;54:196–201.

210. Karchmer T, Jernigan J, Durbin L, et al. Eradication of MRSA colonization with different regimens. Abstracts of the 9th Annual Meeting of the Society for Healthcare Epidemiology of America, April 18–20, 1999, San Francisco. Abstract 65:42.

211. Harbarth S, Dharan S, Liassine N, et al. Randomized, placebo-controlled, double-blind trial to evaluate the efficacy of mupirocin for eradicating carriage of methicillin-resistant *Staphylococcus aureus*. *AAC* 1996;43:1412–1416.

212. Harbarth S, Liassine N, Dharan S, et al. Risk factors for persistent carriage of methicillin-resistant *Staphylococcus aureus*. *Clin Infect Dis* 2000;31:1380–1385.

213. Urth T, Juul G, Skov R, Schonheyder HC. Spread of a methicillin-resistant *Staphylococcus aureus* ST80-IV clone in a Danish community. *Infect Control Hosp Epidemiol* 2005;26:144–149.

214. Vasquez JE, Walker ES, Franzus BW, et al. The epidemiology of mupirocin resistance among methicillin-resistant *Staphylococcus aureus* at a Veterans' Affairs hospital. *Infect Control Hosp Epidemiol* 2000;21:459–464.

215. Miller MA, Dascal A, Portnoy J, Mendelson J. Development of mupirocin resistance among methicillin-resistant *Staphylococcus aureus* after widespread use of nasal mupirocin ointment. *Infect Control Hosp Epidemiol* 1996;17:811–813.

216. Netto dos Santos KR, de Souza FL, Gontijo Filho PP. Emergence of high-level mupirocin resistance in methicillin-resistant *Staphylococcus aureus* isolated from Brazilian university hospitals. *Infect Control Hosp Epidemiol* 1996;17:813–816.

217. Vivoni AM, Santos KR, de Oliveira MP, et al. Mupirocin for controlling methicillin-resistant *Staphylococcus aureus*: lessons from a decade of use at a university hospital. *Infect Control Hosp Epidemiol* 2005;26:662–667.

218. Wertheim HF, Vos MC, Ott A, et al. Mupirocin prophylaxis against nosocomial *Staphylococcus aureus* infections in nonsurgical patients: a randomized study. *Ann Intern Med* 2004;140:419–425.

219. Kalmeijer MD, Coertjens H, Nieuwland-Bollen PM, et al. Surgical site infections in orthopedic surgery: the effect of mupirocin nasal ointment in a double-blind, randomized, placebo-controlled study. *Clin Infect Dis* 2002;35:353–358.

220. Perl TM, Cullen JJ, Wenzel RP, et al. Intranasal mupirocin to prevent postoperative *Staphylococcus aureus* infections. *New Engl J Med* 2002;346:1871–1877.

221. Muto CA, Jernigan JA, Ostrowsky BE, et al. SHEA guideline for preventing nosocomial transmission of multidrug-resistant strains of *Staphylococcus aureus* and *Enterococcus*. *Infect Control Hosp Epidemiol* 2003;24:362–386.

222. Voss A, Widmer AF. No time for handwashing!? handwashing versus alcoholic rub: can we afford 100% compliance? *Infect Control Hosp Epidemiol* 1997;18:205–208.

223. Hugonnet S, Pittet D. Hand hygiene—beliefs or science. *Clin Microbiol Infect* 2000;6:348–354.

224. Boyce JM, Pittet D, Healthcare Infection Control Practices Advisory Committee. Guideline for hand hygiene in health-care settings: recommendations of the Healthcare Infection Control Practices Advisory Committee and the HIC-PAC/SHEA/APIC/IDSA Hand Hygiene Task Force. *Infect Control Hosp Epidemiol* 2002;23:S3–S40.

225. Larson EL, Early E, Cloonan P, et al. An organizational climate intervention associated with increased handwashing and decreased nosocomial infections. *Behavioral Med* 2000;26:14–22.

226. Webster J, Faoagali JL, Cartwright D. Elimination of methicillin-resistant *Staphylococcus aureus* from a neonatal intensive care unit after hand washing with triclosan. *J Paediatrics & Child Health* 1994;30:59–64.

227. Gordin FM, Schultz ME, Huber RA, Gill JA. Reduction in nosocomial transmission of drug-resistant bacteria after introduction of an alcohol-based handrub. *Infect Control Hosp Epidemiol* 2005;26:650–653.

228. MacDonald A, Dinah F, MacKenzie D, Wilson A. Performance feedback of hand hygiene, using alcohol gel as the skin decontaminant, reduces the number of inpatients newly affected by MRSA and antibiotic costs. *J Hosp Infect* 2004;56:56–63.

229. Sunenshine RH, Liedtke LA, Fridkin SK, et al. Management of inpatients colonized or infected with antimicrobial-resistant bacteria in hospitals in the United States. *Infect Control Hosp Epidemiol* 2005;26:138–143.

230. Neely AN, Maley MP. Survival of enterococci and staphylococci on hospital fabrics and plastic. *J Clin Microbiol* 2000;38:724–726.

231. Byers KE, Durbin LJ, Simonton BM, et al. Disinfection of hospital rooms contaminated with vancomycin-resistant *Enterococcus faecium*. *Infect Control Hosp Epidemiol* 1998;19:261–264.

232. Hayden MK, Bonten MJ, Blom DW, et al. Reduction of acquisition of vancomycin-resistant *Enterococcus* after enforcement of routine environmental cleaning measures. *Clin Infect Dis* 2006;42:1552–1560.

233. Perencevich EN, Fisman DN, Lipsitch M, et al. Projected benefits of active surveillance for vancomycin-resistant enterococci in intensive care units. *Clin Infect Dis* 2004;38:1108–1115.

234. Austin DJ, Bonten MJ, Weinstein RA, et al. Vancomycin-resistant enterococci in intensive-care hospital settings: transmission dynamics, persistence, and the impact of infection control programs. *Proceedings of the National Academy of Sciences of the United States of America* 1999;96:6908–6913.

235. Sebille V, Chevret S, Valleron AJ. Modeling the spread of resistant nosocomial pathogens in an intensive-care unit. *Infect Control Hosp Epidemiol* 1997;18:84–92.

236. Muller A, Denizot V, Mouillet S, et al. Lack of correlation between consumption of alcohol-based solutions and adherence to guidelines for hand hygiene. *J Hosp Infect* 2005;59:163–164.

237. Muto CA, Sistrom MG, Farr BM. Hand hygiene rates unaffected by installation of dispensers of a rapidly acting hand antiseptic. *Am J Infect Control* 2000;28:273–276.

238. Pittet D, Hugonnet S, Harbarth S, et al. Effectiveness of a hospital-wide programme to improve compliance with hand hygiene. Infection Control Programme. *Lancet* 2000;356:1307–1312 [erratum on 2196].

239. Nijssen S, Bonten MJ, Weinstein RA. Are active microbiological surveillance and subsequent isolation needed to prevent the spread of methicillin-resistant *Staphylococcus aureus*? *Clin Infect Dis* 2005;40:405–409.

240. Stelfox HT, Bates DW, Redelmeier DA. Safety of patients isolated for infection control. *JAMA* 2003;290:1899–1905.

241. Marshall C, Harrington G, Wolfe R, et al. Acquisition of methicillin-resistant *Staphylococcus aureus* in a large intensive care unit. *Infect Control Hosp Epidemiol* 2003;24:322–326.

242. Cooper BS, Stone SP, Kibbler CC, et al. Isolation measures in the hospital management of methicillin resistant *Staphylococcus aureus* (MRSA): systematic review of the literature. *BMJ* 2004;533–540.

243. Farr BM, Bellingan G. Pro/con clinical debate: isolation precautions for all intensive care unit patients with methicillin-resistant *Staphylococcus aureus* colonization are essential. *Crit Care* 2004;8:153–156.

244. Faoagali JL, Thong ML, Grant D. Ten years' experience with methicillin-resistant *Staphylococcus aureus* in a large Australian hospital. *J Hosp Infect* 1992;20:113–119.

245. Salgado C, Farr B. What proportion of hospital patients colonized with methicillin-resistant *Staphylococcus aureus* are identified by clinical microbiology cultures? *Infect Control Hosp Epidemiol* 2006;27:116–121.

246. Hill A. *A short textbook of medical statistics*. London: Hodder and Stoughton, 1984.

247. Wilson APR, Bellingan G, Singer M. Isolation of patients with MRSA infection. *Lancet* 2005;365:1304–1305.

248. Maki DG, McCormick RD, Zilz MA, et al. An MRSA outbreak in a SICU during universal precautions: new epidemiology for nosocomial MRSA; downside for universal precautions. 3rd Decennial International Conference on Nosocomial Infections, 1990, Atlanta: 26.

249. FH Yap, CD Gomersall, and KS Fung et al. Increase in methicillin-resistant *Staphylococcus aureus* acquisition rate and change in

pathogen pattern associated with an outbreak of severe acute respiratory syndrome *Clin Infect Dis* 2004;39:511–516.

250. Concato J, Shah N, Horwitz RI. Randomized, controlled trials, observational studies, and the hierarchy of research designs. *N Engl J Med* 2000;342:1887–1892.

251. Benson K, Hartz AJ. A comparison of observational studies and randomized, controlled trials. *N Engl J Med* 2000;342:1878–1886.

252. Karlowski TR, Chalmers TC, Frenkel LD, et al. Ascorbic acid for the common cold: a prophylactic and therapeutic trial. *JAMA* 1975;231:1038–1042.

253. McHugh CG, Riley LW. Risk factors and costs associated with methicillin-resistant *Staphylococcus aureus* bloodstream infections. *Infect Control Hosp Epidemiol* 2004;25:425–430.

254. Engemann JJ, Carmeli Y, Cosgrove SE, et al. Adverse clinical and economic outcomes attributable to methicillin resistance among patients with *Staphylococcus aureus* surgical site infection. *Clin Infect Dis* 2003;36:592–598.

255. Chaix C, Durand-Zaleski I, Alberti C, Brun-Buisson C. Control of endemic methicillin-resistant *Staphylococcus aureus*: a cost-benefit analysis in an intensive care unit. *JAMA* 1999;282:1745–1751.

256. Abramson MA, Sexton DJ. Nosocomial methicillin-resistant and methicillin-susceptible *Staphylococcus aureus* primary bacteremia: at what costs? *Infect Control Hosp Epidemiol* 1999;20:408–411.

257. Bjorholt I, Haglind E. Cost-savings achieved by eradication of epidemic methicillin resistant *Staphylococcus aureus* (EMRSA)-16

from a large teaching hospital. *Eur J Clin Microbiol Infect Dis* 2004;23:688–695.

258. Lucet JC, Chevret S, Durand-Zaleski I, et al. Prevalence and risk factors for carriage of methicillin-resistant *Staphylococcus aureus* at admission to the intensive care unit: results of a multicenter study. *Arch Intern Med* 2003;163:181–188.

259. Vriens M, Blok H, Fluit A, et al. Costs associated with a strict policy to eradicate methicillin-resistant *Staphylococcus aureus* in a Dutch University Medical Center: a 10-year survey. *Eur J Clin Microbiol Infect Dis* 2002;21:782–786.

260. Karchmer TB, Durbin LJ, Simonton BM, Farr BM. Cost-effectiveness of active surveillance cultures and contact/droplet precautions for control of methicillin-resistant *Staphylococcus aureus*. *J Hosp Infect* 2002;51:126–132.

261. Papia G, Louie M, Tralla A, et al. Screening high-risk patients for methicillin-resistant *Staphylococcus aureus* on admission to the hospital: is it cost effective? *Infect Control Hosp Epidemiol* 1999;20:473–477.

262. Montecalvo MA, Jarvis WR, Uman J, et al. Costs and savings associated with infection control measures that reduced transmission of vancomycin-resistant enterococci in an endemic setting. *Infect Control Hosp Epidemiol* 2001;22:437–432.

263. Bronstein M, Kaye K, Sexton D. Gown utilization as a measure of cost of methicillin-resistant *Staphylococcus aureus* (MRSA) screening. Abstracts of the 12th Annual Meeting of the Society for Healthcare Epidemiology of America, April 6–9, 2002, Salt Lake City, UT. Abstract 47:51–52.

Healthcare-Associated Respiratory Viral Infections

41

Wing Hong Seto and Wilina Lim

INTRODUCTION

Acute respiratory viral infections are frequent causes of hospital admission, and nosocomial clusters of these diseases are frequent occurrences. Despite the large number of viruses causing these infections and the large number of admissions with such infections, the size of the problem worldwide is not known. Determining the extent of this problem is complicated by the lack of laboratory diagnostic capabilities. However, in recent years, many hospitals have established rapid viral diagnosis capacity. At Queen Mary Hospital in Hong Kong, such capacity has existed since 1995. The number of viral laboratory diagnoses made at this 1,400-bed teaching hospital in Hong Kong during 2003 to 2005 illustrates the magnitude of respiratory viral infections (Table 41-1). As shown, influenza and respiratory syncytial virus (RSV) account for the majority of positive specimens and together account for about 70%. The majority of these patients are children and in adults, many are elderly. It is obvious that the practice of infection control for these patients has its own particular challenges and demands.

This chapter is divided into two sections. The first section provides vital background information on the viruses as it pertains to infection control; the second covers the strategies for infection control.

THE VIRUSES

Although deaths from acute viral respiratory illness gradually decreased until they nearly ended in developed countries, morbidity associated with respiratory illness continues to be a major societal burden. The large number of infectious agents involved makes successful vaccination difficult and development with antivirals for treatment of these infections slow. Implementation of nonpharmaceutical intervention is essential to limit the spread of

TABLE 41-1

NUMBER OF VIRUSES DETECTED BY RAPID TESTS IN QMH 2003–2005

	Adult	Children	Total (%)
Influenza A	420	449	869 (38)
Influenza B	41	142	183 (8)
Parainfluenza (P1, P2, P3)	94	302	396 (17)
Adenovirus	7	232	239 (11)
RSV	135	444	579 (26)
			Total 2,266 (100%)

acute viral respiratory pathogens in hospital settings and community.

Most of the respiratory viral pathogens are subject to marked seasonal influence. Seasonality for a specific agent may be different for different regions, especially when the climates are different. Although the underlying mechanisms still remain largely unexplained, the seasonality for many infectious diseases is stable and well documented [1,2]. Knowledge of seasonal and cyclical variations in the incidence of diseases not only is useful in clinical management of patients but also is essential for the design and implementation of preventive strategies.

To devise effective infection control measures, it is essential to understand factors that affect the spread of respiratory virus pathogens, which include these:

1. Virus concentrations in respiratory secretions.
2. Duration of virus shedding.
3. Ability of the virus to survive in aerosols or on the surface of hands or inanimate environment.
4. Route of infection.
5. Minimal infectious dose.
6. Innate and specific host immunity.
7. Social factors (e.g., crowding, mobility of people).

Influenza

Influenza is a highly transmissible acute respiratory pathogen that can spread rapidly causing local outbreaks or widespread epidemics. It begins with sudden onset of fever with sore throat, dry cough, headache, myalgia, and malaise. The clinical presentation of the infection ranges from asymptomatic infection or mild pharyngitis to pneumonia with fatal outcome. All age groups are at risk for infection with infants and children having the highest infection rates. Infection can be life threatening in the elderly and patients with predisposing heart and chronic chest disease.

Influenza viruses belong to the family *Orthomyxoviridae*. They are divided into types A, B, and C. Influenza A virus gives rise to pandemics. The virus contains 8 segments of RNA corresponding to genes of the virus. The surface of the virus particle has H and N proteins. In influenza virus A, there are 16 subtypes of H and 9 of N. Aquatic birds are the prime reservoir of all subtypes. Swine, horses, and seals also can be infected with influenza virus. Variation occurs frequently in the genes of the influenza viruses, leading to an unstable surface that alters constantly, evading existing human body defenses and causing epidemics and pandemics. The first type of variation occurs as a result of accumulation of point mutation in the H and N genes of surface proteins, called antigenic drift. This change is responsible for the interepidemic outbreaks. A radical change called antigenic shift occurs when genetic materials are swapped between two different strains infecting the same host. The new virus created has led to major pandemic strains, including the

Asian flu H2N2 in 1957 and Hong Kong flu H3N2 in 1968. The Hong Kong flu virus in 1968 had two gene segments changed as compared to the H2N2 virus. The H3 and H2 surface protein differed in more than 60% of their amino acids. The conservation of the other surface protein, the neuraminidase, in the 1968 H3N2 virus may have provided some protection to the population, which had been exposed to H2N2 viruses, and this may explain the lower morbidity and mortality compared with the pandemic in 1957 [3].

The pandemic of 1918 was said to be the greatest medial holocaust on history; it killed more people in a few months than World War I did in four years and more people than anything else in history during the period of one year or less. It originated in the United States and spread to Europe, Africa, and Asia. Within a few cycles of infection, it was apparent that the disease had become more virulent with a 10-fold increase in the death rate among those infected. During the pandemic, it is estimated that 50% of the world population was infected with a total mortality >40–50 million. Deaths occurred mainly in the 20–40 year age group, which is distinct from the experience of all other recorded influenza epidemics. The pandemic was caused by an influenza A H1 virus that is closely related to the virus later found in pigs and that remains an infection of the species to the present time. Recent analysis of lung samples obtained from patients who died from the disease in 1918 shows that the virus appeared to be transmitted unchanged from avian source to humans [4].

The pandemic of Hong Kong flu in 1968 began in China in July, spread to Hong Kong in the same month, reached its maximum intensity in 2 weeks, and lasted some 6 weeks in total. About 15% of the population in Hong Kong was affected, but the mortality rate was low and the clinical symptoms were mild. The epidemic was quickly identified as having been caused by a new virus subtype, designated influenza A H3 [5]. The H3 gene was derived from gene swapping from avian source against which the population had no immunity. However, an antibody to this new virus was identified in blood collected before 1968 in elderly persons alive during the 1898 pandemics, suggesting the two pandemics were caused by related viruses [6].

Influenza is subject to marked seasonal influence and usually has predilection for the winter in temperate climates [7,8]. In the subtropics and tropics, influenza can occur throughout the year, but an increase of influenza is generally observed in late winter/early spring and in the tropics again in the summer months or during the rainy seasons [9,10]. The magnitude of seasonal variation is unpredictable, depending on virus characteristics and herd immunity (Figure 41-1).

Depending on the size of the infecting dose, the incubation period is from 24 to 96 hours. [11]. Viral shedding begins 1 day before the illness onset and continues for 3 to 5 days in adults, with longer periods in persons with severe illness and children [12].

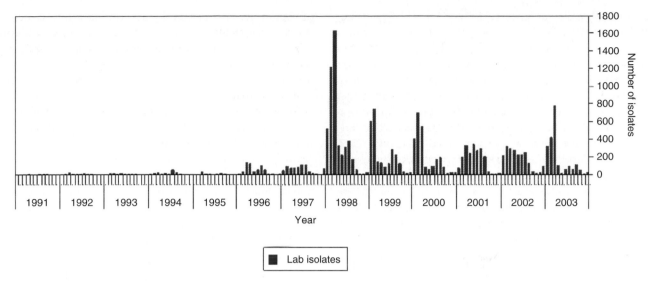

Figure 41-1   Influenza Virus Isolates, Government Virus Unit, Hong Kong, 1991–2003.

Avian Influenza

Avian influenza viruses do not normally infect species other than birds. The first documented influenza A (H5N1) infection in humans occurred in Hong Kong in 1997 with six deaths among 18 reported cases, coinciding with outbreaks among poultry [13]. In February 2003, H5N1 infection again was diagnosed in a father and son who returned from Fujian province China [14]. With unprecedented outbreaks of H5N1 among poultry reported in Southeast Asia and human H5N1 infections starting at the end of 2003 [15], as of June 2006, 224 human infections with H5N1 virus had been confirmed in 10 countries with 127 deaths. So far, transmission of virus from avian to humans appears very inefficient and sustained transmission from human-to-human has not occurred. Human disease caused by H5N1 influenza virus typically presents as a rapidly progressing viral pneumonia, often with evidence of marked lymphopenia, leucopenia, and mild to moderate liver dysfunction. The disease may progress to acute respiratory distress syndrome, multiple organ dysfunction, and death. Evidence is consistent with bird-to-human, possibly environment-to-human and limited, nonsustained human-to-human transmission [16].

As with other enveloped respiratory viruses, influenza viruses could be easily inactivated by heating to 56°C lipid solvents or oxidizing agents [17].

Respiratory Syncytial Virus

RSV is the most important respiratory pathogen in childhood; it is responsible for bronchiolitis and pneumonia in infancy throughout the world. Outbreaks of lower respiratory tract disease in nursing homes and institutions for disabled persons have been reported.

RSV belongs to the family *Paramyxoviridae* and is classified in the genus Pneumovirus. It is an RNA virus with a lipo-protein coat. RSV is a major cause of healthcare-associated infection (HAI) and a particular hazard for premature infants, infants with congenital cardiac and lung disease, and immunodeficient infants, children, and adults. It has been estimated that about 50% of infants will acquire RSV infection during their first year of exposure. Severe RSV disease that requires hospitalization occurs approximately 30% more often among male infants than among female infants. The rate of HAI for infants and children during an RSV season has been reported to range from 26 to 47% in newborn units and for 20–40% for older children [18]. In temperate climates, RSV epidemics occur in late fall, winter, or early spring but are absent during the summer. In contrast, high RSV disease rates occur annually in spring and summer in tropical Hong Kong. The number of RSV isolates begins to rise in March, peaks sharply in April, and remains at a considerably high level until September. Of RSV isolates, 90% are from children under 2 years of age [19].

The incubation period is approximately 5 days, and the illness lasts for 5 days. Patients infected with RSV shed large amounts of virus in their respiratory secretions with a duration of shedding ranging from 1 to 21 days [18]. Virus shedding correlates with severity of disease, and virus transmission has been documented to occur most commonly through contact with infected droplets or fomites. Hospital staff spread the virus by touching secretions or contaminated objects while caring for infected infants. RSV can survive for up to 6 hours on environmental surfaces but can easily be inactivated with alcohol, detergent, or oxidizing agents [20].

Parainfluenza

Human parainfluenza viruses (HPIVs) are common respiratory tract pathogens that can infect persons of any age. They are enveloped RNA viruses with four genetically and antigenically different types, HPIV type 1 to 4 (HPIV1 to 4). HPIV1 and HPIV3 belong to the genus *Respirovirus* within the family *Paramyxovirus*, whereas HPIV2 and HPIV4 belong to the genus *Rubulavirus*. HPIV1 is the principal cause of croup; HPIV3 causes bronchiolitis and pneumonia in infants. HPIV1, 2, and 3 may cause lower respiratory tract infections in young children and immunocompromised hosts, and upper respiratory tract infections in older children and adults [21]. In particular, HPIV1 and HPIV3 have been identified as important causes of outbreaks of respiratory tract infections, especially in institutional settings [22]. In contrast, HPIV4 has been regarded as less clinically important and associated with milder respiratory illness and has rarely been reported to cause major outbreaks of respiratory tract infection.

Parainfluenza viruses can be isolated worldwide throughout the year in temperate and tropical climates [23]. In tropical climates of Hong Kong, these viruses are recovered throughout the year with increased incidence in the winter [24]. This is particularly so for HPIV 1. Interestingly, this also holds true for the incidence of HPIV 3, which is in contrast to the reports from the temperate zone for this virus. In temperate climates, the predilection for diseases by HPIV 1 and 2 is the autumn or winter and for HPIV 3 diseases for the spring or summer [1,23,25]. In some countries, there is evidence of mutual exclusion for HPIV 1 and 2 on the one hand and HPIV 3 on the other [23,24].

HPIV has an incubation period ranging from 3–6 days. The virus can be excreted for 3–10 days following primary infection. It is transmitted through respiratory droplets or person-to-person contact. The virus remains viable on surfaces for several hours and in aerosols for 1 hour. It is readily inactivated by heat, detergents, or oxidizing agents [25].

Respiratory Adenovirus Diseases

Human adenoviruses belong to the family *Adenoviridae*. They are double-stranded, non-enveloped DNA viruses. Adenoviruses cause upper respiratory illnesses including common colds, pharyngitis, and tonsillitis and occur mainly in infants and young children. They are mainly associated with adenovirus types 1 through 7. Severe pneumonia occurs in infants and children. Outbreaks of pharyngo-conjunctival fever in children associated with swimming pools and acute respiratory illness among military recruits have been reported.

Adenoviruses are circulating worldwide around the year. Adenoviruses causing respiratory tract disease are recovered throughout the year in tropical climates of Hong Kong with adenovirus 3 being the most commonly isolated serotype. Decreased incidence is noted in this region in the months of August, September, and October. In moderate climates, the so-called endemic adenoviruses (types 1, 2, 5, and 6) can be detected year-round [26]. In contrast, some marked seasonal prevalence has been reported for the epidemic adenoviruses 3, 4, or 7. For instance, in the 1960s, the highest rates of respiratory adenovirus disease among military recruits in the United States, usually caused by these epidemic adenoviruses, were found in winter and spring. In other countries, however, adenoviruses 3 and 7 epidemics have been described to be most frequent in summer [1,26,27].

The incubation period ranges from 6–9 days, and the virus is first excreted from the respiratory tract. Then it disappears from this site but is found intermittently in fecal specimens for an extended period. The virus can survive for a long time in the environment. It is resistant to detergents and lipid solvents but can be inactivated by heat and oxidizing agents. The mode of transmission is primarily through respiratory droplets or direct hand contacts.

Rhinovirus Disease (Common Cold)

Rhinoviruses belong to the family *Picornaviridae*. They are non-enveloped RNA viruses that cause a typical common cold characterized by rhinorrhea, nasal obstruction, sneezing, pharyngeal discomfort, and cough. Symptoms last from 5 to 7 days. In asthmatic, bronchitic, or immunocompromised individuals, illness may exacerbate asthma or bronchitis or cause lower respiratory tract infection. More than 100 serotypes of rhinovirus cause the common cold. In temperate climates, rhinovirus disease peaks in early autumn (September) and spring [28,29]. After September, the incidence decreases but remains fairly high until the end of the winter and in spring and summer [de Jong, unpublished]. In the tropics, rhinovirus infection coincides with the rainy season in May and June and ends in November and December. Prevalent serotypes change from year to year with multiple serotypes circulating in a given area at any time.

The incubation period of rhinovirus infection is 2–3 days with peak virus shedding coinciding with the acute rhinitis on day 3. The virus can be isolated from 1 day before to 6 days after the onset of cold symptoms. Rhinovirus is present in highest titers in the nose of infected persons and constantly contaminates their hands and the environment. Close personal contact appears necessary for the virus to spread effectively from an infected to susceptible person. In experiments, virus shedding peaked on the third day and fell to low level detectable for up to two weeks [28]. Rhinoviruses are transmitted by direct hand contacts or by large droplets. The rhinovirus is not inactivated by lipid solvents, alcohols, or phenolics but is easily inactivated by heat or oxidizing agents.

Human Metapneumovirus (HMPV)

HMPV is a recently discovered respiratory pathogen of the family *Paramyxoviridae* belonging to the subfamily *Pneumovirinae*. Clinical features associated with HMPV were found to be similar to those of RSV. Clinical symptoms from HMPV-infected children have included nonproductive cough, nasal congestion, wheezing, bronchiolitis, and pneumonia. There is evidence of HMPV infection in approximately 2.2% of patients with influenza-like illness that are negative for RSV and influenza [30]. Studies have found that HMPV-infected children are significantly older (median age 11.5 months) than RSV-positive children (median age 3 months) [34]. Seroepidemiologic data in the Netherlands showed that all children are seropositive for HMPV antibody by 10 years of age [31]. Much like RSV, previous studies, all from temperate regions, have reported HMPV to be a virus with a winter–spring seasonality while in the tropical region such as in Hong Kong, HMPV virus activity is detected in the spring and summer months [32]. There are no clinical data on incubation period, virus shedding, and documented routes of transmission, although HPMV is thought to be transmitted like RSV through contacts and respiratory droplets.

"Classical" Coronavirus Diseases

Human coronaviruses are enveloped RNA viruses of the coronaviridae virus family that cause a cold-like respiratory illness indistinguishable from those caused by other types of respiratory viruses. Coronavirus diagnostics of the "classical" human coronavirus types 229E and OC43 have not often been included in studies of respiratory virus diseases. These viruses were shown to be responsible for up to one-third of common colds [33]. In the United States, France, and Finland, isolation and antibody titre increases are rarely reported outside the period from December through May [34,35]. In children, two peaks of disease in late autumn to early winter and early summer were detected [36]. In the United States, outbreaks of type 229E follow a 2–4-year cycle and outbreaks due to type OC43 occur every other year when the incidence of 229E is low [36]. Rarely do sizeable epidemics of types 229E and OC43 occur in the same year, indicating a seasonal interference phenomenon similar to that observed with HPIVs.

All age groups are susceptible to infection. The incubation period ranges from 2–4 days. Virus shedding lasts for 1–4 days after onset of illness. Classical coronaviruses may be transmitted by droplet nuclei and large-droplet aerosol [37]. Studies show that coronavirus 229E can survive for 3 hours after drying on three different surfaces—aluminum, cotton gauze sponges, and latex gloves—but coronavirus OC43 survived 1 hour or less [37].

Severe Acute Respiratory Syndrome (SARS)

A novel coronavirus identified as the putative cause of SARS in March 2003 was named as SARS-associated coronavirus (SARS-CoV) [38]. The incubation period ranges from 4–5 days. The primary mode of transmission of SARS appeared to be direct mucus membrane contact with infectious droplets and through exposure to fomites. The rate and quantity of viral shedding is low in the initial few days of the illness but rises significantly after 6 days to peak at 6–14 days after onset of illness. Maximal viral shedding

occurred earlier (6–11 days) in respiratory secretions than in feces (9–14 days) but declined more rapidly. This pattern in which maximal viral shedding occurs at the onset of symptoms has not been seen for any other respiratory virus. Because maximal virus shedding appears to reach a maximum 6–14 days after onset, hospital workers are particularly prone to infection because most SARS patients are hospitalized. Because patients are unlikely to be highly infectious in the first few days of illness, early and simple isolation measures including home quarantine likely would be effective. This very characteristic might have played an important part in the eventual containment of the worldwide SARS outbreak because the most infectious patients would have been hospitalized and isolated [39].

Studies demonstrated that SARS CoV contaminates a variety of environmental surfaces in healthcare settings [40]. Surfaces can become contaminated by indirect transfer of SARS-CoV through gloves and gowns. Transmission efficiency appears to be greatest from severely ill patients or those experiencing rapid clinical deterioration, usually during the second week of illness. SARS-CoV can survive in respiratory samples for 5 days at room temperature and up to 3 weeks at 4°C. In diarrheal stool, SARS-CoV can survive for a few days at room temperature [41]. With a high virus load at a concentration of 10^6 TCID$_{50}$/ ml of SARS-CoV, it is notable that fecal droplets containing SARS-CoV remained infectious for 4–5 days. Common disinfectants used in hospital and laboratory settings had been generally found to be effective in virus inactivation [41,42]. Ordinary household detergent, hypochlorite solution, and peroxygen compound at concentrations normally used in the laboratory have been shown to inactivate SARS-CoV within 5 minutes [41].

Obviously, no seasonal pattern can be inferred for SARS at present. It is possible only to compare the dates of the reported detections of the illness with the seasonality of classical coronavirus disease. The first case of SARS was recorded in November 2002 in Guangdong province in China, where the outbreak peaked in February 2003 and disappeared in May 2003. In Hong Kong, the syndrome was first detected in February 2003, outbreaks occurred in March, diminished in magnitude in April, and disappeared by June 2003. These observations are compatible with a seasonal pattern similar to that of the classical coronavirus disease described previously. If so, there is the interesting possibility of seasonal interference between SARS-CoV and the classical coronaviruses, similar to that observed with the HPIVs 1–3 and the classical coronaviruses 229E and OC43.

STRATEGIES FOR INFECTION CONTROL

Understanding the Modes of Transmission

In developing effective strategies for infection control, it is critical to understand the mode of transmission of these pathogens. Because these pathogens infect the lungs and the virus can be dissimilated into the air by coughing, it was assumed that the primary route of transmission was airborne. It is evident now that this is *not* the case. An infected person's cough would produce large droplets of >5μ, because the lungs would be highly congested with fluid, and these large droplets would generally fall to the ground within 1 meter of the patient [43]. Consequently, infection control precautions are necessary only when the healthcare worker comes within 1 meter of the patient. This is the theoretical concept behind the recommendations under "droplet precautions," which will be discussed later.

Some of these respiratory viral diseases (e.g., RSV, HPIVs, and Adenoviruses) emit a vast amount of viral particles in their secretions. These could result in extensive contamination of the patients' environment, and infection control precautions would have to extend beyond the 1 meter perimeter [43]. The isolation measures for these pathogens is designated "contact precautions," which will also be discussed later. Nevertheless, the patient generally does *not* cough out droplets nuclei of <5μ, and, therefore, infectious material is not disseminated for a long distance through the air. Thus, "airborne precautions" are generally not necessary. There are no precise clinical data on transmission of HMPV, but because of its similarity to RSV [44], general consideration is that "contact precautions" are required for infections caused by this agent [32,45].

Presently, none of these acute respiratory viral pathogens is classified as airborne and, as listed in the guideline of the Centers for Disease Control and Prevention (CDC), airborne infections only include pulmonary tuberculosis, varicella, and measles [43]. This fact is important because it means that none of these acute respiratory viral infections requires isolation in a negative pressure isolation room, which often is available only in limited numbers in any hospital. However, it should be noted that these respiratory virus infections may spread by the airborne route under special circumstances described as "opportunistic airborne infections" by Roy et al. [47]. They also stressed that such diseases do *not* require "airborne infection isolation." Rather, one should be alert to those special circumstances in which airborne transmission may be possible and, as in SARS, special precautions such as wearing an N95 respirator are already mandated for high-risk procedures.

Infection Control Measures

The general principles in the infection control measures for these diseases will be discussed together, but special attention will be given to influenzae, avian influenza, and SARS because of the many current issues relate to these diseases.

General Measures

Guidelines for the prevention of transmission of acute respiratory viruses in the hospital are available and should be consulted [47]. The details will not be repeated here, but the key elements will be emphasized.

The key infection control measures that are generally needed for all respiratory viral agents include rigorous hand hygiene, standard precautions, and "cough etiquette." Hand hygiene is extremely important, and every hospital should implement the WHO hand-hygiene guidelines [48]. Data show that the alcohol hand rubs are effective against all respiratory viruses. Standard precautions are the measures adopted for all patients to reduce the risk of blood borne pathogen transmission [43]. For respiratory viral infections, it is particularly important as part of standard precautions that healthcare workers use a surgical mask and eye protection when there is significant risk of contamination from patients with cough. "Cough etiquette" is a measure to contain respiratory secretions from patients with cough [47]. Such patients should be provided with tissues to cover their mouth and nose while coughing. An alternative is to provide ample surgical masks for the patients.

A key element of all of these measures is to obtain compliance from staff and patients. Therefore, staff and patient education must be conducted at all times.

Specific Measures

Specific measures vary, depending on the pathogen (Table 41-2).

Surveillance is extremely useful so that hospitals are alerted to outbreaks circulating in the community. This is helpful for early diagnosis and isolation of patients. A system to alert infection control personnel when there are ≥3 patients with influenzalike illnesses from a single ward also is extremely useful. Immediate assessment of the possibility of an outbreak should be initiated, and early isolation or discharge of patients can be undertaken [47].

Appropriate isolation precautions are discussed in another chapter. The two main precautions for acute viral respiratory infections are droplets precautions and contact precautions. It is important to stress that standard precautions and strict hand hygiene are integral parts of all of these precautions.

The key element of droplets precautions is wearing a surgical mask whenever healthcare workers come within 1 meter of the patient; for contact precautions, the CDC guideline recommends wearing a gown and gloves on entering the patient's room [43]. In the context of respiratory infections, there are variations in the practice of contact precautions, and many hospitals recommend that staff wear a surgical mask, gloves, and a gown only when performing patient care.

The availability of rapid viral diagnosis can be of great help to ward staff and the infection control team. At Queen Mary Hospital, the initiation of such a service has been cost effective [49].

Quarantine is an infection control measure recommended for some severe infectious diseases, but it should be noted that there is *no* such recommendation in any

TABLE 41-2

SPECIAL INFECTION CONTROL PRECAUTIONS FOR ACUTE VIRAL RESPIRATORY DISEASES[a]

Diseases	Usefulness of Surveillance[b]	Isolation Precautions	Vaccination	Availability Other Prophylaxis	Rapid Viral of Diagnosis
Influenza	Yes	Droplets and contact	HCWs of patients at risk	Amantidine and rimantadine for Influenza A	Rapid Flu Kits for A & B
			Persons ≥65 years Children 6–23 months Long-term care residents Chronic lung and cardiac diseases Persons requiring long-term hospital follow-up Pregnant women	Oseltamivir May be used for limiting spread in chronic and long term care facilities high risk patients when vaccination is not possible or fully protective.	Hospitals may need to develop thresholds for routinely testing patients with influenza-like illnesses.
Avian influenza	Presently—rarely occurs in hospitals	Droplets and contact	None	Oseltamivir 75 mg daily for HCWs with unprotected exposure	Yes. Rapid Flu Kits possible for diagnosis; PCR needed for confirmation
SARS	Watch for world alert	Droplets and contact precautions	None	None	PCR available
Adenovirus	None presently recommended	Droplet and contact	None	None	IF/PCR for diagnosis
Respiratory syncytial virus	Yes	Contact, cohorting often needed when in season	None	IV immunoglobalization may be given to premature babies and children with chronic lung diseases	Rapid kit available
Para influenza	Yes	Contact, cohort often needed when in season.	None	None	Usually IF for diagnosis
Rhinovirus	No	Standard[c]	None	None	None PCR available but not routinely used

[a]Hand-hygiene standard precautions and coughing epiquede are to be adopted for all patients.
[b]These includes alert for community outbreaks and clusters detection in the hospital.
[c]Standard precautions only because of insignificant morbidity/mortality of these infections.

guidelines for the present list of acute viral respiratory infections [43]. Quarantine involves the segregation of healthy contacts and was the policy regarding SARS in many countries. Such a drastic measure for SARS was basically carried out for the sake of caution, but the present evidence certainly does not support the need for quarantine. Subclinical infection is virtually nonexistent [51], and even mildly symptomatic patients have not been reported [51]. Furthermore, asymptomatic carriers of the virus have not been identified, and it has been reported that SARS almost exclusively manifests as a florid clinical syndrome [51]. It has been documented that the viral load reaches its peak only in the second week of illness and that transmissibility of the SARS-CoV in the early phase of disease is relatively low [52].

Special Cohorting Precautions

Cohorting is the process of isolating patients with the same diagnosis in the same isolation room. Because significant surge of these viral infections occurs especially in the winter months, cohorting often is necessary.

However, many hospitals often have the problem of having large numbers of patients with respiratory syndromes severe enough for admission, especially among pediatric patients, with insufficient isolation capacity. A possible solution that is practiced in Queen Mary Hospital is to put all of these patients on droplets precautions until there is a clear diagnosis. The steps needed are relatively simple. They include ensuring that all beds are at least 1 meter apart and having healthcare workers wear masks whenever they are within 1 meter of the patient. Patients are advised not to leave their beds without permission, and the common play area commonly seen in pediatric wards is eliminated. Furthermore, there is no sharing of specific patient care equipment, such as stethoscopes, and patient medical records are not placed by the bedside but at the nursing station. When a diagnosis is established, infected patients are taken from this area and placed under the appropriate precautions in the isolation unit. Such cohorting of respiratory illnesses in the pediatric units has been shown to successfully reduce nosocomial respiratory viral infections [53,54]. Similar surges may also be encountered in adults and perhaps such measures may also be adapted with care. However, when toilets are shared, it is important to ensure proper disinfection and adequate hand hygiene after use.

Influenzae

Controversy surrounds the mode of transmission of Influenza, especially with an outbreak report suggesting that it could be airborne [56]. However, recent reviews suggest that the basic mode of transmission is still considered to be droplets [56–58]. Presently, influenzae listed in the CDC guidelines requires droplets precautions [43], and, similarly, the World Health Organization (WHO) recommends that standard precautions and droplet precautions suffice for patients infected with Influenza [59]. However, in a new WHO guideline, both "droplets" and "contact precautions" are recommended [73].

Annual vaccination with trivalent inactivated vaccine is the primary means of prevention and control of seasonal influenza. Antiviral drugs, the amantadine and neuraminidase inhibitors, have been used for chemoprophylaxis of influenza.

There are two main types of attenuated vaccine, namely the inactivated and the live. The CDC recently published its recommendations for influenza prophylaxis [61] and for vaccination of healthcare workers [61]. CDC now recommends that all healthcare workers be vaccinated for influenza unless there are medical contraindications. However, this policy must be taken with caution from an international perspective because in some countries, the mortality for influenzae is not as high as that in the United States. At Queen Mary Hospital, there were only three deaths from influenza from 2003 to 2005 (Table 41-1). Presently, the hospital recommends vaccines for healthcare workers caring for patients in high-risk groups (Table 41-2).

Chemoprophylaxis may be appropriate in certain persons such as those who cannot tolerate the vaccine as in persons with hypersensitivity. Antivirals also can be used if immediate protection is needed because the vaccine requires about 2 weeks before antibodies develop. These agents are especially useful when there is a there is a rapidly growing outbreak in a long-term care facility [62].

The dosages of the drugs for Chemoprophylaxis [60] follow:

Rimantadine or amantadine—Age: 1–9 years, 5 mg per kg per day to max. of 75 mg PO bid; 10–65 years, 100 mg PO bid; >65 years, 100 mg PO q24 h (adjust for decrease in renal function) for 3–5 days or 1–2 days after the disappearance of symptoms.

Oseltamivir 75 mg po bid times 5 days (also approved for treatment of children age 1–12 years, dose 2 mg per kg up to a total of 75 mg bid times 5 days) or Zanamivir 2 inhalations (2 times 5 mg) bid times 5 days.

Avian Influenzae

The WHO has published its interim guideline for infection control measures for avian influenza (AI) [59]. It is a comprehensive guideline that covers many aspects of AI. It is important to point out that the general consensus regarding AI mode of transmission is via droplets. Furthermore, studies had shown that human-to-human spread is possible but a rare event [59]. However, on the side of caution, the WHO has recommended that wherever possible, if facilities are available, airborne precautions may be adopted in view of the high mortality reported and the fact that presently, the number of cases is limited [59]. It should be emphasized, however, that the evidence supports droplets as the mode of transmission, and in practice, droplets precautions should suffice.

The first community outbreak of AI was reported in Hong Kong in 1997 [13] and was successfully controlled with no hospital clusters reported. As an example of how AI can be managed in the hospital, the present protocols for Hong Kong public hospitals are reported in Table 41-3.

Severe Acute Respiratory Syndrome (SARS)

When SARS was first reported, the emotional response was intense and widespread. This is understandable, because it was a new disease with more than 1,700 healthcare workers infected. Nevertheless, this was not the optimal environment for objective information collection and rational precaution determination. Now there has been ample time for proper evaluation of the evidence resulting from that outbreak.

Studies conducted in Hong Kong clearly demonstrated that infection control measures are effective. A case-control study on staff providing direct patient care to 11 proven SARS patients has been reported, comparing the infection control precautions of the 241 noninfected staff with

TABLE 41-3

RECOMMENDED PRECAUTIONS IN HONG KONG PUBLIC HOSPITALS FOR AVIAN INFLUENZA

Standard Precautions for All Patients # Transmission Based Precautions as Indicated

Activity (Based on Risk Assessment)	High-Risk Patient Areas[a] for Caring Suspected or Confirmed Avian Flu	Other Patient Areas	Nonpatient Areas[b]
Enter into isolation room (no patient contact)	N95 respirator/surgical mask[c]	Surgical mask	[c]
Close patient contact (< one meter)	N95 respirator/surgical mask[c] Eye protection Disposable gown	Surgical mask	[c]
Procedures with ■ aerosol-generating potential ■ extensive dispersal of droplets ■ prolonged close contact of dependent patients (for high-risk areas only)	N95 respirator Disposable gown Eye protection Latex gloves Cap	Surgical mask/N95 respirator # Disposable gown Eye protection Latex gloves	[c]
Other activities, no anticipated patient contact	Surgical mask	Surgical mask	

[a]High-risk patient areas refer to triage stations of GOPDs, whole designated clinics, A&E department (triage stations, resuscitation rooms, waiting areas/consultation rooms and isolation room in fever triage cubicles), and isolation wards for confirmed avian influenza patients or for triaging suspected avian influenza cases. All staff working in high-risk patient areas should put on uniform or working clothes.
[b]Individuals with signs and symptoms of respiratory infection should put on surgical mask.
[c]Based on risk assessment.

the 13 infected staff [64]. Four specific measures were specifically studied: (1) the washing of hands and the wearing of (2) masks, (3) gowns, and (4) gloves. The results showed that if proper droplet and contact precautions were undertaken by the staff, as recommended in the CDC guidelines [43], they would be significantly protected. None of the 69 staff reporting the practice of all four measures was infected. In contrast, all 13 infected staff who omitted at least one of the measures ($p < 0.0224$ Fisher's two-tailed) became infected [64].

Although standard infection control measures will prevent transmission of SARS-CoV, the correct practices must be inculcated in a properly organized program for the entire hospital. The SARS outbreak in Hong Kong ultimately infected 405 healthcare workers [51], or 23% of the 1,755 cases. However, at Queen Mary Hospital, only two nurses were infected, and no definite nosocomial infections were reported among patients. Hospital personnel participated fully in the care of SARS patients, admitting a total of 704 patients to the cohort wards during the outbreak period of which at least 52 patients were confirmed cases of SARS. The strategy and infection program for the control of SARS at Queen Mary Hospital have been described elsewhere [65,66] and will not be repeated in this chapter. Nevertheless, the salient strategic features of the program are summarized in Table 41-4. This approach may be a model for others to incorporate into their hospital policy.

Can SARS Be Airborne?

There is much controversy in the literature regarding the transmission of SARS-CoV, and it would be worthwhile to review the scientific data pertaining to airborne transmission of SARS-CoV and to assess the weight of the evidence. There are basically two research studies on this subject published in the reference literature.

The first is a Hong Kong study by Yu et al. [67] that used computerized fluid dynamics modeling to show that SARS-CoV could be transmitted by the airborne route in the Amoy Garden outbreak. It was an elegant study but is basically a simulation, and the level of evidence is not comparable to actual epidemiological comparative studies involving real patients with concomitant controls. The authors correctly point out in their conclusions that their study only "supports the probability of an airborne spread of SARS in the outbreak in Amoy Gardens."

In an editorial regarding the article by Yu et al., Roy et al. [46] stated that "Hydraulic aerosol experiments combined with aerosol and epidemiologic modeling clearly implicated airborne transmission within the apartment complex." However this "should not be considered to represent evidence that airborne infections necessarily cause explosive outbreaks."

It is important to note that Roy et al. also stated that airborne transmission should be classified into

TABLE 41-4
STRATEGIC FEATURES OF THE SARS MANAGEMENT PROGRAMME FOR QUEEN MARY HOSPITAL

Leadership	Intensive Surveillance	Infection Control Program	Education and Communication	Logistics and Staff Welfare

1. Forming SARS task force for the hospital
2. Identifying the professional leadership to lead front-line staff
3. Using only senior staff for direct patient care (only medical staff >6 yrs postgraduate experience to manage SARS patients)
4. No deploying of new staff or volunteers from other hospitals who are unfamiliar with the hospital environment
5. Rapidly decanting non-SARS workload
6. Rapid provision of adequate manpower for clinical care and infection control (e.g., infection control was immediately given 8 additional staff)
	1. Daily telephone follow-up of all hospitalized SARS cases until 10 days after discharge
	2. Contact tracing of all SARS cases contacts for follow-up by department of health
	3. Follow-up of all patients discharged from suspected SARS wards for 10 days
	4. Immediate investigation of even one staff with suspected SARS
	5. Immediate investigation of outbreaks of SARS in the hospital
	6. Staff survey of protocol compliance after all high-risk procedures involving SARS
	7. Informal data reporting by 60 infection control link nurses.
	8. Maintain database
		1. Ensure that strong infection control culture already exists in the hospital
		2. Focus on the basics (hand washing and wearing mask) as obligatory practices in patient care
		3. Have two daily respiratory physician rounds to identify undiagnosed SARS cases in general medical wards for transfer to isolation ward
		4. Eliminate common errors:
		  • Neglecting hand washing after degloving
		  • Using gloves all the time instead of for specific procedures
		  • Washing gloves with alcohol and disinfectant
		  • Double-gloving without washing hands
		  • Use of unnecessary multiple layers of PPEs or those *not* designed for the hospital (e.g., "Barrierman")
		  • Contaminating personal items (e.g., name tags)
		  • Wearing used PPEs outside patient care areas
		  • Careless degowning procedures after use
			1. Direct face-to-face education for all staff by lectures and small group meetings
			2. Demonstrations and drills in usage of PPEs and in high-risk procedures
			3. Daily report of new cases and progress of existing cases for task force core members
			4. Daily newsletter to all hospital staff by the intranet
			5. Hot line for staff advice and counseling
			6. Trouble-shooting sessions with specific departments
			7. Updated guidelines available on the hospital Web site
				1. Formulate triage system for SARS at the emergency department
				2. Ensure sufficient supply of PPEs for all staff
				3. Ensure adequate hand-washing facilities
				4. Provide of shower facilities for all staff while on duty and when going off duty (shower when needed is considered an important infection control practice)
				5. Provide living quarters for staff requiring lodging in the hospital
				6. Provide staff quarantine facilities

obligate, preferential, and opportunistic [46] categories. Obligates are those that under natural conditions spread by the airborne route. Preferentials are those that only predominately spread by air but can also spread through the other routes. Finally, the opportunistics are those that naturally spread by nonairborne routes but under certain special environmental conditions may spread by the airborne route: Roy et al. allocated "SARS to be opportunistically airborne transmission."

The second study is by Booth at al. [68] who had taken air samples in isolation rooms of SARS patients in Toronto. It should be noted that only 1 sample of 10 was positive initially and the other two were detected only after 100-fold concentration. The samples also were positive only by polymerase chain reaction (PCR) indicating viral nucleic material but all cultures were negative, indicating that they are not viable virus able to cause disease. Another method of air sampling also was done in the study, but all 28 samples were negative. The authors rightly pointed out that the data simply "suggest that SARS-CoV could be an opportunistically airborne infection."

In contrast, evidence that SARS-CoV is not airborne transmitted is rather substantial. Many reports indicate a lack of transmission in spite of unprotected extended exposures [69-71]. With the weight of evidence, the general consensus is that SARS-CoV simply does not behave like an airborne-transmitted pathogen.

REFERENCES

1. Noah ND. Cyclical patterns and predictability in infection. *Epidemiol Infect* 1989;102:175-190.
2. Evans AS, ed. *Viral infections of humans: Epidemiology and control* 3rd ed. New York: Plenum Medical Book Company, 1989.
3. Palese P. Influenza: old and mew threats. *Nature Medicine* 2004;12:582-758
4. Tumpey TM, Basler CF, Aguilar PV, et al. Characterization of the reconstructed 1918 Spanish influenza pandemic virus. *Science* 2005;310:77-80
5. Chang WK. National influenza experience in Hong Kong, 1968. *Bull WHO* 1969;41:349-351.
6. Dowdle WR. Influenza A virus recycling revisited. *Bull WHO* 1999;77:820-825.
7. Nguyen-Van-Tam JS. Epidemiology of influenza. In: Fields BN, Knipe DM, Howly PM, eds. *Fields virology*. New York: Raven Press, 1985:207-216.
8. Potter CW. Chronicle of influenza pandemics. In: Nicholson KG, Webster RG, Hay AJ, eds. *Textbook of influenza*. Oxford, England Blackwell Science, 1998:3-18.
9. Dosseh A, Ndiaye K, Spiegel A, et al. Epidemiological and virological influenza survey in Dakar, Senegal: 1996-1998. *Am J Trop Med Hyg* 2000;62:639-643.
10. Chew FT, Doraisingham S, Ling AE, et al. Seasonal trends of viral respiratory tract infections in the tropics. *Epidemiol Infect* 1998;121:121-128.
11. Potter CW. Influenza viruses. In: Zuckerman AJ, Batnavala JE, Pattison JR, eds. *Principles and practice of clinical virology*. 3rd ed. New York: John Wiley &Sons, 1995:229-255.
12. Glezen WP. In: Evans AS, ed. *Viral infections of humans, epidemiology and control* 4th ed. New York: Plenum Medical Book Company.
13. Yuen KY, et al. Clinical features and rapid viral diagnosis of human disease associated with avian influenza A H5N1 virus. *Lancet* 1998;351:467-471.
14. Peiris JSM, et al. Re-emergence of fatal human influenza A subtype H5N1 disease. *Lancet* 2004;363:617-619.
15. Tran TH, et al. Avian influenza A (H5N1) in 10 patients in Vietnam. *N Engl J Med* 2004; 18(350):1179-1188.
16. The Writing Committee of WHO Consultation on Human Influenza A/H5. Avian influenza A(H5N1) infection in human. *NEJM* 2005;353:1374-1385.
17. Harmon MW, Kendal AP . Influenza viruses. In: Schmidt NJ, ed. *Diagnostic procedures for viral, rickettsial and chlamydial infections*. APHA, 1989:631-668.
18. McIntosh K. Respiratory syncytial virus. In: Evans AS, ed. *Viral infections of humans: epidemiology and control*. 4th ed. New York: Plenum Medical Book Company, 1997:691-711.
19. Lo JYC, Lim WW, Yeung FY. Respiratory syncytial virus infection in Hong Kong 1990-1991. *JHKMA* 1994;46:42-45.
20. Tristran DA. Respiratory syncytial virus. In: Murray PR et al., eds. *Manual of clinical microbiology*. 8th ed. ASM Press, 2003:1378-1388.
21. Collins PL, Chanock RM, McIntosh K. Parainfluenza viruses. In: Fields BN, Knipe DM, Howley PM, eds. *Fields virology*. 3rd ed. Philadelphia: Lippincott-Raven Publications, 1996:1205-1241.
22. Fiore AE, Iverson C, Messmer T, et al. Outbreak of pneumonia in a long-term care facility: antecedent human parainfluenza virus 1 infection may predispose to bacterial pneumonia. *J Am Geriatr Soc* 1998;46:1112-1117.
23. Glezen WP, Loda FA, Denny FW. Parainfluenza viruses. In: Evans AS, ed. *Viral infections of humans: epidemiology and control*. 3rd ed. New York: Plenum Medical Book Company, 1989:493-507.
24. Knott AM, Long CE, Hall CB. Parainfluenza viral infections in pediatric outpatients: seasonal patterns and clinical characteristics. *Pediatr Infect Dis J* 1994;13:269-273.
25. Waner JL, Swierkosz EM. Parainfluenza viruses. In: Murray PR, et al, eds. *Manual of clinical microbiology*. 8th ed. ASM: Press, 2003:1368-1377.
26. De Jong JC, Bijlsma K, Wermenbol AG, et al. Detection, typing, and subtyping of enteric adenoviruses 40 and 41 from fecal samples and observation of changing incidences of infections with these types and subtypes. *J Clin Microbiol* 1993;31:1562-1569.
27. Foy HM. Adenoviruses. In: Evans AS, ed. *Viral infections of humans, epidemiology and control*. 3rd ed. New York: Plenum Medical Book Company, 1989:77-94.
28. Gwaltney JM Jr. Rhinoviruses. In: Evans AS, ed. *Viral infections of humans: epidemiology and control*. 3rd ed. New York: Plenum Medical Book Company, 1989:593-615.
29. Couch RB. Rhinoviruses. In: Fields BN, Knipe DM, Howly PM, eds. *Fields virology*. New York: Raven Press, 1985:795-816.
30. Stockton J, Stephenson I, Fleming D, Zambon M. Human metapneumovirus as a cause of community-acquired respiratory illness. *EID* 2005.
31. Mullins JA, Erdman DD, Weinberg GA, et al. Human metapneumovirus infection among children hospitalized with acute respiratory illness. *EID* 2006.
32. Van Den Hoogen BG, De Jong JC, Groen J, et al. A newly discovered human pneumovirus isolated from young children with respiratory tract disease. *Nat Med* 2001;7:719-724.
33. Peiris JSM, Tang WH, Chan KH, et al. children with respiratory disease associated with metapneumovirus in Hong Kong. *EID* 2003;9:628-633.
34. Myint SH. Human coronavirus infections. In: Siddell SG, ed. *The coronaviridae*. New York: Plenum Press, 1995; 389-401.
35. Mäkelä MJ, Puhakka T, Ruuskanen O, et al. Viruses and bacteria in the etiology of the common cold. *J Clin Microbiol* 1998;36:539-542.
36. Monto AS, Sullivan KM. Acute respiratory illness in the community: frequency of illness and the agents involved. *Epidemiol Infect* 1993;110:145-160.
37. Isaacs D, Flowers D, Clarke JR, et al. Epidemiology of coronavirus respiratory infection. *Arch Dis Child* 1983;58:500-503.
38. Sizun J, Yu MWN, Talbot PJ. Survival of human coronavirus 229E and OC43 in suspension and after drying on surfaces: a possible source of hospital-acquired infections. *Journal of Hospital Infection* 2000;46:55-60.
39. Peiris JS, Lai ST, Poon LL, et al. SARS study group: coronavirus as a possible cause of severe acute respiratory syndrome. *Lancet* 2003;361:1319-1325.

40. Cheng PK, Wong DA, Tong LK, et al. Viral shedding patterns of coronavirus in patients with probable severe acute respiratory syndrome. *Lancet* 2004;363:1699–1700.

41. Dowell SF, Simmerman JM, Erdman DD, et al. Severe acute respiratory syndrome coronavirus on hospital surfaces. *Clinical Infectious Diseases* 2004;39:652–657.

42. Lai MY, Cheng PK, Lim WW. Survival of SARS CoV. *CID* 2005;41:e67–e71.

43. Rabenau HF, Kampf G, Cinatl J, Doerr HW. Efficacy of various disinfectants against SARS coronavirus. *Hosp Infect* 2005;61:107–111.

44. Centers for Disease Control. Guideline for isolation precautions in hospitals. *Am J Infect Control* 1996;24:24–52.

45. Crowe JE. Human metapneumovirus as a major cause of human respiratory tract disease. *Pediat Infect Dis J* 2003;23(11): S215–S211.

46. Falsey AR. In: Mnadell GL, Bennett JE, Dolin R, eds. *Human metapneumovisur in principles and practices of infectious diseases.* 6th ed., Philadelphia: Elisevier, 2005:2026–2038.

47. Roy CJ, Milton DK. Airborne transmission of communicable infection: the elusive pathway. *NEJM* 2004;350(17):1710.

48. No author. Guideline for preventing healthcare associated pneumonia, 2003. *MMWR* 2004, 53:RR-3.

49. *WHO guidelines on hand hygiene in health care* (advance draft) (www.who.int/patientsafety/information_centre/who_ghhhcad /en/).

50. Woo PCY, Chiu SS, Seto WH, Peiris M. Cost effectiveness of rapid diagnosis of viral respiratory tract infections in pediatric patients. *JCM* 1997;35(6):1579–1581.

51. Leung GM, Chung PH, Tsang T, et al. SARS-CoV antibody prevalence in all Hong Kong patient contacts. *EID* 2004;10(9):1653–1656.

52. Leung GM, Hedley A Ho L-M, et al. The epidemiology of severe acute respiratory syndrome in the 2003 Hong Kong epidemic: an analysis of all 1755 patients. *Ann Intern Med* 2004;141: 662–673.

53. Peiris JSM, Chu CM, Cheng VCC, et al. Clinical progression and viral load in a community outbreak of coronavirus-associated SARS pneumonia: a prospective study. *Lancet* 2003;361:1767–1772.

54. Karanfil LV, Conion M, Lykens K, et al. Reducing the rate of nosocomially transmitted respiratory syncytial virus. *AJIC,* 1999;27(2):91–96.

55. Mlinaric-Galinovic G, Varda-Brkic. Nosocomial respiratory syncytial virus infections in children's wards. *Virology* 2000;37: 237–246.

56. Moser MR, Bender TR, Margolis HS, et al. An outbreak of influenza aboard a commercial airliner. *Am J Epidemiolo* 1979;110:1–6.

57. Salgado C, Farr B, Hall K, and Hayden F. Influenza in the acute hospital setting. *Lancet Infect Dis* 2002;2:145–155.

58. Buxton Bridges CB, Kuehnert MJ, and Hall CB. Transmission of influenza: implications for control in health care settings. *Clin Infect Dis* 2003;37:1094–1101.

59. Stott DJ, Kerr G, and Carman WF. Nosocomial transmission of influenza. *Occup Med (Lond)* 2002;52:249–253.

60. World Health Organization. *Avian influenza, including influenza A (H5N1) in humans: WHO interim infection control guideline for health care facilities.* (www.wpro.who.int/NR/rdonlyres /EA6D9DF3-688D-4316-91DF-5553E7B1DBCD/0/Infection ControlAIinhumansWHOInterimGuidelinesfor2.pdf) accessed 24 April 2006.

61. No author. Prevention and control of influenza. *MMWR* 2004;53:RR-6.

62. No author. Influenza vaccination of health-care personnel. *MMWR* 2006;55:RR-2.

63. Bowles SK, Lee W, Simor AE, et al. Use of oseltamivir during influenza outbreaks in Ontario nursing homes, 1999–2000. *J Am Geriatr Soc* 2002;50(4):608–618.

64. Bridges CB, Katz JM, Seto WH. Risk of infleunza A (H5N1) infection among health care workers exposed to patients with influenza A (H5N1), Hong Kong.

65. Seto WH, Tsang D, Yung RWH, et al. Effectiveness of "droplets" and "contact precautions" in preventing nosocomial transmission of severe acute respiratory syndrome (SARS). *Lancet* 2003;361:1519–1520.

66. Seto WH, Ching PTY, Ho PL. Infection control for SARS: evidence for efficacy of good practice and description of a successful model. In: Perris M, ed. *Severe acute respiratory syndrome.* Oxford, England: Blackwell Publishing, 2005:176–183.

67. Ho PL, Tang XP, Seto WH. SARS—hospital infection control and admission strategies. *Respirology* 2003;8(suppl):S41–S45.

68. Yu ITS, Yuguo L, Wong TZ, et al. Evidence of airborne transmission of the severe acute respiratory syndrome virus. *NEJM* 2004;350:1731–1739.

69. Booth TF, Kournikakis B, Bastien et al. Detection of airborne severe acute respiratory syndrome (SARS) coronavirus and environmental contamination in SARS outbreak units. *JID* 2005(191):1472–1477.

70. Peck AJ, Newbern, Feikin et al. Lack of SARS transmission and US SARS case-patient. *EID* 2004;10(2):217–224.

71. Park BJ, Peck AJ, Kuehart MJ, et al. Lack of SARS transmission among healthcare workers, United States. *EID* 2004;10(2): 224–248.

72. Chen Y, Chen P, Chang S, et al. Infection control and SARS transmission among healthcare workers, Taiwan. *EID* 2004;10(5):895–897.

73. WHO Interim Infection Prevention and Control Guidelines for Epidemic and Pandemic Prone Acute Respiratory Diseases in Health Care. (In Press).

Blood Borne Pathogen Prevention

42

David K. Henderson

CONTEXT

Blood borne pathogens (BBP) present clearly identifiable occupational hazards to healthcare workers (HCWs). Transmission of so called serum hepatitis to HCWs was detected as early at the 1940s [1]. The past seven decades have provided a clear explication of the various risks associated with handling and processing blood in the healthcare setting. The purpose of this chapter is to identify the BBPs that have been clearly characterized as associated with occupational risks for infection, to describe the factors associated with occupational risk for infection, to discuss other aspects of the epidemiology of occupational infections with BBPs, and to address both primary and secondary prevention/control strategies that have been developed to mitigate the risks for occupational infections with these pathogens. The chapter specifically addresses risks associated with managing patients who are infected with hepatitis B, hepatitis C, hepatitis D, or the human immunodeficiency virus (HIV). The chapter does not discuss issues related to several other potential blood borne agents, including cytomegalovirus, West Nile virus, bovine spongiform encephalopathy/prion disease, hepatitis A virus, the agent called hepatitis French (origin) virus; the blood borne "GB" agents that seem to infrequently cause disease in humans; or the hepatitis G virus. This chapter focuses on the etiology of the major occupationally acquired BBP infections in HCWs, the epidemiology of these viruses in the healthcare setting, and the specific prevention and control strategies that may be relevant to these occupational risks.

ETIOLOGY/PATHOGENS

The agents and selected epidemiological characteristics considered in this chapter as major occupational risks are listed in Table 42 1. Whereas the risks vary substantially by pathogen, all of these agents present risk to HCWs in association with occupational exposures to blood and blood-containing body fluids. Occupational infection with each of these agents is influenced by a host of factors including the relative infectivity of each of the individual pathogens, the occupations and work responsibilities of the individual HCWs under consideration, the prevalences of infection of each of these pathogens in the populations of patients being served, and the individual HCW's attention to detail of and adherence to accepted work-practice standards and accepted infection prevention strategies among numerous others.

An issue that remains perplexing with respect to occupational infections with BBPs is the fact that many HCWs are not aware of precisely what constitutes an occupational exposure. For purposes of this chapter, occupational exposures are considered transcutaneous injuries with blood- (or other blood-containing body fluid-) contaminated devices, mucous membrane contamination with blood (or other blood-containing body fluid); and

	Hepatitis B (HBV)	Hepatitis C (HCV)	Hepatitis D (HDV)	Human Immunodeficiency Virus (HIV)
Occupational risk	Historically extremely common	Becoming increasingly more common	Uncommon	Common
Recommended isolation precautions	Standard precautions	Standard precautions	Standard precautions	Standard precautions
Occupational risk for infection associated with parenteral exposure	6–37% per exposure	1–3% per exposure	Unknown	0.3% per exposure
Major primary prevention strategies	Preventing exposure to blood and blood-containing body fluids Hepatitis B vaccine	Preventing exposure to blood and blood-containing body fluids	Preventing exposure to blood and blood-containing body fluids Hepatitis B vaccine	Preventing exposure to blood and blood-containing body fluids
Efficacy of prophylaxis	Postexposure administration of Hepatitis B vaccine and Hepatitis B immune globulin (HBIG) (see text and Table 42-2)	Postexposure prophylaxis strategies appear to be ineffective; current USPHS recommendations are for no interventions; author suggests consideration be given to either preemptive therapy or watchful waiting strategies (see text) and aggressive early treatment of infection with interferon with or without additional agents	Hepatitis B vaccine and HBIG for persons who are not already infected with hepatitis B; no current options available for HCW who are already chronic carriers of hepatitis B	Postexposure antiretroviral chemoprophylaxis (appears to be efficacious, based on indirect evidence) (see text and Table 42-3)
Controversy/alternative approaches unresolved issues	Need for, and potential efficacy of, booster dose(s) of HBV vaccine for healthcare workers who fail to maintain protective antibody levels	Despite lack of formal recommendations, careful monitoring and early therapeutic intervention appears sensible (see text)	Need for therapeutic management strategies	Many issues poorly understood or poorly delineated (see text)

IG, Immune globulin; HBIG, Hepatitis B immune globulin.

blood-(or other blood-containing body fluid-) contamination of non-intact skin (e.g., chapped, abraded, or integrity compromised by dermatitis) [2].

Hepatitis B Virus (HBV)

As the primary agent responsible for serum hepatitis of the 1930s, 1940s, and 1950s, HBV has long presented the most significant risk for occupational infection to HCWs. Before the development and use of the hepatitis B vaccine, HBV was characterized as the single largest occupational risk for HCWs whose jobs entailed exposure to blood [3].

Several studies have demonstrated definitively that exposure to blood is the single most important risk factor for occupational infection with HBV [4,5]. In an elegant seroepidemiologic survey assessing occupational risk for

HBV infection among HCWs, Denes et al. [6] found that occupational risk for infections increased with practice in an urban location, with the number of years in practice, and with careers in either surgery or pathology. In one of the most definitive studies of its type ever published, Dienstag and Ryan [7] correlated the presence of HBV serological markers in HCWs with (1) frequency of direct contact with blood in the individual's healthcare occupation, (2) years in a healthcare occupation (also identified as a risk for infection among providers who have frequent exposures to blood by Snydman et al.) [8], and (3) practitioner age. Interestingly, several factors that intuitively might have been suggested as likely to be associated with occupational risks for BBP infection including extent of the HCW's contact with patients, years of medical education, documented history of needlestick exposures, past history of receipt of a

TABLE 42-2

STRATEGIES FOR MANAGING OCCUPATIONAL EXPOSURES TO THE HEPATITIS B VIRUS[a]

Exposed Worker's Hepatitis B Vaccination History and Extent to Which Immunologic Status is Understood[b]	Recommended Treatment Strategies[a]		
	Source HBsAg[c] Positive	Source HbsAg[c] Negative	Source Unknown
Never vaccinated	Assess worker's HBV status (Draw anti-HBs anti-HBc)[b,c]; If susceptible, HBIG,[d] 1–2 doses[e]; Begin hepatitis B vaccine series	Assess worker's HBV status (draw anti-HBs,[c] anti-HBc)[a,c], If susceptible, begin hepatitis B vaccine series	Assess worker's HBV status (draw anti-HBs[c], anti-HBc)[a,c]; conduct epidemiological risk assessment (see text); if risk present, and if susceptible, consider HBIG[d]; begin hepatitis B vaccine series
Vaccinated			
Known responder[f] with known positive titer	No treatment needed	No treatment needed	No treatment needed
Known responder[f] with unknown titer	Draw anti-HBs; if titer negative, consider booster; if positive, no treatment needed	Draw anti-HBs	Draw anti-HBs; conduct epidemiological risk assessment; consider booster
Known responder[f] with known negative titer	Draw anti-HBs; administer booster	Draw anti-HBs	Draw anti-HBs; conduct epidemiological risk assessment; consider booster
Known nonresponder[f] with known negative titer	Draw anti-HBs; consider new vaccination series; Administer HBIG, 1–2 doses[e]	Draw anti-HBs	Draw anti-HBs; conduct epidemiological risk assessment; consider booster
Vaccinated but antibody status unknown	Draw anti-HBs; if positive, no treatment; if negative, HBIG, 1 dose; administer booster	Draw anti-HBs; consider booster	Draw anti-HBs; conduct epidemiological risk assessment; if risk present, treat as exposure: HBIG, 1 dose; administer booster

[a]Although this table refers to the management of exposures to hepatitis B, in every instance in which exposure to blood occurs, the clinician managing the exposure should consider the potential for exposure to multiple blood borne pathogens; thus, at a minimum, someone sustaining an exposure to hepatitis B should also have an assessment for potential exposures to hepatitis C and HIV.

[b]Resolved natural infection (associated with anti-HBs and anti-HBc antibody production) produces lifelong immunity.

[c]HBsAg—hepatitis B surface antigen; anti-HBs—antibody against HBsAg; anti-HBc—antibody directed against hepatitis B core antigen (signifies prior natural infection, present in those who have resolved infection and chronic carriers).

[d]HBIG—hepatitis B immune globulin; dose is 0.06 ml/kg; second dose at 4 weeks.

[e]Value of the second dose of HBIG only suggested by one study.

[f]Responder—vaccinated; measurable anti-HBs >10 mIU/ml; nonresponder—vaccinated, but anti-HBs never exceeds 10 mIU/ml.

Modified from

transfusion, and a prior history of having received a gamma-globulin injection, were found not to be associated with serological markers for HBV infection. Among the health-care occupations studied, the highest seroprevalences of HBV markers were found among HCWs in several occupations that are known to have high risks for occupational exposures to blood, including surgeons and surgical house officers, laboratory medicine (clinical pathology) staff, emergency room nurses, and transfusion medicine staff.

Subsequently, Hadler et al. conducted a similarly designed study that also controlled for nonoccupational risk factors [9], again underscoring the findings of Dienstag and Ryan's study and demonstrating that occupational

blood exposure, not patient contact, was associated with risk for serological markers of HBV infection among HCWs. In a retrospective review, West found the risk for HBV infection among HCWs to be four times the risk for the general adult population [10]. He found that surgeons, dialysis personnel, personnel providing care for developmentally disabled individuals, and clinical laboratorians were at 10-fold higher risk for infection and that physicians and dentists were between 5- and 10-fold more likely to have serological markers of prior HBV infection than the general population [10].

In addition to occupational exposure to blood, several additional factors influence the risk for HBV infection in

TABLE 42-3

STRATEGIES FOR MANAGING OCCUPATIONAL EXPOSURES TO THE HEPATITIS C VIRUS[a]

Exposed Worker's Hepatitis C History and Status	Recommended Treatment Strategies[a]		
	Source Anti-HCV[b] Positive	Source Anti-HCV[b] Negative	Source HCV Status Unknown
Hepatitis C status positive	No treatment needed	No treatment needed	No treatment needed
Hepatitis C status negative	Draw anti-HCV, AST, ALT and RT-PCR for HCV RNA[b] to establish negative baseline; repeat PCR at 6–8-week intervals; if negative at 6 months, discontinue follow-up; if RT-PCR becomes repeatedly positive, consider watchful waiting or preemptive therapy strategies (see text)	No treatment needed	Draw anti-HCV, AST, ALT and RT-PCR for HCV RNA[b] to establish negative baseline; conduct epidemiological, risk assessment; if risk present, repeat PCR at 6–8-week intervals; if negative at 6 months, discontinue follow-up; if RT-PCR becomes repeatedly positive, consider watchful waiting or preemptive therapy strategies (see text)
Hepatitis C status unknown	Assess worker's hepatitis C status(draw anti-HCV, AST, ALT[b]); if negative, draw RT-PCR for HCV RNA[b]; if negative,repeat PCR at 6–8-week intervals; if negative at 6 months, discontinue follow-up; if RT-PCR becomes repeatedly positive, consider watchful waiting or preemptive therapy strategies (see text)	No treatment needed	Assess worker's hepatitis C status (draw anti-HCV, AST, ALT[b]) conduct epidemiological risk assessment (see text); if risk present, and if susceptible, draw RT-PCR for HCV RNA[b]; if negative, repeat PCR at 6–8-week intervals; if negative at 6 months, discontinue follow-up; If RT-PCR becomes repeatedly positive, consider watchful waiting or preemptive therapy strategies (see text)

[a]Although this table refers to the management of exposures to hepatitis C, in every instance in which exposure to blood occurs, the clinician managing the exposure should consider the potential for exposure to multiple bloodborne pathogens; thus, at a minimum, someone sustaining an exposure to hepatitis C should also have an assessment for potential exposures to hepatitis B (see Table 42-2) and HIV.
[b]Anti-HCV, antibody against Hepatitis C Virus; ALT, Alanine Aminotransferase; AST, Aspartate Aminotransferase; RT-PCR, reverse transcriptase polymerase chain reaction; HCV RNA, hepatitis C virus ribonucleic acid.
Modified from

HCWs, among them the prevalence of HBV infection in the population being served, practice in urban settings (because the prevalence of infection is higher there than in rural settings), practice involving dialysis patients, and HCWs who provide care for other populations of patients known to be at increased risk for HBV infection (e.g., injecting drug users, men who have sex with men, prison inmates, the developmentally disabled, and/or immigrants from highly endemic areas) [11].

The source-patient's viral burden (i.e., presumably due to an inoculum effect) also influences the risk for transmission. Thus, patients who are hepatitis B "e" antigen positive (who generally have substantially higher circulating viral burdens than those who are "e" antigen negative) present higher levels of risk. HBV infectivity also correlates directly with the levels of hepatitis B virus DNA in the circulation.

The characteristics of the exposure itself influence the risk for acquiring occupational infection. For example, parenteral exposures are associated with increased risks for occupational infection. Conversely, because of the extraordinary levels of viremia in hepatitis B "e" antigen positive patients, even what might be considered trivial inocula of hepatitis B "e" antigen-positive blood may produce infection. Patients who are hepatitis B "e" antigen-positive chronic carriers of HBV may harbor as many as 10^{13} virus particles of HBV per milliliter of blood [3]. Because of these remarkable levels of viremia, miniscule amounts of blood contaminating inanimate objects or environmental surfaces actually may present significant occupational risks for infection. Whereas parenteral exposures account for the large majority of occupational infections with HBV, several episodes document that contaminating mucous membranes also may produce HBV infection [12].

One of the most significant developments in the past 50 years in terms of mitigating risks for occupational infection with BBPs was the development of the HBV vaccine. Studies conducted since the introduction of the HBV vaccine demonstrate its substantial efficacy in preventing occupational infections. For example, a seroprevalence study conducted by Thomas et al. at Johns Hopkins Hospital in Baltimore identified "absence of hepatitis B vaccination" as the only factor independently associated with risk for HBV infection in a large cohort of HCWs [13]. Similarly, Panlilio et al. evaluated a cohort of surgeons for prior HBV infection and found only two factors associated with risk for infection: (1) not having been immunized with the HBV vaccine and (2) having practiced surgery for at least the previous 10 years [14].

Hepatitis C Virus (HCV)

HCV continues to present occupational risks for infection to HCWs for a variety of reasons. The population of patients chronically infected with HCV, particularly among injecting drug users, continues to expand aggressively. Whereas the epidemiology and pathogenesis of HBV infection are understood with a great deal of clarity, our current understanding of the pathogenesis and immunopathogenesis of HCV infection remains far less clear, especially with respect to the early events in the course of the infection. In addition, despite the fact that the pathogen responsible for this disease was identified in 1989 [15], we still have no vaccine for it and have no proof that any intervention is efficacious in preventing infection following occupational exposure to the virus.

Because HCV is known to be a major cause of posttransfusion hepatitis, the thought that HCWs would be at occupational risk for HCV transmission makes implicit sense. Numerous anecdotal case reports of occupational infection have been reported in the literature (summarized in [16]). Whereas, similar to HBV, parenteral inoculation (e.g., needlestick exposure) presents the highest level of risk for occupational HCV infection, inapparent parenteral transmission (including mucous membrane exposures) likely accounts for many of the remaining episodes. To date, all instances of occupational HCV infection have been associated with exposures to blood despite the fact that HCV has been isolated (albeit generally in much lower concentrations) from a variety of other body fluids. With respect to circumstances of occupational exposure, the most frequent type of exposure resulting in HCV infection in the healthcare setting to date has been a needlestick with a hollow-bore needle.

Several serological prevalence studies evaluating HCWs for the presence of antibody directed against HCV have been published. Although these studies have substantial limitations, they demonstrate that HCWs' risk for acquiring occupational (HCVI) infection is only minimally higher than that of volunteer blood donors and approximately

10-fold lower than the comparable occupational risks associated with exposure to HBV in the healthcare setting. Most of these studies were designed as simple seroprevalence surveys, not to investigate risk factors for HCV infection in their respective cohorts. The few studies that were designed to detect risk factors for HCV infection found increasing age [17,18], years of employment in healthcare occupations [17,19,20], a history of blood transfusions [17,21], and a history of prior needlestick injuries [21,22] to be associated with risk for HCV infection (as detected by assays for circulating antibody directed against HCV).

Study and technological limitations cloud the issue of the risk for transmission of HCV associated with single parenteral exposures. The primary technological limitation is the fact that a variety of different tests have been used in these studies to detect prior infection. Some of the published studies used only the first-generation antibody test (that was neither highly sensitive nor specific). Others have used subsequent iterations of the antibody tests that have substantially improved sensitivities and specificities. Some have used direct detection of the HCV genomic material by polymerase chain reaction to detect infection. These studies provide highly disparate estimates of the risk for HCV infection following discrete occupational exposures.

Studies conducted during the past decade have suggested that the detection strategies for HCV infection in these seroprevalence and longitudinal cohort studies may have been relatively insensitive with some studies suggesting that both antibody tests and tests for circulating HCV nucleic acid underestimate the risk. In these studies, the investigators suggest that the most sensitive test for detecting prior infection/exposure to HCV is the measurement of specific cellular immunity directed against this flavivirus [23].

Hepatitis D Virus (HDV)

HDV by itself presents no occupational risk to HCWs. The HDV is an "incomplete" virus that requires co-infection with HBV to produce infection. In addition, although approximately 5% of all HBV carriers are co-infected with HDV, substantial demographic, risk-group, and geographic variations exist. For example, HDV infection is particularly endemic in the Middle East, parts of the Amazon River basin, a few of the Pacific Islands, and southern Italy. Injecting drug users and hemodialysis patients are more likely to be co-infected with HDV than are other groups known to be at risk for HBV infection (e.g., men who have sex with men).

Exposure to HDV represents a risk to those HCWs who are already chronically infected with HBV and to uninfected HCWs who experience an exposure to blood from someone who is chronically infected with both viruses. Occupational HDV infection has been infrequently detected to date, in part because of the requirement for simultaneous infection with HBV, and in part because tests to detect HDV infection are rarely conducted [24,25].

Human Immunodeficiency Virus (HIV)

The introduction of a new BBP—HIV—into the healthcare workplace in the 1980s was associated with significant fear and anxiety on the part of HCWs. Despite the fact that the risk for occupational infection with other BBPs (e.g., HBV) had been common knowledge since the late 1940s, the epidemic of HIV infection in the United States and its association with almost monumental societal fear and anxiety fueled HCWs' concerns. In the years since the widespread introduction of HIV infection into society, we have learned that exposure to blood from an HIV-infected patient is associated with measurable occupational risks for infection, that such occupational infections occur infrequently, and that sensible procedural interventions can reduce the risk for exposure (and therefore infection) with this blood borne retrovirus. We also have learned that postexposure interventions may further reduce the risk for occupational infections.

In the past 25 years, there have been only 57 documented HIV infections in U.S. HCWs, and the majority of those infections occurred in the first 15 years of the epidemic [26]. These definitive episodes are instances in which an HCW sustained an occupational exposure to blood from someone known to be HIV-infected, the HCW had a baseline sample drawn to demonstrate that she or he was not infected at the time of the exposure, was followed by serological evaluation over time, and, in temporal association with the exposure, the HCW developed serological and, in some instances clinical, evidence of HIV infection. In addition to these definitive infections, the U.S. Public Health Service (USPHS) has identified nearly 150 other episodes that could be categorized as possible or probable occupational HIV infections among U.S. HCWs. These latter individuals did not have a baseline serological sample drawn at the time of the occupational exposure to demonstrate absence of infection at the time of the exposure. Despite the fact that these individuals all denied having nonoccupational risks for HIV infection, when one compares the demographics of this population with those of the definitive episodes as described, and the substantial differences in these two populations become apparent, strongly suggesting that confounding community-based risks are present in the possible/probable population [27].

PATHOGENESIS

Transmission of each of the major BBPs identified here has been most closely associated with transcutaneous injuries with sharp objects in the healthcare setting. The preponderance of these exposures have been needlestick injuries with hollow-bore needles; however, a variety of other blood-contaminated sharp objects have been implicated in the transmission of one or more of these infectious diseases. Mucosal exposures to blood also transmit infection. For example, six or seven of the definitive occupational HIV infections described here were associated with mucosal exposures to blood from patients known to harbor HIV infection. Whereas other body fluids may present some risk for occupational infection, the primary risk for all of the pathogens discussed is associated with exposures to blood from infected individuals.

MAGNITUDE OF RISK FOR OCCUPATIONAL INFECTION ASSOCIATED WITH OCCUPATIONAL EXPOSURE

For all of these significant BBPs, the risk for infection associated with a single discrete exposure to blood from a patient known to be infected with one of these viruses depends on a number of variables, including (but not limited to) circulating viral burden in the source patient, inoculum size, significance of the exposure, and the route of exposure, among others. For example, the risk for transmission of HBV following parenteral (e.g., needlestick) occupational exposure ranges from 6–37% per exposure, depending on a variety of factors including the type of exposure, the inoculum size and type, and the source-patient's circulating viral burden and/or hepatitis "e" antigen status [28].

For HCV infection, considering all of the codicils about the different methods that have been used to detect infection (discussed previously), when taken together, these studies suggest that the risk for HCV transmission following a parenteral exposure to blood from a patient known to be infected with HCV is between 1–3% per exposure [16]. Thus, for HCV, the 1–3% risk for transmission per exposure places the occupational risk for transmission of HCV between the infection risk for occupational HIV exposures discussed later and the risk for HBV exposures discussed earlier.

For HIV exposures, >20 longitudinal studies have been conducted attempting to measure the risk for transmission following an individual occupational exposure [29,30]. When data from all of these studies are combined, the risk for transmission of HIV associated with a single percutaneous exposure to blood from a patient known to be HIV-infected is 0.32%, or roughly 1 infection for every 325 percutaneous occupational exposures to blood from an HIV-infected patient [29]. Many of these same studies also attempted to assess the risk for infection associated with mucous membrane exposures to blood from patients known to be HIV infected. Pooling data from these studies, the risk for occupational infection associated with a single mucosal exposure to blood from an HIV-infected patient is estimated to be 0.03%; however, this approximation may be an overestimate because the single infection in this series was actually reported as an anecdotal case-report in the literature [31] before prospective data purportedly had begun to be collected for the longitudinal study. Thus, this episode would have clearly occurred before the prospective study of risk began [30].

For HDV, no prospective studies have been able to measure the risk associated with either a single exposure to blood from a patient harboring HDV or for a single exposure to blood from a patient co-infected with HBV and HDV.

Several other factors likely influence the risk for transmission of these viruses associated with individual exposures. Clearly, inoculum is a major determinant, and the viral inoculum is related both to the volume of material involved in the exposure and the source patient's circulating viral burden. As might be anticipated, studies of needlestick exposures demonstrate that the volume of the exposure increases with the size of the needle causing the injury and the depth of penetration of the needle. In several studies, hollow needles have been shown to be associated with higher inocula of blood than are comparably sized suture needles [32,33].

The amount of virus present in the source material may vary by several logs, depending on the stage of the source patient's illness and the effect of antiviral or immunomodulator. For most, if not all, of these infections, viral burden is likely to be the single best predictor of infection risk.

In 1997, the Centers for Disease Control and Prevention (CDC) published the results from a retrospective case-control study of percutaneous exposures to HIV among HCWs to attempt to define factors associated with transmission risks [34]. The investigators identified four factors to be associated with an increased risk for occupational infection with HIV following percutaneous exposures: deep rather than superficial injuries; injuries with sharp devices that were visibly bloody when compared with devices on which no blood was visible; injuries with sharp devices that had been used in arteries or veins as compared with those that had not been in vascular channels; and injuries associated with source-patients who had preterminal AIDS (defined as source-patients who expired within 2 months of the time of the exposure) than when the sources had earlier stages of infection. Each of these factors is likely a surrogate marker for viral inoculum.

The specific characteristics of the pathogens to which an HCW is exposed also may influence the risk for infection. For example, some strains of HIV may be more aggressive than others (e.g., some strains may produce infection by inducing syncytia more efficiently than others, and some clearly are able to attach to macrophages more efficiently than others). Patients with late stage HIV or HCV infection harbor numerous quasispecies of these viruses, also likely increasing the transmission risk.

A final factor that likely influences the risk for occupational infection relates to host factors in the exposed HCW. Variation in an individual HCW's immunological responses also likely affects the probability of HIV transmission. Three possible outcomes have been postulated to result from occupational exposures to HIV: infection (usually with detectable antibody responses directed against the invading pathogen); no infection with absent immunologic responses; or so-called transient infection that is characterized by measurable and persistent T-cell responses (i.e., directed against HIV peptides and envelope antigens or HCV envelope proteins and absence of protracted or systemic infection and antibody response directed against the infecting virus). With respect to HIV exposures, several populations of exposed but uninfected individuals have been studied to gain these insights, including the steady sexual partners of infected individuals, children born to mothers who are infected with HIV, prostitutes [35,36], and occupationally exposed HCWs [35–44]. Neither the efficacy nor the precise role for this cellular immune response in the overall defense against initial HIV infection is well understood.

PRIMARY PREVENTION—PREVENTING OCCUPATIONAL EXPOSURES

If one examines possible strategies for preventing occupational infections with BBPs, by far the most efficient approach is to implement strategies designed to prevent occupational exposures to blood. Despite the fact that this prevention is, perhaps, counter culture in medicine, the strategy affords the HCW the most cost-effective, most efficient strategy for reducing the risks for occupational infection with all BBPs. In 1987, CDC published its universal precautions guidelines [45]. The recommendations were designed to reduce the risk for exposure to blood and, therefore, to reduce the risk for BBP transmission. Effective use of these precautions will unquestionably reduce cutaneous, mucocutaneous, and percutaneous exposures to blood. Thus, effective implementation of universal/standard precautions will decrease risks for occupational infection with all BBPs.

When one assesses the specific detailed recommendations in these guidelines, the specific components—the effective use of hand-hygiene strategies, the use of appropriate personal protective equipment (e.g., gloves), and the need for attention to the appropriate use and disposal of needles and other sharp objects—the reasons for the efficacy of these precautions becomes readily apparent. A number of additional approaches have been demonstrated as effective in reducing occupational exposures and injuries including the comprehensive education of staff about the attendant occupational risk associated with providing care for patients who have BBP infection, education of staff about the occupational risks that are present and highly prevalent in the healthcare workplace, the need to modify procedures and work practices that are intrinsically associated with risks for occupational exposure, and the need to monitor staff for adherence to standard/universal precautions and other relevant infection control guidelines. Institutions also should develop strategies to be able to monitor the healthcare marketplace for technological advancements that can be implemented to replace existing approaches while simultaneously reducing occupational risks. All healthcare institutions should collect information prospectively about occupational exposures that occur in their institutions and should use these data to drive performance improvement activities to reduce the attendant risks.

Last, the appropriate use of vaccines (e.g., HBV vaccine) already plays a crucial role with respect to HBV in primary prevention of occupational infection with BBPs. When additional vaccines become available (e.g., HCV, HIV), such vaccines would play an increasingly important role in primary prevention.

IMMEDIATE POSTEXPOSURE MANAGEMENT

One of the most important considerations for immediate postexposure management is first to determine that an occupational exposure presenting a risk for transmission of one of these BBPs has actually occurred. To make such a determination, the practitioner must thoroughly evaluate the exposure event, the potential for susceptibility of the exposed HCW (e.g., immunity to HBV, preexisting infection with HBV, HCV, or HIV), and the information available about the patient who was the source for the exposure. If the source-patient's BBP infection status is not known, the source-patient should be tested for all of these BBP infections, making certain that the testing is appropriately conducted within the constraints of relevant state and local laws. Currently, marketed rapid tests for HIV are highly reliable when negative. Positives must be followed up with standard immunoassay and confirmatory tests. In instances in which the source-patient is determined to be infected with one or more of these pathogens, obtaining as much additional information about the source-patient's infection(s) makes implicit sense. Determining the duration of the source-patient's infection, the current therapy for the infection(s), key immunologic and/or virologic parameters for each pathogen, such as viral burden(s), and a variety of other risk factors that relate to each of the pathogens, may help the practitioner understand the significance of the exposure. If information about the source-patient's viral isolates is available (i.e., phenotypic or genotypic information, information about prior resistance), this information should be considered as well. In instances in which such practices are practical, saving a sample of the source-patient's pathogen is entirely sensible. The practitioner responsible for management also should obtain

as much information as possible about additional factors likely to increase the risk for transmission of BBP infections (e.g., if a volume of blood was injected; if the exposure was to a hollow-bore, rather than solid, needle; if the needle was of a large-, rather than small-gauge; if blood was visible on the device causing the injury; or if the device had been placed in one of the source-patient's arteries or veins) [34].

In instances in which source-patient testing is either not possible or readily available, immediately offer prophylaxis; if the HCW elects to take the prophylaxis, sort out the exposure data as quickly as possible. If the source-patient's infection status for these pathogens cannot be discerned, the practitioner should make his or her best epidemiological assessment about the likelihood of exposure and manage the HCW in accord with that assessment. Factors that may be considered in making such an epidemiological assessment include (but are certainly not limited to) the severity of the exposure; the precise circumstances of the exposure; the location where the exposure occurred and the likelihood that pathogens were present; the demographics of the source-patient; and the presence of other epidemiological factors known to be associated with risk for one or more of these infections. Such source-unknown exposures must, of necessity, be managed on a case-by-case basis.

Although determining whether or not an exposure has actually occurred seems straightforward, this determination in actuality is the Achilles-heel of postexposure management. Summary data from the National Clinicians' Post-Exposure Prophylaxis Hotline (PEPLINE) at the University of California at San Francisco have consistently suggested that postexposure prophylaxis often is prescribed and administered for instances in which the PEPLINE professionals felt that an exposure had not occurred [46]. Although these data appear to be improving gradually over time, the number of instances in which post exposure prophylaxis is prescribed for circumstances felt not to represent exposures remains far too high. One reason for the problem of overtreatment may be that the practitioners who ultimately end up managing these exposures (very often emergency room practitioners) often are unfamiliar with the exposure definitions and with the drugs administered for postexposure prophylaxis. Furthermore, because the practitioners often are colleagues of the exposed individuals, they may be more easily influenced by their putatively exposed colleague's anxiety. Institutions should develop systematic procedures and a multidisciplinary team approach to occupational exposures to ensure that these exposures are managed both consistently and with the highest possible quality. Occupational medicine, hospital epidemiology, hospital safety, and the infectious diseases/HIV team should be key members of this team. Qualified, knowledgeable staff should be available 24 hours a day, 7 days a week to assist with the management of these exposures. As part of this multidisciplinary approach, the team should collect information about occupational exposures to blood in their institution to be able to assess their data for common circumstances of exposure or for intrinsic problems with patient-care processes that might be improved to mitigate risk.

Effective exposure management is a healthcare institution's responsibility. Staff need to know precisely what to do when an exposure occurs and precisely when to do it. Access to information about appropriate exposure management procedures must be readily available to all potentially exposed staff and also must be user friendly.

Healthcare institutions are required by law to provide systems for reporting exposures and ensuring rapid access to appropriate postexposure care [47]. Despite the development of elegant strategies to facilitate reporting and management of such exposures, many occupational exposures are never reported. Since the early 1980s, underreporting of these injuries has been identified as a significant problem, and it persists as a major problem well into the 21st century.

We recommend that wounds, punctures, or other skin areas that have had direct contact with blood or body fluids should be initially washed thoroughly with soap and water [2,48]. Some authorities have recommended that antiseptics be used to decontaminate the wound; however, no data actually provide scientific support this recommendation. Flushing and washing the wound should not be delayed until antiseptics can be obtained.

For mucous membrane exposures, we recommend flushing the exposure site aggressively with tap water; eyes should ideally be flushed with sterile water or a commercial eye irrigant; if neither is readily available, clean tap water will suffice.

An important aspect of early postexposure management is counseling. The emotional impact of an occupational exposure to a BBP should never be underemphasized. In addition to ensuring that the staff who are providing care to exposed HCWs are knowledgeable about the epidemiology, risks for transmission, treatment options, and known complications of treatment, institutions also should ensure that staff who sustain these exposures have access to skilled counseling. The clinician providing care for the exposed HCW must be able to provide the exposed staff member understandable, objective information about the risks for infection associated with the type of exposure that the employee has sustained and what is known about the risks and benefits of the various possible treatment options. Clinical staff should guard against minimizing or trivializing the risks and should work hard to express empathy and reassurance. These events are incredibly troubling to the exposed HCW, who may not be able to assimilate all of the information that the clinicians provide. Staff providing care for individuals sustaining these types of exposures should be ready and willing to answer the same questions repeatedly, both for the exposed HCW and her or his spouse or significant other. Regardless of the treatment course elected, the exposed HCW should be

scheduled for a follow-up appointment 48 hours following the initial appointment to assess how she or he is doing and to answer any outstanding questions.

HCWs who are too upset or confused to make a decision about chemoprophylaxis can sometimes be helped by suggesting that treatment be started immediately with the option to stop it later (i.e., "Because some evidence suggests that the timing of the first dose influences the success of treatment, I suggest that you start treatment now and then tomorrow, or even later, if need be, we can decide whether continuing is your best option"). This approach modulates the acute pressure the HCW may feel to make an immediate decision and empowers workers to be able to decide about their own treatments.

Counseling the HIV-exposed HCW should include a clear discussion of several important issues related to occupational exposures and their management: (1) More than 99% of individuals who sustain occupational exposures will not become infected, even if they elect not to take postexposure antiretroviral chemoprophylaxis (PEP); (2) although a great deal of indirect evidence suggesting efficacy for postexposure antiretroviral prophylaxis (discussed later) has been assembled over the years, no agent or combination of agents has been approved as safe and effective by the Food and Drug Administration (FDA) for use in this setting; (3) data about the efficacy and safety of the use of these potentially toxic agents in this setting are far from complete; and (4) exposed HCWs should be counseled to take precautions to prevent secondary transmission, especially during the first 3 months following exposure when seroconversion, including precautions to prevent sexual transmission (e.g., abstinence or condom use), and the avoidance of blood and organ donation and discontinuation of breast-feeding.

Exposed staff should be counseled about the magnitude of risk associated with occupational exposures, the institutional measures that have been put in place to protect the confidentiality of exposed HCWs' medical records, and the typical concerns of sexual partners, co-workers, family, and friends of the exposed worker. Finally, counseling staff should be prepared to answer questions for spouses, significant others, and family who have major concerns about associated risks.

PATHOGEN-SPECIFIC POSTEXPOSURE MANAGEMENT AND FOLLOW-UP

Hepatitis B Virus

A large body of evidence demonstrates that PEP (both active and passive) is effective in preventing infection with HBV following occupational exposures. PEP should be provided to all susceptible HCWs who sustain occupational HBV exposures. As for each of the commonly encountered BBPs, healthcare institutions should establish protocols for providing appropriate management of HBV exposures. As described, management of HBV exposures includes assessing the type, source, and circumstances of the exposure; evaluating the source-patient for clinical, epidemiologic, and laboratory evidence of hepatitis; and evaluating the HBV vaccination history and HBV infection/ immunity status of the exposed HCW. Additionally, institutions should strive to provide prophylactic treatment as soon as possible following occupational HBV exposures. Current recommendations include the administration of both HBV immune globulin and the HBV vaccine series [11] (Table 42-2). Practitioners must be aware that certain BBPs travel together. Simply because a patient is admitted for treatment of complications of HBV infection does not mean that the other pathogens should be ignored. For this reason, even when the source known to harbor HBV, the source-patient should also be tested for HCV and HIV in addition to the current HBV infection status.

The issue of booster doses of HBV vaccine for HCWs who have occupational exposures and who are shown to have undetectable levels of antibody remains controversial. The USPHS does not currently recommend booster doses for HCWs who initially responded to the vaccine but whose antibody levels have declined to the undetectable level. Several studies have addressed the issue of the durability of vaccine-induced immunity. One study suggested that between 30–60% of vaccines had suboptimal levels of antibody 8 years following immunization [49]; however, several other studies have suggested that the vaccine response may be quite durable even 10 years after immunization [50–52]. In fact, productive HBV infection has been relatively rare in vaccine recipients regardless of antibody levels. Nonetheless, some institutions offer booster doses of vaccine to HCWs who have previously responded to HBV vaccination, whose antibody levels have become undetectable, and who remain in jobs associated with risk for blood exposure and HBV infection.

Hepatitis C Virus

For occupational exposures to HCV, the immediate PEP is identical to that described previously for all BBPs. As for known HBV exposures, practitioners must be aware that certain of these BBPs travel together. Thus, even when known to harbor HCV, the source-patient should also be tested for HBV and HIV, in addition to testing for his or her current HCV infection status. Practitioners ordering these tests must be cognizant of the local and state laws relevant to informed consent for these tests. Furthermore, practitioners should be mindful of the fact that the majority of the screening tests are designed to detect antibody directed against some of these pathogens and that these tests clearly do not detect all patients who have been infected previously. Specifically with respect to HCV, detecting antibody against HCV in a source-patient's serum is not an accurate indicator of the individual's infectivity.

The most recent CDC guidelines for managing occupational HCV exposure recommend (1) testing the source-patient for antibody against HCV at the time of exposure; (2) baseline testing of the HCW sustaining the exposure for both antibody against HCV and alanine aminotransferase levels; (3) repeat testing of the HCW (for HCV antibody and alanine aminotransferase levels) at six months following the exposure or at any time when symptoms suggest possible infection; (4) using confirmatory tests, including direct antigen detection, direct genome detection, and supplementary or confirmatory antibody tests (e.g., recombinant immunoblot assay [RIBA]) to investigate positive results of HCV antibody testing in more detail; (5) not providing immunoglobulin, antiviral agents, or immunomodulators as PEP; and (6) providing comprehensive information to the exposed HCW about the magnitude of occupational risks associated with the exposure, the risks for secondary transmission, and strategies known to be effective in preventing exposure to blood and/or transmission of HCV in occupational settings [53].

Some individuals have advocated more aggressive monitoring and interventional strategies [16,54]. One approach is to follow HCWs using periodic monitoring with PCR detection of HCV RNA at some defined interval (e.g., monthly, every 6 weeks, at 3 months following exposure) in addition to the antibody testing described earlier. If an exposed HCW is repeatedly detected as positive for HCV RNA by the PCR (because of frequent false positives in low prevalence settings, one should never rely on a single positive sample), the HCW can be referred to a specialist in the management of HCV for definitive therapy (see the following discussion).

Historically, some investigators advocated the use of immune serum globulin to attempt to decrease the risk for transmission of what has been subsequently identified to be HCV [55–57]. As additional details of the pathogenesis and immunology of HCV infection have been delineated, most experts now agree that postexposure immunoglobulin prophylaxis is of no value. Similarly, no information has provided scientific support for a role for interferon or other immunomodulators administered as true PEP (i.e., in the immediate postexposure period) for occupational HCV exposures. Finally, to date, no agents with specific antiviral activity against HCV have been marketed. Nonetheless, antiviral agents with specific, defined HCV targets (e.g., protease, helicase, and polymerase inhibitors) are in drug development and may ultimately play a role in immediate postexposure prophylaxis (e.g., analogous to antiretrovirals in the management of occupational exposures to HIV discussed later). Currently, in the absence of data purporting efficacy for any of these compounds administered as PEP, no recommendation can be made about their potential use.

Although a clear recommendation for the use of immediate PEP following occupational HCV exposures cannot be made, some postexposure management strategies do show promise. One PEP management strategy that has been adopted by many centers throughout the United States centers on the early treatment of occupational HCV infection. This strategy incorporates the periodic monitoring of exposed HCWs by HCV-PCR combined with early therapy with immunomodulators once infection is confirmed. This strategy was first advocated by Schiff in 1992 [58]. Once occupational infection has been definitively documented, two separate approaches have been advocated: pre-emptive therapy and watchful waiting [16].

The preemptive therapy strategy involves the aggressive initiation of immunomodulator therapy (e.g., interferon, with or without ribavirin) as soon as the diagnosis of occupational HCV infection is established with certainty. The rationale for this strategy is at least in part based on studies documenting the successful treatment of patients with so-called acute HCV infection. In several studies, treatment of patients with "early" HCV infection has been far more successful (i.e., some with efficacies of therapies exceeding 90–95%) [59–64]. In perhaps the largest of these series published to date, Jaeckel et al. treated 44 patients who had acute HCV infection with interferon alpha-2b, initially daily (for 1 month) and then three times a week for 5 months. Of the 44 patients studied, HCV-RNA was undetectable by PCR, and alanine aminotransferase levels were entirely normal in 43/44 patients who were treated, both at the end of their treatments and six months following completion of therapy [62]. Although this study has limitations [16], particularly with respect to generalizing the results to the occupational exposure setting, the success rate is remarkable and substantially exceeds cure rates of even the best studies of the treatment of chronic HCV infection. The 98% "cure rate" observed in this study is extraordinary. In addition to the documented clinical successes of treating acute infection, one can assemble a strong intellectual argument for the preemptive therapy approach primarily because the clinician would be treating the patient when the HCV would have produced a limited number of quasispecies. In fact, a National Institutes of Health (NIH) Consensus Conference published in 2002 argued strongly for the aggressive treatment of individuals who have acute HCV infection [59].

The second approach to the management of occupational HCV infection employs the watchful waiting strategy. Following this strategy, once the definitive diagnosis of occupational HCV infection has been established (by repeatedly detecting HCV-RNA in the circulation of the exposed HCW), the clinician caring for the exposed/infected HCW observes the patient for a defined period of time (e.g., 2–3 months) to see whether the infected HCW spontaneously clears the infection. HCWs who spontaneously resolve their infections obviously would be spared both the potential toxicities and expense of immunomodulator therapy. The rationale for the watchful waiting strategy is discussed shortly.

Although the data describing the success of early interventions in the treatment of patients who have acute HCV infection are undeniably encouraging, there are no data demonstrating that either of these two approaches to managing occupational HCV infections is efficacious, let alone that one approach is advantageous over the other. One anecdotal case-report has documented resolution of HCV infection following early treatment (the HCW became PCR-positive, received immunomodulator treatment, became PCR-negative, and never produced anti-HCV antibody) [65].

Several factors favor the watchful waiting approach to the management of occupational HCV exposures. First, because we have no clear understanding of the early events in the pathogenesis of occupational HCV infection, we need to keep open minds about the factors that do (and might) influence transmission. For example, we do not know what fraction of HCWs who sustain an occupational HCV exposure and subsequently develop PCR evidence of HCV infection will develop a cellular immune response to the insult that allows the individual to clear the infection spontaneously without developing antibody against HCV. Larghi et al. reported that 50% of the individuals exposed to HCV in a point-source epidemic spontaneously resolved their infections without long-term infectious or serologic sequelae [66]. Clearly, clinical scientists need additional insight into the early events in the pathogenesis, immunopathogenesis of, and host immunological response to HCV infection to understand the best strategies for interventions including those involving immunomodulators. Additional support for the watchful waiting approach can be derived from the study by Seeff et al. that found that 20% of patients who acquired transfusion-associated HCV infection spontaneously cleared their infections [67]. This latter finding is perhaps even more striking because individuals who acquire HCV infection from contaminated transfusions presumably receive much higher inocula of virus (and presumably many different quasispecies) than do individuals who become infected from an occupational exposure. Extrapolating from these two studies, administering interferon to 100% of individuals detected by PCR as having circulating HCV-RNA would unnecessarily expose between 20–50% to toxicity with no benefit.

A variety of additional factors qualifies the interpretation of the available data relevant to the management of occupational HCV exposure management [16]. For example, the use of immunomodulating agents as postexposure prophylaxis is substantially different from the use of antiviral agents directed against specific viral targets (e.g., PEP with antiretrovirals for occupational HIV exposures). Finally, administering interferon before the exposed HCW's cellular immune response has matured (i.e., has had time to begin to develop a specific response to the invading pathogen) may be far less effective than waiting until the relevant cells have been activated and expanded (and, thus, the specific response can then be further stimulated by immunomodulators). Even in the absence of definitive scientific support for these approaches, many U.S. healthcare institutions have adopted either the preemptive therapy or watchful waiting strategy for managing occupational HCV exposure [68]. PCR monitoring for viremia, monitoring hepatic function by alanine aminotransferase levels, closely monitoring developing antibody responses, and, finally, levering a decision for intervention from the clinical and chemical data obtained from the actions detailed here represent an entirely sentient approach to this complex management problem.

Human Immunodeficiency Virus

Specific PEP interventions for occupational exposures to the HIV were initially controversial. CDC first published guidelines that included "considerations" with respect to the administration of antiretrovirals for PEP for occupational exposures to HIV in 1990 [69]. Since this initial publication, CDC has published several sets of updated recommendations. The most recent guidelines were published by CDC in 2005 [2].

The rationale for administering postexposure antiretroviral chemoprophylaxis is derived from several disparate sources: (1) *in vitro* studies of the efficacy of antiretrovirals in preventing retroviral infection of susceptibles; (2) studies delineating the early sequence of events in the process of HIV infection of cells that provide a sense of biological plausibility for the efficacy of these agents administered as prophylaxis; (3) studies in relevant animal models of the safety and efficacy of antiretroviral prophylaxis for retroviral infection; (4) clinical studies demonstrating the efficacy of antiretrovirals in preventing vertical transmission; (5) epidemiologic data collected over the past 20 years describing occupational HIV infections in HCWs; and (6) substantial clinical experience over the past 20 years administering these agents in the postexposure setting. Despite the fact that we likely will never have definitive scientific evidence of the efficacy of these agents administered as postexposure prophylaxis, when all of these sources of indirectly relevant data are considered together, they provide substantial rationale for the use of these drugs in this setting. A more detailed discussion of the various aspects of the rationale for administering these agents as chemoprophylaxis for occupational HIV exposures appears.

Laboratory studies conducted in the late 1980s demonstrated that adding nucleoside analogs to the tissue culture milieu could prevent infection of tissue culture cells known to be highly susceptible to HIV infection [70]. These studies provided definitive evidence that reverse transcriptase inhibitors could actually prevent infection of susceptible cells.

Several studies conducted over the past decade have dramatically increased our understanding of the early events in the pathogenesis of HIV infection. This increased clarity has provided additional support for the biological plausibility of postexposure antiretroviral chemoprophylaxis.

These studies suggest that dendritic cells in the mucosa and skin are initial targets for HIV infection and that these cells also play an important role in disseminating HIV to cells in the regional lymph nodes [71]. In animal models, pathogenic retroviruses remain localized with dendritic cells for approximately 24 hours following inoculation with cell-free virus [72]. After 24–48 hours, the cells migrate to regional lymph nodes, resulting in productive infection of the T-cells in these lymph nodes [72].

Thus, our current understanding suggests that HIV infection occurs in a sequence of events, initially involving dendritic cells near the exposure site that subsequently move to and transmit infection to susceptible T-cells in regional lymph nodes. Early antiretroviral intervention appears most likely to prevent infection by preventing infection of susceptible T-cells. Delaying the infection of susceptible T-cells also could allow time for the exposed individual to develop a cellular immune response against HIV (see).

Although several pieces of evidence support the concept that the cellular arm of immunity plays an important role in host defense against HIV, the precise role of the cellular immunity has not been completely elucidated. Among the evidence suggesting a significant role for cellular immunity in host defense against HIV are (1) studies of prostitutes and seronegative sexual partners of HIV-infected individuals that demonstrate HIV-specific cytotoxicity in the uninfected sexual partners, studies of HCWs who have sustained occupational exposure to HIV and did not become infected but did develop cellular cytotoxic responses directed against HIV [35–44], and two anecdotal reports of individuals who sustained exposures (one by receipt of contaminated blood products [73], the other an HCW who sustained a substantial occupational exposure [74] both of whom became PCR-positive for HIV, both of whom cleared their infections [each also received three antiretrovirals], and both of whom developed substantial cellular responses directed against HIV antigens). Neither developed antibody directed against HIV. Interestingly, in two animal PEP models, successful prophylaxis was associated with the presence of effective cellular immune response in both mice and macaques [75,76]. These studies provide reasonably convincing, albeit indirect, evidence for the hypothesis that antiretroviral chemoprophylaxis administered soon after an occupational exposure in concert with a specific cellular immune response directed against HIV envelope antigens may be effective in preventing or inhibiting systemic HIV infection.

Although the initial animal model studies published failed to show any benefit of antiretroviral chemoprophylaxis, subsequent studies in several different models have clearly demonstrated efficacy for PEP. Most of the very early experiments employed intravenous injection of very high inocula. In most of these studies, the inocula were far in excess of what might be anticipated to be associated with a typical occupational exposure.

In one of the most elegant studies published to date, Tsai et al. demonstrated true prophylactic efficacy of phosphonylmethoxypropyladenine (PMPA, Tenofovir®) in a macaque model [77]. In a subsequent study, these same investigators demonstrated that all animals that received postexposure treatment for 28 days remained uninfected; only half of the animals that were treated for 10 days and none of the animals that received only three days of treatment were protected [78]. Similarly, in the latter study, delay in initiating prophylaxis was detrimental in this model. All of the animals that were treated within 24 hours of intravenous simian immunodeficiency virus (SIV) infection remained uninfected, whereas only 50% of the animals that received treatment beginning 48 hours following infection and only 25% of the animals that received treatment beginning 72 hours after exposure were protected [78].

Antiretrovirals also have been shown to be effective in preventing maternal-fetal transmission of HIV during childbirth [79–81]. Several studies have demonstrated the efficacy of single or combinations of agents in preventing neonatal infection. Perhaps even more important, two studies demonstrated efficacy of antiretrovirals in preventing infection when only the child was treated after birth (i.e., PEP efficacy) [82,83]. Although neither of these studies was designed to test the PEP hypothesis, both studies provide compelling evidence that these agents can work to prevent vertical transmission of HIV even well after the exposure has occurred.

Both clinical studies and clinical experience since these agents initially began to be used for PEP in the late 1980s provide additional rational for the use of antiretrovirals as postexposure prophylaxis for occupational HIV exposures. CDC published a retrospective case-control study that was designed to identify factors associated with increased risk for occupational HIV infection. In this study, a number of factors relating to the exposure itself were found to be associated with increased risk; however, the study also found that PEP with zidovudine was associated with an 81% reduction in risk [34,84]. Admittedly, the case-control design is far from the optimal study design to try to demonstrate efficacy of an agent or combination of agents in preventing infection; however, this study provided additional evidence that these agents may be useful in this setting. Antiretroviral chemoprophylaxis for occupational HIV exposures has been in use in the United States since the late 1980s [85], and, although a variety of factors has contributed to the reduction in incidence of occupational HIV infections, at least coincident with the expanded use of antiretroviral chemoprophylaxis, the numbers such infections over the past decade have decreased substantially (Table 42-4). The two anecdotal case-reports of transient infection (in the blood product recipient [73] and in the HCW who sustained an occupational exposure [74]) described earlier also provide indirect anecdotal support for chemoprophylaxis efficacy.

TABLE 42-4
FACTORS LIKELY CONTRIBUTING TO THE OBSERVED DECREASE IN OCCUPATIONAL HIV INFECTIONS IN HEALTHCARE PROVIDERS IN THE UNITED STATES

Decreased reporting of exposures and perhaps of occupational infections to CDC.

Because the risks for occupational infection are now reasonably well defined, less aggressive case-finding for occupational exposures.

The efficacy of primary prevention (i.e., preventing exposures to blood) due to the use of universal/standard precautions, resulting in prevention of infection.

The efficacy of highly active antiretroviral therapy in lowering patients' viral burdens, and, in so doing, reducing the risk for transmission of bloodborne pathogens.

Efficacy of highly active antiretroviral therapy in keeping HIV-infected patients well and out of the hospital.

The efficacy of highly active antiretroviral therapy in decreasing the numbers and types of medically invasive procedures required by HIV-infected patients.

Presumed efficacy of secondary prevention (i.e., the presumed efficacy of antiretroviral postexposure chemoprophylaxis) in reducing the risk for occupational infection.

CURRENT USPHS RECOMMENDATIONS FOR HIV POSTEXPOSURE CHEMOPROPHYLAXIS

A lengthy list of factors influences the selection of antiretroviral drugs for PEP, among them (1) the severity of exposure and the estimated risk of HIV transmission associated with the specific type of exposure that has occurred (e.g., transfusion of a volume of contaminated blood would be associated with a much higher risk for transmission than a needlestick with a solid surgical needle); (2) the source-patient's experience with antiretroviral agents as therapy for her or his infection and the influence this experience has on the likelihood that the source-patient harbors resistant isolates; (3) the source-patient's adherence to his or her current treatment regimen and the influence that this factor has on the likelihood that drug-resistant isolates were present in the circulation at the time the occupational exposure occurred; (4) the known toxicities of the agents proposed for the prophylaxis regimen and the likelihood that the HCW will be able to adhere to the recommended course; (5) the extent to which clinicians have experience administering these agents to uninfected individuals and the known safety profiles of the agent(s); and (6) cost.

Agents from at least five different classes of drugs—nucleoside reverse transcriptase inhibitors, nucleotide reverse transcriptase inhibitors, non-nucleoside reverse transcriptase inhibitors, protease inhibitors, and fusion inhibitors—have been marketed for the treatment of HIV disease, and, thus, are available for use as PEP. In 2006, we unquestionably have the most experience administering agents of the nucleoside analog class for PEP, although we have reasonable clinical experience with agents in three of the other classes of drug. Perhaps only because of its historical role, we have the most experience with the nucleoside analog, zidovudine. Since their marketing, we also have substantial experience using drugs of the protease inhibitor class in the PEP setting. Whereas these agents are extremely potent, they also are associated with a variety of toxicities and complex drug–drug interactions (see).

Recommendations for managing occupational HIV exposures are summarized in Table 42-5. Current recommended drug combinations and their alternatives, with the advantages and disadvantages associated with the various regimens are detailed in Table 42-6. Whereas combinations of antiretroviral drugs have been definitively proven to be more effective than single agents for treating established HIV infection, we do not have such data for the PEP setting. In fact, as noted, because of the way in which we have come to learn about the use of these agents in this setting, we may never have true efficacy data for either individual drugs or combinations.

A major point of controversy involves the issue of whether to offer the basic or expanded regimen, that is, should you offer a third agent—usually a protease inhibitor or a newer non-nucleoside reverse transcriptase inhibitor—as part of the regimen. Historically, CDC has recommended adding the third drug to the regimen when

TABLE 42-5

CURRENT U. S. PUBLIC HEALTH SERVICE GUIDELINES FOR MANAGING OCCUPATIONAL EXPOSURES TO HIV IN HEALTHCARE WORKERS

Percutaneous Exposure Type	Infection Status of Source[a]				
	HIV-Positive Class 1[b]	HIV-Positive Class 2[b]	Source of Unknown HIV Status[c]	Unknown Source[d]	HIV-Negative
Less severe[e]	Recommend basic two-drug PEP	Recommend expanded ≥ three-drug PEP[f]	Generally, no PEP warranted; however, consider basic two-drug PEP[f] for source with HIV risk factors[g]	Generally, no PEP warranted; however, consider basic two-drug PEP[f] in settings in which exposure to HIV-infected persons is likely	No PEP warranted
More severe[h]	Recommend expanded three-drug PEP	Recommend expanded ≥ three-drug PEP	Generally, no PEP warranted; however, consider basic two-drug PEP[f] for source with HIV risk factors[g]	Generally, no PEP warranted; however, consider basic two-drug PEP[f] in settings in which exposure to HIV-infected persons is likely	No PEP warranted
Small volume[i]	Consider basic two-drug PEP	Recommend basic two-drug PEP	Generally, no PEP warranted	Generally, no PEP warranted	No PEP warranted
Large volume[j]	Recommend basic two-drug PEP	Recommend expanded ≥ three-drug PEP	Generally, no PEP warranted; however, consider basic two-drug PEP[f] for source with HIV risk factors[g]	Generally, no PEP warranted; however, consider basic two-drug PEP[f] in settings in which exposure to HIV-infected persons is likely	

[a]Although this table refers to the management of exposures to HIV, in every instance in which exposure to blood occurs, the clinician managing the exposure should consider the potential for exposure to multiple blood borne pathogens; thus, at a minimum, someone sustaining an exposure to HIV should also have an assessment for potential exposures to hepatitis B and hepatitis C.

[b]HIV-positive, class 1—asymptomatic HIV infection or known low viral burden (e.g., <1,500 ribonucleic acid copies/mL). HIV-positive, class 2—symptomatic HIV infection, acquired immunodeficiency syndrome, acute seroconversion, or known high viral load. If drug resistance is a concern, obtain expert consultation. Initiation of PEP should not be delayed pending expert consultation, and, because expert consultation alone cannot substitute for face-to-face counseling, resource should be available to provide immediate evaluation and follow-up care for all exposures.

[c]For example, deceased source patient with no samples available for HIV testing.

[d]For example, a needle from a sharps disposal container or a splash from inappropriately disposed blood.

[e]For example, a solid needle or a superficial injury.

[f]The recommendation consider PEP indicates that PEP is optional; a decision to initiate PEP should be based on a discussion between the exposed person and the treating clinician regarding the risks versus benefits of PEP.

[g]If PEP is offered and administered and the source patient is subsequently determined to be HIV-negative, PEP should be discontinued.

[h]For example, a large-bore, hollow needle, deep puncture, visible blood on the device, or needle used in patient's artery or vein.

[i]For example, a few drops of blood.

[j]For example, a major blood splash.

TABLE 42-6

CURRENT U. S. PUBLIC HEALTH SERVICE RECOMMENDATIONS FOR ANTIRETROVIRAL PROPHYLAXIS REGIMENS FOR MANAGING OCCUPATIONAL EXPOSURES TO HIV IN HEALTHCARE WORKERS

Preferred Basic Regimens	Preferred Dosing	Advantages	Disadvantages
Zidovudine (ZDV) plus Lamivudine (3TC)	ZDV—300 mg twice daily or 200 mg three times daily, with food; total: 600 mg daily; 3TC: 300 mg once daily or 150 mg twice daily □-1; Combivir™: tablet twice daily	Associated with decreased risk for HIV transmission in animals, and vertical transmission studies; also associated with reduced risk in CDC case-control study; largest PEP experience to date is with ZDV; serious toxicities have been uncommon when used for PEP; side effects predictable and manageable with antimotility and antiemetic agents; some experience with this agent administered to HCW during pregnancy □—can be given with lamivudine as a single tablet (Combivir™) twice daily	Side effects predictable, common, and may be protracted (especially nausea, vomiting, diarrhea and fatigue); may result in reduced regimen adherence; because of extensive use of ZDV, source-patient virus resistance to this regimen possible; animal oncogenicity/teratogenicity documented; relevance to human pregnancy unknown
Zidovudine (ZDV) plus Emtricitabine (FTC)	ZDV—300 mg twice daily or 200 mg three times daily, with food; total: 600 mg/day, in 2–3 divided doses; FTC—200 mg (one capsule) once daily	FTC administered once daily; regimen is generally well tolerated; both agents have long intracellular half-lives	Experience with FTC is quite limited in this setting; dermatitis may be more frequent with FTC compared with 3TC; FTC exhibits cross-resistance to 3TC; among non-Caucasians, a small fraction of HIV-infected patients taking FTC for extended periods experience hyperpigmentation with long-term use
Tenofovir (TDF) plus Lamivudine (3TC)	TDF—300 mg once daily; 3TC—300 mg once daily or 150 mg twice daily	TDF—convenient dosing (single pill once daily), TDF effective against isolates resistant to other thymidine analogues; generally well tolerated; 3TC (see above)	TDF—same class warnings as nucleoside reverse transcriptase inhibitors; some drug–drug interactions reported, increased TDF concentrations among persons taking atazanavir and lopinavir/ritonavir; need to monitor patients closely for TDF-associated toxicities; atazanavir dose (when used with TDF)—300 mg plus ritonavir 100 mg once daily
Tenofovir (TDF) plus Emtricitabine (FTC)	TDF—300 mg once daily; FTC—200 mg once daily; also available as combination capsule (Truvada®); one capsule, once daily	TDF—Convenient dosing (single pill once daily); TDF effective against isolates resistant to other thymidine analogues; generally well tolerated; 3TC (see above)	TDF—same class warnings as nucleoside reverse transcriptase inhibitors; some drug–drug interactions reported; although early experience suggests combination is well tolerated, experience is extremely limited with these agents in this setting
Alternative basic regimens			
Lamivudine (3TC) plus Stavudine (d4T)	3TC—300 mg once daily or 150 mg twice daily; d4T—40 mg twice daily (lower doses [e.g., 20–30 mg twice daily] if toxicity occurs; equally effective but less toxic among HIV-infected patients with peripheral neuropathy); dose should be reduced to 30 mg twice daily if body weight is <60 kg	Some evidence (in patients receiving drugs as therapy for HIV infection) that d4T may be at least as equally effective and less toxic in patients who have already developed peripheral neuropathy; 30 mg twice daily if body weight is <60 kg	GI toxicity associated with d4T administration—nausea, vomiting, and diarrhea—can be severe, but occurs relatively uncommonly with d4T. Because both these agents have been widely used in the treatment of HIV infection in the U.S., the possibility that source-patient virus may be resistant to these agents is slightly increased

(continued)

TABLE 42-6
(CONTINUED)

Preferred Basic Regimens	Preferred Dosing	Advantages	Disadvantages
Lamivudine (3TC) plus Didanosine (ddI)	3TC—300 mg once daily or 150 mg twice daily; ddI—chewable/dispersible buffered tablets can be administered on an empty stomach as either 200 mg twice daily or 400 mg once daily. Patients must take at least two of the appropriate strength tablets at each dose to provide adequate buffering and prevent gastric acid degradation of ddI. Dose—adjustment for weight—200 mg twice daily or 400 mg once daily for patients weighing >60 kg and 125 mg twice daily or 250 mg once daily for patients weighing >60 kg	3TC is discussed. ddI has been effective in some settings in which other nucleoside analogues were not effective; resistance profile substantially different	Diarrhea is more common with the buffered preparation than with enteric-coated preparation. ddI administration has been associated with peripheral neuropathy, pancreatitis, and lactic acidosis; some instances of each have been quite severe; must be taken on empty stomach except if administered with TDF. ddI should not be administered to pregnant HCWs, because there are several maternal and fetal deaths associated with the development of lactic acidosis
Emtricitabine (3TC) plus Didanosine (ddI)	FTC—200 mg once daily; ddI—chewable/dispersible buffered tablets can be administered on an empty stomach as either 200 mg twice daily or 400 mg once daily. Patients must take at least two of the appropriate strength tablets at each dose to provide adequate buffering and prevent gastric acid degradation of ddI. Dose—adjustment for weight—200 mg twice daily or 400 mg once daily for patients weighing >60 kg and 125 mg twice daily or 250 mg once daily for patients weighing >60 kg	Both agents are discussed above	Both agents discussed above
Preferred expanded regimen			
One of the preferred basic regimens plus Lopinavir/ Ritonavir (LPV/RTV) (Kaletra®)	LPV/RTV: 400/100 mg (i.e., three capsules taken orally twice daily) (with food)	Kaletra® is a potent HIV protease inhibitor that is generally reasonably well tolerated	As a class, the protease inhibitors are associated with a potential for serious or life-threatening drug interactions. Administration of LPV/RTV may accelerate clearance of certain drugs, including oral contraceptives (requiring alternative contraceptive measures). All protease inhibitors are associated with risks for severe hyperlipidemia; gastrointestinal side effects, particularly diarrhea, are extremely common

TABLE 42-6
(CONTINUED)

Preferred Basic Regimens	Preferred Dosing	Advantages	Disadvantages
		Alternative expanded regimens	
One of the Preferred Basic Regimens plus one of the following agents:			
Atazanavir (Reyataz®; ATV), with or without ritonavir (Norvir®; RTV)	ATV—400 mg once daily; if used in combination with TDF, ATV should be boosted with RTV, preferred dosing of ATV 300 mg plus RTV—100 mg once daily	A potent HIV protease inhibitor that also provides the advantage of once-daily dosing	Protease inhibitor class toxicities, including hyperbilirubinemia and jaundice, the potential for serious or life-threatening drug interactions; should not be administered with proton pump inhibitors; pH dependent absorption—wait for 2 hours before or after administering antacids and buffered medications; if H2-receptor antagonists are administered, wait for dosing until at least 12 hours later to avoid decreasing ATV levels; concerned raised about cardiac electrical problems—use with caution with agents known to induce PR prolongation (e.g., diltiazem)
Fosamprenavir (Lexiva®; FOSAPV), with or without ritonavir (Norvir®; RTV)	FOSAPV—If administered without boosting, 1400 mg twice daily; if boosted, dose is either 1400 mg of FOSAPV once daily plus 200 mg RTV once daily or FOSAPV 700 mg twice daily + RTV 100 mg twice daily	One of a group of highly effective HIV protease inhibitors	Protease inhibitor class toxicities, including multiple drug interactions. Gastrointestinal side effects perhaps just a bit more common. Simultaneous administration of oral contraceptives results in decreased fosamprenavir concentrations. Dermatitis seen frequently, especially when used with low doses of ritonavir. As with a few other antiretrovirals (most commonly the NNRTIs) differentiating between early drug-associated rash and acute seroconversion can be difficult and cause extraordinary concern for the exposed person
Indinavir (Crixivan®; IDV), with or without ritonavir (Norvir®; RTV)	For boosted administration—IDV 800 mg plus RTV 100 mg twice daily; if used alone, IDV 800 mg at 8 hour intervals (a total of 2400 mg/day) administered when stomach is empty to ensure absorption	One of a group of highly effective HIV protease inhibitors	Protease inhibitor class toxicities, including hyperbilirubinemia and jaundice, and the potential for serious or life-threatening drug interactions; nephrolithiasis occurs more frequently with IDV than several other members of the class and can be prevented by having patient drink 8 glasses of fluid/day; should be avoided in late pregnancy; requires acid for absorption; therefore cannot be taken simultaneously with the chewable/dispersible buffered tablet formulation of ddI; if used with this ddI formulation, doses must be separated by at least one hour

(continued)

TABLE 42-6
(CONTINUED)

Preferred Basic Regimens	Preferred Dosing	Advantages	Disadvantages
Saquinavir (Invirase®; SQV) plus ritonavir (Norvir®; RTV)	SQV—1,000 mg plus RTV 100 mg, twice daily	One of a group of highly effective HIV protease inhibitors	Protease inhibitor class toxicities, including hyperbilirubinemia and jaundice, and the potential for serious or life-threatening drug interactions; the large number of pills that are required to be taken may be inconvenient; gastrointestinal side effects may be a bit more common with this regimen
Nelfinavir (Viracept®; NFV)	NFV—1,250 mg (either two 625 mg or five 250 mg tablets), twice daily; should be taken with meals	One of a group of highly effective HIV protease inhibitors	Protease inhibitor class toxicities, including hyperbilirubinemia and jaundice, and the potential for serious or life-threatening drug interactions; the large number of pills that are required to be taken may be inconvenient; gastrointestinal side effects may be a bit more common with this regimen
Efavirenz (Sustiva®; EFV)	EFV—600 mg daily, often optimally administered as the patient is going to sleep	A theoretical advantage is that this agent does not need to be phosphorylated to be active. Convenience of once-daily dosing is a plus.	May be associated with dermatitis (especially early) that can be severe. A few cases have progressed to Stevens-Johnson syndrome; as with other NNRTIs, differentiating between early drug-associated rash and acute seroconversion may be difficult and may cause extraordinary concern for the exposed person. Central nervous system side effects (e.g., dizziness, somnolence, insomnia, or abnormal dreaming) are quite common; severe psychiatric symptoms possible (dosing before bedtime might minimize these side effects). Studies suggest teratogenicity; agent should not be used during pregnancy. Also associated with a potential for serious or life-threatening drug interactions

the risk for transmission is known to be increased, for example, for exposures known to be associated with higher inocula of blood or virus (Table 42-6) [2].

ADVERSE EFFECTS ASSOCIATED WITH POSTEXPOSURE CHEMOPROPHYLAXIS FOR OCCUPATIONAL EXPOSURES TO HIV

Antiretroviral agents are not benign drugs. All of these agents have both known and substantial side effects. One curious finding has been that healthy individuals taking these agents seem to have more and more severe side effects than HIV-infected patients have when they take these agents for therapy. In particular, subjective side effects are remarkably common among HCWs taking PEP for occupational HIV exposures.

Untoward effects have been uniformly associated with each of these agents and each of the varied regimens that have been used for PEP [86,87]. Known or anticipated side effects represent one of several important considerations when selecting a chemoprophylaxis regimen. Toxicities reported with nucleoside analogues include bone marrow suppression (including neutropenia and anemia), nausea, vomiting, diarrhea, abdominal pain, headache, neuropathies, aminotransferase elevations, myalgias, lassitude, malaise, and insomnia. Very severe toxicities including instances of severe pancreatitis, dermatitis, severe hepatic dysfunction, lactic acidosis, or seizures rarely have been reported.

Toxicities associated with the use of protease inhibitors in a chemoprophylaxis regimen include nausea, vomiting, diarrhea, abdominal pain, hyperglycemia, hyperlipidemia, hypercholesterolemia, galactorrhea [88]; hyperprolactinemia [88]; cholestasis [89]; and headache, jaundice, anorexia, altered taste, and/or paresthesias [86]. Less commonly reported side effects associated with protease inhibitor use in chemoprophylaxis include nephrolithiasis [87] and lipodystrophy [90]. Another important issue in the use of the protease inhibitors in chemoprophylaxis regimens is drug–drug interactions that occur extremely commonly. If protease inhibitors are prescribed as part of a chemoprophylaxis regimen, the responsible clinician should evaluate all other drugs currently being taken by the exposed HCW with an eye toward these interactions. For example, simultaneous administration of either rifampin or the nutritional supplement St. John's wort can reduce plasma levels of protease inhibitors well into the subtherapeutic range. Protease inhibitors can potentiate the effects of antihistamines, ergot alkaloids (increasing risk for ergot toxicity, vasospasm, and ischemia), benzodiazepines (increasing risks for central nervous system [CNS] depression), and statins (increasing risk for severe toxicities, such as rhabdomyolysis) and can induce cardiac arrhythmias when administered with diltiazem or cisapride. Another important interaction occurs with oral contraceptives. Protease inhibitors may accelerate their clearance, decreasing their efficacy. For this reason, if protease inhibitors are included in a chemoprophylaxis regimen, women taking the regimen should use alternative contraceptive measures.

Although non-nucleoside reverse transcriptase inhibitors have never been primary choices for PEP, some authorities have advocated their use. This author has generally avoided recommending these agents for a variety of reasons, including the fact that rash is a commonly occurring side effect that could easily be confused with the seroconversion illness. Some instances of dermatitis associated with the use of nevirapine and other agents in this class have been quite severe (e.g., two reported episodes of Stevens-Johnson syndrome) [91], but perhaps the major concern relates to two instances of severe hepatic dysfunction (one requiring hepatic transplantation) and 10 episodes of moderate hepatic toxicity in HCWs who took nevirapine as part of a chemoprophylaxis regimen [91–93]. Concern also has been expressed about the use of efavirenz in pregnancy because of studies suggesting potential for teratogenicity in animal models. Because of its method of metabolism, efavirenz has extensive drug–drug interactions similar to those of the protease inhibitors including

the interactions described previously with antimicrobials, ergots, and benzodiazepines. Other toxicities associated with the use of non-nucleoside reverse transcriptase inhibitors include mild CNS dysfunction (e.g., somnolence, insomnia, difficulty concentrating, abnormal dreams, and dizziness). Nonetheless, because of its substantial potency, CDC has recommended in its most recently published guidelines that efavirenz be included in the list of agents to be considered as the third drug in an alternative expanded regimen [2].

A major lesson learned over the past 15 years is that many, if not most, of these side effects can be anticipated and managed symptomatically prospectively (e.g., acetaminophen for headache and myalgia; prochlorperazine for nausea; antimotility drugs for diarrhea).

FAILURES OF POSTEXPOSURE CHEMOPROPHYLAXIS FOR OCCUPATIONAL HIV EXPOSURES

PEP failures occur. Most of the failures that have been reported involve the use of zidovudine as a single agent (again, perhaps an historical artifact). Additionally, five instances of failure have been reported in association with the use of regimens involving >1 agent (two failures of a 2-drug, three failures of 3-drug, and one failure of 4-drug regimen) [2,94,95]. In the overwhelming majority of these episodes, the source-patient was highly experienced with antiretrovirals and very likely may have harbored resistant isolates. Furthermore, a variety of additional factors may have contributed to chemoprophylaxis failures including exposure to very high inocula; delayed initiation of PEP; failure to achieve adequate drug concentrations; inadequate treatment duration; and so on. Occasionally, what appears to be a chemoprophylaxis failure turns out to be something else. Two publications have detailed episodes that initially were thought to be a result of occupational exposure and infection but with more investigation were found to represent instances of community infection that were entirely unrelated to occupational exposures [96,97].

UNRESOLVED ISSUES

Exposure to Blood from Source-Patients Known or Suspected to Harbor Resistant Isolates of HIV

The basic and expanded CDC drug regimen recommendations represent excellent choices for instances in which the source-patient is unlikely to harbor resistant viral isolates. Drug resistance is most likely among patients who do not consistently adhere to their treatment regimens. When drug resistance is suspected, the clinician providing care should get expert counsel from individuals knowledgeable about HIV therapy to tailor a regimen to which the source-patient's isolates have not been exposed. Basically, the same principles used to select drugs for HIV-infected patients who are failing treatment should be used to craft the chemoprophylaxis regimen [98,99].

Although the responsible clinician should not wait to begin therapy until discussing the patient with an expert in HIV therapy given all of the complexities inherent in selecting antiretroviral drugs, consultation with an expert is highly recommended when legitimate concerns about the possibility of exposure to drug-resistant HIV have arisen. This author recommends beginning an expanded regimen and immediately seeking the counsel of a colleague experienced in tailoring regimens for HIV-infected patients who have resistant isolates. If such expertise is not immediately available, clinicians can call or e-mail the experts at the National Clinicians' Post-Exposure Hotline (PEPLINE) (1-888-HIV-4911 or **www.pepline.ucsf.edu/pepline**).

Managing Occupational Exposure to HIV in Pregnant Staff

The decision to offer a pregnant woman postexposure antiretroviral chemoprophylaxis should be based on the same considerations that apply to all HCWs who have sustained occupational HIV exposures. In counseling the exposed pregnant HCW, the counselor must consider the risks and benefits for the worker and her fetus. Specific issues that should be discussed include the magnitude of risk for HIV transmission to the mother and the fetus associated with the exposure she has sustained, what is known about the potential for teratogenicity and other toxicities associated with the agents being prescribed in the context of the stage of pregnancy, and what is known about the safety and side effects of the specific antiretroviral agents being administered during pregnancy. In general, the data on which to base such discussions are extremely limited. For example, the risk to the fetus of administering a course of postexposure antiretroviral chemoprophylaxis is essentially unknown. Additionally, virtually all marketed antiretroviral agents have the potential for carcinogenicity, teratogenicity, and/or mutagenicity, and a few have been demonstrated to be mutagenic in premarketing animal studies. Furthermore, safety and pharmacology data addressing the risk of administering antiretrovirals to HIV-uninfected pregnant women are extremely limited. Because of the complexity of administering these agents to healthy pregnant women, this is another setting in which the prescriber should seek the counsel of someone who has substantial expertise in using these drugs on a daily basis.

In the final analysis, the HCW herself must make the decision as to whether or not to proceed with postexposure antiretroviral treatment. The role of the clinician providing care has to be to deliver accurate, thorough, balanced, and unbiased counseling.

An almost embarrassing paucity of safety data addresses the risk of administering antiretrovirals to HIV-uninfected pregnant women; similarly, data about the pharmacology of antiretroviral drugs in this setting is extremely limited. Studies evaluating the efficacy of antiretrovirals in preventing vertical HIV provide useful but not directly comparable information about the use of these drugs in the postexposure setting. A large French study identified fetal neurological/mitochondrial toxicity associated with administration of nucleoside analogues in pregnancy. Two infant deaths and six additional instances of probable mitochondrial toxicity were identified in HIV-uninfected offspring of HIV-infected mothers in this large trial [100]. Both deaths were associated with mitochondrial toxicity that led to progressive neurological disease. Interestingly, no fetal deaths attributable to, or associated with, antiretroviral-induced mitochondrial toxicity have been identified among several large U.S. vertical transmission studies. The differences between the French and U.S. experiences remain unclear.

Concern also has been expressed that the didanosine/stavudine (ddI/d4t) regimen also is associated with increased risk in pregnancy. The FDA published a warning about the use of this regimen in the treatment of HIV-infected pregnant women, noting that several instances of severe pancreatitis and lactic acidosis have occurred in pregnant patients, and that some of these episodes were associated with maternal or fetal death (or both) [101]. There are no reports of complications of this severity associated with administration of this combination as PEP. Nonetheless, based on the experience with this regimen in HIV treatment, CDC has decided to recommend against its use for PEP management for pregnant HCWs sustaining occupational HIV exposures.

"Source Unknown" Exposures

Among the most complicated issues with respect to the administration of postexposure antiretroviral chemoprophylaxis are decisions about treatment when the source-patient and/or material is suspected but not known to contain HIV. Each such episode should be handled individually and should be based on a careful risk assessment, including a determination of (1) the probability of HIV infection in the source-patient, (2) the type of exposure and the associated risk of HIV transmission with such an exposure if HIV was, in fact, likely to have been present, and (3) the risks associated with treatment for the HCW. For many such exposures, the risk for HIV transmission is so small as to be considered entirely negligible. In such settings, the risks associated with administration of the antiretrovirals likely outweigh the risks for infection, and treatment should not be recommended. Only in instances in which the risk assessment suggests that the exposure risk outweighs the risks associated with chemoprophylaxis (always a subjective assessment) should treatment proceed, keeping in mind that, if additional data become available suggesting that the risk is lower than initially perceived, the treatment can be discontinued.

Decisions to Administer Chemoprophylaxis When Reporting Has Been Delayed

Based on the data from relevant animal models described previously, treatment should be initiated as soon as possible after exposure. In a number of animal studies, efficacy is reduced when treatment is delayed for more than 24 hours [77], but the relevance of this observation to low-inoculum transcutaneous and transmucosal occupational HIV exposures is completely speculative. Occupational HIV exposures should be considered medical emergencies. Antiretroviral agents should be administered as soon as the rationale for them is apparent. Institutions should use this measure as an HCW safety performance measure, and this issue should become the focus of ongoing institutional performance improvement activities. When definitively indicated, PEP should be started as soon as practical (i.e., within hours rather than days). As noted, if because of the likelihood of resistance, the HCW is pregnant or if the practitioner encounters other complexities, consider initiating the basic or, perhaps more sensibly, the expanded regimen until consultation can be obtained. In instances in which the risk of transmission is high (e.g., an instance in which a surgeon sustains a scalpel cut when the source-patient is known to have a high viral burden), initiate treatment even after a long delay (e.g., even 1 to 2 weeks after the exposure).

Because no data definitively demonstrate the efficacy of PEP, the optimal duration of chemoprophylaxis can obviously not be known. Animal models have provided highly variable results. At the NIH, a four week regimen is used.

Follow-Up for Occupational HIV Exposures

Individuals sustaining occupational exposures should undergo baseline testing at the time of the exposure to demonstrate that they have not been previously infected with the pathogens being considered as occupational risks. In addition to baseline HIV testing, serological testing for a documented occupational exposure is usually performed six weeks, three months, and six months after exposure [2].

Some exposure characteristics may be associated with increased risks for transmission (e.g., injection of a volume of contaminated blood, simultaneous exposure to HIV and HCV). In such instances, extending the testing period makes implicit sense.

Routine follow-up is crucial to effective postexposure management. All HCWs sustaining occupational exposures should be re-evaluated at 48 hours postexposure to get a clear reading on how they are managing their exposures. This author recommends that individuals be seen weekly

if possible while on PEP to make certain that they are tolerating therapy and that they do not have unanswered questions or unresolved issues.

Most (i.e., >80%) instances of documented HCW seroconversions have been associated with the symptoms typical of the acute retroviral infection (fever, lymphadenopathy, pharyngitis, rash, headache, profound fatigue). For this reason, HCWs sustaining occupational exposures should be counseled to return for evaluation and HIV testing if such symptoms occur. Exposed HCWs should be counseled that these symptoms do not always indicate acute HIV infection. A variety of other circumstances (e.g., reactions to nevirapine or other antiretrovirals or other viral infections can produce virtually identical symptoms).

Providers evaluating HCWs who develop symptoms suggesting acute HIV infection must be aware that HIV antibody tests may be negative or indeterminate during the early phases of the illness. Direct tests for the viral genome, viral load tests (quantitative HIV RNA PCR), or viral cultures may be more valuable in making the initial diagnosis. Whereas these latter tests may be of value in differentiating the acute seroconversion illness from other diagnoses, these tests may produce more uncertainty than help in the routine management of occupational exposures and should not be used routinely in follow-up. Positive tests should be repeated to confirm the result.

As noted, HCWs who elect to take chemoprophylaxis after occupational HIV exposures should return 48 hours after the exposure and then, at a minimum of two weeks after the initial return visit. The clinician should consider seeing these individuals weekly while on treatment to assess them carefully for signs and symptoms of drug toxicity and to make certain that their symptoms are being managed appropriately. The visit should include a careful interim history, a focused physical examination, questioning about signs and symptoms of drug toxicity, inquiry as to whether the individual has unanswered questions about the exposure or the treatment, and the collection of specimens for laboratory tests relevant to the antiretrovirals being administered. As a general rule, all patients should have a complete blood count as well as renal and hepatic function tests. If protease inhibitors are included in the HCW's regimen, specimens should be drawn for random blood glucose and a lipid profile. HCWs electing to take PEP also should be counseled to return for re-evaluation if intractable side effects of therapy occur.

A major goal for the provider is to ensure that the exposed HCW completes the course of chemoprophylaxis. At each visit, information should be provided to the exposed HCW about potential drug interactions, emphasizing the drugs that should not be taken with the prophylactic drug regimen. In addition, the clinician should focus on the side effects being experienced by the exposed HCW and should address how to manage them. In addition to the earlier discussion about the symptoms associated with acute HIV infection, HCWs receiving postexposure antiretroviral chemoprophylaxis also should be informed about symptoms suggestive of serious toxicity (e.g., back or abdominal pain, jaundice, pain on urination, or blood in the urine and symptoms of hyperglycemia such as increased thirst or frequent urination).

The most common reason for having HCWs spontaneously discontinue their chemoprophylaxis relates to the myriad side effects associated with these regimens. Common side effects, including nausea and diarrhea, often can be managed successfully with antiemetic and/or antimotility agents without modifying the chemoprophylaxis regimen. Prescribing these drugs prospectively (i.e., at the time the chemoprophylaxis regimen is initiated) often makes implicit sense. HCWs should be told what to expect in side effects and what to do to manage them. Dealing with these problems prospectively will likely increase adherence with the chemoprophylaxis regimens substantially. In instances in which the side effects are not easily managed by antimotility, analgesics, or antiemetics, modifying the dose interval, dose reduction of the prescribed antiretrovirals, or regimen modification may be necessary to make it possible for the HCW to complete the chemoprophylaxis regimen.

Provider-to-Patient Transmission of Blood Borne Pathogens

In general, the risks for provider-to-patient transmission of each of the important BBPs are substantially smaller than the corresponding risk for patient-to-provider transmission. Individuals chronically infected with any of the most prevalent blood borne viruses—HBV, HCV, or HIV—are extremely unlikely to transmit infection during routine patient contact. Nonetheless, instances in which each of these viruses were transmitted from an infected HCW to one or more of her or his patients are well documented in the literature. Because the risks for needlestick transmission of each of the major pathogens differs substantially, a reasonable hypothesis is that the risks for provider-to-patient transmission also varies substantially from pathogen to pathogen. This substantial variation argues for management of providers on a rational, pathogen-by-pathogen basis or, perhaps even more rationally, based on the provider's circulating viral burden.

Hepatitis B

Despite the fact that chronic HBV carriers may have remarkably high levels of circulating viremia, routine aspects of patient care really pose virtually no risk for provider-to-patient HBV transmission. Providers who routinely conduct what CDC has termed exposure-prone invasive procedures do present some risk to their patients for provider-to-patient spread of this BBP. The risk clearly is associated with the provider's HBV circulating viral burden. Thus, providers who have high circulating levels of HBV viral DNA or those who are hepatitis B "e" antigen positive are associated with the highest (albeit still extremely low) levels of risk for provider-to-patient transmission. In a review of articles published in the mid-1990s, CDC reported that 42 different HBV-infected HCWs (most of whom were hepatitis B "e" antigen positive) had been detected as having infected ≥ 1 patients (with >375 patients in these 42 individuals' practices having acquired infection from their providers) [102]. In many of these instances, investigation revealed that the practitioners involved used minimal or, in some instances, inadequate infection control procedures. Only two provider-to-patient HBV clusters have occurred in instances in which the provider was aware of her or his infection and was paying particular attention to infection control procedures that were intended to decrease the risk for transmission. In the first of these two instances, four patients acquired clinical HBV infection from an orthopedic surgeon [103]. In the second cluster, 19 of a thoracic surgery resident's intraoperative patients became infected [104]. Investigation of both of these clusters failed to identify a route of transmission or problem with technique.

The management of HCWs who are chronic HBV carriers is complex. Historically, with the exception of providers who were shown to transmit infection to their patients, no restrictions were put in place for providers who were HBV carriers. In part in response to a cluster of provider-to-patient transmission of HIV discussed subsequently in more detail, in 1991 CDC issued guidelines recommending that HCWs who perform so-called exposure-prone invasive procedures should personally be aware of their HBV infection statuses. These guidelines recommend that HCWs who learn that they are chronically HBV-infected and are HBV "e"-antigen positive should not perform exposure-prone procedures unless they have sought the counsel of an expert review panel and been advised under what circumstances (if any) they would be allowed to perform these procedures [105]. An HCW who is allowed to perform exposure prone procedures must first inform a prospective patient about the HCW's infection status [105]. The Society for Healthcare Epidemiology of America (SHEA) also issued a set of recommendations addressing the management of providers who are chronic carriers of HBV and other BBPs [106]. The guidelines recommend that providers who are HBV "e"-antigen positive take the additional precaution of routinely double gloving. Furthermore, the guidelines suggest that these providers not conduct procedures that have been epidemiologically associated with a risk for provider-to-patient transmission. SHEA further recommends that HBV-infected HCWs should not volunteer their infection status to patients except in circumstances in which the patient sustained an exposure to the provider's blood or other potentially infectious body fluid [106]. The U.S. Congress subsequently mandated that all states either implement the 1991 CDC guidelines or certify that state guidelines were equivalent to them.

The United Kingdom has taken a more conservative approach to the management of practitioners who are chronic HBV carriers. Revised guidelines issued in 1993 require vaccination of all nonimmune HCWs who perform "exposure prone procedures" and postvaccination testing to document a protective response. The guidelines also clearly delineate practice restrictions for providers who are found to be HBV "e" antigen positive chronic carriers [107].

In 1997, several instances of provider-to-patient transmission of HBV from practitioners who were found to be HBV "e"-antigen negative but who were infected with strains of HBV that are "pre-core mutants" (i.e., strains that are genetically unable to express "e"-antigen but still capable of assembling infectious virions and producing high-viral-burden infection) [108]. Some authorities have proposed using the quantitative measure of circulating HBV-DNA as a basis for restricting the practices of infected providers who perform "exposure-prone procedures" [109,110]. In general, whereas most authorities seemed to have embraced this concept, substantial disagreement still exists about where to set the threshold for restriction; some have recommended that a viral burden as low as 100 copies/ml be used, and others have suggested 1,000, 10,000, or even 100,000 as perhaps more appropriate thresholds. Current USPHS guidelines do not address the issue of viral burden as a determinant for practice restrictions.

Hepatitis C

Provider-to-patient HCV transmission has been an extremely uncommon event except in some unusual circumstances. As noted for all of these BBPs, provider-to-patient HCV transmission is extremely unlikely in the setting of routine (i.e., non-invasive) patient care. The risk for provider-to-patient HCV transmission appears to be even smaller than the risk for HBV in this setting, presumably because most individuals chronically infected with HCV have circulating viral loads that are several factors of 10 lower than those of HBV "e"-antigen positive carriers. Despite the low risk for transmission, several instances of provider-to-patient HCV transmission have been reported in the past few years [111–121]. Although the precise mode of transmission for the overwhelming majority of these patients remains unknown, the circumstances surrounding several suggest that transmission was associated with percutaneous exposures. Interestingly, a number of the instances of provider-to-patient HCV transmission have been associated with HCW injecting drug use. The contribution of injection drug use is well documented in a few of these instances (cf. the epidemic of patients associated with an anesthesiologist in Spain who was addicted to opiates who was using some of patients' narcotics and then injecting the patients with the same syringe that he had used, in the process infecting >200 patients [111]). Detection of underlying injection drug use in this setting is difficult at best, so one cannot say for certain the extent to which this behavior may have influenced the other published reports.

Thus, provider-to-patient HCV transmission has been documented only rarely and in only one published episode in the United States. A second instance of HCV transmission from a U.S. provider to a patient has been reported in the lay press but has been described only obliquely in the medical literature. In this latter report, based on a personal communication, the authors report that a "look-back" study of the patients of a cardiac surgeon who according to lay press accounts had transmitted infection to three patients [122] found that the surgeon "likely transmitted HCV to as many as fourteen of the 937 patients who could be evaluated" [121].

In the absence of injection drug use in the HCW, provider-to-patient HCV transmission appears extremely uncommon in association with highly invasive procedures and associated with HCWs who have high circulating HCV viral burdens. To date, because of the paucity of data documenting the occurrence of provider-to-patient HCV transmission, the USPHS has not issued recommendations suggesting that the practices of HCV-infected HCWs be limited in any way. Conversely, public health authorities in the United Kingdom have recommended practice restrictions for HCV-infected providers, specifically noting that HCV-infected providers who have circulating HCV-RNA may not conduct "exposure-prone invasive procedures"; that trainees found to have circulating HCV-RNA should be restricted from starting training in "exposure-prone invasive procedures"; that HCV infected providers who have circulating HCV-RNA who receive antiviral treatment and become HCV-RNA negative for a period of six months can be permitted to return to performing "exposure-prone invasive procedures" (but must be retested in six months to ensure that they remain HCV-RNA negative) [123]. A European conference convened to construct rational guidelines for infected providers could not reach consensus about restrictions for HCV-infected providers, ultimately concluding that, "on balance, it is not recommended that exposure-prone procedures be forbidden for hepatitis C-infected healthcare workers" [124]. Thus, the information accrued to date does not suggest a need for additional intervention. Ultimately, if transmission is detected with more regularity and an intervention becomes appropriate, creating restrictions based on the HCW's viral burden and transmission history may be appropriate. Deciding where to set the threshold for restriction clearly would be a challenge.

Human Immunodeficiency Virus

Four instances of HIV transmission from an infected HCW to ≥1 of her or his patients have been reported in the literature with a total of nine provider-to-patient infections detected in these four instances of transmission [125–131].

One of the four instances of transmission occurred in the United States [126–128], two occurred in France [125,129], and the fourth occurred in Spain [131]. The episodes in the cluster of six infections that were detected in the United States in 1990 were linked to an HIV-infected dentist in Florida. Although these episodes were investigated thoroughly, the precise mechanism of transmission was never identified. The extraordinarily high transmission rate in the U.S. dentist's practice has never been explained. The two French episodes were reported in 1999 and 2000. The initial French episode involved HIV transmission from an HIV-infected orthopedic surgeon to one of his patients [125,130]. The surgeon was not aware of his infection until AIDS was diagnosed in 1994. The one iatrogenic infection that was detected was identified in a retrospective investigation of the surgeon's patients. As in the U.S. dental office episode, the precise mechanism of transmission could not be determined; however, the patient who had become infected had undergone an extremely lengthy procedure at a time that the surgeon very likely had a very high viral burden. The second French episode is more puzzling. In this instance, transmission was thought to have occurred from an infected nurse to a patient despite the fact that the nurse did not conduct any sort of invasive procedure. As with the other episodes, no route of transmission could be delineated. The nurse also was infected with HCV and at the time of the iatrogenic HIV transmission, had both advanced HIV disease and advanced HCV infection [129]. The fourth instance of transmission occurred in Spain and was reported in a news report in the medical literature in 2003 [131]. The details of this episode have never been described in the literature; however, the news report suggests that the transmission occurred during a caesarian section. None of the 250 other patients who had procedures performed by the obstetrician were found to be infected [131].

Given our 25-year experience with this disease, the paucity of episodes that have been detected underscores the fact that the risk HIV transmission from infected providers to patients is extremely low. Following the detection of the cluster in the Florida dentist's practice, the U.S. Public Health Service issued guidelines for providers infected with BBPs [105]. Those guidelines concluded that HCWs who are infected with HIV or HBV and are "e" antigen positive should not perform "exposure-prone procedures" unless they have sought the counsel of an expert review panel and have been advised under what circumstances, if any, they may continue to perform these procedures. The document also noted that the circumstances under which infected practitioners were permitted to continue performing exposure-prone procedures would include prospectively notifying patients of the practitioner's infection status before the procedure. After the guidelines were published, the U.S. Congress passed a statute (P.L. 102–141) mandating that all states adopt the CDC (or equivalent) guidelines. Subsequently, the CDC director at that time wrote a letter to all state health departments, emphasizing that the states, not the CDC, would certify the equivalency of the individual state's guidelines. He also concluded that, in his view, exposure-prone procedures would best be determined on a case-by-case basis, taking into consideration the specific procedure and the skill, technique, and possible impairment of the infected HCW. Many states created their own guidelines and certified them as equivalent. Thus, as a result, substantial variability exists in state guidelines. Whereas the U.S. guidelines are state based, the U.K. guidelines state that HIV-infected providers may not conduct exposure-prone invasive procedures [132].

Curiously, none of the U.S. guidelines take intos consideration that fact that the risk for provider-to-patient transmission of each of these BBPs almost certainly is associated with the provider's viral burden. In an era in which many HIV-infected patients have their circulating viral burden suppressed below detectable levels, in which a substantial fraction of patients who have chronic HCV infection can be either cured or have their infections substantially suppressed, and that includes promising new therapies for chronic HBV infection, this important factor should certainly be considered in the recommendations for managing infected providers. Whereas the United Kingdom, the European consortium, and the Netherlands all have included viral burden in assessing risks associated with HBV-infected providers, no one has attempted to do this with HCV or HIV. The 1991 USPHS guidelines clearly need updating. Until these guidelines are brought to currency, this author i recommends basing practice restrictions on evidence suggesting (1) that an infected HCW is impaired, (2) that the HCW does not adhere to accepted infection-control procedures, (3) that a documented risk for transmission has been established for the pathogen and procedure under consideration, or (4) that BBP transmission to a patient has occurred or is suspected to have occurred (modified from reference [106]).

REFERENCES

1. Leibowitz S, Greenwald L, Cohen I, et al. Serum hepatitis in a blood bank worker. *JAMA* 1949;140:1331–1333.
2. Panlilio AL, Cardo DM, Grohskopf LA, et al. Updated U.S. Public Health Service guidelines for the management of occupational exposures to HIV and recommendations for postexposure prophylaxis. *MMWR Recomm Rep* 2005 30;54(RR-9):1–17.
3. Hadler SC. Hepatitis B virus infection and health care workers. *Vaccine* 1990;8:S24–S28.
4. Pattison CP, Maynard JE, Berquist KR, Webster HM. Epidemiology of hepatitis B in hospital personnel. *Am J Epidemiol* 1975;101:59–64.
5. Williams SV, Huff JC, Feinglass EJ, et al. Epidemic viral hepatitis, type B, in hospital personnel. *Am J Med* 1974;57:904–911.
6. Denes AE, Smith JL, Maynard JE, et al. Hepatitis B infection in physicians: results of a nationwide seroepidemiologic survey. *JAMA* 1978;239(3):210–212.
7. Dienstag JL, Ryan DM. Occupational exposure to hepatitis B virus in hospital personnel: Infection or immunization. *Am J Epidemiol* 1982;115:26–39.
8. Snydman DR, Muñoz A, Werner BG, et al. A multivariate analysis of risk factors for hepatitis B virus infection among hospital employees screened for vaccination. *Am J Epidemiol* 1984;120:684–693.

9. Hadler SC, Doto IL, Maynard JE, et al. Occupational risk of hepatitis B infection in hospital workers. *Infection Control* 1985;6:24–31.

10. West DJ. The risk of hepatitis B infection among health professionals in the United States: a review. *Am J Med Sci* 1984;287(2):26–33.

11. Centers for Disease Control. Protection against viral hepatitis: recommendations of the Immunization Practices Advisory Committee (ACIP). *MMWR.* 1990;39:1–26.

12. Francis DP, Maynard JE. The transmission and outcome of hepatitis A, B, and non-A, non-B: a review. *Epidemiol Rev* 1979;1:17–31.

13. Thomas DL, Factor SH, Kelen GD, et al. Viral hepatitis in health care personnel at The Johns Hopkins Hospital: the seroprevalence of, and risk factors for, hepatitis B virus and hepatitis C virus infection. *Arch Intern Med* 1993;153(14):1705–1712.

14. Panlilio AL, Shapiro CN, Schable CA, et al. Serosurvey of human immunodeficiency virus, hepatitis B virus, and hepatitis C virus infection among hospital-based surgeons. *J Am Coll Surg* 1995;180(1):16–24.

15. Choo QL, Kuo G, Weiner AJ, et al. Isolation of a cDNA clone derived from a blood-borne non-A, non-B viral hepatitis genome. *Science* 1989;244(4902):359–362.

16. Henderson DK. Managing occupational risks for hepatitis C transmission in the health care setting. *Clin Microbiol Rev* 2003;16(3):546–568.

17. Puro V, Petrosillo N, Ippolito G, et al. Occupational hepatitis C virus infection in Italian health care workers. *Am J Public Health* 1995;85:1272–1275.

18. Shapiro C, Tokars J, Chamberland M, The American Academy of Orthopaedic Surgeons Serosurvey Study Committee. Use of the hepatitis-B vaccine and infection with hepatitis B and C among orthopaedic surgeons. *J Bone Joint Surg Am* 1996; 78-A:1791–1800.

19. Jadoul M, Akrout M, Cornu C, van Ypersele de Strihou C. Prevalence of hepatitis C antibodies in health-care workers. *Lancet* 1994;344:339.

20. Klein RS, Freeman K, Taylor PE, Stevens CE. Occupational risk for hepatitis C virus infection among New York City dentists. *Lancet* 1991;338:1539–1542.

21. Polish L, Tong M, Co R, et al. Risk factors for hepatitis C virus infection among health care personnel in a community hospital. *Am J Infect Control* 1993;21:196–200.

22. Campello C, Majori S, Poli A, et al. Prevalence of HCV antibodies in health-care workers from norhern Italy. *Infection* 1992;20:224–226.

23. Takaki A, Wiese M, Maertens G, et al. Cellular immune responses persist and humoral responses decrease two decades after recovery from a single-source outbreak of hepatitis C *Nat Med* 2000;6(5):578–582.

24. Lettau LA, Alfred HJ, Glew RII, et al. Nosocomial transmission of delta hepatitis. *Ann Intern Med* 1986;104:631–635.

25. Marinucci G, Valeri L, Di Giacomo C, Morganti D. Spread of delta in a group of haemodialysis carriers of HBsAg. In: Verme G, Bonino F, Rizzetto M, ed. *Viral hepatitis and delta infection.* New York: Alan R. Liss, 1983:151–154.

26. Do AN, Ciesielski CA, Metler RP, et al. Occupationally acquired human immunodeficiency virus (HIV) infection: national case surveillance data during 20 years of the HIV epidemic in the United States. *Infect Control Hosp Epidemiol* 2003;24(2):86–96.

27. Beekmann SE, Fahey BJ, Gerberding JL, Henderson DK. Risky business: using necessarily imprecise casualty counts to estimate occupational risks for HIV-1 infection. *Infect Control Hosp Epidemiol* 1990;11(7):371–379.

28. Werner BJ, Grady GF. Accidental hepatitis-B-surface- antigen-positive inoculations: use of "e" antigen to estimate infectivity. *Ann Intern Med* 1982;97:367–369.

29. Henderson DK, Gerberding JL. Healthcare worker issues, including occupational and nonoccupational postexposure management. In: Dolin RM, and Saag MS, eds. *AIDS Therapy.* 2nd ed. New York: Churchill Livingstone, 2002:327–346.

30. Ippolito G, Puro V, Heptonstall J, et al. Occupational human immunodeficiency virus infection in health care workers: worldwide cases through September 1997. *Clin Infect Dis* 1999;28(2):365–383.

31. Gioananni P, Sinicco A, Cariti G, et al. HIV infection acquired by a nurse. *Eur J Epidemiol* 1988;4:119–120.

32. Bennett NT, Howard RJ. Quantity of blood inoculated in a needlestick injury from suture needles. *J Am Coll Surg* 1994;178(2):107–110.

33. Mast E, Alter M, Holland P, Purcell R. Evaluation of assays for antibody to hepatitis E virus by a serum panel. *Hepatology* 1998;27:857–861.

34. Cardo DM, Culver DH, Ciesielski CA, et al. A case-control study of HIV seroconversion in health care workers after percutaneous exposure. *N Engl J Med* 1997;337(21):1485–1490.

35. Rowland-Jones S, Sutton J, Ariyoshi K, et al. HIV-specific cytotoxic T-cells in HIV-exposed but uninfected Gambian women. *Nat Med* 1995;1(1):59–64.

36. Rowland-Jones S, Dong T, Krausa P, et al. The role of cytotoxic T-cells in HIV infection. *Dev Biol Stand* 1998;92:209–214.

37. Cheynier R, Langlade-Demoyen P, Marescot MR, et al. Cytotoxic T lymphocyte responses in the peripheral blood of children born to human immunodeficiency virus-1-infected mothers. *Eur J Immunol* 1992;22(9):2211–2217.

38. Clerici M, Giorgi JV, Chou CC, et al. Cell-mediated immune response to human immunodeficiency virus (HIV) type 1 in seronegative homosexual men with recent sexual exposure to HIV-1. *J Infect Dis.* 1992;165(6):1012–1019.

39. Clerici M, Levin JM, Kessler HA, et al. HIV-specific T-helper activity in seronegative health care workers exposed to contaminated blood. *JAMA* 1994;271(1):42–46.

40. Kelker IIC, Seidlin M, Vogler M, Valentine FT. Lymphocytes from some long-term seronegative heterosexual partners of HIV-infected individuals proliferate in response to HIV antigens *AIDS Res Hum Retroviruses* 1992;8(8):1355–1359.

41. Mazzoli S, Trabattoni D, Lo Caputo S, et al. HIV-specific mucosal and cellular immunity in HIV-seronegative partners of HIV-seropositive individuals. *Nat Med* 1997;3(11):1250–1257.

42. Pinto LA, Landay AL, Berzofsky JA, et al. Immune response to human immunodeficiency virus (HIV) in healthcare workers occupationally exposed to HIV-contaminated blood. *Am J Med* 1997;102(5B):21–24.

43. Pinto LA, Sullivan J, Berzofsky JA, et al. ENV specific cytotoxic T lymphocyte responses in HIV seronegative health care workers occupationally exposed to HIV-contaminated body fluids. *J Clin Invest* 1995;96(2):867–876.

44. Ranki A, Mattinen S, Yarchoan R, et al. T-cell response towards HIV in infected individuals with and without zidovudine therapy, and in HIV-exposed sexual partners. *AIDS* 1989;3(2): 63–69.

45. Centers for Disease Control. Recommendations for prevention of HIV transmission in health-care settings. *MMWR Morb Mortal Wkly Rep* 1987;36 (Suppl 2):1S–18S.

46. Bangsberg D, Goldschmidt RH. Postexposure prophylaxis for occupational exposure to HIV. *JAMA* 1999;282(17):1623–1624.

47. Department of Labor OSHA. Occupational exposure to bloodborne pathogens; final rule. *Federal Register* 1991;56:64175–182.

48. Gerberding JL, Henderson DK. Design of rational infection control policies for human immunodeficiency virus infection. *J Infect Dis* 1987;156:861–864.

49. Hadler SC, Margolis HS. Hepatitis B immunization: vaccine types, efficacy, and indications for immunization. *Curr Clin Top Infect Dis* 1992;12:282–308.

50. Bulkow L, Wainwright R, McMahon B, Parkinson A. Increases in levels of antibody to hepatitis B surface antigen in an immunized population. *Clin Infect Dis* 1998;26:933–937.

51. Mahoney FJ, Stewart K, Hu H, et al. Progress toward the elimination of hepatitis B virus transmission among health care workers in the United States. *Arch Intern Med* 1997;147:2601–2605.

52. Wainwright RB, Bulkow LR, Parkinson AJ, et al. Protection provided by hepatitis B vaccine in a Yupik Eskimo population—results of a 10-year study. *J Infect Dis* 1997;175(3):674–677.

53. Centers for Disease Control and Prevention. Updated U.S. Public Health Service Guidelines for the Management of Occupational Exposures to HBV, HCV, and HIV and Recommendations for Postexposure Prophylaxis. *MMWR Morb Mortal Wkly Rep* 2001;50(RR-11):1–52.

54. Schiff E, de Medina M, Hill M, Johnson G. Prevalence of anti-HCV in the VA dental environment form 1979–1981. *Hepatology* 1990;12:849. [Abstract].

55. Knodell RG, Conrad ME, Ginsberg AL, Bell CJ. Efficacy of prophylactic gamma-globulin in preventing non-A, non-B post-transfusion hepatitis. *Lancet* 1976;1:557–561.

56. Sanchez-Quijano A, Pineda JA, Lissen E, et al. Prevention of post-transfusion non-A, non-B hepatitis by non-specific immunoglobulin in heart surgery patients. *Lancet* 1988;1:1245–1249.

57. Seeff LB, Zimmerman HJ, Wright EC, et al. A randomized, double blind controlled trial of the efficacy of immune serum globulin for the prevention of post-transfusion hepatitis. *Gastroenterology* 1977;72:111–121.

58. Schiff ER. Hepatitis C among health care providers: risk factors and possible prophylaxis. *Hepatology* 1992;16:1300–1301.

59. Alberti A, Boccato S, Vario A, Benvegnu L. Therapy of acute hepatitis C. *Hepatology*. 2002;36(5 suppl):S195–S200.

60. Calleri G, Colombatto P, Gozzelino M, et al. Natural beta interferon in acute type-C hepatitis patients: a randomized controlled trial. *Ital J Gastroenterol Hepatol* 1998;30(2):181–184.

61. Hoey J, Wooltorton E. Early treatment of acute hepatitis C infection may lead to cure. *CMAJ* 2001;165(11):1527.

62. Jaeckel E, Cornberg M, Wedemeyer H, et al. Treatment of acute hepatitis C with interferon alfa-2b. *N Engl J Med* 2001;345(20):1452–1457.

63. Jaeckel E, Manns MP. The course and therapy of acute hepatitis C viral infection: is a prevention of its becoming chronic possible? *Z Gastroenterol* 2000;38(5):387–395.

64. Vogel W. Treatment of acute hepatitis C virus infection. *J Hepatol* 1999;31(suppl 1):189–192.

65. Morand P, Dutertre N, Minazzi H, et al. Lack of seroconversion in a health care worker after polymerase chain reaction-documented acute hepatitis C resulting from a needlestick injury. *Clin Infect Dis* 2001;33(5):727–729.

66. Larghi A, Zuin M, Crosignani A, et al. Outcome of an outbreak of acute hepatitis C among healthy volunteers participating in pharmacokinetics studies, Part 1. *Hepatology* 2002;36(4):993–1000.

67. Seeff LB, Hollinger FB, Alter HJ, et al. Long-term mortality and morbidity of transfusion-associated non-A, non-B, and type C hepatitis: a National Heart, Lung, and Blood Institute collaborative study. *Hepatology* 2001;33(2):455–463.

68. Alvarado-Ramy F, Alter MJ, Bower W, et al. Management of occupational exposures to hepatitis C virus: current practice and controversies. *Infect Control Hosp Epidemiol* 2001;22(1):53–55.

69. Centers for Disease Control. Public Health Service statement on management of occupational exposure to human immunodeficiency virus, including considerations regarding zidovudine postexposure use. *MMWR Morbid Mortal Wkly Rep* 1990;39(RR-1):1–14.

70. Mitsuya H, Jarrett RF, Matsukura M, et al. Long-term inhibition of human T-lymphotropic virus type III/lymphadenopathy-associated virus (human immunodeficiency virus) DNA synthesis and RNA expression in T cells protected by 2'3'dideoxynucleosides *in vitro*. *Proc Natl Acad Sci* 1987;84:2033–2037.

71. Blauvelt A, Glushakova S, Margolis LB. HIV-infected human Langerhans cells transmit infection to human lymphoid tissue *ex vivo*. *AIDS* 2000;14(6):647–651.

72. Spira AI, Marx PA, Patterson BK, et al. Cellular targets of infection and route of viral dissemination after an intravaginal inoculation of simian immunodeficiency virus into rhesus macaques. *J Exp Med* 1996;183(1):215–225.

73. Katzenstein TL, Dickmeiss E, Aladdin H, et al. Failure to develop HIV infection after receipt of HIV-contaminated blood and postexposure prophylaxis. *Ann Intern Med* 2000;133(1):31–34.

74. Puro V, Calcagno G, Anselmo M, et al. Transient detection of plasma HIV-1 RNA during postexposure prophylaxis. *Infect Control Hosp Epidemiol* 2000;21(8):529–531.

75. Putkonen P, Makitalo B, Bottiger D, et al. Protection of human immunodeficiency virus type 2-exposed seronegative macaques from mucosal simian immunodeficiency virus transmission. *J Virol* 1997;71(7):4981–4984.

76. Ruprecht RM, Bronson R. Chemoprevention of retroviral infection: success is determined by virus inoculum strength and cellular immunity. *DNA Cell Biol* 1994;13(1):59–66.

77. Tsai CC, Emau P, Follis KE, et al. Effectiveness of postinoculation (R)-9-(2-phosphonylmethoxypropyl) adenine treatment for prevention of persistent simian immunodeficiency virus SIVmne infection depends critically on timing of initiation and duration of treatment. *J Virol* 1998;72(5):4265–4273.

78. Tsai CC, Follis KE, Beck TW, et al. Effects of (R)-9-(2-phosphonylmethoxypropyl) adenine monotherapy on chronic SIV infection in macaques. *AIDS Res Hum Retroviruses* 1997;13(8):707–712.

79. Blanche S, et al. Zidovudine-lamivudine for prevention of mother to child HIV-1 Transmission. 6th Annual Conference on Retroviruses and Opportunistic Infections 1999 Chicago, IL. 1999: Abstract 267.

80. Connor EM, Mofenson LM. Zidovudine for the reduction of perinatal human immunodeficiency virus transmission: pediatric AIDS Clinical Trials Group Protocol 076—results and treatment recommendations. *Pediatr Infect Dis J* 1995;14(6):536–541.

81. Connor EM, Sperling RS, Gelber R, et al. Reduction of maternal-infant transmission of human immunodeficiency virus type 1 with zidovudine treatment. *N Engl J Med* 1994;331(18):1173–1180.

82. Bulterys M, Orloff S, Abrams E, et al. Impact of zidovudine postperinatal exposure prophylaxis on vertical HIV-1 transmission: a prospective cohort study in four US cities. Global strategies for the prevention of HIV Transmission from Mothers to Infants, September 1–6 1999; Toronto, Ontario. Abstract 15.

83. Wade NA, Birkhead GS, Warren BL, et al. Abbreviated regimens of zidovudine prophylaxis and perinatal transmission of the human immunodeficiency virus. *N Engl J Med* 1998;339(20):1409–1414.

84. Centers for Disease Control and Prevention. Case-control study of HIV seroconversion in health-care workers after percutaneous exposure to HIV-infected blood—France, United Kingdom, and United States, January 1988–August 1994. *MMWR Morb Mortal Wkly Rep* 1995;44(50):929–933.

85. Henderson DK, Gerberding JL. Prophylactic zidovudine after occupational exposure to the human immunodeficiency virus: an interim analysis. *J Infect Dis* 1989;160(2):321–327.

86. Lee LM, Henderson DK. Tolerability of postexposure antiretroviral prophylaxis for occupational exposures to HIV. *Drug Saf* 2001;24(8):587–597.

87. Wang SA, Panlilio AL, Doi PA, et al. Experience of healthcare workers taking postexposure prophylaxis after occupational HIV exposures: findings of the HIV Postexposure Prophylaxis Registry. *Infect Control Hosp Epidemiol* 2000;21(12):780–785.

88. Luzzati R, Crosato IM, Mascioli M, et al. Galactorrhoea and hyperprolactinemia associated with HIV postexposure chemoprophylaxis. *AIDS* 2002;16(9):1306–1307.

89. Trape M, Barnosky S. Nelfinavir in expanded postexposure prophylaxis causing acute hepatitis with cholestatic features: two case reports. *Infect Control Hosp Epidemiol* 2001;22(6):333–334.

90. Spenatto N, Viraben R. Early lipodystrophy occurring during post-exposure prophylaxis. *Sex Transm Infect* 1998;74(6):455.

91. Centers for Disease Control and Prevention. Serious adverse events attributed to nevirapine regimens for postexposure prophylaxis after HIV exposures—worldwide, 1997–2000. *MMWR Morb Mortal Wkly Rep* 2001;49(51):1153–1156.

92. Johnson S, Chan J, Bennett CL. Hepatotoxicity after prophylaxis with a nevirapine-containing antiretroviral regimen. *Ann Intern Med* 2002;137(2):146–147.

93. Sha BE, Proia LA, Kessler HA. Adverse effects associated with use of nevirapine in HIV postexposure prophylaxis for 2 health care workers. *JAMA* 2000;284(21):2723.

94. Hawkins DA, Asboe D, Barlow K, Evans B. Seroconversion to HIV-1 following a needlestick injury despite combination postexposure prophylaxis. *J Infect* 2001;43(1):12–15.

95. Perdue B, Wolderufael D, Mellors J, Quinn T, J. M. HIV-1 transmission by a needle-stick injury despite rapid initiation of four-drug postexposure prophylaxis. 6th Conference on Retroviruses and Opportunistic Infections; 1999 January 31-February 4, 1999; Chicago, IL; 1999. p. Abstract 210:107.

96. Jochimsen EM, Luo CC, Beltrami JF, et al. Investigations of possible failures of postexposure prophylaxis following occupational exposures to human immunodeficiency virus. *Arch Intern Med* 1999;159(19):2361–2363.

97. Lucey D, Milum S, Lindquist C, et al. Pseudofailure of zidovudine prophylaxis after a human immunodeficiency virus-positive needlestick. *J Infect Dis* 1990;162(5):1211–1212.

98. Dybul M, Fauci AS, Bartlett JG, et al. Guidelines for using antiretroviral agents among HIV-infected adults and adolescents, part 2. *Ann Intern Med* 2002;137(5):381–433.

99. Dybul M, Fauci AS, Bartlett JG, et al. Guidelines for using antiretroviral agents among HIV-infected adults and adolescents: recommendations of the Panel on Clinical Practices for Treatment of HIV. *MMWR Recomm Rep* 2002;51(RR-7): 1–55.

100. Blanche S, Tardieu M, Rustin P, et al. Persistent mitochondrial dysfunction and perinatal exposure to antiretroviral nucleoside analogues. *Lancet* 1999;354(9184):1084–1089.

101. Smyth AC. Important drug warning (www.fda.gov/medwatch/safety/2001/pregwarnfinalbms.pdf, www.fda.gov/medwatch/safety/2001/safety01.htm#zerit, www.fda.gov/bbs/topics/ANSWERS/ANS01063.html) accessed 26 June 2006.

102. Bell D, Shapiro CN, Chamberland ME, CA. C. Preventing bloodborne pathogen transmission from health-care workers to patients: the CDC perspective. *Surg Clin North Amer* 1995;75:1189–1203.

103. Johnston B, Langille D, LeBlanc J, et al. Transmission of hepatitis B related to orthopedic surgery. *Infect Control Hosp Epidemiol* 1994;15:352 (abstract).

104. Harpaz R, Von Seidlein L, Averhoff FM, et al. Transmission of hepatitis B virus to multiple patients from a surgeon without evidence of inadequate infection control. *N Engl J Med* 1996;334(9):549–554.

105. Centers for Disease Control. Recommendations for preventing transmission of human immunodeficiency virus and hepatitis B virus to patients during exposure-prone invasive procedures. *MMWR Morb Mortal Wkly Rep* 1991;40(RR-8):1–9.

106. AIDS/Tuberculosis Subcommittee of the Society for Healthcare Epidemiology of America. Management of healthcare workers infected with hepatitis B virus, hepatitis C virus, human immunodeficiency virus, or other bloodborne pathogens. *Infect Control Hosp Epidemiol* 1997;18(5):349–363.

107. U.K. Department of Health, U.K. Advisory Group on Hepatitis. *Protecting health care workers and patients from hepatitis B.* Heywood Lancashire, England: U.K. Department of Health, 1993.

108. The Incident Investigation Teams and Others. Transmission of hepatitis B to patients from four infected surgeons without hepatitis B e antigen. *N Engl J Med* 1997;336:178–184.

109. Noone P, Symington I, Carman W. Hepatitis B and health-care workers. *Lancet* 1997;350:219.

110. Poole C. Hepatitis B and health-care workers. *Lancet* 1997;350: 218.

111. Bosch X. Hepatitis C outbreak astounds Spain. *Lancet* 1998;351: 1415.

112. Brown P. Surgeon infects patient with hepatitis C. *BMJ* 1999;319(7219):1219.

113. Cody SH, Nainan OV, Garfein RS, et al. Hepatitis C virus transmission from an anesthesiologist to a patient. *Arch Intern Med* 2002;162(3):345–350.

114. Duckworth GJ, Heptonstall J, Aitken C. Transmission of hepatitis C virus from a surgeon to a patient. *Commun Dis Public Health* 1999;2(3):188–192.

115. Esteban JI, Gomez J, Martell M, et al. Transmission of hepatitis C virus by a cardiac surgeon. *N Engl J Med* 1996;334(9):555–560.

116. Public Health Laboratory Service. Hepatitis C transmission from health care worker to patient. *PHLS Communicable Disease Report* 1995;5(26):121.

117. Public Health Laboratory Service. Transmission of hepatitis C virus from surgeon to patient prompts lookback. *Commun Dis Rep CDR Wkly* 1999;9(44):387.

118. Public Health Laboratory Service. Hepatitis C lookback exercise. *Commun Dis Rep CDR Wkly* 2000;10(23):203–206.

119. Ross RS, Viazov S, Roggendorf M. Phylogenetic analysis indicates transmission of hepatitis C virus from an infected orthopedic surgeon to a patient. *J Med Virol* 2002;66(4):461–467.

120. Ross RS, Viazov S, Thormahlen M, et al. Risk of hepatitis C virus transmission from an infected gynecologist to patients: results of a 7-year retrospective investigation. *Arch Intern Med* 2002;162(7):805–810.

121. Williams IT, Perz JF, Bell BP. Viral hepatitis transmission in ambulatory health care settings. *Clin Infect Dis* 2004;38(11):1592–1598.

122. Rabin R. Officials: surgeon likely infected at least 3 patients. *Newsday* 2000 March 27.

123. Department of Health. *HIV infected health care workers.* London: U.K. Department of Health 2002; 28876.

124. Gunson RN, Shouval D, Roggendorf M, et al. Hepatitis B virus (HBV) and hepatitis C virus (HCV) infections in health care workers (HCWs): guidelines for prevention of transmission of HBV and HCV from HCW to patients. *J Clin Virol* 2003;27(3):213–230.

125. Blanchard A, Ferris S, Chamaret S, et al. Molecular evidence for nosocomial transmission of human immunodeficiency virus from a surgeon to one of his patients. *J Virol* 1998;72(5):4537–4540.

126. Centers for Disease Control. Possible transmission of human immunodeficiency virus to a patient during an invasive dental procedure. *MMWR Morb Mortal Wkly Rep* 1990;39(29):489–493.

127. Centers for Disease Control. Update: transmission of HIV infection during an invasive dental procedure—Florida. *MMWR Morb Mortal Wkly Rep* 1991;40(2):21–33.

128. Cieslelski C, Marianos D, Ou C-Y, et al. Transmission of human immunodeficiency virus in a dental practice. *Ann Intern Med* 1992;116(10):798–805.

129. Goujon CP, Schneider VM, Grofti J, et al. Phylogenetic analyses indicate an atypical nurse-to-patient transmission of human immunodeficiency virus type 1. *J Virol* 2000;74(6):2525–2532.

130. Lot F, Seguier JC, Fegueux S, et al. Probable transmission of HIV from an orthopedic surgeon to a patient in France. *Ann Intern Med* 1999;130(1):1–6.

131. Bosch X. Second case of doctor-to-patient HIV transmission. *Lancet Infect Dis* 2003;3(5):261.

132. Department of Health. *HIV infected health care workers: guidance on management and patient notification.* London, England: U.K. Department of Health; 2005 (269675).

Healthcare-Associated Fungal Infections*

43

Douglas C. Chang, David B. Blossom, and Scott K. Fridkin

INTRODUCTION

Over the past several decades, advances in medical and surgical therapy have changed the type of patients cared for in today's healthcare facilities. In addition, advances in immunosuppressive agents, treatments for malignancy, chemotherapeutic agents, and bone marrow, stem cell and solid organ transplantation have resulted in many immunocompromised individuals. Also, care provided in specialized units, including parenteral nutrition, broad-spectrum antimicrobials, and mechanical ventilation, have helped treat patients suffering from previously devastating diseases and provided life to neonates previously thought to be nonviable. These successes have resulted in more severely ill, immunocompromised patients who are highly susceptible to infections caused by fungi previously considered to be of low virulence or "nonpathogenic."

Fungal infections among these patients often are severe and difficult to diagnose and treat. Fungi are eukaryotic and more complex than bacteria; an appreciation of the unique features of nosocomial fungal infections is needed among clinicians, epidemiologists, and infection control personnel (ICPs) to best implement measures to prevent these infections. This chapter reviews the epidemiology of healthcare-associated infections (HAIs) caused by fungi, including surveillance, prevention, control, advances in diagnostics, antifungal susceptibility testing, and fungal typing.

MOLD

Invasive Aspergillosis

Clinical Disease and Diagnosis of Invasive Aspergillosis

In the immunocompetent person, *Aspergillus* spp. can cause localized infection of the lungs or sinuses. In the immunocompromised patient, however, these pathogens often cause invasive disease of the lungs or sinuses and, because of their tendency to invade blood vessels, often spread to distant organs (Table 43-1). Clinical manifestations depend somewhat on the susceptibility of the host population under evaluation. In addition, *Aspergillus* spp. outbreaks have involved infections of not only the upper and lower respiratory tracts (the usual portals of entry) but also the skin and postoperative sites including vascular prostheses. From an infection control standpoint, the recognition of clinically significant cultures of mold is the cornerstone of an effective strategy to detect and prevent nosocomial invasive mold infections including aspergillosis.

Diagnosis usually is suggested by compatible but nonspecific symptoms and signs in highly susceptible hosts (e.g., those with severe or prolonged neutropenia, those taking immunosuppressive medications including solid-organ transplant recipients, and those with graft versus host disease [GVHD]). Imaging studies often are essential to establishing a diagnosis. However, plain chest radiographs are nonspecific because findings compatible with

*The use of product names in this manuscript does not imply their endorsement by the U.S. Department of Health and Human Services. The findings and conclusions in this report are those of the author(s) and do not necessarily represent the views of the Centers for Disease Control and Prevention.

TABLE 43-1

FREQUENT SITES OF INFECTIONS AND COMMON PATHOGENS FOR HEALTHCARE-ASSOCIATED INVASIVE FUNGAL INFECTIONS

Site of Infection	Fungal Pathogens
Bloodstream (CVC-related)	Candida species
	Rhodotorula species
	Trichosporon asahii
	Trichosporon mucoides
Bloodstream (regardless of CVC)	Aspergillus terreus
	Acremonium species
	Candida species
	Fusarium species
	Scedosporium species
Central nervous system	Aspergillus fumigatus
	Scedosporium species
Eye	Acremonium species
	Aspergillus species (A. fumigatus, A. nidulans, A. ustus, A. versicolor)
	Candida species
	Fusarium species
	Scedosporium species
	Zygomycetes (Rhizopus, Rhizomucor, Absidia)
Gastrointestinal tract	Candida species
Lungs	Aspergillus species (A. fumigatus, A. nidulans, A. niger, A. versicolor)
	Zygomycetes (Rhizopus, Rhizomucor, Absidia)
	Scedosporium species
Skin/soft tissue	Acremonium species
	Aspergillus species (A. fumigatus, A. nidulans, A. ustus, A. versicolor)
	Fusarium species
	Scedosporium species
	Zygomycetes (Rhizopus, Rhizomucor, Absidia)
Sinuses	Aspergillus species (A. flavus, A. fumigatus)
	Zygomycetes (Rhizopus, Rhizomucor, Absidia)

CVC, central venous catheter.

aspergillosis overlap with other etiologies. Chest computerized tomography (CT) scan is more helpful; compatible findings by CT scan usually precede those of plain films and specific findings such as the halo sign [1] and air-crescent sign are more specific for *Aspergillus* spp. infection than findings on plain films [2]. In contrast, sinus, sputum, and even bronchoalveolar lavage (BAL) fluid cultures occasionally yield *Aspergillus* spp., but this often reflects colonization rather than infection [3]. Among patients who are bone marrow transplant recipients and those who are neutropenic, the positive predictive value of these cultures can be 75–80% [4] but is likely much less among immunocompetent patients. Positron emission tomography (PET)

can prove useful for the diagnosis and staging of invasive fungal infections but currently remains a research tool [5].

For any given patient, a respiratory culture growing an *Aspergillus* spp. can represent true disease or colonization. From a clinical standpoint, this culture needs to be evaluated in the context of the clinical signs and symptoms and supporting diagnostic evidence for invasive disease. Ultimately, the clinical diagnosis can be confirmed only by histopathologic evidence or recovery from an involved organ. Additional challenges exist from an infection control standpoint, however; the culture also could need to be evaluated in the context of possible nosocomial acquisition regardless of whether the patient is colonized or infected.

The nonspecific presentation of invasive mold infections has spurred interest in new laboratory methods for diagnosing these infections. Briefly, several categories of nonculture based tests could be useful to the clinician in diagnosing invasive mold infections, especially aspergillosis [6]. Measurement of (1,3)-beta-D (β-D) glucan in blood can be useful as a preliminary screening tool for invasive aspergillosis despite the fact that this antigen can be detected with a number of other fungi. The Food and Drug Administration (FDA) approved a commercially available test for this antigen, Fungitell™ (Associates of Cape Cod, Inc., East Falmouth, Masachusetts), for invasive fungal infections in 2004. Fungitell™ appears to be promising for detecting most medically important fungi including *Aspergillus* and *Candida* spp., but the test does not detect Zygomycetes and has limited detection of *Cryptococcus* spp. due to the absence or low levels of (1,3)-β-D-glucan in these fungi. In addition, research on the detection of *Aspergillus* DNA through polymerase chain reaction (PCR) techniques is ongoing but these techniques are currently limited to research settings.

Techniques to detect circulating galactomannan, an antigen expressed by *Aspergillus* spp., in serum using a commercial enzyme immunoassay (Platelia Aspergillus EIA, Bio-Rad Laboratories, Redmond, Washington) could be more frequently encountered. This serum test was FDA-approved for use in the United States for invasive aspergillosis in 2003 but is being used more extensively in Europe. This test and the (1,3)-β-D glucan assay could provide laboratory evidence needed by clinicians to determine whether to treat a patient for invasive aspergillosis, and the European Organization for Research and Treatment of Cancer/National Institute of Allergy and Infectious Diseases Mycoses Study Group (EORTC/MSG) will likely incorporate it in the next revision of the diagnostic criteria for invasive aspergillosis [7].

Despite the fact that the galactomannan assay is validated only for serum samples, specimens of other body fluids including urine, BAL, and cerebrospinal fluid, are increasingly used to detect galactomannan. Although the test often is positive (at times more often than routine culture), its use in nonserum samples is discouraged [8]. Moreover, until more experience with these types of tests is gained, the use of nonculture-based diagnostics as part of the infection control assessment should be avoided. Likewise, by themselves, these test results should not constitute sufficient evidence of invasive disease for surveillance purposes.

Risk Factors for Invasive Aspergillosis

Invasive mold infections, including invasive aspergillosis, usually occur in immunosuppressed persons. The groups at greatest risk remain those undergoing hematopoeitic stem cell transplant (HSCT) and those receiving cytotoxic chemotherapy.

Allogeneic HSCT recipients are at high risk for invasive aspergillosis because of disruption of mucosal barriers, delayed engraftment, GVHD, and the use of steroids and broad-spectrum antibacterial agents [9–12]. During the early period after transplant, neutropenia due to the conditioning regimen is the major risk factor for fungal infection whereas immunosuppressive therapy for GVHD is the major risk factor during the postengraftment period [13]. Solid organ transplant recipients are other patients at risk for invasive aspergillosis. The percent of solid organ transplant recipients developing invasive aspergillosis is highest among lung recipients (6–13%), the next highest among heart and liver transplant recipients (1–8%) [14–17], and the lowest among kidney recipients [18].

ICPs should be mindful that other immunosuppressed patients also are at risk for invasive aspergillosis: Those with chronic lung diseases (i.e., chronic obstructive pulmonary disease), acquired immunodeficiency syndrome (AIDS), chronic granulomatous disease, and other hereditary immunodeficiency syndromes as well as those taking immunosuppressive medications such as corticosteroids. There have been recent reports of invasive aspergillosis in patients receiving infliximab, an agent approved in the late 1990s for use in treating Crohn's disease and rheumatoid arthritis [19–21]. The extent to which infliximab or other antitumor necrosis factor (TNF) therapies increase risk of fungal infection remains to be established. In these immunosuppressed groups, as well as HSCT and solid organ transplant recipients, it could be difficult to prevent environmental exposures to mold because these patients either are managed predominantly in the community or have prolonged periods of risk in nonhospital settings.

Impact and Incidence of Invasive Aspergillosis

Aspergillus spp. infections cause substantial morbidity and mortality. A study using the U.S. National Hospital Discharge Data from the 1990s estimated that >10,000 aspergillosis-related discharges occurred annually [22]. These hospitalizations resulted in 1,970 deaths and $633.1 million in costs [22]. In addition, the excess length of stay was ~12 days and excess cost was $50,000 compared with patients without aspergillosis [22]. This large study used an administrative database and lacked the ability to determine the proportion that were HAIs. Despite advances in antifungal therapy, mortality rates reported for invasive aspergillosis remain high at 30–50% [23,24].

The incidence of invasive aspergillosis is estimated to be in the range of 5% to >20% in high-risk groups [25]. Aspergillosis has been estimated to occur after 6–11% of allogeneic HSCT [10,26,27]. Some studies suggest that the incidence of *Aspergillus* infection among allogeneic HSCT could have increased in the 1990s [12,26] perhaps due to more frequent use of high-risk donor sources and more intense immunosuppression. Recent data suggest diagnoses during the postengraftment period could be occurring more frequently [10,12,13,27–31]. Explanation for this increase in disease observed in the postengraftment period could include decreased duration of the neutropenia, increased use of HLA-mismatched transplants that increase risk for GVHD, and increased survival past the early transplant period. The risk of invasive aspergillosis among autologous HSCT is lower compared to the risk in allogeneic transplantation; reports describe incidence rates of about 1–2% [10].

Assessing the incidence of invasive aspergillosis is difficult for a variety of reasons. The lack of a consistent case definition and absence of effective surveillance mechanisms make it difficult to compare incidence rates from different studies. This problem is not unique to aspergillosis but applies to other invasive mold infections as well. With the adoption of an international consensus definition for opportunistic invasive fungal infections for multicenter clinical trials in HSCT or cancer patients, the situation could be improving [7]. Multicenter epidemiologic studies such as those coordinated by the Transplant Associated Infection Surveillance Network (TransNet) have likewise adopted these definitions, which require evidence of histopathologic or microbiologic evidence of tissue invasion to classify a patient as having "proven" disease; in the past, diagnosis of invasive aspergillosis and other invasive fungal infections could have required neither. Because these strict definitions require the use of more invasive diagnostic procedures that may not be performed in all patients, incidence estimates likely will underestimate the true burden of disease.

Differences Among Aspergillus Species

The most common species associated with infection is *Aspergillus fumigatus* followed by *Aspergillus flavus* (Table 43-1). Other species can cause disease but less commonly, including, but not limited to, *A. amstelodami*, *A. avenaceus*, *A. candidus*, *Aspergillus carneus*, *A. caesiellus*, *A. clavatus*, *A. glaucus*, *A. granulosus*, *A. lentulus*, *A. nidulans*, *A. niger*, *A. oryzae*, *A. quadrilineatus*, *A. restrictus*, *A. sydowi*, *A. terreus*, *A. ustus*, and *A. versicolor*. Some recent reports have documented a shift in pathogen profile to a profile with more non*fumigatus* species of *Aspergillus*. One *Aspergillus* sp. of concern is *A. terreus*, which has increased or is almost as frequent as *A. fumigatus* in some institutions [32–35].

Infections due to *A. terreus* are concerning because these isolates demonstrate in vitro resistance to amphotericin B, and these infections often respond poorly to treatment [33,34,36,37]. *A. terreus* has been isolated from showerheads, hospital water systems, and potted plants [38,39]. While most bloodstream isolates of *Aspergillus* represent pseudofungemia, *A. terreus* (as well as other fungi such as *Fusarium*, *Scedosporium*, and *Acremonium* spp.) often has caused true fungemia, so detection by recovery in blood culture often represents true disease [35,40–42]. The emergence of *A. terreus* could be due in part to improved means of laboratory recovery, altered microbial flora among patients with prior exposure to amphotericin B, and/or other unmeasured environmental factors.

Outbreaks of Aspergillus, Likely Sources, and Routes of Exposure

Infection with *Aspergillus* spp. requires an exposure to the fungus from the environment in a susceptible host. It often is impossible to link specific exposures to disease, especially in sporadic episodes. Regardless, an understanding of the sources and routes of exposure associated with nosocomial aspergillosis, based largely on reports from outbreak investigations, has contributed to the rational basis for development of evidence-based preventive measures (Table 43-2).

Inhalation of *Aspergillus* spp. conidia from contaminated air is thought to be the primary means of acquiring aspergillosis. Conidia are able to remain viable for prolonged periods of time and can be disturbed from soil, where they are commonly found, and other contaminated material dispersed into the air. Because fungal conidia are relatively small, they can be suspended in air for extended periods and subsequently inhaled by individuals. When conidia eventually settle, they can contaminate environmental surfaces in the hospital.

The best evidence implicating contaminated air as a source of exposure comes from multiple outbreaks temporally associated with demolition, renovation, and construction projects [43–64]. These projects have been both within or adjacent to the healthcare facility. Malfunctions of hospital ventilation systems, which can allow contaminated air into patient areas, also have been implicated in the development of nosocomial fungal infections during construction [53,60,63,65,66]. A hospital ventilation system can malfunction in multiple ways due to gaps between filters and framework [60], inappropriate air pressurization allowing flow of air from dirty to clean areas [63,65], and improper maintenance of high-efficiency particulate air (HEPA) filters. Lutz et al. recently found direct contamination of an air-handling system by using a confined space video camera to identify moisture and contaminated insulating material in ductwork downstream of final filters associated with an operating theater after an outbreak of postsurgical infections [66]. Contaminated air also has been reported as a result of improperly sealed windows [50,63], use of fire-proofing material [67], presence of false ceilings [43,48,51,68–70], and insulating material [66,70,71].

Dust particles disturbed during demolition, renovation, and construction could subsequently contaminate other surfaces in the healthcare setting. In one *Aspergillus* outbreak, a fire that had destroyed a building near the hospital was thought to have dispersed conidia through an open window, contaminating a hall carpet, which was believed to be the ongoing source of infection [72]. Wound infections due to *Aspergillus* species have been traced to the outside of packages of dressing supplies in a central supply area that were contaminated during construction [44]. Two outbreaks of pseudofungemia associated with construction have occurred when laboratory specimens were contaminated [69,73]. In one of these pseudo-outbreaks, a breakdown in specimen-processing protocols was noted [69].

Attempts to correlate conidial air concentrations with disease or colonization have provided mixed results. One study found a correlation between incidence of invasive aspergillosis in immunocompromised patients and indoor air concentration of conidia [68]. However, two longitudinal studies found no correlation between concentration and sporadic episodes [74,75]. As a result, there is no established consensus on the safe concentration of airborne conidia [76,77].

Much debate surrounds the role of hospital water systems as a source for airborne molds, including but not limited to *Aspergillus* spp. [38,78–80]. *Aspergillus* spp. have been isolated from hospital and municipal water supplies in several countries including the United States [38,80–84]. Air sampling showing increased conidial counts after using a shower suggests that conidia present in the shower head or on the walls or floor of bathrooms can be released during showering. It also has been shown that cleaning floors in patient shower facilities in a bone-marrow transplant unit reduced mean air concentrations of molds, including *Aspergillus* spp. [79]. Even though inhalation of conidia-laden aerosols from water sources is plausible, potable water systems are not considered a well-recognized source for disease because the link between disease and the isolation of *Aspergillus* spp. conidia from water is not firmly established.

Other routes of exposure besides inhalation, such as contact transmission from contaminated fomites, are possible. Molecular strain typing supported a link between a cluster of cutaneous *A. flavus* infections in neonatal intensive care unit patients to contaminated adhesive tape used for umbilical catheters [85]. In addition, direct inoculation from *Aspergillus* spp. conidia contaminating dressing materials has resulted in a cluster of surgical and burn wound infections [44].

Other environmental sources of human infection have been less commonly reported. One study in France showed that infecting *Aspergillus* spp. were present in foods, such as pepper, tea, and dried soup, served in a hematology

TABLE 43-2

SELECTED PUBLISHED OUTBREAKS OF *ASPERGILLUS SPP.* IN HEALTHCARE FACILITIES, 1990–2005

Author (Year, Country) [Ref.]	Patient Population	Number	Primary Site(s)	Species	Probable Source[a]	Control Measures Recommended or Applied
Panackal et al. (2003, US) [57]	Renal transplant	7	LRTI	A. fumigatus	Construction	Impermeable barriers, HEPA filters in HVAC system, N95 respirator use during patient transport, reduce traffic, designated elevator for construction workers
Myoken et al. (2003, Japan) [277]	Hematology	6	Stomatitis	A. flavus	Undetermined	Not reported
Lutz et al. (2003, US) [66]	Surgical	6	SSI	A. fumigatus, A. flavus	Air-handling system, moist insulation	Remediation of air-handling unit: remove interior insulation, coat units with fungicide, clean diffusers
Pegues et al. (2002, US) [88]	Transplant ICU	3	SSI, LRTI	A. fumigatus	Debriding and dressing wounds	Disruption of wound minimized, wound covered
Hahn et al. (2002, US) [278]	Hematology–oncology	10	LRTI	A. flavus, A. niger	Contaminated wall insulation from non-BMT wing	Impermeable barriers, wall insulation, decontaminated HEPA filters in non-BMT wing
Oren et al. (2001, Isreal) [56]	Hemeatology–oncology	10	LRTI	Not reported	Construction	Prophylaxis with low-dose systemic and inhaled or systemic amphotericin B, patients located in special ward with HEPA-filtered air
Lai (2001, US) [52]	Hematology–oncology	3	LRTI	A. flavus	Construction?	BMT unit closed for 2 weeks, air intake ducts cleaned, filters and prefilters replaced; impermeable barriers installed, alarm installed and air pressure made negative in stairwell leading to construction site, edge guards around doors to anterooms, carpeting replaced by vinyl flooring, special unit that allowed breathing filtered air during patient transport
Burwen (2001, US) [46]	Hematology–oncology	6	LRTI	A. flavus	Construction	High-risk patients identified and located in rooms with HEPA or laminar airflow
Thio et al. (2000, US) [127]	Hematology–oncology	21	LRTI	A. flavus	Connected hospital with higher air pressure than unit	Elective admissions stopped, plants and produce prohibited in patient rooms, doors connecting to adjacent hospital engineered to close automatically, all surfaces wet wiped or mopped, pressure relationships maximized, doors to individual patient rooms kept closed, N95 masks for neutropenic patients used during transport, windows resealed, employee entrance near construction area closed

(continued)

TABLE 43-2
(CONTINUED)

Author (Year, Country) [Ref.]	Patient Population	Number	Primary Site(s)	Species	Probable Source[a]	Control Measures Recommended or Applied
Gaspar et al. (1999, Spain) [47]	Hematology–oncology	11	LRTI	Not reported	Construction	Construction area sealed, patients relocated
Tabbara and al Jabarti (1998, Saudi Arabia) [61]	Cataract surgery	5	Eye infection	A. fumigatus	Construction	Not reported
Singer et al. (1998, Germany) [279]	NICU	4	Skin infection	A. fumigatus, A. flavus	Latex finger stall attached to penis to collect urine samples from male preterms	Removal of finger stalls
Loo et al. (1996, Canada) [54]	Hematology–oncology	36	LRTI, sinusitis	A. flavus, A. fumigatus	Construction	Portable HEPA-filter units: walls, doors, baseboards, vents, and above false ceiling painted with copper-8-quinolinolate formulated paint; windows sealed; perforated ceiling tiles replaced with nonperforated, vinyl-faced aluminum tiles; horizontal dust-accumulating blinds replaced with roller shades; patient relocated temporarily
Leenders et al. (1996, Netherlands) [280]	Hematology–oncology	5	LRTI, sinusitis, eye infection, mastoiditis	A. fumigatus, A. flavus	No single source	Policies for maintaining HEPA-filtered rooms reinforced, windows kept closed at all times
Bryce et al. (1996, Canada) [44]	Surgical and burn units	4	Skin infection	Not reported	Construction, contaminated packages of dressing supplies	Construction area sealed, supply room damp dusted and vacuumed, boxes and supplies wiped with cloth with buffered bleach
Tang et al. (1994, UK) [281]	Renal transplant unit	2	LRTI	A. fumigatus	Construction	Impermeable barriers
Iwen et al. (1994, US) [50]	Hematology–oncology	5	LRTI	A. fumigatus, A. flavus	Construction	Multiple measures taken prior to construction, environmental monitoring with gravity air-settling plates during construction-guiding additional measures

Study	Setting	No.	Type of infection	Organism	Probable source[a]	Remedial measures
Buffington et al. (1994, US) [45]	Hematology–oncology	7	LRTI	A. fumigatus, A. flavus	Construction	HEPA filters, proper pressure relationships, physical barriers, area decontamination
Tritz, Woods (1993, US) [282]	Hematology–oncology	4	LRTI	A. terreus, A. fumigatus	Not reported	Not reported
Flynn et al. (1993, US) [65]	Hematology–oncology; medical ICU	4	LRTI	A. terreus	Construction: improper air pressure relationships	Positive pressure and unidirectional airflow in ICU reestablished
Richet et al. (1992, US) [283]	Open heart surgery	6	SSI	A. fumigatus	Undetermined	Not reported
Pla et al. (1992, Spain) [284]	Liver transplant	2	SSI	A. fumigatus	Contaminated operating room?	Not reported
Loosveld et al. (1992, Netherlands) [285]	Hematology–oncology	6	LRTI	A. fumigatus	Cracked plasterwork?	Plastering renovated; HEPA filters installed in each room; cleaning procedures intensified
Humphreys et al. (1991, UK) [71]	General ICU	6	LRTI	A. fumigatus, A. flavus	Perforated metal ceiling with contaminated insulation	ICU cleaned extensively, patients temporarily relocated, old ICU replaced by new ICU with enhanced ventilation system and without false ceilings
Arnow et al. (1991, US) [68]	Hematology–oncology; solid-organ transplant	15	LRTI	A. flavus, A. fumigatus	Contaminated air filters	Air-handling unit remediated, contaminated air filters removed, surfaces in patient areas damp-wiped, carpet removed
Weber et al. (1990, US) [62]	Hematology–oncology	18	LRTI	Not reported	Construction	Not reported
Mehta (1990, India) [286]	Open heart surgery	4	Endocarditis	A. fumigatus	Air-handling system; broad spectrum antibiotics	V filters and cooling coils scrubbed weekly, filters replaced with series of prefilters and HEPA filters, air changes increased, broad spectrum antibiotics restricted

SSI, surgical site infection; LRTI, lower respiratory tract infection; HEPA, high-efficiency particulate air; HVAC, heating, ventilation, and air conditioning; NICU, neonatal intensive care unit.
[a]Construction can constitute activities that include demolition or renovation.

unit [86]. Massive contamination of spices, such as pepper, by *A. flavus* and *A. fumigatus* has been linked to infection in hospitalized neutropenic patients [87]. These infections, however, were believed to be acquired through inhalation, not ingestion. Consequently, the importance of contaminated food as a source of infection has yet to be well established.

Potted plants and flowers have been found to be contaminated with *Aspergillus* spp. and are suggested as sources of conidia in the air of homes and hospitals. Lass-Flor et al. recently reported that isolates from four patients infected with *A. terreus* were identical to isolates from in-hospital plants by molecular typing [39]. One study found that one patient could have served as the environmental source during the debridement and dressing of his wounds, causing airborne transmission and subsequent wound infection in a neighboring transplant recipient although such transmission likely extremely rare [88].

Hospital Versus Community Acquisition of Invasive Aspergillosis

Although invasive aspergillosis often manifests itself during hospitalization when patients are profoundly immuno-suppressed, exposure can occur outside the hospital. The relative importance of exposures from sources within the hospital or from the community is debatable; such knowledge is important for recommending prevention and control measures appropriate for different settings. Determining whether *Aspergillus* spp. infections are nosocomial is difficult for several reasons, one of which is that its incubation period is unknown. Thus, there is no agreement on how to define HAI episodes, and definitions are by necessity somewhat arbitrary. For example, investigators have used 3 [89], 4 [90], and 7 days [54] after hospitalization. Paterson et al. defined an HAI as one that occurred >7 days after admission to hospital or <14 days after discharge; accordingly, more than 70% of aspergillosis episodes during a 2-year period of hospital construction at their institution was acquired outside the hospital [91]. There is further evidence that most sporadic episodes are community acquired. Among allogeneic HSCT recipients, there appears to be a shift toward later onset aspergillosis after transplantation [10,12,13,27–31]. These later onset episodes often develop in persons long after hospital discharge.

Molecular epidemiology has improved our understanding of where *Aspergillus* spp. infections are acquired. Chazalet et al. used retriction fragment polymorphism (RFLP) analysis to fingerprint >700 isolates of *A. fumigatus* [92]. These isolates were obtained from 70 patients with invasive aspergillosis and from their hospitals' environment. Based on the theory that the isolation of an indistinguishable strain from a patient and from the immediate hospital environment is suggestive of nosocomial acquisition, 40% of the patients evaluated in this study had an HAI. It is important to note, however, that Chazalet et al.

calculated that they had sampled and typed <20% of the population of strains present in the four hospitals studied.

Zygomycosis, Including Mucormycosis

Although much less common than nosocomial *Aspergillus* infections, HAIs caused by other molds have been increasingly reported over the past decade [33,34,93]. The next most frequently encountered infections include the Zygomycoses, which are caused by molds of the class Zygomycetes. Similar to *Aspergillus* spp., Zygomycetes are found in soil and decaying organic matter worldwide. Pathogens within this class include members of the order Mucorales (which cause mucormycosis), more often of the genera *Absidia*, *Rhizopus* and *Rhizomucor*, and are than the other genera within the order Mucorales including *Cunninghamella*, *Apophysomyces*, *Saksenaea*, *Syncephalastrum*, or *Cokeromyces*. Disease most often occurs in severely immunocompromised persons but can occur in persons with only diabetes or recent corticosteroid therapy. Classically, persons in diabetic ketoacidosis are susceptible to infection because the acidic environment amplifies the mold's ability to use iron. Persons on deferoxamine also are susceptible because the mold is able to access the iron bound to the deferoxamine better than the iron bound to normal hemoglobin [94]. The most common manifestations of zygomycosis are pulmonary and rhinocerebral infection, yet cutaneous infection associated with preexisting skin or soft tissue breakdown also can occur (Table 43-1).

Nosocomial cutaneous zygomycosis outbreaks, specifically with *R. arrhizus* and *R. microsporus* var *rhizopodiformis*, have been associated with contaminated wooden tongue depressors and elasticized adhesive bandages [95–98]. A pseudo-outbreak linked to wooden sticks used in the laboratory also has been described [99]. In a recent outbreak, there were two reports of cutaneous *R. arrhizus* infections at stomas, the source of which were karaya gum, a nonsterile product, used as an ostomy bag adhesive [100]. While nosocomial cutaneous infections by zygomycetes are more commonly described, there also have been reports of nosocomial pulmonary or bloodstream infections (BSIs) [101–103]. One outbreak of rhinocerebral and disseminated zygomycosis was associated with air handler intake vents located near a hospital heliport [104]. Mortality due to zygomycosis varies by infection site, but overall mortality has improved from 84% in the 1950s before the introduction of amphotericin B to 47% in the 1990s [105].

Voriconazole, a second-generation triazole, has become the initial therapy of choice for invasive aspergillosis since 2002 and has demonstrated appropriateness as an alternative agent to amphotericin B in patients with neutropenia and persistent fever. Voriconazole has also become an attractive option for prophylaxis in severely immunocompromised patients [24,106,107]. It is important to recognize, however, that voriconazole has poor activity against zygomycotic infections [24]. Several healthcare facilities have documented increases in zygomycosis since the availability of voriconazole [106,108–111]. This increase could not be entirely attributable to voriconazole but to an unrelated temporal fluctuation in the environmental reservoir or an increase over time of the patients' underlying susceptibility to infection. Marr et al. reported that twice as many transplant recipients developed zygomycosis during 1995–1999 compared to 1985–1989 [112]. Similar increases occurred for aspergillosis and fusariosis, suggesting that the increase could have more to do with patient susceptibility than selection pressure for zygomycosis.

The TransNet reported preliminary data pooled from 16 centers illustrating an increase in the number of reported zygomycosis since 2001 despite stable numbers of fusariosis and declining numbers of aspergillosis. However, these data require proper adjustment (e.g., calculation of incidence by risk categories) to reflect true trends in incidence. The question remains as to whether the rate of zygomycosis is increasing because patients are surviving longer to become infected with a zygomycete or because the microbial floras among patients are being altered. Regardless, clinicians are likely to see more episodes of zygomycosis in the coming years, particularly among recipients of transplants and patients with cancer.

Other Mold Infections

Mold infections caused by *Fusarium* spp., *Scedosporium* spp., *S apiosermum* (*Ps. boydii*), and *S. prolificans* also are notable because they appear to be resistant to the polyene antifungal agents and can result in breakthrough infections in high-risk patients exposed to amphotericin B. *Fusarium* spp. are found in soil and can cause a range of infections in humans from superficial or locally invasive skin infections to disseminated infections involving the bloodstream, sinuses, and lower respiratory tract (Table 43-1). Although the environment outside the hospital is thought to be the reservoir for most exposures, some evidence points to the involvement of water including a hospital water distribution system [80,113]. A recent study involving 9 HSCT centers reported fungemia and skin manifestations in 44% and 75% of patients with fusariosis, respectively [114]. The most frequent species causing infections in humans includes members of the *Fusarium solani* spp. complex, *Fusarium oxysporum* spp. complex, and *Fusarium moniliforme* [112,114,115]. Breakthrough infections have been reported during amphotericin B therapy, to which *Fusarium* spp. have in vitro resistance as it appears to have triazoles. The use of voriconazole as salvage therapy has been reported with some success, but immune reconstitution should be central to therapy because persistant neutropenia is the main predictor of poor outcome [114]. Overall, the mortality rate of *Fusarium* infection among HSCT recipients usually exceeds 80% at 90 days after infection onset [112,114].

Scedosporium apiospermum and *Scedosporium prolificans* are being increasingly recognized as causes of disseminated infection, often including pulmonary and central nervous system disease (Table 43-1). The combination of a severely immunosuppressed host, a predilection for dissemination, and a lack of effective antifungal therapy results in almost universally fatal outcomes. Like *A. terreus* and *Fusarium* spp., *Scedosporium* prolificans is capable of adventititous sporulation (sporulation in tissue), allowing hematogenous spread and frequent dissemination. A detailed review of infections among solid organ and HSCT recipients identified dissemination in >50% of *Scedosporium* infections; fungemia was common and occurred in >50% of them infections [116]. Blood cultures positive for these molds among patients with leukemia or HSCT recipients should be considered clinically relevant. A review of 29 cancer patients with blood cultures positive for molds found that 80% of blood cultures from which *S. prolificans* or *S. apiospermum* was recovered represented definite or probable fungemia compared with 4% (1/24) cultures in which other fungi (*Aureobasidium pullulans* and *Paecilomyces*, *Alternaria*, *Trichoderma*, *Bipolaris*, and *Chaetomium* spp.) were recovered [117].

Although it is difficult to know whether the recent appreciation of *Scedosporium* spp. as a pathogen is the result of improved laboratory practices or a patient population that is more susceptible, several factors suggest the latter. *Scedosporium* spp. are resistant to amphotericin B. Moreover, *S. prolificans* are considered to be resistant to all triazoles and echinocandins, whereas *S. apiospermum* appears to be susceptible to extended-spectrum triazoles (e.g., voriconazole and posaconazole) [118]. Husain et al. noted that in recent years, these infections have been appearing later in the posttransplantation period (i.e., median of 6 months after transplantation) and could be related to amphotericin B or triazole prophylaxis [116]. However, prolonged survival, delays in GVHD onset, and other factors could be more important in the later occurrence of these infections. Because these infections are rare, the relative importance that increasing amounts of antifungal prophylaxis will have on their incidence is unlikely to be determined.

Environmental Sampling and Molecular Typing of Mold

Because certain molds including a variety of *Aspergillus* spp. are widespread and commonly found in the hospital environment, interpreting the results of environmental sampling often is difficult. Isolation of the same mold species from the patient and an environmental source could be coincidental rather than proof that the sampled environment was the source of the pathogen. Isolation of a particular mold species from an environmental source, therefore, is at best suggestive, and other potential environmental sources should not be immediately dismissed. Furthermore, current sampling and analytical methods often are insensitive. Thus, failure to identify a particular mold species from a specific environmental source cannot rule it out as a potential source. As a general rule, environmental cultures during an outbreak investigation can be helpful only if they are directed by epidemiologic data.

Environmental sampling can be problematic because it often is not conducted until an increase in infections has been detected. Therefore, temporal continuity and baseline concentrations to determine whether an outbreak is associated with increased exposure levels are almost always unavailable. If environmental sampling is attempted, careful consideration of a number of factors is needed, ideally in consultation with someone experienced in sampling for mold. For air sampling, these factors include characteristics of the target species that could influence the choice of appropriate sampler and analytical method, sampling period to best represent probable human exposure (e.g., minutes, hours, or days), sample volume that should be large enough to be representative but not exceed the capability of the instrument, and sampling medium [119,120]. Although attractive due to the low cost, gravity sediment methods (e.g., an open petri dish) are limited because they are not volumetric, provide qualitative rather than quantitative results, preferentially select large particles, and are less sensitive than volumetric methods [119].

Culture-based methods often underestimate variety and concentrations of molds in the air [120]. Methods to measure conidia counts that do not rely on culture also are problematic because *Aspergillus* conidia cannot be differentiated from *Penicillium* conidia and cannot be identified to the species level. In addition to air samples, samples of dust settled on surfaces and of suspected contaminated materials can be helpful. Compared to swab cultures, contact plates [119] and vacuuming methods could be preferable because they allow quantification (e.g., colony-forming units per square centimeter) and can be a good historical representation of past airborne molds because air samples collected under quiescent conditions can underestimate exposure levels due to settling.

Molecular epidemiology assumes that when several isolates are found to be genetically indistinguishable using molecular typing methods with a sufficiently high discriminatory power, they are derived from a recent common ancestor [121]. However, although molecular typing of fungi, such as *Aspergillus* spp., has improved, traditional epidemiological data are still needed to interpret the results. The indications for molecularly typing molds associated with invasive disease remain undefined.

Molecular typing methods designed to determine the relatedness of particular strains have improved. For *Aspergillus* spp., the molecular typing methods reported to have had some success include (1) isoenzyme analysis, (2) RFLP analysis, which includes restriction endonuclease analysis and hybridization with single genes, tandemly repeated genes, and dispersed repetitive DNA probes, and (3) PCR-based procedures using randomly amplified polymorphic DNA (RAPD) (also termed arbitrarily primed PCR [AP-PCR]), sequence-specific polymorphic DNA, and analysis of polymorphic microsatellite markers [122]. No consensus on the use of typing methods for *Aspergillus* spp. exists. These tests should be used in conjunction with specialty reference laboratories. Ideally, samples from nonoutbreak patients and areas of the hospital should be collected and typed together with the outbreak strains.

Surveillance for Invasive Mold Infection

Surveillance strategies for invasive mold HAIs, including aspergillosis, traditionally have focused on identifying pulmonary disease. The Healthcare Infection Control Practices Advisory Committee (HICPAC) of the Centers of Disease Control and Prevention (CDC) strongly recommends taking several routine steps supported by experimental, clinical, and/or epidemiologic studies and by strong theoretical rationale. These steps include (1) maintaining a high index of suspicion for healthcare-associated invasive mold infection in severely immunocompromised patients (Table 43-3) and (2) establishing a system by which the facility's infection control personnel are promptly informed when *Aspergillus* spp. is isolated from cultures of specimens from a patient's respiratory tract and by periodically reviewing the hospital's microbiologic, histopathologic, and postmortem data (Table 43-3) [77]. Currently, there is good evidence that routine, periodic cultures of the nasopharynx or nares of asymptomatic patients at high risk for disease are not informative of nosocomial transmission and should be discouraged. Likewise routine, periodic cultures of equipment or devices used for respiratory therapy, pulmonary function testing, and delivery of inhalation anesthesia in the HSCT unit or of dust in rooms of HSCT recipients are discouraged.

ICP need to balance the costs of and time involved in performing ongoing surveillance with the likelihood for detecting any disease. Any ongoing surveillance usually can be limited to the high-risk population, which can change periodically as new programs are added or removed from the hospital. In addition, heightened surveillance should be encouraged during periods of potential increased exposure (e.g., during renovation, construction, and destruction). This includes expanding either the scope of baseline surveillance to include new patients (postoperative patients or those with less severe but significant immunosuppression) or new data sources (Table 43-3).

CDC and infection control staff in New Orleans outlined a strategy for a reasonable approach to detecting invasive mold infections among immunosuppressed persons during a period of extensive exposure to indoor molds in the aftermath of Hurricane Katrina [123]. These definitions were modified from the EORTC/MSG criteria and could be useful to ICP performing surveillance for invasive mold infections in healthcare settings during periods of increased

TABLE 43-3

FACTORS TO CONSIDER IN DEVISING A SURVEILLANCE STRATEGY FOR NOSOCOMIAL MOLD INFECTIONS

Surveillance Aspects	Considerations
Patients of concern: Identify groups of patients at greatest risk for invasive mold infections	Transplant recipients, including organ and hematopoietic stem cell, within 6 months of transplant and/or during periods of substantial immunosuppression Neutropenia (neutrophil count $<500/\mu L$) from any cause including neoplasm and cancer chemotherapy CD4+ lymphocyte count $<200/\mu L$ from any cause including HIV infection Ongoing cancer chemotherapy, corticosteroid and other immunosuppressive drug therapy, and immunosuppressive diseases, such as leukemia or lymphoma
Data sources: Consider expanding access to selected data sources during the finite period of concern (e.g., demolition)	Microbiology reports should be performed at least weekly, and infection control personnel should be notified of positive results for *Aspergillus* spp., *Fusarium* spp., *Scedosporium* spp., *Rhizopus* spp., *Rhizomucor* spp., and *Absidia* spp. or other molds isolated from culture. Because the utility of subtyping isolates to assist in ascertainment of possible healthcare-related transmission is largely determined by the epidemiology of a suspected outbreak, microbiology laboratories should retain all mold isolates known to cause invasive disease to facilitate investigations during period immediately postremediation. Histopathologic and postmortem data should be reviewed at least monthly for reports for morphological terms suggestive of an infection such as "fungal elements" or "hyphae." If possible, chest radiographs and CT scans should be reviewed at least weekly (e.g., specialty care ward) for entries that specify findings consistent with fungal pneumonia or aspergillosis such as the halo sign, air-crescent sign, and cavity within an area of consolidation. Consider enlisting assistance of radiologist to log all patients with these findings for 6 months. Consider receiving printouts from inpatient pharmacy on all voriconazole and amphotericin-B starts if available as possible "cases." These drugs are the most commonly prescribed for invasive mold infections and were used for candidemia as empiric therapy in 2005 less often than for mold infections. The staff of wards housing high-risk patients, such as oncology and pulmonology wards and intensive care units, should be interviewed regularly to identify patients with possible invasive mold infections.
Nosocomial: When ≥ 1 invasive mold infection is identified, consider the following in determining whether infections are nosocomial	The more characteristics present, the higher is the likelihood of the infections being acquired in the healthcare setting: Patient was hospitalized for >2 weeks or was discharged for <2 weeks after a long hospitalization before symptoms began. Patient had frequent hospitalizations in the preceding 6 months. Symptoms occurred within 4 weeks of another suspected healthcare-associated mold infection. Two suspected healthcare-associated mold infections occurred in the same area of the hospital.

μL, microliter.

concern or in populations at high risk for invasive mold HAIs (Tables 43-4 and 43-5). An investigation should be conducted if one or more episodes of hospital-acquired invasive mold infections are detected.

Prevention and Control of Mold of Invasive Mold Infection

Several standardized approaches to eliminating exposure to indoor mold should be applied in inpatient healthcare settings. HICPAC outlines preventive measures and estimates the level of evidence-based support for each recommendation (Table 43-6, footnote a). Patient-care areas should be cleaned on a regular basis, and Environmental Protection Agency (EPA)–registered disinfectants should be used in accordance with the manufacturer's instructions to clean environmental surfaces (category IC) [76]. There is no evidence, however, that special measures, such as the use of fungicides on carpeting in general patient care areas, reduce fungal exposure (unresolved category) [76]. Similarly, there is no clear indication of the need for routinely sampling air, water, and environmental surfaces in healthcare facilities (category IB) [76]. Fungi are ubiquitous, and interpretation of fungi sampling data continues to be a challenge [124].

Because most patients are at minimal risk for invasive disease with molds and because exposures are difficult to

TABLE 43-4

SURVEILLANCE DEFINITIONS OF COMMONLY ENCOUNTERED INVASIVE MOLD INFECTIONS AMONG IMMUNOSUPPRESSED PATIENTS BASED ON CRITERIA OUTLINED IN THE REVISED EORTC/MSG DEFINITIONS FOR INVASIVE FUNGAL DISEASES

Infection Site	Definition
Pneumonia (Lower Respiratory Tract Mold Infection-LRT-MI)	**Proven LRT-MI:** Patient with EITHER 1. Biopsy or needle aspirate of lung tissue showing histopathologic or cytopathologic evidence of hyphae and associated tissue damage 2. Positive culture result from normally sterile site (e.g., pleural fluid, tissue) (excluding BAL, sinus cavity, urine) *and* that is clinically consistent with an invasive mold disease process (with or without evidence on radiograph) **Probable LRT-MI:** Patient with at least ONE HOST FACTOR (Table 43-5) AND either CLINICAL CRITERIA: 1. CT imaging showing air-crescent sign cavity, wedge-shaped infiltrate, or well-defined nodule ±, a "halo sign 2. New nonspecific focal infiltrate *and* ≥1 of the following (unless microbial criteria are met): • Hemoptysis • Pleural rub • Pleural pain AND at least ONE of the MICROBIOLOGIC CRITERIA 1. Sputum or BAL culture positive for mold or direct microscopic evidence of hyphal forms 2. Positive *Aspergillus* antigen from BAL or ≥1 serum samples 3. Positive glucan assay (beta-D-glucan) ≥1 serum sample **Possible LRT-MI:** Same as Probable LRT-MI except NO MICROBIOLOGIC CRITERIA, AND other potential causes have been excluded
Sinonasal infection (Upper Respiratory Tract Mold Infection-URT-MI)	**Proven URT-MI:** Patient with: 1. Biopsy or needle aspirate of sinus tissue showing histopathologic or cytopathologic evidence of hyphae and associated tissue damage 2. Positive culture result for a sample obtained by sterile procedure from upper respiratory tract and clinically or radiologically abnormal site consistent with infection **Probable URT-MI:** Patient with at least ONE HOST FACTOR (Table 43-5) AND BOTH CLINICAL CRITERIA: 1. Imaging studies (e.g., CT or radiograph imaging showing "erosion of sinus walls," "extentsion of infection to neighboring structures," or "extensive skull base destruction") 2. Any ONE of the following: • Acute localized pain (especially radiating to the eye) • Nose ulceration or eschar of nasal mucoas ± epistaxis • Extension of paranasal sinus across bony barriers including the orbit AND the following MICROBIOLOGIC CRITERION 1. Sinus aspirate culture positive for mold or direct microscopic evidence of hyphal elements **Possible URT-MI:** Same as Probable URT-MI except NO MICROBIOLOGIC CRITERIA, AND other potential causes have been excluded.
Central Nervous System Mold Infection (CNS-MI)	**Proven CNS-MI:** Patient with EITHER 1. Biopsy or needle aspirate of CNS tissue showing histopathologic or cytopathologic evidence of hyphae and associated tissue damage 2. Positive culture result for a sample obtained by sterile procedure from CNS and clinically or radiologically abnormal site consistent with infection

TABLE 43-4
(CONTINUED)

Infection Site	Definition
	Probable CNS-MI: Patient with at least ONE HOST FACTOR (Table 43-5) AND either CLINICAL CRITERIA: 1. Radiographic evidence showing meningeal enhancement (i.e., CT or MRI imaging showing "meningitis extending from a perinasal, auricular, or vertebreal process") 2. Focal lesions on imaging of the head. AND at least ONE of the following MICROBIOLOGIC CRITERIA 1. Non-sterile site culture (BAL, sputum) positive for mold or direct microscopic evidence of mold 2. Positive *Aspergillus* antigen from BAL, pleural fluid, CSF, or ≥ 1 serum samples 3. Positive glucan assay (beta-D-glucan) from ≥ 1 serum sample
	Possible CNS-MI: Same as Probable CNS-MI except NO MICROBIOLOGIC CRITERIA, AND other potential causes have been excluded
Skin Mold Infection (SKIN-MI)	**Proven SKIN-MI:** Patient with 1. Biopsy or needle aspirate of skin/soft tissue showing histopathologic or cytopathologic evidence of hyphae and associated tissue damage 2. Positive culture result for a sample obtained by sterile procedure from soft tissue and clinically or radiologically abnormal site consistent with infection.
	Probable SKIN-MI: Patient with at least ONE HOST FACTOR (Table 43-5) AND the following CLINICAL CRITERIA: 1. Papular or nodular skin lesions without any other explanation AND the following MICROBIOLOGIC CRITERIA 2. Non-sterile site culture (swab, debridement, aspirate) positive for mold or direct microscopic evidence of hyphal forms
	Possible SKIN-MI: Same as Probable except NO MICROBIOLOGIC CRITERIA, AND other potential causes have been excluded
EYE Mold Infection (EYE-MI)	**Proven EYE-MI:** Patient with 1. Biopsy or needle aspirate of vitreous fluid or cornea showing histopathologic or cytopathologic evidence of hyphae and associated tissue damage, or 2. Positive culture result from a sample of vitreous and clinically or radiologically abnormal site consistent with infection.
	Probable EYE-MI: Patient with at least ONE HOST FACTOR (Table 43-5) AND the following CLINICAL CRITERIA: 1. Intraocular findings suggesting endophthalmitis (i.e., as determined by ophthalmologic examination) AND the following MICROBIOLOGIC CRITERION 2. Non-sterile site culture (swab) positive for mold or direct microscopic evidence of hypal forms
	Possible EYE-MI: Same as Probable EYE except NO MICROBIOLOGIC CRITERIA, AND other potential causes have been excluded
Fungemia (BSI-MI)	**Proven BSI-MI:** Patient with blood culture that yields a mold (e.g., *Fusarium* spp., *Scedosporium* spp.) in the context of a compatible infectious disease process (i.e., contamination has been excluded)

EORTC/MSG, European Organization for Research and Treatment of Cancer/National Institute of Allergy and Infectious Diseases Mycoses Study Group; BAL, bronchoalveolar lavage; CSF, cerebrospinal fluid.
(Modified from [313]).

TABLE 43-5

HOST FACTORS FROM THE EORTC/MSG REVISED DEFINITIONS FOR INVASIVE FUNGAL INFECTIONS

1. Recent history of neutropenia (<500 neutrophils/μL for >10 days) in previous 3 weeks
2. Receipt of allogeneic stem cell transplant recipient
3. Prolonged use of corticosteroids (excluding patient with allergic bronchopulmonary aspergillosis) at an average minimum dose of 0.3 mg/kg/day prednisone equivalent for >3 weeks
4. Treatment with other recognized T-cell immune suppressants, such as cyclosporine, TNF-α blockers, specific monoclonal antibodies (alemtuzumab), nucleoside analogues during the past 90 days
5. Inherited severe immunodeficiency (e.g., chronic granulomatous disease, severe combined immunodeficiency)

EORTC/MSG, European Organization for Research and Treatment of Cancer/National Institute of Allergy and Infectious Diseases Mycoses Study Group.
(Adapted from [313]).

prevent, preventive measures to limit mold exposure should focus on patient populations at highest risk for such disease. The CDC guidelines for preventing nosocomial pulmonary aspergillosis (Table 43-6) [77] focus on allogeneic HSCT recipients as one group of patients at high risk for respiratory exposure. The establishment of a protected environment for these patients includes providing a sealed room with ≥12 air changes per hour [125–127], using HEPA filtration of incoming air [56,128], and maintaining positive pressure relative to the hallway [129]. Whether similar measures to prevent exposure are required for other populations of patients, such as patients who received autologous HSCT and solid-organ transplants, remains unresolved [77].

Severely immunocompromised patients, including allogeneic patients with HSCT, are at particularly high risk of acquiring *Aspergillus* spp. infections during periods of hospital demolition, construction, renovation, and repair [55]. Before initiating any of these projects, a multidisciplinary team including infection control staff should estimate the level of risk they will create [76]. Both the construction team and the healthcare staff in immunocompromised patient-care areas should be educated about preventive measures (category 1B) [76]. One of the most important elements of infection control is to construct barriers to prevent dust exposure. If the project is outside the hospital, windows should be sealed to prevent air intrusion (category 1B) [76]. For internal projects, the air-handling system in work zones adjacent to patient-care areas should be set to negative pressure (category 1B). Barrier materials that are impermeable to fungal spores should be used, and breaches in the barrier should be repaired [76]. In addition, pedestrian traffic should be restricted or redirected from patient-care areas. When severely immunocompromised patients need to leave their rooms (e.g., for diagnostic procedures), they should wear high-efficiency respiratory protection devices to decrease their risk of inhalation of fungal elements (category II) [77].

If a patient develops an *Aspergillus* spp. infection, the episode should be investigated to determine whether it is healthcare associated or community acquired. In an outbreak situation, the collection of environmental cultures can be useful. Various techniques discussed previously can be used to type the *Aspergillus* spp. to suggest an environmental source. In addition, ventilation deficiencies should be investigated and repaired [77].

Considerable research also is being done to decrease the severity of clinical disease from mold in high-risk patient populations. These efforts range from shortening the window of susceptibility due to neutropenia with growth factors such as granulocyte colony-stimulating factor (G-CSF) [130] to improving the early detection of mold infections [131,132]. Similarly, the role of prophylactic antifungals for patients deemed at highest risk for invasive fungal diseases, such as recipients of HSCT, is still being defined [133].

The hospital water supply remains to be established as an important source of *Aspergillus* spp. HAIs. As such, current HICPAC guidelines do not offer specific guidance for avoiding water exposures to prevent aspergillosis [76,77]. Some experts have proposed measures to prevent nosocomial waterborne infection with *Aspergillus* spp. [134]: minimizing patient exposure to tap water (e.g., using sterile water and avoiding showering) and intensively monitoring water supplies when infections occur [134]. If more evidence showing the importance of water as a source of exposure is obtained, recommendations can change.

YEAST

Candidiasis

Clinical Disease and Diagnosis of Candidiasis

The clinical manifestations of *Candida* spp. infections are quite variable. Although immunocompetent hosts can suffer from *Candida* dermatitis, oral candidiasis, and *Candida* vulvovaginitis, these diseases tend to be more severe in the immunosuppressed. In most circumstances,

TABLE 43-6

SUMMARY OF SELECTED PREVENTION AND CONTROL MEASURES FOR HEALTHCARE-ASSOCIATED PULMONARY ASPERGILLOSIS [77]

Recommendation	Category[a]
Staff education, especially healthcare personnel about infection control procedures for aspergillus	II
Surveillance	
Maintain high index of suspicion in immunocompromised (ANC <500/mm^3 for two weeks, <100/mm^3 for one week)	IA
Periodically review microbiologic, histopathologic, and postmortem data	II
Do not perform routine nasopharyngeal cultures of high-risk patients	IB
Do not perform routine cultures of equipment in the HSCT unit	IB
Determine the role of air sampling during construction or renovation	unresolved
Perform surveillance of room ventilation	IB
New construction of specialized care units for high-risk patients	
Create PE for allogeneic HSCT recipients that minimizes fungal spore counts by HEPA filtration of incoming air, directed room airflow, positive air pressure, proper seals, and high (≥12) air changes per hour	IB, IC
Do not use LAF routinely in PE	IB
Determine the role of PE for autologous HSCT recipients	unresolved
Determine the role of PE for solid-organ transplants	unresolved
Existing facilities with no cases of healthcare-associated aspergillus cases	
Place allogeneic HSCT recipients in appropriate PE	IB
Maintain air-handling systems in PE	IB, IC
Develop a water damage response plan	IB
Use proper dusting method for HSCT recipients	IB
Eliminate carpeting in hallways or rooms with HSCT recipients	IB
Remove upholstered furniture in rooms with HSCT recipients	II
Minimize time during which HSCT recipients are outside room and wear mask	II
Coordinate infection control strategies with other hospital personnel	IB
Eliminate flowers or plants in areas for HSCT recipients	II
Develop plan to prevent aspergillus exposure during construction and renovation activities.	IA
During construction, erect barriers and direct pedestrian traffic away from patient care areas	IB
Determine the role of PE for autologous HSCT recipients	unresolved
Determine the role of PE for solid-organ transplants	unresolved
Actions following a case of healthcare-associated aspergillus	
Begin a retrospective review and prospective search for other cases	II
Determine whether there is a ventilation deficiency	IB
Do epidemiologic investigation and contact state/local health department	IB
Decontaminate structural materials with antifungal biocide	IB
Chemoprophylaxis	
Administer prophylactic antifungal by inhalation to HSCT recipients	unresolved
Develop strategies to prevent recurrence of pulmonary aspergillosis in HSCT recipients	unresolved

ANC, absolute neutrophil count; HSCT, hematopoietic stem cell transplant; PE, protective environment; HEPA, high-efficiency particulate air filter; LAF, laminar air flow.
[a]Each recommendation is categorized as follows:
IA-Strongly recommended for implementation and strongly supported by well-designed experimental, clinical, epidemiologic studies.
IB-Strongly recommended for implementation and supported by certain clinical or epidemiologic studies and by strong theoretical rationale.
IC-Required for implementation as mandated by federal and/or state regulation or standard.
II-Suggested for implementation and supported by suggestive clinical or epidemiologic studies or by strong theoretical rationale.
Unresolved-Insufficient evidence or consensus regarding efficacy exists.

the presence of *Candida* spp. in the urine or sputum does not represent infection. Candidemia, on the other hand, almost always represents infection and is a condition with the potential for serious complications, including Candida spp. endocarditis and disseminated candidiasis.

Diagnosis of a *Candida* spp. infection depends on the suspected site. Infections of the skin or oral or vaginal mucosa can be diagnosed by recognizing the clinical pattern and the demonstration of fungal elements on potassium hydroxide (KOH) preparation. Infections of the respiratory tract, urine, or bloodstream can be confirmed by culture. Disseminated candidiasis is diagnosed by culture of biopsy material or demonstration of *Candida* spp. in histologic specimens from >1 site.

Risk Factors for Invasive Candidiasis

A variety of risk factors for candidemia exists (Table 43-7) [135]. Colonization by *Candida* spp. is the leading risk factor for infection in many series [135]. Colonization of multiple sites is an independent risk factor for developing invasive disease [136–138]. In different patient populations, including neutropenic and non-neutropenic patients, bloodstream and invasive infections could be preceded by *Candida* spp. colonization or superficial infection with a genotypically indistinguishable strain [139–143]. Approximately 5–15% of hospitalized patients is already colonized on admission; however, as exposure to risk factors for colonization accumulate during hospitalization, the percentage increases over time. Among intensive care unit (ICU) patients, it has been estimated that between 50–86% become colonized during their stay [143–147]. However, only a small percentage of these proceed to develop disease. Surveillance cultures are sometimes obtained, but their clinical significance is not known [144,148].

Other important risk factors include the receipt of antibiotics and/or neutropenia as well as the presence of vascular access devices. In general, the more antibiotic agents used, the broader the antibacterial spectrum, and the longer the duration of treatment, the higher is the risk of invasive candidiasis [135,138]. It is suspected that the risk is higher for cephalosporins and antibiotics with anti anaerobic activity [135,149–151]. Neutropenia is a well-recognized risk factor, not only for invasive candidiasis but also for other fungal infections [135–137,152,153]. Vascular access devices, often multiple, are required to manage ICU patients. The proportion of catheter-related candidemia ranges from 35–80% [135]. These catheters are used increasingly in non-ICU settings, including ambulatory care and home settings. Overall, it is important to note that factors associated with candidemia are no longer limited to the ICU. The diversity of elements listed in Table 43-7 highlights the extension of risk to other patient populations.

Epidemiology and Impact of Canadidemia

Infections due to *Candida* spp. represent the most important group of fungal HAIs; they cause substantial morbidity and mortality in hospitalized patients. Candidemia is the third or fourth most common cause of bloodstream infection among hospitalized patients [154,155]. Its incidence at single centers varies greatly, ranging from 0.3 to 28 per 10,000 admissions worldwide (Table 43-8). The attributable mortality for candidemia has been estimated to be as high as 49% [156]. Data from a multicenter study from Baltimore and Connecticut measured a lower attributable mortality rate of 19–24%, depending on the patients' ages [157]. When extrapolated to the entire United States, the annual number of excess deaths due to candidemia is estimated to be 4,256–5,376, and the excess hospital costs were estimated at $44–$320 million [155].

Candidemia is not limited to the ICU, although ICU patients are at high risk secondary to the presence of

TABLE 43-7
RISK FACTORS FOR CANDIDEMIA

Candida colonization	Surgery
From ≥1 body sites other than blood	Chemotherapy
Increase>4 log in stools	Steroids
Candiduria	H2 blockers
Rectal swabs	Multiple transfusion
Antibiotics	Renal failure
Prolonged use	Mechanical ventilation
Multiple antibiotics	Intubation
Broadspectrum antibiotics	Duration
Vascular access	Increased length of stay
Arterial catheter	Severity of disease
Swan-Ganz catheter	Prior bacteremia
Hickman catheter	Leukemia
Central venous catheter	Mismatched donor
Bladder catheter	Acute graft-versus-host disease
Neutropenia	Increased APACHE II or III score
Prolonged	Low birthweight for neonates
<500/μL or <100/μL	Age (>40 years; <32 weeks)
Parenteral nutrition	
Prolonged use	
Lipid use	
Antifungal prophylaxis (absence; for *C. krusei*, and *C. glabrata* vs.other strains)	

(Adapted from [135]).

TABLE 43-8

INCIDENCE OF CANDIDEMIA IN GENERAL PATIENT POPULATION REPORTS FROM SINGLE CENTERS COMPLETED 1995–2006, WORLDWIDE

Author [Ref.]	Country	Study Years	Overall Incidence of *Candida* BSI	Overall *C. albicans* (%)	Overall Mortality (%)
Karlowsky et al. [287]	Canada	1976–96	N/A	55.0	52.0
Luzatti et al. [288]	Italy	1992–97	1.14/10,000 patient-days	54.0	45.0
Viudes et al. [289]	Spain	1995–97	7.6/10,000 admissions	46.0	44.1
Malani et al. [182]	United States	1988–99	N/A	N/A	N/A
Garbino et al. [290]	Switzerland	1989–2000	0.3/10,000 patient-days	66.0	44.0
Alonso-Valle et al. [291]	Spain	1995–99	8.1/10,000 admissions	44.0	45.0
Hsueh et al. [292]	Taiwan	1981–2000	28/10,000 discharges in 2000	50.0	60.6 [in 2000]
McMullan et al. [293]	Ireland	1984–2000	N/A	60.7	N/A
San Miguel et al. [294]	Spain	1988–2000	6/10,000 admissions	51.0	N/A
Doczi et al. [295]	Hungary	1996–2000	2-4.1/10,000 admissions	77.0	N/A
Schelenz, Gransden et al. [187]	England	1995–2001	3/10,000 admissions	64.0	35.2

BSI, bloodstream infections; N/A, not available.
(Modified from [161]).

central venous catheters and have been the focus of epidemiological study in the recent past. Data from the CDC's National Nosocomial Infections Surveillance (NNIS) system found that *Candida albicans* BSIs in ICUs decreased overall from more than 8 BSIs per 10,000 central venous catheter (CVC) days in 1989 to less than 3 BSIs per 10,000 CVC-days in 1999, whereas *Candida glabrata* BSIs increased [158]. Results of another large multicenter study involving 49 U.S. hospitals were that BSIs due to *Candida* spp. increased from 8% in 1995 to 12% in 2002 [154]. Further data from the U.S. National Center for Health Statistics indicate that the number of patients discharged with sepsis caused by fungi tripled from 1979 to 2000 and that candidemia was the most likely cause of fungal sepsis in hospitalized patients [159]. One possible explanation for these apparently disparate findings is that advances in medical therapy have increased the number of patients susceptible to *Candida* spp. BSI. Furthermore, the established risk factors for candidemia, including prior colonization, use of central venous catheters and broadspectrum antimicrobials, mucosal surface disruption (e.g., surgery, hypotension, or the presence of cytotoxins), and neutropenia are no longer limited to ICU patients (Table 43-7) [135]. In fact, a U.S. population-based study found that only one-third of patients with candidemia had disease onset in the ICU and about one-quarter was actually diagnosed before admission (although these patients could have been colonized during their previous hospitalization) [160].

A recent, comprehensive review of candidemia trends found *Candida* BSI to be stable in most reports during the decade spanning 1995 to 2005 in different parts of the world [161]. This finding was documented by all three survey types: general patient population from single-

and multicenter surveys and specific population surveys. However, almost one third of the reports from the general patient population indicated an increasing trend, whereas one third of the specific population reports indicated a decreasing trend [161]. This finding suggests that in these specific patient populations (e.g., ICU patients in whom the incidence of *Candida* BSIs often are the highest), antifungal prophylaxis measures can be showing an impact on incidence.

Four *Candida* spp., including *C. albicans*, *C. glabrata*, *C. parapsilosis*, and *C. tropicalis*, account for ~95% of all *Candida* BSIs [160,162,163]. The remaining 5% is caused by different species, such as *C. krusei*, *C. lusitaniae*, *C. guilliermondii*, *C. dubliniensis*, *C. rugosa*, and others [118, 164]. Reports of these unusual causes of infection are being reported increasingly and some are noted to occur in HAI clusters [165–173].

Candida albicans continues to be the most commonly isolated species, but the proportion of nonalbicans *Candida* BSIs could be increasing. In fact, nonalbicans *Candida* BSIs in some centers from multiple countries are now >50% [152,158,165,174–194]. In some instances, this increase has been attributed to the use of azole for prophylaxis and treatment of fungal infections among certain groups of patients at high risk for *Candida* BSIs. Fluconazole became widely available in the early 1990s. Several reports have documented a shift in the species of *Candida* that cause candidemia when fluconazole use is increased [152,195]. One cancer center using fluconazole prophylaxis has reported higher numbers of *C. krusei* and *C. glabrata* in the 1990s compared with historical figures [152].

In one study of ICUs in 311 U.S. hospitals, *C. glabrata* BSIs per 10,000 CVC-days increased from about 0.2 in 1989 to more than 0.5 in 1999 [158]. An increase in

C. glabrata infections is concerning because the infection can rapidly acquire resistance to azoles after exposure to them [158,163]. In contrast, another large multicenter U.S. study found that percentage of *C. albicans* and *C. parapsilosis* increased from 1995 to 2002 whereas the percentage of *C. tropicalis* and *C. glabrata* decreased [154].

One factor that could influence different pathogen profiles can be geographic differences in fluconazole susceptibility in vitro among *C. glabrata* strains causing BSIs. For example, Pfaller et al. described geographic differences in fluconazole susceptibility trend, both internationally and within the United States; susceptibility was highest in the Asia–Pacific region (80.5%) and lowest in North America (64%) and Latin America (62.1%) [196]. Whether increased azole use is causing a shift from *C. albicans* remains controversial, and many variables that confound such evaluations exist.

Less Common Yeast Pathogens

A wide variety of less common yeast pathogens including *Trichosporon* spp., *Rhodotorula* spp., *Pichia anomala* (Candida pelliculosa), and *Malassezia* spp. [118,197–207] can cause invasive infection in an immunocompromised host. Of particular concern are opportunistic yeasts that pose challenges due to antifungal resistance [118]. *Trichosporon* spp. is the most commonly reported noncandidal yeast infection with reported mortality rates >80% [115,197–201,208–219]. Clinical failures with amphotericin B and fluconazole have been reported [115,200,201,209,216]. Isolates that are multidrug resistant to amphotericin, flucytosine, and fluconazole have been reported [219,220]. However, newer triazoles appear to be more active than fluconazole against *Trichosporon* spp, and successful treatment with voriconazole has been reported [209,210, 219–222].

Rhodotorula spp. are emerging as important pathogens [207,223–228] Although typically a commensal of skin, nails, and mucous membranes, this species has been reported to cause fungemia, central venous catheter and ocular infections, peritonitis, endocarditis, and meningitis [207,223–228]. Clinical isolates appear to be susceptible to amphotericin B, flucytosine, and newer triazoles, but reported minimum inhibitory concentrations (MICs) for fluconazole, caspofungin, and micafungin are high [205–207,229].

Antifungal Susceptibility Testing of Candida

Compared with other fungi, treatment of candidiasis can be better guided by in vitro susceptibility testing. Because the susceptibilities of *Candida* spp. in general are predictable based on species identification, it is currently not recommended to routinely test all *Candida* isolates for susceptibility [230]. Infectious Diseases Society of America (IDSA) guidelines recommend that susceptibility testing is most helpful in treating deep infection due to *nonalbicans* species of *Candida* [230]. If the patient has been treated previously with an azole antifungal agent, the possibility of microbiologic resistance must be considered.

Although the Clinical and Laboratory Standards Institute (formerly the National Committee for Clinical Laboratory Standards) has established standards for *Candida* spp., interpretative breakpoints exist only for fluconazole, itraconazole, and voriconazole [231–233]. Evidence supporting the association between MIC and clinical outcome for invasive candidal disease is not extensive; for example, fluconazole breakpoints were based predominantly on mucosal candidiasis data. One other limitation of testing for *Candida* spp. is the variability in interpretating the results (e.g., misinterpretation of trailing growth at high drug concentrations) [234].

Based on in vitro susceptibility testing performed on BSI isolates from around the world, *C. albicans*, *C. tropicalis*, and *C. parapsilosis* are considered to be generally susceptible to current antifungal agents [160,162]. Some strains of *C. lusitaniae* can be resistant to polyene agents (amphotericin B and nystatin) although they remain susceptible to triazoles (fluconazole, itraconazole, voriconazole, posaconazole, and ravuconazole) [162,235]. *C. krusei* is intrinsically resistant to fluconazole and often demonstrates decreased susceptibility to amphotericin B and flucytosine, although it remains susceptible to caspofungin, voirconazole, posaconazole, and ravuconazole [118]. *C. rugosa* has demonstrated decreased susceptibility to amphotericin B, nystatin, and fluconazole [118]. This property and its propensity to colonize skin could help explain how this species has caused several difficult-to-control outbreaks of infection in hospitals [166,167]. *C. glabrata* has emerged as an important problem, ranking second or third most frequently isolated after *C. albicans* in some institutions. Although it is generally susceptible to fluconazole, this species can easily develop acquired resistance, particularly in patients who have received prior fluconazole prophylaxis or treatment [158,163].

Outbreaks of *Candida*

Molecular epidemiology has been instrumental in establishing the gastrointestinal tract as the most important endogenous reservoir for *Candida* spp. infections [141,236–239]. Although the majority of episodes of nosocomial candidemia is likely of endogenous origin, outbreaks of *Candida* spp. infections can occur from exogenous transmission. A wide array of *Candida* spp. has been implicated as the cause of HAI outbreaks worldwide (Table 43-9). *Candida* spp. also are able to colonize a variety of fluids, and there have been several reports of transmission via contaminated infusates and biomedical devices (Table 43-9). In many instances, advances in molecular typing have been used to confirm the source of these outbreaks [172,238–242]. However, transmission of *Candida* spp. from one patient

TABLE 43-9
SELECTED PUBLISHED OUTBREAKS OF NOSOCOMIAL *CANDIDA* SPP. INFECTIONS

Author (Year, Country) [Ref.]	Patient Population	No.	Primary Site	Species	Probable Source	Control Measures Recommended or Applied
Plouffe et al. (1977, US) [296]	Surgery	14	Candidemia	*C. parapsilosis*	Contaminated IV fluids	Vacuum system cleaned
Solomon et al. (1984, US) [297]	Medicine	5	Candidemia	*C. parapsilosis*	Contaminated vacuum pump	Use of vacuum pump stopped
Burnie et al. (1985, England) [298]	ICU	14	Candidemia	*C. albicans*	Cross-infection	Strict cross-infection control strategies
McCray et al. (1986, US) [299]	Ophthalmalogy	13	Endopthalmitis	*C. parapsilosis*	Contaminated ocular irrigating solution	Solution recall
Berger et al. (1988, Germany) [300]	Hematology	12	Mixed	*C. krusei*	Bottle of contaminated lemon juice in hospital kitchen	Bottle elimination
Vaudry et al. (1988, Canada) [301]	NICU	3	Candidemia	*C. albicans*	Cross-infection	No intervention
Isenberg et al. (1989, US) [302]	Surgical	8	Sternal wound infections	*C. tropicalis*	Scrub nurse	Removal from cardiac team
Moro et al. (1990, Italy) [303]	ICU	8	Candidemia	*C. albicans*	Parenteral nutrition	Adherence to standard protocols for compounding and administering parenteral nutrition
Sherertz et al. (1992, US) [304]	NICU	5	Candidemia	*C albicans* (3), *C. tropicalis* (1) *C. parapsilosis*	Syringe fluids, TPN	Single use of syringes
Finkelstein et al. (1993, Israel) [305]	NICU	6	Candidemia	*C. tropicalis*	Cross-infection	Strict hand washing and contact isolation of cases
Johnston et al. (1994, Canada) [306]	Surgery	5	Prosthetic valve endocarditis	*C. parapsilosis*	Intraoperative contamination of cardiac bypass equipment	Decontamination of equipment
Reagan et al. (1995, US) [307]	NICU	7	Candidemia	*C. albicans*	No specific source	Not specified
Diekema et al. (1997, US) [308]	Surgery	4	Prosthetic valve endocarditis	*C. parapsilosis*	Glove tears during surgery	Change to more durable gloves
D'Antonio et al. (1998, Italy) [309]	Hematology/oncology	3	Candidemia	*C. inconspicua*	Cross-infection	No intervention
Huang et al. (1998, Taiwan) [268]	NICU	9	Candidemia	*C. albicans*	Cross-infection	Strict hand washing
Levin et al. (1998, Brazil) [269]	Oncology	6	Candidemia	*C. parapsilosis*	Implantable central venous catheters	Improved central venous catheter management
Huang et al. (1999, Taiwan) [267]	NICU	17	Candidemia	*C. parapsilosis*	Cross-infection	Strict hand washing with alcoholic chlorhexidine handrub
Nedret Koc et al. (2002, Turkey) [310]	ID clinic	9	Candidemia	*C. glabrata*	Contaminated bottles for milk feed	Bottle sterilization process fixed

(continued)

TABLE 43-9
(CONTINUED)

Author (Year, Country) [Ref.]	Patient Population	No.	Primary Site	Species	Probable Source	Control Measures Recommended or Applied
Chowdhary et al. (2003, India) [311]	NICU	16	Candidemia	*C. tropicalis*	Linens	Strict hand washing and contact isolation of cases
Colombo et al. (2003, Brazil) [166]	Hospital	6	Candidemia	*C. rugosa*	Not identified	No intervention
Barchiesi et al. (2004, Italy) [266]	Pediatric oncology		Candidemia	*C. parapsilosis*	Cross-infection	Not specified
Clark et al. (2004, US) [262]	Hospital	22	Candidemia	*C. parapsilosis*	Multiple	Improved hand hygiene
Posteraro et al. (2004, Italy) [270]	Pediatric oncology	3	Candidemia	*C parapsilosis*	Cross-infection	No intervention
Jang et al. (2005, Korea) [312]	SICU	34	Candiduria	*C. tropicalis*	Urine disposal route	Improvement in urine disposal system

ICU, intensive care unit; NICU, neonatal intensive care unit; TPN, total parenteral nutrition; SICU, surgical intensive care unit.

to another via the hands of healthcare workers is most commonly reported (Table 43-9). *Candida* spp. can survive on environmental surfaces and increase the likelihood of cross-transmission.

Control and Prevention of Nosocomial Yeast Infections

All of the established risk factors for developing nosocomial bacterial BSIs also apply to candidemia, and established prevention guidelines for preventing BSIs should be applied routinely to prevent candidemia as well (See Chapters 29, 37, 38, 42). CDC's HICPAC has no specific guidelines for candidemia prevention in hospitalized patients except for the approaches outlined in the Guidelines for the Prevention of Intravascular Catheter-Related Infections [243,244]. Regardless, several factors should be considered if a persistent problem with *Candida* BSIs or other forms of nosocomial candidiasis is detected in a healthcare setting.

Reducing Gastrointestinal Colonization with Candida

Colonization with *Candida* spp. is the overriding risk factor associated with developing nosocomial candidiasis. Removing the endogenous reservoir should reduce a patient's risk for subsequent disease substantially. Using systemic antifungals (i.e., prophylaxis) before any evidence of active disease is one well-studied method that can accomplish this. Mounting evidence on the efficacy of preventing candidemia in the subset of patients at highest risk for invasive disease has led the HICPAC and IDSA to make specific

recommendations for the HSCT and neutropenic population [245,246]. Because candidiasis usually occurs in the period after transplant but before engraftment, fluconazole should be started on the day of HSCT and continued at least until engraftment [245]. The appropriate duration of prophylaxis is not known, but at least one study has shown a survival benefit when prophylaxis is extended for at least 75 days [247,248]. Because autologous recipients generally have a lower risk for invasive fungal infection than allogeneic recipients have, only autologous recipients with particular conditions (underlying hematologic malignancies, prolonged neutropenia and mucosal damage from intense conditioning regimens or graft manipulation, and recent treatment with fludarabine or 2-CDA) should receive antifungal prophylaxis [245].

Patients who receive solid organ transplants, especially these undergoing orthotopic liver transplantation, also have been identified as being at high risk for invasive candidiasis [249,250]. Various therapies, including amphotericin B deoxycholate, itraconazole, liposomal amphotericin B, and fluconazole have been studied as prophylactic regimens posttransplantation [246]. At this time, the IDSA recommends that only patients with liver transplant who have ≥2 risk factors for invasive fungal disease [251] receive antifungal prophylaxis during the early postoperative period [230]. Prophylaxis in patients receiving liver transplants who are considered low risk and patients receiving pancreas, small-bowel, or other solid organ transplantations is not currently recommended [230].

Prophylaxis could be warranted in ICU patients with high incidence of invasive candidiasis when aggressive infection-control procedures are failing to reduce rates [230, 252,253]. The use of prophylaxis in ICU patients with only low risks of candidiasis could be inappropriate due to the increased risk of adverse drug events and selection of resistant organisms [254]. For example, infections with *Candida* spp. exhibiting reduced susceptibility to fluconazole (e.g., *C. glabrata* or *C. krusei*) could increase as a consequence of the introduction of fluconazole prophylaxis [194,255,256].

A patient population in which the role of antifungal prophylaxis is under increasing study is the neonatal ICU population, specifically extremely low-birth-weight infants (<1,000 grams). Although several studies have documented decreased rates of infection with antifungal prophylaxis [257–260], no consensus on the specific subset of patients in which this approach should be used [261] exists among practitioners. Fewer studies have evaluated this approach in surgical ICU patients. A recent meta-analysis evaluating these studies determined no overall survival benefit among treated patients compared with untreated patients [256].

Preventing Cross-Transmission of Yeast

Currently, standard precautions should be used for all patients with candidemia [243]. Although transmission via healthcare workers' hands could be the pathway for some acquisition of *Candida* spp., most candidemia is thought to be derived from the patient's own flora, so enhanced precautions to prevent person-to-person spread are not justified. Local authorities' identification of an organism of epidemiologic concern (e.g., a particular *Candida* spp. of high virulence or resistance) could justify contact precautions. However, outbreaks of candidemia involving cross-transmission have been associated with sub standard hand hygiene and have been interrupted by improved compliance with standard precautions [262]. Efforts to improve hand hygiene, such as those described in HICPAC guidelines [244], therefore, are relevant to preventing and controlling candidemia. Use of waterless antiseptic agents (e.g., alcohol-based solutions) has gained acceptance, and studies have shown that alcohol-based hand washes are effective against *Candida* spp. [158,263], but efficacy can vary based on the concentration of alcohol in the products, amount of contact time, and burden of yeast present [264,265]. Other hand-hygiene antiseptic agents (e.g., chlorhexidine [2% and 4% aqueous], iodine compounds, iodophors, and phenol derivatives) also have activity against fungi [244].

Molecular Typing of Yeast

Molecular epidemiology has proven useful for implicating the gastrointestinal tract as the most important endogenous reservoir for *Candida* spp. infections [141,236–239] documenting transmission via hands of healthcare workers [262,266–270] and for confirming the source (e.g.,

contaminated infusates, biomedical devices) during outbreak investigations [172,238–242]. In addition, molecular typing methods have documented that strains of *Candida* spp. surviving on environmental surfaces within the hospital can be acquired by patients there [172,271].

Molecular typing methods are rapidly evolving. A variety of methods has been described in detail elsewhere [272, 273]. Techniques used in the past include those based on RFLP with Southern blot hybridization, electrophoretic karyotyping, multilocus enzyme electrophoresis, and PCR-based techniques (e.g., random amplified polymorphic DNA). Newer techniques such as multilocus sequence typing (MLST) and microsatellite typing have performed at least comparably to other established DNA fingerprinting techniques for *C. albicans* [274–276]. MLST is emerging as a powerful tool for subtyping *C. albicans* because it has a high degree of resolution, can characterize large numbers of isolates rapidly, and does not require subjective interpretation of banding patterns [274–276]. MLST also is available for *C. glabrata* and *C. tropicalis*. Other methods, including use of microarrays, which offer the hope of reproducible, high throughput typing, are under development.

REFERENCES

1. Yella LK, Krishan P, Gillege V, Pinto PS. The CT Halo Sign. *Radiology* 2004;230:109–10.
2. Yella LK, Krishnan P, Gillego V. The air crescent sign. A clue to the etiology of chronic necrotizing pneumonia. *Chest* 2005; 127:395–97.
3. Yu VL, Muder RR, Poorsattar A. Significance of isolation of *Aspergillus* from the respiratory tract in diagnosis of invasive pulmonary aspergillosis: Results from a three-year prospective study. *Am J Med* 1986;81:249–54.
4. Horvath JA, Dummer S. The use of respiratory-tract cultures in the diagnosis of invasive pulmonary aspergillosis. *Am J Med* 1996; 100:171–78.
5. Hot A et al. Positron emission scanning with 18-FDG for the diagnosis of invasive fungal infections (IFI). In: 46th Interscience Conference on Antimicrobial Agents and Chemotherapy. San Francisco: 2006: [abstract].
6. Hope WW, Walsh TJ, Denning DW. Laboratory diagnosis of invasive aspergillosis. *Lancet Infect Dis* 2005;5:609–22.
7. Ascioglu S et al. Defining opportunistic invasive fungal infections in immunocompromised patients with cancer and hematopoietic stem cell transplants: An international consensus. *Clin Infect Dis* 2002;34:7–14.
8. Klont RR, Mennink-Kersten MA, Verweij PE. Utility of Aspergillus antigen detection in specimens other than serum specimens. *Clin Infect Dis* 2004;39:1467–74.
9. Baddley JW et al. Invasive mold infections in allogeneic bone marrow transplant recipients. *Clin Infect Dis* 2001;32:1319–24.
10. Jantunen E et al. Incidence and risk factors for invasive fungal infections in allogeneic BMT recipients. *Bone Marrow Transplant* 1997;19:801–8.
11. Morrison VA, Haake RJ, Weisdorf DJ. Non-Candida fungal infections after bone marrow transplantation: Risk factors and outcome. *Am J Med* 1994;96:497–503.
12. Wald A et al. Epidemiology of Aspergillus infections in a large cohort of patients undergoing bone marrow transplantation. *J Infect Dis* 1997;175:1459–66.
13. Bhatti Z et al. Review of epidemiology, diagnosis, and treatment of invasive mould infections in allogeneic hematopoietic stem cell transplant recipients. *Mycopathologia* 2006;162:1–15.

14. Minari A et al. The incidence of invasive aspergillosis among solid organ transplant recipients and implications for prophylaxis in lung transplants. *Transpl Infect Dis* 2002;4:195–200.

15. Montoya JG et al. Infectious complications among 620 consecutive heart transplant patients at Stanford University Medical Center. *Clin Infect Dis* 2001;33:629–40.

16. Paterson DL, Singh N. Invasive aspergillosis in transplant recipients. *Medicine* (Baltimore) 1999;78:123–38.

17. Singh N, Husain S. Aspergillus infections after lung transplantation: Clinical differences in type of transplant and implications for management. *J Heart Lung Transplant* 2003;22:258–66.

18. Hagerty JA et al. Fungal infections in solid organ transplant patients. *Surg Infect (Larchmt)* 2003;4:263–71.

19. De Rosa FG et al. Invasive pulmonary aspergillosis soon after therapy with infliximab, a tumor necrosis factor-alpha-neutralizing antibody: A possible healthcare-associated case? *Infect Control Hosp Epidemiol* 2003;24:477–82.

20. Warris A, Bjorneklett A, Gaustad P. Invasive pulmonary aspergillosis associated with infliximab therapy. *N Engl J Med* 2001; 344:1099–1100.

21. Bongartz T, et al. Anti-TNF antibody therapy in rheumatoid arthritis and the risk of serious infections and malignancies: Systematic review and meta-analysis of rare harmful effects in randomized controlled trials. *JAMA* 2006;295:2275–85.

22. Dasbach EJ, Davies GM, Teutsch SM. Burden of aspergillosis-related hospitalizations in the United States. *Clin Infect Dis* 2000;31:1524–28.

23. Denning DW. Therapeutic outcome in invasive aspergillosis. *Clin Infect Dis* 1996;23:608–15.

24. Herbrecht R et al. Voriconazole versus amphotericin B for primary therapy of invasive aspergillosis. *N Engl J Med* 2002;347: 408–15.

25. Denning DW. Invasive aspergillosis. *Clin Infect Dis* 1998;26:781–805.

26. Marr KA et al. Invasive aspergillosis in allogeneic stem cell transplant recipients: Changes in epidemiology and risk factors. *Blood* 2002;100:4358–66.

27. Martino R et al. Invasive fungal infections after allogeneic peripheral blood stem cell transplantation: Incidence and risk factors in 395 patients. *Br J Haematol* 2002;116:475–82.

28. Grow WB et al. Late onset of invasive aspergillus infection in bone marrow transplant patients at a university hospital. *Bone Marrow Transplant* 2002;29:15–19.

29. Shaukat A et al. Invasive filamentous fungal infections in allogeneic hematopoietic stem cell transplant recipients after recovery from neutropenia: Clinical, radiologic, and pathologic characteristics. *Mycopathologia* 2005;159:181–88.

30. McWhinney PH et al. Progress in the diagnosis and management of aspergillosis in bone marrow transplantation: 13 years' experience. *Clin Infect Dis* 1993;17:397–404.

31. Yuen KY et al. Stage-specific manifestation of mold infections in bone marrow transplant recipients: Risk factors and clinical significance of positive concentrated smears. *Clin Infect Dis* 1997; 25:37–42.

32. Hachem RY et al. Aspergillus terreus: An emerging amphotericin B-resistant opportunistic mold in patients with hematologic malignancies. *Cancer* 2004;101:1594–1600.

33. Baddley JW et al. Epidemiology of Aspergillus terreus at a university hospital. *J Clin Microbiol* 2003;41:5525–29.

34. Iwen PC et al. Invasive pulmonary aspergillosis due to Aspergillus terreus: 12-year experience and review of the literature. *Clin Infect Dis* 1998;26:1092–97.

35. Perfect JR et al. The impact of culture isolation of Aspergillus species: A hospital-based survey of aspergillosis. *Clin Infect Dis* 2001;33:1824–33.

36. Lass-Florl C et al. In-vitro testing of susceptibility to amphotericin B is a reliable predictor of clinical outcome in invasive aspergillosis. *J Antimicrob Chemother* 1998;42:497–502.

37. Sutton DA et al. In vitro amphotericin B resistance in clinical isolates of Aspergillus terreus, with a head-to-head comparison to voriconazole. *J Clin Microbiol* 1999;37:2343–45.

38. Anaissie EJ et al. Pathogenic Aspergillus species recovered from a hospital water system: A 3-year prospective study. *Clin Infect Dis* 2002;34:780–89.

39. Lass-Florl C et al. Aspergillus terreus infections in haematological malignancies: Molecular epidemiology suggests association with in-hospital plants. *J Hosp Infect* 2000;46:31–35.

40. Kontoyiannis DP et al. Significance of aspergillemia in patients with cancer: A 10-year study. *Clin Infect Dis* 2000;31:188–89.

41. Schett G et al. Endocarditis and aortal embolization caused by Aspergillus terreus in a patient with acute lymphoblastic leukemia in remission: Diagnosis by peripheral-blood culture. *J Clin Microbiol* 1998;36:3347–51.

42. Walsh TJ et al. Experimental pulmonary aspergillosis due to Aspergillus terreus: Pathogenesis and treatment of an emerging fungal pathogen resistant to amphotericin B. *J Infect Dis* 2003; 188:305–19.

43. Arnow PM et al. Pumonary aspergillosis during hospital renovation. *Am Rev Respir Dis* 1978;118:49–53.

44. Bryce EA et al. An outbreak of cutaneous aspergillosis in a tertiary-care hospital. *Infect Control Hosp Epidemiol* 1996;17:170–72.

45. Buffington J et al. Investigation of an epidemic of invasive aspergillosis: Utility of molecular typing with the use of random amplified polymorphic DNA probes. *Pediatr Infect Dis J* 1994;13:386–93.

46. Burwen DR et al. Invasive aspergillosis outbreak on a hematology-oncology ward. *Infect Control Hosp Epidemiol* 2001; 22:45–48.

47. Gaspar C et al. [Outbreak of invasive pulmonary mycosis in neutropenic hematologic patients in relation to remodeling construction work]. *Enferm Infecc Microbiol Clin* 1999;17:113–18.

48. Grossman ME et al. Primary cutaneous aspergillosis in six leukemic children. *J Am Acad Dermatol* 1985;12:313–18.

49. Hopkins CC, Weber DJ, Rubin RH. Invasive aspergillus infection: Possible non ward common source within the hospital environment. *J Hosp Infect* 1989;13:19–25.

50. Iwen PC et al. Airborne fungal spore monitoring in a protective environment during hospital construction, and correlation with an outbreak of invasive aspergillosis. *Infect Control Hosp Epidemiol* 1994;15:303–6.

51. Krasinski K et al. Nosocomial fungal infection during hospital renovation. *Infect Control* 1985;6:278–82.

52. Lai KK. A cluster of invasive aspergillosis in a bone marrow transplant unit related to construction and the utility of air sampling. *Am J Infect Control* 2001;29:333–37.

53. Lentino JR et al. Nosocomial aspergillosis: A retrospective review of airborne disease secondary to road construction and contaminated air conditioners. *Am J Epidemiol* 1982;116:430–37.

54. Loo VG et al. Control of construction-associated nosocomial aspergillosis in an antiquated hematology unit. *Infect Control Hosp Epidemiol* 1996;17:360–64.

55. Opal SM et al. Efficacy of infection control measures during a nosocomial outbreak of disseminated aspergillosis associated with hospital construction. *J Infect Dis* 1986;153:634–37.

56. Oren I et al. Invasive pulmonary aspergillosis in neutropenic patients during hospital construction: Before and after chemoprophylaxis and institution of HEPA filters. *Am J Hematol* 2001; 66:257–62.

57. Panackal AA et al. Outbreak of invasive aspergillosis among renal transplant recipients. *Transplantation* 2003;75:1050–53.

58. Ruutu P et al. Invasive pulmonary aspergillosis: A diagnostic and therapeutic problem: Clinical experience with eight haematologic patients. *Scand J Infect Dis* 1987;19:569–75.

59. Ruutu P et al. An outbreak of invasive aspergillosis in a haematologic unit. *Scand J Infect Dis* 1987;19:347–51.

60. Sarubbi FA Jr et al. Increased recovery of Aspergillus flavus from respiratory specimens during hospital construction. *Am Rev Respir Dis* 1982;125:33–38.

61. Tabbara KF, al Jabarti AL, Hospital construction-associated outbreak of ocular aspergillosis after cataract surgery. *Ophthalmology* 1998;105:522–26.

62. Weber SF et al. Interaction of granulocytopenia and construction activity as risk factors for nosocomial invasive filamentous fungal disease in patients with hematologic disorders. *Infect Control Hosp Epidemiol* 1990;11:235–42.

63. Weems JJ Jr et al. Construction activity: An independent risk factor for invasive aspergillosis and zygomycosis in patients with hematologic malignancy. *Infect Control* 1987;8:71–75.

64. Vonberg RP, Gastmeier P. Nosocomial aspergillosis in outbreak settings. *J Hosp Infect* 2006;63:246–54.

65. Flynn PM et al. Aspergillus terreus during hospital renovation. *Infect Control Hosp Epidemiol* 1993;14:363–65.

66. Lutz BD et al. Outbreak of invasive Aspergillus infection in surgical patients, associated with a contaminated air-handling system. *Clin Infect Dis* 2003;37:786–93.

67. Aisner J et al. Aspergillus infections in cancer patients: Association with fireproofing materials in a new hospital. *JAMA* 1976;235:411–12.

68. Arnow PM et al. Endemic and epidemic aspergillosis associated with in-hospital replication of Aspergillus organisms. *J Infect Dis* 1991;164:998–1002.

69. Hruszkewycz V et al. A cluster of pseudofungemia associated with hospital renovation adjacent to the microbiology laboratory. *Infect Control Hosp Epidemiol* 1992;13:147–50.

70. Perraud M et al. Invasive nosocomial pulmonary aspergillosis: Risk factors and hospital building works. *Epidemiol Infect* 1987;99:407–12.

71. Humphreys H et al. An outbreak of aspergillosis in a general ITU. *J Hosp Infect* 1991;18:167–77.

72. Gerson SL et al. Aspergillosis due to carpet contamination. *Infect Control Hosp Epidemiol* 1994;15:221–23.

73. Laurel VL et al. Pseudoepidemic of Aspergillus niger infections traced to specimen contamination in the microbiology laboratory. *J Clin Microbiol* 1999;37:1612–16.

74. Hospenthal DR, Kwon-Chung KJ, Bennett JE. Concentrations of airborne Aspergillus compared to the incidence of invasive aspergillosis. Lack of correlation. *Med Mycol* 1998;36:165–68.

75. Leenders AC et al. Density and molecular epidemiology of Aspergillus in air and relationship to outbreaks of Aspergillus infection. *J Clin Microbiol* 1999;37:1752–57.

76. Sehulster L, Chinn RY. Guidelines for environmental infection control in health-care facilities: Recommendations of CDC and the Healthcare Infection Control Practices Advisory Committee (HICPAC). *MMWR Recomm Rep* 2003;52(RR-10).1–42.

77. Tablan OC, Anderson LJ, Besser R, et al. Guidelines for preventing health-care-associated pneumonia, 2003: Recommendations of CDC and the Healthcare Infection Control Practices Advisory Committee. *MMWR Recomm Rep* 2004;53(RR-3):1–36.

78. Anaissie EJ, Costa SF. Nosocomial aspergillosis is waterborne. *Clin Infect Dis* 2001;33:1546–48.

79. Anaissie EJ et al. Cleaning patient shower facilities: A novel approach to reducing patient exposure to aerosolized Aspergillus species and other opportunistic molds. *Clin Infect Dis* 2002;35:E86–88.

80. Anaissie EJ et al. Pathogenic molds (including Aspergillus species) in hospital water distribution systems: A 3-year prospective study and clinical implications for patients with hematologic malignancies. *Blood* 2003;101:2542–46.

81. Arvanitidou M et al. The occurrence of fungi in hospital and community potable waters. *Lett Appl Microbiol* 1999;29:81–84.

82. Arvanitidou M et al. High level of recovery of fungi from water and dialysate in haemodialysis units. *J Hosp Infect* 2000;45:225–30.

83. Warris A et al. Recovery of filamentous fungi from water in a paediatric bone marrow transplantation unit. *J Hosp Infect* 2001;47:143–48.

84. Warris A et al. Contamination of hospital water with Aspergillus fumigatus and other molds. *Clin Infect Dis* 2002;34:1159–60.

85. James MJ et al. Use of a repetitive DNA probe to type clinical and environmental isolates of Aspergillus flavus from a cluster of cutaneous infections in a neonatal intensive care unit. *J Clin Microbiol* 2000;38:3612–18.

86. Bouakline A et al. Fungal contamination of food in hematology units. *J Clin Microbiol* 2000;38:4272–73.

87. De Bock R et al. Aspergillus in pepper. *Lancet* 1989;2:331–32.

88. Pegues DA et al. Cluster of cases of invasive aspergillosis in a transplant intensive care unit: Evidence of person-to-person airborne transmission. *Clin Infect Dis* 2002;34:412–16.

89. Sopena N, Sabria M. Multicenter study of hospital-acquired pneumonia in non-ICU patients. *Chest* 2005;127:213–19.

90. Bocquet P et al. [The epidemiological surveillance network for nosocomial invasive aspergillosis of the Assistance Publique-Hopitaux de Paris]. *Ann Med Interne* (Paris) 1995;146:79–83.

91. Patterson JE et al. Hospital epidemiologic surveillance for invasive aspergillosis: Patient demographics and the utility of antigen detection. *Infect Control Hosp Epidemiol* 1997;18:104–8.

92. Chazalet V et al. Molecular typing of environmental and patient isolates of Aspergillus fumigatus from various hospital settings. *J Clin Microbiol* 1998;36:1494–1500.

93. Walsh TJ et al. Infections due to emerging and uncommon medically important fungal pathogens. *Clin Microbiol Infect* 2004;10:48–66.

94. Mandell GL et al. *Mandell, Douglas, and Bennett: Principles and Practice of Infectious Diseases.* 6th ed. Philadelphia: Elsevier, 2005.

95. Everett ED, Pearson S, Rogers W. Rhizopus surgical wound infection with elasticized adhesive tape dressings. *Arch Surg* 1979;114:738–39.

96. Holzel H et al. Rhizopus microsporus in wooden tongue depressors: A major threat or minor inconvenience? *J Hosp Infect* 1998;38:113–18.

97. Mead JH et al. Cutaneous Rhizopus infection: Occurrence as a postoperative complication associated with an elasticized adhesive dressing. *JAMA* 1979;242:272–74.

98. Mitchell SJ et al. Nosocomial infection with Rhizopus microsporus in preterm infants: Association with wooden tongue depressors. *Lancet* 1996;348.441–43.

99. Verweij PE et al. Wooden sticks as the source of a pseudoepidemic of infection with Rhizopus microsporus var. rhizopodiformis among immunocompromised patients. *J Clin Microbiol* 1997;35:2422–23.

100. LeMaile-Williams M et al. Outbreak of cutaneous infections with Rhizopus arrhizus associated with Karaya ostomy bags. *Clin Infect Dis* in press.

101. Hayes D Jr. Nosocomial pulmonary Rhizopus diagnosed by bronchoalveolar lavage with cytology in a child with acute lymphoblastic leukemia. *Pediatr Hematol Oncol* 2006;23:323–27.

102. Passos XS et al. Nosocomial invasive infection caused by Cunninghamella bertholletiae: Case report. *Mycopathologia* 2006;161:33–35.

103. Passamonte PM, Dix JD. Nosocomial pulmonary mucormycosis with fatal massive hemoptysis. *Am J Med Sci* 1985;289:65–67.

104. Abzug MJ et al. Heliport associated nosocomial mucormycoses. *Infect Control Hosp Epidemiol* 1992;13:325–26.

105. Roden MM et al. Epidemiology and outcome of zygomycosis: A review of 929 reported cases. *Clin Infect Dis* 2005;41:634–53.

106. Vigouroux S et al. Zygomycosis after prolonged use of voriconazole in immunocompromised patients with hematologic disease: Attention required. *Clin Infect Dis* 2005;40:e35–37.

107. Walsh TJ et al. Voriconazole compared with liposomal amphotericin B for empirical antifungal therapy in patients with neutropenia and persistent fever. *N Engl J Med* 2002;346:225–34.

108. Imhof A et al. Breakthrough fungal infections in stem cell transplant recipients receiving voriconazole. *Clin Infect Dis* 2004;39:743–76.

109. Kontoyiannis DP et al. Zygomycosis in a tertiary-care cancer center in the era of Aspergillus-active antifungal therapy: A case-control observational study of 27 recent cases. *J Infect Dis* 2005;191:1350–60.

110. Marty FM, Cosimi LA, Baden LR. Breakthrough zygomycosis after voriconazole treatment in recipients of hematopoietic stem-cell transplants. *N Engl J Med* 2004;350:950–52.

111. Siwek GT et al. Invasive zygomycosis in hematopoietic stem cell transplant recipients receiving voriconazole prophylaxis. *Clin Infect Dis* 2004;39:584–87.

112. Marr KA et al. Epidemiology and outcome of mould infections in hematopoietic stem cell transplant recipients. *Clin Infect Dis* 2002;34:909–17.

113. Anaissie EJ et al. Fusariosis associated with pathogenic fusarium species colonization of a hospital water system: A new paradigm for the epidemiology of opportunistic mold infections. *Clin Infect Dis* 2001;33:1871–78.

114. Nucci M et al. Fusarium infection in hematopoietic stem cell transplant recipients. *Clin Infect Dis* 2004;38:1237–42.

115. Fleming RV, Walsh TJ, Anaissie EJ. Emerging and less common fungal pathogens. *Infect Dis Clin North Am* 2002;16.915–33.

116. Husain S et al. Infections due to Scedosporium apiospermum and Scedosporium prolificans in transplant recipients: Clinical

characteristics and impact of antifungal agent therapy on outcome. *Clin Infect Dis* 2005;40:89–99.

117. Lionakis MS et al. The significance of blood cultures positive for emerging saprophytic moulds in cancer patients. *Clin Microbiol Infect* 2004;10:922–25.

118. Pfaller MA, Diekema DJ. Rare and emerging opportunistic fungal pathogens: Concern for resistance beyond Candida albicans and Aspergillus fumigatus. *J Clin Microbiol* 2004;42:4419–31.

119. Morris G et al. Sampling of Aspergillus spores in air. *J Hosp Infect* 2000;44:81–92.

120. Martinez KF, Rao CY, Burton NC. Exposure assessment and analysis for biological agents. *Grana* 2004;43:93–208.

121. Blanc DS. The use of molecular typing for epidemiological surveillance and investigation of endemic nosocomial infections. *Infect Genet Evol* 2004;4:193–97.

122. Warnock DW, Hajjeh RA, Lasker BA. Epidemiology and prevention of invasive aspergillosis. *Curr Infect Dis Rep* 2001;3:507–16.

123. Brandt M et al. Mold prevention strategies and possible health effects in the aftermath of hurricanes and major floods. *MMWR Recomm Rep* 2006;55(RR-8):1–27.

124. Tovey ER, Green BJ. Measuring environmental fungal exposure. *Med Mycol* 2005;43:S67–70.

125. Sherertz RJ et al. Impact of air filtration on nosocomial Aspergillus infections: Unique risk of bone marrow transplant recipients. *Am J Med* 1987;83:709–18.

126. Rice N, Streifel A, Vesley D. An evaluation of hospital special-ventilation-room pressures. *Infect Control Hosp Epidemiol* 2001;22:19–23.

127. Thio CL et al. Refinements of environmental assessment during an outbreak investigation of invasive aspergillosis in a leukemia and bone marrow transplant unit. *Infect Control Hosp Epidemiol* 2000;21:18–23.

128. Kruger WH et al. Effective protection of allogeneic stem cell recipients against Aspergillosis by HEPA air filtration during a period of construction—A prospective survey. *J Hematother Stem Cell Res* 2003;12:301–7.

129. Humphreys H. Positive-pressure isolation and the prevention of invasive aspergillosis: What is the evidence? *J Hosp Infect* 2004;56:93–100.

130. Hubel K, Engert A. Clinical applications of granulocyte colony-stimulating factor: An update and summary. *Ann Hematol* 2003;82:207–13.

131. Maertens J et al. Galactomannan and computed tomography-based preemptive antifungal therapy in neutropenic patients at high risk for invasive fungal infection: A prospective feasibility study. *Clin Infect Dis* 2005;41:1242–50.

132. Florent M et al. Prospective evaluation of a polymerase chain reaction-ELISA targeted to Aspergillus fumigatus and Aspergillus flavus for the early diagnosis of invasive aspergillosis in patients with hematological malignancies. *J Infect Dis* 2006;193:741–47.

133. Bow EJ. Long-term antifungal prophylaxis in high-risk hematopoietic stem cell transplant recipients. *Med Mycol* 2005;43: S277–87.

134. Anaissie EJ, Penzak SR, Dignani MC. The hospital water supply as a source of nosocomial infections: A plea for action. *Arch Intern Med* 2002;162:1483–92.

135. Eggimann P, Garbino J, Pittet D. Epidemiology of Candida species infections in critically ill non-immunosuppressed patients. *Lancet Infect Dis* 2003;3:685–702.

136. Karabinis A et al. Risk factors for candidemia in cancer patients: A case-control study. *J Clin Microbiol* 1988;26:429–32.

137. Richet HM et al. Risk factors for candidemia in patients with acute lymphocytic leukemia. *Rev Infect Dis* 1991;13:211–15.

138. Wey SB et al. Hospital-acquired candidemia: The attributable mortality and excess length of stay. *Arch Intern Med* 1988;148: 2642–45.

139. Klempp-Selb B, Rimek D, Kappe R. Karyotyping of Candida albicans and Candida glabrata from patients with Candida sepsis. *Mycoses* 2000;43:159–63.

140. Pittet D et al. Contour-clamped homogeneous electric field gel electrophoresis as a powerful epidemiologic tool in yeast infections. *Am J Med* 1991;91:256S–263S.

141. Reagan DR et al. Characterization of the sequence of colonization and nosocomial candidemia using DNA fingerprinting and a DNA probe. *J Clin Microbiol* 1990;28:2733–38.

142. Reef SE et al. Nonperinatal nosocomial transmission of Candida albicans in a neonatal intensive care unit: Prospective study. *J Clin Microbiol* 1998;36:1255–59.

143. Saiman L et al. Risk factors for candidemia in neonatal intensive care unit patients: The National Epidemiology of Mycosis Survey study group. *Pediatr Infect Dis J* 2000;19:319–24.

144. Blot SI et al. Effects of nosocomial candidemia on outcomes of critically ill patients. *Am J Med* 2002;113:480–85.

145. Borzotta AP, Beardsley K. Candida infections in critically ill trauma patients: A retrospective case-control study. *Arch Surg* 1999;134:657–65.

146. Calandra T et al. Clinical significance of Candida isolated from peritoneum in surgical patients. *Lancet* 1989;2:1437–40.

147. Petri MG et al. Epidemiology of invasive mycosis in ICU patients: A prospective multicenter study in 435 non-neutropenic patients. Paul-Ehrlich Society for Chemotherapy, Divisions of Mycology and Pneumonia Research. *Intensive Care Med* 1997;23:317–25.

148. Blumberg HM et al. Risk factors for candidal bloodstream infections in surgical intensive care unit patients: The NEMIS prospective multicenter study: The National Epidemiology of Mycosis Survey. *Clin Infect Dis* 2001;33:177–86.

149. Kennedy MJ, Volz PA. Effect of various antibiotics on gastrointestinal colonization and dissemination by Candida albicans. *Sabouraudia* 1985;23:265–73.

150. Pappu-Katikaneni LD, Rao KP, Banister E. Gastrointestinal colonization with yeast species and Candida septicemia in very low birth weight infants. *Mycoses* 1990;33:20–23.

151. Samonis G et al. Prospective evaluation of effects of broad-spectrum antibiotics on gastrointestinal yeast colonization of humans. *Antimicrob Agents Chemother* 1993;37:51–53.

152. Abi-Said D et al. The epidemiology of hematogenous candidiasis caused by different Candida species. *Clin Infect Dis* 1997;24: 1122–28.

153. Nucci M, Colombo AL. Risk factors for breakthrough candidemia. *Eur J Clin Microbiol Infect Dis* 2002;21:209–11.

154. Wisplinghoff H et al. Nosocomial bloodstream infections in US hospitals: Analysis of 24,179 cases from a prospective nationwide surveillance study. *Clin Infect Dis* 2004;39:309–17.

155. Morgan J et al. Excess mortality, hospital stay, and cost due to candidemia: A case-control study using data from population-based candidemia surveillance. *Infect Control Hosp Epidemiol* 2005;26:540–47.

156. Gudlaugsson O et al. Attributable mortality of nosocomial candidemia, revisited. *Clin Infect Dis* 2003;37:1172–77.

157. Fridkin SK et al. Changing incidence of Candida bloodstream infections among NICU patients in the United States: 1995–2004. *Pediatrics* 2006;117:1680–87.

158. Trick WE et al. Secular trend of hospital-acquired candidemia among intensive care unit patients in the United States during 1989–1999. *Clin Infect Dis* 2002;35:627–30.

159. Martin GS et al. The epidemiology of sepsis in the United States from 1979 through 2000. *N Engl J Med* 2003;348:1546–54.

160. Hajjeh RA et al. Incidence of bloodstream infections due to Candida species and in vitro susceptibilities of isolates collected from 1998 to 2000 in a population-based active surveillance program. *J Clin Microbiol* 2004;42:1519–27.

161. Morgan J. Global trends in candidemia: Review of reports from 1995–2005. *Curr Infect Dis Rep* 2005;7:429–39.

162. Ostrosky-Zeichner L et al. Antifungal susceptibility survey of 2,000 bloodstream Candida isolates in the United States. *Antimicrob Agents Chemother* 2003;47:3149–54.

163. Pfaller MA, Diekema DJ. Twelve years of fluconazole in clinical practice: Global trends in species distribution and fluconazole susceptibility of bloodstream isolates of Candida. *Clin Microbiol Infect* 2004;10:11–23.

164. Pfaller MA et al. In vitro susceptibilities of rare Candida bloodstream isolates to ravuconazole and three comparative antifungal agents. *Diagn Microbiol Infect Dis* 2004;48:101–5.

165. Baran J Jr, Muckatira B, Khatib R. Candidemia before and during the fluconazole era: Prevalence, type of species and approach to treatment in a tertiary care community hospital. *Scand J Infect Dis* 2001;33:137–39.

166. Colombo AL. Outbreak of Candida rugosa candidemia: An emerging pathogen that may be refractory to amphotericin B therapy. *Diagn Microbiol Infect Dis* 2003;46:253–57.

167. Dube MP et al. Fungemia and colonization with nystatin-resistant Candida rugosa in a burn unit. *Clin Infect Dis* 1994;18: 77–82.

168. Hawkins JL, Baddour LM. Candida lusitaniae infections in the era of fluconazole availability. *Clin Infect Dis* 2003;36:e14–18.

169. Jabra-Rizk MA et al. Prevalence of Candida dubliniensis fungemia at a large teaching hospital. *Clin Infect Dis* 2005;41: 1064–67.

170. Krcmery V Jr et al. Nosocomial Candida krusei fungemia in cancer patients: Report of 10 cases and review. *J Chemother* 1999;11:131–36.

171. Mardani M et al. Nosocomial Candida guilliermondii fungemia in cancer patients. *Infect Control Hosp Epidemiol* 2000;21:336–37.

172. Sanchez V et al. Epidemiology of nosocomial acquisition of Candida lusitaniae. *J Clin Microbiol* 1992;30:3005–8.

173. Tietz HJ, Czaika V, Sterry W. Case report: Osteomyelitis caused by high resistant Candida guilliermondii. *Mycoses* 1999;42:577–80.

174. Anaissie EJ et al. Predictors of adverse outcome in cancer patients with candidemia. *Am J Med* 1998;104:238–45.

175. Fraser VJ et al. Candidemia in a tertiary care hospital: Epidemiology, risk factors, and predictors of mortality. *Clin Infect Dis* 1992; 15:414–21.

176. Girmenia C, Martino P. Fluconazole and the changing epidemiology of candidemia. *Clin Infect Dis* 1998;27:232–34.

177. Horn R et al. Fungemia in a cancer hospital: Changing frequency, earlier onset, and results of therapy. *Rev Infect Dis* 1985;7:646–55.

178. Safdar A et al. Prospective study of Candida species in patients at a comprehensive cancer center. *Antimicrob Agents Chemother* 2001;45:2129–33.

179. Viscoli C et al. Candidemia in cancer patients: A prospective, multicenter surveillance study by the Invasive Fungal Infection Group (IFIG) of the European Organization for Research and Treatment of Cancer (EORTC). *Clin Infect Dis* 1999;28:1071–79.

180. Wingard JR et al. Association of Torulopsis glabrata infections with fluconazole prophylaxis in neutropenic bone marrow transplant patients. *Antimicrob Agents Chemother* 1993;37:1847–49.

181. Hope W, Morton A, Eisen DP. Increase in prevalence of nosocomial non-Candida albicans candidaemia and the association of Candida krusei with fluconazole use. *J Hosp Infect* 2002;50:56–65.

182. Malani PN et al. Trends in species causing fungaemia in a tertiary care medical centre over 12 years. *Mycoses* 2001;44:446–49.

183. Debusk CH et al. Candidemia: Current epidemiologic characteristics and a long-term follow-up of the survivors. *Scand J Infect Dis* 1994;26:697–703.

184. Mathews MS, Samuel PR, Suresh M. Emergence of Candida tropicalis as the major cause of fungaemia in India. *Mycoses* 2001; 44:278–80.

185. Sandven P et al. Constant low rate of fungemia in norway, 1991 to 1996: The Norwegian Yeast Study Group. *J Clin Microbiol* 1998; 36:3455–59.

186. Krcmery V Jr, Kovacicova G. Longitudinal 10 year prospective survey of fungaemia in Slovak Republic: Trends in etiology in 310 episodes. Slovak Fungaemia study group. *Diagn Microbiol Infect Dis* 2000;36:7–11.

187. Schelenz S, Gransden WR. Candidaemia in a London teaching hospital: Analysis of 128 cases over a 7-year period. *Mycoses* 2003; 46:390–96.

188. Tortorano AM et al. Epidemiology of candidaemia in Europe: Results of 28-month European Confederation of Medical Mycology (ECMM) hospital-based surveillance study. *Eur J Clin Microbiol Infect Dis* 2004;23:317–22.

189. Beck-Sague C, Jarvis WR. Secular trends in the epidemiology of nosocomial fungal infections in the United States, 1980–1990: National Nosocomial Infections Surveillance System. *J Infect Dis* 1993;167:1247–51.

190. Diekema DJ et al. Epidemiology of candidemia: 3-year results from the emerging infections and the epidemiology of Iowa organisms study. *J Clin Microbiol* 2002;40:1298–1302.

191. Edgeworth JD, Treacher DF, Eykyn SJ. A 25-year study of nosocomial bacteremia in an adult intensive care unit. *Crit Care Med* 1999;27:1421–28.

192. Kao AS et al. The epidemiology of candidemia in two United States cities: Results of a population-based active surveillance. *Clin Infect Dis* 1999;29:1164–70.

193. Macphail GL et al. Epidemiology, treatment and outcome of candidemia: A five-year review at three Canadian hospitals. *Mycoses* 2002;45:141–45.

194. Pfaller MA et al. National surveillance of nosocomial blood stream infection due to Candida albicans: Frequency of occurrence and antifungal susceptibility in the SCOPE Program. *Diagn Microbiol Infect Dis* 1998;31:327–32.

195. Gleason TG et al. Emerging evidence of selection of fluconazole-tolerant fungi in surgical intensive care units. *Arch Surg* 1997;132: 1197–1202.

196. Pfaller MA et al. Geographic variation in the susceptibilities of invasive isolates of Candida glabrata to seven systemically active antifungal agents: A global assessment from the ARTEMIS Antifungal Surveillance Program conducted in 2001 and 2002. *J Clin Microbiol* 2004;42:3142–46.

197. Erer B et al. Trichosporon beigelii: A life-threatening pathogen in immunocompromised hosts. *Bone Marrow Transplant* 2000;25: 745–49.

198. Hoy J et al. Trichosporon beigelii infection: A review. *Rev Infect Dis* 1986;8:959–67.

199. Krcmery V Jr et al. Hematogenous trichosporonosis in cancer patients: Report of 12 cases including 5 during prophylaxis with itraconazol. *Support Care Cancer* 1999;7:39–43.

200. Walsh TJ et al. Trichosporon beigelii, an emerging pathogen resistant to amphotericin B. *J Clin Microbiol* 1990;28:1616–22.

201. Walsh TJ et al. Trichosporonosis in patients with neoplastic disease. *Medicine* (Baltimore), 1986;65:268–79.

202. Alter SJ, Farley J. Development of Hansenula anomala infection in a child receiving fluconazole therapy. *Pediatr Infect Dis J* 1994; 13:158–59.

203. Chang HJ et al. An epidemic of Malassezia pachydermatis in an intensive care nursery associated with colonization of health care workers' pet dogs. *N Engl J Med* 1998;338:706–11.

204. Mickelsen PA et al. Clinical and microbiological features of infection with Malassezia pachydermatis in high-risk infants. *J Infect Dis* 1988;157:1163–68.

205. Diekema DJ et al. Activities of caspofungin, itraconazole, posaconazole, ravuconazole, voriconazole, and amphotericin B against 448 recent clinical isolates of filamentous fungi. *J Clin Microbiol* 2003;41:3623–26.

206. Galan-Sanchez F et al. Microbiological characteristics and susceptibility patterns of strains of Rhodotorula isolated from clinical samples. *Mycopathologia* 1999;145:109–12.

207. Zaas AK et al. Risk of fungemia due to Rhodotorula and antifungal susceptibility testing of Rhodotorula isolates. *J Clin Microbiol* 2003;41:5233–35.

208. Ramos JM et al. Clinical case of endocarditis due to Trichosporon inkin and antifungal susceptibility profile of the organism. *J Clin Microbiol* 2004;42:2341–44.

209. Antachopoulos C et al. Fungemia due to Trichosporon asahii in a neutropenic child refractory to amphotericin B: Clearance with voriconazole. *J Pediatr Hematol Oncol* 2005;27:283–85.

210. Girmenia C et al. Invasive infections caused by Trichosporon species and Geotrichum capitatum in patients with hematological malignancies: A retrospective multicenter study from Italy and review of the literature. *J Clin Microbiol* 2005;43:1818–28.

211. Krzossok S et al. Trichosporon asahii infection of a dialysis PTFE arteriovenous graft. *Clin Nephrol* 2004;62:66–68.

212. Yang R et al. Disseminated trichosporonosis in China. *Mycoses* 2003;46:519–23.

213. Marty FM et al. Disseminated trichosporonosis caused by Trichosporon loubieri. *J Clin Microbiol* 2003;41:5317–20.

214. Yildiran A et al. Disseminated Trichosporon asahii infection in a preterm. *Am J Perinatol* 2003;20:269–71.

215. Nettles RE et al. Successful treatment of Trichosporon mucoides infection with fluconazole in a heart and kidney transplant recipient. *Clin Infect Dis* 2003;36:E63–66.

216. Meyer MH et al. Chronic disseminated Trichosporon asahii infection in a leukemic child. *Clin Infect Dis* 2002;35:e22–25.

217. Gokahmetoglu S et al. Case reports: Trichosporon mucoides infection in three premature newborns. *Mycoses* 2002;45:123–25.

218. Panagopoulou P et al. Trichosporon asahii: An unusual cause of invasive infection in neonates. *Pediatr Infect Dis J* 2002; 21:169–70.

219. Wolf DG et al. Multidrug-resistant Trichosporon asahii infection of nongranulocytopenic patients in three intensive care units. *J Clin Microbiol* 2001;39:4420–25.

220. Falk R et al. Multidrug-resistant Trichosporon asahii isolates are susceptible to voriconazole. *J Clin Microbiol* 2003;41:911.

221. Paphitou NI et al. In vitro antifungal susceptibilities of Trichosporon species. *Antimicrob Agents Chemother* 2002;46:1144–46.

222. Fournier S et al. Use of voriconazole to successfully treat disseminated Trichosporon asahii infection in a patient with acute myeloid leukaemia. *Eur J Clin Microbiol Infect Dis* 2002; 21:892–96.

223. Braun DK, Kauffman CA. Rhodotorula fungaemia: A life-threatening complication of indwelling central venous catheters. *Mycoses* 1992;35:305–8.

224. Eisenberg ES et al. Rhodotorula rubra peritonitis in patients undergoing continuous ambulatory peritoneal dialysis. *Am J Med* 1983;75:349–52.

225. Guerra R et al. Rhodotorula glutinis keratitis. *Int Ophthalmol* 1992;16:187–90.

226. Hsueh PR et al. Catheter-related sepsis due to Rhodotorula glutinis. *J Clin Microbiol* 2003;41:857–59.

227. Lanzafame M et al. Rhodotorula glutinis-related meningitis. *J Clin Microbiol* 2001;39:410.

228. Maeder M et al. Aortic homograft endocarditis caused by Rhodotorula mucilaginosa. *Infection* 2003;31:181–83.

229. Diekema DJ et al. Activities of available and investigational antifungal agents against rhodotorula species. *J Clin Microbiol* 2005;43:476–78.

230. Pappas PG et al. Guidelines for treatment of candidiasis. *Clin Infect Dis* 2004;38:161–89.

231. (no author). Development of in vitro susceptibility testing criteria and quality control parameters. Approved guideline. Villanova, PA: Clinical and Laboratory Standards Institute, 2001.

232. (no author) Reference method for broth dilution antifungal susceptibility testing of filamentous fungi: Approved standard. NCCLS document M38-A. Villanova, PA: Clinical and Laboratory Standards Institute, 2002.

233. (no author) Reference method for broth dilution antifungal susceptibility testing of yeasts: Approved standard, 2nd ed. NCCLS document M27-A2. Villanova, PA: Clinical and Laboratory Standards Institute, 2002.

234. Arthington-Skaggs BA et al. Comparison of visual and spectrophotometric methods of broth microdilution MIC end point determination and evaluation of a sterol quantitation method for in vitro susceptibility testing of fluconazole and itraconazole against trailing and nontrailing Candida isolates. *Antimicrob Agents Chemother* 2002;46:2477–81.

235. Rex JH et al. Practice guidelines for the treatment of candidiasis. Infectious Diseases Society of America. *Clin Infect Dis* 2000; 30:662–78.

236. Voss A et al. Investigation of the sequence of colonization and candidemia in nonneutropenic patients. *J Clin Microbiol* 1994; 32:975–80.

237. Pfaller MA et al. Strain variation and antifungal susceptibility among bloodstream isolates of Candida species from 21 different medical institutions. *Clin Infect Dis* 1995;21:1507–9.

238. Cormican MG, Hollis RJ, Pfaller MA. DNA macrorestriction profiles and antifungal susceptibility of Candida (Torulopsis) glabrata. *Diagn Microbiol Infect Dis* 1996;25:83–87.

239. Marco F et al. Elucidating the origins of nosocomial infections with Candida albicans by DNA fingerprinting with the complex probe Ca3. *J Clin Microbiol* 1999;37:2817–28.

240. Doebbeling BN et al. Restriction fragment analysis of a Candida tropicalis outbreak of sternal wound infections. *J Clin Microbiol* 1991;29:1268–70.

241. Lupetti A et al. Horizontal transmission of Candida parapsilosis candidemia in a neonatal intensive care unit. *J Clin Microbiol* 2002;40:2363–69.

242. Vazquez JA et al. Nosocomial acquisition of Candida albicans: An epidemiologic study. *J Infect Dis* 1993;168:195–201.

243. O'Grady NP et al. Guidelines for the prevention of intravascular catheter-related infections. *Infect Control Hosp Epidemiol* 2002;23:759–69.

244. Boyce JM, Pittet D. Guideline for hand hygiene in healthcare settings: Recommendations of the Healthcare Infection Control Practices Advisory Committee and the HICPAC/ SHEA/APIC/IDSA Hand Hygiene Task Force. Society for Healthcare Epidemiology of America/Association for Professionals in Infection Control/Infectious Diseases Society of America. *MMWR Recomm Rep* 2002;51(RR-16):1–45.

245. Dykewicz CA. Guidelines for preventing opportunistic infections among hematopoietic stem cell transplant recipients: Focus on community respiratory virus infections. *Biol Blood Marrow Transplant* 2001;7:19S–22S.

246. Hughes WT et al. 2002 guidelines for the use of antimicrobial agents in neutropenic patients with cancer. *Clin Infect Dis* 2002; 34:730–51.

247. Marr KA et al. Prolonged fluconazole prophylaxis is associated with persistent protection against candidiasis-related death in allogeneic marrow transplant recipients: Long-term follow-up of a randomized, placebo-controlled trial. *Blood* 2000;96:2055–61.

248. Slavin MA et al. Efficacy and safety of fluconazole prophylaxis for fungal infections after marrow transplantation—A prospective, randomized, double-blind study. *J Infect Dis* 1995;171:1545–52.

249. Hadley S, Karchmer AW. Fungal infections in solid organ transplant recipients. *Infect Dis Clin North Am* 1995;9:1045–74.

250. Karchmer AW et al. Fungal infections complicating orthotopic liver transplantation. *Trans Am Clin Climatol Assoc* 1994;106: 38–48.

251. Collins LA et al. Risk factors for invasive fungal infections complicating orthotopic liver transplantation. *J Infect Dis* 1994; 170:644–52.

252. Eggimann P et al. Fluconazole prophylaxis prevents intra-abdominal candidiasis in high-risk surgical patients. *Crit Care Med* 1999;27:1066–72.

253. Pelz RK et al. Double-blind placebo-controlled trial of fluconazole to prevent candidal infections in critically ill surgical patients. *Ann Surg* 2001;233:542–48.

254. Rex JH, Sobel JD. Prophylactic antifungal therapy in the intensive care unit. *Clin Infect Dis* 2001;32:1191–1200.

255. Shorr AF et al. Fluconazole prophylaxis in critically ill surgical patients: A meta-analysis. *Crit Care Med* 2005;33:1928–36.

256. Vardakas KZ et al. Antifungal prophylaxis with azoles in high-risk, surgical intensive care unit patients: A meta-analysis of randomized, placebo-controlled trials. *Crit Care Med* 2006;34: 1216–24.

257. Kaufman DA et al. Patterns of fungal colonization in preterm infants weighing less than 1000 grams at birth. *Pediatr Infect Dis J* 2006;25:733–37.

258. Kicklighter SD et al. Fluconazole for prophylaxis against candidal rectal colonization in the very low birth weight infant. *Pediatrics* 2001;107:293–98.

259. Manzoni P et al. Prophylactic fluconazole is effective in preventing fungal colonization and fungal systemic infections in preterm neonates: A single-center, 6-year, retrospective cohort study. *Pediatrics* 2006;117:e22–32.

260. Bertini G et al. Fluconazole prophylaxis prevents invasive fungal infection in high-risk, very low birth weight infants. *J Pediatr* 2005;147:162–65.

261. Benjamin DK Jr et al. Neonatal candidiasis among extremely low birth weight infants: Risk factors, mortality rates, and neurodevelopmental outcomes at 18 to 22 months. *Pediatrics* 2006;117:84–92.

262. Clark TA et al. Epidemiologic and molecular characterization of an outbreak of Candida parapsilosis bloodstream infections in a community hospital. *J Clin Microbiol* 2004;42:4468–72.

263. Mody L et al. Introduction of a waterless alcohol-based hand rub in a long-term-care facility. *Infect Control Hosp Epidemiol* 2003;24: 165–71.

264. Kampf G et al. Spectrum of antimicrobial activity and user acceptability of the hand disinfectant agent Sterillium Gel. *J Hosp Infect* 2002;52:141–47.

265. Kampf G, Meyer B, Goroncy-Bermes P. Comparison of two test methods for the determination of sufficient antimicrobial activity

of three commonly used alcohol-based hand rubs for hygienic hand disinfection. *J Hosp Infect* 2003;55:220–25.

266. Barchiesi F et al. Outbreak of fungemia due to Candida parapsilosis in a pediatric oncology unit. *Diagn Microbiol Infect Dis* 2004;49:269–71.

267. Huang YC et al. Outbreak of Candida parapsilosis fungemia in neonatal intensive care units: Clinical implications and genotyping analysis. *Infection* 1999;27:97–102.

268. Huang YC et al. Outbreak of Candida albicans fungaemia in a neonatal intensive care unit. *Scand J Infect Dis* 1998;30:137–42.

269. Levin AS et al. Candida parapsilosis fungemia associated with implantable and semi implantable central venous catheters and the hands of healthcare workers. *Diagn Microbiol Infect Dis* 1998;30:243–49.

270. Posteraro B et al. Candida parapsilosis bloodstream infection in pediatric oncology patients: Results of an epidemiologic investigation. *Infect Control Hosp Epidemiol* 2004;25:641–45.

271. Sanchez V et al. Nosocomial acquisition of Candida parapsilosis: An epidemiologic study. *Am J Med* 1993;94:577–82.

272. Soll DR. The ins and outs of DNA fingerprinting the infectious fungi. *Clin Microbiol Rev* 2000;13:332–70

273. Gil-Lamaignere C et al. Molecular typing for fungi—A critical review of the possibilities and limitations of currently and future methods. *Clin Microbiol Infect* 2003;9:172–85.

274. Bougnoux ME et al. Collaborative consensus for optimized multilocus sequence typing of Candida albicans. *J Clin Microbiol* 2003;41:5265–66.

275. Chowdhary A et al. Comparison of multilocus sequence typing and Ca3 fingerprinting for molecular subtyping epidemiologically-related clinical isolates of Candida albicans. *Med Mycol* 2006;44:405–17.

276. Robles JC et al. Multilocus sequence typing is a reliable alternative method to DNA fingerprinting for discriminating among strains of Candida albicans. *J Clin Microbiol* 2004;42:2480–88.

277. Myoken Y et al. Molecular epidemiology of invasive stomatitis due to Aspergillus flavus in patients with acute leukemia. *J Oral Pathol Med* 2003;32:215–18.

278. Hahn T et al. Efficacy of high-efficiency particulate air filtration in preventing aspergillosis in immunocompromised patients with hematologic malignancies. *Infect Control Hosp Epidemiol* 2002;23:525–31.

279. Singer S et al. Outbreak of systemic aspergillosis in a neonatal intensive care unit. *Mycoses* 1998;41:223–27

280. Leenders A et al. Molecular epidemiology of apparent outbreak of invasive aspergillosis in a hematology ward. *J Clin Microbiol* 1996;34:345–51.

281. Tang CM et al. Molecular epidemiological study of invasive pulmonary aspergillosis in a renal transplantation unit. *Eur J Clin Microbiol Infect Dis* 1994;13:318–21.

282. Tritz DM, Woods GL. Fatal disseminated infection with Aspergillus terreus in immunocompromised hosts. *Clin Infect Dis* 1993;16:118–22.

283. Richet HM et al. Aspergillus fumigatus sternal wound infections in patients undergoing open heart surgery. *Am J Epidemiol* 1992;135:48–58.

284. Pla MP et al. Surgical wound infection by Aspergillus fumigatus in liver transplant recipients. *Diagn Microbiol Infect Dis* 1992;15:703–6.

285. Loosveld OJ et al. Invasive Aspergillus infections in patients with a malignancy: Description of an outbreak and overview of the literature. *Neth J Med* 1992;40:62–68.

286. Mehta G. Aspergillus endocarditis after open heart surgery: An epidemiological investigation. *J Hosp Infect* 1990;15:245–53.

287. Karlowsky JA et al. Candidemia in a Canadian tertiary care hospital from 1976 to 1996. *Diagn Microbiol Infect Dis* 1997;29:5–9.

288. Luzzati R et al. Nosocomial candidemia in non-neutropenic patients at an Italian tertiary care hospital. *Eur J Clin Microbiol Infect Dis* 2000;19:602–7.

289. Viudes A et al. Candidemia at a tertiary-care hospital: Epidemiology, treatment, clinical outcome and risk factors for death. *Eur J Clin Microbiol Infect Dis* 2002;21:767–74.

290. Garbino J et al. Secular trends of candidemia over 12 years in adult patients at a tertiary care hospital. *Medicine* (Baltimore), 2002;81:425–33.

291. Alonso-Valle H et al. Candidemia in a tertiary care hospital: Epidemiology and factors influencing mortality. *Eur J Clin Microbiol Infect Dis* 2003;22:254–57.

292. Hsueh PR et al. Emergence of nosocomial candidemia at a teaching hospital in Taiwan from 1981 to 2000: Increased susceptibility of Candida species to fluconazole. *Microb Drug Resist* 2002;8:311–19.

293. McMullan R et al. Trends in the epidemiology of Candida bloodstream infections in Northern Ireland between January 1984 and December 2000. *J Infect* 2002;45:25–28.

294. San Miguel LG et al. Secular trends of candidemia in a large tertiary-care hospital from 1988 to 2000: Emergence of Candida parapsilosis. *Infect Control Hosp Epidemiol* 2005;26:548–52.

295. Doczi I et al. Aetiology and antifungal susceptibility of yeast bloodstream infections in a Hungarian university hospital between 1996 and 2000. *J Med Microbiol* 2002;51:677–81.

296. Plouffe JF et al. Nosocomial outbreak of Candida parapsilosis fungemia related to intravenous infusions. *Arch Intern Med* 1977;137:1686–89.

297. Solomon SL et al. An outbreak of Candida parapsilosis bloodstream infections in patients receiving parenteral nutrition. *J Infect Dis* 1984;149:98–102.

298. Burnie JP et al. Outbreak of systemic Candida albicans in intensive care unit caused by cross infection. *Br Med J* (Clin Res Ed) 1985;290:746–48.

299. McCray E et al. Outbreak of Candida parapsilosis endophthalmitis after cataract extraction and intraocular lens implantation. *J Clin Microbiol* 1986;24:625–28.

300. Berger C et al. [A Candida krusei epidemic in a hematology department]. *Schweiz Med Wochenschr* 1988;118:37–41.

301. Vaudry WL, Tierney AJ, Wenman WM. Investigation of a cluster of systemic Candida albicans infections in a neonatal intensive care unit. *J Infect Dis* 1988;158:1375–79.

302. Isenberg HD et al. Single-source outbreak of Candida tropicalis complicating coronary bypass surgery. *J Clin Microbiol* 1989;27:2426–28.

303. Moro ML et al. Nosocomial outbreak of systemic candidosis associated with parenteral nutrition. *Infect Control Hosp Epidemiol* 1990;11:27–35.

304. Sherertz RJ et al. Outbreak of Candida bloodstream infections associated with retrograde medication administration in a neonatal intensive care unit. *J Pediatr* 1992;120:455–61.

305. Finkelstein R et al. Outbreak of Candida tropicalis fungemia in a neonatal intensive care unit. *Infect Control Hosp Epidemiol* 1993;14:587–90.

306. Johnston BL, Schlech WF III, Marrie TJ. An outbreak of Candida parapsilosis prosthetic valve endocarditis following cardiac surgery. *J Hosp Infect* 1994;28:103–12.

307. Reagan DR et al. Evidence of nosocomial spread of Candida albicans causing bloodstream infection in a neonatal intensive care unit. *Diagn Microbiol Infect Dis* 1995;21:191–94.

308. Diekema DJ et al. An outbreak of Candida parapsilosis prosthetic valve endocarditis. *Diagn Microbiol Infect Dis* 1997;29:147–53.

309. D'Antonio D et al. A nosocomial cluster of Candida inconspicua infections in patients with hematological malignancies. *J Clin Microbiol* 1998;36:792–95.

310. Nedret Koc A et al. Outbreak of nosocomial fungemia caused by Candida glabrata. *Mycoses* 2002;45:470–75.

311. Chowdhary A et al. An outbreak of candidemia due to Candida tropicalis in a neonatal intensive care unit. *Mycoses* 2003;46:287–92.

312. Jang SJ et al. PFGE-based epidemiological study of an outbreak of Candida tropicalis candiduria: The importance of medical waste as a reservoir of nosocomial infection. *Jpn J Infect Dis* 2005;58:263–67.

313. De Pauw B, Walsh TJ, conveners. Defining invasive fungal infections: New Directions. Paper presented at 45th Interscience Conference on Antimicrobial Agents and Chemotherapy, Washington DC, December 18, 2005.

Infection in Transplant Recipients

44

Robert H. Rubin

Clinical transplantation has undergone an extraordinary transformation over the past four decades evolving from an interesting experiment in human immunobiology to the most practical means of rehabilitating individuals with end-stage kidney, heart, liver, lung, and bone marrow disease. Despite these advances, the major barriers to success remain the same: (1) rejection for solid organ transplant recipients and graft-vs-host disease (GVHD) for bone marrow transplant recipients, both examples of allogeneic reactions, and (2) infection. These two are closely linked; indeed, the therapeutic prescription for the transplant patient may be said to have two components: (1) an immunosuppressive program to prevent and/or treat rejection and GVHD and (2) an antimicrobial program to make it safe. Any manipulation or intervention that decreases the risk of infection will then permit the use of more intensive immunosuppression that will result in better control of rejection or GVHD; any manipulation or intervention that decreases the risk of these allogeneic reactions will decrease the risk of infection. The end result is the need to individualize therapy rather than use fixed regimens; (e.g., duration of antimicrobial therapy is "long enough," with this being determined by microbial burden, clinical response, the intensity of the immunosuppression required, and the potential consequences of infection relapse [1–3]. See Figures 44-1, 44-2).

The transplant recipient remains a highly unusual patient because of the need for lifelong immunosuppression, the presence of chronic immunomodulating viral infection, ongoing rejection, and a susceptibility to a variety of microbial invaders.

These organisms can be divided into three general categories: (1) true pathogens, (2) sometime pathogens, and (3) nonpathogens. True pathogens (the classic plagues of mankind [e.g., influenza, plague, typhoid] have the genetic makeup necessary to cross fascial planes, produce damaging toxins, and invade normal tissue. Sometime pathogens are found primarily on mucocutaneous surfaces, where they are not harmful (e.g., *Staphylococcus aureus*, *E. coli*, *Bacteroides fragilis*); however, if there is a break in the integrity of these tissues, they can easily cause lethal disease. Nonpathogens are ubiquitous in the environment (e.g., *Aspergillus species*, *Nocardia species*, *Cryptococcus neoformans*) and rarely produce clinical disease in the nonimmunosuppressed host. The term opportunistic infection is used to describe invasive infection due to nonpathogens or invasive/disseminated infection due to organisms that cause a trivial infection in normal hosts (e.g., candidal vaginitis vs. disseminated candidiasis [1,2]).

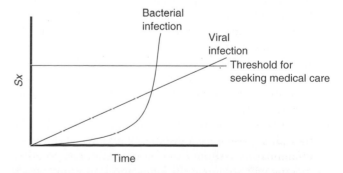

Figure 44-1 Progression of symptoms in patients with bacterial vs. viral infection. Note the rapid change in the deterioration, so there is relatively little time available to reverse the process once the threshold level of symptoms is reached.

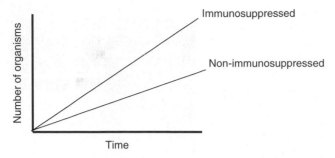

Figure 44-2 Effect of the immunosuppressed state on the microbial burden. The continuous increase in organisms means that the prognosis has to be guarded, more extensive antimicrobial therapy is needed, and the chance for both toxicity and resistance are increased. If the infection in question is transmissible, the increased microbial burden will increase the efficacy of transmission.

In sum, a unique set of challenges is created in the transplant recipient [1–3]:

1. The potential sources of infection are almost limitless, including endogenous organisms, the allograft itself, and the air, water, and food the patient encounters. Immunosuppressive therapy renders the transplant recipient susceptible to microbial species and inoculum sizes that would have little impact on the normal host.

2. Chronic immunosuppression, persistent infection with immunomodulating viruses (e.g., cytomegalovirus, Epstein-Barr, and the hepatitis viruses) that themselves are modulated by the exogenous immunosuppressive therapy, and the presence of foreign tissue in which the expression of cell surface antigens (such as major histocompatibility complex [MHC] antigens) are determined by infectious agents and by cytokines elaborated in response to microbial invasion. The clinical syndromes produced by these interactions are unprecedented in clinical medicine.

3. The nature of the infections that commonly occur in these patients (particularly certain viruses, fungi, and certain bacteria [e.g., *Mycobacterium tuberculosis*, *Nocardia species*, *Listeria monocytogenes*, and *Salmonella species*]) requires intensive antimicrobial therapy. The microbial burden is significantly higher in these patients, thereby increasing the duration of therapy required and, hence, the possibility of drug toxicities and the development of drug resistance. Antimicrobial agents as a general rule are associated with a high incidence of drug interactions, particularly with cyclosporine and tacrolimus, the cornerstones of modern immunosuppressive therapy.

4. The prevention of infection is an important goal in the transplant patient for a number of reasons: The blunted inflammatory response caused by immunosuppressive therapy will attenuate the signs and symptoms associated with microbial invasion until relatively late in the course. Not surprising, important prognostic factors for infections occurring in the transplant patient are the rapidity of diagnosis and the institution of appropriate therapy.

Approximately 75% of transplant patients develop clinically significant infection. Not only are the opportunistic infections present, but also more severe clinical syndromes due to common pathogens (e.g., influenza and other community-acquired viral infections, legionellosis, and viral induced malignancies—EBV induced lymphoproliferative disease, squamous cell carcinomas from papillomavirus, and hepatocellular carcinomas) are the rule [1,2].

RISK OF INFECTION IN THE TRANSPLANT RECIPIENT

The risk of infection in the transplant patient is largely determined by the interaction among four factors: (1) the presence of anatomic/technical abnormalities, (2) an excessive exposure to environmental pathogens, particularly within the hospital, (3) the net state of immunosuppression, and (4) Darwinian pressures.

ANATOMIC/TECHNICAL ABNORMALITIES IN THE PATHOGENESIS OF INFECTION

Anatomic/technical factors can be divided into two categories: (1) those related to surgical misadventures at the time of the transplant that result in the creation of devitalized tissue, fluid collections, and/or ongoing urine or bile leaks; unless these abnormalities are promptly eliminated, secondary infection is inevitable, and (2) perioperative abridgement of mucocutaneous surfaces by vascular access devices, endotracheal tubes, drainage devices, and bladder catheters, which are associated with secondary infection unless they are cared for impeccably. Early removal of these devices is indicated whenever possible. The incidence of such infections is related to the nature of the transplant (small bowel = liver > lung = pancreas > heart > kidney), the complexity of the surgery, and the duration of time that "devices" that compromise the integrity of the skin and mucosal surfaces are required. Transplantation is one of the most unforgiving forms of surgery with a technical abnormality signaling a high risk for superinfection. Although any undrained fluid can be a problem, hematoma is a particular problem as a source of iron, a particularly important growth factor for *Listeria, the Zygomycetes*, and other microbes [1–3]. See Figure 44-3.

ENVIRONMENTAL FACTORS

Although community-acquired infections can be an important issue for transplant patients, the more important

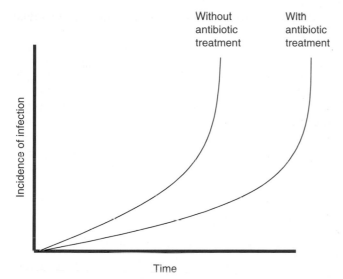

Without antibiotic treatment   With antibiotic treatment

Incidence of infection

Time

Figure 44-3 Infection in the face of a technical/anatomic abnormality. Without antibiotics there is a progressive increase in the prevalence of infection. Antibiotics shift the curve to the right. If the anatomic abnormality can be corrected during this extra time period, then antibiotics are useful. If no change in the anatomic abnormality is accomplished then, resistance is *induced*. The most effective therapy in this situation is to combine repair of the underlying problem in conjunction with antimicrobial therapy.

exposures are those that occur in the hospital where two important patterns—domiciliary and nondomiciliary—can be demonstrated. The term domiciliary is used to describe acquisition of organisms from the potable water and/or contaminated air, which occurs on the transplant ward or in the patient's room. Outbreaks in which infection is acquired in a domiciliary mode are usually characterized by clustering of cases in time and space and are therefore relatively easy to recognize. Domiciliary outbreaks of *Pseudomonas aeruginosa* (and other gram negative organisms), *Legionella*, and *Aspergillus* spp. infection are well documented [1–5].

Nondomiciliary infection is acquired when the patient travels within the hospital for an essential procedure and is exposed to excessive levels of potential opportunistic pathogens present in the air, usually associated with construction, and/or areas of moisture that favor the growth of such molds as *Aspergillus*, *Fusarium*, and *Scedosporium* spp. Thus, invasive infection due to the molds, particularly *Aspergillus* species, has been well documented in radiology and endoscopy suites, in holding areas outside cardiac catheterization laboratories, the operating room, and a hospital area that is undergoing renovation. Nondomiciliary infection is probably more common than domiciliary infection, but because of the lack of clustering of cases in time and space can be more difficult to detect. The best clue to the presence of an environmental hazard is the occurrence of infection due to one of these opportunistic organisms when the net state of immunosuppression is not, under normal circumstances, great enough to allow

such an infection to occur unless an environmental hazard is present [1–4].

A not infrequent problem is the person-to-person spread of respiratory viruses within the hospital. For example, when influenza is present in a community, great effort is needed to protect immunocompromised patients because vaccine and treatment with the neuroiminidase inhibitors are far less effective than in the immunologically normal patients. Transplant patients with influenza have a higher rate of both viral pneumonia and bacterial superinfection. Experience with the severe acute respiratory syndrome (SARS) and other viruses confirm that the impact of such infection is greater than that seen in the general population. Unfortunately, management of such problems is difficult, and prevention via a "quarantine" effort is greatly to be preferred [1–4].

An essential point to be emphasized is that immunosuppressed patients such as transplant recipients are like "sentinel chickens," reflecting any excess traffic in microbes in the hospital environment (particularly with agents that cause opportunistic respiratory infection). Constant surveillance of infection among transplant patients is essential. In addition, in institutions undergoing major construction, transplant patients will benefit greatly from being housed in areas where the air quality is maintained by high-efficiency particulate air filters and from an ongoing assessment of routes of transport within the hospital [1,2,6].

THE NET STATE OF IMMUNOSUPPRESSION

The net state of immunosuppression is a complex function determined by the interaction of a number of factors: host defense deficits caused by the underlying disease process (e.g., diabetes, systemic lupus erythematosis) and attempts at treating it with immunosuppression before transplant (e.g., chronic hepatitis, biliary cirrhosis, inflammatory lung disease); the dose, duration, and temporal sequence of immunosuppressive therapies administered; the presence or absence of damage to the mucocutaneous surfaces of the body (the primary host defense barriers to invasive infection); neutropenia, especially with an absolute granulocyte count $<100/mm^3$ that is persisting; the presence of such metabolic abnormalities as protein-calorie malnutrition, uremia, or hyperglycemia; and the presence of infection with one or more of the immunomodulating viruses (e.g., cytomegalovirus, Epstein-Barr virus, human herpesvirus-6, hepatitis viruses B or C, and the human immunodeficiency virus) [1,2,7].

The major determinant of the net state of immunosuppression is the nature of the immunosuppressive therapy. However, two other observations underline the principle that other factors are important as well: >90% of opportunistic infections in transplant patients occur in individuals with chronic viral infection with the 10% exceptions almost invariably due to excessive environmental exposure; if the transplant population is stratified into two groups on the basis of a serum albumin > or <2.5 g/dl, those with the lower value have a 10-fold higher risk of life-threatening infection [1,2].

There is a semi-quantitative relationship between the patient's net state of immunosuppression and the environmental hazards that are encountered. If the patient's net state of immunosuppression is great enough, even trivial exposures to relatively avirulent organisms (nonpathogens) can produce life-threatening infection; conversely, if the exposure is great enough, even immunologically normal individuals can succumb to the infectious challenge [1,2].

DARWINIAN PRESSURES IN THE TRANSPLANT PATIENT

Several forms of Darwinian pressure affect the nature of infection in the transplant recipient. First, previous antimicrobial exposure, the normal flora on the skin, in the gut, and in the upper respiratory tract—is very much influenced by previous antimicrobial therapy, with an increase of the microbial burden of resistant bacteria and *Candida* species being an end result. Because these sites are the reservoirs from which invasive infection is derived, the clinician is obligated to modify antimicrobial regimens for initial therapy. Second is the availability of nutrients and growth factors. A number of organisms are very responsive to these Darwinian pressures: The availability of iron will greatly increase the possibility of infection with such organisms as the *Zygomycetes, Listeria,* and *Staphylococcus aureus.* Thus, the occurrence of wound infection following the transplant operation is several times greater if bleeding has complicated the procedure. Hyperglycemia will greatly increase the level of *Candida* colonization on the skin, in the gut, the pharynx, and the female genital tract. A relatively minor break in the integrity of these tissues (e.g., vascular access device, placement of drains and catheters) will lead to significant clinical *Candida* spp. infection because of the high organism load that is present. The third pressure is the presence of devitalized tissue and/or foreign body. If these are not corrected, antimicrobial therapy will lead only to microbial resistance because the ecologic niche is unchanged and more resistant flora will emerge, causing resistant infection [1–3].

Successful antimicrobial therapy in these patients, then, requires attention to Darwinian factors, a term that encompasses past exposures to antibiotics as part of this effort. Overgrowth of microbes is potentiated by metabolic derangement (e.g., *Candida* spp. overgrowth) and the presence of excessive amounts of growth factors (e.g., iron and the zygomcytes). It is then a small step to invasive infection [1–3].

1. If immediate therapy is necessary (to deal with a potential therapeutic emergency before microbiologic

information is available), the previous antimicrobial regimen should be avoided with broader spectrum therapy initiated until precise information as to the organism and its susceptibility are known at which time adjustment of the therapeutic regimen can be safely carried out.

2. Correction of metabolic abnormalities should be accomplished as quickly as possible to increase the efficacy of the therapeutic program.

3. Antimicrobial therapy is best carried out in conjunction with repair of the technical/anatomic abnormalities that led to the infection in the first place (Figure 44-1).

4. A frequent consideration in the management of infection in the transplant patient is duration of therapy. On the one hand, dose and duration of therapy are important issues in achieving cure as opposed to just selecting resistant organisms. On the other hand, longer durations of therapy can be associated with toxicity. Therefore, the appropriate answer to the question of How long to treat is "long enough." In the transplant patient, such factors as surgery, increasing levels of immunosuppressive therapy, and the presence of blood or hemolysis argue for the need for prolonged therapy. Our approach is to treat until all laboratory and clinical evidence of infection are gone and then add a "buffer" period, the duration of which depends on the nature of the infection, anatomic site, and the consequences of relapse, should it occur. Fixed regimens of antimicrobial therapy have no place in the management of transplant patients [1–3].

TIMETABLE OF INFECTION AFTER ORGAN TRANSPLANTATION

The general pattern of infection is the same in all forms of organ transplantation, reflecting the use of similar immunosuppressive programs in all of these patients (Figure 44-4). Thus, a timetable can be defined (Figure 44-2) delineating when in the posttransplantation course a particular form of infection is likely to occur; that is, although a given infectious disease clinical syndrome, such as pneumonia, can occur at any point in the posttransplantation period, the microbial etiologies are very different in the different time periods. Application of this timetable to the clinical management of transplant recipients is useful in at least three different ways: in arriving at a differential diagnosis of the causes of a particular clinical presentation; in designing directed, cost-effective antimicrobial preventative strategies; and in recognizing epidemiologic hazards. Exceptions to the timetable are usually due to previously unrecognized environmental exposure, often within the hospital environment. In the organ transplant patient, the timetable is conveniently divided into three different time periods; the first month post-transplantation, the period 1 to 6 months post-transplantation, and the late period, more than six months post-transplantation [1–3,7].

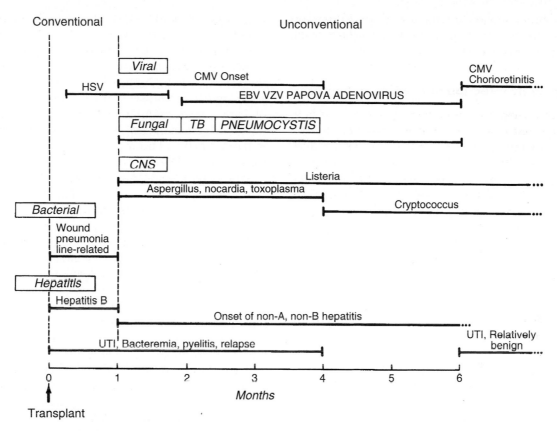

Figure 44-4   Timetable of Infection following Organ Transplant. Infection in the Transplant Patient: Lessons from the bedside. Reprinted with permission from Rubin RH, Wolfson JS, Cosimi AB, et al. Infection in the renal transplant recipient. *Am J Med* 1981;70:405–411.

INFECTION IN THE FIRST MONTH POST-TRANSPLANTATION

In the first month post-transplantation, there are three major causes of clinically important infection: (1) infection that was present in the recipient before the transplantation procedure and that was exacerbated by the surgery, anesthesia, the physical manipulations required, or the initiation of immunosuppression; (2) active infection conveyed with the allograft; and (3) the same wound-, catheter-, vascular access-related infection and pneumonia seen in nonimmunosuppressed patients subjected to comparable amounts of surgery.

Importance of Infection in the Recipient Before Transplantation

A cardinal rule of clinical transplantation is that all infectious processes should be under control before the transplantation procedure. Thus, before transplantation, every attempt must be made to identify and eradicate infection, such as tuberculosis, localized and systemic fungal infection, and strongyloidiasis (with particular infections to be considered based on a careful epidemiologic history). In patients awaiting heart, lung, and/or liver transplantation,

acquisition of infection during an extended stay in intensive care units is quite common. The nature of these infections are as expected: vascular access bloodstream infection, infection related to the presence of ventricular assist devices, aspiration pneumonia, and so on [1–3].

In recent years, a relatively new entity, *Pneumocystis* pneumonia, has been encountered as have cryptococcosis and other opportunistic infections in the first few weeks following transplantation. In this instance, pretransplant immunosuppression was creating an environment appropriate for opportunistic infection, often in the setting of a desperate attempt to control the primary disease and thus avoid transplantation. These patients are coming to transplantation with active infection that is far more difficult to treat in the face of a fresh transplant [1].

As heart, lung, and liver transplantation are being used to treat an ever-increasing number of diseases, acute bacterial and fungal infection of clinical importance may be acquired during the wait for emergency transplantation. Examples include aspiration pneumonia in the patient his unable to protect his airway due to advanced hepatic encephalopathy; pneumonia and vascular sepsis in the patient with end-stage cardiac disease who is intubated and receiving life support from vasopressors delivered through central venous access and cardiac assist devices;

and bronchopulmonary infection or colonization with antibiotic-resistant gram-negative bacilli in the patient with end-stage pulmonary disease [1–5].

Importance of Infection in the Organ Donor

Infection to a recipient can be transmitted with an allograft. Of greatest concern is viral infection: the human immunodeficiency virus (HIV), hepatitis B virus (HBV), hepatitis C virus (HCV), and cytomegalovirus (CMV) are all transferred with near 100% efficiency with transplantation [8–10]. As a result, pretransplant serologies provide a great help in avoiding such transmission. An important point that merits emphasis is that only "pedigreed" blood samples should be used. Transmission of HIV and HBV have been well documented in instances in which massive transfusions have been administered in an attempt to salvage a trauma victim before brain death is pronounced. At that point, a blood sample will reflect transfused blood and will be falsely negative, but the allograft itself will still carry infection to recipients [8–12].

Other infectious agents transmitted from the donor include systemic fungal and mycobacterial infection, fortunately an uncommon event [8,12–14]. In contrast, the protozoan *Toxooplasma gondii* is a potential hazard primarily in patients undergoing cardiac transplantation. Transplantation of a heart from a donor seropositive for toxoplasmosis into a seronegative recipient is associated with >50% incidence of *T. gondii* myocarditis and disseminated infection. Accordingly, prophylaxis with trimethoprim-sulfamethoxazole or pyrimethamine and a sulfonamide is indicated for these individuals. Other forms of organ transplantation do not require antitoxoplasmosis prophylaxis [15–25].

A more difficult problem is the identification of immediately preterminal contamination of organs due to acute infection developing while the potential donor is in the intensive care unit. For example, unsuspected *Pseudomonas aeruginosa* bacteremia in an afebrile donor resulted in the infection of the two kidneys that were being transplanted. Both of these kidneys required emergency removal because of massive bleeding; examination of them revealed ruptured mycotic aneurysms at the suture line of the arterial anastamosis. Less commonly, organs may be secondarily contaminated during the harvesting process or during the transplant operation [1–3].

Technical Complications as a Risk Factor for Infection

The concept that technical complications lead to significant infectious problems applies to the perioperative period and the operation itself. Poor management of the airway leads to aspiration pneumonia; inadequate attention to vascular access devices, particularly central venous catheters, leads to septicemia; and drainage catheters can lead to infection of

normally sterile sites. Infection occurring as a consequence of technical mishaps accounts for >95% of the infections that occur in the first month post-transplantation. The consequences of such infections can be far greater than in the normal host; for example, although transient vascular access–related candidemia carries a risk of visceral seeding of <10% in the nonimmunosuppressed patient, in the transplant patient the risk is >50%, and antifungal therapy is mandatory (in addition to removal of the contaminated vascular access device) [1–3,5,26–28].

Wound infection is the most important treatable infection occurring in the first month after transplantation. Its incidence is directly related to whether or not the transplant operation is free of vascular compromise and the creation of devitalized tissue, wound hematomas, fluid collections, and the need for re-exploration or prolonged use of drainage catheters. The particular technical challenges of liver transplantation, with a biliary anastomosis that is susceptible to ischemic injury, as well as four vascular anastomoses (superior and inferior vena cava, portal vein, and hepatic artery) all performed in patients with coagulopathies explain the high rate of intraabdominal infection that dominates the first month post-transplantation in these patients. Indeed, the major difference between liver transplant recipients and other allograft recipients is the higher incidence of technically related infection in and around the area of surgery [1–3,29,30].

There is considerable variability in the choice of perioperative antibiotics to prevent wound infection among different transplant centers. Two principles merit emphasis whatever the antimicrobial regimen is: (1) antimicrobial prophylaxis is not a substitute for technically impeccable surgery and (2) antimicrobial choice should be directed toward prevention of wound infection, not systemic sepsis. The author's center uses cefazolin for <72 hours, which has provided adequate protection without creating intensive pressure for the selection of resistant flora. In the special case of liver transplantation, some centers opt for the use of an elaborate program of nonabsorbable antimicrobials aimed at decreasing the amount of aerobic gram-negative flora and yeast colonizing in the gastrointestinal tract and then use a perioperative drug, such as cefotaxime, that leaves the anaerobic flora (and hence "colonization resistance") intact. The author's group does attempt to eliminate yeast from the gastrointestinal tract but does not use the rest of the program. With these regimens, the post-transplantation intraabdominal infection rate of <5% has been achieved. Such results are primarily a testimony to the expert surgery being performed with the antibiotics playing an ancillary role [1–3,31–34].

Opportunistic Infection in the First Month Post-Transplantation

Noteworthy in this discussion of infections in the first month after organ transplantation is the absence of opportunistic infection. Indeed, in this one-month "golden period," the net state of immunosuppression should not be great enough to permit infection with such organisms as *Pneumocystis, Listeria, Legionella,* or *Aspergillus.* This observation leads to two conclusions: the major determinant of the net state of immunosuppression is the duration of immunosuppressive therapy ("the area under the curve") rather than the daily dose (indeed, the daily doses of immunosuppression are at their highest in this time period). Thus, the occurrence of opportunistic infection in the first month is an important clue to the presence of either an unsuspected environmental hazard or the presence of opportunistic infection pretransplant due to efforts to use immunosuppressive therapy to reverse the underlying disease [1–3].

INFECTION ONE TO SIX MONTHS POST-TRANSPLANTATION

In general, this is the period of greatest vulnerability to infection for the transplant recipient. Not only is sustained immunosuppressive therapy exerting an increasing effect, but also this is the time period when the immunomodulating viruses (cytomegalovirus [CMV], human herpesvirus-6 [HHV-6], Epstein-Barr virus [EBV], hepatitis viruses B and C [HBV and HCV], and the human immunodeficiency virus [HIV]) become important. In this period, the net state of immunosuppression is significantly increased because of these two factors. Clinically, the infections that are important fit into two general categories: (1) the direct effects of one or more of these viruses, for example, two-thirds of the fevers occurring in this time period are due to the direct effects of CMV alone, and (2) opportunistic infection occurs not because of unusual environmental exposures but is attributable to the increased net state of immunosuppression [1–3,6,35].

Impact of Viral Infection on the Transplant Recipient

When clinical infection due to viral pathogens occurs in nonimmunosuppressed patients, the patient usually recovers or succumbs to the direct effects of the virus (although chronic infection can occur with HBV and HCV). In the transplant recipient, the direct effects of viral invasion and proliferation are frequently superseded by the indirect effects. Thus, the consequences of viral infection in this patient population can be particularly broad [1–3,36,37]:

1. The direct production of such infectious disease syndromes as fever, mononucleosis, pneumonia, encephalitis, enterocolitis, and hepatitis.
2. The indirect effects of viral infection, which include the following:
    The production of a state of immunosuppression in addition to that induced by the antirejection

therapy being administered so that the patient is at increased risk of invasive infection with such opportunistic pathogens as *Pneumocystis, Listeria,* and *Aspergillus* in the absence of an excessive epidemiologic exposure.
    The initiation of a series of events that lead to allograft injury.
    The participation of these viruses in the process of oncogenesis.

Effects of Immunosuppressive Therapy on the Occurrence of Infection

The major determinants of the net state of immunosuppression are the dose, duration, and temporal sequence in which the immunosuppressive regimen is administered. Of all the drugs used in transplant patients, corticosteroids have the most global effects, and the thrust of modern antirejection efforts is "steroid sparing" therapy in which other drugs that exert their effects through other mechanisms can be used to achieve the desired level of immunocompromise but with reduced adverse events [1–3,38].

The effects of corticosteroids can be divided into two categories: an immunosuppressive effect and an anti-inflammatory one. The key immunosuppressive effect of corticosteroids is the inhibition of T-cell activation and proliferation (thus blocking clonal expansion in response to antigenic stimulation). This is accomplished through the suppression of interleukin-2 and other proinflammatory cytokines. The end result is a striking inhibition of cell-mediated immunity. The infections promoted by this impairment include herpes group viruses, the hepatitis viruses, the fungi and mycobacteria, and bacteria that persist intracellularly (e.g., *Listeria* and *Salmonella*) [1–3,39].

The anti-inflammatory effects of corticosteroids include the following: inhibition of proinflammatory cytokines; inhibition of the ability of polymorphonuclear leukocytes to accumulate at sites of infection and inflammation; inhibition of the proinflammatory arachidonic acid metabolites (prostaglandins, thromboxane, leukotrienes, and platelet activating factor); inhibition of mediators of vasodilation, including the inducible form of nitric oxide synthase, thus decreasing macrophage nitric oxide production, endothelial permeability, and microvascular leak [1–3,38,39].

From an infectious disease point of view, the most important adverse effects of corticosteroids have to do with their inhibition of the inflammatory response to microbial invasion. The consequences of this suppressed inflammatory response are twofold: the signs and symptoms of infection, as well as the X-ray findings, will be greatly blunted until late in the clinical course, and the microbial burden at the site of infection is likely to be far higher than that observed in normal hosts [1–3,38,39].

The standard of care for organ transplant recipients is a multidrug regimen consisting of a calcineurin inhibitor (cyclosporine or tacrolimus), prednisone, and either azathioprine or mycophenolate. In addition, antithymocyte globulin (ATG, a polyclonal anti-T cell drug) or OKT3 (a monoclonal anti-T cell drug) can be used as induction therapy or to treat steroid-resistant rejection. The calcineurin inhibitors are the cornerstones of modern antirejection therapy. These exert their effects through a complex signaling pathway that results in the inhibition of the transcriptional activation of genes required for T-cell activation, proliferation, and function. This results in the inhibition of a large number of proinflammatory cytokines, with the most important of these effects being the blockade of essential functions of interleukin-2 (IL-2). The infectious disease consequences of these drugs are direct results of these mechanisms: a dose-related inhibition of microbial specific T-cell cytotoxic activity, thus promoting the herpes group viruses, fungal, mycobacterial, and other intracellular infections. The key toxicities of the calcineurin inhibitors are injury to the kidneys and hypertension [1–3,38,40,41].

Azathioprine and mycophenolate should be thought of as mediating their immunosuppressive effects by depleting purine stores and inhibiting RNA and DNA synthesis. Actively dividing lymphocytes are particularly susceptible to these effects. In recent years, the rate-limiting step in the metabolism of azathioprine has been shown to be the function of the enzyme thiopurine methyltransferase with significant genetic heterogeneity in the activity of this enzyme. Thus, it is likely that there have been important effects of this enzyme in clinical transplantation due to drug over- or underdose and that azathioprine is probably a more useful drug than was recognized. The toxicities of these two drugs are very different: bone marrow and hepatic toxicity for azthioprine and gastrointestinal toxicity (diarrhea and cramps) for mycophenolate [1,38,42].

ATG and OKT3 are the most potent therapies for steroid resistant rejection. The administration of these agents is associated with fever and rigors due to "cytokine storm." These side effects are important not only because of the patient's discomfort but also because of secondary effects on herpes viruses. Reactivation of latent viruses due to tumor necrosis factor (TNF) release plays an important role in the pathogenesis of herpes group virus infection, particularly CMV and EBV. Interest in the anti-IL-2 monoclonal antibodies in part is related to the lack of the initial cytokine release seen with ATG or OKT3. However, the clinical roles of these newer antibodies (daclizumab and basilixmab) in transplantation are still being defined [2,43,44].

The final immunosuppressive therapy to be considered here is rapamycin (sirolimus), which has a mechanism of action separate from cyclosporine and tacrolimus. Whereas cyclosporine and tacrolimus initiate their effects by binding to specific cell surface immunophilins, rapamycin's targets include RAFT1/FRAP proteins in mammalian cells, which are associated with cell cycle phase G_1. Rapamycin is less potent than the other drugs in terms of inhibition of cytokine synthesis but has potentially useful activity in inhibiting immunoglobulin synthesis and growth factor synthesis, potentially useful effects in protecting against chronic allograft injury. At present, the primary use of rapamycin is in combination with cyclosporine, thus permitting lower doses of cyclosporine with less renal toxicity [45–47]. Major difficulties in the use of rapamycin include pulmonary toxicity, aphthous ulcers, and significant drug–drug interactions [48–50].

Infection More Than 6 Months Post-Transplantation

Patients with functioning allografts more than 6 months post-transplantation can be divided into three general categories in terms of their infectious disease problems [1–3]:

1. Approximately 75% of patients have good allograft function and are being maintained on minimal immunosuppression. Their infectious disease problems are largely related to exposures within the community and are of three types:

    Community-acquired respiratory infections, with influenza, respiratory syncytial virus, parainfluenza, and other viruses having a particular impact on these patients. In general, the rate of both viral pneumonia and secondary bacterial pneumonia associated with these infections is higher than that in the general population; that is, the etiology is the same, but the incidence of severe disease is increased. It is not surprising, then, that such unusual pulmonary processes as SARS and *Legionella* will have a greater impact on the transplant patient than the general population.

    Community-acquired gastrointestinal infection after the ingestion of contaminated food or water, due to *Salmonella* species, *L. monocytogenes*, *Campylobacter jejuni*, and others. In general, the duration of disease and the incidence of bacteremia and metastatic infection are longer/greater in the transplant patient than for individuals in the general population [1].

    Exposure in the community to one of the geographically restricted systemic mycoses or tuberculosis, which, as previously stated, has a higher incidence of systemic spread than in the general population.

    Because therapies of these infections are not ideal, transplant recipients are cautioned to avoid exotic travel or undue exposure to infection within the community. Disease prevention with vaccine administration is less successful in transplant patients as well, making the avoidance of exposure particularly important.

2. A few individuals, ~5% to 15% of the group, will acquire progressive organ dysfunction, malignancy, or full-blown acquired immunodeficiency syndrome (AIDS) due to chronic viral infection. Thus, CMV chorioretinitis (unless intensively treated with ganciclovir) proceeds inexorably to blindness; hepatitis B and C can cause end-stage liver disease and contribute to the development

of hepatocellular carcinoma; EBV can initiate posttransplantation lymphoproliferative disorder (PTLD); and HIV infection progresses to AIDS—all occurring at a more rapid and higher rate than in any populations other than those individuals with progressive immune deficiency due to HIV infection unrelated to transplantation.

3. A few individuals, again ~5% to 15% of transplant patients, will have had a poor result from their transplant (relatively poor allograft function because of repeated episodes of acute or chronic rejection). Typically, these patients have required higher than normal doses of immunosuppressive drugs for prolonged periods and often suffer with chronic immunomodulating viral infection. They are at the highest risk for life-threatening opportunistic infection. These "chronic n'er do wells" are at particular risk for *Pneumocystis* pneumonia, cryptococcosis, listeriosis, and nocardiosis. If their overall clinical state cannot be reversed, consideration should be given to chronic prophylaxis with trimethoprim–sulfamethoxazole (TMP-SMX) and fluconazole. Recurrent CMV infection, squamous cell carcinomas, or herpes simplex infections may necessitate long-term antiviral or chemotherapeutic approaches in these individuals [1].

INFECTIONS OF PARTICULAR IMPORTANCE IN THE TRANSPLANT RECIPIENT

Cytomegalovirus

Cytomegalovirus is the single most important cause of infectious disease morbidity and mortality in transplant patients with evidence of active viral replication being found in 50% to 75% of transplant recipients. Three patterns of CMV transmission, each with a different risk for clinically overt disease, may be observed [1–3,51–62]:

1. *Primary CMV infection* occurs when latently infected cells from a CMV-seropositive donor (D+) are administered to a CMV-seronegative recipient (R−). More than 90% of the time, those cells are contained in the allograft; occasionally, viable leukocytes in blood transfusions can transmit the virus. Approximately 60% of individuals at risk for primary CMV infection become clinically ill. D + R− transplants account for 10% to 15% of all transplants (D-R- transplants account for a similar number) [51–62].

2. *Reactivation CMV infection* occurs when a CMV-seropositive individual (D±R+) reactivates endogenous latent virus. When conventional cyclosporine (or FK-506)-based immunosuppression is used in transplant patients, the incidence of clinical disease is ~10%; when antilymphocyte antibody therapy is used in the first 5 to 7 days post-transplantation as "induction" therapy, the incidence of clinical disease is 24%; and when antilymphocyte antibody therapy (either ATG or OKT3) is used to treat allograft rejection, >60% of seropositive individuals not receiving effective antiviral prophylaxis become ill from CMV infection. Approximately 70% to 80% of patients coming to transplantation are CMV seropositive [51–62].

3. *Superinfection with CMV* occurs when a CMV-seropositive recipient (R+) receives an allograft from a seropositive donor (D+) and the virus that is reactivated is of donor origin. Although the database for making this statement is quite incomplete, there is the general impression that the rate of clinical disease is somewhat higher in patients with superinfection as opposed to reactivation infection. An estimated 25% to 35% of transplant patients have CMV superinfection [1,31,38,39].

Whatever form of CMV infection is operative, clinically overt infectious disease syndromes classically present in the time period 1 to 4 months post-transplantation. Three exceptions to this pattern may be observed. First, an individual who is still CMV seronegative after this period can acquire primary CMV disease because of acquisition of the virus in the community after intimate contact. Second, an occasional seropositive patient with severe bacterial infection, such as urosepsis or bacteremic pneumococcal disease, can acquire symptomatic CMV disease 3 to 4 weeks later because of cytokine release (the "second wave phenomenon"), particularly release of TNF release during the septic episode. Third, late CMV disease can occur many months post-transplant due to incomplete protection from prophylactic antiviral therapy. In this instance, the incubation period is greatly prolonged as a partial effect of the antiviral regimen, thus delaying the onset of CMV disease [1–3,63–73].

The general pattern of clinical disease due to CMV is similar in all forms of organ transplantation with one notable exception: The organ transplanted is far more vulnerable than are native organs—for example, CMV hepatitis is a significant problem only in liver transplant patients, CMV myocarditis in heart transplant patients, and CMV pancreatitis in pancreas transplant patients—whereas the attack rate for CMV pneumonia is many times higher in lung and heart–lung transplant patients [1,30]. The spectrum of clinical illness produced by CMV includes asymptomatic shedding of virus (most common in patients with reactivation infection), a mononucleosis-like illness that has been termed the *CMV syndrome*, and life-threatening disease affecting such organs as the lungs and the gastrointestinal tract [1–3].

The role of proinflammatory cytokines has been well studied in recent years. TNF-alpha appears to be the mediator of reactivation of the virus from latency. Other inflammatory mediators appear to be responsible for inflammatory symptoms that are part of the direct effects of the virus as well as the indirect effects. Presently, another piece of the pathogenic puzzle has been elucidated. Toll-like receptors (TLR) are stimulated by pattern recognition of unique motifs of different pathogens. This leads to the induction of antimicrobial activity and an inflammatory cytokine response through the activation of intracellular signaling pathways. The TLR-pathogen interaction plays a key role in the functioning of innate immunity. Ten different TLRs have been identified in humans, and extensive genetic polymorphisms have been shown to occur with increasing evidence that the nature of the TLR-pathogen infection is a major determinant of the clinical syndrome that is operative in particular patients [74–78].

The CMV syndrome typically refers to a prolonged episode of otherwise unexplained fever associated with constitutional symptoms in concert with such laboratory abnormalities as leukopenia (with or without thrombocytopenia), a mild atypical lymphocytosis (usually <10% of the circulating leukocytes and often not seen), and a mild, usually transient hepatitis. Severe CMV disease consists of severe leukopenia and thrombocytopenia, pneumonia, gastrointestinal ulcerations and perforation, and, in the liver transplant patient, severe hepatitis. Not infrequently, opportunistic superinfection with other pathogens further complicates the course of severe CMV infection. CMV chorioretinitis is a late manifestation of systemic CMV infection, presenting 4 months or more post-transplantation. Chorioretinitis may follow earlier clinical manifestations of CMV infection or be the first manifestation of CMV disease [1,30]. A unique clinical syndrome of interstitial pneumonitis is observed in the bone marrow transplant recipient after marrow engraftment. Although many of these forms of pneumonitis are idiopathic, up to 50% are observed in CMV seropositive recipients and are preventable with empiric antiviral therapy. This disease likely reflects both CMV infection and the emerging T-cell, cytotoxic response to CMV antigens. Both in bone marrow transplants and solid-organ transplants, the degree of MHC mismatch appears to contribute to the incidence and severity of disease [79–82].

The most valuable diagnostic test for managing clinical CMV disease is the demonstration of viremia (although invasive biopsies of tissue are even more specific but are usually not available until relatively late in the disease course). Viremia is usually present as early as 5 to 7 days before the onset of clinical disease and continues until effective treatment is initiated. At present, quantitative polymerase chain reaction (PCR) and the CMV antigenemia assays are quite useful with a sensitivity and specificity of >90%. Demonstration of "shed" virus in respiratory secretions and urine may be found in many transplant patients and, hence, correlates poorly with clinical events. Similarly, serial measurements of antibody not only correlate poorly with clinical events ("diagnostic rises" in antibody titers or the appearance of IgM antibody) but also are too delayed to allow for use in clinical decision making. Hence, the major use of antibody testing is to characterize

donor and recipient at the time of transplant in an effort to guide preventative strategies.

Although still somewhat controversial, there is increasing evidence that CMV contributes to the pathogenesis of allograft injury (as well as to GVHD in bone marrow transplant patients). CMV infection has been particularly linked to accelerated coronary artery atherosclerosis in cardiac allograft recipients, to bronchiolitis obliterans in lung transplant recipients, to certain forms of hepatic injury in liver transplant patients, and to an unusual glomerulopathy in renal transplant patients, as well as to more conventional patterns of rejection. The problem has been that each of these lesions has also been observed in patients without viral infection. Cytokines elaborated in the course of CMV infection (and other processes) affect the display of histocompatibility antigens and thus modulate the immune response to the allograft. A similar array of proinflammatory cytokines are elaborated in response to rejection, infection, and key forms of infection. Thus, CMV is not the only way to cause these reactions but is just a common way. A report in which allograft dysfunction was successfully treated with the antiviral drug ganciclovir, not increased immunosuppression, is particularly interesting in this regard [83–86].

As discussed previously, the nature of the immunosuppressive therapy administered has a major influence on the course of CMV infection. TNF and other proinflammatory cytokines play a key role in reactivating CMV from latency, the critical first step in the pathogenesis of CMV-related events. The excessive rate of CMV infection induced by antilymphocyte antibody administration has now been shown to be largely related to the release of TNF. It is clear that the occasional cases of CMV disease that follow other circumstances in which TNF is released (e.g., severe allograft rejection and urosepsis) are due to the same mechanism [1–3].

The proposed linkage between rejection and CMV disease appears to be mediated by cytokines as well and seems to be *bidirectional:* in addition to the TNF–CMV activation mechanism, it is now apparent that gamma-interferon (and presumably other cytokines) elaborated in response to CMV infection upregulate the display of histocompatibility antigens on the allograft, thus promoting rejection [1]. Finally, CMV disease appears to be a significant risk factor in the occurrence of EBV-related PTLD with a greater than 7-fold increase in PTLD in patients with CMV, probably because of the effects of growth factors and cytokines elaborated in the course of the CMV infection but also because GVHD, allograft rejection, and immune suppression are major activators of latent viral infection [1–3].

Given the myriad of effects due to CMV, considerable effort has been directed at controlling it. Intravenous ganciclovir, at a dose of 5 mg/kg twice daily (with dosage correction in the face of renal dysfunction), for 2 to 3 weeks is quite effective in treating symptomatic disease. Relapse,

TABLE 44-1

ESTIMATED EFFICACIES OF DIFFERENT PROPHYLACTIC ANTIVIRAL STRATEGIES AGAINST CYTOMEGALOVIRUS (CMV) INFECTION IN DIFFERENT FORMS OF ORGAN TRANSPLANTATION[a]

Type of Transplant	Form of CMV Infection	Antimicrobial Strategy Used	Estimated Efficacy
Kidney	Primary	CMV hyperimmune globulin	2+
		High-dose acyclovir	2+
		CMV hyperimmune globulin + moderate-dose acyclovir	3+
	Secondary[b]	High-dose acyclovir	3+
		CMV hyperimmune globulin + moderate-dose acyclovir	3+
Heart or lung	Primary	High-dose ganciclovir (1 mo)	0
	Secondary[a]	High-dose ganciclovir (1 mo)	4+
Liver	Primary	CMV hyperimmune globulin	0
	Secondary[a]	CMV hyperimmune globulin	3+

[a]Unless otherwise noted, the regimens outlined were administered for a minimum of 3 mo. Only semiquantitative assessments of efficacy are given because of the recognition that the type of immunosuppression used will have a major effect on the efficacy of each of these regimens.

[b]Patients were not differentiated in the studies as to whether they had reactivation or superinfection; all patients seropositive for CMV before transplantation are grouped together.

Modified from Rubin RH, Tolkoff-Rubin NE. Antimicrobial strategies in the care of organ transplant recipients. *Antimicrob Agents Chemother* 1993;37:619–624.

which may develop several times after seemingly effective treatment, occurs in ~10% of seropositive individuals and in >60% of those with primary infection. MHC antigen mismatch will significantly add to the occurrence of relapse. Based on apparent success in several cases with multiple relapses, we now routinely add oral ganciclovir at a dose of 2 to 3 g/day or valganciclovir for 10 weeks to the conventional intravenous course of therapy for those with primary infection [1–3]. Far less clear is the appropriate way to prevent CMV disease, which would be preferable to the treatment of tissue invasive disease.

Two forms of *preemptive* therapy have been described: (1) monitoring patients for preclinical viremia and treating on that basis without any prophylaxis and (2) the administration of ganciclovir during antilymphocyte antibody therapy. Both offer considerable protection, and the concept of linking a particular antimicrobial strategy to the type of immunosuppression used is especially appealing [1–3,87,88]. See Table 44-1.

Human Herpesvirus-6

HHV-6 is a β herpesvirus closely related to CMV (66% DNA sequence homology). HHV-6 infects and replicates within a wide array of leukocytes, most notably CD4 positive lymphocytes. An important effect of HHV-6 replication is the elaboration of proinflammatory cytokines, most importantly TNF and interferon-χ. Primary HHV-6 infection usually occurs in the first year of life; as a consequence, 90% of adults harbor latent infection (and are seropositive). In normal children, HHV-6 is the cause of a febrile

exanthema known as roseola. The consequences of HHV-6 reactivation and subsequent replication, particularly in the immunocompromised host, are several: mononucleosis syndrome with and without hepatitis and/or interstitial pneumonia, bone marrow suppression, and encephalitis. Dual infection with CMV and HHV-6 is common, and it has been suggested that such patients are sicker than those with single virus replication. Diagnosis of HHV-6 is best done with a PCR or antigenemia assay. It is likely that many of the direct and indirect effects of HHV-6 are similar to those seen with CMV and a clearer view of the impact of HHV-6 infection will emerge over the next few years. HHV-6 is susceptible to both ganciclovir and foscarnet, and it is probable that antiviral programs designed for one of these is modulating the course of other herpes group viruses [89–93].

Epstein-Barr Virus

Active EBV replication is present in 20% to 30% of organ transplant patients on maintenance immunosuppression (slightly higher than the general population), rising to >80% during antilymphocyte antibody therapy of acute rejection. Although a mononucleosis-like syndrome (usually heterophile negative in this patient population) comparable to that produced by CMV has been shown to be due to EBV in some patients, the critical impact of EBV is in its role in the pathogenesis of PTLD [1].

PTLD is a B-cell lymphoproliferative process that ranges in severity from a benign polyclonal process that responds to a decrease in immunosuppressive therapy

($\pm$ antiviral therapy) to a highly malignant monoclonal process resistant to all forms of treatment. It is frequently totally extranodal in presentation with brain involvement, invasion of the allograft, gastrointestinal tract disease, and liver invasion being not uncommon. The pathogenesis of this process is related to the effects of immunosuppressive therapy on the usual mechanisms for preventing the outgrowth of EBV-infected, immortalized B cells. As with CMV, the cornerstone of this defense is virus-specific, MHC-restricted, cytotoxic T cells, which destroy the EBV-infected B cells. Cyclosporine and FK-506 have a dose-related inhibitory effect on this defense and, thus, on the incidence of PTLD. OKT3 and ATG contribute to the pathogenesis of PTLD at two levels: they inhibit the surveillance mechanism, but, even more important, as with CMV, are their potent effects in reactivating latent EBV, thus increasing the potential for outgrowth of immortalized B cells. Other risk factors for PTLD include primary EBV infection, high levels of virus replicating in the oropharynx, and, as previously discussed, preceding CMV disease [1,94].

Other than decreasing immunosuppression, which will result in regression of 20–30% of these processes, therapy of PTLD remains unclear. Most groups use high-dose acyclovir or ganciclovir in hope that EBV is still driving the process, although evidence that infection susceptible to antiviral therapy is present at the time of development of PTLD is lacking. Patients not responding to these measures are usually treated with an anti-B cell antibody. For refractory patients, some combination of chemotherapy, radiation therapy, and surgery usually is prescribed with disappointing results. Other experimental therapies include interferon, an anti–B-cell antibody, and, perhaps most interesting, the adoptive transfer of activated cytotoxic T cells [95–100].

Clearly, this process would best be prevented. Both antivirals commonly used in transplant patients, ganciclovir and acyclovir, can inhibit EBV replication. The critical question is whether this will interrupt the pathogenesis of PTLD either directly through effects on EBV replication or indirectly through effects on CMV [1,95–100].

Viral Hepatitis

The course of both HBV and HCV infection is accelerated in these immunosuppressed patients compared with the general population, with both progressive liver failure and cirrhosis with hepatocellular carcinoma occurring as consequences of these infections (see Chapter 42). With modern serologic testing, it is now uncommon for patients to acquire HBV infection at the time of transplantation from either the donor of the organ or from blood. This is fortunate because the acquisition of HBV at the time of transplantation has a relatively high incidence of acute hepatic failure. The bigger problem clinically is the question of disease progression in HBV-infected individuals after transplantation. By 10 years post-transplantation, more than half of these individuals will have progressed to end-stage liver disease or hepatocellular carcinoma [1,101–103].

Both HBV and HCV are modulated by the immunosuppressive therapy, particularly corticosteroids, which appear to have a direct stimulatory effect on the level of virus replication. In HBV infection, this is manifest by a rapid increase in HBV DNA polymerase activity, HBeAg levels, HBV DNA, and HBsAg levels. These findings are in contrast to the gradual decrease in HBV production that often is observed in viral carriers not receiving immunosuppressive therapy [1–3].

Hepatitis B has a particularly detrimental effect on liver transplant recipients. Recurrent HBV infection occurs in 80–90% of patients undergoing liver transplantation, and 1-year survival in these patients has been 50–60% (significantly less than the 80% to 85% survival seen in other patient groups). Recurrent disease is rare in patients being transplanted for fulminant hepatic failure due to HBV or in those with simultaneous delta virus infection. The range of clinical disease that results from recurrent HBV infection is quite broad: mild, persistent hepatitis to aggressive, chronic hepatitis and fulminant liver failure [1,104–108].

Two major advances have had a significant effect on the outcome of transplantation in patients with chronic HBV infection: (1) the effectiveness of long-term immunoprophylaxis with anti-HBs hyperimmune globulin and (2) the potency of lamivudine as an anti-HBV drug. The administration of 10,000 units of hyperimmune anti-HBV immunoglobulin during the anhepatic phase followed by daily administration for 6 days and then administration at $\sim$3- to 6-week intervals to maintain the anti-hepatitis B surface antigen titer at >1:100 IU appears to provide significant protection against recurrent liver disease and to increase patient survival. However, the indefinite need for this therapy adds $15,000 to $25,000 to the first-year costs (and continues to be a significant cost thereafter) [1].

Lamivudine is a nucleoside analogue that is a powerful inhibitor of the HBV polymerase/reverse transcriptase. This drug has been extremely effective in lowering HBV levels and improving hepatic function in the full range of HBV clinical syndromes, including the devastating fibrosing, cholestatic hepatitis form of HBV disease. The major disadvantage of lamivudine is the emergence of drug resistance in the virus (usually in a highly conserved region of the reverse transcriptase called the YMDD motif). These mutants begin to emerge approximately 1 year after the drug is initiated with an increasing incidence over time. The higher the viral load, the more likely and the more quickly resistance mutants will emerge. After the first year of therapy, 15–30% of patients receiving lamividine will have resistant virus; this rises to ≥40% after two years of therapy. It is clear that combination drug therapy or the combination of hyperimmune globulin with antiviral(s) will be necessary to control this infection [1–3,107–114].

HCV is the cause of >80% of end-stage liver disease and is the most common indication for liver transplantation in much of the world. Both transfusion and transplantation are highly efficient means of transmitting HCV to another individual. In liver transplant recipients who are infected with HCV, re-infection of the allograft is the rule. Re-infection is accomplished by HCV-infected peripheral blood mononuclear cells [115–117].

A series of risk factors has been defined in patients with HCV re-infection that are correlated with increased morbidity and mortality: viral load—the higher the viral load, the greater is the risk of serious disease and/or the more accelerated the course; intensity of immunosuppression—especially excessive amounts of corticosteroids (both pulse doses to treat acute rejection and sustained high daily doses to prevent rejection); ideally, patients with HCV infection are maintained on "steroid sparing regimens." In addition to steroids, OKT3 therapy and mycophenolate use have been associated with significant increases in HCV viral load; allograft rejection—cytokines, chemokines, and growth factors produced in the rejection process will increase viral load; the additional immunosuppression required to control the rejection process will likewise add to the viral burden; HCV genotype—genotype 1b infection is associated with higher viral loads, a more accelerated course, and a poorer response to interferon-based therapeutic regimens; the presence of quasispecies—the greater the heterogeneity in the virus present, the greater difficulty the patient has in containing the infection; CMV viremia—there is a bidirectional effect between HCV and CMV, with chemokines and cytokines produced in response to one virus causing an increase in the level in the other virus; iron overload—which decreases the patient's cytotoxic T cell response to HCV, thus allowing the viral burden to increase; donor and recipient class II HLA matching—associated with re-infection and allograft injury; and, finally, donor tumor necrosis factor gene—the donor TNF-α promoter genotype may influence the inflammatory response to HCV infection of the graft and the extent of subsequent allograft injury [118–130].

A potentially devastating consequence of HCV infection in the transplant recipient is an uncommon clinical syndrome, fibrosing cholestatic hepatitis. Also seen with HBV infection, this is a syndrome characterized by high levels of circulating virus, rapidly progressive hepatic failure, mildly elevated serum aminotransferase levels, and a pathologic picture of extensive periportal fibrosis, intense cholestasis, minimal inflammatory infiltrate, and no cirrhosis. The hepatocytes are choked with exceedingly high levels of virus, causing direct hepatocyte injury. This entity requires decreased immunosuppression and intensive antiviral therapy [133–143].

An additional potential complication of HCV infection is glomerulonephritis. The most common form of this is membranoproliferative glomerulonephritis with or without mixed cryoglobulinemia. Less common forms of renal injury associated with HCV are membranous glomerulonephritis, acute and chronic transplant glomerulopathy, and thrombotic microangiopathy with anticardiolipin antibody; management of these complications centers on antiviral therapy [137–143].

The presently available therapy of HCV includes a dramatic decrease of immunosuppressive therapy, control of CMV infection if it is present, and antiviral therapy. The best therapy currently available is the combination of ribovirin and pegolated versions of interferon-α (conventional interferon-α plus ribovirin regimens yield a 50% response with the pegolated form even better). Side effects are unfortunately common with such treatment: Interferon use is associated with fever, malaise, bone marrow dysfunction, and risk of rejection, and ribovirin can cause hemolytic anemia [144–150].

Approximately 5% of all organ donors are anti-HCV positive, with approximately half of these being positive by PCR assay for circulating viral RNA. Organs from PCR-positive individuals are extremely efficient at transmitting virus to the recipient. Given the relatively slow pace of HCV illness and the continuing shortage of donors, there has been great controversy about whether to accept anti-HCV-positive donors. Reserving these organs for anti HCV-positive recipients results in superinfection with donor-strain HCV. The policy at the author's center is to reserve organs from anti-HCV-positive donors for critically ill heart and liver patients, for highly sensitized renal patients, and for older patients (with potentially shorter life spans during which the hepatitis would progress). Even in these circumstances, ethical considerations require full disclosure to the individuals involved regarding the potential consequences of such an action [1–3].

Mycobacterial Infections

Infection due to *M. tuberculosis* has been less of a problem after transplantation than might have been predicted. Despite immunosuppressive therapy, reactivation and dissemination of *M. tuberculosis* have been exceedingly uncommon in individuals whose only evidence of dormant tuberculosis is a positive tuberculin test. Conversely, patients with (1) a history of active tuberculosis (treated or untreated), (2) an abnormal chest radiograph, (3) noncaucasian racial background, (4) protein-calorie malnutrition, or (5) another immunosuppressing illness, in addition to a positive tuberculin test, are at significant risk for reactivating their tuberculosis. The approach at the author's center is to reserve antituberculous prophylaxis for those with added risk factors in addition to a positive tuberculin skin test. We have now followed more than 100 "low-risk" individuals post-transplantation for periods of up to 10 years without a single case of reactivation despite the positive tuberculin reaction; the high background rate of hepatocellular dysfunction in these patients makes the use of isoniazid or rifampin challenging; and antituberculous drugs affect the pharmacokinetic profile of cyclosporine and tacrolimus, rendering the use of these drugs more difficult as well [1–3].

Atypical mycobacterial infection also may be observed in transplant recipients: Local or disseminated disease due to *Mycobacterium kansasii* and progressive skin infection due to *Mycobacterium marinum*, *Mycobacterium haemophilum*, and *Mycobacterium chelonei* has been reported. These infections typically present initially at sites of cutaneous injury. Management usually involves surgery and chemotherapy based on *in vitro* antimicrobial susceptibility testing [1–3].

Fungal Infections

The fungal infections that affect transplant recipients can be divided into two general categories: (1) disseminated primary or reactivated infection with one of the geographically restricted systemic mycoses (histoplasmosis, blastomycosis, and coccidioidomycosis), and (2) invasive opportunistic infections with such organisms as *Candida* species, *Aspergillus* species, *C. neoformans*, and the Mucoraceae. The first category of disease should be considered in patients with a history of recent or remote travel to an endemic region who present with one of the following clinical syndromes: subacute respiratory illness, with focal, disseminated, or miliary infiltrates on chest radiograph; a nonspecific, systemic, febrile illness; unexplained pancytopenia; and an illness in which metastatic aspects of the infection predominate (e.g., mucocutaneous manifestations of histoplasmosis and blastomycosis or central nervous system manifestations in coccidioidomycosis or histoplasmosis) [1–3].

The opportunistic fungal infections have a far greater impact on the transplant patient than do the endemic mycoses. Primary infection, usually of the lungs but occasionally of the nasal sinuses, may occur in patients who inhale air contaminated with *Aspergillus* species, *C. neoformans*, or, particularly in diabetic patients, Mucoraceae. In addition, secondary infection of wounds and hematomas and intravenous lines by *Candida* or *Aspergillus* species may occur. Evidence of metastatic infection may follow either primary or secondary fungal infection with the skin and central nervous system being common sites of presentation. Fungal infection is a particular concern at the bronchial anastomotic site of lung transplant recipients with chronic infection and occasional dehiscence developing [1–3].

A revolutionary change in antifungal therapy has occurred in recent years. Although the only useful drug for many years was amphotericin deoxycholate, today there are three major classes of effective drugs available [1]:

1. Lipid associated amphotericin preparations. These maintain the broad spectrum antifungal activity of the parent molecule while decreasing the incidence and severity of the two major toxicities: the acute "cytokine storm" with fever, rigors, malaise, and even hypotension, and progressive renal dysfunction.

2. The azoles. Although oral ketoconazole has been available for more than 20 years, its unreliable bioavailability (requiring an acid pH in the stomach) and its undesirable pharmacologic properties—poor penetration into the central nervous system (CNS) and urinary tract; and its hepatic toxicity and its effects on cytochrome P450 metabolism—have made this a drug of minimal utility for systemic therapy. Fluconazole was a major advance in antifungal therapy with excellent bioavailability permitting both oral and parenteral therapy with penetration into the CNS, eye, and urinary tract and with minimal toxicity. The only limitation to fluconazole use has been its spectrum of activity—*Cryptococcus neoformans*, *Candida species*, and *Coccidioides imitis*—but not the molds. With the extensive use of fluconazole, there have been small incremental increases in resistance among *Candida* spp. requiring attention when prescribing. Itraconazole has a desirable spectrum of activity (including *Aspergillus* and *Histoplasma*) but shares the undesirable pharmacologic properties of ketoconazole, and its use is largely restricted to "wrap-up" therapy. Newer azoles such as voriconazole and posiconazole offer further advantages. Voriconazole is now the drug of choice for invasive aspergillosis and other infections caused by moulds and is a useful drug in the management of fluconazole-resistant *Candida* spp. infections. Posiconazole has a similar spectrum as voriconazole, and has become the drug of choice for mucormycosis [1].

   Adverse effects of azoles are few, including hepatic dysfunction, skin rash, and drug–drug interactions. Voriconazole can cause visual disturbances that clear with cessation of the drug.

3. Echinocandins. These act by inhibiting glucan synthase activity, thus affecting cell wall synthesis. Caspofungin, the first of the echinocandins to be approved, have been shown to be useful in the treatment of invasive aspergillosis and systemic candidiasis. The most important question to be answered is the possibility of improved results with combination therapy. For example, the echinocandins, because of their effects on cell wall synthesis, have been called "the penicillins" of antifungal therapy with the hypothesis that they may improve the penetration of other drugs (e.g., an azole) and thus improve the ability to treat invasive fungal infection [1].

Pneumocystis Jirovici

Long considered a protozoan, *P. jirovici* has been shown by molecular taxonomic studies to be more appropriately regarded as a fungus. Regardless of this detail of classification, effective therapy thus far has been provided by drugs having antiprotozoan (as opposed to antifungal) profiles. The incidence of *Pneumocystis* pneumonia in organ transplant patients not receiving anti-*Pneumocystis* prophylaxis is 10–15%. Traditionally, such infections have been regarded as immunosuppression-induced reactivation of infection acquired in childhood. However, the possibility of immunosuppressed person-to-immunosuppressed person spread (possibly by an aerosolized route) exists. It is the policy at the author's center, therefore, to isolate patients with P. carinii pneumonia from other immunosuppressed patients, including transplant recipients [1–3].

In transplant recipients, *Pneumocystis* infection typically occurs either in the period 1 to 6 months posttransplantation, often in association with CMV infection, or in the late period, typically in the subgroup of patients with poor allograft function, excessive immunosuppression, and chronic viral infection [1–3].

When *Pneumocystis* pneumonia does develop, it is a subacute disease characterized by fever, nonproductive cough, and progressive dyspnea with hypoxemia occurring over several days, and the presence of an interstitial infiltrate on chest radiograph. Administration of low-dose TMP-SMX (one single-strength tablet at bedtime) is effective in the prevention of *Pneumocystis* pneumonia and is routinely used in our transplant recipients. Alternative therapies are less effective but include monthly aerosolized or intravenous pentamidine, atovaquone, and clindamycin with pyrimethamine. Because treatment of confirmed *Pneumocystis* pneumonia with high-dose TMP-SMX or parenteral pentamidine in transplant recipients is associated with a high rate of side effects, particularly bone marrow and renal toxicity, the importance of prevention cannot be overemphasized [1–3].

PRINCIPLES OF ANTIMICROBIAL THERAPY IN TRANSPLANT RECIPIENTS

The Importance of Drug–Drug Interactions in Prescribing Antimicrobial Treatment in Transplant Patients

Interactions between the calcineurin inhibitors and certain antimicrobial agents are common and important in the transplant patient. Both cyclosporine and tacrolimus are metabolized by hepatic cytochrome P450 enzymes, which account for two of the three types of drug interactions observed [1–3]:

1. Antimicrobial agents (most notably rifampin, nafcillin, and isoniazid) can upregulate the metabolism of the calcineurin inhibitors, resulting in lower blood levels for a given dose of drug and a high risk for insufficient immunosuppression and resulting allograft rejection.
2. Antimicrobial agents, most notably the macrolides (erythromycin > clarithromycin > azithromycin) and azoles (ketoconazole > itraconazole, voriconazole > fluconazole) can downregulate the metabolism of the calcineurin inhibitors. This results in higher blood levels for a given dose of drug and a high risk for overimmunosuppression, infection, and nephrotoxicity.

3. Antimicrobial agents given in appropriate doses to patients with therapeutic (not toxic) blood levels of the calcineurin inhibitors can develop nephrotoxicity quite quickly in the absence of any change in blood levels. There are three variants of this phenomenon:
   a. Dose-related. Whereas 1 single strength tablet of trimethoprim-sulfamethoxazole or 250 mg of ciprofloxacin is well tolerated, higher doses have a dose-related increased risk of renal dysfunction.
   b. "Accelerated nephrotoxicity." Drugs such as amphotericin or aminoglycosides, which commonly produce nephrotoxicity with sustained exposure, now manifest nephrotoxicity at a far lower dose.
   c. "Idiopathic nephrotoxicity." Single doses of gentmicin, amphotericin, and intravenous trimethoprim-sulfamethoxazole in the face of therapeutic levels of cyclosporine or tacrolimus have been documented to produce oliguric renal failure in some patients.

Sirolimus (rapamycin) has been a particular problem with most transplant centers not administering sirolimus and voriconazole to a transplant recipient. Recently, it has been shown that a sirolimus dose reduced by 90% will permit coadministration of the two drugs [50].

Problem-Directed Prophylactic Strategies

Antimicrobial therapy in transplant recipients presents several challenges. Many of the antimicrobial agents are themselves toxic and that toxicity frequently is exacerbated by cyclosporine and tacrolimus, the cornerstones of current immunosuppressive regimens. Prolonged courses of therapy with these toxic agents are required to achieve adequate treatment of clinically overt disease. Once disease has occurred, the infected tissue may become vulnerable to infection from other organisms (secondary infections).

The only way to avoid these difficulties is to shift the emphasis of infectious disease management of the transplant recipient to the prevention of infectious complications. This principle has led to development of prophylactic strategies directed toward specific problems, such as prevention of urinary tract infection in the renal transplant patient, prevention of procedure-related complications in the liver transplant recipient, prevention of toxoplasmosis in the heart transplant recipient, and prevention of *Pneumcystis* infection in all transplant recipients. All of these strategies have proved to be useful and cost-effective approaches to disease prevention [1–3].

The practice of routine prophylaxis is best illustrated by the use of TMP-SMX (one single-strength tablet daily) for 6 months or longer after transplantation. This practice presents a large series of common infections without perturbing the anaerobic flora of the gastrointestinal tract. Among the infections generally prevented are those due to P. jirovici, T. gondii, L. monocytogenes, N. asteroides, susceptible organisms involved in urinary tract infections due to *Enterobacteriaceae*; sinopulmonary infections due to *S. pneumoniae* and *H. influenzae*; and gastrointestinal infections due to *Salmonella* and *Shigella* species. Four aspects of patient care are altered by the routine use of TMP-SMX: (1) infections, when they occur, are rarely due to these pathogens, (2) the presence of these pathogens in a compliant patient suggests an increased epidemiologic exposure or excessive immune suppression (e.g., high-dose steroids, drug-induced neutropenia, CMV infection), (3) in the absence of increased risk, technical/anatomic factors (obstruction, hematoma, lymphocele, indwelling stent, anastomotic leak) must be considered, and (4) infections, when they occur, are usually due to antibiotic-resistant, often nosocomially acquired, organisms. Initial clinical evaluations and therapies must be aggressive (e.g., invasive procedures, broad-spectrum antibiotics) to identify and reverse the infectious process and any predisposing factors and to obtain appropriate microbiologic data to guide further therapies [1–3].

Two examples of the limitations of prophylaxis are relevant. The use of daily quinolone prophylaxis in renal transplant recipients successfully prevents urinary tract infections in the absence of mechanical obstruction. However, a 10–14% incidence of *Pneumocystis* pneumonia is observed in these individuals. The routine use of fluconazole prophylaxis successfully prevents infections due to susceptible yeasts. However, these patients and these institutions experience, over time, a shift to colonization and infection with resistant yeasts (e.g., *Candida glabrata, Candida krusei*) and filamentous fungi (e.g., *Aspergillus and Mucorales* species) Thus, individualized antifungal strategies (for those at greatest risk because of prolonged antibiotic use or those already colonized) may be preferred [1–3].

Preemptive Therapy

A newer mode of antimicrobial therapy, called preemptive therapy, has been described. Traditionally, antimicrobial therapy has been administered either prophylactically to a large number of patients at risk of disease before there is evidence of infection to prevent serious disease in a few or therapeutically to the few in whom tissue invasion and clinically overt disease are present. Typically, prophylactic regimens involve the administration of a nontoxic drug, often with less-than-ideal antimicrobial activity, for a prolonged period of time, whereas therapeutic regimens use the most effective medications, often at toxic doses, for shorter periods of time. Preemptive therapy combines the most desirable aspects of these two options: administration of highly effective therapy over a short period of time to a relatively small number of patients who are at risk of serious infection. The short duration of therapy reduces the potential toxicity, and clinical and laboratory markers may be used to determine predictors of serious infection. For example, preemptive therapy with low-dose ganciclovir administered in conjunction with OKT3 therapy to CMV-seropositive renal transplant

recipients appears to be a promising approach to the prevention of CMV disease. Similarly, the early use of fluconazole to eradicate asymptomatic candiduria in renal transplant recipients and to prevent progression to urinary tract obstruction and pyelonephritis and the use of fluconazole in association with surgical manipulation of a pulmonary nodule due to *Cryptococcus* to prevent cryptococcal meningitis are other examples of preemptive therapy [1–3].

FUTURE TRENDS

Given the therapeutic constraints imposed by the necessary immunosuppressive regimen and the devastation that infection may cause in the transplant recipient, appropriate emphasis is increasingly being placed on evaluation of predictors of serious infection. New technologies, including molecular hybridization and PCR, may allow the cost-effective screening and detection of at-risk individuals most in need of preemptive treatments. Development of clinical epidemiologic databases and appropriate laboratory markers will permit further major advances beyond the preemptive approach to infection in this ever-increasing and challenging population of patients.

REFERENCES

1. Rubin RH. *Infection in the organ transplant recipient.* New York:, 2002.
2. Rubin R, Ikonen T, et al. The therapeutic prescription for the organ transplant recipient: the linkage of immunosuppression and antimicrobial strategies. *Trans Infect Dis* 1999;1:29–39.
3. Fishman JA and Rubin RH. Infection in organ-transplant recipients. *N Engl J Med* 1998;338(24):1741–1751.
4. Hopkins CC, Weber DJ, et al. Invasive aspergillus infection: possible non-ward common source within the hospital environment. *J Hosp Infect* 1989;13(1):19–25.
5. Johnson R, Rubin R. Respiratory disease in kidney and liver transplant recipients. In: Shelhamer J, Pizzo P, Parrillo J, Masure H, eds. *Respiratory disease in the immunosuppressed host.* Philadelphia: JB Lippincott, 1991; 567–594.
6. Rubin RH. The compromised host as sentinel chicken. *N Engl J Med* 1987;317(18):1151–1153 [editorial].
7. Rubin RH, Wolfson JS, et al. Infection in the renal transplant recipient. *Am J Med* 1981;70(2):405–411.
8. Gottesdiener KM. Transplanted infections: donor-to-host transmission with the allograft. *Ann Intern Med,* 1989;110(12):1001–1016.
9. Nelson PW, Delmonico FL, et al. Unsuspected donor pseudomonas infection causing arterial disruption after renal transplantation. *Transplantation* 1984;37(3):313–314.
10. Rubin RH. Infectious disease complications of renal transplantation. *Kidney Int* 1993;44(1):221–236 [clinical conference].
11. Simonds RJ, Holmberg SD, et al. Transmission of human immunodeficiency virus type 1 from a seronegative organ and tissue donor. *N Engl J Med* 1992;326(11):726–732 [comments].
12. Rubin RH, Tolkoff-Rubin NE. The problem of human immunodeficiency virus (HIV) infection and transplantation. *Transpl Int* 1988;1(1):36–42.
13. Limaye AP, Connolly PA, et al. Transmission of Histoplasma capsulatum by organ transplantation. *N Engl J Med* 2000;343(16):1163–1166.
14. Ooi BS, Chen BT, et al. Survival of a patient transplanted with a kidney infected with Cryptococcus neoformans. *Transplantation* 1971;11(4):428–429.

15. Ryning FW, McLeod R, et al. Probable transmission of Toxoplasma gondii by organ transplantation. *Ann Intern Med* 1979;90(1):47–49.
16. Luft BJ, Naot Y, et al. Primary and reactivated toxoplasma infection in patients with cardiac transplants. Clinical spectrum and problems in diagnosis in a defined population. *Ann Intern Med* 1983;99(1):27–31.
17. Rose AG, Uys CJ, et al. Toxoplasmosis of donor and recipient hearts after heterotopic cardiac transplantation. *Arch Pathol Lab Med* 1983;107(7):368–373.
18. McGregor CG, Fleck DG, et al. Disseminated toxoplasmosis in cardiac transplantation. *J Clin Pathol* 1984;37(1):74–77.
19. Nagington J, Martin AL. Toxoplasmosis and heart transplantation. *Lancet* 1983;2(8351):679 [letter].
20. Hakim M, Esmore D, et al. Toxoplasmosis in cardiac transplantation. *Br Med J (Clin Res Ed)* 1986;292(6528):1108.
21. Britt RH, Enzmann DR, et al. Intracranial infection in cardiac transplant recipients. *Ann Neurol* 1981;9(2):107–119.
22. Luft BJ, Billingham M, et al. Endomyocardial biopsy in the diagnosis of toxoplasmic myocarditis. *Transplant Proc* 1986;18(6):1871–1873.
23. Michaels MG, Wald ER, et al. Toxoplasmosis in pediatric recipients of heart transplants. *Clin Infect Dis* 1992;14(4):848–851.
24. Wreghitt TG, Gray JJ, et al. Efficacy of pyrimethamine for the prevention of donor-acquired Toxoplasma gondii infection in heart and heart-lung transplant patients. *Transpl Int* 1992;5(4):197–200.
25. Conti DJ, Rubin RH. Infection of the central nervous system in organ transplant recipients. *Neurol Clin* 1988;6(2):241–260.
26. Hibberd PL and Rubin RH. Clinical aspects of fungal infection in organ transplant recipients. *Clin Infect Dis* 1994;19 (suppl 1):S33–S40.
27. Paya CV. Fungal infections in solid-organ transplantation. *Clin Infect Dis* 1993;16(5):677–688.
28. Hadley S, Karchmer AW. Fungal infections in solid organ transplant recipients. *Infect Dis Clin North Am* 1995;9(4):1045–1074.
29. Belzer F. Technical complications after renal transplantation. In: Morris P, ed. *Kidney transplantation: principles and practice.* New York: Academic Press, 1979:267–284.
30. Kusne S, Dummer JS, et al. Infections after liver transplantation. an analysis of 101 consecutive cases. *Medicine (Baltimore)* 1988;67(2):132–143.
31. Rosman C, Klompmaker IJ, et al. The efficacy of selective bowel decontamination as infection prevention after liver transplantation. *Transplant Proc* 1990;22(4):1554–1555.
32. Castaldo P, Stratta RJ, et al. Clinical spectrum of fungal infections after orthotopic liver transplantation. *Arch Surg* 1991 126(2):149–156.
33. Arnow PM, Furmaga K, et al. Microbiological efficacy and pharmacokinetics of prophylactic antibiotics in liver transplant patients. *Antimicrob Agents Chemother* 1992; 36(10):2125–2130.
34. Arnow PM. Prevention of bacterial infection in the transplant recipient: the role of selective bowel decontamination. *Infect Dis Clin North Am* 1995; 9(4):849–862.
35. Fishman JA, Rubin RH. Infection in organ-transplant recipients *N Engl J Med* 1998; 338(24).1741–1751 [comments].
36. Rubin RH. Impact of cytomegalovirus infection on organ transplant recipients. *Rev Infect Dis.* 1990; 12(suppl 7):S754–S66.
37. Rubin RH. Infectious disease complications of renal transplantation. *Kidney Int* 1993; 44(1):221–236 [clinical conference].
38. Tolkoff-Rubin N, Rubin R. The purine antagonists: azathioprine and mycophenolate mofetil. In: Austen K, Burakoff S, Rosen F, Strom T, eds. *Therapeutic Immunology,* Cambridge: Blackwell Science, 2000.
39. Miner JN, Brown M. Glucocorticoid action. In: Austen K, Burakoff S, Rosen F, Strom T, eds. *Therapeutic Immunology.* 2nd ed. Cambridge: Blackwell Science, 2001:103–116.
40. Kahan BD. Cyclosporine *N Engl J Med* 1989; 321(25):1725–1738. [see comments].
41. Schreiber SL. Chemistry and biology of the immunophilins and their immunosuppressive ligands. *Science* 1991; 251(4991): 283–287.
42. Sebbag L, Boucher P, et al. Thiopurine S-methyltransferase gene polymorphism is predictive of azathioprine-induced myelosuppression in heart transplant recipients. *Transplantation* 2000; 69(7):1524–1527.
43. Cosimi A. Antilymphocyte globulin—a final look. In: Moris P, Tilney N, eds. *Progress in Transplantation.* 2nd ed. Edinburgh: Churchill Livingstone, 1985:167–188.
44. Ortho Multicenter Transplant Group. A randomized clinical trial of OKT3 monoclonal antibody for acute rejection of cadaveric renal transplants. *N Engl J Med* 1985; 313(6):337–342.
45. Gregory CR, Huie P, et al. Rapamycin inhibits arterial intimal thickening caused by both alloimmune and mechanical injury: its effect on cellular, growth factor, and cytokine response in injured vessels. *Transplantation* 1993, 55(6):1409–1418.
46. Poon M, Marx SO, et al. Rapamycin inhibits vascular smooth muscle cell migration. *J Clin Invest* 1996; 98(10):2277–2283.
47. Dominguez J, Mahalati K, et al. Conversion to rapamycin immunosuppression in renal transplant recipients: report of an initial experience *Transplantation* 2000; 70(8):1244–1247 [in process citation].
48. Garrean S, Massad MG, et al. Sirolimus-associated interstitial pneumonitis in solid organ transplant recipients. *Clin Transplant* 2005; 19(5):698–703.
49. Morelon E, Stern M, et al. Characteristics of sirolimus-associated interstitial pneumonitis in renal transplant patients. *Transplantation* 2001; 72(5):787–790.
50. Marty FM, Lowry CM, et al. Voriconazole and sirolimus coadministration after allogeneic hematopoietic stem cell transplantation. *Biol Blood Marrow Transplant* 2006; 12(5):552–559.
51. Rubin RH. Impact of cytomegalovirus infection on organ transplant recipients. *Rev Infect Dis* 1990; 12(suppl 7):S754–S766.
52. Cheeseman SH, Rubin RH, et al. Controlled clinical trial of prophylactic human-leukocyte interferon in renal transplantation: effects on cytomegalovirus and herpes simplex virus infections. *N Engl J Med* 1979; 300(24):1345–1349.
53. Betts RF, Freeman RB, et al. Transmission of cytomegalovirus infection with renal allograft. *Kidney Int* 1975; 8(6):385–392.
54. Ho M, Suwansirikul S, et al. The transplanted kidney as a source of cytomegalovirus infection. *N Engl J Med* 1975; 293(22):1109–1112.
55. Suwansirikul S, Rao N, et al. Primary and secondary cytomegalovirus infection. *Arch Intern Med* 1977; 137(8):1026–1029.
56. Rubin RH, Cosimi AB, et al. Infectious disease syndromes attributable to cytomegalovirus and their significance among renal transplant recipients. *Transplantation* 1977; 24(6):458–464.
57. Chou SW. Acquisition of donor strains of cytomegalovirus by renal transplant recipients. *N Engl J Med* 1986; 314(22). 1418–1423.
58. Grundy JE, Lui SF, et al. Symptomatic cytomegalovirus infection in seropositive kidney recipients: reinfection with donor virus rather than reactivation of recipient virus. *Lancet* 1988; 2(8603):132–135.
59. Rubin R, Colvin R. The impact of CMV infections on renal transplantation. In: Racusen L, Solez K, Burdick J, eds. *Kidney transplant rejection.* New York: Marcel Dekker. 1998:605–626.
60. Tolkoff-Rubin NE, Rubin RH. Recent advances in the diagnosis and management of infection in the organ transplant recipient. *Semin Nephrol* 2000; 20(2):148–163.
61. Chou SW, Norman DJ. The influence of donor factors other than serologic status on transmission of cytomegalovirus to transplant recipients. *Transplantation* 1988; 46(1):89–93.
62. Betts RF. Cytomegalovirus infection in transplant patients. *Prog Med Virol* 1982; 28:44–64.
63. Greaves RF, Mocarski ES. Defective growth correlates with reduced accumulation of a viral DNA replication protein after low-multiplicity infection by a human cytomegalovirus ie1 mutant. *J Virol* 1998; 72(1):366–379.
64. Reinke P, Prosch S, et al. Mechanisms of human cytomegalovirus (HCMV) (re)activation and its impact on organ transplant patients. *Trans Infect Dis* 1999; 1:157–164.
65. Fietze E, Prosch S, et al. Cytomegalovirus infection in transplant recipients: the role of tumor necrosis factor. *Transplantation* 1994; 58(6):675–680.

66. Stein J, Volk HD, et al. Tumour necrosis factor alpha stimulates the activity of the human cytomegalovirus major immediate early enhancer/promoter in immature monocytic cells, part 11. *J Gen Virol* 1993; 74:2333–2338.

67. Prosch S, Staak K, et al. Stimulation of the human cytomegalovirus IE enhancer/promoter in HL-60 cells by TNF—alpha is mediated via induction of NFkB. *Virology* 1995; 208:107–116.

68. Docke WD, Prosch S, et al. Cytomegalovirus reactivation and tumour necrosis factor. *Lancet* 1994; 343(8892):268–269.

69. Mutimer D, Mirza D, et al. Enhanced (cytomegalovirus) viral replication associated with septic bacterial complications in liver transplant recipients. *Transplantation* 1997; 63(10):1411–1415.

70. Mutimer DJ, Shaw J, et al. Enhanced (cytomegalovirus) viral replication after transplantation for fulminant hepatic failure. *Liver Transpl Surg* 1997;3(5):506–512 [comments].

71. Kutza AS, Muhl E, et al. High incidence of active cytomegalovirus infection among septic patients. *Clin Infect Dis* 1998;26(5):1076–1082 [comments].

72. Ho M. Cytomegalovirus infection in patients with bacterial sepsis. *Clin Infect Dis* 1998;26(5):1083–1084 [editorial;comment].

73. Nordoy I, Muller F, et al. The role of the tumor necrosis factor system and interleukin-10 during cytomegalovirus infection in renal transplant recipients. *J Infect Dis* 2000;181(1):51–57.

74. Janssens S, Beyaert R. Role of Toll-like receptors in pathogen recognition. *Clin Microbiol Rev* 2003;16(4):637–646.

75. Arbour NC, Lorenz E, et al. TLR4 mutations are associated with endotoxin hyporesponsiveness in humans. *Nat Genet* 2000;25(2):187–191.

76. Compton T, Kurt-Jones EA, et al. Human cytomegalovirus activates inflammatory cytokine responses via CD14 and Toll-like receptor 2. *J Virol* 2003;77(8):4588–4596.

77. Beutler B. Innate immunity: an overview. *Mol Immunol* 2004;40(12):845–859.

78. Kijpittayarit S, Eid AJ, Brown RA, et al. Toll-like receptor 2 influences the pathogenesis of cytomegalovirus infection in humans. *J Infect Dis* [In press].

79. Gleaves CA, Smith TF, et al. Comparison of standard tube and shell vial cell culture techniques for the detection of cytomegalovirus in clinical specimens. *J Clin Microbiol* 1985;21(2):217–221.

80. Swenson PD, Kaplan MH. Rapid detection of cytomegalovirus in cell culture by indirect immunoperoxidase staining with monoclonal antibody to an early nuclear antigen. *J Clin Microbiol* 1985;21(5):669–673.

81. Paya CV, Wold AD, et al. Detection of cytomegalovirus infections in specimens other than urine by the shell vial assay and conventional tube cell cultures. *J Clin Microbiol* 1987;25(5):755–757.

82. Marsano L, Perrillo RP, et al. Comparison of culture and serology for the diagnosis of cytomegalovirus infection in kidney and liver transplant recipients. *J Infect Dis* 1990;161(3):454–461.

83. de Otero J, Gavalda J, et al. Cytomegalovirus disease as a risk factor for graft loss and death after orthotopic liver transplantation. *Clin Infect Dis* 1998;26(4):865–870 [see comments].

84. Rubin RH. Cytomegalovirus disease and allograft loss after organ transplantation. *Clin Infect Dis* 1998;26(4):871–873 [editorial; comment].

85. Grattan MT, Moreno-Cabral CE, et al. Cytomegalovirus infection is associated with cardiac allograft rejection and atherosclerosis. *JAMA* 1989;261(24):3561–3566.

86. Rubin RH. The indirect effects of cytomegalovirus infection on the outcome of organ transplantation. *JAMA* 1989;261(24):3607–3609.

87. Turgeon N, Fishman JA, et al. Effect of oral acyclovir or ganciclovir therapy after preemptive intravenous ganciclovir therapy to prevent cytomegalovirus disease in cytomegalovirus seropositive renal and liver transplant recipients receiving antilymphocyte antibody therapy. *Transplantation* 1998;66(12):1780–1786.

88. Kusne S, Grossi P, et al. Cytomegalovirus PP65 antigenemia monitoring as a guide for preemptive therapy: a cost effective strategy for prevention of cytomegalovirus disease in adult liver transplant recipients. *Transplantation* 1999;68(8):1125–1131.

89. Singh N, Paterson DL. Encephalitis caused by human herpesvirus-6 in transplant recipients: relevance of a novel neurotropic virus. *Transplantation* 2000;69(12):2474–2479.

90. Dockrell DH, Smith TF, et al. Human herpesvirus 6. *Mayo Clin Proc* 1999;74(2):163–170.

91. Griffiths PD, Ait-Khaled M, et al. Human herpesviruses 6 and 7 as potential pathogens after liver transplant: prospective comparison with the effect of cytomegalovirus. *J Med Virol* 1999;59(4):496–501.

92. Tong CY, Bakran A, et al. Association of human herpesvirus 7 with cytomegalovirus disease in renal transplant recipients. *Transplantation* 2000;70(1):213–216.

93. Brennan DC, Storch GA, et al. The prevalence of human herpesvirus-7 in renal transplant recipients is unaffected by oral or intravenous ganciclovir. *J Infect Dis* 2000;181(5):1557–1561.

94. Herbert D, Sullivan E. Malignancy and post-transplant lymphoproliferative disorder (PTLD) in pediatric renal transplant recipients: a report of the North American Pediatric Transplant Cooperative Study Group (NAPRTCS). *Pediatric Transplant* 1998;2:57.

95. Paya CV, Fung JJ, et al. Epstein-Barr virus-induced posttransplant lymphoproliferative disorders. *Transplantation* 1999;68(10):1517–1525.

96. Harris NL, Ferry JA, et al. Posttransplant lymphoproliferative disorders: summary of Society for Hematopathology Workshop. *Semin Diagn Pathol* 1997;14(1):8–14.

97. Preiksaitis JK. Epstein-Barr virus infection and malignancy in solid organ transplant recipients: strategies for prevention and treatment. *Transpl Infect Dis* 2001;3(2):56–59.

98. Preiksaitis JK, Diaz-Mitoma F, et al. Quantitative oropharyngeal Epstein-Barr virus shedding in renal and cardiac transplant recipients: relationship to immunosuppressive therapy, serologic responses, and the risk of posttransplant lymphoproliferative disorder. *J Infect Dis* 1992;166(5):986–994.

99. Pagano JS. Epstein-Barr virus: culprit or consort? [see comments]. *N Engl J Med* 1992;327(24):1750–1752 [editorial; comment].

100. Cohen JI. The biology of Epstein-Barr virus: lessons learned from the virus and the host. *Curr Opin Immunol* 1999;11(4):365–370.

101. Dusheiko G, Song E, et al. Natural history of hepatitis B virus infection in renal transplant recipients—a fifteen-year follow-up. *Hepatology* 1983;3(3):330–336.

102. Weir MR, Kirkman RL, et al. Liver disease in recipients of long-functioning renal allografts. *Kidney Int* 1985;8(5):839–844.

103. Rao KV, Andersen RC. Long-term results and complications in renal transplant recipients: observations in the second decade. *Transplantation* 1988;45(1):45–52.

104. Debure A, Degos F, et al. Liver diseases and hepatic complications in renal transplant patients. *Adv Nephrol Necker Hosp* 1988;17:375–400.

105. Rao KV, Kasiske BL, et al. Variability in the morphological spectrum and clinical outcome of chronic liver disease in hepatitis B-positive and B-negative renal transplant recipients. *Transplantation* 1991;51(2):391–396.

106. Luketic VA, Shiffman ML, et al. Primary hepatocellular carcinoma after orthotopic liver transplantation for chronic hepatitis B infection. *Ann Intern Med* 1991;114(3):212–213.

107. Samuel D, Bismuth A, et al. Passive immunoprophylaxis after liver transplantation in HBsAg-positive patients. *Lancet* 1991;337(8745):813–815.

108. Grazi GL, Mazziotti A, et al. Liver transplantation in HBsAg-positive HBV-DNA—negative cirrhotics: immunoprophylaxis and long-term outcome. *Liver Transpl Surg* 1996; 2(6):418–425.

109. Shields PL, Owsianka A, et al. Selection of hepatitis B surface "escape" mutants during passive immune prophylaxis following liver transplantation: potential impact of genetic changes on polymerase protein function. *Gut* 1999;45(2):306–309.

110. Al Faraidy K, Yoshida EM, et al. Alteration of the dismal natural history of fibrosing cholestatic hepatitis secondary to hepatitis B virus with the use of lamivudine. *Transplantation* 1999;64(6):926–928.

111. Ben-Ari Z, Shmueli D, et al. Beneficial effect of lamivudine in recurrent hepatitis B after liver transplantation. *Transplantation* 1997;63(3):393–396.

112. Nery JR, Weppler D, et al. Efficacy of lamivudine in controlling hepatitis B virus recurrence after liver transplantation. *Transplantation* 1998;65(12):1615–1621.

113. Perrillo R, Rakela J, et al. Multicenter study of lamivudine therapy for hepatitis B after liver transplantation. *Hepatology* 1999;29(5):1581–1586.

114. Mutimer D, Pillay D, et al. High pre-treatment serum hepatitis B virus titre predicts failure of lamivudine prophylaxis and graft re-infection after liver transplantation. *J Hepatol* 1999;30(4):715–721.

115. Katkov W, Rubin R. Liver disease in the organ transplant recipient: etiology, clinical impact, and clinical management. *Transplant Rev* 1991;5:200–208.

116. McCaughan G, Zekry A. Effects of immunosuppression and organ transplantation on the natural history and immunopathogenesis of hepatitis C virus infection. *Transplant Infect Dis* 2000;2:166–185.

117. Alter HJ, Purcell RH, et al. Detection of antibody to hepatitis C virus in prospectively followed transfusion recipients with acute and chronic non-A, non-B hepatitis. *N Engl J Med* 1989;321(22):1494–1500.

118. Charlton M, Seaberg E, et al. Predictors of patient and graft survival following liver transplantation for hepatitis C. *Hepatology* 1998;28(3):823–830.

119. Rosen HR, Martin, P. Hepatitis C infection in patients undergoing liver retransplantation. *Transplantation* 1998;66(12):1612–1616.

120. Feray C, Caccamo L, et al. European collaborative study on factors influencing outcome after liver transplantation for hepatitis C. *Gastroenterology* 1999;117(3):619–625.

121. Magy N, Cribier B, et al. Effects of corticosteroids on HCV infection. *Int J Immunopharmacol* 1999;21(4):253–261.

122. Papatheodoridis GV, Barton SG, et al. Longitudinal variation in hepatitis C virus (HCV) viraemia and early course of HCV infection after liver transplantation for HCV cirrhosis: the role of different immunosuppressive regimens. *Gut* 1999;45(3):427–434 [see comments].

123. Charlton M, Seaberg, E. Impact of immunosuppression and acute rejection on recurrence of hepatitis C: results of the National Institute of Diabetes and Digestive and Kidney Diseases Liver Transplantation Database. *Liver Transpl Surg* 1999;5(4 suppl 1):S107–S114.

124. Rostaing L, Izopet J, et al. Changes in hepatitis C virus RNA viremia concentrations in long-term renal transplant patients after introduction of mycophenolate mofetil. *Transplantation* 2000;69(5):991–914.

125. Rosen HR, Shackleton CR, et al. Use of OKT3 is associated with early and severe recurrence of hepatitis C after liver transplantation. *Am J Gastroenterol* 1997;92(9):1453–1457 [see comments].

126. Prieto M, Berenguer M, et al. High incidence of allograft cirrhosis in hepatitis C virus genotype 1b infection following transplantation: relationship with rejection episodes. *Hepatology* 1999;29(1):250–256.

127. Cotler SJ, Gaur LK, et al. Donor-recipient sharing of HLA class II alleles predicts earlier recurrence and accelerated progression of hepatitis C following liver transplantation. *Tissue Antigens* 1998;52(5):435–443.

128. Neumann AU, Lam NP, et al. Differences in viral dynamics between genotypes 1 and 2 of hepatitis C virus. *J Infect Dis* 2000;182(1):28–35.

129. Pessoa MG, Bzowej N, et al. Evolution of hepatitis C virus quasispecies in patients with severe cholestatic hepatitis after liver transplantation. *Hepatology* 1999;30(6):1513–1520.

130. Rosen HR, Chou S, et al. Cytomegalovirus viremia: risk factor for allograft cirrhosis after liver transplantation for hepatitis C. *Transplantation* 1997;64(5):721–726.

131. Singh N, Zeevi A, et al. Late onset cytomegalovirus disease in liver transplant recipients: de novo reactivation in recurrent hepatitis C virus hepatitis. *Transpl Int* 1998;11(4):308–311.

132. Weiss G, Umlauft F, et al. Associations between cellular immune effector function, iron metabolism, and disease activity in patients with chronic hepatitis C virus infection. *J Infect Dis* 1999;180(5):1452–1458.

133. Rosen HR, Lentz JJ, et al. Donor polymorphism of tumor necrosis factor gene: relationship with variable severity of hepatitis C recurrence after liver transplantation. *Transplantation* 1999;68(12):1898–1902.

134. Toth CM, Pascual M, et al. Hepatitis C virus-associated fibrosing cholestatic hepatitis after renal transplantation: response to interferon-alpha therapy. *Transplantation* 1998;66(9):1254–1258.

135. Delladetsima JK, Boletis JN, et al. Fibrosing cholestatic hepatitis in renal transplant recipients with hepatitis C virus infection. *Liver Transpl Surg* 1999;5(4):294–300.

136. Abraczinskas D, Chung R. Allograft dysfunction and hyperbilirubinemia in a liver transplant recipient. *Transplant Infect Dis* 2000;2:186–193.

137. Davis CL, Gretch DR, et al. Hepatitis C–associated glomerular disease in liver transplant recipients. *Liver Transpl Surg* 1995;1(3):166–175.

138. Morales JM., Campistol JM, et al. Glomerular diseases in patients with hepatitis C virus infection after renal transplantation. *Curr Opin Nephrol Hypertens* 1997;6(6):511–515.

139. Hestin D, Guillemin F, et al. Pretransplant hepatitis C virus infection: a predictor of proteinuria after renal transplantation. *Transplantation* 1998;65(5):741–744.

140. Pascual M, Thadhani R, et al. Nephrotic syndrome after liver transplantation in a patient with hepatitis C virus-associated glomerulonephritis. *Transplantation* 1997;64(7):1073–1076.

141. Morales JM, Pascual-Capdevila J, et al. Membranous glomerulonephritis associated with hepatitis C virus infection in renal transplant patients. *Transplantation* 1997;63(11):1634–1639.

142. Cantarell MC, Charco R, et al. Outcome of hepatitis C virus-associated membranoproliferative glomerulonephritis after liver transplantation. *Transplantation* 1999;68(8):1131–1134 [see comments].

143. Baid S, Cosimi, AB et al. Renal disease associated with hepatitis C infection after kidney and liver transplantation. *Transplantation* 2000;70(2):255–261.

144. no author. Management of hepatitis C. *NIH Consens Statement* 1997;15(3):1–41.

145. Sheiner PA, Boros P, et al. The efficacy of prophylactic interferon alfa-2b in preventing recurrent hepatitis C after liver transplantation. *Hepatology* 1998;28(3):831–838.

146. Cattral MS, Hemming AW, et al. Outcome of long-term ribavirin therapy for recurrent hepatitis C after liver transplantation. *Transplantation* 1999;67(9):1277–2780.

147. Bizollon T, Palazzo U, et al. Pilot study of the combination of interferon alfa and ribavirin as therapy of recurrent hepatitis C after liver transplantation *Hepatology* 1997;26(2):500–504 [see comments].

148. Muramatsu S, Ku Y, et al. Successful rescue of severe recurrent hepatitis C with interferon and ribavirin in a liver transplant patient. *Transplantation* 2000;69(9):1956–1958.

149. Zeuzem S, Feinman SV, et al. Peginterferon Alfa-2a in patients with chronic hepatitis C. *N Engl J Med* 2000;343(23):1666–1672.

150. Heathcote EJ, Shiffman ML, et al. Peginterferon Alfa-2a in patients with chronic hepatitis C and cirrhosis. *N Engl J Med* 2000;343(23):1673–1680.

Miscellaneous Procedure-Related Infections

45

Sharon F. Welbel and Robert A. Weinstein

Technical, computer, and radiologic advances over the past 10–20 years have facilitated dramatic growth in the fields of diagnostic and therapeutic procedures. With miles of vascular network, dozens of extravascular spaces, and several organ systems, any patient is a candidate for a staggering array of such interventions. Although many of these procedures can provide information that is essential for sophisticated patient care, supplant more traumatic interventions, and are critical for life support, most procedures also bypass natural host defenses and place patients at increased risk of healthcare-associated infection (HAI) [1,2]. It is not surprising, then, that the introduction of any new procedure often is followed closely by case-reports of procedure-associated infections. Occasionally, epidemiologic experiments of nature in the form of HAI outbreaks provide more detailed information on specific procedure-related hazards, which eventually could be subjected to prospective study. This chapter discusses a variety of procedure-associated infections that have been highlighted by retrospective or prospective investigations and that have not been discussed elsewhere in this book.

Because of the seemingly eclectic contents of this chapter, it is important to recognize from the outset that the procedures to be discussed have certain themes in common. First, all of the procedures are exquisitely vulnerable to these possibilities: inexperienced operators; breaks in aseptic technique; contaminated, inadequately disinfected, and/or technically difficult-to-clean equipment; and

ineffective antiseptics. Second, many procedure-related infection problems unfortunately reemerge as new generations of healthcare workers (HCWs) rediscover these vulnerabilities and/or are being newly recognized in developing countries that have fewer resources to devote to infection control, hence the importance of reviewing hazards that at first glance could appear remote [3]. Third, various procedures involving many different sites have as a common path of infection the bloodstream, although the risk of infection differs depending on whether bloodstream contamination is transient or persistent as well as on host- and organism-specific factors. Fourth, risks of biofilm formation on surfaces of many different devices that enter normally sterile body sites and the value of anti-infective coatings (e.g., antimicrobials, antiseptics, and heavy or precious metals) for such devices are being studied actively. Finally, many procedures bear the burden that the specific risks have not been defined sufficiently to determine whether certain preventive measures, such as the use of prophylactic antimicrobial therapy, are mandated.

INFECTIONS FROM PROCEDURES INVOLVING THE VASCULAR SYSTEM

Needleless Devices

HCWs always have been at risk of needlestick injuries, but quantifying the actual number of percutaneous needlestick injuries (NSIs) sustained by U.S. HCWs is difficult. Panlilio et al. combined data for 1997 and 1998 from the National Surveillance System for Healthcare Workers (NaSH) and the Exposure Prevention Information Network (EPINet) and adjusted the data for underreporting. The investigators estimated that the number of percutaneous NSIs sustained annually by U.S. HCWs is 304,325 [4]. This is in contrast to the 1,728 percutaneous NSIs reported in 2003 by 48 U.S. healthcare facilities to the EPINet surveillance program. The overall annual percutaneous NSI rate for all network hospitals in 2003 was 23.87 per 100 occupied beds [5]. Clearly, the risk of transmission of blood borne pathogens, such as human immunodeficiency virus (HIV), Hepatitis B virus (HBV), and Hepatitis C virus (HCV), still exists. The current federal standard for addressing NSIs among HCWs is the blood-borne pathogens standard promulgated by the Occupational Safety and Health Administration (OSHA) [6]. This standard requires that engineering controls and work practices eliminate or minimize HCW exposure to blood. One means of accomplishing this goal is to use needleless systems.

Since the introduction of needleless systems, decreased rates of occupational needlestick exposures have been documented [7–9]. Protected-needle intravenous (IV) systems also have decreased NSIs related to IV connectors by 62–88% [10,11]. Unfortunately, the devices are not routinely activated, which appears to be related to inadequate training [9].

The impact for the patient is less clear. A study to determine risk factors for bloodstream infections (BSIs) in patients receiving home intravenous infusion therapy [12] revealed that receipt of total parenteral nutrition and intralipid therapy through a needleless system was a BSI risk factor. The results of a survey on the subject of injection caps demonstrated that positive cultures were significantly more common from needleless devices than from protected-needle devices. It was concluded that when injection caps are manipulated, nutrient-rich solutions can remain in the caps of the needleless devices and become contaminated. Another study that assessed needleless systems used with Hickman catheters suggested that such systems can be associated with increased rates of catheter-related BSI [13]. The investigators cultured luminal fluid from Hickman catheters of hematology patients and found that these catheters with the needleless system were twice as likely to show luminal contamination compared with catheters without the system. Four BSIs in patients with the needleless device had peripheral blood and luminal fluid cultures that yielded concordant bacterial strains based on results of pulsed-field electrophoresis and restriction fragment polymorphism studies. Do et al. described an increased BSI rate with the use of a needleless intravenous system in a home care setting when caps were changed every 7 days and a subsequent decrease in BSIs when the needleless device end cap was changed every 2 days, suggesting that the mechanism for BSI could involve contamination

from the end cap [14]. Kellerman et al. reported an 80% increase in BSIs related to central venous catheters (CVC) in pediatric hematology oncology patients receiving home health care after introduction of a needleless device for CVC access [15]. At another institution, a significant increase in the BSI rate in a surgical intensive care unit (ICU) and an organ transplant unit was associated with the introduction of a needleless intravenous system. This was attributed to nurses' lack of familiarity with the device and deviation from the manufacturers' recommended practices [16]. Finally, another study that investigated risk factors associated with an increased rate of BSIs in pediatric ICU found that exposure to the IVAC first-generation needleless device (IVAC, San Diego, California) was an independent BSI risk factor. The BSI rate returned to baseline after institution of a policy to replace the entire IVAC device, valve, and end-cap every 24 hours [17].

The association between needleless devices and infection seems to relate to lack of familiarity with the device and/or its mechanics. Some investigators have investigated the mechanics of needleless devices to determine whether new technology added to the device could reduce infection risk. Menyhay and Maki reported on a simulation study that compared the efficacy of conventional alcohol disinfection of the membranous septum of needleless luer-activated valved connectors before access with the use of a novel antiseptic-barrier cap that, when threaded onto the connector, places a chlorhexidine-impregnated sponge in continuous contact with the membranous surface [18]. After removal of the cap, there is no need to disinfect the surface with alcohol before accessing it. After contaminating, disinfecting, and then culturing the connectors, the authors demonstrated that if the membranous septum of a needleless luer-activated connector is heavily contaminated, conventional disinfection with 70% alcohol did not reliably prevent entry of microorganisms. In contrast, the antiseptic-barrier cap provided a high level of protection. Another study considered a recently developed needleless closed luer access device (CLAD) (Q-Syte, Becton Dickinson, Sandy, Utah). Devices were contaminated with bacteria and then disinfected with 70% isopropyl alcohol followed by flushing with 0.9% saline. Although devices had been accessed up to 70 times, no microorganisms were found even when challenge microorganisms were detected on the syringe tip after activation and on the compression seals before decontamination, suggesting that the Q-Syte CLAD can be activated up to 70 times with no increase risk of microbial contamination within the fluid pathway [19]. Needleless systems are now almost universally used; the benefit to the HCW and the risk to the patient have been demonstrated. Education is a key intervention to prevent patient infections with devices new to an institution. Novel interventions as mentioned previously will need to be studied further to assess their benefit and cost. The luer-activated valved connector, which allows a chlorhexidine-impregnated sponge to do the work, could be particularly helpful because it does not depend on the action of an HCW for disinfection.

Finally, the tourniquet could function as a possible vehicle for cross-contamination of pathogens such as methicillin-resistant *Staphylococcus aureus* (MRSA). Leitch et al. examined the contamination rate of phlebotomy tourniquets with MRSA. The investigators found that the tourniquets were contaminated with MRSA 25% of the time; they believed that the contamination occurred via the phlebotomists' hands, not the patients' skin [20]. The practice for tourniquet use varies widely from single patient use to disposal upon the discretion of the phlebotomist. Given that multidrug-resistant organisms, such as community-acquired MRSA, now are ubiquitous, the need for practices such as discarding or disinfecting tourniquets with alcohol wipe between uses to prevent tourniquets from harboring pathogens must be considered and evaluated.

Leeches

Despite the popular appeal of highly sharpened, disposable phlebotomy needles for diagnostic bloodletting, leeches have, in fact, resurfaced as a specialized part of the reconstructive and microvascular surgeons' armamentarium (e.g., for salvage of congested flaps [21]). However, as with many other advances discussed in this chapter, leeches have an infectious risk [22]. *Aeromonas hydrophila*, normal gut flora of the leech, has caused wound infections in 2.4–20.0% of microsurgical procedures using leeches [23,24]. *Aeromonas* sp. meningitis also has been associated with leech therapy [25]. In an attempt to decrease infectious complications of leeches, one group tried unsuccessfully to sterilize the gut of leeches [26]. Some investigators believe that aquariums filled with tap water to house leeches could contribute to the *Aeromonas* sp. problem [27]. Infection with *Serratia marcescens* also has been linked to leech therapy [28]. Understanding the nature of the leech's contamination (gut flora and surrounding environment) could help direct control efforts and prophylactic antimicrobial therapy.

Cardiac Catheterization

Serious local and systemic infections can result from cardiac catheterization procedures, particularly when contaminated instruments or ineffective antiseptics (e.g., dilute aqueous benzalkonium chloride) are used inadvertently or when breaks in technique occur in the cardiac catheterization laboratory. The major pathogens are staphylococci and gram-negative bacteria.

Up to 50% of patients undergoing cardiac catheterization could experience an increase in temperature of $>1°C$ ($1.8°F$) within 24 hours after catheterization. Their fever, however, has been attributed to the use of angiocardiographic contrast material rather than to infection. In fact, bacterial endocarditis has been reported very rarely

in large studies evaluating the complications of cardiac catheterization, and individual examples could have been due to initially undetected concurrent infection. The BSI rate after procedures in the cardiac catheter laboratory range from 0.11–18.00%. In a study of more than 22,000 patients undergoing invasive, nonsurgical, coronary procedures from 1991–1998, BSIs occurred in 0.11% at a median of 1.7 days after the procedure; in $>4,000$ patients undergoing coronary intervention, bacterial infections occurred in 0.64% and septic complications in 0.24% [29,30]. However, in 147 consecutive patients undergoing complex percutaneous coronary interventions (PCI), positive blood cultures were found in 18% immediately after the procedure and in 12% at 12 hours after the procedure [31].

Some studies reporting transient BSIs obtained blood cultures from the intravascular catheter or from the vessel from which the catheter had been removed. It is possible that some of the isolates represented contamination of the external part of the catheter or the site of insertion and that the incidence of BSI was actually less frequent. A study designed to assess this possibility obtained blood for culture by using standard techniques from a vein distant from the site of catheter manipulation [32]. Venous blood cultures of 106 patients, most whom had valvular heart disease, were obtained in this manner during cardiac catheterization, and all were sterile. Of 38 samples drawn through the catheter that was placed in the heart or aorta during the procedure, 3 grew diphtheroids or microaerophilic streptococci. The researchers concluded that the contamination of the hub end of the catheter with normal skin flora led to an overestimation of the BSI incidence. Removal of organisms by lung filtration also could have accounted, in part, for the failure to isolate organisms from distal sites. In either instance, it is clear that some contamination of the catheterization field had occurred.

Coronary stent placement, a newer procedure, now is routinely practiced yet has been linked to few reports of coronary stent infections. When such infections do occur, mortality and morbidity is high (Table 45-1). Once a stent has been placed, it is not removable; therefore, illuminating risk factors for stent infection is paramount [33–37].

Retrospective and prospective studies have illuminated various risk factors for PCI-associated BSI. These factors include difficult vascular access, multiple skin punctures, repeated catheterizations at the same vascular access site, extended procedure duration, use of multiple percutaneous transluminal coronary angioplasty (PTCA)-balloons, deferred removal of the arterial sheath, presence of congestive heart failure, and patient's age >60 years [29,30,38]. We should focus on nonpatient factors such as timely removal of the arterial sheath after percutaneous transluminal angioplasty to decrease HAI rates in the cardiac catheter laboratory. In addition, catheterization-associated infection should be infrequent with rigorous application of strict aseptic technique and adoption of the working principle that cardiac catheterization is a

TABLE 45-1

PUBLISHED CASE REPORTS OF CORONARY STENT INFECTIONS (ADAPTED WITH PERMISSION FROM [33])

Age in Years/Gender	Stent Type	Symptoms	Time of Presentation After Initial Procedure	Vessel; Complications	Diagnostic Tool	Organism	Therapy	Outcome
66/f	Palmaz-Schatz	Fever	4 weeks	RCA; abscess, pericardial empyema	TEE	S. aureus	IV antibiotics, stent removal	Death
49/m	Palmaz-Schatz	Fever	1 week	LAD; false aneurysm	Coronary angiogram	P. aeruginosa	IV antibiotics, surgery	Death
38/m	Palmaz-Schatz	Fever, chest pain	4 days	LCX; false aneurysm	CT scan, coronary angiogram	P. aeruginosa	IV antibiotics, debridement, stent removal	Survival
54/m	AVE microstent	AMI, fever	4 days	LAD; vessel destruction	None	S. aureus	None	Death
67/m	Not specified	Fever, chest pain, AMI	4 days	LCX; abscess	CT scan	S. aureus	IV antibiotics	Survival
72/m	NIR	Fever, chest pain	18 days	LAD; false aneurysm	Coronary angiogram	S. aureus	IV antibiotics, debridement, partial stent removal	Survival
55/m	Jostent Flex	Fever, chest pain	14 days	RCA; pericarditis	TEE	CNRS Candida spp.	IV antibiotics, IV antimycotics, stent removal	Survival
53/m	Jomed covered stent	Fever	2 days	Vein graft; abcess	TTE, TEE	S. aureus	IV antibiotics, abcess drainage	Death
56/m	Cypher (sirolimus-eluting stent)	Fever	4 days	LAD; mycotic aneurysm	Coronary angiogram	S. aureus	IV antibiotics	Survival
80/m	Jomed heparin coated	Fever, chills	5 days	LAD	CT scan	S. aureus	IV antibiotics	Survival

AMI, acute myocardial infarction; CNRS, coagulase-negative oxacillin-resistant staphylococci; CT, computed tomography; IV, intravenous; LAD, left anterior descending coronary artery; LCX, left circumflex coronary artery; MRI, magnetic resonance imaging; RCA, right coronary artery; TEE, transeseophageal echocardiography; TTE, transthoracic echocardiography.

surgical procedure. The Laboratory Performance Standards Committee of the Society for Cardiovascular Angiography and Interventions (SCAI) has published an updated guideline that addresses the increased utilization of the catheterization laboratory as an interventional suite with device implantation. The guide is divided into sections on the patient, laboratory personnel, and laboratory environment [39]. The guidelines can be accessed at **www.scai.org**.

Indwelling Arterial Catheters

Indwelling arterial catheters are used regularly in patients who require pressure monitoring or repeated blood gas determination (see Chapter 37). Although they provide information that is essential for patient care and eliminate the need for potentially traumatic repeated arterial punctures, such catheters also provide a continuing portal of entry for microbial invasion of the bloodstream. The reported incidence of arterial catheter colonization and infection varies depending on the catheter-tip culture technique used. Colonization incidence reports vary from 27% (49 episodes per 1,000 catheter-days) to 4% (11.7 episodes per 1,000 catheter-day) [40,41]. The source-organisms have not always been evaluated, and no direct relation with patient disease has been established, but the incidence of colonization of radial catheters (in contrast to umbilical catheters) did appear to be related to longer durations of catheterization (>4 days) [42]. Inflammation at the catheter site and the use of a cutdown procedure to place the catheter also appear to be associated with an increased infection risk [43–46] (see Chapter 37). A prospective study of 95 patients (130 catheters) in a medical–surgical ICU found a 4% risk of arterial cannula-related septicemia; 12% of all sepsis in this unit was the result of intra-arterial catheters [47]. These BSIs were caused by gram-negative bacilli, enterococci, or Candida organisms.

There are no national guideline recommendations for arterial catheter site insertion [48]. Intuitively, it seems that a femoral catheter would engender a greater risk of infection than a radial site, but few studies have demonstrated this. One study by Lorente et al. attempted to answer this question [49]; the authors performed a prospective observational study of all consecutive patients (2,018 patients with 2,049 arterial catheters) admitted to a medical–surgical ICU over 3 years. Multivariate analysis revealed that the catheter-related local infection rate was significantly higher for femoral than radial access (odds ratio [OR], 1.5; 95% confidence interval, 1.10–2.1). The catheter-related BSI rate also was higher (femoral 1.92/1,000 catheter-days versus radial 0.25/1,000 catheter-days) (OR, 1.9; 95% confidence interval, 1.15–3.4.). Other studies investigating arterial catheter infection rates have not found a difference between the rate of radial or femoral site infections or of BSIs [50–52].

In addition to choosing the best site to decrease infection risk, the best aseptic techniques must be used. Rijnders et al. studied colonization rates of arterial catheter tips and found no difference in the incidence of arterial catheter colonization when the catheter was inserted under maximal sterile barrier precautions, defined as an HCW wearing sterile gloves and a sterile gown, a mask, and a cap with the use of a large sterile sheet; skin was disinfected with 0.5% chlorhexidine in 70% alcohol versus the standard of care group in which hand washing was done, sterile gloves were worn, and the same skin disinfection was applied [46]. However, similar studies of CVC insertions have shown definite infection control value of maximal barrier precautions whose benefit could be operator dependent (e.g., of more benefit with less experienced inserters). Arterial catheters are frequently accessed for blood sampling, so perhaps the focus for decreasing the rate of infection should be on protecting the catheter hub during manipulation [48,53].

The infectious complications of arterial catheters also have been studied in neonates. In different centers, the incidence of colonization of indwelling umbilical artery catheters has varied from 6–60% [54–57]. Unexpectedly, however, the incidence of colonization fails to increase with duration of catheterization, which suggests that catheters become contaminated initially or soon after insertion through the umbilical stump, an area that is heavily colonized and impossible to sterilize completely by local or systemic antibiotics. Indeed, the same organisms usually are isolated from both the umbilical cord and catheter in any individual patient. The most frequent contaminants are staphylococci, streptococci, and gram-negative bacilli, particularly Pseudomonas, Proteus, Escherichia coli, and Klebsiella. The clinical significance of umbilical catheter colonization is difficult to assess because the incidence of sepsis in most studies has been low. When serial prospective blood cultures have been obtained from umbilical catheterized neonates, however, transient catheter-related BSI has been noted. In a prospective study of temporary (2–4 hours) umbilical catheterization for exchange transfusion, investigators documented a 60% incidence of catheter contamination and a 10% incidence of transient BSI due to Staphylococcus epidermidis (and, in one patient, Proteus) that occurred 4–6 hours after transfusion; this study suggests that the risk of BSI from umbilical catheterization could be highest during catheter insertion and removal [58]. This study and others found that prophylactic systemic antibiotics failed to reduce the incidence of catheter contamination and BSI. At present, systemic antibiotic prophylaxis does not appear to be beneficial during umbilical catheterization; instead, attention should be focused on meticulous cord preparation and care. Other infectious complications of umbilical arterial catheters include mycotic aneurysm or pseudoaneurysm with or without hemoperitoneum [59–61].

Pulmonary artery catheters that are inserted through a Teflon® introducer and are mostly heparin bonded have similar rates of infection as do CVCs, but flow-directed pulmonary artery catheters carry the added risk of right-sided endocarditis related to endocardial trauma and septic thrombosis of the great vein or pulmonary artery. One autopsy study found that 7% of 55 patients had endocarditis in association with these catheters [62]. Studies that used multivariate analysis have identified a number of risk factors for infection associated with the use of pulmonary artery catheters [63]. Strong independent predictors of an increased risk of catheter colonization were the use of catheters in neonates and in younger children, the placement of the catheter without using maximal barrier precautions, the placement in an internal jugular (rather than a subclavian) vein, the heavy cutaneous colonization at the insertion site, and a prolonged catheterization—particularly >3 days [41,64–67].

Transducers

Pressure-monitoring devices are used regularly to monitor cardiovascular pressures of critically ill patients. Guidelines for preventing infections related to intravascular pressure monitoring have been formulated and updated by the Centers for Disease Control and Prevention (CDC) [68]. Reusable transducers have been sources of HAIs in outbreaks of gram-negative BSI, candidemia, and dialysis-associated hepatitis [69]. However, disposable pressure transducers can be safely used without change for 4 days, even in busy ICUs [70]. Currently, it is recommended that disposable transducer assemblies be used and replaced every 96 hours [48].

Circulatory Assist Devices

Left ventricular assist devices (LVAD) are used to maintain a patient's circulation while awaiting cardiac transplantation (see Chapter 38). The frequently used Heartmate (Thoratec Corporation, Pleasanton, California) LVAD consists of a titanium-encased blood pump, an inflow cannula from the left ventricular apex, and an outflow cannula to the ascending aorta. Two porcine valves maintain unidirectional flow. The pump is placed into either a preperitoneal pocket or the abdominal cavity. A driveline connects the device to an external power source via an exit site in the abdominal wall (Figure 45-1). These devices have supplanted the totally artificial heart whose morbidity and mortality are associated with wound infection [70]. Although LVADs may be life saving, infection has been one of its most common complications [71–75]. Infections associated with LVADs include device-related BSI, exit site infections, mediastinitis, and infections at the entrance site of the transcutaneous power cables. One of the more common and difficult problems is a result of the tunneled driveline that connects data between the pump and the extracorporeal controller unit and can result in deep driveline tract, pocket, and device infections. Infectious complications of LVADs are particularly important because they could preclude subsequent

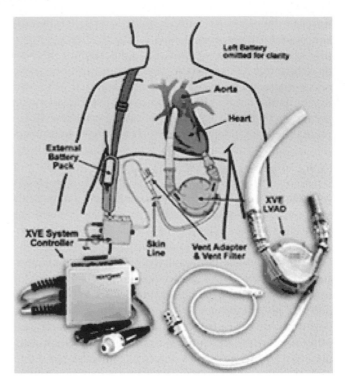

Figure 45-1   Heartmate left ventricular assist device (with verbal permission from Thoratec Corporation, Pleasanton, California).

heart transplantation [73–77]. In a retrospective analysis of experience with LVADs over an 8-year period, 32% (14/44) of patients did not receive a donor organ because of LVAD-related infection. However, in another retrospective analysis of 14 patients who required an LVAD despite four device-related infections in 3 patients, all 14 patients underwent transplantation that was not delayed because of infection [78]. Others have found the same results [79].

In a particularly robust 9-year retrospective study, investigators found 76 patients who underwent LVAD implantation with the pneumatically or electrically driven Heartmate LVAD as a bridge to cardiac transplantation [73]. Forty-six LVAD-related infections developed in 38 patients for an incidence of 4.9 LVAD-related infections per 1,000 LVAD-days. Twenty-nine LVAD-related BSIs were found in 24 patients for an incidence of 3.1 LVAD-related BSI per 1,000 LVAD-days; persistent sepsis with multiorgan failure caused by LVAD-related infection was the cause of death in 3 patients who did not survive to transplantation. Seven patients who were treated for LVAD-related infection died due to a new infectious complication in the early posttransplantion period versus one death among patients without LVAD-related infection. The driveline exit site appeared to be the major portal of entry in 18/30 episodes of LVAD-related BSI. The most common pathogens were *Staphylococcus epidermidis* (38%) and *S. aureus* (24%). Of the LVAD recipients, 84% survived to transplantation. Diabetes mellitus was a risk factor for LVAD-related BSI, and longer device support time was associated with LVAD-related infection. Conversely, patients who received continuous antimicrobial therapy from the time of initial diagnosis until transplantation or death had fewer episodes of relapse of infection, of LVAD superinfecions, and of LVAD support times as opposed to patients who received 2–6-week courses of treatment. Another group found 6.2 surgical site infections (SSI) per 1,000 LVAD-days in 36 LVADs implanted in 35 patients [74]. The Heartmate was used for all patients. Three patients developed deep soft-tissue infections (8.3 infections per 100 LVAD implantations) and 6 patients had organ/space infections (16.7 infections per 100 LVAD implantations). Two patients developed mediastinitis; 26% of patients had infections associated with gram-positive bacteria. Of 35 patients, 30 (86%) underwent successful heart transplantation. Three patients had clinical signs of sepsis despite negative cultures. Hemodialysis was the only infection risk factor identified. Finally, a study comparing different LVADs looked at infection rates of the Jarvik 2000 permanent LVAD (Jarvik Heart, Inc., New York) and the Heartmate single-lead vented, electrical LVAD (Thoratec Corporation, Pleasanton, California). The Heartmate group had an infection rate of 0.43 infections/100 patient-days versus 0.08 infections/100 patient-days for the Jarvik group. The Jarvik 2000 LVAD is an axial flow pump designed for permanent use. It has a novel power supply that is a small percutaneous retroauricular skull-mounted pedestal. The investigators believe that the percutaneous, immobile pedestal protected the patients from infection. However, the Jarvik 2000 cannot completely replace left-ventricular function and cannot be used in all patients who need mechanical support [80].

LVADs are associated with a significant risk of infection but still could be superior to medical management alone. Homan et al. prospectively randomized patients to receive LVADs or optimal medical management (OMM) for end-stage heart failure. They found that survival with LVAD (68 patients) was superior to OMM for (61 patients) a 47% decrease death risk ($p < 0.001$) [81].

Uncommon infectious complications of LVADs also have been described. Kotschet et al. described two patients with severe postpartum cardiomyopathy who developed a left ventricular pseudoarneuysm after device removal; the patients had bacteremia during device support [82]. Others have reported fungal infection of the inflow and outflow valves that led to LVAD malfunction and death [83].

Some newer interventions could help to prevent or heal LVAD-related infections. The previously described driveline infections can be difficult to manage. Yuh et al. presented a patient with a deep driveline infection who was successfully treated with a vacuum-assisted closure system [77]. The patient was found to have an abscess within the driveline tract that grew *Pseudomonas* sp. A vacuum-assisted closure system applied to the wound after debridement was wrapped around the exposed driveline, which was left within the opened tract until adequate healing had occurred. Another possible intervention is an antimicrobial-coated driveline

to prevent early infections. Choi et al. evaluated the ability of an LVAD driveline impregnated with chlorhexidine, triclosan, and silver sulfadiazine to resist bacterial and fungal colonization by placing driveline segments onto agar plates inoculated with *S. aureus*, *S. epidermidis*, *Enterobacter aerogenes*, *Pseudomonas aeruginosa*, and *Candida albicans* [84]. Antimicrobial activity was demonstrated against all organisms for >14 days, and for >21 days for gram-positive bacteria. *In vivo* efficacy was tested using rats; 100% of control segments were colonized versus 13% of the test explants. To date, Thoratec has not incorporated this technology [personal communication, October 2006] but has published infection control guidelines for the Heartmate XVE Left Ventricular Assist System. The guidelines were first created by the REMATCH Trial Surgical Working Group and then were updated by the Park City Trial Surgical Working Group in February 2004. They can be accessed at **www.Thoratec.com**.

TRANSFUSION-ASSOCIATED INFECTIONS

Blood Transfusion and Bacteremia

The three main postulated mechanisms of bacterial contamination of blood products are the use of nonsterile tubing or collection bags due to improper manufacturing, bacteria from the donor's skin or blood, and unsterile handling during preparation and/or storage [85]. Now that systematic blood donor programs have greatly reduced the frequency of transfusion transmitted viral infections by carefully screening donors and using nucleic acid testing (for HIV and HCV), transfusion-associated bacterial contamination is the most frequent transfusion-transmitted infection. The first case reports of transfusion-related sepsis appeared in the 1940s and 1950s and involved shock syndromes produced by transfusion of cold-stored blood contaminated with psychrophilic organisms able to survive and grow at 4°C (30°F), such as *Achromobacter* and some *Pseudomonas* species. Prospective microbiologic studies soon followed these reports and documented a contamination rate of 1–6% in banked blood [86]. Most contaminants were normal skin flora, presumably introduced with fragments of donor skin cored out during phlebotomy. Such contaminants usually were present in extremely low concentrations (several logarithmic factors below the level of ~100 organisms per milliliter of blood associated with transfusion sepsis), and multiplication of organisms during storage seemed unlikely because of the long lag phase produced by refrigeration and of the antibacterial action of blood. Indeed, retrospective studies failed to document any clinical illness associated with the transfusion of blood that contained low-level skin flora contamination [87]. Nevertheless, asymptomatic patients or patients with nonspecific gastrointestinal symptoms on rare occasions still could be a source of bacterial contamination, especially of *Yersinia enterocolitica*-contaminated red blood cell transfusions. Infections due to this contamination have been associated with a high mortality rate, particularly with units stored >25 days at 1–6°C (34–43°F). The donors presumably had asymptomatic bacteremia at the time of donation. An example of bacterial contamination of blood components during collection or processing is illustrated by an outbreak of *Serratia marcescens* traced to the use of blood bags intrinsically contaminated during manufacturing [88].

Investigators more recently sought to determine the risk of bacterial contamination of blood components by combining data reported to the CDC from blood collection facilities and transfusion services affiliated with the American Red Cross, American Association of Blood Banks (AABB), and Department of Defense blood programs from 1998–2000. A *case* was defined as any transfusion reaction meeting clinical criteria in which the same bacterial species was cultured from a blood component and from recipient blood and molecular typing confirmed the organism pair as identical. There were 34 cases and 9 deaths. The rate of transfusion-transmitted bacteremia (in events per million units) was 9.98 for single-donor platelets, 10.64 for pooled platelets, and 0.21 for red blood cells (RBC) units; for fatal reactions, the rates were 1.94, 2.22, and 0.13, respectively. Patients at greatest risk for death received components containing gram-negative organisms (OR, 7.5; 95% CI, 1.3–64.2) [89].

The French BACTHEM study assessed transfusion-associated bacterial contamination determinants using a matched case-control study design. Cases were derived from a database of patients presenting during a 3-year period with a transfusion-related adverse event reported to the French blood agency as a suspected case of transfusion-associated bacterial contamination. Of the 158 cases of suspected transfusion-associated bacterial contamination reported during the study period, 41 cases and 82 matched controls were included. The bacteria were gram negatives (42%), gram-positive cocci (28%), gram-positive rods (21%), and others (9%). The overall incidence rate of contamination was 6.9 per million units issued. The risk of contamination was >12 times higher after platelet pool transfusion and 5.5 times higher after aphaeresis platelet transfusion than after RBC transfusion. Gram-negative rods accounted for nearly 50% of the bacterial species involved and for six deaths. Risk factors included patients receiving RBC for pancytopenia, platelets for thrombocytopenia and pancytopenia, immunosuppressive treatment, shelf life more >1 day for platelets or 8 days for red blood cells, and >20 previous donations by donors [90].

Blood Transfusion and Parasitemia

The frequent use of blood transfusions and the increased travel to-from countries where malaria is endemic have led to an increased occurrence of transfusion-related malaria. During the period 1911–1950, ~350 episodes of transfusion-associated malaria were reported worldwide. In contrast, during the period 1950–1972, the number of reported episodes was >2,000 [91]. In the United States, 101 episodes of transfusion-induced malaria were reported during 1957–1994 [92,93]. The United States still has two–three episodes of transfusion-transmitted malaria per year [94,95].

Based on worldwide incidence data, *Plasmodium malariae* appears to be the most common cause of transfusion-associated malaria, accounting for almost 50% of episodes. *Plasmodium vivax* and *Plasmodium falciparum* are second and third in worldwide incidence, respectively. This ordering probably reflects the fact that although *P. malariae* infection can persist in an asymptomatic donor for many years, the longevity of *P. vivax* malaria in humans rarely exceeds 3 years and that of *P. falciparum* rarely 1 year. Hence, there is higher chance for an asymptomatic donor infected with *P. malariae* to escape detection and become the source of a contaminated transfusion.

The AABB adopted recommended guidelines for the selection of blood donors to prevent transmission of malaria in 1970, but they were relaxed in 1974 [92, 93]. In the changes added to the 24th edition of the Standards for Blood Banks and Transfusion Services (effective November 1, 2006), prospective donors who have a definite history of malaria are deferred for 3 years after becoming asymptomatic. Individuals who have lived for ≥5 consecutive years in areas considered malaria endemic by the CDC are deferred 3 years after departure from the area(s). Because platelet and leukocyte preparations also have been incriminated in the transmission of malaria, the guidelines must be applied to potential donors of any formed elements of blood.

Chagas' disease (American trypanosomiasis) is prevalent through South and Central America. The potential for blood-borne transmission is high because some infected individuals can become asymptomatic but still have persistent parasitemia for 10–30 years. After 10 days of storage the infectivity of blood contaminated with this parasite declines, but storage is not a useful method for preventing transmission; moreover, the parasite is viable in whole blood and RBC stored at 4°C (30°F) for ≥21 days. Serologic screening blood of donors has become mandatory in many South American countries. The problem of transfusion-associated Chagas' disease also has become an issue for U.S. blood banks, secondary to increased immigration and to more potentially infectious U.S. blood donors. It is estimated that about 100,000 infected people live in the United States [96], and estimates of *T. cruzi* seroprevalence in U.S. blood donors range from 0.01–0.20%. Six episodes of transfusion-transmitted Chagas' disease have been reported in the United States since the mid-1980s [97,98]. Anyone with a history of Chagas' disease must be permanently prevented from donating blood [99].

Toxoplasmosis also can be transmitted via blood transfusion. One prospective survey of thalassemia patients who were frequently transfused detected subclinical toxoplasmosis at a rate comparable to that seen in a control group and therefore was considered to be evidence against the transmission of toxoplasmosis by transfusion [100]. Another study found, however, that patients treated for acute leukemia acquired toxoplasmosis after leukocyte transfusions from donors with chronic myelogenous leukemia; serologic data retrospectively obtained from donors revealed elevated anti-*Toxoplasma* antibody titers [101]. This inferential evidence for transfusion-associated toxoplasmosis is supported by the findings that the disease can be transmitted between animals and by transfusion, that *Toxoplasma* organisms retain their viability in stored blood for 50 days, and that organisms can be recovered from the blood buffy-coat layers of patients with toxoplasmosis. Because it seems likely that toxoplasmosis can be transmitted if large concentrations of leukocytes are transfused and all of the leukocyte donors had chronic myelogenous leukemia, it is recommended that blood or leukocytes from patients with leukemia not be used especially because recipients' host defenses usually are severely compromised.

As the rate of human *Babesia microti* has risen in the United States, so has transfusion-transmitted *Babesia*. Donations from a group of blood donors in *Babesia*-endemic areas of Connecticut were seropositive 1.4% of the time, and >50% of those had demonstrable parasitemia [102]. More than 40 U.S. episodes of *Babesia microti* infection acquired by blood transfusion have been reported, including one in an infant [103–105]. However, symptoms secondary to disease with *Babesia microti* can be mild in immunocompetent people, and the true incidence of the infection is unknown. Donors with a history of babesiosis are indefinitely restricted from donating blood because of the possibility of ongoing asymptomatic parasitemia [99].

Because of the many Americans serving in Iraq, there has been the concern for transmission of Leishmanaiasis. As a result, there is a 1-year donor deferral for military personnel serving in Iraq.

As molecular technology, such as polymerase chain reaction, becomes more sophisticated and available, we could be better equipped to efficiently identify parasites in donated blood and prevent transfusion-associated transmission [106,107].

Platelet Transfusion

Approximately 9 million platelet-unit concentrates are estimated to be transfused in the United States each year and 1 in 1,000–3,000 platelet units is estimated to be contaminated with bacteria, resulting in possible transfusion-associated sepsis [108,109]. In fact, the largest prospective study of transfusion-transmitted bacterial infection in the United States confirms that the incidence of bacterial contamination of platelets ranges from 0.04–1.00 [89]. As

noted, screening for viral pathogens in blood has greatly improved, and the risk of platelet-associated transfusion sepsis is about 24fold higher than the transfusion risk for HCV and 28fold higher than the transmission risk for HIV [110]. In fact, transfusion-transmitted bacterial contamination of platelets is the most common cause of fatalities related to transfusion-transmitted disease in developed countries. It is estimated that the risk of bacterial-related death after the transfusion of a platelet unit ranges from 1:7500 to 1:500,000 [111,112].

Because it is now recommended that platelets be stored at room temperature (20–24°C/68–75°F) to increase *in vivo* half-life, concern over the true incidence of intrinsic contamination and the possible proliferation of contaminants during storage is justified. Of interest platelets, historically have been stored at 4°C (39°F). In 1969, Murphy and Gardner demonstrated that platelet storage at 22°C (72°F) led to improved *in vivo* viability and function as compared to storage at 13°, 20°, and 37°C (55°, 68°, 99°F) [113]. These observations led to the current practice of storing platelets at room temperature for up to 5 days. It seems reasonable to assume that platelet concentrates are as susceptible to contamination during collection as is blood, which is routinely found to have a 1–6% incidence of low-level contamination. Moreover, platelet concentrates, unlike blood, have no protective antibacterial activity, and platelet transfusions are frequently obtained by pooling the contributions of several donors, which additionally increases the risk of contamination. Despite this seemingly negative picture, most bacterial contaminants isolated from platelet concentrates have been normal skin flora, such as *S. epidermidis* and diphtheroids, present in extremely low concentrations. Even in the highly susceptible patient populations that normally receive platelet transfusions, such contaminants have failed to produce any documented adverse reactions [114–116]. However, there has been at least one report of a Gram-positive organism causing septic shock in a young woman. This was an episode of *Streptococcus bovis* septicemia found to be secondary to contaminated donor platelets. The donor had undergone colonoscopy 2 months before the platelet transfusion [117].

Although meticulous blood-banking techniques and the widespread use of closed collection systems have made platelet transfusion relatively safe, the occurrence of outbreaks emphasizes the possibility of sporadic, significant contamination of platelets. One outbreak involved seven episodes of *Salmonella choleraesuis* sepsis traced to platelet transfusions from a blood donor with clinically unapparent *Salmonella* sp. osteomyelitis and intermittent asymptomatic bacteremia [118]. A long incubation period in this outbreak—that is, a mean interval of 9 days between the transfusion with contaminated platelets and the signs of sepsis—was caused by coincidental administration of antibiotics at the time of platelet transfusion in several patients and delayed recognition of platelets as the vehicle of infection. A second outbreak involved two episodes of transfusion-induced *Enterobacter cloacae* sepsis [114]. An investigation revealed that 20% of the platelet pools prepared in the affected hospital were contaminated. Although most of the contaminants were nonpathogens present only in low concentrations, 6/258 platelet pools grew *E. cloacae*. The source of these unusual contaminants was not discovered. A third outbreak with *Serratia* sp. was traced to contaminated evacuated tubes used after blood collection [119]. In a fourth outbreak [120], a cluster of four patients at a university hospital received platelets contaminated with *Bacillus cereus*, *Pseudomonas aeruginosa*, or *S. epidermidis* during a 34-day period. The patient with platelet transfusion-related *Pseudomonas* sepsis died; the remaining patients survived. The investigators surmised that the most likely explanation for the outbreak was contamination of the platelets at the time of phlebotomy. In addition, the four contaminated platelet units were significantly older (mean age, 4.8 days) than 106 randomly selected individual platelet units (mean age, 3.7 days; $p = 0.04$). The hospital increased its surveillance, probably after the one patient died, which could have fostered the discovery of the contaminated platelet pools. More recently, two episodes of *Salmonella* sp. sepsis, one fatal, from platelet transfusions linked to an asymptomatic bacteremic donor presumably infected during handling his pet boa constrictor was reported, and in 2004 two fatal episodes of transfusion-associated sepsis occurred in platelet recipients [112,121]. One patient, a 74-year-old man with leukemia, had received a transfusion consisting of a pool of five platelet unit concentrates. The pooled platelet unit had been tested for bacterial contamination with a reagent strip test (Multistix® BayerDiagnostics, Tarrytown, New York) before transfusion to determine the pH level, a means for detecting the presence of bacteria. The pH test result was within the accepted range for quality control of the clinic's blood bank. After the transfusion, the patient's blood grew *S. aureus*, and the patient died 21 days after hospital admission. The same organism was cultured from the leftover platelet unit bag and was indistinguishable by pulsed-field gel electrophoresis (PFGE). The second patient was a 79-year-old man who had received a transfusion of pheresis platelets for thrombocytopenia after coronary artery bypass surgery. The platelets were tested for bacterial contamination with liquid culture media (BacT/Alert®, Bio Merieux Inc., Durham, North Carolina) and found to be negative after 5 days of incubation. Approximately 1 hour after transfusion, the patient deteriorated and died 72 hours later. *S. lugdunensis* was cultured from the patient's blood and the leftover platelet bag and were identical by PFGE. These last two episodes highlight some of the opportunities for platelet contamination and difficulties with contamination recognition. Blood collection centers culture single-donor platelets, but pooling platelets is done immediately before transfusion; therefore, the hospital is responsible for the bacterial testing of these units. Because of the logistic problem with culturing and providing platelets on a timely

manner, some hospitals use nonculture-based methods such as the pH indicators (used in one of the case-patients just described). Non–culture based methods can result in false-negative results as can culture technique.

If the possibility of transfusion-associated bacterial sepsis is considered (e.g., hypotension or fever occur), the transfusion should be stopped immediately, the reaction should be reported to the hospital blood bank, and an investigation should be initiated. The platelet bag and its contents should be returned to the blood bank for inspection, bag defects, and Gram stain and culture of contents. The patient should have blood cultures drawn. The blood supplier also should be notified of possible bacterial contamination in order to recall and culture blood components from the same donation to prevent additional potential morbidity and mortality.

Clearly, we need to use current technology to better prevent and detect bacterial contamination of blood products so that we can improve safety for patients and possibly extend the shelf life of platelets. It is possible that using pathogen inactivation techniques and a spore-based biosensor to detect low levels of bacteria in real time (e.g., the label-free exponential signal-amplification system [LEXAS], which exploits the spore's ability to produce fluorescence when sensing neighboring bacterial cell), could extend shelf life [122,123]. Since March 1, 2004, all platelets have been tested for bacterial contamination before transfusion as required by both the College of American Pathologists and the standards of the AABB [99].

Even when all precautions are taken, transfusion reactions frequently are unrecognized. HCWs must be aware of the risk of bacterial contamination of blood products, particularly platelets because it is often not considered in the differential diagnosis at the time of transfusion reaction due to the similarity of signs and symptoms to those expected from sepsis from other causes [120]. To assess clinician experience with transfusion-associated bacterial infections and knowledge of the new AABB standard, the Infectious Diseases Society of America (IDSA) surveyed U.S. infectious disease consultants via e-mail and fax during July 27–August 24, 2004. The survey went to all 870 infectious disease consultant members of the Emerging Infections Network, a sentinel provider network of ISDA [124]. Completed surveys were received from 46% (399/870) members. Forty-eight (12%) respondents recalled consulting on 85 reactions to blood transfusions potentially caused by bacterial contamination in which 10 reactions were fatal. In 31% (26) of episodes, contamination was confirmed by positive cultures of the recipient's blood and transfused unit. Of respondents, 20% (78) indicated that they were familiar with the new AABB standard for bacterial detection in platelets.

Unfortunately, several interventions to decrease blood contamination have not been successful; it is possible that in one study, expanding the screening questions was not effective in identifying blood donors who may harbor

Y. enterocolitica [125]. Reducing storage time could reduce contamination but would also reduce platelet supply, and the use of single-donor platelets rather than pooled platelet concentrates has not consistently been shown to decrease the incidence of septic platelet transfusion reactions [89].

To improve bacterial testing and reporting, the AABB provided additional guidance on standardized definitions for test results, investigation and management of implicated units and associated cocomponents, and laboratory testing of detected organisms [126]. Transfusion-related fatalities should be reported to the Food and Drug Administration, Center for Biologic and Evaluation Research (fatalities2@cber.fda.gov, phone: 1-301-827-6220, fax: 1-301-827-6748).

Albumin Infusion

Because of faith in commercial manufacturing practices and the extremely low incidence of reactions to albumin infusion, most physicians consider commercial human serum albumin to be a completely safe product. Years ago, however, a nationwide outbreak of albumin-related *P. cepacia* sepsis emphasized that any commercial product, particularly any blood component, is susceptible to contamination [127]. In addition to emphasizing the risk of infection associated with the infusion of a nonformed blood component, it is worthwhile to note that the albumin outbreak illustrates several general problems in the detection and evaluation of low-frequency contamination of commercial products. First, HAIs caused by low-frequency contaminants can be difficult to distinguish from endemic problems in any one institution. In the initial reporting hospital, the infusion-related infections became apparent only because of the enormous quantity of albumin used. Second, because commercial products usually are prepared and sterilized in bulk lots, being able to trace the distribution of individual suspect lots is important. Third, sterility of an infusion product cannot be ascertained by visual inspection. Despite *P. cepacia* concentrations of approximately 100 organisms per milliliter, the contaminated albumin was completely clear. Finally, sampling schemes currently used for product quality control can miss some contaminants when present in low frequency, and endotoxin could escape terminal filtration and be missed by currently used pyrogen tests.

Emerging and Reemerging Organisms Associated with Blood Transfusion

Newer technology and improvement in the blood collection, handling, and transfusion process have created a safe blood supply. Emerging and reemerging pathogens that are not yet easily identified either in the donor, as with asymptomatic disease, or in the product itself, could pose a threat to transfusion recipients [128]. Mumps, which has reemerged particularly in the 18–25-year-old group, is asymptomatic in 20% of people, and 50% of the time the symptoms are nonspecific. Although transfusion-acquired mumps virus has never been observed, viremia is known to occur and therefore has the potential for transfusion transmission of mumps to transfusion recipients from donors with unrecognized infection and asymptomatic viremia. Members of the AABB Transfusion-Transmitted Diseases (TTD) Committee and representatives of the U.S. Food and Drug Administration (FDA) have made available recommendations for the prevention of transfusion-associated mumps [129]. West Nile Virus (WNV) is another pathogen that can cause asymptomatic viremia and has been transmitted via blood transfusions. Since 2003, all blood donated in the United States has been screened via nuclear acid testing (NAT) of donor pools for presence of WNV. The WNV Task Force, which includes representatives from AABB, CDC, FDA, U. S. Deparment of Defense, the American Red Cross, America's Blood Centers, Canadian Blood Services and United Blood Services, initiated an electronic data network in 2006 to enhance identification and tracking. The WNV Biovigilance Network collates data on blood donors with suspected infection in the United States and Canada. Data are collected from blood donor screening by nucleic acid testing. The data from the network demonstrates the magnitude of this potential problem; until September 12, 2006, the network had detected 216 confirmed positive donations and 137 with pending interpretation. Updated data can be found at **www.aabb.org**. Finally, the recognition of mad cow disease and varient Creutzfeldt-Jacob disease (vCJD) has led to policy preventing blood donation if the prospective donor had a 3-year stay in certain countries including Great Britain from 1980–1996 or has had a blood transfusion in certain European counties from January 1, 1980, to the present. Although no episodes of transfusion-related transmission have been reported because vCJD is most probably due to a prion, a theoretical risk of transmission exists.

INFECTION HAZARDS ASSOCIATED WITH ANESTHESIA

Severe bacterial infections have been well documented in association with the use of contaminated equipment for local and spinal anesthesia and of contaminated anesthesia machines for delivery of general anesthesia.

Anesthetic Agents

Propofol (Diprivan, Stuart Pharmaceutical, Wilmington, Delaware) is an oil-based anesthetic agent that is not an antimicrobially preserved product under USP standards and can be stored at 4–22°C (40–72°F) (Diprivan injection, 2005 package insert). An investigation of seven outbreaks of postoperative infection or acute febrile illness revealed an association with the receipt of propofol. The extrinsic contamination of propofol due to poor aseptic technique by anesthesia personnel compounded by the ability of the oil-based product to support the growth of contaminants or the use of the same syringe for multiple patients was thought to be the cause of these outbreaks [130]. Infection control practitioners must maintain surveillance for infections due to propofol, which also has been approved for use as a sedative agent in the ICU. In addition, it could be necessary for practitioners to investigate the manner in which such products are handled to ensure that aseptic technique is being used. Products that do not contain preservatives or antimicrobials but have the ability to support microbial growth because of the products' properties should not be used in multidose vials.

Surgical-Specific Anesthesia/Analgesia

Continuous peripheral nerve block (CPNB) is effective for postoperative analgesia after orthopedic surgery. However, this procedure that uses a catheter also has been the cause of infection. Patients scheduled to undergo orthopedic surgery performed with a CPNB were prospectively evaluated in a 1-year multicenter study. Cultures from 28.7% of the catheters were positive, and risk factors for local inflammation or infection included postoperative monitoring in the ICU, catheter duration >48 hours, male gender, and absence of antibiotic prophylaxis [131]. Another study evaluated 211 catheters for CPNB and found that 57% of 208 catheters had positive bacterial colonization after 48 hours. The most frequent organisms were *S. epidermidis* (71%), *Enterococcus* (10%), and *Klebsiella* (4%). Three transitory BSIs likely related to the catheter occurred. After 6 weeks, no septic complications were noted [132]. As with most device-related infections, duration is a risk factor, and gram-positive organisms predominate. HCWs must consider this with all such procedures.

It is difficult to provide anesthesia for a prostate biopsy that requires two or more needle punctures through a highly contaminated rectum. Obek et al. prospectively evaluated 100 patients who underwent transrectal ultrasound guided prostate biopsy [133]. The patients were randomized to receive a periprostatic nerve block or no anesthesia. High fever and hospitalization were more frequent in the nerve block group; bacteriuria in postbiopsy urine cultures was significantly more common in the anesthesia group. Prospective randomized trials will be necessary to determine the optimum antibiotic prophylaxis regimen in patients undergoing biopsy with a periprostatic nerve block.

Endotracheal Intubation

A potential hazard of anesthesia is the occurrence of BSI secondary to the passage of an endotracheal tube. The organisms isolated from the blood usually are α-hemolytic streptococci, both aerobic and anaerobic diphtheroids, and other anaerobic organisms that normally colonize the upper respiratory tract. A higher incidence of BSI after nasotracheal intubation could occur, however, than after the less traumatic orotracheal route [134], but antibiotic prophylaxis is not recommended for either route.

Prolonged nasotracheal (or nasogastric) intubation has been associated with a 2–5% incidence of sinusitis, which may be occult [135,136]. The maxillary and sphenoid sinuses are most commonly involved [135], and frequent pathogens include *S. aureus*, *Enterobacter*, *P. aeruginosa*, *Hemophilus*, pneumococci, and anaerobes [136]. Sterile and occasionally infected middle ear effusions also are common in patients receiving endotracheal intubation and mechanical ventilation [137]. The CDC guidelines for preventing healthcare-associated pneumonia now recommend using orotracheal rather than nasotracheal tubes in patients who receive mechanically assisted ventilation; using noninvasive ventilation to reduce the need for and duration of endotracheal intubation; changing the breathing circuits of ventilators when they malfunction or are visibly contaminated; and, when feasible, using an endotracheal tube with a dorsal lumen to allow drainage of respiratory secretions [138].

The laryngeal mask airway (LMA) is a reusable device for maintaining the patency of a patient's airway during general anesthesia; it consists of an inflatable silicone mask and rubber connecting tube that is generally reusable. Because of the concern for the accumulation of proteinaceous material on LMAs and therefore the potential for transmitting organisms including prions even after disinfection, a number of investigators have quantified the amount of protein contamination after sterilization and found protein deposits even after sterilization that increased with device use [139–141]. Whether the remaining protein deposits pose a risk to patients is unknown, but they clearly represent a concern for potential transmission of pathogens that could be difficult to recognize as sporadic episodes at different institutions and at different times. As new devices made of new materials come to the market, it is incumbent upon the manufacturer to recommend safe cleaning practices and upon the infection control practitioner to pay close attention to such developments.

Endotracheal intubation also can place the HCW at risk because of exposure to oral and respiratory secretions at the time of intubation. Severe acute respiratory syndrome (SARS) is an example of a transmissible disease that can cause significant morbidity and mortality. In fact, one investigation found a higher risk of developing SARS for physicians and nurses performing endotracheal intubation [142]. The outbreak inspired the creation of infection control guidelines for anesthesiology in Canada. These guidelines address routine precautions for non-SARS patients in the operating room, management of SARS patients in the operating room, and emergency tracheal intubation of SARS patients outside the operating room. The guidelines were developed in consultation with anesthesiologists, intensivists, infection control staff, and respiratory therapists and provide a good example of the dynamic state of emerging pathogens and the value of a prompt response by a multidisciplinary team [143].

INFECTIONS OF THE CENTRAL NERVOUS SYSTEM: RESERVOIRS AND SHUNTS

Serious infection can complicate the insertion or prolonged use of two very important neurosurgical devices: the Ommaya-type subcutaneous reservoir used for administering intrathecal therapy for fungal or neoplastic meningitis and the ventricular shunt used for decompression of hydrocephalus (see Chapter 31). Infectious complications have been observed frequently after the insertion or chronic use of subcutaneous intraventricular reservoirs [144–146]. The use of valved catheters for the treatment of hydrocephalus (i.e., to shunt cerecro-spinal fluid [CSF] from the lateral ventricle of the brain to the superior vena cava, the right atrium, or the peritoneum) also has been complicated by a high incidence of infections. In a number of studies, the overall incidence of shunt infections has ranged from 6–23% [147]. Most of these infections are caused by *S. aureus* and *S. epidermidis* and occurred within 2 weeks to 2 months after surgery; this incidence emphasizes the importance of intraoperative and perioperative wound or shunt contamination in the pathogenesis of shunt infection. Shunt infections uncommonly are caused by other organisms such as vancomycin-resistant *Enterococcus faecium* or Group B *streptococcus* [148,149] The equal risk of infection in patients with ventriculoatrial or ventriculoperitoneal shunts suggests that transient BSI is a less likely cause of such infections because ventriculoperitoneal shunts are not exposed to the bloodstream [150].

The antimicrobial treatment of shunt infections that complicate hydrocephalus usually is unsatisfactory unless the shunt is removed [151]. Adherence of slime-producing, coagulase-negative staphylococci to shunt material could be only one reason for failure of antimicrobial therapy [152]. Although <10% of patients has the infection eradicated by systemic antimicrobial therapy alone, those treated with combinations of systemic and intraventricular antibiotics can have 30–90% cure rates [153]. Repeated administration of intraventricular antibiotics has its own complications, however, and when infection is widespread, the treatment of choice appears to be the administration of appropriate systemic antibiotics and the complete removal of the shunt and insertion of a new one at another site [154]. Even after appropriate therapy and presumed successful treatment of a CSF shunt infection, reinfection can occur [155]. Preferably, some time should elapse between the removal of the infected shunt and the insertion of a new one. Despite this discouraging picture, many of the antibiotics previously used to treat shunt infections have been supplanted by newer agents that could prove to be more efficacious. In addition, the epidemiologic characteristics of shunt infections (e.g., perioperative acquisition of organisms) and the narrow spectrum of shunt pathogens suggest that the use of prophylactic antimicrobials and antibiotic-impregnated cerebrospinal fluid shunt catheters at the time of shunt surgery could prove beneficial [156,157]. Two meta-analyses [158,159] evaluating the use of perioperative antimicrobial prophylaxis suggested that the use of prophylactic antibiotics is associated with a significant reduction in subsequent CSF shunt infection. Both studies demonstrated a ~50% reduction in infection risk. Only a few of the studies included in these two meta-analyses reached statistical significance by themselves, which could be due to lack of power at least in part. A third meta-analysis that included randomized or quasi-randomized controlled trials also found the use of systemic antibiotic prophylaxis to be associated with a decrease in shunt infection. In addition, the study evaluated the effectiveness of antibiotic-impregnated catheters to prevent shunt infections and found that too was associated with a decrease in shunt infection [160].

Epidural catheters used for anesthesia or pain management and spinal cord and/or dorsal column stimulators used for pain management also have the potential to cause device-related infections. Few reported episodes of discitis or meningitis are associated with spinal anesthesia. There are, however, some case-reports including one of *Streptococcus bovis* discitis after spinal anesthesia for cesarean delivery, *Streptococcus* sp. meningitis after epidural anesthesia, and *Streptococcus salivarius* meningitis after spinal anesthesia [161–163]. No specific risk factors were identified. Proper aseptic technique is the mainstay for preventing such infections.

A prospective, randomized, controlled trial to assess the efficacy of a chlorhexidine dressing in reducing the microbial flora at the insertion site of epidural catheters found that the use of the antiseptic at the catheter wound site reduced catheter colonization [164]. The trial authors hypothesized that this could reduce the risk of epidural catheter-related infection. A meta-analysis also supports the use of chlorhexine-impregnated dressing to reduce the risk of epidural catheter bacterial colonization and infection. Analysis of eight randomized controlled clinical trials comparing a single type of chlorhexidine-impregnated dressing with placebo and with povidine-iodined concludes that the chlorhexidine-impregnated dressing reduced the risk of epidural (3.6% vs. 35%; OR 0.07; 95% confidence interval, 0.02–0.31, $p = 0.0005$) exit site bacterial colonization and was associated with a trend toward reduction in central nervous system (CNS) infections. Local cutaneous reactions to chlorhexidine-impregnated dressing were reported in 5.6% of patients in three studies; 96% of the reactions occurred in neonatal patients [165].

TRANSIENT BSI FROM NONVASCULAR PROCEDURES

The occurrence of transient BSI associated with relatively noninvasive manipulation of colonized mucosa is well recognized [166]. Such BSIs usually last no longer than 5–15 minutes, at its peak can shower 100 organisms per milliliter of blood (although the peak concentration is almost always much less), and is largely asymptomatic. Hundreds of studies have reported on BSIs after oral treatments alone [167]. This section discusses BSIs after diagnostic gastrointestinal procedures, genitourinary instrumentation, and bronchoscopy; BSIs after endotracheal intubation and invasive vascular procedures were covered earlier in this chapter. Table 45-2 presents a summary of the characteristics of BSIs associated with selected nonvascular procedures.

Gastrointestinal Procedures

BSI has been reported as a sequelae to a variety of gastrointestinal procedures, including sigmoidoscopy, colonoscopy, barium enema, esophagoscopy, biopsy of mucosal masses, injection sclerotherapy of esophageal varices, endoscopic retrograde cholangiopancreatography (ERCP), liver biopsy, esophageal dilatation, and rectal examination. Routine antibiotic prophylaxis is recommended only for high-risk patients before sigmoidoscopy or colonoscopy [168]. Host factors also can influence the incidence and outcome of procedure-related BSI. Rare episodes of symptomatic barium enema septicemia in patients with impaired host defenses (acute leukemia) and in patients with active inflammatory bowel disease have been reported.

Although the role of antibiotic prophylaxis for endoscopy procedures is not always certain, other preventive measures, particularly careful disinfection of endoscopes and good aseptic technique, are of definite importance [169]. Many anecdotal reports and outbreaks have highlight the importance of such measures [170–178]. In one report, two episodes of *Pseudomonas* sp. sepsis in leukemic patients undergoing esophagoscopy with mucosal biopsy were traced to exogenous bacteria introduced during biopsy. Cultures of the esophagoscope and of the endoscopy room revealed widespread contamination with enteric organisms, including *P. aeruginosa*, and it was shown that routine handling of the instruments ignored aseptic technique [176]. In addition, several series of ERCP-related BSI [170–172,174] highlight the multiple sources of contamination in the endoscopy suite, particularly the lens irrigation bottles, and the difficulty in disinfecting the levers and many small-bore channels in these sophisticated instruments even when automatic washers are used. In fact, the automatic endoscope "sterilizers" are at times the source of endoscope contamination, particularly by *P. aeruginosa*. Significant sporadic problems can be easily overlooked for prolonged periods even with established infection control programs. The poor level of endoscope

TABLE 45-2

CHARACTERISTICS OF TRANSIENT BACTEREMIA ASSOCIATED WITH SELECTED PROCEDURES

Involved System	Maximum Incidence of Bacteremia (%)
Dental	90
Urologic	80
Airway	30
Gastrointestinal	15
Obsteric-gynecologic	4
Concentration of bacteria (cfu) per milliliter	<20–130
Duration of bacteremia (min after procedure)	10–30
Predominant bacterias	Anaerobes, enterococci, enteric gram-negative bacilli; occasionally, *Streptococcus pneumoniae*
Symptoms	Usually none; fever more common with urologic-related bacteremia

CFU, colony forming units.

disinfection in many hospitals occur despite established guidelines and the many reported outbreaks [179–181]. Still, there is no recommendation for routinely culturing endoscopes. Interestingly, almost all of the ERCP-related episodes are due to *P. aeruginosa*, most to one particular serotype, 010, that is either very prevalent or has an undisclosed source related to ERCP procedures. Most of the ERCP patients are at particular risk because of obstructions in the biliary and pancreatic ducts that can trap contaminated injectate. Any patient undergoing ERCP who has suspected ductal obstruction should receive antimicrobial prophylaxis [168]. BSI also has been documented in patients who need esophageal dilation of a stricture and in slerotheapy of esophageal varicies [182–184]. However, endoscopic variceal ligation (EVL) has for the most part supplanted esophageal sclerotherapy; still at least six studies have documented BSI associated with EVL (1–25% of the time) [185–190]. Although it is an invasive procedure, percutaneous liver biopsy usually is not associated with infection risk. Ultrasound-guided procedures have a mechanical advantage and can impact positively to prevent infection. A prospective cohort study of 500 patients who underwent an ultrasound-guided liver biopsy identified no infectious complications [191]. Antibiotic prophylaxis with liver biopsy is not warranted at present [168].

Nasogastric feeding and enteral nutrition have been associated with BSI and with diarrhea and feeding intolerance, particularly in neonates, due to contamination introduced during collection, preparation, and/or administration of formula or human milk [192,193].

Urologic and Gynecologic Instrumentation

An association among urethral instrumentation, fever, and BSI has been recognized for many years. In various studies, the incidence of BSIs associated with urologic procedures has been 2–80%, with the greatest BSI risk in patients with preexisting urinary tract infections (UTIs), patients undergoing transurethral resection of the prostate, and patients with prostatitis that is evident on histologic section of biopsy specimens [194]. Similar organisms in 50–67% of patients in whom BSI develops after instrumentation have been recovered from both preinstrumentation urine cultures and postinstrumentation blood cultures. The available evidence suggests that the sources of the other 33–50% of postinstrumentation BSIs include occult prostatitis, the introduction of normal urethral flora, and the contamination of equipment or irrigating fluids before or during instrumentation. Careful evaluation and treatment of genitourinary tract infection should occur before instrumentation [195]; appropriate disinfection of equipment and careful aseptic technique are mandatory. Endometrial biopsy and chorionic villus sampling have been associated rarely with BSI or *candidemia* [196–198].

Pulmonary Procedures

Fever and BSI have been documented in patients after rigid-tube and fiberoptic bronchoscopy.

Procedure-Related BSI Conclusions

Two conclusions can be drawn from the studies of procedure-related BSIs just cited: The equipment used for the procedures should be adequately disinfected/sterilized before every use, and the operator should observe proper aseptic technique. Beyond this, it is apparent that carefully planned, prospective, multicenter studies are needed to assess the incidence and clinical significance of procedure-related transient BSI to determine which hosts are at risk of associated sepsis or infection at distal sites; to determine whether specific risks for certain procedures can be sufficiently defined to justify preventive measures, such as antibiotic prophylaxis; and to determine which prophylactic regimens would be most efficacious. Although such studies cannot ever be conducted, the procedures will continue, and we have tried to note situations in which it seems reasonable to "cover" patients [166]. In this regard, it should be noted that for years dental patients with valvular heart disease have received endocarditis prophylaxis, largely on an empiric basis [199], although the specific regimens [200] and even the mechanisms by which prophylaxis could protect [201,202] have been called into question. The 1997 guidelines of the American Heart Association relaxed recommendations [203].

ADDITIONAL PROCEDURES ASSOCIATED WITH INFECTIONS

Interventional Radiology

Percutaneous radiologically guided placement of biopsy needles, catheters, and stents for diagnosis and therapy has become commonplace since the mid-1980s [204]. Infectious complications—primarily BSI, organ perforation, and catheter site infection—vary according to the particular procedure, patient risk factors, and experience of the operator and hospital but are no more frequent than those following more invasive procedures [204]. The use of prophylactic antibiotics for interventional radiographic procedures depends on the situation [205]. In addition, when infection is suspected clinically, therapeutic antibiotics should be administered before a procedure.

Laparoscopic Surgery

Laparoscopic surgery, particularly laparoscopic cholecystectomy, is now one of the most common surgical procedures performed in the United States. Recovery is much faster than after conventional surgery. SSIs have been lower with laparoscopic chelecystectomy [206,207]. Because the biliary tract is normally sterile, antimicrobial prophylaxis in biliary surgery has been recommended only for high-risk patients—defined as those who are >60 years of age or who have had either common duct stones, bile duct obstruction, recent acute cholecystitis, or prior operations on the biliary tract. Until risk stratification data exist for patients undergoing laparoscopic cholecystectomy, antimicrobial prophylaxis standards followed for the same procedure done through a traditional incision can be used [195]. A number of studies have concluded that there is no need for prophylactic antibiotis before laparoscopic surgery in low-risk patients [208–214].

Cystoscopy

In addition to the risk of BSI associated with cystoscopy, a significant risk of UTI is associated with it. Several remarkably similar outbreaks have been reported in which the use of dilute aqueous quaternary ammonium compounds as cystoscope disinfectants was associated with procedure-related UTIs with *Pseudomonas* species, particular *P. cepacia* (see Chapter 30). In these outbreaks, the quaternary ammonium compounds either were ineffective in decontaminating the equipment or were themselves actually harboring viable bacteria while being used as disinfectants [215].

Although the risk of infection associated with the use of dilute aqueous quaternary ammonium compounds has been known at least since the mid-1970s, many hospital personnel persist in using these compounds as antiseptics and disinfectants. Such use has most likely resulted in many outbreaks of hospital-associated UTI and BSIs with occasional outbreaks of hospital-associated respiratory tract or SSIs. To help decrease the risk of hospital-associated UTI after cystoscopy, it is important that the equipment be thoroughly cleaned and properly disinfected between uses.

Ureteral Stents

Ureteral stents often are necessary for upper urinary tract drainage but can cause significant patient morbidity including infection. Urologic stents were first developed in 1978 and now include softer biomaterials that are more resistant to encrustation and infections. Chew et al. reviewed the potential use of newer stent materials, coatings, and other innovations, such as the potential for drug-eluting stents [216]. Others have investigated the bacteriology of UTI associated with indwelling J ureteral stents and found that they carry a significant risk of bacteriuria and stent colonization but that the sensitivity of a urine culture could be low, and a negative culture does not rule out a colonized stent. The most common isolates were *Escherichia coli*, *Enterococcus* spp., *Staphylococcus* spp., *Pseudomonas*, and *Candida* spp., and stent isolates were more resistant to antibiotics than the organism isolated before stent insertion [217,218]. With new devices and device material, we must find ways to accommodate and enhance surveillance to identify possible new mechanisms of infection and infection transmission.

Bronchoscopy and Endoscopy

An estimated 497,000 bronchoscopy procedures were performed in the United States in 1996 [219]. Several outbreaks have highlighted the problems of pulmonary infection and false-positive culture results because of inadequately cleaned fiberoptic bronchoscopes [220,221]. Especially worrisome is a report of the failure of povidone-iodine to kill *Mycobacterium tuberculosis* (*M. tuberculosis*) on bronchoscopes [222]. Preparations of this agent intended for skin degerming often are used inadvisably for decontaminating equipment. This experience has reemphasized the need for higher-level disinfection (e.g., with glutaraldehyde) and/or sterilization of these scopes, especially after use on patients who could have tuberculosis [223]. Even with high-level disinfection, *M. tuberculosis* has been found in bronchoscopy specimen cultures in 3 patients; specimens of all 3 patients were collected by the same bronchoscope. Only the first patient had clinical evidence of disease with *M. tuberculosis*. Although the hospital's procedures for disinfection, corresponded with most guidelines, the bronchoscope showed patient debris after disinfection, indicating that the manual cleaning was inadequate and was not approved for reprocessing in the hospital's automated endoscope reprocessor system [224]. Failure to perform leak testing led to failure to discover a hole in the sheath of a bronchoscope, which led to inadequate disinfection and transmission of *M. tuberculosis* to patients via the bronchoscope resulting in infection and pseudoinfections [225].

Other pseudo-outbreaks related to bronchoscopes that were inadequately disinfected or damaged have been reported [226–228]. Others report infection or pseudoinfection due to contaminated bronchoscopes [229]. One outbreak was believed to be a result of a manufacturing defect of the biopsy-port caps, and another was due to incorrect connectors joining the bronchoscope suction channel to the STERIS SYSTEM 1® (STERIS Corp., Mentor, Ohio) processor, obstructing peracetic acid flow through the bronchoscope lumen [230,231]. Infection and pseudoinfection from bronchoscopic procedures reflect a number of problems including ineffective cleaning due to poor technique, damaged equipment, difficult-to-clean accessories, ineffective reprocessing equipment (because of errors and the use of improper connectors, and ineffective disinfectants), use of tap water to rinse the scopes, inappropriate storage (e.g., coiling the scopes), and lack of familiarity with national recommendations for reprocessing. Srinivasan et al. distributed a survey to practicing bronchoscopists regarding infection control issues related to bronchoscopy and specific reprocessing recommendations [232]. Medical directors of bronchoscopy suites or attending bronchoscopists completed 46 surveys. Of the respondents, 65% were not familiar with national reprocessing recommendations, and 39% did not know what reprocessing procedure was used at their own institution. In addition, some parts of the bronchoscopes (e.g., reusable spring-operated suction valves) could require autoclaving if they become heavily contaminated with microbes that are relatively resistant to disinfection such as mycobacteria [233].

Cholangits is a complication associated with ERCP, and outbreaks have been the result of such procedures [234]. Despite negative surveillance cultures of the endoscopes, one outbreak of multidrug-resistant *Pseudomonas aeruginosa* cholangitis after ERCP was reported [235].

Endoscopic ultrasound (EUS) also has been examined for risk of infection after ERCP; one evaluation of an ambulatory endoscopy center found few infections [236]. Prophylactic antibiotics should be given before EUS of pancreatic cystic lesions [168].

Bronchoscopic and gastrointestinal endoscopic procedure-related infection and pseudoinfection are ongoing problems whose full impact is yet to be defined. Because infection can be associated with an endoscope exposed to microorganisms either from the environment or from a previous patient use, several organizations have published guidelines on infection control for flexible endoscopes [237–239]. In spite of the many adverse reports noted and published guidelines, various suboptimal procedures for disinfecting endoscopes are being practiced (Table 45-3) [240–243]. Even if institutions using endoscopes followed the manufacturer's guidelines for disinfecting scopes, it is becoming more evident that perhaps it is not always possible to clean such devices, most likely because of their complex designs. When "inspection endoscopes" were used to examine the conditions of the

TABLE 45-3

STEPS IN THE DISINFECTION PROCESS AND MECHANISMS FOR FAILURE (ADAPTED FROM [250] WITH PERMISSION)

Disinfection Component	Reasons for Component	Mechanisms for Failure
Cleaning	Reduce bioburden Remove interfering substances: blood, salt	Inadequate policies Inadequate staff training Ineffective disinfectant
Appropriate disinfectant	Inactivate contaminating microbes (demonstrated efficacy and effectiveness)	Inadequate concentration Inadequate duration
Contact between disinfectant and contaminating microbes	Kill	AER: failure to use channel connectors AER: wrong channel connectors Occluded lumen Torn or damaged lumen
Sterilization of biopsy forceps	Eliminate contaminating microbes	Inadequate policies Inadequate staff training
Rinse	Remove potentially toxic chemicals (e.g., glutaraldehyde, hydrogen peroxide)	Mucous membrane damage (e.g., colitis)
Prevention of recontamination	Prevent contamination with environmental microbes	Tap water rinse without subsequent alcohol rinse Failure to air-dry scope Contaminated AER Placement of scope in contaminated container

AER, automatic endoscope reprocessor.

working and suction channels of 241 flexible gastrointestinal endoscopes at 80 healthcare facilities [244], it was found that 47% (38/80) of facilities had at least one patient-ready endoscope whose suction or biopsy channels were visibly encrusted with debris, and 11% (26/241) of endoscopes had severely scratched channels that provided pockets for debris. Only 5.4% (3/56) of facilities that attempted to dry their endoscopes between procedures were successful. Because high-level disinfectants require clean surfaces, flexible endoscopes must be carefully cleaned of all mucus, blood, and other biologic materials before subjecting them to a high-level disinfectant [239,245]. To further complicate endoscope care, automated machines developed for endoscope reprocessing have been flawed [229,246–249]. Users should adhere carefully to the manufacturer's protocols but also should be aware of the possibility that colonization of the washer holding tanks is not reversible despite use of the manufacturer's recommended disinfection protocol. Surveillance for endoscope-related infection and pseudoinfection is important, and infection control practitioners must educate their endoscope users (e.g., endoscopy suite personnel and physicians) about problems discussed in this section; the users also must be vigilant to monitor best practice for a complicated cleaning procedure because there are many opportunities for inadequate disinfection. As Weber and Rutala noted, preventing outbreaks from endoscopes requires cleaning to precede disinfection or sterilization, avoiding ineffective or inadequate concentrations of disinfectants, contacting all internal and external surfaces with the disinfectant,

and attaching all channel connectors according to the manufacturer's directions when an automated endoscope reprocessor is used. Following disinfection, a sterile water rinse followed by forced-air drying or a tap water rinse followed by forced-air drying and a 70% alcohol rinse must be used to prevent recontamination. The disinfected endoscope must be stored in a manner to prevent recontamination [250].

Arthrocentesis and Thoracentesis

Although septic arthritis is caused most commonly by hematogenous spread of organisms, sporadic episodes of *Staphylococcal* spp. arthritis and, at times, gram-negative bacillary arthritis have followed several days after invasive joint manipulations. During the mid-1960s, CDC investigated a cluster of infection episodes of staphylococcal arthritis that the occurred 1–7 days after outpatient arthrocentesis or intraarticular injection of steroids. Epidemiologic evidence suggested that the physician who had performed these procedures was a disseminator of the epidemic strain, and microbiologic investigation showed that areas of chronic dermatitis on the physician's hands harbored the epidemic organism. A similar cluster of staphylococcal arthritis in which the infections occurred 5–6 days after arthrographic examination of the knee joint and 3–4 days after knee surgery was traced epidemiologically to the surgeon who had performed these procedures who was a nasal carrier of staphylococci. In 1987, 10 episodes of *Serratia* spp. septic arthritis were traced to contaminated benzalkonium chloride antiseptic used in a physician's office [251].

Other diagnostic taps such as thoracentesis [252] also have been associated with HAIs. This emphasizes the fact that all invasive procedures should be performed only under strict aseptic conditions with careful skin antisepsis by an appropriately scrubbed and gloved operator using sterile equipment. Although the relative rarity of centesis-associated infections can be considered testimony that good technique usually is observed in hospitals and clinics, the lack of such infections also could be evidence of the capacity of the local tissue response to limit bacterial invasion in uncompromised hosts [253]. When procedures are performed in patients with compromised host defenses or on tissues that could have diminished ability to limit bacterial invasion (e.g., rheumatoid joints), the risk of procedure-associated infections can be considerable, which emphasizes the need for continued vigilance.

Peritoneal Manipulation

Infectious complications of laparoscopy and amniocentesis are rare, presumably because of careful technique, sterile equipment, local host defense mechanisms, and patients' frequently healthy nature. In fact, high-level disinfection of peritoneoscopes with glutaraldehyde instead of gas sterilization has appeared acceptable. In a retrospective analysis of polymicrobial bacterial ascites in 1,578 abdominal paracenteses, only 1 episode of clinical peritonitis developed, presumably due to entry of the bowel by the paracentesis needle [254].

Artificial Insemination

Artificial insemination has transmitted a variety of infections and mandates careful adherence to protocol for screening candidates [255]. Artificial insemination could have resulted in HIV-1 infection of a woman inseminated with her HIV-infected husband's semen in spite of attempts to remove the virus from semen. The CDC recommends against insemination with semen from HIV-infected men [256]. Although there are no updates to the CDC recommendations, some centers do practice insemination with isolated and virologically tested spermatozoa for couples with an HIV-infected male partner [257–259]. However, an episode of HIV-1 transmission through artificial insemination was reported from an infertility clinic in India [260].

Ophthalmologic Examination

Manipulation of the conjunctiva and cornea can occur during tonometry, instillation of eye drops, and manual ophthalmologic examination. Such manipulation can result in conjunctivitis and other eye infections. The infection most commonly transmitted is epidemic keratoconjunctivitis, a highly contagious, frequently iatrogenic disease usually caused by adenovirus type 8 [261]. Transmission of the virus occurs through fomites, such as inadequately disinfected tonometers or contaminated eye droppers and by indirect person-to-person spread from HCW hands. Similar modes of transmission have been implicated in outbreaks of other viral and bacterial eye infections. Although proper care of equipment and conscientious hand hygiene between patient contacts is remarkably effective in halting the transmission of such pathogens, some manufacturer recommendations for disinfection could be inadequate [262], and ongoing community outbreaks could require extrastringent triage and infection control to limit nosocomial spread [263].

REFERENCES

1. Schroeder SA, Marton KI, Strom BL. Frequency and morbidity of invasive procedures: Report of a pilot study from two teaching hospitals. *Arch Intern Med* 1978;138:1809.
2. Wenzel RP, Osterman CA, Donowitz LG, et al. Identification of procedure-related nosocomial infections in high-risk patients. *Rev Infect Dis* 1981;3:701.
3. Rosenthal V, Maki D, Salomao R, et al. Device-associated nosocomial infections in 55 intensive care units of 8 developing countries. *Ann Intern Med* 2006;145:582–591.
4. Panlilio A, Orelien J, Srivastava P, et al. Estimate of the annual number of percutaneous injuries among hospital-based healthcare workers in the United States, 1997–1998. *Infect Control Hosp Epidemiol* 2004;25:556–62.
5. Perry J, Parker G, Jagger J. EPINet Report: 2003 percutaneous injury rates. *Advances in Exposure Prevention Bol* 2005; 7(4).
6. Department of Labor, Occupational Safety and Health Adminstration. Occupational exposure to bloodborne pathogens, needlestick and other sharps injuries: Final rule. *Federal Register* 2001;66:5318–25.
7. Ippolito G, De Carli G, Puro V, et al. Device-specific risk of needlestick injury in Italian healthcare workers. *JAMA* 1994;272:607–10.
8. Centers for Disease Control and Prevention. Evaluation of safety devices for preventing percutaneous injuries in health-care workers during phlebotomy procedures—Minneapolis-St. Paul, New York City, and San Francisco, 1993–1995. *MMWR* 1997;46:21–25.
9. Chamberland M, Alvarado-Ramy F, Beltrami E, Short L, et al. A comprehensive approach to percutaneous injury prevention during phlebotomy: Results of a multicenter study, 1993–1995. *Infect Control Hosp Epidemiol* 2003;24:97–104.
10. Yassi A, McGill M, Khokhar J. Efficacy and cost-effectiveness of a needleless intravenous access system. *Am J Infect Control* 1995;23:57–64.
11. Lawrence L, Delclos L, Felknor A, et al. The effectiveness of an intravenous connection system: An assessment by injury rate and user satisfaction. *Infect Control Hosp Epidemiol* 1997;18:175–82.
12. Danzig LE, Short LJ, Collins K, et al. Bloodstream infections associated with a needleless intravenous infusion system in patients receiving home infusion therapy. *JAMA* 1995;273:1882–84.
13. Maki DG, Stolz S, McCormick R, et al. Possible association of a commercial needleless system with central venous catheter-related bacteremia. In: *Proceedings of Programs and abstracts of the thirty-fourth interscience conference on antimicrobial agents and chemotherapy, October 1994, Orlando, Florida.* Washington, DC: American Society for Microbiology, 1994:195 [abstract].
14. Do A, Ray B, Banerjee S, et al. Bloodstream infection associated with needleless device use and the importance of infection-control practices in the home health care setting. *J Infect Dis* 1999;179:442–48.

15. Kellerman S, Shay D, Howard J, et al. Bloodstream infections in home infusion patients: The influence of race and needleless intravascular access devices. *J Pediatr* 1996;129:711–17.

16. Cookson S, Ihrig M, O'Mara E, et al. Increased bloodstream infection rates in surgical patients associated with variation from recommended use and care following implementation of a needleless device. *Infect Control Hosp Epidemiol* 1998;19:23–27.

17. McDonald LC, Banerjee SN, Jarvis WR. Line-associated bloodstream infections in pediatric intensive care-unit patients associated with a needleless device and intermittent intravenous therapy. *Infect Control Hosp Epidemiol* 1998;19:772–77.

18. Menyhay SZ, Maki DG. Disinfection of needleless catheter connectors and access ports with alcohol may not prevent microbial entry: The promise of a novel antiseptic-barrier cap. *Infect Control Hosp Epidemiol* 2006;27:23–27.

19. Adams D, Karpanen T, Worthington T, et al. Infection risk associated with a closed luer access device. *J Hosp Infect* 2006;62:353–57.

20. Leitch A, McCormick I, Gunn I, Gillespie T. Reducing the potential for phlebotomy tourniquets to act as a reservoir for methicillin-resistant *Staphylococcus aureus*. *J Hosp Infect* 2006;63:428–31.

21. Adams SL. The medicinal leech. *Ann Intern Med* 1988;109:399.

22. Abrutyn E. Hospital-associated infection from leeches. *Ann Intern Med* 1988;109:356.

23. Mercer NS, Beere DM, Bornemisza AJ, Thomas P. Medical leeches as sources of wound infection. *Br Med J* 1987;294:937.

24. Ardehali B, Hand K, Nduka C, et al. Delayed leech-borne infection with *Aeromonas hydrophilia* in escharotic wound. *J Plast Reconstr Aesthet Surg* 2006;59:94–95.

25. Ouderkirk JP, Bekhor D, Turett GS, Murali R. Aeromonas meningitis complicating medicinal leech therapy. *Clin Infect Dis* 2004;38:e36–37.

26. Mackay DR, Manders EK, Saggers GC, et al. Aeromonas species isolated from medicinal leeches. *Ann Plast Surg* 1999;42:275–79.

27. Sartor C, Limouzin-Perotti F, Legre R, et al. Nosocomial Infections with *Aeromonas hydorphila* from leeches. *Clin Infect Dis* 2002;35:E1–5.

28. Pereira JA, Greig JR, Liddy H, et al. Leech-borne *Serratia marcescens* infection following complex hand injury. *Br J Plast Surg* 1998;51:640–41.

29. Munoz P, Blanco J, Rdorquez-Creixems M, et al. Bloodstream infections after invasive nonsurgical cardiology procedures. *Arch Intern Med* 2001;16:2110–15.

30. Samore M, Wessolossky M, Lewis S, et al. Frequency risk factors, and outcome for bacteremia after percutaneous transluminal coronary angioplasty. *Am J Cardiol* 1997;79:873–77.

31. Ramsdale D, Aziz S, Newall N, et al. Bacteremia following complex percutaneous coronary intervention. *J Invas Cardiol* 2004;16:632–34.

32. Sande MA, Levinson ME, Lukas DS, Kaye D. Bacteremia associated with cardiac catheterization. *N Engl J Med* 1969;281:1104.

33. Kaufmann B, Kaiser C, Pfisterer M, Boneti P. Coronary stent infection: A rare but severe complication of percutaneous coronary intervention. *Swiss Med Wkly* 2005;135:483–87.

34. Hoffman M, Baruch R, Kaplan E, et al. Coronary stent bacterial infection with multiple organ septic emboli. *Eur J Intern Med* 2005;16:123–25.

35. Bouchart F, Dubar A, Bessou J, et al. *Pseudomonas aeruginosa* coronary stent infection. *Ann Thorac Surg* 1997;64:1810–13.

36. Singh H, Singh C, Aggarwal N, et al. Mycotic aneurysm of left anterior descending artery after sirolimus-eluting stent implantation: A case report. *Catheter Cardiovasc Interv* 2005;65:282–85.

37. Marcu C, Balf D, Donohue T. Post-infectious pseudoaneurysm after coronary angioplasty using drug eluting stents. *Heart Lung Circ* 2005;14:85–86.

38. Banai S, Selister V, Keren A, et al. Prospective study of bacteremia after cardiac catheterization. *Am J Cardiol* 2003;92:1004–7.

39. Chambers C, Eisenhauer M, McNicol L, et al. Members of the Catheterization Lab Performance Standards Committee for the Society for Cardiovascular Angiography and Interventions. Infection control guidelines for the cardiac catheterization laboratory: Society guidelines revisited. *Catheter Cardiovasc Interv* 2006;67:78–86.

40. Thomas F, Burke J, Parker J, et al. The risk of infection related to radial vs. femoral sites for arterial catheterization. *Crit Care Med* 1983;11:807–12.

41. Gardner R, Schwartz R, Wong H, Burke J. Percutaneous indwelling radial-artery catheters for monitoring cardiovascular function: Prospective study of the risk of thrombosis and infection. *N Engl J Med* 1974;290:1227–31.

42. Raad I, Umphrey I, Khan A, et al. The duration of placement as a predictor of peripheral and pulmonary arterial catheter infections. *J Hosp Infect* 1993;23:17–26.

43. El-Hamamsy I, Durrleman N, Stevens L, et al. Incidence and outcome of radial artery infections following cardiac surgery. *Ann Thorac Surg* 2003;76:801–4.

44. Raad I, Abi-Said D, Carrasco C, et al. The risk of infection associated with intra-arterial catheters for cancer chemotherapy. *Infect Control Hosp Epidemiol* 1998;19:640–42.

45. Traore O, Liotier J, Souweine B. Prospective study of arterial and central venous catheter colonization and of arterial and central venous catheter-related bacteremia in intensive care units. *Crit Care Med* 2005;33:1437–39.

46. Rijnders Bart J, Winjngaerden E, Wilmer A, Peetermans W. Use of full sterile barrier precautions during insertion of arterial catheters: A randomized trial. *Clin Infect Dis* 2003;36:743–48.

47. Band JD, Maki DG. Infections caused by arterial catheters used for hemodynamic monitoring. *Am J Med* 1979;67:735–41.

48. Centers for Disease Control and Prevention. Guidelines for the prevention of intravascular catheter-related infections. *MMWR* 2002;51(RR-10);1–26.

49. Lorente, L, Santacreu R, Martin M, et al. Arterial catheter-related infection of 2,949 catheters. *Crit Care* 2006;10:R83.

50. Furaro S, Gauthier M, Lacroix J, et al. Arterial catheter-related infections in children. *Am J Dis Child* 1991;145:1037–42.

51. Lorent L, Villegas J, Martin MM, et al. Catheter-related infection in critically ill patients. *Inten Care Med* 2004;30:1681–84.

52. Thomas F, Burke JP, Parker J, et al. The risk of infection related to radial vs. femoral sites for arterial catheterization. *Crit Care Med* 1983;11:807–12.

53. Lorente, L, Santacreu R, Martin M, et al. Arterial catheter-related infection of 2,949 catheters. *Crit Care Med* 2006;10:R83.

54. Adam RD, Edwards LD, Becker CC, Schrom HM. Semiquantitative cultures and routine tip cultures on umbilical catheters. *J Pediatr* 1982;100:123.

55. Bard H et al. Prophylactic antibiotics in chronic umbilical artery catheterization in respiratory distress syndrome. *Arch Dis Child* 1973;48:630.

56. Krauss AN, Albert RF, Kannan MM. Contamination of umbilical catheters in the newborn infant. *J Pediatr* 1970;77:965.

57. Powers WF, Tooley WH. Contamination of umbilical vessel catheters. *Pediatrics* 1971;48:470.

58. Anagnostakis D et al. Risk of infection associated with umbilical vein catheterization. *J Pediatr* 1975;86:759.

59. Deliege R, Cneude F, Barbier C, et al. Ruptured mycotic aneurysm with hemoperitoneum: An unusual septic complication of umbilical arterial catheter. *Arch Pediatr* 2003;10:716–18.

60. Roy N, Azakiea A, Moon-Grady A, et al. Mycotic aneurysm of the descending thoracic aorta in a 2-kg neonate. *Ann Thorac Surg* 2005;80:726–29.

61. Wyers M, McAlister WH. Umbilical artery catheter use complicated by pseudoaneurysm of the aorta. *Pediatr Radiol* 2002;32:199–201.

62. Rowley KM, Clubb KS, Smith GJW, Cabin HS. Right-sided infective endocarditis as a consequence of flow directed pulmonary artery catheterization. *N Engl J Med* 1984;311:1152.

63. Mermel LA, Maki DG. Infectious complications of Swan-Ganz pulmonary artery catheters. *Am J Respir Crit Care Med* 1994;149:1020–36.

64. Damen J, Ver Der Twell I. Positive tip cultures and related risk factors associated with intravascular catheterization in pediatric cardiac patients. *Crit Care Med* 1988;16:221–28.

65. Mermel LA, McCormick RD, Springman SR, Maki DG. The pathogenesis and epidemiology of catheter-related infection with pulmonary artery Swan-Ganz catheters: a prospective study utilizing molecular subtyping. *Am J Med* 1991;38:197S–205S.

66. Rello J, Coll P, Net A, Prats G. Infection of pulmonary artery catheters: Epidemiologic characteristics and multivariate analysis of risk factors. *Chest* 1993;103; 132–36.

67. Maki DG, Stolz SS, Wheeler S, Mermel LA. A prospective, randomized trial of gauze and two polyurethane dressings for site care of pulmonary artery catheters: Implications for catheter management. *Crit Care Med* 1994;22:1729–37.

68. Weinstein RA, Stamm WE, Kramer L, Corey L. Pressure monitoring devices: Overlooked source of nosocomial infection. *JAMA* 1976;236:936.

69. Luskin RL et al. Extended use of disposable pressure transducers. *JAMA* 1986;255:916.

70. Kormos RL, Borovetz HS, Armitage JM, et al. Evolving experience with mechanical circulatory support. *Ann Surg* 1991;214:471–77.

71. Pennington DG, McBride LR, Peigh PS, et al. Eight years' experience with bridging to cardiac transplantation. *J Thorac Cardiovasc Surg* 1994;107:472–81.

72. Farrar DJ, Hill DJ. Univentricular and biventricular thoratec VAD support as a bridge to transplantation. *Ann Thorac Surg* 1993;55:276–82.

73. Simon D, Fischer S, Grossman A, et al. Left ventricular assist device-related infection: Treatment and outcome. *Clin Infect Dis* 2005;40:1108–15.

74. Malani P, Dyke D, Pagani F, Chenoweth C. Nososcomial infections in left ventricular assist device recipients. *Clin Infect Dis* 2002;34:1295–300.

75. Bentz B, Hupcey J, Polomano R, Boehmer J. A retrospective study of left ventricular assist device-related infections. *J Cardiovasc Manag* 2004;15:9–16.

76. Mill CA, Pae WE, Pierce WS. Combined registry for the clinical use of mechanical ventricular assist pumps and the total artificial heart in conjunction with heart transplantation: Fourth official report. *J Heart Transplant* 1989;9:453–58.

77. Yuh D, Albaugh M, Ullrich S, Conte J. Treatment of ventricular assist device driveline infection with vacuum-assisted closure system. *Ann Thorac Surg* 2005;80:1493–95.

78. Myers TJ, McGee MG, Zeluff BJ, et al. Frequency and significance of infections in patients receiving prolonged LVAD support. *ASAIO Trans* 1991;37:M283–85.

79. Fisher S, Trenholme G, Costanzo MR, Piccione W. Infectious complications of left ventricular assist device recipients. *Clin Infect Dis* 1997;24:18–23.

80. Siegenthaler M, Martin J, Pernice K, et al. The Jarvik 2000 is associated with less infections than the HeartMate left ventricular assist device. *Eur J Cardiothorac Surg* 2003;23:748–54.

81. Holman W, Park S, Long J, et al. Infection in permanent circulatory support: Experience from the REMATCH trial. *J Heart Lung Transplant* 2004;23:1359–65.

82. Kotschet E, Aggarwal A, Esmore D, Kaye D. Left ventricular apical infection and rupture complication left ventricular assist device explantation in 2 women with postpartum cardiomyopathy. *J Heart Lung Transplant* 2005;24:350–54.

83. Babone A, Pini D, Grossi P, et al. Aspergillus left ventricular assist device endocarditis. *Ital Heart J* 2004;5:876–80.

84. Choi L, Choudhri AF, Pillarisetty VG, et al. Development of an infection-resistant LVAD driveline: A novel approach to the prevention of device-related infections. *J Heart Lung Transplant* 1999;18:1103–10.

85. Hogman C, Engstrand L. Seriopus bacterial complications from blood components—How do they occur? *Transfus Med* 1998;8:1–3.

86. James JD. Bacterial contamination of preserved blood. *Vox Sang* 1959;4:177.

87. Braude Al, Sanford JP, Bartlett JE, Mallery OT. Effects and clinical significance of bacterial contaminants in transfused blood. *J Lab Clin Med* 1952;39:902.

88. Heltberg O, Skov F, Grener-Smidt P, et al. Nosocomial epidemic of *Serratia marcescens* septicemia ascribed to contaminated blood transfusion bags. *Transfusion* 1993;33:221–27.

89. Kuehnert M, Roth V, Haley N, et al. Transfusion-transmitted bacterial infection in the United States, 1998 through 2000. *Transfusion* 2001;41:1493–99.

90. Perez P, Salmi L, Follea G, et al. Determinants of transfusion-associated bacterial contamination: Results of the French BACTHEM case-control study. *Transfusion* 2001;41:862–72.

91. Chwatt U. Blood transfusion and tropical disease. *Tropical Disease Bulletin* 1972;69:825.

92. Dover AS, Schultz MG. Transfusion-induced malaria. *Transfusion* 1971;11:353.

93. Guerrero IC, Weniger BC, Schultz MG. Transfusion malaria in the United States, 1972–1981. *Ann Intern Med* 1983;99:221.

94. Busch M, Kleinman S, Nemo G. Current and emerging infectious risks of blood transfusions. *JAMA* 2003;289:959–62.

95. Tejura B, Sass D, Fischer R, et al. Transfusion-associated falciparum malaria successfully treated with red blood cell exchange transfusion. *Am J Med Sci* 2000;320:337–41.

96. Schmunis GA. *Trypanosoma cruzi*, the etiological agent of Chagas' disease as a contaminant of blood supplies: A problem of endemic and non-endemic countries. *Transfusion* 1991;31:547–57.

97. Leiby D. Parasites and other emergent infectious agents. In: Stramer S, ed. *Blood safety in the new millennium*. Bethesda, MD: American Association of Blood Banks, 2001:55–78.

98. Leiby D, Read E, Lenes B, et al. Seroepidemiology of *Trypanosoma cruzi*, etiologic agent of Chagas' disease, in U.S. blood donors. *J Infect Dis* 1997;176:1047–52.

99. American Association of Blood Banks. *Standards for blood banks and transfusion services*. Bethesda, MD: AABB, 2004.

100. Kimball AC, Kean BH, Kellner A. The risk of transmitting toxoplasmosis by blood transfusion. *Transfusion* 1965;5:447.

101. Siegel SE et al. Transmission of toxoplasmosis by leukocyte transfusion. *Blood* 1971;37:388.

102. Leiby D, Chung A, Gill J, et al. Demonstrable parasitemia among Connecticut blood donors with antibodies to *Babesia microti*. *Transfusion* 2005;45:1894–1910.

103. Herwaldt B, Neitzel D, Gorlin J, et al. Transmission of *Babesia microti* in Minnesota through four blood donations from the same donor over a 6-month period. *Transfusion* 2002;42:1154–58.

104. Kjemtrup A, Lee B, Fritz C, et al. Investigation of transfusion transmission of a WA1-type babesial parasite to a premature infant in California. *Transfusion* 2002;42:1482–87.

105. Dobroszycki J, Herwaldt B, Boctor F, et al. A cluster of transfusion-associated babesiosis cases traced to a single asymptomatic donor. *JAMA*. 1999; 10;281:927–30.

106. Shehata N, Kohli M, Detsky A. The cost-effectiveness of screening blood donors for malaria by PCR. *Transfusion* 2004;44:217–28.

107. Seed C, Kitchen A, Davis T. The current status and potential role of laboratory testing to prevent transfusion-transmitted malaria. *Transfus Med Rev* 2005;19:229–40.

108. Sullivan MT, Wallace EL. Blood collection and transfusion in the United States in 1999. *Transfusion* 2005;5:141–48

109. Yomtovian R, Lazarus M, Goodnough L, et al. A prospective microbiologic surveillance program to detect and prevent the transfusion of bacterially contaminated platelets. *Transfusion* 1993;33:902–9.

110. Strong D, Katz L. Blood-bank testing for infectious diseases: How safe is blood transfusion? *Trends Mol Med* 2002;8:355–58.

111. Brecher ME, Hay SN. Improving platelet safety: Bacterial contamination of platelets. *Curr Hemoatol Rep* 2004;3:121–27.

112. Centers for Disease Control and Prevention. Fatal bacterial infections associated with platelet transfusions—United States, 2004. *MMWR* 2005;54:168–70.

113. Murphy S, Gardner FH. Effect of storage temperature on maintenance of platelet viability-deleterious effect of refrigerated storage. *N Engl J Med* 1969;280:1094–98.

114. Buchholtz DH et al. Bacterial proliferation in platelets stored at room temperature. *N Engl J Med* 1971;285:429.

115. Cunningham M, Cash JD. Bacterial contamination and platelet concentrates stored at 20°C. *J Clin Pathol* 1973;26:401.

116. Te Boekhorst PA, Beckers EA, Bos MC, et al. Clinical significance of bacteriologic screening in platelet concentrates. *Transfusion* 2005;45:514–9.

117. Chang A, Kirsch C, Mobashery N, et al. *Streptococcus bovis* septic shock due to contaminated transfused platelets. *Am. J. Hematol* 2004;77:282–86.

118. Rhame FS et al. *Salmonella* septicemia from platelet transfusions. *Ann Intern Med* 1973;78:633.

119. Blajchman MA et al. Platelet transfusion-induced *Serratia marcescens* sepsis due to vacuum tube contamination. *Transfusion* 1979;19:39.

120. Zaza S, Tokars JI, Yomtovian R, et al. Bacterial contamination of platelets at a university hospital: Increased identification due to intensified surveillance. *Infect Control Hosp Epidemiol* 1994;15:82–87.

121. Jafari M, Forsberg J, Gilcher R, et al. Salmonella sepsis caused by a platelet transfusion from a donor with a pet snake. *N Engl J Med* 2002;347:1075–78.

122. Wollowitz S. Fundamentals of psoralen-based Helinx technology for inactivation of infectious pathogens on leukocytes in platelets and plasma. *Semin Hematol* 2001;38 (Suppl 11):4–11.

123. Rotman B, Cote M. Application of a real-time biosensor to detect bacteria in platelet concentrates. *Biochem Biophys Res Commun* 2003;300:197–200.

124. Executive Committee of the Infectious Diseases Society of America Emerging Infections Network. The emerging infections network: A new venture for the Infectious Diseases Society of America. *Clin Infect Dis* 1997;25:34–36.

125. Grossman B, Kollins P, Lau P, et al. Screening blood donors for gastrointestinal illness: A strategy to eliminate carriers of *Yersinia enterocolitica*. *Transfusion* 1991;31:500–1.

126. American Association of Blood Banks. *Guidance on implementation of new bacteria and reduction standard*. Bulletin 04–07. Bethesda, MD: AABB, 2004.

127. Steere AC et al. *Pseudomonas* species bacteremia caused by contaminated normal human serum albumin. *J Infect Dis* 1977;135:729.

128. Chamberland ME. Emerging infectious agents: Do they pose a risk to the safety of transfused blood and blood products. *Clin Infec Dis* 2002;34:797–805.

129. American Association of Blood Banks. *Association Bulletin 6-04*, April 26, 2006.

130. Bennett SN, McNeil MM, Bland LA, et al. Postoperative infections traced to contamination of an intravenous anesthetic, propofol. *N Engl J Med* 1995;333:147–54.

131. Capdevila X, Pirat P, Bringuier S, et al; French Study Group on Continuous Peripheral Nerve Blocks: Continuous peripheral nerve blocks in hospital wards after orthopedic surgery: A multicenter prospective analysis of the quality of postoperative analgesia and complications in 1,416 patients. *Anesthesiology* 2005;103:1035–45.

132. Cuvillon P, Ripart J, Lalourcey L, et al. The continuous femoral nerve block catheter for postoperative analgesia: Bacterial colonization, infectious rate and adverse effects. *Anetsh Analg* 2001;93:1045–49.

133. Obek C, Onal B, Ozkan B, et al. Is periprostatic local anesthesia for transrectal ultrasound guided prostate biopsy associated with increased infectious or hemorrhagic complications? A prospective randomized trial. *J UROL* 2002;168:558–61.

134. Berry FA, Blankenbaker WL, Ball CG. A comparison of bacteremia occurring with nasotracheal and orotracheal intubation. *Anesth Analg* 1973;52:873.

135. Fassoulaki A, Pamouktsoglou P. Prolonged nasotracheal intubation and its association with inflammation of paranasal sinuses. *Anesth Analg* 1989;69:50.

136. Linden BE, Aguilar EA, Allen SJ. Sinusitis in the nasotracheally intubated patient. *Arch Otolaryngol Head Neck Surg* 1988;114:860.

137. Lucks D, Consiglio A, Stankiewicz J, O'Keefe P. Incidence and microbiological etiology of middle ear effusion complicating endotracheal intubation and mechanical ventilation. *J Infect Dis* 1988;157:368.

138. Centers for Disease Control and Prevention. Guidelines for preventing health-care-associated pneumonia, 2003. *MMWR Recomm Rep* 2004;53(RR-3):1–36.

139. Bannon L, Brimacombe J, Nixon T, Keller C. Repeat autoclaving does not remove protein deposits from the classic laryngeal mask airway. *Eur J Anaesthesiol* 2005;22:515–17.

140. Greenwood J, Green N, Power G. Protein contamination of the laryngeal mask airway and its relationship to re-use. *Anaesth Intensive Care* 2006;34:343–46.

141. Richards E, Brimacombe J, Laupau W, Keller C. Protein cross-contamination during batch cleaning and autoclaving of the ProSeal laryngeal mask airway. *Anaesthesia* 2006;61:431–3.

142. Fowler R, Guest C, Lapinsky S, et al. Transmission of severe acute respiratory syndrome during intubation and mechanical ventilation. *Am J Respir Crit Care Med* 2004;169:1177–78.

143. Peng P, Wong D, Bevan D, Gardam M. Infection control and anesthesia: Lessons learned from the Toronto SARS outbreak. *Can J Anes* 2003;50:987–97.

144. Diamond RD, Bennett JE. A subcutaneous reservoir for intrathecal therapy of fungal meningitis. *N Engl J Med* 1974;288:186.

145. Lishner M et al. Complications associated with Ommaya reservoirs in patients with cancer. *Arch Intern Med* 1990;150:173.

146. Trump DL, Grossman SA, Thompson G, Murray K. CSF infections complicating the management of neoplastic meningitis. *Arch Intern Med* 1982;142:583.

147. Luthardt T. Bacterial infections in ventriculo-auricular shunt systems. *Dev Med Child Neurol Suppl* 1970;12:105.

148. Baysallar M, Izci Y, Avci IY, et al. A case of ventricular drainage infection with a rare pathogen in cerebrospinal fluid: Vancomycin-resistant *Enterococcus faecium*. *Microb Drug Resist* 2006;12:59–62.

149. McAdams RM, Simone S, Grant G, Digeronimo RJ. Ventricular peritoneal shunt infection resulting from group B streptococcus. *Pediatr Crit Care Med* 2006;77:586–8.

150. Schoenbaum SC, Gardner P, Shillito J. Infections of cerebrospinal fluid shunts. *J Infect Dis* 1975;131:543.

151. James H, Walsh JW, Wilson HD, et al. Prospective randomized study of therapy in cerebrospinal fluid shunt infections. *Neurosurgery* 1980;7:459–63.

152. Younger JJ et al. Coagulase-negative staphylococci isolated from cerebrospinal fluid shunts: Importance of slime production, species identification, and shunt removal to clinical outcome. *J Infect Dis* 1987;156:548.

153. McLaurin RL, Frane PT. Treatment of infections of cerebrospinal fluid shunts. *Rev Infect Dis* 1987;9:595.

154. Guertin SR. Cerebrospinal fluid shunts: Evaluation, complications, and crisis management. *Pediatr Clin North Am* 1987;34:203.

155. Kestle JR, Garton HJ, Whitehead WE, et al. Management of shunt infections: A multicenter pilot study. *Neurosurg* 2006;105(3suppl):177–81.

156. Pattavilakom A, Kotasnas D, Korman T, et al. Duration of *in vivo* antimicrobial activity of antibiotic-impregnated cerebrospinal fluid catheters. *Neurosurgery* 2006;58:930–35.

157. Sciubba D, Stuart R, McGirt M, et al. Effect of antibiotic-impregnated shunt catheters in decreasing the incidence of shunt infection in the treatment of hydrocephalus. *J Neurosurg* 2005;103(2suppl):131–36.

158. Langley JM, LeBlanc JC, Drake J, Milner R. Efficacy of antimicrobial prophylaxis in placement of cerebrospinal fluid shunts: Meta-analysis. *Clin Infect Dis* 1993;17:98–103.

159. Haines SJ, Walters BC. Antibiotic prophylaxis for cerebrospinal fluid shunts: A meta analysis. *Neurosurgery* 1994;34:87–92.

160. Ratilal B, Costa J, Sampaio C. Antibiotic prophylaxis for surgical introduction of intracranial ventricular shunts. *Cochrane Database Syst Rev* 2006;3.CD005365.

161. Bajwa Z, Ho C, Grush A, et al. Discitis associated with pregnancy and spinal anesthesia. *Anesth Analg* 2002;94:415–16.

162. Baer ET. Post-dural puncture bacterial meningitis. *Anesthesiology* 2006;105:381–93.

163. Conangla G, Rodriquez L, Alonso-Tarres C, et al. *Streptococcus salivarius* meningitis after spinal anesthesia. *Neurologia* 2004;19:331–33.

164. Shapiro JM, Bond EL, Garman JK. Use of a chlorhexidine dressing to reduce microbial colonization of epidural catheters. *Anesthesiology* 1990;73:625–31.

165. Ho KM, Litton E. Use of chlorhexidine-impregnated dressing to prevent vascular and epidural catheter colonization and infection: A meta-analysis. *J Antimicrob Chemother* 2006;58:281–87.

166. Everett ED, Hirschmann JV. Transient bacteremia and endocarditis prophylaxis: a review. *Medicine* 1977;56:61.

167. Crawford JJ et al. Bacteremia after tooth extractions studied with the aid of prereduced anaerobically sterilized culture media. *Appl Microbiol* 1974;27:927.

168. (no author) Guidelines for antibiotic prophylaxis for gastrointestinal endoscopy. *Gastrointes Endosc* 2003;58:475–82.

169. Nelson DB. Infection control during gastrointestinal endoscopy. *J Lab Clin Med* 2003;141:159–67.

170. Allen JI, Allen MO, Wlson MA, et al. *Pseudomonas* infection of the biliary system resulting from use of a contaminated endoscope. *Gastroenterology* 1987;92:759–63.

171. Classen DC, Jacobson JA, Burke JP, et al. Serious *Pseudomonas* infections associated with endoscopic retrograde cholangiopancreatography. *Am J Med* 1988;84:590–6.

172. Cryan EM, Falkiner FR, Mulvhill TE, et al. *Pseudomonas aeruginosa* cross-infection following endoscopic retrograde cholangiopancreatography. *J Hosp Infect* 1984;5:371–6.

173. Doherty DE et al. *Pseudomonas aeruginosa* sepsis following retrograde cholangiopancreatography (ERCP). *Dig Dis Sci* 1982;27:169–70.

174. Earnshaw JJ, Clark AW, Thom BT. Outbreak of *Pseudomonas aeruginosa* following endoscopic retrograde cholangiopancreatography. *J Hosp Infect* 1985;6:95–7.

175. Elson CO, Hattori K, Blackstone MO. Polymicrobial sepsis following endoscopic retrograde and cholangiopancreatography. *Gastroenterology* 1975;69:507–10.

176. Greene WH et al. Esophagoscopy as a source of *P. aeruginosa* sepsis in patients with acute leukemia: The need for sterilization of endoscopes. *Gastroenterology* 1974;67:912–9.

177. Low DE, Micflikier AB, Kennedy JK, Stiver HG. Infectious complications of endoscopic retrograde cholangiopancreatography: A prospective assessment. *Arch Intern Med* 1980;140:1076–7.

178. Spach DH, Silverstein FE, Stamm WE. Transmission of infection by gastrointestinal endoscopy and bronchoscopy. *Ann Intern Med* 1993;118:117–28.

179. Nelson D, Jarvis W, Rutala W, et al. Society for Healthcare Epidemiology of America: Multi-society guideline for reprocessing flexible gastrointestinal endoscopes. *Infec Control Hosp Epidemiol* 2003;24:532–37.

180. Alvarado C, Reichelderfer M. APIC guidelines for infection prevention and control in flexible endoscopy. *Am J Infect Control* 2000;28:138–55.

181. Ogoshi K, Reprocessing of gastrointestinal endoscopic accessories. *J Gastroenterol Hepatol* 2000;15 (suppl):G82–85

182. Zuccaro G, Richeter J, Rice T, et al. Viridans streptococcal bacteremia after esophageal stricture dilation. *Gastrointest Endosc* 1998;48:568–73.

183. Nelson D, Sanderson S, and Azar M. Bacteremia with esophageal dilation. *Gastrointest Endosc* 1998;48:563–67.

184. Hirota W, Wortmann G, Maydonovitch C, et al. The effect of oral decontamination with clindamycin palmitate on the incidence of bacteremia after esophageal dilation. A prospective trial. *Gastrointest Endosc* 1999;50:475–79.

185. Lo G, Lai K, Shen M, Chang C. A comparison of the incidence of transient bacteremia and infectious sequelae after sclerotherapy and rubber band ligation of bleeding esophageal varices. *Gastrointest Endosc* 1994;40:675–79.

186. Lo G, Lai K, Cheng J, et al. A prospective, randomized trial of sclerotherapy versus ligation in the management of bleeding esophageal varices. *Hepatology* 1995;22:466–71.

187. Tseng C, Green R, Burke S, et al. Bacteremia after endoscopic band ligation of esophageal varices. *Gastrointest Endosc* 1992;38:336–37.

188. Berner J, Gaing A, Sharma R, et al. Sequelae after esophageal variceal ligation and sclerotherapy: A prospective randomized study. *Am J Gastroenterol* 1994;89:852–58.

189. Rohr M, Siqueira E, Brant C, et al. Prospective study of bacteremia rate after elastic band ligation and sclerotherapy of esophageal varices in patients with hepatosplenic schistosomiasis. *Gastrointest Endosc* 1997;46:321–23.

190. Lin OS, Wu S, Chen Y, Soon M. Bacterial peritonitis after elective endoscopic variceal ligation: A prospective study. *Am J Gastroenterol* 2000;95:214–17.

191. Beddy P, Lyburn I, Geoghegan T, et al. Outpatient liver biopsy: A prospective evaluation of 500 cases. *Gut* 2006 (October)?

192. Botsford KB et al. Gram-negative bacilli in human milk feedings: Quantitation and clinical consequences for premature infants. *J Pediatr* 1986;109:707.

193. Levy J. Enteral nutrition: An increasingly recognized cause of nosocomial bloodstream infection. *Infect Control Hosp Epidemiol* 1989;10:395–7.

194. Sullivan NM, Sutter VL, Carter WT, et al. Bacteremia after genitourinary tract manipulation. *Appl Microbiol* 1972;23:1101–6.

195. Dellinger EP, Gross PA, Barrett TL, et al. Quality standard for antimicrobial prophylaxis in surgical procedures. *Clin Infect Dis* 1994;18:422–27.

196. Barela A, Kleinman GE, Goldich IM, et al. Septic shock with renal failure after chorionic villus sampling. *Am J Obstet Gynecol* 1986;154:1100–2.

197. Livengood CH, Land MR, Addison WA. Endometrial biopsy, bacteremia, and endocarditis, risk. *Obstet Gynecol* 1985;65:678–81.

198. Paz A, Gonen R, Potasman I. Candida sepsis following transcervical chorionic villi sampling. *Infect Dis Obstet Gynecol* 2001;9:147–48.

199. Durack D. Prevention of infective endocarditis. *N Engl J Med* 1995;332:38–44.

200. Oakley C, Somerville W. Prevention of infective endocarditis. *Br Heart J* 1981;45:233.

201. Hess J, Holloway Y, Dankert J. Incidence of postextraction bacteremia under penicillin cover in children with cardiac disease. *Pediatrics* 1983;71:554.

202. Lowy FD et al. Effect of penicillin on the adherence of *Streptococcus sanguis in vitro* and in the rabbit model of endocarditis. *J Clin Invest* 1983;71:668.

203. Dajani AS, Taubert KA, Wilson W, et al. Prevention of bacterial endocarditis: Recommendations by the American Heart Association. *JAMA* 1997;277:1794–1801.

204. Mueller PR, van Sonnenberg E. Interventional radiology in the chest and abdomen. *N Engl J Med* 1990;322:1364–74.

205. Hunter DW, Simmons RL, Hulbert JC. Antibiotics for radiologic interventional procedures. *Radiology* 1988;166:571.

206. Chuang S, Lee K, Chang W, et al. Risk factors for wound infection after cholecystectomy. *J Formos Med Assoc* 2004;103:607–12.

207. Boni L, Benevento A, Rovera F, et al. Infective complications in laparoscopic surgery. *Surg Infect* 2006;7 (suppl 2):S109–11.

208. Chang W, Lee K, Chuang S, et al. The impact of prophylactic antibiotics on postoperative infection complication in elective laparoscopic sholecystectomy: A prospective randomized study. *Am J Surg* 2006;191:721–25.

209. Kuthe S, Kaman L, Verma G, Singh R. Evaluation of the role for prophylactic antibiotics in elective laparoscopic cholecystectomy: A prospective randomized trial. *Trop Gastroenterol* 2006;27:54–57.

210. Catarci M, Mancini S, Gentileschi P, et al. Antibiotic prophylaxis in elective laparoscopic cholecystectomy. Lack of need or lack of evidence? *Surg Endosc* 2004;18:638–41.

211. Koc M, Zulfikaroglu B, Kece C, Ozalp N. A prospective randomized study of prophylactic antibiotics in elective laparoscopic cholecystectomy. *Surg Endosc* 2003;17:1716–18.

212. Mahatharadol V. A reevaluation of antibiotic prophylaxis in laparoscopic cholecystectomy: A randomized controlled trial. *J Med Assoc Thai* 2001;84:105–8.

213. Dixon RE, Kaslow RA, Mackel DC, et al. The need for antibiotic prophylaxis in elective laparoscopic cholecystectomy: A prospective randomized study. *Arch Surg* 2000;131:67–70.

214. McGuckin M, Shea J, Schwartz J. Infection and antimicrobial use in laparoscopic cholecystectomy. *Infect Control Hosp Epidemiol* 1999;20:624–26.

215. Dixon RE et al. Aqueous quaternary ammonium antiseptics and disinfectants: Use and mis-use. *JAMA* 1976;236:2415–7.

216. Chew B, Denstedt J. Technology insight: Novel ureteral stent materials and designs. *Nat Clin Pract Urol* 2004;1:44–48.

217. Kehinde E, Rotimi V, Al-Hunayan A, et al. Bacteriology of urinary tract infection associated with indwelling J ureteral stents. *J Endourol* 2004;18:891–96.

218. Paz A, Amiel G, Pick N, et al. Febrile complications following insertion of 100 double-J ureteral stents. *J Endourol* 2005;19:147–50.

219. Center for Disease Control and Prevention. Vital and health statistics: Ambulatory and inpatient procedures in the United States, 1996. DHHS publication 99–1710. Hyattsville, MD: US Department of Health and Human Services, National Center for Health Statistics, 1998.

220. Hoffman KK, Weber DJ, Rutala WA. Pseudoepidemic of *Rhodotorula rubra* in patients undergoing fiberoptic bronchoscopy. *Infect Control Hosp Epidemiol* 1989;10:511–xx.

221. Bennett S, Peterson D, Johnson D, et al. Bronchoscopy-associated *Mycobacterium xenopi* pseudoinfections. *Am J Respir Crit Care Med* 1994;150:245–50.

222. Nelson KE, Larson PA, Schraufnagel DE, Jackson J. Transmission of tuberculosis by flexible fiberbronchoscopes. *Am Rev Respir Dis* 1983;127:97.

223. Favero MS. Sterilization, disinfection and antisepsis in the hospital. In: *Manual of clinical microbiology*. 4th ed. Washington, DC: American Society for Microbiology, 1985:129–37.

224. Larson J, Lambert L Stricof R, et al. Potential nosocomail exposure to *Mycobacterium tuberculosis* from a bronchoscope. *Infect Control Hosp Epidemiol* 2003;24:825–30.

225. Ramsey A, Oemig T, Davis J, et al. An outbreak of bronchoscopy-related *Mycobacterium tuberculosis* infections due to lack of bronchoscope leak testing. *Chest* 2002;121:976–81.

226. Silva C, Magalhaes V, Pereira C, et al. Pseudo-outbreak of *Pseudomonas aeruginosa* and *Serratia marcescans* related to bronchoscopes. *Infect Control Hosp Epidemiol* 2003;24:195–97.

227. Corne P, Godreuil S, Jean-Pierre H, et al. Unusual implication of biopsy forceps in outbreaks of *Pseudomonas aeruginosa* infections and pseudo-infections related to bronchoscopy. *J Hosp Infect* 2005;61:20–26.

228. Cetre J, Nicolle M, Salord H, et al. Outbreaks of contaminated broncho-alveolar lavage related to intrinsically defective bronchoscopes. *J Hosp Infect* 2005;61:39–45.

229. Bou R, Aguilar A, Perpinan J, et al. Nosocomial outbreak of *Pseudomonas aeruginoasa* infections related to a flexible bronchoscope. *J Hosp Infect* 2006;64:129–35.

230. Sorin M, Segal-Maurer S, Mariano N, et al. Nosocomial transmission of Impipenem-resistant *Pseudomonas aeruginosa* following bronchoscopy associated with improper connection to the STERIS SYSTEM 1 processor. *Infect Control Hosp Epidemiol* 2001;22:409–13.

231. Kirschke D, Jones T, Craig A, et al. *Pseudomonas aeruginosa* and *Serratia marcescens* contamination associated with a manufacturing defect in bronchoscopes. *N Engl J Med* 2003;348:214–20.

232. Srinivasan A, Worlfenden LL, Song X, et al. Bronchoscope reprocessing and infection prevention and control: Bronchoscopy-specific guidelines are needed. *Chest* 2004;125:307–14.

233. Wheeler PW, Lancaster D, Kaiser AB. Bronchopulmonary cross-colonization and infection related to mycobacterial contamination of suction valves of bronchoscopes. *J Infect Dis* 1989;159:954–8.

234. Ozden I, Tekant Y, Bilge O, et al. Endoscopic and radiologic interventions as the leading causes of severe cholangitis in a tertiary referral center. *Am J Surg* 2005;189:702–6.

235. Graser T, Reiner S, Malczynski M, et al. Multidrug-resistant *Pseudomonas aeruginosa* cholangitis after endoscopic retrograde cholangiopancreatography: Failure of routine endoscope cultures to prevent an outbreak. *Infect Control Hosp Epidemiol* 2004;25.856–59.

236. Mahnke D, Chen Y, Antillon M, et al. A prospective study of complications of endoscopic retrograde cholangiopancreatography and endoscopic ultrasound in an ambulatory endoscopy center. *Clin Gastroenterol Hepatol* 2006;4:924–30.

237. Mehta A, Prakash U, Garland R, et al. American College of Chest Physicians and American Association for Bronchology consensus statement: Prevention of flexible bronchoscopy-associated infection. *Chest* 2005;128:1742–55.

238. Culver D, Gordon S, Mehta A. Infection control in the bronchoscopy suite: A review of outbreaks and guidelines for prevention. *Am J Resp Crit Care Med* 2003;167:1050–1056.

239. Martin MA, Reichelderfer M, Association for Professionals in Infection Control and Epidemiology, Inc., 1991, 1992, and 1993 APIC Guidelines Committee. APIC guideline for infection prevention and control in flexible endoscopy. *Am J Infect Control* 1994;22:19–38.

240. Rutala WA, Clontz E, Weber DJ, Hoffmann KK. Disinfection practices for endoscopes and other semicritical items. *Infect Control Hosp Epidemiol* 1991;12:282–88.

241. Favero MS. Strategies for disinfection and sterilization of endoscopes: The gap between basic principles and actual practice. *Infect Control Hosp Epidemiol* 1991;12:279–81.

242. Cheung R, Ortiz D, DiMarino A. GI endoscopic reprocessing practices in the United States. *Gastrointest Endosc* 1999;50:362–68.

243. Moses F, Lee J. Current GI endoscope disinfection and QA practices. *Dig Dis Sci* 2004;49:1791–97.

244. McCracken JE. Endoscopy revels debris, fluid, and damage in patient-ready GI endoscopes. *Infect Control and Sterilization Techn* 1995;1:32–43.

245. Kinney T, Kozarek R, Raltz S, Attia F. Contamination of single-use biopsy forceps: A prospective *in vitro* analysis. *Gastrointest Endosc* 2002;56:209–12.

246. Maloney S, Welbel S, Daves B, et al. *Mycobacterium abscessus* pseudoinfection traced to an automated endoscope washer: Utility of epidemiologic and laboratory investigation. *J Infect Dis* 1994;169:1166–69.

247. Centers for Disease Control and Prevention. Nosocomial infection and pseudoinfection from contaminated endoscopes and bronchoscopes: Wisconsin and Missouri. *MMWR* 1991;40:675–78.

248. Alvardo CJ, Stolz SM, Maki DG. Nosocomial infections from contaminated endoscopes: A flawed automated endoscope washer: An investigation using molecular epidemiology. *Am J Med* 1991;91(suppl 3B):272S–80S.

249. Fraser V, Jones M, Murray P, et al. Contamination of flexible bronchoscopes with *Mycobacterium chelonae* linked to an automated bronchoscope disinfection machine. *Am Rev Respir Dis* 1992;145:853–55.

250. Weber D, Rutula W. Lessons from outbreaks associated with bronchoscopy. *Infect Cont Hosp Epidem* 200;22:403–8.

251. Nakashima AK, McCarthy MA, Martone WJ, Anderson RL. Epidemic septic arthritis caused by *Serratia marcescens* and associated with benzalkonium chloride antiseptic. *J Clin Microbiol* 1987;25:1014–8.

252. Bayer AS, Nelson SC, Galpin JE. et al. Necrotizing pneumonia and empyema due to *Clostridium perfringens*. *Am J Med* 1975;59.851–6.

253. Dann TC. Routine skin preparation before injection: An unnecessary procedure. *Lancet* 1969;2:96–8.

254. Runyon BA, Hoefs JC, Canawati HN. Polymicrobial bacterascites: A unique entity in the spectrum of infected ascitic fluid. *Arch Intern Med* 1986;146:2173–6.

255. Mascola L, Guinan ME. Screening to reduce transmission of sexually transmitted diseases in semen used for artificial insemination. *N Engl J Med* 1986;314:1354–9.

256. Centers for Disease Control and Prevention. HIV-1 infection and artificial insemination with processed semen. *MMWR* 1990;39:249, 255–56.

257. Bujan L, Pasquier C, Labeyrie E, et al. Insemination with isolated and virologically tested spermatozoa is a safe way for human immunodeficiency type 1 virus-serodiscordant couples with an infected male partner to have a child. *Fertil Steril* 2004;82:857–62.

258. Sauer M. Sperm washing techniques address the fertility needs of HIV-seropositive men: A clinical review. *Reprod Biomed Online* 2005;10:135–40.

259. Lowenstein L, Lightman A, Draz Z, et al. Insemination from HIV-positive males. *Harefuah* 2005;144:319–21, 383.

260. Bhatacharya N, Guha S, Neogi D. First report in India of HIV transmission through artificial insemination. *Indian J Pathol Microbiol* 2003;46:106–7.

261. Hendley JO. Epidemic keratoconjunctivitis and hand washing. *N Engl J Med* 1973;289:1368–9.

262. Koo D, Bouvier B., Wesley M, et al. Epidemic keratoconjunctivitis in a university medical center ophthalmology clinic: Need for re-evaluation of the design and disinfection of instruments. *Infect Control Hosp Epidemiol* 1989;10:547–52.

263. Warren D, Nelson KE, Farrar JA, et al. A large outbreak of epidemic keratoconjunctivitis: Problems in control of nosocomial spread. *J Infect Dis* 1989;160:938–43.

Public Reporting of Healthcare-Associated Infection Rates

46

Michael Edmond

The movement to mandate that hospitals publicly disclose information on rates of healthcare associated infections (HAIs) has gained momentum rapidly. In 2003, Illinois and Pennsylvania became the first states to enact legislation that mandated reporting. Since then, eight additional states have enacted legislation, and the vast majority of remaining states are evaluating the issue in their legislative bodies.

The incidence and impact of HAIs are primarily driven by progress in medical care. The development of invasive diagnostic and therapeutic modalities, which have revolutionized medical care, bypass anatomic and physiologic barriers and markedly increase the risk of HAIs. This is compounded by the increase in severity of illness in inpatients along with an increased proportion of these patients who are immunosuppressed via their underlying diseases or transplantation, or cytotoxic therapies. Problems in the healthcare delivery system have contributed to the problem as well. The decreasing profitability of hospitals has caused some to decrease funding for infection control programs, and the nursing shortage has had an impact on the quality of care delivered. Thus, for a myriad of reasons, the incidence of HAIs remains problematic.

Over the past few years, the once hidden magnitude of HAIs has been exposed by the popular press. In response to this and a grassroots campaign by Consumers Union, the organization that publishes *Consumer Reports* [1], states are enacting legislation mandating the reporting of HAIs and disclosure of infection rates to the public.

The concept of mandatory reporting of HAIs and other healthcare quality issues converges well with the emergence of consumer-driven health care, the newest paradigm to attempt to control healthcare costs. Unlike managed care that controls costs by limiting the supply of health care, consumer-driven health care attempts to control costs by limiting the demand for health care. This is accomplished through the use of health savings accounts and the provision of incentives for healthcare consumers to seek involvement in decisions about their health and their health care [2]. Thus, the well-informed consumer is an integral feature of consumer-driven health care.

Whether public reporting of healthcare quality data is effective remains unknown. In a systematic review of the literature performed by the Centers for Disease Control and Prevention (CDC), the authors found that few rigorous studies adequately addressed the issue of effectiveness and no conclusions could be drawn [3]. They also noted that no studies have addressed public reporting of HAIs.

HEALTHCARE-ASSOCIATED INFECTIONS: THE SCOPE OF THE PROBLEM

With any public policy issue, it is important to estimate the impact of the problem for which legislation is intended to address. It is estimated that 2 million persons [4], or 5–10% of hospitalized patients in the United States, develop HAIs each year [5,6]. These infections account for an estimated 90,000 deaths and have an attributable cost of $4.5 billion [7].

From the standpoint of public policy, it is important to point out that the focus should be on HAIs that are preventable because interventions and policies will have no impact on infections that cannot be prevented—but what fraction of HAIs can be prevented? In the only recent study designed to answer this question, Harbarth et al. performed a meta-analysis of 24 multimodal intervention studies to decrease HAIs reported in the medical literature from 1990–2002. They determined that the preventable proportion of HAIs ranges from 10–70%, with the best overall estimate at 20–30%[8]. Unfortunately, when HAIs are discussed in the popular press, it is seldom pointed out that many of these infections cannot be prevented, leading to unrealistic expectations on the part of healthcare consumers.

Table 46-1 illustrates the potential impact of mandatory reporting of HAIs. Each year, 7% of Americans are hospitalized [9]. If 5–10% of inpatients develop HAIs and 10–70% of these HAIs are preventable, the annual incidence of preventable HAIs is 0.0035% to 0.245%. Applied to 2006 census data (U.S. population 298 million) [10], we can estimate that the number of persons affected by preventable HAIs in the United States ranges

from approximately 100,000 to 1.5 million yearly. Finally, by estimating the effect of a mandatory reporting and disclosure program at a range of 10–50% reduction in HAIs, we can determine that the estimated number of persons who will be affected ranges from approximately 10,000 to 700,000 annually.

ASSUMPTIONS UNDERLYING THE POLICY OF MANDATORY REPORTING AND DISCLOSURE

The mandatory reporting movement is predicated on 10 assumptions (Table 46-2), all of which must be true for a completely successful outcome. However, at the present time there is little reason to believe that all of these assumptions are true, as discussed, and for some, data are not currently available to either confirm or refute.

1. *Transparency, open exchange of information, and accountability are important societal values.* At the heart of the consumer movement is the desire to diminish information asymmetry so that consumers are able to select providers of high-quality care. Consumer advocates argue that consumers currently do not have the data necessary to make decisions regarding their health care. Thus, release of HAI rates by all hospitals should empower consumers. When hospitals attempt to block disclosure, they risk the loss of trust by their patients because of the assumption made by many that the hospital must have something to hide. Conversely, when hospitals disclose their quality data, they pursue a transparent approach that demonstrates

TABLE 46-1

POTENTIAL ANNUAL, NATIONAL IMPACT OF MANDATORY REPORTING AND DISCLOSURE OF HEALTHCARE-ASSOCIATED INFECTIONS (HAIs)

	Estimate	Number of Persons Affected
U.S. population	298,000,000	
Proportion of population hospitalized annually	7%	20,860,000
Proportion of inpatients developing an HAI	5–10%	1,043,000–2,086,000
Proportion of HAIs that are preventable	10–70%	104,300–1,460,200
Effectiveness of mandatory reporting (% reduction in preventable HAIs)	10–50%	10,430–730,100

TABLE 46-2

ASSUMPTIONS UNDERLYING MANDATORY REPORTING AND PUBLIC DISCLOSURE OF HEALTHCARE-ASSOCIATED INFECTION (HAI) RATES

1. Transparency, open exchange of information, and accountability are important societal values.
2. HAIs are preventable.
3. Valid data on HAI rates will be produced.
4. Consumers make rational decisions about choices in health care.
5. Consumers will understand and use data on HAI rates.
6. Consumers are able to choose their site of medical care and are willing to change their site of care.
7. Consumers who use HAI rate data will make decisions that will improve the quality of their care.
8. Market forces will provide incentive for hospitals to lower HAI rates.
9. Positive outcomes will outweigh negative unintended consequences.
10. Health care is a commodity.

accountability to the public and honors the public's right to know.

2. *HAIs are preventable.* While the medical literature is replete with examples of how to prevent HAIs through best practices and technological advances, the proportion of HAIs that can be prevented remains unknown. As noted, Harbarth et al. estimated the proportion of HAIs that are preventable at 10–70%. However, some newer studies demonstrating the ability to dramatically reduce nosocomial bloodstream infections [11,12] may be pushing the preventable proportion of HAIs to the higher end of that range.

3. *Valid HAI data will be produced.* Given the complexities of surveillance and the difficulties in risk adjustment, delivering valid data to consumers will not be easy. Careful attention must be directed to surveillance methodology. This will require standardization of HAI case definitions, surveillance strategies, and data sources. Moreover, the data must be risk adjusted to account for the severity of illness and the complexity of care offered at each hospital. Without risk adjustment, hospitals with the sickest patients will appear to be providing lower quality care simply on the basis of higher crude HAI rates. Standardization and risk adjustment are imperative to produce meaningful interhospital comparisons. While this can be addressed in mandatory reporting legislation, arriving at valid risk adjustment remains extraordinarily difficult.

4. *Consumers make rational decisions about choices in health care.* In other words, do consumers make decisions regarding their health care that maximize their welfare? There has been little research focused on how patients reach such decisions; however, it seems likely that the more urgent the required treatment, the less likely that the patient will proceed with a rational, well-planned investigation of the options with regard to where to seek treatment. In the setting of a major health crisis, patients rely on the recommendations of their physicians, family members, and friends, and often need to reach decisions relatively quickly. A well-publicized, illustrative anecdote is the decision by former President Bill Clinton to have coronary artery bypass graft (CABG) surgery at the hospital in the State of New York with the highest mortality rate for that procedure [13].

5. *Consumers will understand and use reported data on HAI rates.* It is important to realize that reports on healthcare quality are designed by experts and policy makers whose understanding of the healthcare system informs their decision on the specific indicators that should be used to measure quality. However, the end user of the data, the consumer, may not be able to work backward from the indicator to the bigger picture of quality [14]. Overall, consumers have a poor understanding of quality of care indicators, and this is worse in patients with low socioeconomic status. A significant proportion of the population does not have the reading proficiency to understand quality report cards [15]. Moreover, consumers do not use indicators which they do not understand [16].

Given that HAI rates are among the newest metrics to be released to consumers, it is unknown at this point how frequently these specific data are used by consumers. However, two recent reviews concluded that consumers rarely seek out this information and that it has a modest impact on medical decision making [17,18].

A national survey of 2,102 adults in 2004 by the Kaiser Family Foundation assessed how consumers access and use healthcare quality information [19]. Only 19% of those surveyed stated that they had used quality information in the last year to make a healthcare decision. When asked which sources of information on hospital quality they are very likely to use, 65% of respondents reported friends, family, and co-workers, and 65% also reported their doctor or nurse. However, fewer said they would consult a Web site (37%), order a booklet (20%), contact a state agency (18%), or use a newspaper or magazine (16%). When asked which sources of information would have "a lot of influence" in selecting a new doctor, 61% reported their physician and 52% friends or family, but only 37% would use patient surveys; 17% would contact a government agency, 14% would use insurance company data, and only 10% would visit a Web site.

When asked if they would prefer a hospital that is familiar or one that is more highly rated, 61% of respondents preferred a hospital that is familiar. Similarly, when asked if they would prefer a surgeon who has treated family or friends versus a surgeon who is more highly rated, respondents were nearly evenly split.

In a survey of 474 patients who had undergone CABG surgery in Pennsylvania, a state that publishes a report card on CABG mortality, only 12% of the patients were aware of the quality report before surgery and only 2% stated that it had impacted their choice of surgeon [20]. A recent survey of 510 Medicare patients who underwent surgery found that only 11% looked for information to compare hospitals and 48% stated they would not use hospital performance data if they required surgery in the future [21]. Last, a survey of 1,500 persons in New York state found that 18.5% used available data on healthcare quality in medical decision making [22].

Although the public's desire to access healthcare quality data may change as consumers become more educated, more data become available, and more individuals have access to and are more comfortable with online information sources, at the present time it appears that a minority of individuals are interested in these data and prefer the recommendations of their healthcare providers, family, and friends.

6. *Consumers are able to choose their site of care and are willing to change their site of care.* Many patients are unable to choose their site of care due to their health insurance plan. Twenty-four percent of Americans are enrolled in health maintenance organizations (HMOs), and 95% of covered workers are enrolled in a managed care plan (HMO, preferred provider organization, or point-of-service plan) [23].

Thus, a significant proportion of the population has little choice in healthcare venue or may have some choice that comes with financial penalty.

A recent analysis of New York CABG quality data from 1989–2002 showed that public reporting of hospital performance had no impact on changes in market share for hospitals [24]. However, it could be argued that even if patients are unwilling to use healthcare quality reports or change their site of care, third-party payers will use the data to direct their members to hospitals that demonstrate higher quality. There is also little evidence to date, however, to support that argument [24–27]. It also could be argued that if public reporting is effective in improving the overall quality of care in a given state, even patients who are unwilling to change their site of care may experience a benefit [28].

7. *Consumers who use data reported on HAIs will make decisions that will improve their care.* This assumption depends on two other assumptions: that comparative data on hospital HAI rates are valid and that healthcare consumers can and will change their site of care in response to the reported data.

8. *Market forces will provide incentive for hospitals to improve quality.* Public reporting can theoretically improve quality in four ways: (1) remediation (hospitals make a concerted effort to improve quality), (2) restriction (licensing and accreditation organizations use the data to restrict provision of care by poor performers), (3) removal (poor performers discontinue providing services), and (4) stimulation of competition between providers on the basis of improving quality to improve market share.

Most of the data that support these assumptions come from observational studies. Some have cited the 21% reduction in CABG mortality in New York following public reporting of mortality rates as evidence of the positive effect of market forces [29] However, others believe that the decline in mortality was due to other factors, such as the avoidance of surgery on high-risk patients. Nonetheless, some low-volume surgeons with high mortality rates stopped performing CABGs after mortality rates were published [30]. One experimental study in Wisconsin compared the number of quality improvement activities in hospitals that had publicly reported quality data to those who received private reports on their performance without public reporting to those who had neither private nor public reporting. Hospitals with publicly reported quality data performed significantly more quality improvement activities than did the other two groups of hospitals [31]. The difference was even greater when the subset of hospitals that had received poor quality ratings were compared.

9. *Positive outcomes will outweigh negative unintended consequences.* The impacts of public reporting of HAIs are myriad. If the data are collected via nonstandardized methodologies, comparing the resulting HAI rates from hospitals will not be meaningful. This may lead consumers to make choices that are not congruent with their wishes. Even if data were collected appropriately, without adequate risk adjustment, those hospitals that care for the sickest patients will appear to have higher HAI rates. In addition, Marshall et al. have described seven other unintended consequences of public reporting on the quality of medical care [32]:

- *Tunnel vision.* This occurs when quality improvement efforts are concentrated on areas being measured to the detriment of other important areas. For example, a hospital might focus efforts on the area of bloodstream infection (BSI) because this infection rate is publicly reported, while ignoring rising rates of ventilator-associated pneumonias that are not required to be publicly reported.

- *Suboptimization.* This is defined as pursuing narrow organizational objectives at the expense of strategic coordination. In a hospital placing great emphasis on decreasing nosocomial BSIs, multiple groups (e.g., infection control, performance improvement, unit nurses) may each develop competing interventions to reduce infections that duplicate work and data collection. This type of problem could be avoided by developing a multidisciplinary team that involves members of all the stakeholder groups.

- *Myopia.* Hospitals may concentrate on short-term issues and lose sight of the long-term outcomes. This unintended consequence is particularly worrisome. Given the high stakes associated with mandatory disclosure of HAI rates, hospitals with high rates should be motivated to improve infection control activities, an obvious desirable outcome. However, some hospitals, especially those with particularly high rates, may seek solutions that are not appropriate in a desperate attempt to rapidly lower HAI rates. Of greatest concern is that hospitals will resort to antimicrobial prophylaxis for patients with commonly used medical devices (urinary catheters, central venous catheters, and mechanical ventilators). This will almost surely yield a short-term result in lower HAI rates, but the long-term consequences of rapidly accelerating antimicrobial resistance associated with such practices could be very problematic.

- *Convergence.* Convergence is defined as placing more emphasis on being exposed as an outlier than on efforts to perform in an outstanding fashion. Hospitals could aim for average or median HAI rates instead of pushing to drive their rates to the absolute minimum, which should be the goal.

- *Ossification.* This occurs when organizations avoid experimentation with new approaches out of fear of poor performance. This may be particularly problematic in academic medical centers where innovative approaches to decrease HAIs may be discouraged due to concerns that HAIs may increase.

- *Gaming.* Hospitals game the system when they alter behavior to gain strategic advantage. For example, quality indicators that are measured via administrative data can be affected by coached changes in the coding of diagnoses because risk adjustment depends on the coding of co-morbid conditions.

- *Misrepresentation.* Unfortunately, with public reporting comes an inherent incentive for hospitals to structure their surveillance activities to produce a system with suboptimal sensitivity. In the absence of mandatory reporting, it is in the best interest of hospitals to maximally detect HAIs for quality improvement purposes and to decrease unreimbursed costs of care associated with infections. However, in the setting of mandatory reporting and disclosure, it may be overall more economically advantageous for hospitals to detect fewer HAIs because disclosure of high infection rates may lead patients to seek care elsewhere. It is important to note that in the hypothetical case of two hospitals that have identical HAI rates, the hospital with the best surveillance system will appear to have a higher infection rate, a phenomenon known as surveillance bias.

In addition, it is important to consider the opportunity cost of public reporting. Given that public reporting is an unfunded mandate in almost all states that have enacted laws and that hospital budgets are a zero-sum game, diversion of resources from other programs and problems is of great concern.

Some striking examples of unintended consequences have been associated with public reporting of health quality data. A recent large, multicenter study compared patients in Michigan (where there is no public reporting for percutaneous coronary intervention [PCI] outcomes) to those in New York (where outcome reporting is mandated) [33]. The Michigan patients had a higher incidence of co-morbidities, a higher incidence of high-risk indications for PCI, and an observed mortality rate that was nearly 2-fold higher. When multivariate analysis was used to control for co-morbidities, there was no significant difference in mortality rates between the two states. The authors of this study postulated that the difference in mortality rates may have been due to physicians in New York avoiding PCI on high-risk patients due to fear of increasing their publicly reported mortality rates.

A separate study surveyed all interventional cardiologists in New York, and 65% responded [34]. Of those responding, 79% disclosed that the public reporting of mortality statistics influenced their decision on whether to perform PCI on individual patients, and 83% believed that some patients may not receive PCI because of public reporting of mortality rates. Two surveys of cardiothoracic surgeons in states reporting mortality rates following CABG revealed similar findings. In a survey of Pennsylvania surgeons, 63% reported they were less willing to operate on severely ill patients following public reporting [35]. When surgeons in New York were surveyed, 62% reported refusing to operate on high-risk patients due to public reporting of mortality rates [36].

Another phenomenon noted after public reporting started was that CABGs were performed on 19% fewer African Americans and Hispanics in New York [37]. These racial disparities lasted for 9 years. It is thought that the surgeons assumed that racial minorities were at higher risk for poor outcomes and thus avoided performing surgery on them.

In summary, with regard to CABG and PCI, several unintended consequences emerged. These included denial of aggressive therapy to high-risk patients, punishing physicians willing to treat high-risk patients, and racial profiling. As Hughes and Mackay note, the real question regarding the impact of public reporting is whether it results in better delivery of health care or in better risk avoidance via shifting of high-risk patients to other practitioners or hospitals [38].

10. *Health care is a commodity.* In the United States, unlike many other countries, health care is treated as a commodity rather than as a basic human right. The unfortunate downside of this is that a large segment of the U.S. population is unable to purchase it health care because they lack the resources. Public reporting of quality indicators stems from and reinforces the commodity concept.

Minority and low-income persons are overrepresented among those without health insurance. Some unique issues with regard to public reporting apply to these groups. Metrics addressing quality of health care typically emphasize diseases, procedures, and health status rather than more relevant issues to the underserved (e.g., proximity of services, availability of appointments, financial barriers, and navigability of bureaucracy) [39]. These patients are least likely to be able to choose their healthcare venue. In addition, vulnerable populations may be affected by unintended consequences. These include the avoidance of minority and low-income patients because they may decrease quality scores, the opportunity costs that affect these patients and increase their marginalization, and damage to institutions that care for a disproportionate number of vulnerable patients.

An inherent flaw in the U.S. healthcare system is that some nonemergency services for the uninsured are a discretionary component of hospitals' budgets at a time when fiscal stress is increasing in hospitals due to decreasing revenues and unfunded mandated programs. In 2004, one-third of U.S. hospitals posted an operating budget deficit [40]. Because ultimately a hospital's finances are a zero-sum game, we must examine the opportunity cost of mandatory reporting and disclosure. This raises important questions: From where will these resources be diverted? How can we ensure that an improvement in healthcare for those able to afford it does not result in denying it to those who cannot?

OPTIONS FOR REPORTING

The ideal mandatory reporting and disclosure program is characterized by four important characteristics:

1. The accuracy of data collection is maximized.
2. The methodology for data collection and analysis is standardized in all hospitals to be compared.
3. The costs to hospitals and state agencies are minimized.

4. The end product delivered is valid, easy to access, useful to consumers, and fair to hospitals.

To meet surveillance needs of individual hospitals, how HAI data are collected is not especially important provided that it is consistent. However, interhospital comparisons are impossible when hospitals use different methodologies [41]. Thus, requiring hospitals to report their data without a mandated methodology would do little to inform consumers and likely mislead them. In addition, there must be mechanisms to adjust the rates for risk factors and severity of illness; otherwise, hospitals that care for the sickest patients will appear to be poor performers when compared to hospitals that offer lower levels of care.

At the present time, there is no standard methodology used by U.S. hospitals to define or detect HAIs. Each hospital can choose which type of infection (e.g., urinary tract infection [UTI], BSI, pneumonia, surgical site infection [SSI]) to track, how to define the infection, and the methods to use to determine which patients have the infection.

The CDC's National Healthcare Safety Network (NHSN, formerly the National Nosocomial Infections Surveillance [NNIS] system) offers an excellent approach with standardized infection definitions utilizing multiple sources of data that are applied in a specified fashion [42]. However, only 5% of U.S. hospitals participate in the surveillance system [43], and the remaining 95% are free to track HAIs in any manner they choose.

Despite being the oldest, most highly developed, and the only U.S. national HAI surveillance system, an important problem with NHSN is that the sensitivity for detection of HAIs is suboptimal. For the major infections, the sensitivity is 59% for catheter-associated UTI, 67% for SSIs, 68% for nosocomial pneumonia, and 85% for nosocomial BSIs [44]. Moreover, with the added pressure of public disclosure, underreporting of HAIs may become even more problematic.

As states evaluate mandatory reporting legislation, several questions must be addressed: Which indicators will be included? What data sources will be used? What populations will be surveyed? How will the data be risk adjusted? How will the results be validated?

INDICATORS

To date, consumer advocates have focused on public reporting of outcome indicators. Although SSIs, ventilator-associated pneumonia (VAP), and central line-associated BSIs are relatively infrequent events, their impact in terms of morbidity, mortality, and cost are great. While nosocomial UTIs are associated with low mortality risk and are relatively inexpensive, they occur at higher frequency than the other infections. Validated definitions for each of these infections have been developed by CDC.

Because surveillance for BSIs is triggered by a positive blood culture and the case definition is relatively simple to apply, surveillance for these infections is straightforward. On the other hand, case definitions for VAP are complicated. The major difficulty with surgical site infection surveillance relates to case ascertainment. Because at least 50% of these infections occur after hospital discharge, capturing all SSIs is difficult, particularly in hospitals that do not have a centralized medical record or an electronic medical record. Thus, the validity of SSI rates may be questionable. Acknowledging the pitfalls associated with SSI surveillance, CDC's Healthcare Infection Control Practices Advisory Committee (HICPAC) recommends central line-related BSIs and SSIs as the best outcome indicators for public reporting [45].

It is important to note that as the interest in avoidance of HAIs has increased, in part due to an increased level of interest by healthcare consumers, analysis of surveillance data is becoming more intense. In an effort to prevent infections, each case identified via surveillance may undergo scrutiny by clinicians who may question the diagnosis from a clinical perspective. However, surveillance definitions are typically not developed for use by clinicians in making decisions regarding therapy. This was demonstrated in a study of VAP in trauma patients in which Miller et al. found that 31% of patients without pneumonia as clinically defined by bronchoalveolar lavage criteria were classified as having pneumonia using CDC definitions [46].

More recently, process indicators have gained attention. In general, process measures are practices proven to decrease HAI incidence. Thus, they provide direct measures of performance that have been linked to outcomes. Berenholtz et al. demonstrated spectacular decreases in catheter-related BSIs in a surgical ICU by focusing on the process of central venous catheter insertion. Other examples include head-of-bed elevation to prevent nosocomial pneumonia, avoidance of vascular catheters in the femoral area to prevent BSI, hand hygiene, and influenza vaccination of healthcare workers. As compared to outcome measures, process indicators are easier to define and measure and do not require risk adjustment. Monitoring these indicators can be accomplished by personnel with less training than outcome measures, which can require complex definitions and the review of multiple data sources. Feedback of process indicators has been shown to more forcefully drive compliance with best practices than does feedback of outcomes indicators [47]. The major disadvantage of process indicators is that they are less meaningful to consumers. The CDC's HICPAC recommends that states include both outcomes and process measures in their mandatory reporting programs.

SOURCES OF DATA

Clinical data from multiple sources (e.g., physician notes, laboratory data, radiology reports) collected by trained infection control practitioners in real time via active surveillance remains the gold standard data source. Through

NNIS, there is more than three decades of U.S. experience with this methodology. Unfortunately, such data acquisition is labor intensive and costly. For this reason, most hospitals have limited surveillance for HAIs to their intensive care units and to selected surgical procedures.

Use of administrative claims data as a surrogate for clinical data collected via concurrent surveillance has been advocated by some and forms the basis for public reporting in Pennsylvania. The primary advantage of identifying HAIs via these data are low cost and high efficiency because the data already exist for every hospital discharge, and electronic reports searching for ICD-9 codes of interest can be generated rapidly. However, the use of coding data, which were designed for billing, not clinical purposes, is very problematic. Use of administrative data for HAI detection shifts case ascertainment from trained infection control practitioners (ICPs) to medical records abstractors with little medical knowledge. Thus, surveillance using these data is highly prone to misclassification bias.

Another problem is that this coding does not distinguish between conditions present on admission and those that develop after admission, which makes coding for complications of care, including HAIs, problematic. Moreover, the codes for complications are vaguely defined, often depend on physician documentation, and require interpretation by the coder, all of which produce variability in rates of complications among hospitals [48]. In a review of nearly 500 inpatient records from two different states, McCarthy et al. found that for surgical patients, 31% of the coded complications had no objective clinical evidence in the medical record to support the diagnosis; for medical patients, 44% of the complications lacked evidence [49]. An Italian study evaluated the use of ICD-9 codes for SSI surveillance and found that depending on the codes used, sensitivity for detection of infection ranged from 10–21% [50].

A recent study from a children's hospital in Pennsylvania compared active surveillance by ICPs to identification of HAIs via administrative data [51]. Active surveillance by ICPs had a sensitivity of 76%, positive predictive value of 100%, and a negative predictive value of 99%, whereas administrative data had a sensitivity of 61%, positive predictive value of 20%, and a negative predictive value of 99%. When cases were identified by administrative data only, further review revealed that 90% were misclassified because the infection originated before hospital admission, no infection was present, or no device predisposing the patient to infection had been in situ. One potential improvement in the use of ICD-9 codes would be to note whether each condition coded was present at admission ("date stamping") [52], which is currently required only in California and New York [53].

LEGISLATIVE ACTIVITY

Fourteen states have now enacted laws regarding mandatory reporting of HAIs (Table 46-3) with many differences in data sources, metrics to be reported, and mechanisms for reporting and release to the public. Four additional states (Alaska, Indiana, Texas, and Utah) have passed proposals to study the issue and recommend legislative actions. Twenty-one other states considered bills in their 2006 legislative sessions.

Many states evaluating legislation have adopted the Consumer's Union Model Hospital Infections Disclosure Act. This requires acute care hospitals to report quarterly to their state health departments infection rates for SSIs, VAP, nosocomial central line-related BSI, nosocomial UTIs, and other nosocomial infections at the discretion of the state's health department. It is recommended that patient race, ethnicity, and primary language be reported to assess racial and language disparities. The act requires state health departments to create an advisory committee with representatives from public and private hospitals, direct care nurses, physicians, epidemiologists with HAI expertise, academic researchers, consumer organizations, health insurers, health maintenance organizations, and purchasers of health insurance (e.g., employers). In addition, the act requires the state health department and advisory committee to validate the HAI rates and publish an annual report with comparative risk-adjusted HAI rates available to the public via Web site.

The advantages of the Consumers Union bill are that it focuses on the major HAIs and mandates risk adjustment and validation. The disadvantages are that it requires hospital-wide surveillance, which is resource intensive, and mandates the formation of a large advisory committee, which dilutes the expertise of healthcare epidemiologists and ICPs.

To achieve the goals of the Model Hospital Infections Disclosure Act as proposed by Consumers Union, most hospitals would need to significantly increase the resources provided to their infection control programs. A recent survey of acute care hospitals in Virginia revealed that 64% of hospitals had only one ICP full-time equivalent (FTE) and at 86% of hospitals, the ICPs had other major responsibilities [54]. Moreover, had Virginia mandated reporting of all HAIs, an estimated 160 ICPs would have been required statewide at an estimated cost of $11.5 million yearly.

Virginia, Colorado, and Tennessee chose to use an existing surveillance network, NHSN, to avoid the costs of establishing a surveillance system de novo and to be able to benchmark its hospitals against other hospitals nationally. Hospitals will submit raw HAI data to CDC and then report their risk-adjusted infection rates to the state department of health. Colorado's law also requires hospitals to submit their infection data to NHSN. Most of the states have developed an advisory committee to assist in the analysis of data and the methodology for public disclosure and most will post comparative data on HAI rates on a public Web site. Few of the states have made provisions for validation of the data or funding to offset costs. Some states have built in a delay (up to three years)

TABLE 46-3
STATE LAWS ENACTED REGARDING REPORTING OF NOSOCOMIAL INFECTIONS

State	Year	Data Source/Venues Targeted	Metrics Reported	Reporting & Release Mechanisms
Illinois	2003	Administrative claims and clinical data; applies to hospitals and ambulatory surgery centers	Class I SSI, VAP, CL-BSI occurring during hospitalization	Mandatory quarterly reports to the Department of Public Health which then submits to the General Assembly a summary report to be published on its Web site.
Pennsylvania	2003	Administrative claims data; applies to hospitals	All HAI	Data are reported to the PA Health Care Cost Containment Council, which releases data to the public.
Florida	2004	Data source not specified, although current report available online utilizes administrative claims data; applies to health care facilities	Not specified	A Web site maintained by the Agency for Health Care Administration (**www.FloridaCompareCare.gov**) reports facility rates for infections due to medical care and postoperative sepsis, along with process indicators from the Surgical Infection Prevention Project.
Missouri	2004	Data source not specified; applies to hospitals and ambulatory surgery centers	Class I SSI, VAP, CL-BSI	Data collection, analysis and reporting rules to be recommended by an advisory committee. Department of Health to publish a quarterly report on its Web site.
Nevada	2005	Data source not specified; applies to medical facilities	SSI, VAP, CL-BSI, nosocomial UTI	Hospitals report to the Health Division of the Department of Human Resources. No provision for public disclosure.
New York	2005	Clinical data; applies to general hospitals	CL-BSI and SSI occurring in critical care units	Hospitals are required to report no more frequently than every 6 months; the commissioner of health shall establish a state wide database of all reported hospital-acquired infection information organized so that consumers, hospitals, healthcare professionals, purchasers, and payers may compare hospitals to each other, to regional and statewide averages and, when available, to national data.
Virginia	2005	Clinical data using CDC definitions for nosocomial infections; applies to acute care hospitals	Infections and target populations to be determined by the State Board of Health	Acute care hospitals required to report selected indicators to the National Healthcare Safety Network and forward adjusted infection rates to the State Health Department; data may be released to the public on request.
Colorado	2006	Applies to hospitals, ambulatory surgery centers, dialysis centers	Cardiac SSI, orthopedic SSI, CL-BSI; physicians are required to report cardiac and orthopedic SSIs identified postdischarge	Acute care hospitals required to report selected indicators to the National Healthcare Safety Network. The Department of Public Health will include risk-adjusted infection rates in an annual report to be distributed widely, published on its Web site and released to the public on request.
Connecticut	2006	Data sources to be determined by an advisory committee; applies to hospitals	Metrics to be determined by an advisory committee	Annual report on infection rates produced by the Department of Public Health will be posted on the department's Web site.
Maryland	2006	Data sources to be determined by the Maryland Health Care Commission; applies to hospitals and ambulatory surgery centers	Metrics to be determined by the Maryland Health Care Commission	Reporting and release mechanisms to be determined by the Maryland Health Care Commission.

TABLE 46-3
(CONTINUED)

State	Year	Data Source/Venues Targeted	Metrics Reported	Reporting & Release Mechanisms
New Hampshire	2006	Data source not specified; applies to hospitals	CL-BSI, VAP, SSI, adherence rates of central line insertion practices, surgical antimicrobial prophylaxis, coverage rates of influenza vaccination for health care personnel and patients	Hospitals report to the State Department of Health and Human Resources no more frequently than quarterly. The department's Web site will report infection rates both exclusive and inclusive of adjustments for potential differences in risk factors for each reporting hospital; an analysis of trends in the prevention and control of infection rates in hospitals across the state; regional and, if available, national comparisons for the purpose of comparing individual hospital performance, and a narrative describing lessons for safety and quality improvement.
South Carolina	2006	Clinical data; applies to hospitals	SSI, VAP, CL-BSI, other infections decided by the Department of Health and Environmental Control in consultation with an advisory committee	Hospitals submit reports at least every 6 months to the Department of Health and Environmental Control, which then publishes an annual report on its Web site.
Tennessee	2006	Clinical data using CDC definitions for HAIs; applies to hospitals with an average daily census ≥25 inpatients and outpatient facilities performing on average ≥25 procedures daily	CL-BSI in ICUs, excluding burn units and level 1 trauma units; SSI for CABG	Acute care hospitals required to report selected indicators to the National Healthcare Safety Network. Hospital-specific CL-BSI rates to be reported on the Department of Health's Web site for hospitals with >30 central line insertions per year, updated every 6 months with the most recent 4 quarters of data. For CABG SSI, only an aggregate statewide rate will be released.
Vermont	2006	Data source not specified; applies to hospitals	Metrics that are "valid, reliable, and useful, including comparisons to appropriate industry benchmarks" to be determined by the health commissioner in consultation with representatives of specified groups	Data on HAI rates to be included along with other quality metrics in hospital community reports.

SSI, surgical site infections; VAP, ventilator-associated pneumonia; CL-BSI, central line associated bloodstream infection; HAI, healthcare-associated infections.

before data submission is required to allow hospitals to gain experience with the surveillance methodology.

Nevada's law is unique in that it mandates reporting of HAIs, but the data are not disclosed to the public. While this approach may be effective in improving the quality of care, it does not meet the needs of the consumer in acquiring the data needed to choose their site of care. Also, without public disclosure, hospitals may not be viewed as being held accountable to the public.

There has been some interest in the establishment of federal legislation on mandatory reporting and disclosure to establish a single national standard rather than have states develop varying standards. The National Quality Forum is currently in the process of developing national standards for reporting of HAIs, and a Congressional hearing explored the issue recently.

CONCLUSION

In the end, the benefit to the healthcare consumer due to the transparency provided by mandatory reporting and disclosure of HAIs should trump the risk to hospitals' reputations and finances, and states are increasingly enacting laws to ensure this. This is an excellent incentive for hospitals to commit resources to prevent HAIs. However, standardization of methodology for detecting infections, accurate risk adjustment, and validation of reported infection rates is paramount in providing consumers with reliable data. Last, the impact of such legislation, including intended and unintended consequences, should be evaluated after implementation.

REFERENCES

1. Consumers Union. Stop Hospital Infections.org (www .consumersunion.org/campaigns/stophospitalinfections/about .html) accessed 10 april 2006.
2. Bachman RF. Consumer-driven health care: the future is now. *Benefits Q* 2004;20:15–22.
3. McKibben L, Fowler G, Horan T, Brennan PJ. Ensuring rational public reporting systems for health care-associated infections: systematic literature review and evaluation recommendations. *Am J Infect Control* 2006;34:142–149.
4. Center for Disease Control and Prevention. Public health focus: surveillance, prevention and control of nosocomial infections. *MMWR Morb Mortal Wkly Rep* 1992;41:783–787.
5. Haley RW, Culver DH, White JW, et al. The nationwide nosocomial infection rate: a new need for vital statistics. *Am J Epidemiol* 1985;121:159–167.
6. Ducel G, Fabry J, Nicolle L, eds. *Prevention of hospital-acquired infections.* 2nd ed. Geneva: World Health Organization, 2002. (www.who.int/csr/resources/publications/drugresist/en /whocdscsreph200212.pdf) accessed 10 April 2006.
7. Centers for Disease Control and Prevention. Healthcare-associated infections. (www.cdc.gov/ncidod/dhqp/healthDis.html) accessed 10 April 2006.
8. Harbarth S, Sax H, Gastmeier P. The preventable proportion of nosocomial infections: an overview of published reports. *J Hosp Infect* 2003;54:258–266.
9. Roberts M. Hospital admission rates—1987 and 1998 (http: //www.meps.ahrq.gov/mepsweb/data_files/publications/st9/ stat09.pdf#xml=http://207.188.212.220/cgi-bin/texis/webinator/ search/pdfhi.txt?query=hospital+admission+rates&pr= MEPSFULLSITE&prox=page&rorder=500&rprox=500&rdfreq= 500&rwfreq=500&sufs=0&order=r&cg=&id= 4663bc6ebb) accessed 10 April 2006.
10. U.S. Census Bureau. U.S. and world population clocks (www. census.gov/main/www/popclock.html) accessed 10 April 2006.
11. Berenholtz SM, Pronovost PJ, Lipsett PA, et al. Eliminating catheter-related bloodstream infections in the intensive care unit. *Crit Care Med* 2004;32:2014–2020.
12. Centers for Disease Control and Prevention. Reduction in central line–associated bloodstream infections among patients in intensive care units—Pennsylvania, April 2001–March 2005. *MMWR Morb Mortal Wkly Rep* 2005; 54:1013–1016.
13. Altman LK. Clinton surgery puts attention on death rate. *New York Times* 6 September 2004;6:Sec A:1.
14. Jewett JJ, Hibbard JH. Comprehension of quality care indicators: differences among privately insured, publicly insured, and uninsured. *Health Care Financ Rev* 1996;18:75–94.
15. Hochhauser M. Can consumers understand managed care report cards? *Manag Care Interface* 1998;11:91–95.
16. Hibbard JH, Jewett JJ. Will quality reports cards help consumers? *Health Aff* 1997;16:218–228.
17. Schauffler HH, Mordavsky JK. Consumer reports in health care: do they make a difference? *Ann Rev Pub Health* 2001;22:69–89.
18. Marshall MN, Shekelle PG, Leatherman S, Brook RH. The public release of performance data: what do we expect to gain? a review of the evidence. *JAMA* 2000;283:1866–1874.
19. The Kaiser Family Foundation, Agency for Healthcare Research and Quality, Harvard School of Public Health. National survey on consumers' experiences with patient safety and quality information (www.kff.org/kaiserpolls/upload/National-Survey -on-Consumers-Experiences-With-Patient-Safety-and-Quality -Information-Survey-Summary-and-Chartpack.pdf accessed 9 April 2006.
20. Schneider EC, Epstein AM. Influence of cardiac-surgery performance reports on referral practices and access to care: a survey of cardiovascular specialists. *N Engl J Med* 1996;335: 251–256.
21. Schwartz LM, Woloshin S, Birkmeyer JD. How do elderly patients decide where to go for major surgery? telephone interview survey. *BMJ* 2005;331:821.
22. Boscarino JA, Adams RE. Public perceptions of quality care and provider profiling in New York: implications for improving quality care and public health. *J Public Health Management Practice* 2004;10:241–250.
23. Kaiser Family Foundation. Trends and indicators in the changing health care marketplace (www.kff.org/insurance/7031/print -sec2.cfm) accessed 9 april 2006. [online] 2005 [cited 2006 April 9]. Available from: URL:
24. Jha AK, Epstein AM. The predictive accuracy of the New York state coronary artery bypass surgery report-card system. *Health Affairs* 2006;25:844–855.
25. Mukamel DB, Mushlin AI, Weimer D, et al. Do quality report cards play a role in HMOs' contracting practices? evidence from New York state. *Health Serv Res* 2000;35:319–332.
26. Mukamel DB, Weimer DL, Zwanziger J, Mushlin AI. Quality of cardiac surgeons and managed care contracting practices. *Health Serv Res* 2002;37:1129–1144.
27. Erickson LC, Torchiana DF, Schnieder EC, et al. The relationship between managed care insurance and use of lower-mortality hospitals for CABG surgery. *JAMA* 2000;283:1976–1982.
28. Werner RM, Asch DA. The unintended consequences of publicly reporting quality information. *JAMA* 2005;293:1239–1244.
29. Hannan EL, Kilburn H Jr, Racz M, et al. Improving the outcomes of coronary artery bypass surgery in New York State. *JAMA* 1994;271:761–766.
30. Chassin MR, Hannan EL, DeBuono BA. Benefits and hazards of reporting medical outcomes publicly. *N Engl J Med* 1996;334:394–398.
31. Hibbard JH, Stockard J, Tusler M. Does publicizing hospital performance stimulate quality improvement efforts? *Health Affairs* 2004;22:84–94.
32. Marshall MN, Romano PS, Davies HTO. How do we maximize the impact of the public reporting of quality of care? *Int J Qual Health Care* 2004;16(suppl 1):i57–i63.
33. Moscucci M, Eagle KA, Share D, et al. Public reporting and case selection for percutaneous coronary interventions: an analysis from two large multicenter percutaneous coronary intervention databases. *J Am Coll Cardiol* 2005;45:1759–1765.
34. Narins CR, Dozier AM, Ling FS, Zareba W. The influence of public reporting of outcome data on medical decision making by physicians. *Arch Intern Med* 2005;165:83–87.
35. Schneider EC, Epstein AM. Influence of cardiac-surgery performance reports on referral practices and access to care: a survey of cardiovascular specialists. *N Engl J Med* 1996;335: 251–256.
36. Burack JH, Impellizzeri P, Homel P, Cunningham JN Jr. Public reporting of surgical mortality: a survey of New York State cardiothoracic surgeons *Ann Thorac Surg.* 1999;68:1195–1200.
37. Werner RM, Asch DA, Polsky D. Racial profiling: the unintended consequences of coronary artery bypass graft report cards. *Circulation* 2005;111:1257–1263.
38. Hughes CF, Mackay P. Sea change: public reporting and the safety and quality of the Australian health care system. *Med J Aust* 2006;184(10 suppl):S44–S47.
39. Davies HTO, Washington AE, Bindman AB. Health care report cards: implications for vulnerable patient groups and the organizations providing them care. *J Health Polit Policy Law* 2002;27:379–399.
40. American Hospital Association. The state of America's hospitals—taking the pulse (http://www.aha.org/aha/resource-and-trends/ trendwatch/2007chartbook.html) accessed 8 June 2006.
41. Braun BI, Kritchevsky SB, Kusek L, et al. Comparing bloodstream infection rates: the effect of indicator specifications in the evaluation of processes and indicators in infection control (EPIC) study. *Infect Control Hosp Epidemiol* 2006;27:14–22.

42. Cardo DM, Brennan PJ, Peaden D Jr, Khabbaz R. Mandatory reporting of hospital-acquired infections: steps for success. *J Law Med Ethics* 2005;33(4 suppl):86–88.

43. Gaynes R, Richards C, Edwards J, et al. Feeding back surveillance data to prevent hospital-acquired infections. *Emerg Infect Dis* 2001; 7:295–298.

44. Emori TG, Edwards JR, Culver DH, et al. Accuracy of reporting nosocomial infections in intensive-care-unit patients to the National Nosocomial Infections Surveillance System: a pilot study. *Infect Control Hosp Epidemiol* 1998;19:308–316.

45. McKibben L, Horan T, Tokars JI, et al. Guidance on public reporting of healthcare-associated infections: recommendations of the Healthcare Infection Control Practices Advisory Committee. *Am J Infect Control* 2005;33:217–226.

46. Miller PR, Johnson JC III, Karchmer T, et al. National Nosocomial Infection Surveillance System: from benchmark to bedside in trauma patients. *J Trauma* 2006;60:98–103.

47. Berhe M, Edmond MB, Bearman G. Measurement and feedback of infection control process measures in the intensive care unit: impact on compliance. *Am J Infect Control* 2006;34: 537–539.

48. Romano PS, Chan BK, Schembri ME, Rainwater JA. Can administrative data be used to compare postoperative complication rates across hospitals? *Med Care* 2002;40:856–867.

49. McCarthy EP, Iezzoni LI, Davis RB, et al. Does clinical evidence support ICD-9-CM diagnosis coding of complications? *Med Care* 2000;38:868–876.

50. Moro ML, Morsillo F. Can hospital discharge diagnoses be used for surveillance of surgical-site infections? *J Hosp Infect* 2004;56:239–241.

51. Sherman ER, Heydon KH, St. Johns KH, et al. Administrative data fail to accurately identify cases of healthcare-associated infection. *Infect Control Hosp Epidemiol* 2006;27:322–337.

52. Naessens JM, Huschka TR. Distinguishing hospital complications of care from pre-existing conditions. *Int J Qual Health Care* 2004;16(suppl 1):i27–i35.

53. Glance LG, Dick AW, Osler TM, Mukamel DB. Does date stamping ICD-9-CM codes increase the value of clinical information in administrative data? *Health Serv Res* 2006;41:231–251.

54. Edmond MB, White-Russell MB, Ober J, et al. A statewide survey of nosocomial infection surveillance in acute care hospitals. *Am J Infect Control* 2005;33:480–482.

Patient Safety

47

Moi Lin Ling

INTRODUCTION

With the release of the Institute of Medicine's (IOM) report on patient safety, *To Err Is Human*, several healthcare organizations have responded with the development of patient safety programs. Patient safety refers to the freedom from injury or illness resulting from processes in healthcare [1]. Many patient care processes are interlinked through varied systems involving multiple handoffs. The possibility of medical errors increases with the level of complexity of care. This is not surprising because medicine remains very much an inexact, hands-on endeavor. Patients are at greater risk than nonpatients, and medical interventions are by their nature high-risk procedures with a rather narrow margin for error.

An error is defined as an unintended act, either by omission or commission, or an act that does not achieve its intended outcome [1]. This may either be a near miss or an incident in which the error results in an adverse outcome for the patient. Healthcare organizations are highly complex systems with thousands of interlinked processes that can go wrong. A healthcare-associated infection (HAI) is one of the possible outcomes of processes that did not turn out right. Other incidents considered as healthcare errors include incorrect diagnosis, inappropriate use of tests or treatments, wrong site surgery, medication errors, transfusion mistakes, patient falls, decubitus ulcers, phlebitis associated with intravenous lines, preventable suicides, and so on.

The IOM report estimated that healthcare errors occur in about 3–4% patients with approximately 2 million HAIs occurring annually in United States with an average of each intensive care unit (ICU) patient experiencing two errors a day [1]. HAIs represent a major cause of death and disability worldwide [2]. The World Health Organization (WHO) estimates that more than 1.4 million people worldwide suffer from HAIs at any one time. It also is estimated that 2 million HAIs occur in the United States annually with

about 80,000 deaths; in England, an estimated 5,000 HAI deaths occur annually. The economic burden is heavy at an estimated annual cost of US\$ 4,500–5,700 million a year in the United States and £1,000 million annually to the National Health Service in the United Kingdom [2].

The Swiss cheese model of system accidents proposed by James Reason [3] gives a good explanation as to how system issues play a key role in patient safety. Defenses, barriers, and safeguards have many holes just like slices of Swiss cheese. Although these systems are to prevent errors, ironically, errors will lead to bad outcomes if the holes are lined up in a manner to allow an adverse event to pass through unstopped. It is not difficult to appreciate this; we are all too familiar with the many system factors that contribute to an HAI. A key process in prevention of surgical site infection (SSI) is the timely delivery of appropriate antimicrobials to a patient at anesthesia induction [4]. This process has many interlinked steps to contribute to a successful timely delivery of SSI prophylaxis: (1) the development of evidence-based guidelines on prophylaxis regime, (2) the collaboration of the anesthesiologist with the surgeon in adhering to the guidelines, (3) the availability of the appropriate antimicrobial at time of need, and (4) the act of administering it by the anesthesiologist at time of induction. A break in any part of this process will lead to noncompliance with the guidelines and then to possible SSI development.

Errors occur because of basic flaws in the systems of a healthcare organization. Hence, in contrast to previous error reviews that assumed that these were the result of bad behavior, incompetence, negligence, or corporate greed, a new approach in the review of incidents is process review in an attempt to identify gaps in the system that need improvement.

Therefore, to improve patient safety, the prevention of errors points to designing safer systems of care. The second IOM report, *Crossing the Quality Chasm*, recommended that a quality healthcare system be characterized as one that is safe, effective, patient centered, timely, efficient, and equitable [5]. The key challenge will be the redesign of health care organizations to meet these expected characteristics.

BUILDING THE SAFETY CULTURE

Safety culture has been said to be the greatest challenge in the healthcare system: "The biggest challenge to moving toward a safer health care system is changing the culture from one of blaming individuals for errors to one in which errors are treated not as personal failures but as opportunities to improve the system and prevent harm" [5]. The safety culture refers to a state in which there is a willingness to report all safety events and near misses without fear of retribution but with an understanding of accountability [1]. Staff have the ability to speak up when they have concerns. Having the understanding that each is accountable for the safety in the organization, staff want to work in teams to help each perform his or her part well. To allay all fear and anxiety and remove the blame and shame culture, the systems approach is used to analyze safety issues. In this approach, processes are examined to appreciate how they may lead to errors instead of focusing on individual blame. An integrated system is required to support the safe behavior. The organization sets the philosophy and values for an integrated pattern of behavior. Open communication about safety concerns and a nonpunitive environment can come about only when the leaders of the organization make it possible. In building a learning organization, which learns from errors, an organizational change has to happen. Structure, processes, goals, and rewards will have to be aligned with improving patient safety. The patient safety triangle is an illustration that helps appreciate how the patient safety culture can be developed (Figure 47-1).

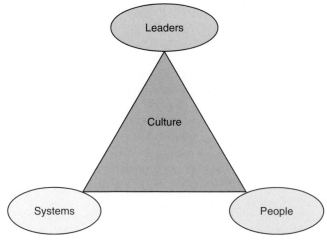

Figure 47-1 The interrelationships between infection control, patient safety, and quality.

The Role of Leaders

Leaders play a key role in developing and shaping the safety culture. They lead the change and are responsible for setting the direction for an organization. Following the example of the Joint Commission on Accreditation of Healthcare Organizations' (JCAHO) annual patient safety goals [6], setting annual goals to include patient safety helps the organization to express its commitment to building a safe environment for its patients. Leaders also lead by setting examples. Its commitment of leaders to patient safety will have to be expressed in action. Resources will have to be provided to enable the program to succeed. Healthcare organizations committed to safety need to appoint a patient safety officer, usually someone of a senior-level position within the organization who will work with both administrative and clinical leaders [7]. This person must have a strong partnership with the chief executive officer to successfully develop and deploy a comprehensive patient safety program as he plays a significant role in supervising the patient safety program. In addition to personnel, other resources may be required (e.g., budget set aside to improve the systems, enable access to safety devices or equipment). The tone is set when senior management conducts a safety walkabout on a regular basis. These executive walkabouts have been demonstrated to be successful in not only building staff confidence in management but, more importantly, engaging staff in giving contributory feedback or suggestions for making a safer environment [8]. Greater synergy is present when the infection control professional joins the patient safety walkabout, which will help to foster closer relationships between the infection control team and the ground staff.

The Patient Safety Triangle: Systems

Systems influence safety. A reporting system of incidents made easy or user friendly helps to ensure good reporting of incidents and near misses. Anonymous reporting has been used to encourage reporting of near misses. The database of incidents from the reporting system is a wealth of information where learning points may be gathered to build a better and safer workplace. Equally important to tracking and monitoring indicators from this database is the analysis of selected critical events or sentinel events. The root cause analysis methodology is a quality tool used in analyzing these sentinel events. The steps for this analysis as recommended by JCAHO may be summarized [9] as follows:

1. Organize a team.
2. Define the problem using brainstorming.
3. Study the problem.
4. Determine what happened.
5. Identify contributing process factors.
6. Explore and identify risk-reduction strategies.
7. Formulate recommendations for improvement actions.

8. Implement improvement plan.
9. Develop measures of effectiveness.
10. Evaluate implementation of improvement efforts.

The final step of evaluation of implementation of improvement measures is an equally important step not to be ignored. This is aided in a system of required feedback on effectiveness of measures implemented within a set time frame by the authority receiving the sentinel event reports.

Fallibility is part and parcel of the human condition. We may not be able to change the human condition, but we are able to change conditions under which people work. Design management entails designing work so that it is easy to do it right but very difficult or almost impossible to do it wrong. Design management is part of change management. Several methods may be adopted:

■ Reduce reliance on memory (e.g., the use of posters to illustrate the 7 steps in hand hygiene).
■ Reduce or simplify steps in processes.
■ Use standardization (e.g., standardize the device for phlebotomy in an effort to reduce sharps and needlestick injuries and ensuring good-quality blood specimens).
■ Use constraints and forcing functions to achieve desired behavior (e.g., only consultants/attendings may prescribe the use of vancomycin [to avoid inappropriate use of vancomycin in an effort to control the incidence of vancomycin-resistant enterocci (VRE)]).
■ Use protocols and checklists (e.g., the checklist used in the Institute for Healthcare Improvement [IHI] 100K Lives Ventilator bundle comprising four components: (1) elevation of the head of the bed to between 30°–45°, (2) daily "sedation vacation", (3) daily assessment of readiness to extubate, peptic ulcer disease (PUD) prophylaxis, and (4) deep vein thrombosis prophylaxis (unless contraindicated) [10].
■ Recognize fatigue's effect on performance (e.g., restrict the number of work hours for junior doctors).
■ Require education and training for safety (e.g., mandate infection control training for all staff so that they are familiar with isolation precautions, hand hygiene).
■ Promote teamwork (e.g., the close collaboration of infection control liaison officers and the infection control team).
■ Reduce known sources of confusion (e.g., have a clear central source of information on infection control guidelines on the intranet for easy access by staff in a major outbreak [SARS, influenza pandemic]).

Although infection control has increased through the years with emphasis on policies and procedures, the use of both the system reviews approach and quality improvement technique can help the organization to move on to achieve a higher level of quality of patient care.

The Patient Safety Triangle: People

People and their behavior determine the safety culture. Healthcare workers (HCWs) have the innate ability to care and express concern for their patients. Closely related to the system issues discussed previously, habits and attitudes may require some modification to help HCWs comply with safe practices. A good example is the practice of hand hygiene. Although there is clear evidence that this is an important and evidence-based practice that limits the transmission of pathogens, the compliance of hand hygiene has not reached a desirable level whether at the best centers or after a hand-hygiene campaign [9–13]. Behavioral change needs to take place. This comes about with the creation of awareness of the problem through education, presentations, posters, seminars, and example setting by leaders in the organization. The public demonstration of examples or role models has been shown to be an effective intervention in improving hand-hygiene compliance [14]. The practice of Patient Safety Leadership Walkrounds™ is another good demonstration of key leaders setting examples [8].

Patients as partners also play a vital part in building patient safety. After all, they are the ones with the greatest interest in making sure the program works because their safety is the issue at stake. Bringing them into the program as partners in safety and quality may appear to be a nonconventional practice; in infection control however, patients and their family members can play a key role in ensuring that HCWs know and comply with the necessary infection control precautions. Their part in pointing out noncompliance or reminding staff of safe practices can bring compliance to the desired level.

Building a patient safety culture may be a long, arduous process. However, adopting a systematic approach will help to bring the organization to a higher level of safety. An initial assessment of existing safety culture helps to know the baseline from which one is starting and from which action plans are made to effect change [15]. More and more healthcare organizations are now conducting regular organizational culture surveys to measure attitudes and practices to determine success in their programs [16]. The Agency of Healthcare Research and Quality (AHRQ) *Hospital Survey on Patient Safety* is one example of such survey tools when the following dimensions of patient safety culture are measured [17]:

1. Supervisor/manager expectations and actions promoting patient safety.
2. Organizational learning—continuous improvement.
3. Teamwork within units.
4. Communication openness.
5. Feedback and communication about error.
6. Nonpunitive response to error.
7. Staffing.
8. Hospital management support for patient safety.
9. Teamwork across hospital units.
10. Hospital handoffs and transitions.

Leaders also need to determine priorities for change. This may be done during the regular annual review of organizational goals. Incorporating patient safety goals as part of the organizational goals helps management to keep this clearly visible on the radar screen. In addition, the review needs to lead to actions formulated to effect the necessary change (e.g., quality and safety framework may need to be modified or help systems need to be created). Last, a regular review of progress made in accomplishing the goals helps to complete the cycle of change.

QUALITY, INFECTION CONTROL, AND PATIENT SAFETY

Both patient safety and infection control share the objective of protecting the patient from harm. However, infection control has a larger scope of safety. It includes staff safety or occupational health issues. There is considerable overlap between patient safety and infection control (Figure 47-2). Infection control is a quality program.

Quality improvement, a science of process management, will help us not only deliver quality care but also enhance patient care. Quality improvement focuses on streamlining, aligning, and improving systems and processes with the goal of eliminating inappropriate variation in process steps and documenting continuous improvement or outcomes [18] (Figures 47-3 and 47-4). Quality improvement uses the application of known systematic methods with means of analysis and measurement to reach a objective conclusions to improve a process. Effective process management will lead to the desired outcomes. This has been seen clearly in good infection control programs in which surveillance, if correctly applied, plays a large part in guiding the organization in assessing its systems in ensuring safety for patients, staff, and the organization. As defined by U.S. Centers for Disease Control and Prevention, surveillance is the ongoing systematic collection, analysis, and interpretation of health data essential to the planning, implementation, and evaluation of public health practice, closely integrated with the timely dissemination of these data to those who need to know [19]. These steps demonstrating surveillance

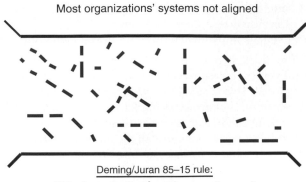

Most organizations' systems not aligned

Deming/Juran 85–15 rule:
85% of organizations' problems are the result of inefficient processes or systems; 15% by human factors

Figure 47-3   Problems in an organization's processes or systems.

as a data-driven process are similar to the principles of plan, do, check, and act (PDCA) of the quality improvement model [20]. Planning the change involves modifying the current process in patient care practices in some way or perhaps redesigning it completely. A pilot study is usually performed to test the effectiveness of the intervention. This is then closely monitored through continual tracking of the indicators to determine whether the new process has a level of performance and/or random variation that is superior to that displayed by the previous process. Finally, if the pilot is successful, the intervention is implemented on a wider scale; if it is unsuccessful, modification is made and testing is done again using another PDCA cycle.

Variation is inevitable in practices. However, it is the inappropriate variation that should be removed because it is a quality waste leading to cost. Quality improvement aims at eliminating inappropriate variation through process management with resultant cost savings. Hence, quality controls cost. This effective approach in achieving quality is a workable winning strategy, especially for organizations facing the constant challenge of balancing resources. When applied to infection control programs, the impact is magnified as can be seen in both the physical and cost outcomes.

One of the contributory factors for success in using the improvement model is the inclusion of process

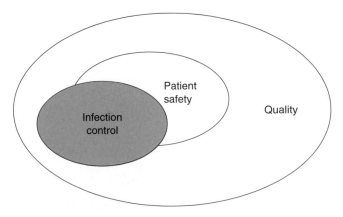

Figure 47-2   Overlap between patient safety and infection control.

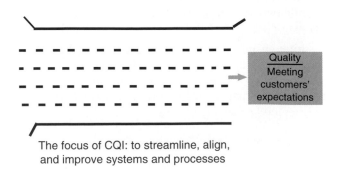

The focus of CQI: to streamline, align, and improve systems and processes

Figure 47-4   Focus of continuous quality improvement.

owners in the improvement process. These process owners have the body knowledge concerning their processes and, hence, will invariably give useful insight to the cause of a problem and good suggestions for improvement. When applied to infection control programs, this powerful technique will help make the quantum leap in the program. Quality improvement teams are formed in response to an identified problem. Process owners use quality tools (e.g., flowcharts, fishbone diagrams, or Pareto charts) in the diagnostic phase of the project to analyze the problem. Testing change using several rapid PDCA cycles helps to ensure success in the implementation of the improvement measures. One can improve only if one is able to measure. Hence, indicator tracking is a key component in any quality improvement program. This process encompasses all components of surveillance: data collection, analysis, interpretation, and feedback. Quality tools such as run charts and statistical process control (SPC) charts have helped other industries in discerning random variation from special cause variation [21,22]. These are excellent objective tools in data analysis and, when used in infection control surveillance, will help the infection control practitioner to respond appropriately to the variation seen and, hence, will assist in better time management. Time and energy can then be directed to teaching, policy development or review, and quality improvement projects. The synergy within these quality improvement teams helps to bring about effective change.

CONCLUSION

The strong interrelationships among patient safety, infection control, and quality call for close collaboration for optimal results. The application of quality improvement techniques and principles, will greatly enhance infection control programs to achieve the goal of ensuring patient safety and a better quality of care to patients while they are in our facilities.

REFERENCES

1. Institute of Medicine, Committee on Quality in Health Care in America. *To err is human: building a safer health system.* Washington, DC: The National Academy Press, 1999.

2. World Alliance for Patient Safety. WHO guidelines on hand hygiene in health care: a summary: clean hands are safer hands (advanced draft). Geneva: World Health Organization, 2005.

3. Reason J. Human error: models and management. *BMJ* 2000;320:768–770.

4. Mangram AJ, Horan TC, Pearson ML, et al. The Hospital Infection Control Practices Advisory Committee. Guideline for prevention of surgical site infection, 1999. *Infect Control Hosp Epidemiol* 1999;20:247–278.

5. Institute of Medicine, Committee on Quality in Health Care in America. *Crossing the quality chasm: a new health system for the 21st Century.* Washington, DC: The National Academy Press, 2001.

6. Joint Commission on Accreditation of Healthcare Organizations. National patient safety goals (www.jointcommission.org/PatientSafety/NationalPatientSafetyGoals/).

7. Gandhi TK, Graydon-Baker E, Barnes JN, et al. Creating an integrated patient safety team. *Jt Comm J Qual Improv* 2003;29:383–390.

8. Frankel A, Graydon-Baker E, Neppl C, et al. Patient safety leadership walkrounds™. *Joint Comm J Quality Saf.* 2003;29(1):16–26.

9. Joint Commission on Accreditation of Healthcare Organizations. *Root cause analysis in health care: tools and techniques.* Oakbrook Terrace, IL: JCAHO, 2000:7.

10. Institute for Healthcare Improvement. 100k lives campaign: prevention of ventilator-associated pneumonia (www.ihi.org/IHI/Programs/Campaign/).

11. Dubbert PM, Dolce J, Richter W, et al. Increasing ICU staff handwashing: effects of education and group feedback. *Infect Control Hosp Epidemiol* 1990;11:191–193.

12. Coignard B, Grandbastien B, Berrouane Y, et al. Handwashing quality impact of a special program. *Infect Control Hosp Epidemiol* 1998;19:510–513.

13. McGuckin M, Waterman R, Prten L, et al. Patient education model for increasing handwashing compliance. *Am J Infect Control* 1999;27:309–314.

14. Pittet D, Hugonnet S, Harbath S, et al. Effectiveness of a hospital wide program to improve compliance with hand hygiene. *Lancet* 2000;356:1307–1312.

15. Nieva VF, Sorra J. Safety culture assessment: a tool for improving patient safety in healthcare organizations. *Qual Saf Health Care* 2003;12(suppl II):ii17–ii23.

16. Singer SJ, Gaba DM, Geppert JJ, et al. The culture of safety: results of an organization-wide survey in 13 California hospitals. *Qual Saf Health Care* 2003;12:112–118.

17. Agency of Healthcare Research and Quality (AHRQ). Hospital survey on patient safety (www.ahrq.gov/qual/hospculture/).

18. Ling ML, Ching TY, Seto WH. *A handbook of infection control for the Asian healthcare worker.* 2nd ed. Singapore: Elsevier Pte Ltd, 2004.

19. Centers for Disease Control and Prevention. *CDC surveillance update.* Atlanta: Centers for Disease Control, 1988.

20. Langley GJ, Nolan KM, Nolan TW, et al. *The Improvement model: a practical approach to enhancing organizational performance.* New York; Josey-Bass, 1996.

21. Brassard M, Ritter D. *The memory jogger™ II: healthcare edition. a pocket guide of tools for continuous improvement and effective planning.* Goal/QPC: Methuen, MA.

22. Guthrie B, Love T, Fahey T, et al. Control, compare and communicate: designing control charts to summarize efficiently data from multiple quality indicators. *Qual Saf Health Care* 2005; 14:450–454.

Index

Note: Page numbers followed by *f* indicate figures; those followed by *t* indicate tables.